Conceptual Review of

Pharmacology for NBE

Covering 3200 Qs with Explanations, 100+ IBQs & 500+ Colored Illustrations/Images

References and Updates from Harrison's 20/e, CMDT 2019, Goodman Gilman's 13/e, & Standard Journals

Fifth Edition

Ranjan Kumar Patel
MD Pharmacology
Ex Faculty UCMS and GTB Hospital, Delhi

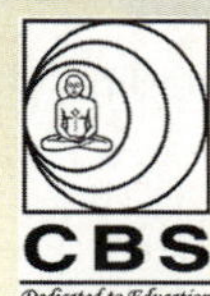

CBS Publishers & Distributors Pvt Ltd

• New Delhi • Bengaluru • Chennai • Kochi • Kolkata • Mumbai
• Hyderabad • Nagpur • Patna • Pune • Vijayawada

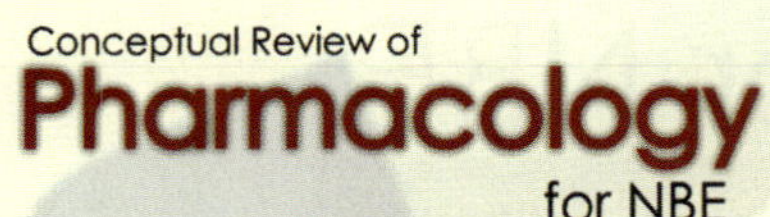

ISBN: 978-93-89941-96-8

Fifth Edition: 2020

Fourth Edition: 2019-20

Third Edition: 2018

Published by **Satish Kumar Jain** and produced by **Varun Jain** for

CBS Publishers & Distributors Pvt Ltd

4819/XI Prahlad Street, 24 Ansari Road, Daryaganj, New Delhi 110 002, India.
Ph: +91-11-23289259, 23266861, 23266867 Website: www.cbspd.com
Fax: 011-23243014
e-mail: delhi@cbspd.com; cbspubs@airtelmail.in.
Corporate Office: 204 FIE, Industrial Area, Patparganj, Delhi 110 092
Ph: +91-11-4934 4934 Fax: 4934 4935
e-mail: feedback@cbspd.com; bhupesharora@cbspd.com

Branches

- **Bengaluru:** Seema House 2975, 17th Cross, K.R. Road
  Banasankari 2nd Stage, Bengaluru 560 070, Karnataka
  Ph: +91-80-26771678/79 Fax: +91-80-26771680 e-mail: bangalore@cbspd.com
- **Chennai:** 7, Subbaraya Street, Shenoy Nagar, Chennai 600 030, Tamil Nadu
  Ph: +91-44-26680620, 26681266 Fax: +91-44-42032115 e-mail: chennai@cbspd.com
- **Kochi:** 68/1534, 35, 36-Power House Road, Opp. KSEB, Cochin-682018, Kochi, Kerala
  Ph: +91-484-4059061-65 Fax: +91-484-4059065 e-mail: kochi@cbspd.com
- **Kolkata:** 6/B, Ground Floor, Rameswar Shaw Road, Kolkata-700 014, West Bengal
  Ph: +91-33-22891126, 22891127, 22891128 e-mail: kolkata@cbspd.com
- **Mumbai:** 83-C, Dr E Moses Road, Worli, Mumbai-400018, Maharashtra
  Ph: +91-22-24902340/41 Fax: +91-22-24902342 e-mail: mumbai@cbspd.com

Representatives

- **Hyderabad** +91-9885175004
- **Patna** +91-9334159340
- **Pune** +91-9623451994
- **Vijayawada** +91-9000660880

Printed at: Rashtriya Printers, 27/487, Zulfe Bengal Industrial Area, Dilshad Garden, Delhi-110095

Dedicated to

My twin stars Additri and Aaryahi

From Publisher's Desk

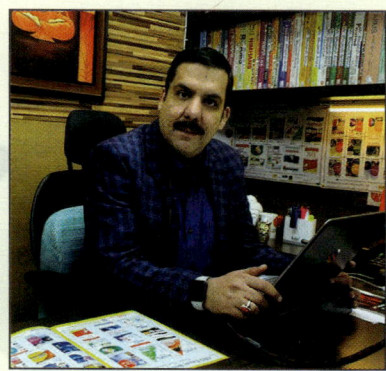

Dear Readers,

I extend my warm welcome and convey my heartfelt thanks for appreciating the CBS Exam Books for another successful year. It has been an amazing journey so far and I am highly grateful for your support and cooperation to help us achieve various milestones in this whole span of time. The mission with which we started in the year 2015 was to bring nothing but the best of everything to our target audience and today I can proudly say that we have maintained that standard and are committed to continue the same in future as well.

Every single title under the banner of CBS Exam Books has been developed and nurtured like an infant. The authors and our entire team work day and night to bring the best in everything for you. Be it content, presentation, social media contests and offers, we strive to meet your expectations with every passing year. Your trust has motivated us to maintain and upgrade ourselves during this period. I am extremely thankful to all our authors who are the real pillars of the complete series of CBS Exam Books. The contributions of our esteemed authors have laid the foundations of CBS Exam Books.

At this juncture, I can recall these lines by Drake,

"Sometimes it's the journey that teaches you a lot about your destination".

We have grown and changed with the passage of time to upgrade our ways of providing our readers with maximum benefits and help them manage their time and efforts in effective manner. Previous year was the year of great achievements. Let me show you a glimpse of our successful journey:

- Most of the titles of CBS Exam Books received wide acceptance and recognition by the readers of proving their usefulness and supremacy. To mention a few, SARP Anatomy, CRISP, Surgery Sixer, Complete Review of Pathology, Conceptual Review of Pharmacology, SOCH, Forensic Medicine, Complete Review of Medicine, Conceptual Review of PSM, MICRONS, My PGMEE Notes, AIIMS MedEasy, and PRIMEs. With your constant support and our consistent efforts, I am sure that we will together witness an exponential acceptance of all CBS Exam Books in coming future as well.
- The presence of CBS Exam Books has broadened through our various social media platforms. We have received great appreciation for our regular Facebook activities such as online test series, giveaways, scientific content for knowledge enhancement, authors' live sessions, and various contests, like Bid 2 Win, Fastest Finger First, Book Fair and Facebook Community Awards. Join us on all these platforms to avail and enjoy our exciting offers and benefits.

A book is incomplete if it does not have the right readers. We value you and your feedback. Please share your feedback and suggestions directly with me at **bhupesharora@cbspd.com.** We promise to deliver in our books, what you desire to see.

I would like to sum up with these eternal lines of Robert Frost:

Woods are lovely dark and deep,
But I have promises to keep.
And miles to go before I sleep,
And miles to go before I sleep!
Wishing you success in all your endeavors!

Bhupesh Arora
Vice President – Publishing & Marketing
(PGMEE and Nursing Division)
Email: bhupesharora@cbspd.com
Mobile: (+91) 9555590180

Preface

Dear students,

I would like to thank all of you for the fantabulous response that you have given to the previous editions. Your reviews and feedback about first, second, third and fourth editions made me ecstatic and at the same time fueled me to give you an even better **fifth edition**.

As compared to the fourth edition, I have added several recent guidelines regarding New Drugs 2019 list with changes that have taken place in pharmacotherapy in the year 2019. For the first time Recently Changed AIIMS Pattern Questions Review 2019 and recently-conducted 2020 examination papers (Recent Pattern Questions 2020-2019, AIIMS November and May 2019, JIPMER November and May 2019 and PGI May 2019) have been added to ace your preparation practice before upcoming AIIMS examination.

In the chapter **'Cardiovascular System'**, I have added **ACLS Guidelines 2017** for management of cardiac arrest, tachycardia and bradycardia. Apart from this, **Changes in ACC/AHA Guidelines in management of CHF and dyslipidemia** have also been incorporated. In the topic of **'Antimicrobials'**, the **Recent Changes in regimens for management of TB, HIV, leprosy, etc**. have been discussed in details. Many changes have been incorporated wherever needed, based on CMDT 2019, Goodman Gilman 13th Edition and recent journals.

Sincere attention has been paid on the feedback sent by the students and the important suggestions have been incorporated in this edition like—**'Classification of Drugs'** is now given in every topic so that you can revise the drugs at one place. A **drug chart on ANS** separately available with the book will prove quite handy for frequent revision.

The backbone of the first edition was concepts, which continue to be there even in this edition. Every topic begins with the relevant part from preclinical subjects, like anatomy, physiology, pathology, biochemistry and microbiology, and then finally, drugs come into picture making a web of correlation. The correlation is well explained in the **Conceptual Boxes**, which tell you why a drug is used. After all details of drugs are covered, the **Clinical Boxes** will guide you through the medicine aspect of treatment as to understand where drugs stand as compared to nondrug strategies of management. These clinical boxes tell you how and when a drug is used. With every topic, a separate box of **Recent Advances** has been given to guide you through the future trends in treatment; in recent exams new drugs and even drugs under trials have been asked.

MCQs of recent exams are cherry on the cake that will keep you abreast with the changing pattern. MCQs of JIPMER and NIMHANS are also included, so that students preparing for these exams are also benefited. The question section begins with AIIMS and recent exam questions, which are segregated subtopic wise so that you can solve them after you are through a particular subtopic. However, the other questions of PGI, JIPMER and NIMHANS are not segregated and you can practice them after you are done with complete topics. Finally, as **Image-based Questions** are the current toast of the town, I have given them at the end of each chapter for your practice.

Mnemonics have been included to make learning easier in remembering different aspects related to drugs. **One Liners** in the beginning of each chapter cover the most important points, which will give you a quick revision source, a day before exam. **'Annexures'**, after every chapter, contain the **Updated Drugs of Choice and New Drugs Approved by FDA** for quick revision.

I have done my part by bringing the world of pharmacology onto your palms and now all depends on how you utilize this book. Study plans for mastering pharmacology are present on my Facebook Group **"Dr Ranjan's Pharmacology–Discussion and Updates"**. The other important aspects are—**Regular Updates** and **Doubt Discussion** in this group.

I have tried my level best to make this book simple, concise and error free. However, if there are any errors you can notify the same to me through my email ID. I would like to thank all the students who have contributed to book with their suggestions, doubts, etc. and this is the reason why I say that this is a book **"Of the students, By the students and For the students."**

Thank You!

Ranjan Kumar Patel
Email: ranjankumarpatel@yahoo.com

Acknowledgements

The foundation of a career is laid down during the school days and hence I would like to begin with thanking all my teachers in DAV Public School, Bandhabahal, Jharsuguda, Odisha. I convey my special thanks to BK Singh sir for shaping my mathematics and science during my school days.

I would like to thank my parents and sister who have always been there to support me in my ups and downs. I have never seen God, but if at all He is There then He cannot be better than Parents.

I would also like to thank Dr SK Bhattacharya, ex HOD, Department of Pharmacology, UCMS and GTB Hospital, Delhi and present HOD, Department of Pharmacology, Hindu Rao Hospital Associated Medical College, for his immense support during my postgraduation days. I have learnt not only pharmacology from him, but also an art to remain grounded always in life.

Besides, I would like to thank all other assistant professors in UCMS and GTB hospital, Dr Seema, Dr Rachna and Dr Sumita for their constant encouragement and support. I cannot forget my juniors and friends in Department of Pharmacology, UCMS and GTB Hospital Delhi. Tons of thanks to Dr Vijay Chamle, Dr Umesh Suranagi, Dr Mahindra, Dr Dinesh, Dr Chetan Bhangale, Dr Abhishek, Dr Chandrapal, Dr Rupanwita Ghosh, Dr Tripti Rastogi, Dr Vijayalakshmi, Dr Verrana Karadi, Dr Suresh, Dr Ankit Bharadwaj, Dr Sengovettel, Dr Durga Prasad and Dr Keshav Gupta.

I would like to thank Dr KS Anand HOD Department of Neurology at Dr RML Hospital, Delhi for his immense support who is most kind and a gem of a person I have ever met in my life. I would also like to thank Dr BK Bajaj and Dr Jyoti for their support and inspiration while I was a JR.

Faculty members, friends and seniors who have been instrumental in my life will always remain in my heart. I would like to thank all of them for their immense support and love; K Santosh Kumar, Deepak Jaiswal, Rajesh Sharma, Dr Harmeet Goel, Dr Vivek Jain, Dr Devesh Mishra, Dr Gobind Rai Garg, Dr Sparsh Gupta, Dr Deepak Marwah, Dr Amit Sharma, Dr Akhilesh Jhamad, Dr Thameem Saif, Dr Rajesh Kaushal, Dr Apurv Mehra, Dr Apurva Sastry, Dr Praveen Kumar, Dr Rebecca James, Dr Rajeshwar Gudadhe, Dr Raja Mahendran, Dr Dharmendra, Dr Deepak Gupta, Dr Utsav Bansal, Dr Shrikant Verma, Dr Satbir Singh, Rahul and Hansraj.

Finally, I would like to thank all my students from the bottom of my heart for the love and respect they have given me for these years. That's the real fuel that keeps me going.

My special thanks are due to **Mr Satish Kumar Jain** (Chairman) and **Mr Varun Jain** (Managing Director), M/s CBS Publishers and Distributors Pvt Ltd for their wholehearted support in publication of this book. I have no words to describe the role, efforts, inputs and initiatives undertaken by **Mr Bhupesh Arora** (Vice President – Publishing & Marketing, PGMEE and Nursing Division) for helping and motivating me.

I sincerely thank the entire CBS team for bringing out the book with utmost care and attractive presentation. I would like to thank Dr Mrinalini Bakshi (Editorial Head & Content Strategist) for her editorial support and Ms Nitasha Arora (Production Head & Content Strategist), Dr Anju Dhir (Project Manager & Senior Scientific Coordinator), Mr Shivendu Bhushan Pandey (Senior Editor), Mr Ashutosh Pathak (Senior Proof Reader) and all the production team members Mr Chaman Lal, Mr Prakash Gaur, Mr Phool Kumar, Mr Bunty Kashyap, Ms Tahira Parveen, Ms Manorama, Ms Babita Verma, Mr Chander Mani, Mr Raju Sharma, Mr Manoj Chaudhary, Mr Vikram Chaudhary, Mr Manoj Malakar, Mr Arun Kumar and Mr Rahul Negi for devoting laborious hours in designing and typesetting of the book.

Contents

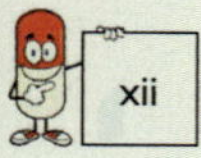

NEW DRUGS 2019

New drug	Mechanism of action	Use
Esketamine nasal spray	NMDA antagonist	Resistant depression
Netarsudil + Latanoprost FDC ophthalmic solution	Netarsudil is a rho kinase inhibitor and latanoprost is a prostaglandin F2alpha analog	Open angle glaucoma
Trastuzumab + Hyaluronidase FDC	Hyaluronidase increases absorption rate of trastuzumab	Her2 positive breast cancer
Triclabendazole	Benzimidazole which inhibits microtubules	Liver flukes
Caplacizumab	Anti von Willebrand factor monoclonal antibody which blocks adhesion of platelets to blood vessels	Acquired thrombocytopenic purpura
Parabotulinum toxin A	Inhibits release of acetylcholine	Temporary improvement in glabellar lines associated with corrugator and/or procerus muscle activity in adults
Brexanolone	GABA-A receptor modulator	Postpartum depression
Tafamidis meglumine	Oral transthyretin stabilizer	Cardiomyopathy of wild type or hereditary transthyretin-mediated amyloidosis (ATTR-CM)
Risankizumab	Anti IL-23 monoclonal antibody	Plaque psoriasis
Onasemnogene abeparvovec	Adeno-associated virus vector-based gene therapy	Spinal muscular atrophy (SMA) in children <2 years
Polatuzumab vedotin	Immunotoxin made up of polatuzumab (anti CD 79b MAb) and vedotin (toxin)	Used along with bendamustine and rituximab for treatment of diffuse large B cell lymphoma
Venetoclax and Obinutuzumab FDC	Venetoclax is a BCL-2 inhibitor and Obinutuzumab is an anti CD 20 monoclonal antibody	Chronic lymphocytic leukemia and small lymphocytic lymphoma
Ramucirumab	Anti VEGFR monoclonal antibody	Hepatocellular carcinoma in patients having alpha fetoprotein levels >400 ng/mL, despite being treated with sorafenib
Amifampridine	Potassium channel blocker	Lambert Eaton myasthenic syndrome in patients of 6–17 years age
Dengvaxia	Recombinant live tetravalent dengue vaccine	Prevention of dengue caused by serotypes 1–4 only in age group 9–16 years with laboratory confirmed previous dengue infection
Ruxilotinib	JAK 1 and 2 inhibitor	Treatment of steroid resistant acute GVHD in age group more than 12 years
Certolizumab	Anti TNF alpha drug	Treatment of active non-radiographic axial spondyloarthritis with objective signs of inflammation
Romosozumab	Antisclerostin monoclonal antibody	Osteoporosis in postmenopausal females with high risk of fracture
Cladribine	Purine analog	Relapsing form of multiple sclerosis
Siponimod	Sphingosine 1-phosphate receptor modulator	Relapsing form of multiple sclerosis
Avelumab plus Axitinib	Avelumab is an anti-programmed death ligand 1 monoclonal antibody and axitinib is a VEGFR tyrosine kinase inhibitor	Combination therapy has been approved for treatment of renal cell carcinoma
Pembrolizumab	Pembrolizumab is an anti-programmed death ligand 1 receptor monoclonal antibody	Renal cell carcinoma Advanced endometrial carcinoma Squamous cell cancer of esophagus Small and non-small cell lung cancer
Intranasal midazolam spray	GABA A receptor agonist	Acute repetitive seizures in age group >12 years of age

Contd...

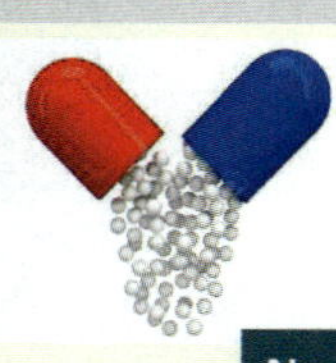

New drug	Mechanism of action	Use
Solriamfetol	Dopamine and norepinephrine reuptake inhibitor	Excessive sleepiness associated with narcolepsy and obstructive sleep apnea
Alpelisib	Phosphatidylinositol 3 kinase (PI3K) inhibitor	Treatment of ER+ breast cancer in postmenopausal females with PI3KCA mutation in combination with fluvestrant
Atezolizumab	Anti-programmed death cell ligand 1 monoclonal antibody	Used along with paclitaxel for treatment of triple negative breast cancer which is unresectable or locally advanced
Erdafitinib	Fibroblast growth factor receptor tyrosine kinase inhibitor	Locally advanced or metastatic urothelial carcinoma
Apremilast	Phosphodiesterase-4 inhibitor	Oral ulcers associated with Behçet's syndrome
Oral semaglutide	It is the first oral GLP-1 agonist. It is to be taken exactly 30 minutes before the first food of the day. Sodium caprylate is added to semaglutide to increase its intestinal absorption.	Type II diabetes mellitus
Tenapanor	• Sodium/hydrogen exchanger 3 (NHE3) inhibitor. • NHE3 is an antiporter that absorbs sodium in the intestine in exchange for proton. Hence its inhibition increases sodium in intestine that draws water.	IBS associated with constipation
Relebactam	Beta lactamase inhibitor	Approved to be used with imipenem + cilastatin for treatment of complicated UTI and intra-abdominal infections
Fedratinib	Oral Janus Associated Kinase 2 (JAK2) and FMS-like tyrosine kinase 3 (FLT3) inhibitor	Myelofibrosis
Selinexor	• Nuclear export inhibitor • By inhibition of export of tumor suppressor proteins from nucleus of cancer cells, it induces apoptosis of cancer cells.	Resistant multiple myeloma
Nintedanib	Multiple tyrosine kinase inhibitor	Systemic sclerosis associated interstitial lung disease
Pretomanid	Mycolic acid synthesis inhibitor	Approved for treatment of XDR TB along with bedaquiline and linezolid
Lefamulin	Protein synthesis inhibitor which acts by inhibiting peptidyl transferase	Community acquired pneumonia
Upadacitinib	Oral JAK inhibitor	Methotrexate resistant rheumatoid arthritis
Ixekizumab	Anti-IL17A monoclonal antibody	Active ankylosing spondylitis
Pitolisant	Histamine-3 (H3) receptor antagonist/inverse agonist	Narcolepsy
Istradefylline	Adenosine A2A receptor antagonist	On-off phenomena seen with levodopa
Bremelanotide	Melanocortin peptide receptors agonist	Hypoactive sexual desire disorder in premenopausal females
Darolutamide	Androgen receptor inhibitor	Non-metastatic castration resistant prostate cancer
Entrectinib	Multiple kinase (RTL, ROS1, ALK) inhibitor	ROS1 positive metastatic non-small cell lung cancer
Pexidartinib	Multi-kinase inhibitor	Symptomatic tenosynovial giant cell tumor
Brolucizumab	Vascular endothelial growth factor (VEGF) inhibitor	Neovascular (Wet) Age-Related Macular Degeneration (AMD)

Contd...

New drug	Mechanism of action	Use
Afamelanotide	Alpha-MSH analog that stimulates melanocortin 1 receptor (MC1-R)	Indicated to increase pain free light exposure in adult patients with a history of phototoxic reactions from erythropoietic protoporphyria
Lasmiditan	5-HT 1F receptor agonist	Treatment of acute migraine attack
Luspatercept	Promotes erythroid maturation	Treatment of anemia in patients of beta thalassemia
Zanubrutinib	Bruton's tyrosine kinase inhibitor	Mantle cell lymphoma (MCL)
Cefiderocol	Cephalosporin antibiotic	Complicated urinary tract infections
Crizanlizumab	Selectin blocker	Indicated to reduce the frequency of vaso-occlusive crises in sickle cell disease
Givosiran	Aminolevulinate synthase 1-directed small interfering RNA	Acute hepatic porphyria
Cenobamate	Sodium channel blocker and a GABA-A receptor modulator	Partial seizures
Voxelotor	Hemoglobin S polymerization inhibitor	Sickle cell disease
Golodirsen	Antisense oligonucleotide	Duchenne muscular dystrophy
Lumateperone	Atypical antipsychotic	Schizophrenia
Lemborexant	Orexin receptor antagonist	Insomnia
Ubrogepant	CGRP receptor antagonist	Acute migraine attack

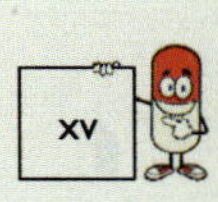

Latest Exam Questions 2020-2019

1. Recent Pattern Questions 2020
2. AIIMS November 2019
3. AIIMS May 2019
4. JIPMER November 2019
5. JIPMER May 2019
6. PGI May 2019

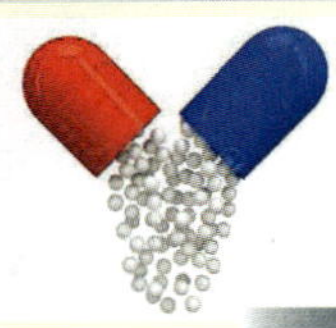

RECENT PATTERN QUESTIONS 2020

General Pharmacology

1. **Drug acting via tyrosine kinase receptor is**
   a. TRH b. TSH
   c. Insulin d. MSH
2. **Most potent drug in the DRC is**

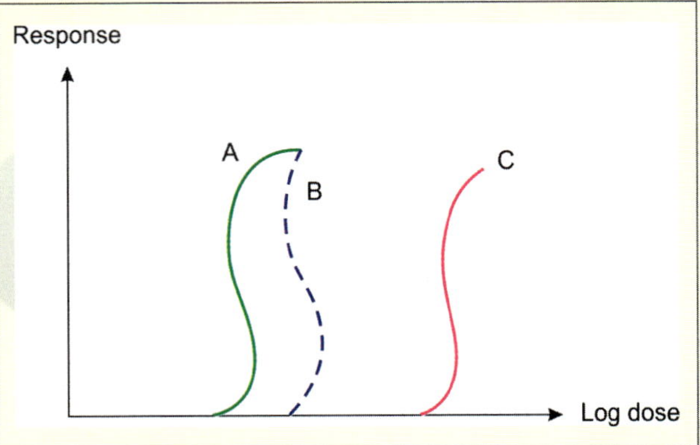

   a. Only A b. Only B
   c. Only C d. Only A+B
3. **True about non-competitive inhibition is**
   a. K_m remains same, V_{max} decreases
   b. K_m increases, V_{max} remains same
   c. K_m decreases, V_{max} increases
   d. K_m increases, V_{max} increases

Autonomic Nervous System

4. **A patient with diabetes and COPD developed post-operative urinary retention. Which of the following drugs can be used for short term treatment to relieve the symptoms of this person?**
   a. Bethanechol
   b. Methacholine
   c. Terazosin
   d. Tamsulosin
5. **A person was given a muscle relaxant that competitively blocks nicotinic receptors. Which of the following drug is used for reversal of muscle relaxation after surgery?**
   a. Neostigmine b. Carbachol
   c. Succinylcholine d. Physostigmine
6. **Anti-glaucoma drug that acts by increasing uveoscleral outflow via ciliary muscles is**
   a. Latanoprost b. Timolol
   c. Pilocarpine d. Dorzolamide

Cardiovascular System

7. **Which of the following antihypertensive drug is avoided in patients with high serum uric acid levels?**
   a. Prazosin b. Enalapril
   c. Hydrochlorothiazide d. Atenolol
8. **Which of the following antiarrhythmic drug is contraindicated in a patient with interstitial lung disease?**
   a. Amiodarone b. Sotalol
   c. Quinidine d. Lignocaine
9. **Which of the following is a late inward sodium channel blocker?**
   a. Ivabradine b. Ranolazine
   c. Trimetazidine d. Fasudil

Diuretics

10. **At a high altitude of 3000 m, a person complains of breathlessness. All of the following can be used for management of this person except:**
    a. Intravenous digoxin b. Oxygen supplementation
    c. Immediate descent d. Acetazolamide

Central Nervous System

11. **A patient on lithium therapy developed hypertension. He was started on thiazides for hypertension. After few days, he developed coarse tremors and other symptoms suggestive of lithium toxicity. Explain the likely mechanism of this interaction.**
    a. Thiazides inhibits the metabolism of lithium
    b. Thiazides act as an add on drug to lithium
    c. Thiazides increase the tubular reabsorption of lithium
    d. Thiazides cause loss of water thereby increased lithium levels
12. **A female patient was on lithium therapy for bipolar disorder for 6 months. She kept the fast for few days due to religious reasons and presented with seizures, coarse tremors, confusion and weakness of limbs. Which of the following should be done to diagnose her condition?**
    a. Serum electrolytes b. Serum lithium levels
    c. ECG d. MRI
13. **A woman sleeping in the night develops pain and funny feelings like insect crawling in the legs, which is relieved by shaking her legs. Which of the following drug is used as first line?**
    a. Pramipexole b. Gabapentin
    c. Vit B12 d. Iron tablets
14. **A patient was recently started on fluphenazine. Few weeks later, he developed tremors, rigidity, bradykinesia and excessive salivation. First line of management for this patient is**
    a. Selegiline b. Trihexyphenidyl
    c. Pramipexole d. Amantadine
15. **A patient of biliary colic presented to hospital. Intern gave an injection and the pain worsened. Which is the most likely injection given?**
    a. Morphine b. Diclofenac
    c. Nefopam d. Etoricoxib

Antimicrobials

16. **Which of the following fluoroquinolone contraindicated in liver disease?**
    a. Levofloxacin b. Pefloxacin
    c. Ofloxacin d. Lomefloxacin
17. **Drug of choice for invasive aspergillosis is**
    a. Posaconazole b. Voriconazole
    c. Liposomal AMB d. Caspofungin

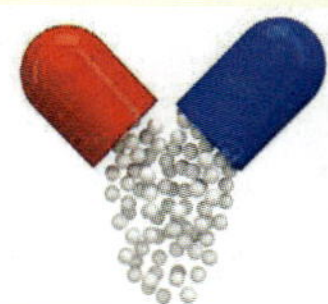

18. **Which of the following drug acts by inhibiting the transcription of DNA to RNA?**
    a. Rifampicin b. Nitrofurantoin
    c. Ciprofloxacin d. Novobiocin
19. **Which of the following antimicrobials should not be given to a chronic asthmatic patient managed on theophylline therapy?**
    a. Erythromycin b. Cefotaxime
    c. Cotrimoxazole d. Amoxicillin
20. **Beta lactamase confers resistance by:**
    a. Alteration of penicillin binding protein
    b. Drug efflux
    c. Break down of drug structure
    d. Alteration in 50s ribosome structure
21. **Which of the following drugs is used as nail lacquer for onychomycosis?**
    a. Fluconazole b. Ciclopirox
    c. Itraconazole d. Terbinafine

Anticancer Drugs

22. **Which of the following drugs act by inhibiting DNA replication?**
    a. 6 Mercaptopurine b. Actinomycin D
    c. Mitomycin C d. Asparaginase

Endocrinology

23. **Which of the following is used as a first line drug in postmenopausal osteoporosis?**
    a. Estrogen b. Bisphosphonates
    c. Raloxifene d. Combined OCP

Autacoids

24. **Pegloticase is used for treatment of**
    a. Ankylosing spondylosis
    b. CPPD
    c. Chronic tophaceous gout
    d. Refractory Rheumatoid arthritis
25. **A patient diagnosed with Rheumatoid arthritis was on medications. After 2 years, he developed blurring of vision and was found to have corneal opacity. Which drug is most likely to cause this?**
    a. Sulfasalazine b. Chloroquine
    c. Methotrexate d. Leflunomide
26. **A boy is planning to travel by bus. Which of the following drug can be used to prevent motion sickness in this person?**
    a. Promethazine b. Cetirizine
    c. Loratadine d. Fexofenadine

Respiratory System

27. **Theophylline causes diuresis because of**
    a. PDE4 inhibition
    b. Adenosine A1 receptor antagonism
    c. Beta 2 agonists
    d. PDE 3 inhibition

Gastrointestinal System

28. **Which of the following is not a prokinetic?**
    a. 5HT4 agonist b. D2 blocker
    c. Macrolides d. Diphenoxylate

Blood

29. **Which of the following factor is targeted by warfarin by inhibiting activity of gamma carboxylase**
    a. VIII b. V
    c. II d. XI

AIIMS NOVEMBER 2019

Single Best Response Questions

30. **Which of the following is not used in heart failure?**
    a. Metoprolol
    b. Trimetazidine
    c. Sacubitril
    d. Nesiritide
31. **All of the following can cause miosis except:**
    a. Organophosphates
    b. Belladonna
    c. Morphine
    d. Pilocarpine
32. **Pegloticase is used in:**
    a. Chronic gout
    b. Paralytic ileus
    c. Psoriatic arthritis
    d. Rheumatoid arthritis
33. **GPCR not acting through secondary messenger via potassium channels is:**
    a. Muscarinic M2 receptor b. Dopamine D2 receptor
    c. Serotonin 5 HT1 receptor d. Angiotensin 1 receptor
34. **A patient was given ampicillin 2 g intravenously. After that, the person developed rash on skin, hypotension and difficulty in breathing. This patient should be managed by:**
    a. 0.5 mL of 1:1000 adrenaline by intramuscular route
    b. 0.5 mL of 1:1000 adrenaline by intravenous route
    c 0.5 mL of 1:10000 adrenaline by intramuscular route
    d. 0.5 mL of 1:10000 adrenaline by intravenous route
35. **All of the following can be used to decrease IOP in glaucoma except:**
    a. Mannitol
    b. Methazolamide
    c. Clonidine
    d. Dexamethasone
36. **Prucalopride is a:**
    a. 5HT4 agonist
    b. 5HT2b agonist
    c. 5HT2b antagonist d. 5HT1a partial agonist
37. **Z track technique is used for:**
    a. Monitoring of lithium therapy
    b. Monitoring of carbamazepine therapy
    c. Administration of long acting depot antipsychotics
    d. Administration of nicotine patches

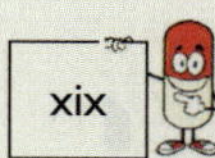

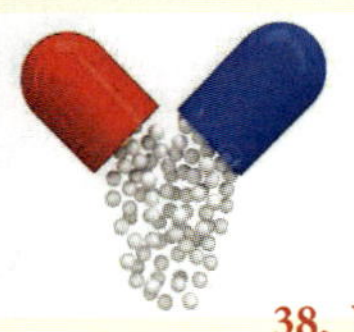

38. **Which of the following is a schedule X drug?**
   a. Thalidomide b Colistin
   c. Ketamine d. Halothane
39. **Which of the following is used for the treatment of pauci-bacillary leprosy?**
   a. 2 drugs for 6 months b. 2 drugs for 12 months
   c. 3 drugs for 6 months d. 3 drugs for 12 months
40. **Route of administration of LMWH for prophylaxis of thrombosis in a patient who had undergone surgery few hours back is:**
   a. Subcutaneous b. Intravenous
   c. Inhalational d. Intramuscular
41. **Doc of bacterial vaginosis in pregnancy is:**
   a. Clindamycin b. Metronidazole
   c. Erythromycin d. Rovamycin
42. **Which of the following is clinical use of intravaginally?**
   a. Radical cure of Plasmodium vivax
   b. Prophylaxis of malaria in pregnancy
   c. Treatment of severe falciparum malaria
   d. Treatment of endemic malaria in children <2 years
43. **Which of the following statements about tedizolid is true?**
   a. Peripheral neuropathy is a common adverse effect
   b. It is active against gram positive organisms
   c. It has poor oral bioavailability
   d. Major mode of elimination is renal excretion
44. **Non-pulsatile dose of GnRH agonist is used in all of the following conditions except:**
   a. Endometriosis
   b. Male infertility
   c. Central precocious puberty
   d. Prostate cancer
45. **A nurse got accidental prick from the HIV infected needle. Which of the following statements is false regarding the management of this nurse?**
   a. Zidovudine used as monotherapy in post-exposure prophylaxis
   b. Washing hands with soap and water is advised
   c. Baseline viral markers of health care personnel should be done at the time of prick
   d. Follow up viral markers of health care personnel should be measured at 6 weeks
46. **A patient was schedule for surgery. Before giving anesthesia, he was administered glycopyrrolate. What is rationale of giving glycopyrrolate before anesthesia?**
   a. To allay anxiety b. To decrease secretions
   c. As inducing agent d. For muscle relaxation
47. **Inhibition of which presynaptic ion channels will decrease release of acetylcholine from the nerve terminal:**
   a. Voltage gated sodium channel
   b. Voltage gated calcium channel
   c. Voltage gated potassium channel
   d. Leaky chloride channels
48. **Tramadol mechanism of action other than μ receptor agonism is:**
   a. Anticholinergic b. Antihistaminic
   c. Serotonin and norepinephrine reuptake inhibition
   d. Serotonin and dopamine reuptake inhibition
49. **A 10 years old child presents with easily pluckable hair and black dots on the scalp as given in the picture. The drug of choice for the condition is:**

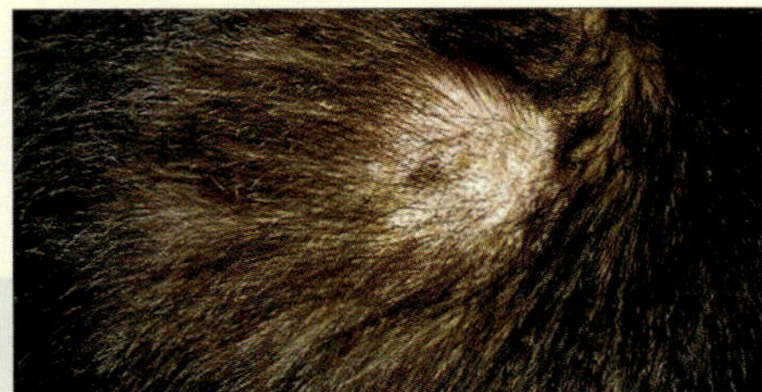

   a. Griseofulvin b. Ciclopirox olamine
   c. Fluconazole d. Amphotericin B

Match The Following

50. **Match the following drugs their mechanism of action:**

Colum A	Column B
1. Omalizumab	a. Anti-CD 6
2. Itolizumab	b. Anti-IgG1
3. Daclizumab	c. Anti-CD 25
4. Belimumab	d. Anti-B lymphocyte stimulator
	e. Anti-Ig E

Assertion Reasoning Type

51. **Assertion: In a patient admitted in hospital for community acquired pneumonia, combination therapy of beta lactams and azithromycin is given.**
   Reason: This combination covers gram positive organisms and anaerobes.
   a. Both assertion and reason are true and reason is correct explanation of assertion
   b. Both assertion and reason are true and reason is not the correct explanation of assertion
   c. Assertion is true but reason is false
   d. Assertion is false but reason is true
   e. Both assertion and reason are false

Multiple True/False Type

52. **Which of the following is True or False regarding drugs used for viral infections?**
   a. Treatment with ribavirin is considered better than sofosbuvir
   b. Ombitasvir is inhibitor of protein synthesis
   c. Imiquimod is used for Condyloma acuminate
   d. Simeprevir inhibits protease of hepatitis C
   e. Oseltamivir is used for swine flu
53. **A patient presented to emergency with overdose of some drug. There were increased salivation and increased bronchial secretions. On examination, blood pressure was 88/60 mm Hg. RBC esterase level is 50. What should be the treatment of this person?**
   a. Neostigmine
   b. Atropine
   c. Flumazenil
   d. Physostigmine
   e. PAM

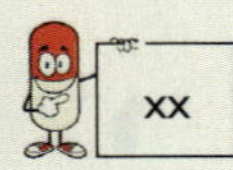

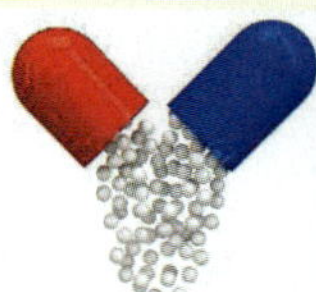

54. **Which of the following statements regarding foscarnet are T/F:**
   a. It is used for resistant CMV (True)
   b. Renal toxicity is seen (True)
   c. It is activated by viral thymidine kinase (False)
   d. Regular monitoring of serum electrolytes is required (True)
   e. It can cause genital ulceration (True)

AIIMS MAY 2019

55. **SGLT-2 inhibitors are recently used for type 2 diabetes mellitus. Which of the following are the rare but serious side effect?**
   a. Ketoacidosis b. Fournier gangrene
   c. Urosepsis d. Angioedema
   1. a, b and c are correct
   2. a and c are correct
   3. b and d are correct
   4. All four options are correct

56. **Match the following drugs with side-effects:**

Drugs	Side-effects
1. Amiodarone	a. Optic neuritis
2. Digoxin	b. Cataract
3. Systemic steroids	c. Yellow vision
4. Hydroxychloroquine	d. Retinopathy
	e. Angle closure Glaucoma
	f. Blepharoconjunctivitis
	g. Corneal microdeposits
	h. Maculopathy

57. **Propranolol is drug of choice for:**
   a. Ulcerated infantile hemangioma
   b. Lymphangioma circumscriptum
   c. Capillary malformation
   d. Pyogenic granuloma

58. **Match the antimicrobial drug preferred for the organism:**

Antimicrobial drug	Organism
1. Praziquantel	a. A. lumbricoides
2. Mebendazole	b. Tape worm
3. Nitazoxanide	c. Filariasis
4. DEC	d. Leishmaniasis
	e. Giardiasis
	f. S. hematobium

59. **Match the following drugs and antidotes:**

Drugs	Antidotes
1. Paracetamol	a. Amyl nitrite
2. Nicotine	b. N acetyl cysteine
3. Morphine	c. Diazepam
4. HCN	d. Bupropion
	e. Nalorphine
	f. Trimethadione

60. **Cl. difficile associated diarrhea is mostly due to:**
   a. Aminopenicillins
   b. Fluoroquinolones
   c. Carbapenems
   d. Macrolide

61. **Drugs used in postpartum hemorrhage are:**
   a. Misoprostol
   b. Dinoprostone
   c. Prostaglandin F2 alpha
   d. Oxytocin
   1. a, b and c are correct 2. a and c are correct
   3. b and d are correct 4. All four options are correct

62. **There was outbreak of MRSA in hospital and it was found that the nurse had MRSA in her nares. How will you treat her?**
   a. Bacitracin ointment b. Intranasal colistin
   c. Oral vancomycin d. Intravenous cefazolin

63. **Chlorpromazine is an antipsychotic that also acts as an anxiolytic and produces adverse effects like sedation, dry mouth and hypotension. All these actions are due to which receptors.**
   a. D1, D2 and 5HT2 b M1, M2 and A1, A2
   c. GABA and beta receptors d. H1
   1. a, b and d correct 2. b and d correct
   3. a and c correct 4. a, b, c and d correct

64. **Match the following anesthetic agents with their side-effects:**

Anesthetic agent	Side-effect
1. Propofol	a. Rigid chest syndrome
2. Fentanyl	b. Pulmonary vasoconstriction
3. Midazolam	c. Egg allergy
4. Nitrous oxide	d. Hypotension
	e. Dissociative anesthesia
	f. Adrenal insufficiency

65. **A bank employee felt depressed, no interest in activities came to AIIMS OPD and was started with escitalopram. Which of these side effects cannot be explained with escitalopram?**
   a. Vivid dreams b. Sialorrhea
   c. Anorgasmia d. Nausea vomiting

66. **Assertion: Larger doses of acyclovir is recommended for treating genital herpes in HIV.**

   Reason: Severe/frequent recurrences are seen in HIV patients.
   a. Both Assertion and Reason are independently true statements and the Reason is correct explanation for the Assertion
   b. Both Assertion and Reason are independently true statements, but the Reason is not the correct explanation for the Assertion
   c. Assertion is independently true statement, but reason is independently a false statement
   d. Assertion is independently false statement, but reason is independently a true statement
   e. Both Assertion and Reason are independently false statements

67. **Which of the following is correct regarding digoxin?**
   a. Earliest side effect is nausea and vomiting
   b. Causes nonspecific color vision
   c. Hypokalemia is associated with digoxin toxicity
   d. It causes hypomagnesemia
   1. a, b and c are correct 2. a and c are correct
   3. b and d are correct 4. All four options are correct

68. **The pH of gastric acid is 1-2 and pH of intestine is 6. PKa of weak acids like paracetamol is 9.5, and phenobarbitone is 7.2 and weak base diazepam is 3.3. Which of the following statements are true/false?**
   a. Paracetamol is present in nonionizable form and hence easily absorbed from stomach
   b. No drugs are absorbed from large intestine because of small surface area
   c. Phenobarbitone is absorbed more in small intestine than stomach as it has more blood supply
   d. Drugs which decrease the transit time like drugs causing diarrhea increase absorption
   e. Diazepam is absorbed in small intestine

69. **Consider the following statements regarding P falciparum. Which are true/false?**
   a. Cases of drug resistance have not been reported in India
   b. Chloroquine, sulfamethoxazole and pyrimethamine have given good results
   c. Quinine, doxycycline and clindamycin are effective in Rx.
   d. Artemether and lumefantrine is effective
   e. Artesunate is not used as monotherapy

70. **Theme and Focus: Seizure**
   Answer option list:
   a. IV phenobarbitone b. Rectal diazepam
   c. Intraosseous midazolam d. IV Phenytoin
   e. Nasal carbamazepine f. Oral valproate

   Lead in Question: A one and half year-old baby comes to OPD with generalized convulsive episode which lasts for 45 min. On duty Senior Resident asked junior resident to start an IV line and left.
   - If IV access is not possible at that time by the junior resident; what is the next step?
   - The SR comes back and finds out that the status is still not improved after initial management but does observe that the IV line is accessed. What is the next line of management now?

71. **A 53 years old is found to be hypertensive stage 2 without any co morbidities. Which drug will you start?**
   a. Furosemide b. Chlorthalidone
   c. Spironolactone d. Triamterene

72. **Which of the following will lead to change in biological activity of the hormone given in picture?**

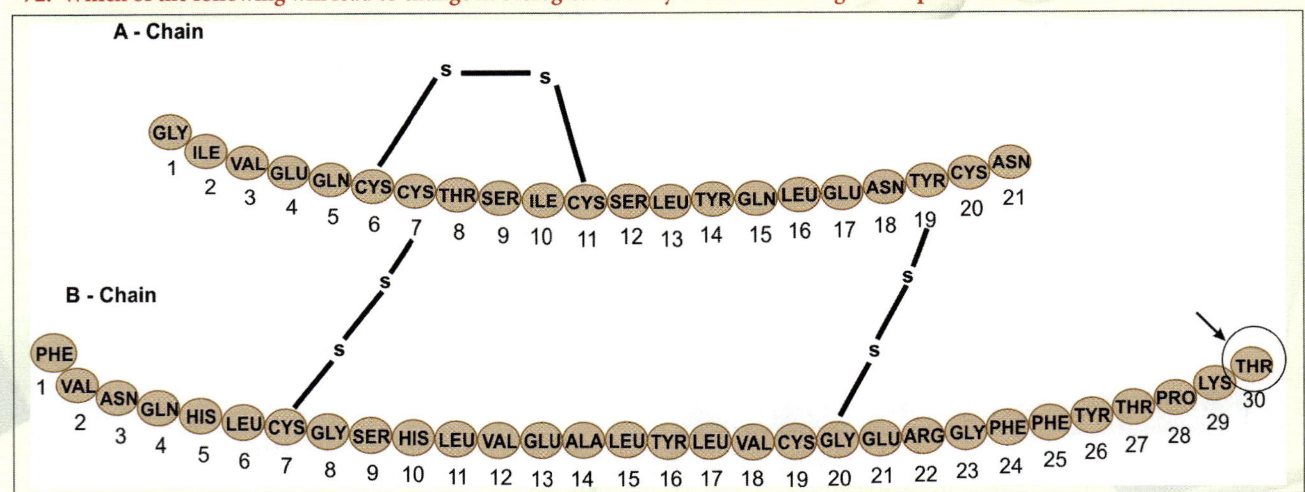

   a. Change in 1 to 4 amino acids in chain A
   b. Break in intra strand disulfide bond in chain A
   c. Change of 28 and 29 amino acid in chain B
   d. Change in 14 and 16 amino acid in chain A

73. **Which of the mentioned drugs most commonly causes acute liver failure?**
   a. Warfarin b. Tetracycline
   c. Paracetamol d. Valproate

74. **Strain used for Mw vaccine is:**
   a. M. indicus pranii b. M. welchii
   c. M. bovis d. M. vaccae

JIPMER NOVEMBER 2019

75. **Protein synthesis inhibitor used in CML is**
   a. Panobinosta
   b. Bortezomib
   c. Carfilzomib
   d. Omacetaxine

76. **The following adverse effect is associated with bedaquiline therapy:**
   a. QT prolongation b. Hearing loss
   c. Renal failure d. Thrombocytopenia

77. **Which of the following drug is not metabolized by plasma esterases?**
   a. Esmolol b. Clevidipine
   c. Mepivacaine d. Remifentanil

78. **Following is a beta 2 agonist used by athletes to increase performance due to its anabolic action?**
   a. Clenbuterol
   b. Albuterol
   c. Colterol
   d. Prenalterol

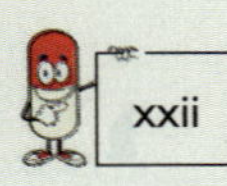

79. **Which of the following drug is used in malignant ascites?**
   a. Ramucirumab b. Catumaxomab
   c. Trastuzumab d. Cetuximab

80. **Which of the following antimicrobial contains additional MAO inhibitory property**
   a. Polymyxin B b. Linezolid
   c. Colistin d. Quinupristin

81. **Which of the following statement is FALSE about dronabinol**
   a. It is a synthetic cannabinoid
   b. It acts as antagonist at cannabinoid 2 receptors
   c. It acts as appetite stimulant in AIDS patients
   d. It is used for the treatment of nausea and vomiting associated with cancer chemotherapy

82. **Longest acting bisphosphonate is**
   a. Alendronate b. Risedronate
   c. Zoledronate d. Pamidronate

83. **Mechanism of action of bisphosphonates is**
   a. Inhibit osteoclast apoptosis
   b. Inhibit farnesyl pyrophosphate synthase
   c. Decrease osteoprotegerin
   d. Stimulate osteoblast

84. **Shortest acting opioid is**
   a. Fentanyl b. Alfentanil
   c. Remifentanil d. Sufentanil

85. **Anaerobic bacteria are intrinsically resistant to the following antimicrobial drug?**
   a. Ampicillin b. Meropenem
   c. Aminoglycosides d. Metronidazole

86. **The dose of the following drug should be decreased in patients with Crigler-Najjar syndrome?**
   a. Irinotecan b. Topotecan
   c. Ceftizoxime d. Thiazides

87. **Among the following antimicrobial drugs, which is not a peptide?**
   a. Vancomycin b. Telavancin
   c. Cycloserine d. Daptomycin

88. **A patient presented with bradycardia and hypotension after overdose of metoprolol. The drug of choice for this patient is**
   a. Atropine b. Glucagon
   c. Adrenaline d. Nor-adrenaline

89. **Hemodialysis is not useful in poisoning due to**
   a. Lithium b. Digoxin
   c. Carbamazepine d. Aminophylline

90. **Dose of which of the following drug should be reduced when used concomitantly with febuxostat**
   a. 6-Thioguanine b. Azathioprine
   c. 5-Fluorouracil d. Methotrexate

91. **Therapeutic plasma level of phenytoin are**
   a. 5-10 mcg/mL b. 10-20 mcg/mL
   c. 20-50 mcg/mL d. 50-100 mcg/mL

92. **Which of the following drug follows time dependent killing?**
   a. Beta lactams
   b. Aminoglycosides
   c. Fluoroquinolones
   d. Metronidazole

93. **A patient on haloperidol starts developing dystonia and akathisia. What is next best drug for this person?**
   a. Chlorpromazine b. Lurasidone
   c. Fluphenazine d. Lithium

JIPMER MAY 2019

94. **Bile acid resins causes ...% decrease in LDL and ...% increase in HDL.**
   a. 10-15% and 3-5% b. 15-25% and 3-5%
   c. 3-5% and 15-30% d. 25-35% and 5-10%

95. **Which of the following statements is false regarding bedaquiline?**
   a. Inhibits mycobacterial cell wall synthesis
   b. Causes QT prolongation
   c. Half-life is very long
   d. Indicated for MDR TB

96. **Raxibacumab is used in:**
   a. Anthrax b. Pontiac fever
   c. Listeria d. Clostridium

97. **Which of the following statement is true regarding atazanavir?**
   a. Effective against only HIV-1
   b. Resistance is due to mutation in codon 50 isoleucine to valine substitution
   c. ↓ Cholesterol and TG levels
   d. Combination with ritonavir do not have any advantage

98. **Mechanism of resistance of tetracyclines is due to:**
   a. Drug efflux mechanism
   b. Both drug influx and drug efflux mechanisms
   c. DNA methylation
   d. Cell wall alteration

99. **Initial drug to start with newly detected hypertension in a 42 years old male with calcium stones (nephrolithiasis) is:**
   a. Furosemide
   b. Spironolactone
   c. Atenolol
   d. Thiazides

100. **Diplopia with dizziness are side effects of which of the following drug combination?**
   a. Phenytoin and carbamazepine
   b. Lamotrigine and carbamazepine
   c. Gabapentin with phenytoin
   d. Valproate and topiramate

101. **Dose of fosfomycin in a 40 years patient who is weighing 60 kg:**
   a. 6 gm single dose b. 6 mg/kg single dose
   c. 3 gm single dose d. 3 mg/kg single dose

102. **Which statin is not metabolized by CYP3A4?**
   a. Lovastatin b. Simvastatin
   c. Atorvastatin d. Pravastatin

103. **Acetylcholine receptors has 5 subunits:**
   a. a_2, β_1, δ and k b. α_1, β_2, δ and k
   c. α_2, β_1, δ and e d. α_1, β_2, δ and e

104. **Which drug has anti-inflammatory and also has immune-modulator actions?**
   a. Fluoroquinolones b. Macrolides
   c. Tetracyclines d. Acyclovir

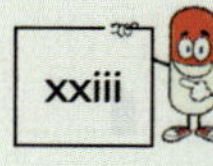

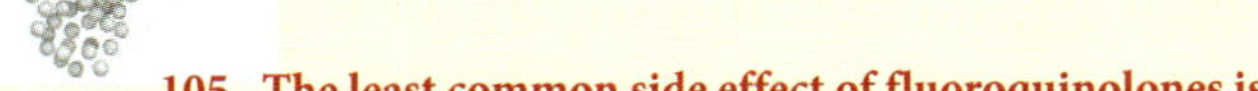

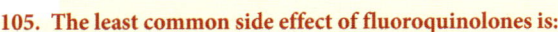

105. **The least common side effect of fluoroquinolones is:**
   a. Abdominal discomfort b. Hypoglycemia
   c. QT prolongation d. Hallucinations

106. **Which of the following combinations can result in severe toxicity due to inhibition of cytochrome 450 enzyme?**
   a. Amiodarone + Cimetidine
   b. Carbamazepine + Phenytoin
   c. Atorvastatin + Itraconazole
   d. Phenytoin + Rifampin

107. **Which of the following decreases defibrillation threshold?**
   a. Amiodarone b. Verapamil
   c. Sotalol d. Diltiazem

108. **All are true regarding isavuconazonium sulfate except:**
   a. Effective against yeasts, molds and dimorphic fungi
   b. Acts through blocking cytoplasmic proteins
   c. Approved for aspergillosis and mucormycosis
   d. Devoid of nephrotoxicity

109. **Which of the following is relatively contraindicated in chronic kidney disease?**
   a. Rivaroxaban b. Apixaban
   c. Edoxaban d. Dabigatran

110. **Erectile dysfunction (Hypogonadism) is caused by:**
   a. Antihistamines b. Leukotriene antagonists
   c. Thyroxine d. Insulin glargine

111. **Deprescription of PPIs can be done in all except:**
   a. 40-year-old with Barrett's esophagus
   b. 40-year-old with one episode of variceal bleeding
   c. 45-year-old with NSAID induced ulcer
   d. Stress ulcer in ICU patient

112. **Half-life of basiliximab is:**
   a. 7 days b. 7 hours
   c. 15 days d. 24 hours

113. **Colistin is not active against:**
   a. Pseudomonas aeruginosa
   b. Serratia
   c. Klebsiella pneumoniae d. Burkholderia

114. **Regarding artemisinin pharmacokinetics all are true except:**
   a. Dose adjustment not required in hepatic or renal failure
   b. Has a long half-life
   c. Oral bioavailability is around 30%
   d. Autoinducers

115. **A patient on blinatumomab for refractory B cell ALL is now resistant to the drug. Which drug to be used?**
   a. Vorinostat b. Brentuximab
   c. Pembrolizumab d. Tisagenlecleucel

116. **Which of the following drugs is most useful for acute severe depression and has good side effect profile?**
   a. RIMAs b. SSRIs
   c. Tricyclics d. MAO-inhibitors

117. **Which of the following drug do not act via NF-κB:**
   a. Sunitinib b. Emetine
   c. Diltiazem d. Bortezomib

118. **Which of the following is the most beta-1 selective antagonist?**
   a. Acebutolol b. Atenolol
   c. Metoprolo d. Bisoprolol

119. **All are TNF alpha inhibitors except:**
   a. Alemtuzumab b. Infliximab
   c. Adalimumab d. Etanercept

120. **Denosumab is used in:**
   a. Osteomalacia b. Osteoarthritis
   c. Osteoporosis d. Osteosarcoma

PGI MAY 2019

121. **Which of the following statement(s) is/are true about bioavailability:**
   a. Bioavailability of an orally administered drug is calculated by comparing the area under curve after oral and IV drug administration
   b. Studies in zero phase of clinical trials
   c. Can be determined by plasma level and urinary excretion
   d. Low oral bioavailability always and necessarily means low absorption
   e. It is the fraction of drug reaching the systemic circulation

122. **Which of the following drug(s) is/are T-type calcium channel blocker:**
   a. Verapamil b. Diltiazem
   c. Nifedipine d. Mibefradil
   e. Ethosuximide

123. **Regarding first order kinetics, true statement(s) is/are:**
   a. Rate of elimination is directly proportional to drug concentration
   b. Plasma half-life is independent of drug concentration
   c. Clearance is proportional to dose of drug
   d. Constant fraction of drug is eliminated over time
   e. Constant amount of drug is eliminated over time

124. **Which of the following inhibit Iodide trapping:**
   a. Vegetables of Brassica family
   b. Perchlorates
   c. Carbimazole
   d. Excessive iodide intake
   e. Para-amino salicylic acid

125. **Which among the following drugs can cause Gynecomastia:**
   a. Valproate b. Omeprazole
   c. Calcium channel blockers
   d. Penicillamine
   e. Amiodarone

126. **Which of the following agent(s) is/are a racemic mixture of two enantiomers with different pharmacodynamics and pharmacokinetic properties:**
   a. Phenytoin
   b. Esomeprazole
   c. Digoxin
   d. Epinephrine
   e. Verapamil

127. **Which of the following(s) is/are example of Type-A adverse drug reaction:**
   a. Anaphylaxis due to penicillin
   b. Beta-blocker: Bradycardia
   c. Carcinogenicity of diethylstilbestrol
   d. Aplastic anemia with chloramphenicol
   e. Deafness from aminoglycoside overdose

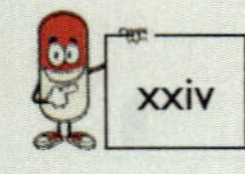

128. Which of the following is/are true regarding pseudocholinesterase except:

a. Also called Acetyl cholinesterase
b. Also called butyrylcholinesterase
c. Hydrolyses succinylcholine
d. Synthesized in the liver
e. Found in plasma

129. Toxic effect(s) of cisplatin include(s):

a. Neurotoxicity
b. Nephrotoxicity
c. Ototoxicity
d. Neuropathy
e. Cardiac toxicity

130. Drug(s), which is/are used for moderate severe psoriasis, act on IL-12 and IL-23 drug(s) is/are:

a. Ustekinumab
b. Efalizumab
c. Abatacept
d. Secukinumab
e. Guselkumab

131. Which of the following is/are true about thiazide diuretics:

a. Act by blocking sodium channel in interstitium
b. Lead to decrease in absorption of sodium and chloride in Distal tubule
c. Retain responsiveness even if GFR is decreased
d. Can cause hypoglycemia
e. Act on ascending loop of Henle

132. Which of the following drug(s) has been approved by FDA to be used in the treatment of cystic fibrosis with G551D mutation:

a. Lumacaftor
b. Ivacaftor
c. Tezacaftor
d. Crofelemer
e. Ataluren

133. All are CNS stimulants except:

a. Methylphenidate
b. Atomoxetine
c. Amphetamine
d. Pentazocine
e. Clonidine

134. Which of the following drug acts by inhibiting alpha IIb beta 3-integrin:

a. Eptifibatide
b. Tirofiban
c. Abciximab
d. Rivaroxaban
e. Ticagrelor

135. Which of the following antibiotics cause time dependent killing:

a. Macrolides
b. Aminoglycosides
c. Vancomycin
d. Linezolid
e. β-lactams

136. Drug(s), which is/are metabolized by *CYP3A4 isoenzyme:*

a. Verapamil
b. Amiodarone
c. Statins
d. Cyclosporine
e. Phenytoin

137. Medical treatment of Multiple myeloma include(s):

a. Daratumumab
b. Rituximab
c. Lenalidomide
d. Bortezomib
e. Bendamustine

138. Drugs which DONOT cause significant hypoglycemia at overdose:

a. Metformin
b. Sulfonylurea
c. Insulin
d. Sitagliptin
e. Pioglitazone

139. Fentanyl, which is used in cancer pain management, is characterized by:

a. Synthetic opioid
b. 100 times more potent than morphine
c. Acts on dorsal horn cells
d. Metabolized into inactive metabolite norfentanyl
e. μ agonist

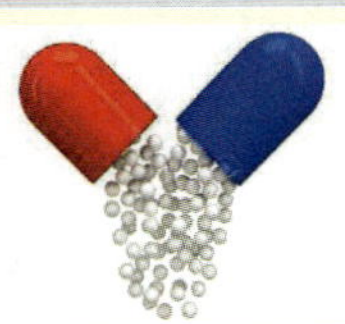

Answers with Explanations

RECENT PATTERN QUESTIONS 2020

General Pharmacology

1. Ans. (c) Insulin

(Ref: Goodman Gilman 13th E/P40)

- Important examples of tyrosine kinase receptors are receptors for insulin, IGF1 and various growth factors like EGF, VEGF and PDGF.
- Receptors for TRH and TSH are Gs subtype of GPCR
- Receptor for MSH is also known as melanocortin 1 receptor is a Gs subtype of GPCR.

2. Ans. (a) Only A

(Ref: Goodman Gilman 13th E/P34)

- Potency of a drug in DRC can be determined from the position of DRC on dose axis, as potency is inversely proportional to dose.
- Hence it can be said that DRC on left are more potent and DRC on right are less potent.
- Since DRC of A is most left here, it is the most potent drug.

3. Ans. (a) K_m remains same, V_{max} decreases

(Ref: Goodman Gilman 13th E/P35)

Competitive antagonism	Non-competitive antagonism
At same site	At different sites
DRC shifts to right side	Slope of DRC decreases
Efficacy and V_{max} does not change	Efficacy and V_{max} decreases
Dose and K_m increases as potency decreases	Dose, potency and K_m does not change

Autonomic Nervous System

4. Ans. (d) Tamsulosin

(Ref: https://clinicaltrials.gov/ct2/show/NCT02486653)

- Bethanechol is primarily used for its stimulatory action on bladder and GIT.
- It is used for treatment of urine retention seen in postoperative period or associated with diabetic neuropathy. It can be used for treatment of gastroparesis and adynamic ileus as well. However, it can cause bronchoconstriction and is contraindicated in asthma and COPD.
- Methacholine has more cardiac stimulatory effects and hence is not preferred for the above mentioned uses. It is used for diagnosis of bronchial asthma in bronchial challenge test.
- Terazosin being a non-selective alpha 1 blocker is used for treatment of hypertension and hypertension associated with BPH.
- Tamsulosin being a selective alpha1a blocker is preferred for treatment of BPH. It is under trial for prevention of postoperative urine retention. Hence tamsulosin is the best answer in this question.

5. Ans. (a) Neostigmine

(Ref: Goodman Gilman 13th E/P184)

- **Neostigmine** is used for reversal of muscle relaxant effect produced by nondepolarizing muscle relaxants (NDMR), which competitively block nicotinic receptors.
- **Sugammadex** is a chelating agent that removes NDMRs from the synapse. It is specifically used for reversal of muscle relaxation produced by rocuronium and vecuronium.

6. Ans. (a) Latanoprost

(Ref: KDT 8th E/P169)

- **Latanoprost** is a prostaglandin F2alpha analog that increases uveoscleral outflow of aqueous by increasing permeability of ciliary muscles or episcleral vessels.
- Timolol is a beta blocker that acts by decreasing aqueous production.
- Pilocarpine is a miotic agent that increases trabecular outflow.
- Dorzolamide is a carbonic anhydrase inhibitor that decreases aqueous production.

Cardiovascular System

7. Ans. (c) Hydrochlorothiazide

(Ref: Goodman Gilman 13th E/P455)

- Thiazides can competitively block uric acid excretion in the proximal convoluted tubule and hence cause hyperuricemia.
- Thus, thiazides like hydrochlorothiazide should not be given to patients with high serum uric acid levels.

8. Ans. (a) Amiodarone

(Ref: Goodman Gilman 13th E/P564)

- **Amiodarone** can cause **pulmonary fibrosis** and risk is increased in case of underlying lung disease and hence is contraindicated in patients with interstitial lung disease.
- Pulmonary fibrosis can be rapidly progressive and fatal and hence chest X-ray and pulmonary function tests should be conducted regularly. Plasma concentration does not have good correlation with pulmonary fibrosis.

9. Ans. (b) Ranolazine

(Ref: Goodman Gilman 13th E/P500)

- **Ranolazine** primarily acts by **inhibiting late sodium current** in the myocardial cells. This decreases intramyocardial sodium and leads to activation of sodium calcium exchanger, which pumps sodium in and calcium out. A decrease in calcium decreases myocardial contraction and oxygen demand.
- Secondary mechanisms are **inhibition of fatty acid oxidation** and **beta-1 receptors**.

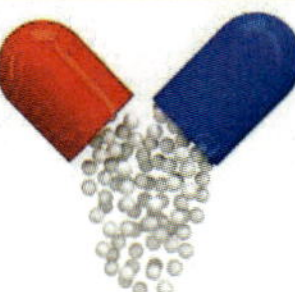

Diuretics

10. Ans. (a) Intravenous digoxin

(Ref: CMDT 2019/P1577)

- High altitude pulmonary edema is usually seen at heights of 3000 meters and above.
- This is a case of high altitude pulmonary edema where immediate descent to at least 610 meters should be done and oxygen is administered. Nifedipine can be used for treatment in case there is no response to initial management.
- Acetazolamide is not used for treatment, but can be used for prophylaxis of high altitude pulmonary edema associated with neurological symptoms of mountain sickness or cerebral edema.
- Intravenous digoxin is used for treatment of cardiogenic pulmonary edema but not for noncardiogenic pulmonary edema as in this case.

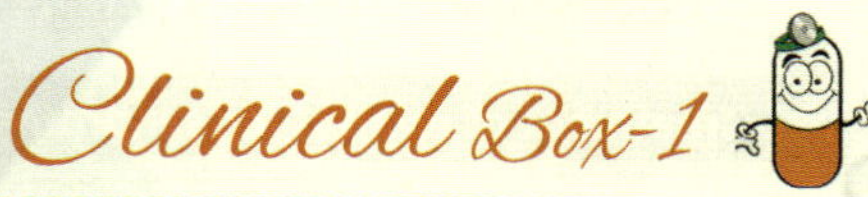

Treatment of High Altitude Illness

Initial management begins with immediate descent of minimum 610 meters and in case immediate descent is not possible, then hyperbaric chambers can be used. Oxygen must be administered to keep oxygen saturation of at least 90%. Then pharmacologic therapy can be given as given below.

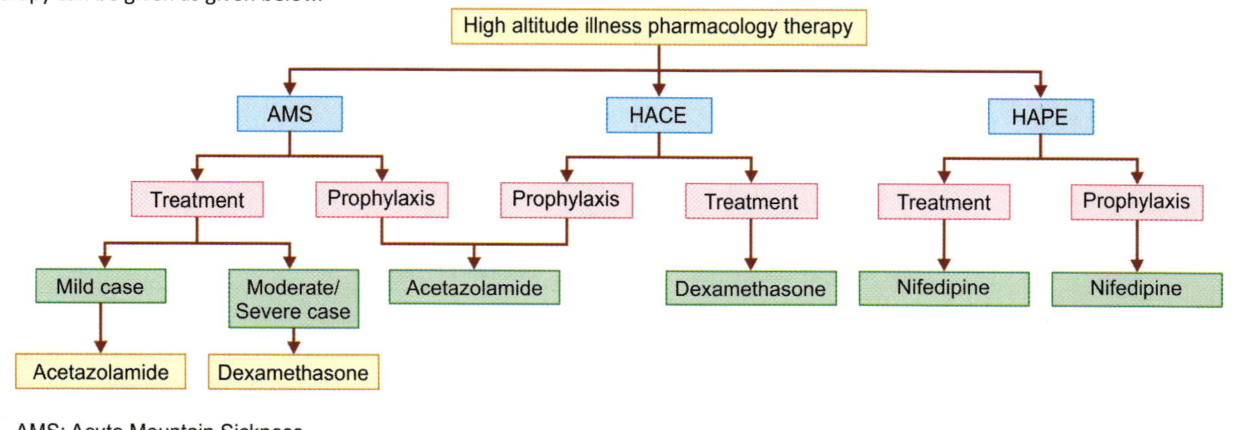

Note: In case of HAPE, PDE-5 inhibitor like sildenafil can be used as an alternative.

Central Nervous System

11. Ans. (c) Thiazides increase tubular reabsorption of lithium

(Ref: Goodman Gilman 13th E/P295)

- Lithium and sodium have similar characteristics and hence in case of sodium loss from the body caused by fasting, vomiting, diarrhoea or diuretics like thiazides, there can be an increased tubular reabsorption of lithium.
- Hence there can be an increased risk of lithium toxicity.

Effect of diuretics on lithium clearance	
Carbonic anhydrase inhibitors Mannitol	Increases clearance of lithium
Thiazides > Potassium sparing diuretics	Decrease clearance by increasing tubular reabsorption
Loop diuretics	No effect on lithium clearance

12. Ans. (a) Serum electrolytes

(Ref: Goodman Gilman 13th E/P295)

- Lithium and sodium have similar characteristics and hence in case of sodium loss from the body **caused by fasting**, vomiting, diarrhoea or diuretics like thiazides, there can be an increased tubular reabsorption of lithium.
- Hence it is appropriate here to test the serum electrolyte level first to diagnose hyponatremia.

13. Ans. (d) Iron tablets

(Ref: CMDT 2019/P1030)

- Restless leg syndrome is associated with abnormal sensation in legs, which improves with leg movement. The symptoms mentioned in the question are consistent with restless leg syndrome.
- Iron tablets should be given as first line in case of iron deficiency and if serum ferritin level is ≤75 mcg/L.

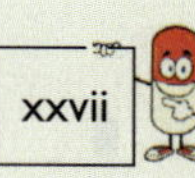

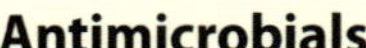

- In case there is no response to iron tablets or there is no iron deficiency, then the **first line becomes dopamine agonists (pramipexole, ropinirole and rotigotine) or GABA releasing drugs (pregabalin and gabapentin)**. Overall dopamine agonists are more effective and are considered drugs of choice. But with increasing dose of dopamine agonists, the effect decreases; a phenomenon known as augmentation.
- In case patient does not respond to above mentioned drugs, then **levodopa** or an **opioid** (**oxycodone, methadone, tramadol**) is used i.e. in resistant cases.
- Thus, the best answer here is pramipexole.

Treatment of restless leg syndrome

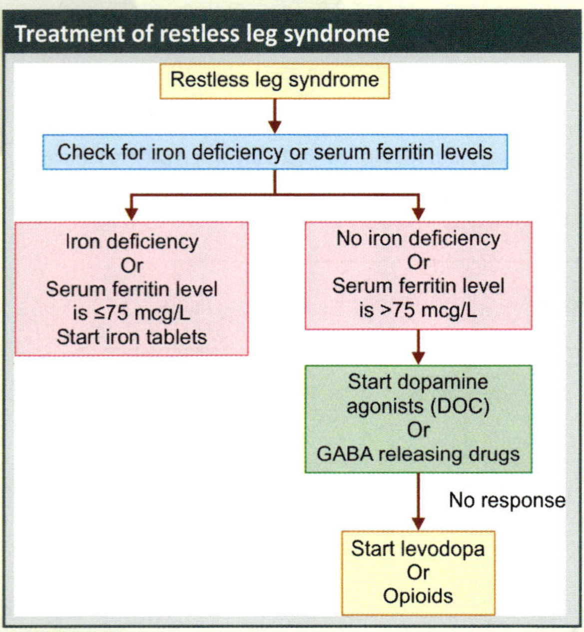

Note: Intravenous iron is used in case serum ferritin level is <100 mcg/L or there is malabsorption state or intolerance to oral iron.

14. Ans. (b) Trihexyphenidyl

(Ref: Goodman Gilman 13th E/P291)

- Mentioned symptoms in the question are consistent with drug induced Parkinsonism that can be seen with antipsychotics like fluphenazine.
- Anticholinergics like **trihexyphenidyl** (benzhexol), benztropine and biperiden are drugs of choice.
- Alternatives are antihistaminics with maximum anticholinergic effects i.e. promethazine, diphenhydramine and dimenhydrinate.
- Amantadine can also be used as an alternative.

15. Ans. (a) Morphine

(Ref: Goodman Gilman 13th E/P368)

- Opioids like morphine can constrict sphincter of Oddi and hence can worsen pain of biliary colic.
- The first line drugs for biliary colic are NSAIDs like ketorolac, diclofenac, ibuprofen etc.

Antimicrobials

16. Ans. (b) Pefloxacin

(Ref: KDT 8th E/P763)

- Most fluoroquinolones are excreted by kidney except moxifloxacin and pefloxacin.
- Hence both these drugs are safe in renal failure and contraindicated in liver failure.
- Trovafloxacin was banned due to hepatotoxicity.

17. Ans. (b) Voriconazole

(Ref: Goodman Gilman 13th E/P1095)

- Voriconazole is more effective than amphotericin B against invasive aspergillosis.
- Hence voriconazole is the drug of choice and amphotericin B can be used as an alternative.

18. Ans. (a) Rifampicin

(Ref: Goodman Gilman 13th E/P1068)

- Rifampicin blocks DNA dependent RNA polymerase and hence inhibits transcription of DNA to RNA.
- Nitrofurantoin produces free radicals which damage DNA of bacteria.
- Ciprofloxacin and novobiocin inhibit DNA gyrase or topoisomerase IV and thus block DNA synthesis.

19. Ans. (a) Erythromycin

(Ref: Goodman Gilman 13th E/P1056)

- Theophylline is metabolized by CYP1A2, which is blocked by erythromycin, as it is an enzyme inhibitor.
- Hence erythromycin can precipitate theophylline toxicity; this is important as theophylline has a low therapeutic index.

20. Ans. (c) Break down of drug structure

(Ref: Goodman Gilman 13th E/P1023)

Resistance to Penicillins

Resistance to penicillins can be seen by four mechanisms described below.

1. **Beta lactamase production**
   Beta lactamase breaks down the beta lactam structure in penicillins. Beta lactamase can be classified by **Ambler's molecular classification and Bush's functional classification.**
2. **Alteration of penicillin binding protein (PBP)**
   - An alteration in the PBP is responsible for resistance particularly in gram positive organism staphylococcus.
   - A **high molecular weight PBP** results in resistance of **staphylococcus aureus to methicillin (MRSA)** and it is **plasmid mediated**. Thus, resistance to penicillins in staphylococcus is due to penicillinase and to PRPs like methicillin is due to altered PBP mediated by **Mec A gene**.
3. **Decreased porin production**
   - Porins are the gateway for entry of beta lactams in to the gram negative organisms.

- **Pseudomonas** can selectively decrease porin production and deny entry to the penicillins.

4. Drug efflux

- Microorganisms can develop drug efflux active pumps, which can pump drug out against concentration gradient.
- This mechanism is present in gram negative organisms like **pseudomonas, E. coli and gonococcus.**

21. Ans. (b) Ciclopirox

(Ref: Goodman Gilman 13th E/P1281)

Drugs used for treatment of onychomycosis

Oral	Topical
Terbinafine – Preferred for dermatophytes Itraconazole – Preferred for candida Fluconazole – It is an alternative Griseofulvin – It is not preferred due to resistance	**Ciclopirox lacquer** Efinaconazole solution Tavaborole solution

Note: Oral drugs are more effective and hence preferred to topical drugs. Topical drugs are effective only in mild to moderate cases i.e. without nail matrix involvement.

Anticancer Drugs

22. Ans. (a) 6 Mercaptopurine

(Ref: Goodman Gilman 13th E/P1184)

- Purine analogs like 6 mercaptopurine inhibit de novo purine synthesis and also inhibit DNA synthesis by getting incorporated in to nucleic acids.
- Actinomycin D inhibits RNA synthesis by inhibiting RNA polymerase.
- Mitomycin C primarily acts by alkylating DNA.
- Asparaginase acts by depleting asparagine, which leads to lymphocyte toxicity.

Endocrinology

23. Ans. (b) Bisphosphonates

(Ref: Goodman Gilman 13th E/P898)

- Oral bisphosphonates like alendronate and risedronate are preferred first line drugs for treatment of postmenopausal osteoporosis. In case of intolerance or contraindication to oral drugs, intravenous zoledronate is used.
- In patients with intolerance to both oral and intravenous bisphosphonates, alternatives like denosumab, romosozumab, teriparatide and raloxifene can be used.
- In case of high risk of fracture (osteoporosis without fragility fracture or osteoporosis with fragility fracture + BMD, T score > –2.5) denosumab is preferred.
- In case of very high risk of fracture (T score ≤ –3.5 or T score ≤ –2.5 + fragility fracture or severe/multiple vertebral fractures) anabolic drugs like teriparatide > abaloparatide or romosozumab is preferred.
- Raloxifene can also be used as an alternative and is preferred in females with high risk of breast cancer. Bazedoxifene can also be used but is less preferred than raloxifene for treatment of osteoporosis. Bazedoxifene conjugated estrogen is used in menopausal females to treat hot flashes and prevent osteoporosis.
- Calcitonin though can be used is less preferred due to poor efficacy and risk of cancers.

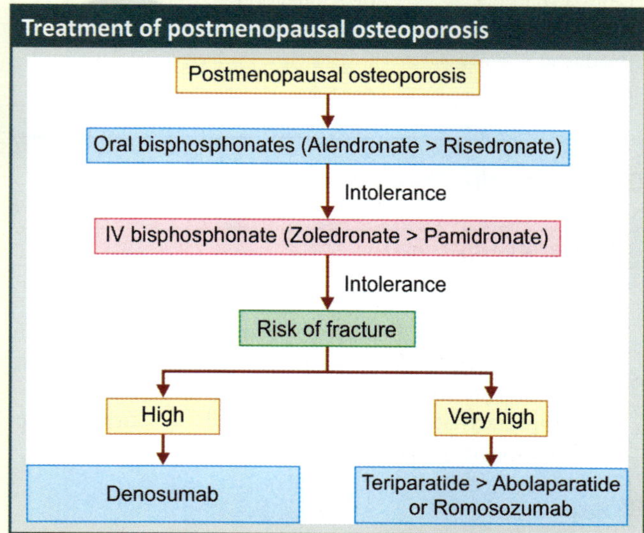

Autacoids

24. Ans. (c) Chronic tophaceous gout

(Ref: Goodman Gilman 13th E/P705)

- Uricase analog pegloticase is reserved for treatment of severe/refractory chronic gout, whereas rasburicase is used for treatment of tumor lysis syndrome.
- Common side-effects associated are anaphylaxis and hemolysis in G6PD deficiency.
- Another drawback of these drugs is production of autoantibodies which can limit efficacy.

25. Ans. (b) Chloroquine

(Ref: KDT 8th E/P880)

- Ocular toxicity in the form of retinopathy and corneal deposits can be seen with chloroquine on prolonged use.
- The risk is high with doses >250 mg daily. Ophthalmological examination once in a year is advised for patients on chloroquine.

26. Ans. (a) Promethazine

(Ref: Goodman Gilman 13th E/P718)

- Anticholinergic drug scopolamine is the drug of choice for motion sickness. It is given by transdermal route as a patch, 4-5 hours before travel.
- Antihistaminics with significant anticholinergic effect like **promethazine**, diphenhydramine and dimenhydrinate can also be used.

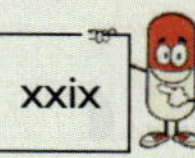

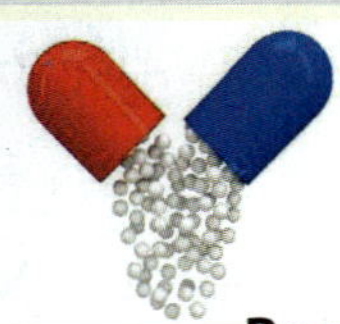

Respiratory System

27. Ans. (b) Adenosine A1 receptor antagonism

(Ref: Goodman Gilman 13th E/P735)

Side-effects of theophylline

Seizure Diuresis	Adenosine A1 receptor antagonism
Nausea vomiting GIT upset Headache	PDE-4 inhibition
Arrhythmia	Adenosine A1 receptor antagonism PDE-3 inhibition

Gastrointestinal System

28. Ans. (d) Diphenoxylate

(Ref: Goodman Gilman 13th E/P924)

- 5HT4 agonists (Mosapride, Prucalopride), D2 blockers (Metoclopramide, Domperidone) and macrolides (erythromycin) are used as prokinetics.
- Diphenoxylate is an opioid used for treatment of nonsecretory diarrhoea.

Blood

29. Ans. (c) II

(Ref: Goodman Gilman 13th E/P592)

- Warfarin inhibits synthesis of coagulation factors II, VII, IX and X.
- It also inhibits synthesis of anticoagulant protein C and S.
- Factor VII is shortest acting and first to disappear, whereas factor II is longest acting and last to disappear after starting warfarin.

AIIMS NOVEMBER 2019

Single Best Response Questions

30. Ans. (b) Trimetazidine

(Ref: Goodman Gilman 13th E/P501)

- **Trimetazidine** is a partial fatty acid oxidase (PFOX) inhibitor which inhibits free fatty acid oxidation in heart (major source of ATP in heart). Hence heart compensates by increasing glycolysis to generate ATP. Since glycolysis has lesser oxygen requirement, there is an overall decrease in myocardial oxygen demand, which is beneficial in ischemia. It can cause agranulocytosis, thrombocytopenia and increases risk of movement disorders (Parkinson's disease) in elderly. Hence it is reserved as a second line drug for treatment of **stable angina**.
- Beta blockers like **metoprolol,** bisoprolol, carvedilol and nebivolol are approved for treatment of chronic CHF.
- **Sacubitril** is a neutral endopeptidase inhibitor approved for treatment of chronic CHF in combination with valsartan.
- **Nesiritide** is a BNP analog approved for treatment of resistant pulmonary edema associated with acute CHF.

31. Ans. (b) Belladonna

(Ref: Goodman Gilman 13th E/P153)

- Belladonna plant (Atropa belladonna) is source for anticholinergic compounds like atropine and scopolamine. Hence belladonna poisoning can produce anticholinergic symptoms like mydriasis.
- Pilocarpine and organophosphates are cholinergic drugs and hence produce miosis.
- Opioids like morphine produce miosis; pethidine though produces mydriasis due to anticholinergic effect.

32. Ans. (a) Chronic gout

(Ref: Goodman Gilman 13th E/P705)

- Pegloticase is a pegylated uricase and rasburicase is an uricase analog. Both drugs act by metabolizing uric acid into water soluble compound allantoin that is excreted by kidney.
- **Pegloticase** is used for treatment of **severe or drug resistant chronic gout** by intravenous route. The drawback is autoantibody production that can neutralize pegloticase and decrease its efficacy. This antibody production is more against rasburicase and hence is not used in gout. Rasburicase is rather used for treatment of hyperuricemia seen with tumor lysis syndrome.
- Side-effects associated are anaphylaxis and hemolysis in G6PD deficiency.

33. Ans. (d) Angiotensin 1 receptor

- Gi and Go subtype of GPCRs act by opening potassium channels.
- Among the given options M2, D2 and 5HT1 are Gi/o subtype of GPCRs and hence act by opening potassium channels. Apart from that Gi subtype decrease cyclic AMP and Go subtype decrease calcium.
- Angiotensin 1 receptor on the other hand is a Gq subtype of GPCR which acts by increasing calcium via IP3.
- Gs subtype act by increasing cyclic AMP which phosphorylates proteins.
- Some examples of different subtype of GPCRs is given in the table below.

Gs	Gq	Gi/o
Beta 1, 2 and 3	Alpha 1	Alpha 2
	M 1, 3 and 5	M2
H2	H1	H3
5HT 4	5HT 2	5HT 1
		Cannabinoid receptors
D1		D2

34. Ans. (a) 0.5 mL of 1:1000 adrenaline by intramuscular route

(Ref: CMDT 2018/P885)

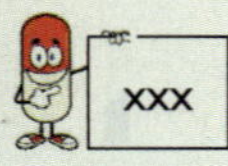

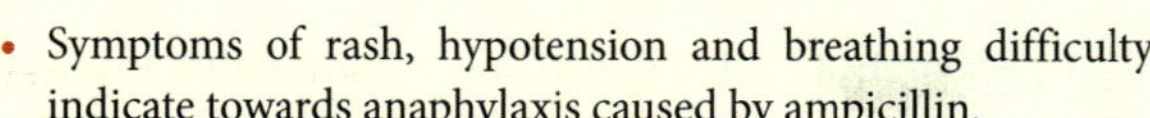

- Symptoms of rash, hypotension and breathing difficulty indicate towards anaphylaxis caused by ampicillin.
- In anaphylaxis the drug of choice is epinephrine 0.3–0.5 mL by intramuscular route at 1:1000 dilution (0.3–0.5 mg). Intravenous epinephrine 2.5 mL at 1:10,000 (0.25 mg) is used in case of severe anaphylactic shock only.
- Other supportive drugs used in anaphylaxis are steroids, bronchodilators and antihistamines.

35. Ans. (d) Dexamethasone

(Ref: Goodman Gilman 13th E/P1259)

- Mannitol, carbonic anhydrase inhibitors like methazolamide, alpha 2 agonist like brimonidine and apraclonidine (clonidine derivative), beta blockers like timolol, prostaglandin analogs like latanoprost and miotics like pilocarpine are used to decrease IOP in glaucoma.
- Dexamethasone on the other hand can rather increase IOP.

36. Ans. (a) 5HT4 agonist

(Ref: Goodman Gilman 13th E/P924)

- Prucalopride is a 5HT4 agonist which is approved for treatment of laxative resistant chronic constipation in females.
- Other drugs in this class are cisapride, tegaserod and mosapride. Cisapride and tegaserod have been banned due to risk of QT prolongation.

5HT1A partial agonist	• Buspirone • Ipsapirone
5HT 1B/1D agonist	• Sumatriptan • Rizatriptan • Eletriptan • Frovatriptan
5HT 1F agonist	• Lasmiditan
5HT 2A/2C antagonist	• Methysergide • Ketanserin
5HT 2C agonist	• Lorcaserin
5HT3 antagonist	• Ondansetron • Palonosetron • Alosetron
5HT 4 agonist	• Cisapride • Mosapride • Prucalopride • Tegaserod

37. Ans. (c) Administration of long acting depot antipsychotics

Guidelines for administration of long acting antipsychotic depot injections (LAAI)

- LAAIs are given to patient with psychosis or mania who have poor compliance to oral treatment.
- A test dose is given for all drugs except olanzapine, risperidone, paliperidone and aripiprazole.
- Route of administration is by intramuscular route with maximum permissible volume as as follows:

Deltoid	2 mL
Dorsogluteal	4 mL
Ventrogluteal (Safest site)	4 mL
Rectus femoris	5 mL
Vastus lateralis	5 mL

- Z track technique is used for injection in to all sites, except deltoid. The skin is stretched laterally from the intended site of injection and then insert the needle at 90° angle. After 10 seconds of injecting the drug, skin is released to allow the displaced tissue to cover the needle track. It is done to maximize absorption in to muscles by preventing the drug from moving back to subcutaneous tissue.
- Z track technique is also used to inject iron.

38. Ans. (c) Ketamine

(Ref: Drugs and cosmetics rule 1945)

- Schedule X drugs are psychotropic drugs which need special licensing for manufacturing and sale. The drugs in schedule X are given below.

Schedule X drugs	• Amobarbital Glutethimide • Pentobarbital • **Ketamine** • Amphetamine • Meprobamate Phencyclidine • Methamphetamine • Phenometrazine • Methylphenidate • Ethchlorvynol

- Some important drug schedules

Schedule A	Gives specimens of prescribed forms required for obtaining drug licenses, permits, certificates etc.
Schedule B	Includes fees for test or analysis by central drug laboratory, e.g. determination of LD50 in mice.
Schedule C	Includes biologicals and special products like sera, vaccines, toxin, antitoxin, insulin etc.
Schedule D	Provides conditions regarding exemption regarding import of drugs. E.g. fortified milk with vitamins, lactose, ginger, pepper, Cummins etc.
Schedule E	Gives list of poisonous substances under Ayurvedic and Unani system of medicine. E.g. bhang, datura, snake poison etc.
Schedule F	Includes requirement for functioning and operation of blood bank.
Schedule FF	Lays down standards for ophthalmic preparations.

Contd...

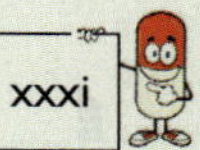

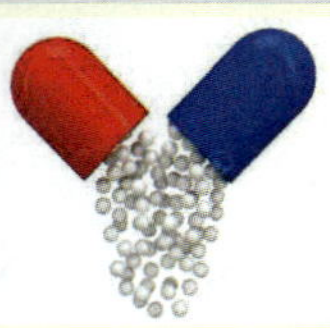

Schedule G	List of drugs that requires a mandatory text on label "Caution: It is dangerous to take this preparation, except under medical supervision". E.g. antihistaminics, metformin, insulin, anticancer drugs, antiepileptics etc.
Schedule H	List of drugs that can be sold only when a prescription is produced. Most drugs belong to this category. The drug label must display the text "Rx" and "Schedule H drug. Warning: To be sold by retail on the prescription of a Registered Medical practitioner only".
Schedule H1	Introduced in 2013 to deal with unauthorized sale of antibiotics. Drugs are labelled with "Rx" in red.
Schedule J	Contains list of various diseases and conditions which no drug should claim to prevent or cure e.g. AIDS, deafness, blindness, diabetes, paralysis etc.
Schedule K	Drugs under this schedule are exempted from the provisions of chapter IV of the act. E.g. antimalarials, paracetamol, gripe water etc.
Schedule M	Includes Good Manufacturing Practices and requirement of premises, plant and equipment for manufacture of pharmaceutical products.
Schedule N	Gives list of minimum requirements for the efficient running of a pharmacy.
Schedule O	Deals with provisions applicable to disinfectant fluids.
Schedule P	It is about drug expiry period i.e. maximum period till which drug can be used with intact potency.
Schedule P1	Specifies the pack size of certain drugs like aspirin should have a pack size of 14 tablets.
Schedule Q	Gives the list of dyes, colors and pigments permitted to be used in cosmetics and soaps.
Schedule R	Gives standards for mechanical contraceptives like condoms.
Schedule R1	Gives standard for medical devices.
Schedule S	Prescribes standards for cosmetics.
Schedule T	Lays down Good Manufacturing Practices for Ayurvedic, Siddha and Unani medicines.
Schedule U and U1	Gives the particulars to be shown in manufacturing records.
Schedule V	Gives details of standards for patent and proprietary medicines.
Schedule W	List of drugs marketed under generic names only.
Schedule X	List of narcotic and psychotropic drugs which need special license for manufacture and sale. Drugs are labelled with "NRx" and prescription copy should be retained by the retailer for minimum of 2 years.
Schedule Y	Guidelines on clinical trials, import and manufacture of new drugs.

Contd...

- Note: 1. OTC (Over The Counter) drugs don't require a prescription and are drugs which don't belong to schedule G, H and X.
- 2. Drugs under schedule G, H and X cannot be directly advertised to the patient.

39. Ans. (c) 3 drugs for 6 months

(Ref: WHO leprosy guidelines 2018)

- The number of drugs used for treatment of both paucibacillary and multibacillary leprosy is same i.e. Rifampicin, Dapsone and clofazimine (3).
- However the duration of treatment of paucibacillary leprosy is of 6 months and multibacillary leprosy is of 12 months.

40. Ans. (a) Subcutaneous

(Ref: Goodman Gilman 13th E/P589)

- LMWH and fondaparinux can be used by subcutaneous route once a day for both treatment and prophylaxis of thrombosis.
- Unfractionated heparin can be used by subcutaneous route twice a day for prophylaxis and by intravenous route four times a day for treatment of thrombosis.

41. Ans. (b) Metronidazole

(Ref: Goodman Gilman 13th E/P1061 and CDC)

- Metronidazole, tinidazole and clindamycin are preferred antibiotics for treatment of bacterial vaginosis, however the single best drug of choice is metronidazole.

First line	Second line
• **Metronidazole (DOC) 500 mg orally BD for 7 days** • Metronidazole gel 0.75% 5 g intravaginally once a day for 5 days • Clindamycin cream 2% 5 g intravaginally once a day for 7 days	• Tinidazole 2 g orally OD FOR 2 days • Tinidazole 1 g orally OD for 5 days • Clindamycin 300 mg orally BD for 7 days • Clindamycin ovules 100 mg OD intravaginally for 3 days

42. Ans. (a) Radical cure of plasmodium vivax

(Ref: FDA)

Tafenoquine

- Tafenoquine also acts on hypnozoite stage, i.e. exoerythrocytic tissue stage and prevents relapse of malaria in vivax and ovale.

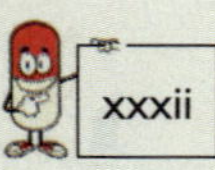

- **It is used for radical cure of malaria caused by vivax and ovale.** Unlike primaquine which needs to be given for 14 days, 300 mg of tafenoquine is given once on the first or second day of therapy with other drugs like chloroquine.
- Side-effects associated are hemolysis in G6PD deficiency, methemoglobinemia, and neuropsychiatric side-effects.
- Pregnancy, lactation and age group less than 16 years are absolute contraindication.

43. Ans. (b) It is active against gram positive organisms

(Ref: Goodman Gilman 13th E/P1058)

- Oxazolidinediones like linezolid and tedizolid have good spectrum against **gram positive organisms** like staphylococcus, streptococcus, enterococcus etc.
- Linezolid and tedizolid have **good oral absorption** and bioavailability of 100% and 80% respectively. Linezolid is excreted primarily by kidney, whereas **tedizolid by liver**.
- Tedizolid is longer acting and more active against gram positives as compared to linezolid. Hence linezolid is given by oral or intravenous route by BD dosing and tedizolid by oral or intravenous route by OD dosing.
- Linezolid can cause bone marrow suppression (thrombocytopenia predominantly) and hence platelet count should be monitored. Tedizolid causes lesser bone marrow suppression.
- Linezolid also causes mitochondrial toxicity, which presents as peripheral neuropathy, optic neuritis and lactic acidosis. **These side-effects are not seen with tedizolid.**

44. Ans. (b) Male infertility

(Ref: Goodman Gilman 13th E/P781)

- GnRH agonists can be used by pulsatile and non-pulsatile or continuous dosing.
- By pulsatile dosing they increase release of LH/FSH and cause ovulation, spermatogenesis and increase synthesis estrogen and testosterone. Hence used for treatment of anovulation, oligospermia (male infertility), delayed puberty and sexual infantilism.
- By continuous dosing they decrease synthesis of estrogen and testosterone. Hence used for treatment of estrogen and testosterone dependent conditions like ER positive breast cancer, endometriosis, uterine fibroids and prostate cancer.

45. Ans. (a) Zidovudine used as monotherapy in post-exposure prophylaxis

(Ref: NACO guidelines 2018)

- Post exposure prophylaxis should be given within 2 hours and can be given till 72 hours after exposure.
- First line regimen is tenofovir + lamivudine for 28 days or lopinavir + ritonavir for 28 days. Thus single drug regimen is not used.

46. Ans. (b) To decrease secretions

(Ref: Goodman Gilman 13th E/P157)

- Glycopyrrolate is used prior to anesthesia to decrease salivary, tracheobronchial and pharyngeal secretions.
- It can also be used after surgery to prevent the cholinergic effects of neostigmine that is used to reverse effect of muscle relaxants.
- It is also used to decrease drooling in patients of Parkinson's disease and as an antispasmodic agent.

47. Ans. (b) Voltage gated calcium channels

(Ref: Goodman Gilman 13th E/P128)

- **Presynaptic membrane:** Depolarization of presynaptic membrane activates voltage gated calcium channels, which increases entry of calcium in to presynaptic neuron. Calcium facilitates movement of vesicle and fusion of vesicular membrane with presynaptic membrane, which is followed by exocytosis/release of acetylcholine. Aminoglycosides can block presynaptic calcium channels and decrease release of acetylcholine.
- **Postsynaptic membrane:** Once acetylcholine is released it can act on muscarinic receptors or nicotinic receptors present on postsynaptic membrane.

48. Ans. (c) Serotonin and norepinephrine reuptake inhibition

(Ref: Goodman Gilman 13th E/P 374)

- Tramadol is a synthetic codeine analog used for treatment of mild to moderate acute pain. It is used along with acetaminophen in an FDC for analgesia.
- Thus, it is not effective in chronic or severe pain.
- It is a racemic mixture of enantiomers. Apart from μ receptor agonism, it is also an agonist at alpha 2 receptor and inhibits reuptake of serotonin and norepinephrine.

Dextro (+) enantiomer	μ agonist and inhibits serotonin reuptake
Levo (-) enantiomer	Alpha 2 agonist and inhibits norepinephrine reuptake

- It can cause seizures, however causes lesser respiratory depression and constipation as compared to other opioids.
- Other opioids with action other than opioid receptor agonism are:

Meperidine	Anticholinergic MAO inhibition (By metabolite normeperidine)
Tapentadol	MAO inhibition

49. Ans. (a) Griseofulvin

(Ref: Goodman Gilman 13th E/P1098)

- The given condition in the picture is black dot tinea capitis.
- The drug of choice for treatment of tinea capitis is griseofulvin.

Match the Following

50. Ans. 1-e, 2-a, 3-c and 4-d

(Ref: Goodman Gilman 13th E)

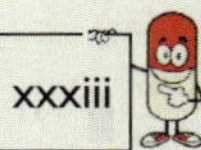

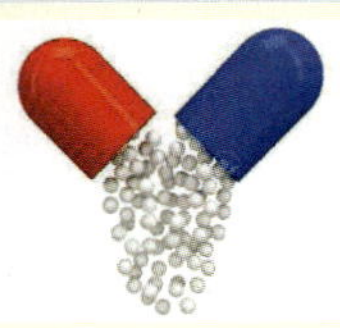

- Omalizumab is an anti IgE monoclonal antibody approved for treatment of severe persistent bronchial asthma.
- Itolizumab is an anti CD6 monoclonal antibody approved for treatment of plaque psoriasis.
- Daclizumab is an anti CD25 monoclonal antibody used for treatment of ultiple sclerosis.
- Belimumab is an anti B lymphocyte stimulator monoclonal antibody approved for treatment of SLE.

Assertion Reasoning Type

51. Ans. (c) Assertion is true but reason is false

(Ref: Goodman Gilman 13th E/P1055)

- In case of a hospitalized patient with community acquired pneumonia, beta lactams are used to cover gram positives like pneumococcus and macrolides are used to cover atypical organisms like mycoplasma, chlamydia and legionella.

Multiple True/False Type

52. Ans. True-c, d and e; False- a and b

(Ref: Goodman Gilman 13th E)

- Direct Acting Antivirals like sofosbuvir are better than the older drugs like ribavirin and interferon alpha.
- Ombitasvir is an inhibitor of NS5A, which results in block of viral replication, assembly and release. Protein synthesis is blocked by ribavirin.
- Imiquimod is used by topical route for treatment of condyloma acuminata.
- Simeprevir is an inhibitor of NS3/4 A or protease, which results in in block of viral maturation.
- Oseltamivir is the drug of choice for influenza A, influenza B and bird flu.

53. Ans. (b) Atropine, (e) PAM

(Ref: Goodman Gilman 13th E/P170)

- The symptoms given in the question are suggestive of cholinergic poisoning. A significant decrease in RBC esterase (Normal is around 100) confirms it as a case of organophosphate poisoning.
- Hence atropine and pralidoxime should be used.

54. Ans. True-a, b, d and e; False -c

(Ref: Goodman Gilman 13th E/P1112)

- Foscarnet is drug of choice for treatment of resistant HSV, VZV and CMV.
- It can cause nephrotoxicity, which can be decreased by preloading of normal saline.
- It does not require activation by thymidylate kinase. Rather nucleoside analogs like acyclovir require activation.
- It can cause hypo/hyper calcemia, hypo/hyper phosphatemia, hypokalemia and hypomagnesemia. Hence regular serum electrolyte monitoring is required.
- It can cause genital ulceration as well.

AIIMS MAY 2019

55. Ans. (1) a, b and c are correct

(Ref: FDA, Goodman Gilman 13th E/P880)

Side-effects of SGLT-2 Inhibitors

Common	Rare
Urinary tract infection (Most common) Hypotension Dehydration Polyuria Raised LDL	**Diabetic ketoacidosis** **Fournier gangrene** **Urosepsis** Acute renal injury Hyperkalemia Pancreatitis Venous thromboembolism Fracture Bladder and breast cancer (Dapagliflozin) Increased lower limb amputation (Canagliflozin)

Note: Angioedema is a side-effect of DPP-4 inhibitors.

- **Diabetic ketoacidosis** seen in diabetes mellitus usually is a result of absolute insulin deficiency which results in decreased glucose utilization and hyperglycemia. Insulin deficiency stimulates hormone sensitive lipase which leads to free fatty acid release from adipocytes and production of ketone bodies in the liver. This leads to hyperglycemia diabetic ketoacidosis.
- However, in case of SGLT-2 induced ketoacidosis the scenario is somewhat different. In patients of type 1 diabetes mellitus or insulin deficient type 2 diabetes mellitus, due to normalization of blood glucose level by SGLT-2 inhibitors, patient decrease the dose of insulin. This triggers the same pathway as described above but is associated with euglycemia.
- **Fournier gangrene** (infective necrosis of the perineal, perianal and genital tissues) is a rare and severe condition associated with diabetes mellitus. However the incidence increases with the use of SGLT-2 inhibitors. This might be associated with increased UTI with SGLT-2 inhibitors.
- **Urosepsis** i.e. spread of urinary tract infection to blood is also a rare side-effect. What is striking is that, UTI is mycotic, but urosepsis is commonly caused by *E. coli*.

Mnemonics

Side-effects of SGLT-2 Inhibitors

D: Diabetic ketoacidosis
A: Acute kidney injury
P: Pancreatitis
A: Amputation of lower limbs (Canagliflozin)
G: Gangrene (Fournier)
L: Low BP
I: Infection of urinary tract and urosepsis
F: Fracture

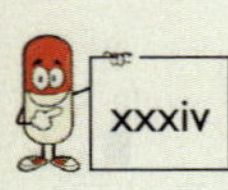

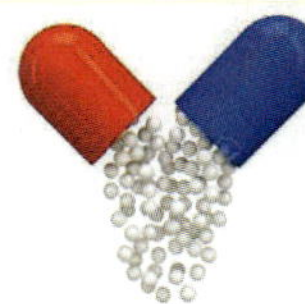

56. Ans. 1-g, 2-c, 3-b and 4-d

(Ref: Goodman Gilman 13th Edition)

Side-effects which are Correct Match

- Amiodarone can cause whorl like corneal microdeposits called as cornea verticillata or vortex keratopathy.
- Digoxin can cause yellow vision or xanthopsia.
- Systemic steroids cause cataract, whereas topical steroids cause glaucoma.
- Hydroxychloroquine can cause bull's eye retinopathy.

Other Side-effects

- Optic neuritis is caused by drugs like ethambutol and linezolid.
- Primary angle closure glaucoma is caused by anticholinergics or drugs with anticholinergic effect like tricyclic antidepressants, antipsychotics and antihistaminics. Secondary angle closure glaucoma is caused by sulfonamide group drugs like topiramate, carbonic anhydrase inhibitors and sulfonamide antibiotics.
- Allergic blepharoconjunctivitis is caused by topical timolol.
- Maculopathy is caused by drugs like latanoprost.

57. Ans. (a) Ulcerated infantile hemangioma

(Ref: Katzung 14th E/P169, file:///E:/Journals % 20 and % 20 guidelines % 202018/Infantile % 20 hemangioma. pdf)

Infantile Hemangioma

- **Infantile hemangiomas** are most common tumors of childhood, which appears as localized blanching or erythema before 4 weeks of age. Then it can grow in size till 1 years of age and become elevated with a rubbery feel.
- Then it can begin to involute spontaneously at 1 year of age and usually it completely disappears by 4 years of age.
- Types of infantile hemangioma

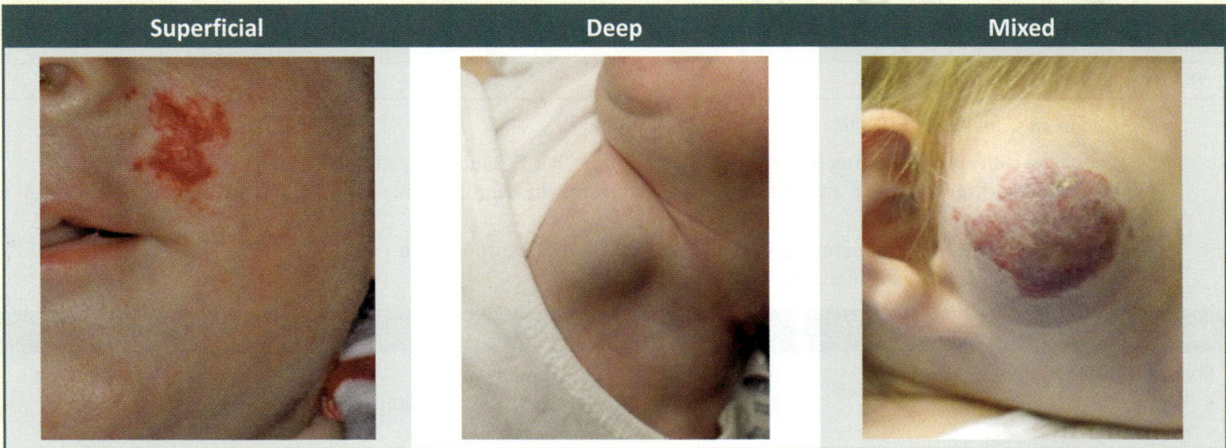

- Since these hemangioma involutes spontaneously treatment is usually not required. However, in some cases, due to complications like ulceration (most common) followed by others like visual impairment, CHF, auditory impairment, etc.

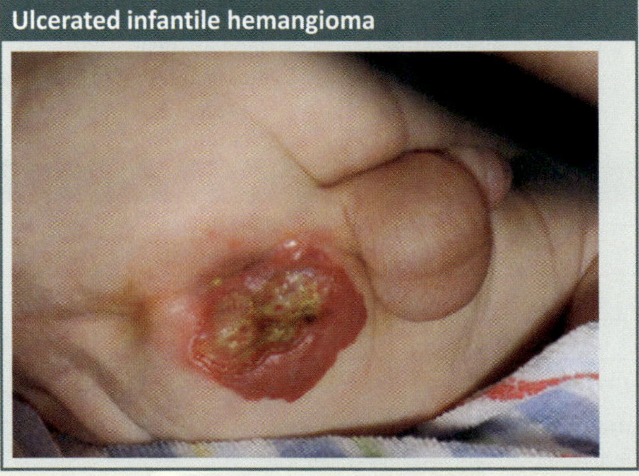

- The treatment of ulcer includes wound care, antibiotics and analgesics. Apart from these **propranolol** > topical timolol and systemic steroids have been effective. In nonresponsive cases pulsed dye laser therapy is used.

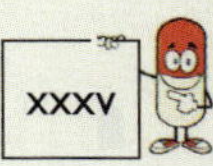

Other Options

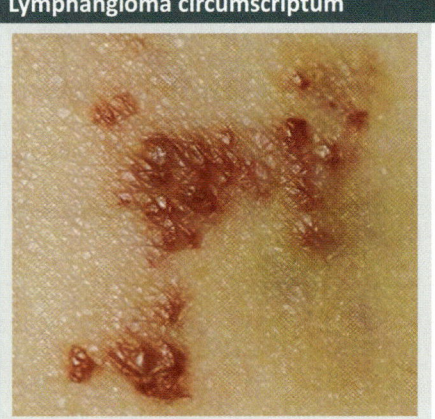

Lymphangioma circumscriptum	Capillary malformation	Pyogenic granuloma
	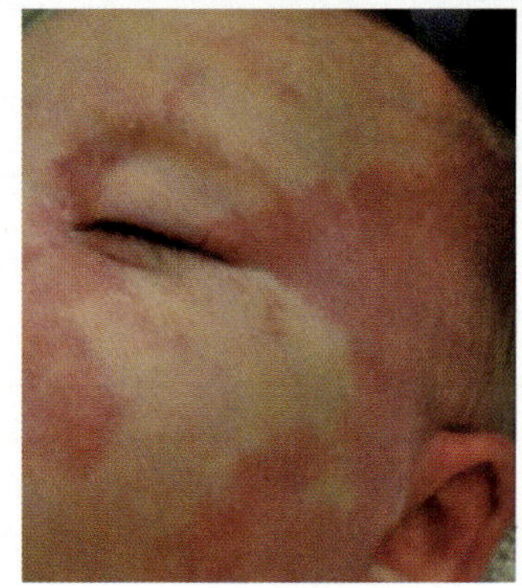	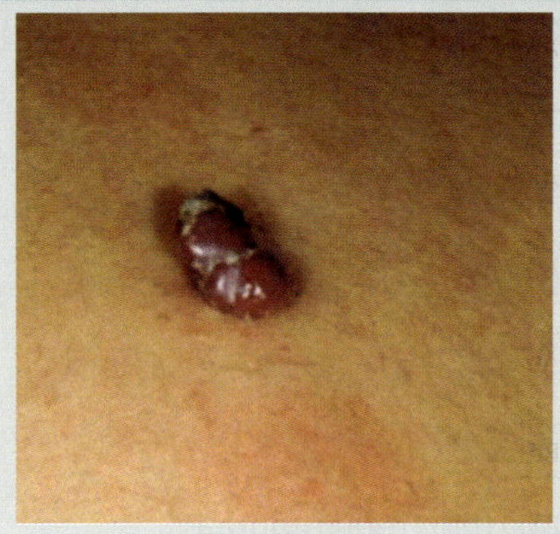
Lymphangioma circumscriptum is a congenital lymphatic malformation which presents as clusters of translucent vesicles. Treatment consists of surgical excision, laser therapy, sclerotherapy, electrocoagulation and cryosurgery.	Capillary malformation is a congenital vascular malformation which presents as flat red cutaneous patches with irregular borders on the face and neck usually. The mainstay of treatment is laser therapy.	Pyogenic granulomas are similar to infantile hemangioma in presentation but are smaller and pedunculated. They have a higher risk of bleeding. Although topical timolol or steroids are used the evidence is limited.

58. Ans. 1-b, 2-a, 3-e and 4-c

(Ref: Goodman Gilman 13th E/P1008)

- Praziquantel is the preferred drug for cestodes or tape worms like T. solium, T. saginata. H. nana, D. latum etc.
- Albendazole and mebendazole are preferred for soil transmitted helminths like round worm (A. lumbricoides), whip worm (T. trichiura) and hook worm.
- Nitazoxanide is used for treatment of protozoa like giardia and cryptosporidium.
- DEC is the drug of choice for filariasis.

Nematodes: Drug of choice					
Soil transmitted helminths • Round worm (A. lumbricoides) • Hook worm • Whip worm Trichinella spiralis Enterobius vermicularis	}	Albendazole> Mebendazole	Thread worm Onchocerca Volvulus	}	Ivermectin
			Filariasis Loa Loa	}	DEC
			Dracunculiasis	}	Metronidazole
Cestodes: Drug of choice					
Neurocysticercosis Echinococcus	}	Albendazole	(Tape worms) Intestinal T. solium T. saginata H. nana D. latum	}	Praziquantel
Trematodes: Drug of choice					
Liver Fluke	}	Triclabendazole	Lung fluke Schistosoma	}	Praziquantel

59. Ans. 1-b, 2-f, 3-e and 4-a

(Ref: Goodman Gilman 13th E/P63)

- N acetyl cysteine is the drug of choice for paracetamol poisoning. It acts by inhibiting toxic metabolite of paracetamol, i.e. NPQI and by regenerating glutathione.
- Nicotine poisoning can cause seizure for which antiepileptic like trimethadione can be used. Bupropion is used in smoking dependence; it is not nicotine antidote.
- Current drugs preferred for morphine toxicity are naloxone and nalmefene; previously nalorphine was also used.
- HCN or hydrogen cyanide toxicity is treated with drugs like amyl nitrite, hydroxocobalamin and sodium thiosulphate.

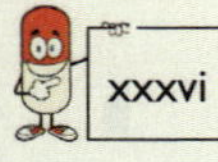

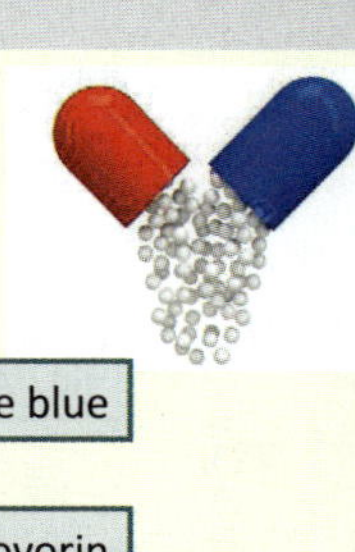

Drug of Choice for Poisoning and Drug Toxicity

Poisoning / Toxicity	Drug of Choice
Acetaminophen	Acetylcysteine
Amphetamine Toxicity	Urine acidification (Ammonium chloride)
Antihistaminics	Physostigmine
Antipsychotics Bicarbonate	TCA
Atropine (Belladonna) Poisoning	Physostigmine
Beta blockers	Glucagon
Benzodiazepine Poisoning	Flumazenil
CCB Toxicity	Calcium gluconate
Cyanide Toxicity	(Lilly Kit) 1. I/V Hydroxocobalamin Or I/V Amyl Nitrite Plus 2. IV Sodium Thiosulphate
Digoxin Toxicity	Digibind (Anti digoxin antibodies)
Ergot Alkaloids	1. Nitroprusside Or 2. Nitroglycerine
Ethylene glycol Methanol	Fomepizole
Heparin Toxicity	Protamine Sulfate
Iron	Deferoxamine
Isoniazid	Pyridoxine (Vitamin B6)
MAO Inhibitors	1. Nitroprusside Or 2. Esmolol
Methemoglobinemia	I/V Methylene blue
Methotrexate	Leucovorin
Methylxanthines	Propranolol
Mushroom Poisoning	1. Amanita Muscaria – Physostigmine 2. Boletus, Clitocybe, Inocybe – Atropine
Nicotinic agonist poisoning 1. Nicotine 2. Lobeline	Cholinesterase Reactivators
Organophosphate poisoning Carbamate poisoning	Atropine
Opioid toxicity	Naloxone > Nalorphine
Salicylates	1. Urine Alkalization Or 2. Dialysis (High Levels)
Serotonin Syndrome	Cyproheptadine
Sulfonylurea induced hypoglycemia	Octreotide
Sympatholytics	1. α_2 agonists – Dopamine and NE 2. β blockers – Glucagon
Sympathomimetics 1. α_1 agonists – Phentolamine 2. β_1 agonists – Propranolol 3. Non Selective (Cocaine, Amphetamine, Ephedrine) – Labetalol	
Valproate hyperammonemia	Carnitine
Warfarin toxicity	Vitamin K

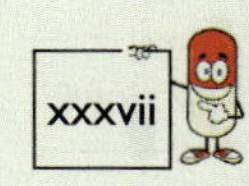

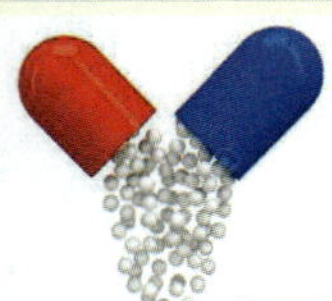

60. Ans. (a) Aminopenicillins

(Ref: Harrison 20th E/P964)

Pseudomembranous enterocolitis (Updated guidelines)

- Pseudomembranous enterocolitis is caused by gram positive bacteria clostridium difficile. The precipitating factor is suppression of normal microbiota of colon by prolonged use of antibiotics like cephalosporins, aminopenicillins, fluoroquinolones and clindamycin. The most common cause currently are **3rd generation cephalosporins like ceftriaxone followed by aminopenicillins**.
- The only FDA approved drugs for treatment are oral **vancomycin** and oral **fidaxomicin**. Other drugs that can be used off label are metronidazole, rifaximin, nitazoxanide, bacitracin, tigecycline and fusidic acid.

Doses of drugs used:

- Vancomycin R1 (Regimen 1): Oral vancomycin 125 mg QID for 10 days
- Vancomycin R2 (Regimen 2): Oral vancomycin 125 mg: QID for 10-14 days → BD for 7 days → OD for 7 days → Every 2-3 days once for 2-8 weeks. This is a prolonged tapered and pulsed regimen.
- Fidaxomicin: 200 mg BD for 10 days
- Rifaximin: 400 mg TDS for 20 days

- In an **initial episode** oral vancomycin is the current drug of choice for treatment of mild/moderate/severe cases. In severe complicated or fulminant cases oral vancomycin + intravenous metronidazole is used. If the patient dose not respond to drugs in fulminant cases, then colectomy is done to save life of the patients. Oral metronidazole as single agent is used in mild/moderate cases only if other drugs like vancomycin or fidaxomicin is not available.
- In patients with **first recurrence** oral vancomycin R1 is used if patient was on metronidazole and oral vancomycin R2 is used if patient was on oral vancomycin R1. The other alternative in first recurrence is oral fidaxomicin. In case of a **second recurrence** oral vancomycin R2 or oral vancomycin R1 + oral rifaximin or oral fidaxomicin can be used. In case of **third recurrence** fecal microbiota transplantation is done. To prevent recurrence along with antibiotics, bezlotoxumab (anti-clostridium difficile toxin B monoclonal antibody) can be used.

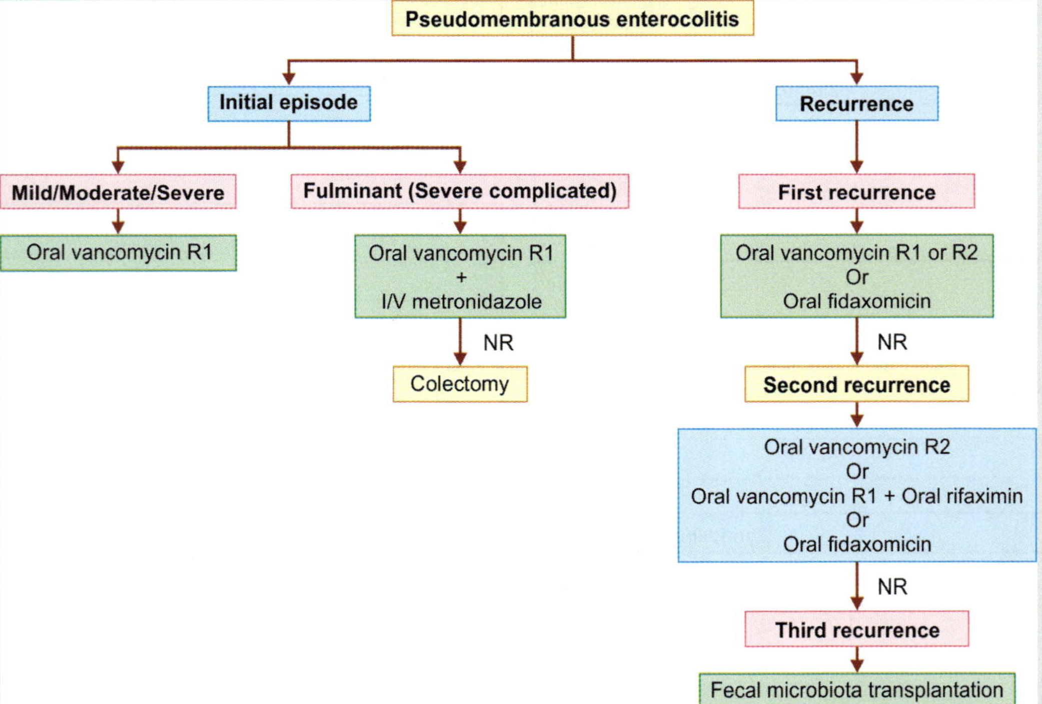

61. Ans. (4) All four options are correct

(Ref: William's Obstetrics)

Drugs used in Postpartum Hemorrhage

- Oxytocin by intravenous or intramuscular route is the drug of choice for treatment of postpartum hemorrhage.

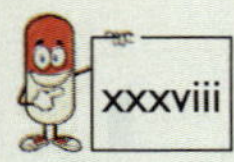

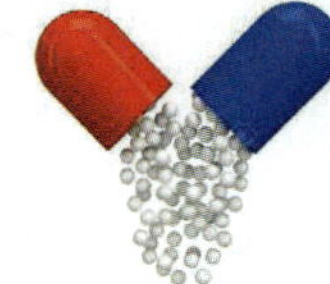

- In case there is no response to oxytocin, ergot alkaloids like methylergonovine (methergine) or ergonovine, prostaglandin F2 alpha (Carboprost), prostaglandin E2 (Dinoprostone, Sulprostone) and prostaglandin E1 (Misoprostol) can be used.
- Methergine, ergonovine and carboprost are given by intramuscular route and are highly effective drugs.
- Dinoprostone is given by rectal or vaginal route, whereas sulprostone by intravenous route. These are also highly effective drugs.
- Misoprostol can be given by intravenous or rectal route. It is least effective drug.

Treatment of postpartum hemorrhage

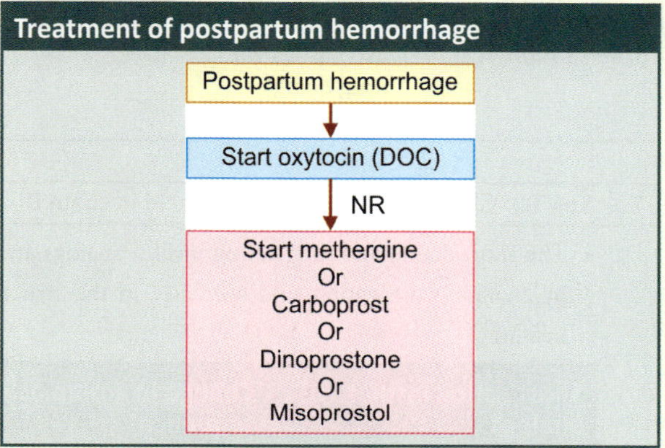

62. Ans. (a) Bacitracin ointment

(Ref: Goodman Gilman 13th E/P1062)

- Patients infected with staphylococcus often harbor it most commonly in anterior nares and serves as source for infections in hospitals.
- Hence for any patient infected with staphylococcus should be given topical mupirocin (DOC) to prevent nasal carriage. Chlorhexidine bath is used to prevent colonization in other body sites.
- An alternative to mupirocin is topical bacitracin, which is less effective.

63. And. (2) b and d are correct

(Ref: Goodman Gilman 13th E/P292)

- Tricyclic antidepressants, **typical antipsychotics (chlorpromazine)** and atypical antipsychotics produce side-effects due to block of a common group of receptors like H1, 5HT2, Alpha1 and Muscarinic receptors.

Receptor block	Associated side-effect
Muscarinic	Constipation Dry mouth Arrhythmia
H1	Sedation
H1 and 5HT2	Obesity
Alpha1	Postural hypotension

64. Ans. 1-c, 2-a, 3-d and 4-b

(Ref: Goodman Gilman 13th Edition)

Side-effects which are Correct Match

- Propofol is a highly lipid soluble compound and hence is combined with soybean oil, glycerol and egg phospholipid. Hence it carries a risk of egg allergy.
- Fentanyl can cause severe rigidity of chest muscles known as wooden or rigid chest syndrome.
- Midazolam can cause vasodilation and result in hypotension.
- Nitrous oxide can cause pulmonary vasoconstriction and hence is avoided in patients with pulmonary hypertension.

Other side-effects

- Dissociative anesthesia is a side-effect of ketamine.
- Adrenal insufficiency is caused by etomidate.

65. Ans. (b) Sialorrhea

(Ref: Goodman Gilman 13th E/P 273)

- Side-effects of SSRIs are due to an elevated serotonin levels in the body at different places, which stimulates different types of serotonin receptors.

Receptor subtype	Side-effect
5HT2 in brain	• Anxiety • Insomnia • Irritability • Vivid dreams
5HT2 in spinal cord	• Erectile dysfunction • Anorgasmia • Delayed ejaculation
5HT3 in CTZ area	• Nausea and vomiting
5HT4 in GIT	• Loose stools

66. Ans. (a) Both Assertion and Reason are independently true statements and the Reason is correct explanation for the Assertion

(Ref: Harrison 20th E/P1352)

- In immunocompetent patients, acyclovir is given 200 mg 5 times a day.
- In HIV patients, acyclovir is given 400 mg 4 times a day. The dose is higher as the risk of recurrence is higher in immunocompromised patients.

67. Ans. (2) a and c are correct

(Ref: Goodman Gilman 13th E/P539)

- GIT related side-effects like nausea and vomiting are the earliest to be seen in digoxin toxicity.
- Digoxin causes specifically yellow color vision or xanthopsia.
- Hypokalemia increases digoxin binding to Na/K ATPase pumps and hence increases risk of toxicity.
- Digoxin causes hyperkalemia but hypomagnesemia is not seen. Rather hypomagnesemia increases risk of digoxin toxicity.

68. Ans. True: a, c and e, False: b and d

(Ref: Goodman Gilman 13th E/P14)

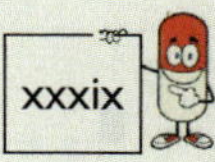

- For drug absorption unionization (lipid solubility) of drug and surface area of the organ are important. Thus, drugs with high unionization present in an organ with large surface area will have higher absorption.
- When the medium is same drugs are unionized and when medium is different drugs are ionized.
- Thus, both weakly acidic drugs like phenobarbital and paracetamol will be in unionized form in the stomach and will get absorbed in stomach. But for both maximum absorption will happen in small intestine due to considerably larger surface area of small intestine as compared to stomach.
- Diazepam on the other hand being a weak base will be more unionized in small intestine and there it will get absorbed.
- Drug absorption in large intestine is lesser due to unsuitable epithelium for absorption and small surface area. But it is not that no drug absorption takes place; hence option b is false.
- Drugs that increase motility of GIT decrease transit time of drug in GIT and hence faster movement of drug in GIT will decrease absorption.

69. Ans. True: c, d and e; False: a and b

(Ref: NVBD Malaria guidelines)

- P. falciparum is universally resistant to chloroquine in India and hence chloroquine is not used. Hence both option a and b are false.
- Artemisinin group drugs, quinine, tetracycline, doxycycline, clindamycin and lumefantrine are effective drugs for P. falciparum. Hence option c and d are true.
- Artemisinin group drugs are short acting drugs and hence never used alone, rather used with other drugs to prevent resistance. Hence option e is true.

70. Ans. (b) Rectal diazepam and (d) IV phenytoin

(Ref: Rudolph Pediatrics 21st E/P8701)

- This is a case of status epilepticus, where an IV line should be established and benzodiazepines like intravenous diazepam or lorazepam should be started followed by intravenous phenytoin. In case there is no response to phenytoin, then intravenous phenobarbitone is given.
- But in this case an IV line was not established and hence rectal diazepam is a suitable alternative to intravenous benzodiazepines.
- Since the child did not respond to rectal diazepam, the next best step is to start intravenous phenytoin.

71. Ans. (b) Chlorthalidone

(Ref: Goodman Gilman 13th E/P508)

Hypertension stage	Blood pressure	Treatment
Prehypertension	120/80 to 139/89	Lifestyle modification
Hypertension stage 1	140/90 to 159/99	First line drugs like ACE inhibitors/ARB, CCB or Thiazides
Hypertension stage 2	>160/100	First line drugs like ACE inhibitors/ARB, CCB or **Thiazides**
HTN urgency	>220/125 without end organ damage	Clonidine (DOC) Captopril Nifedipine
HTN emergency	High blood pressure with end organ damage	IV Nicardipine (DOC)
Resistant hypertension	Resistance to at least 3 drugs with 1 drug being a diuretic	Spironolactone (DOC)

Contd...

72. Ans. (c) Change of 28 and 29 amino acid in chain B

- The short acting and long acting insulin analogs are made by changing the amino acid sequence in the structure of insulin.

Short acting insulin analogs	Change in amino acid sequence
Lispro	Interchange of lysine and proline in 28 and 29 position of chain B
Aspart	Change of proline with aspartic acid in 28 position of chain B
Glulisine	Change of lysine with glutamic acid in 29 position of chain B and change of asparagine with lysine in 3 position of chain B

Long acting insulin analogs	Change in amino acid sequence
Glargine	Addition of two arginine with threonine in 30 position of chain B and change of asparagine with glycine in 21 position of chain A
Detemir	Addition of saturated fatty acid to lysine in 29 position of chain B
Degludec	Removal of threonine in 30 position of chain B and addition of glutamic acid and hexadecenoic acid to lysine in 29 position of chain B

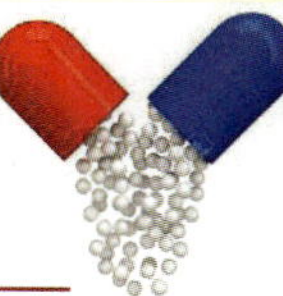

73. **Ans. (c) Paracetamol**

(Ref: Goodman Gilman 13th E/P696)

- All mentioned drugs can cause hepatotoxicity and liver failure, but the most common drug overall implicated in drug poisoning and suicidal attempts is paracetamol.
- Hence liver failure is most commonly seen with paracetamol. In case of fulminant liver failure liver transplantation is required.

74. **Ans. (a) M. indicus pranii**

(Ref: https://www.ncbi.nlm.nih.gov/pmc/articles/PMC5422320/pdf/btt-11-055.pdf)

- Mw mycobacterium, currently known as M. indicus pranii is a cultivable mycobacterium that is used to produce vaccine against leprosy.
- This vaccine is effective for treatment of leprosy, category II TB and anogenital warts.

JIPMER NOVEMBER 2019

75. **Ans. (d) Omacetaxine**

(Ref: Goodman Gilman 13th E/P1227)

- Omacetaxine is an inhibitor of synthesis of short-lived proteins like BCR-ABL protein which is involved in the pathogenesis of CML.
- Other three drugs in the options are proteasome inhibitors.

76. **Ans. (a) QT prolongation**

(Ref: Goodman Gilman 13th E/P1077)

- Recent drugs for TB like bedaquiline and delamanid can cause QT prolongation and hence are contraindicated in patients with arrhythmia.

77. **Ans. (c) Mepivacaine**

(Ref: Goodman Gilman 13th E/P415)

- Drugs metabolized by plasma esterase are
  - Succinylcholine
  - Mivacurium
  - Procaine
  - Cocaine
  - Heroin
  - Esmolol
  - Clevidipine
  - Remifentanil
- Drugs metabolized in plasma are very short acting.

78. **Ans. (a) Clenbuterol**

(Ref: Kenneth's Autonomic pharmacology/P200)

- Clenbuterol is a beta 2 agonist abuses by athletes to increase muscle mass and decrease fat.
- It is a banned substance by the doping agencies.

79. **Ans. (b) Catumaxomab**

(Ref: Goodman Gilman 13th E/P661)

- Catumaxomab is a bispecific monoclonal antibody that targets EPCAM and CD 3.
- It is approved for treatment of malignant ascites.

80. **Ans. (b) Linezolid**

(Ref: Goodman Gilman 13th E/P1075)

- Linezolid is a weak inhibitor of MAO and hence can have interactions with other drugs that increase serotonin levels like SSRI, MAO inhibitors and TCAs.

81. **Ans. (b) It acts as antagonist at cannabinoid 2 receptors**

(Ref: Goodman Gilman 13th E/P937)

- Dronabinol is a natural cannabinoid present in marijuana plant, that can be derived from it or can also be synthesized chemically. Nabilone is a synthetic cannabinoid.
- Both act by stimulating cannabinoid-1 receptors in CTZ area and medullary vomiting center.
- It is used as an antiemetic and appetite stimulant in cancer patients.
- Side-effects are usually related to a decrease release in norepinephrine causing hypotension, tachycardia and conjunctival congestion (blood shot eyes).

82. **Ans. (c) Zoledronate**

(Ref: CMDT 2019/P1173)

- Zoledronate is the most potent as well as longest acting bisphosphonate. It is given by intravenous route once in a year.
- Dosing of bisphosphonates

Zoledronate	Once in a year
Pamidronate	Once in 3-6 months
Risedronate Ibandronate	Once in a month
Alendronate	Once in a week

83. **Ans. (b) Inhibit farnesyl pyrophosphate synthase**

(Ref: Katzung 13th E/P755)

- Bisphosphonates are structurally derived from pyrophosphate, which can bind to hydroxyapatite in bones and taken up by osteoclasts. Overall bisphosphonates block ruffled border formation in osteoclasts and also induce apoptosis.
- The first-generation bisphosphonates (etidronate, clodronate, tiludronate) are more identical to pyrophosphate with minimal changes and hence get incorporated in to terminal pyrophosphate moiety of ATP. This results in synthesis of an ATP that cannot be used as a source of energy and leads to apoptosis of osteoclasts.
- The second generation (alendronate, pamidronate) and third generation (zoledronate, risedronate) are structurally more different from pyrophosphate, as they have a nitrogen group attached. These drugs inhibit **farnesyl pyrophosphate synthase** and thus block mevalonic acid pathway i.e. synthesis of cholesterol and other lipids. This blocks posttranslational modification of proteins required for survival of osteoclasts and results in osteoclast apoptosis.
- Block of farnesyl pyrophosphate synthase leads to accumulation of isopentenyl pyrophosphate that increases release of TNF-alpha, which causes acute phase reaction associated with bisphosphonates.

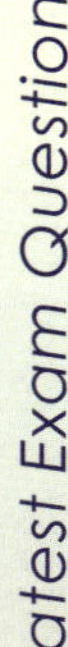

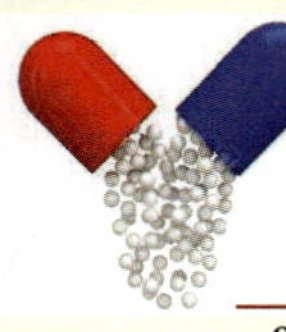

84. **Ans. (c) Remifentanil**

(Ref: Goodman Gilman 13th E/P374)

- Remifentanil is metabolized by plasma esterase and hence is the shortest acting opioid. It is also the fastest acting opioid.
- Because of above mentioned reasons it is opioid of choice in day care surgery.

85. **Ans. (c) Aminoglycosides**

(Ref: Goodman Gilman 13th E/P1040)

- Aminoglycosides entry in to gram negatives is by an energy dependent process and requires ATP/oxygen.
- Hence aminoglycosides can never enter in to anaerobes and are not effective.

86. **Ans. (a) Irinotecan**

(Ref: Goodman Gilman 13th E/P1190)

- Irinotecan and atazanavir like drugs are metabolized by glucuronidation and hence are poorly metabolized in patients of Crigler-Najjar syndrome.
- Thus, there is an increased risk of toxicity in Crigler-Najjar syndrome and hence both these drugs should not be used.

87. **Ans. (c) Cycloserine**

(Ref: Goodman Gilman 13th E/P1059)

Antibiotics which are peptides are:

- Lipopeptide – Daptomycin
- Glycopeptides – Vancomycin, Dalbavancin, Telavancin, Oritavancin

88. **Ans. (b) Glucagon**

(Ref: Goodman Gilman 13th E/P864)

- Beta block beta-1 receptors (Gs subtype of GPCR) and decrease cyclic AMP in myocardial cells.
- Hence glucagon is used for treatment of beta blocker toxicity, glucagon increases cyclic AMP synthesis.

89. **Ans. (b) Digoxin**

(Ref: Goodman Gilman 13th E/P540)

- Digoxin has a high volume of distribution and hence cannot be removed by dialysis.
- Anti-digoxin antibody digibind is used for treatment of digoxin toxicity treatment.

90. **Ans. (b) Azathioprine**

(Ref: Goodman Gilman 13th E/P705)

- Purine analog 6 – Mercaptopurine and azathioprine (prodrug of 6 – MP) are metabolized by xanthine oxidase.
- Hence xanthine oxidase inhibitors like allopurinol/oxypurinol/febuxostat inhibit metabolism of above mentioned purine analogs and cause toxicity.
- Thus dose of these purine analogs is decreased by 75%.

91. **Ans. (b) 10-20 mcg/mL**

(Ref: Adam's Neurology 10th E/P345)

92. **Ans. (a) Beta lactams**

(Ref: Katzung 13th E/P879)

93. **Ans. (b) Lurasidone**

(Ref: Goodman Gilman 13th E/P281)

- Being on a typical antipsychotic, haloperidol, patient has developed extrapyramidal side-effects.
- Hence it should be stopped and an atypical antipsychotic like lurasidone should be started.

JIPMER MAY 2019

94. **Ans. (b) 15-25% and 3-5%**

(Ref: Goodman Gilman 13th E/P610-617)

Hypolipidemic drugs	Effect on lipoproteins
Statins	HDL – Increases by 5-10% LDL – Decreases • High intensity statins - >50% • Moderate intensity statins – 30-50% • Low intensity statins - <30%
Bile acid binding resins	HDL – Increases by 3-5% LDL – Decreases by 15-25%
Niacin	HDL – Increases by 30-40% LDL – Decreases by 25% Triglycerides – Decreases by 35-50%
Fibric acid derivatives	HDL – Increases by 15% LDL – No change or increases Triglyceride – Decreases by 50%
Ezetimibe	LDL – Decreases by 15-20%
PCSK-9 Inhibitors Evolocumab and Alirocumab	LDL – Decreases by 60-70%
Lomitapide	LDL – Decreases LDL by 50%
Mipomersen	LDL – Decreases by 30-5%

95. **Ans. (a) Inhibits mycobacterial cell wall synthesis**

(Ref: Goodman Gilman 13th E/P1076)

- Bedaquiline acts by inhibiting mycobacterial ATP synthase, whereas delamanid/pretomanid/isoniazid/ethionamide inhibit cell wall synthesis by inhibiting mycolic acid synthesis.
- Bedaquiline and delamanid can cause QT prolongation and hence are contraindicated in patients with arrhythmia.
- Bedaquiline is sequestered in tissues and hence has a prolonged half-life of 165 days.
- It is indicated for treatment of MDR TB with additional resistance and for treatment of XDR TB.

96. **Ans. (a) Anthrax**

(Ref: Goodman Gilman 13th E/P662)

- Raxibacumab is an anti-B. anthracis protective antigen monoclonal antibody approved for prevention of inhalational anthrax.

Antimicrobial monoclonal antibodies		
Monoclonal antibodies	**Target**	**Use**
Raxibacumab	B. anthracis	Prevention of inhalational anthrax
Obiltoxaximab	B. anthracis exotoxin	Prevention of inhalational anthrax
Bezlotoxumab	C. difficile toxin B	C. difficile infection (Pseudomembranous enterocolitis)
Palivizumab	Respiratory Syncytial Virus (RSV)	Prevention of bronchiolitis caused by RSV

97. Ans. (c) ↓ Cholesterol and TG levels

(Ref: Goodman Gilman 13th E/P1147)

- All protease inhibitors including atazanavir are active against both HIV 1 and 2.
- I50L substitution (substitution of leucine to isoleucine due to mutation in codon 50) gives resistance to atazanavir but increases susceptibility to other protease inhibitors.
- All protease inhibitors can cause dyslipidemia except atazanavir, which rather decreases cholesterol and triglyceride)
- All protease inhibitors including atazanavir is combined with atazanavir to boost the half-life. Only exception is nelfinavir.

98. Ans. (b) Both drug influx and drug efflux mechanisms

(Ref: Goodman Gilman 13th E/P1049)

Resistance to tetracyclines can be seen due to

- **Drug efflux**
- **Impaired drug influx**
- Enzymatic inactivation
- Production of 30s ribosomal protective protein

99. Ans. (d) Thiazides

(Ref: Goodman Gilman 13th E/P455)

- Thiazides decrease calcium excretion and urine and hence can be used for treatment of calcium nephrolithiasis.
- Thus, for a patient of hypertension and nephrolithiasis the preferred drug would be thiazides.
- Loop diuretics like furosemide increase calcium excretion and hence can cause calcium nephrolithiasis.

100. Ans. (a) Phenytoin and carbamazepine

(Ref: Goodman Gilman 13th E/P310, 314)

- Phenytoin and carbamazepine can cause diplopia, ataxia and dizziness as side-effects.
- On appearance of these side-effects therapeutic drug monitoring is done and dose is adjusted.

101. Ans. (c) 3 gm single dose

(Ref: Goodman Gilman 13th E/P1019)

- Fosfomycin is used as 3 gm single dose for treatment of uncomplicated UTI.
- For complicated UTI 3mg 3 doses on alternate days is given.
- For prophylaxis of UTI 3 gm once every 10 days is given.

102. Ans. (d) Pravastatin

(Ref: Goodman Gilman 13th E/P611)

- All statins are metabolized by CYP3A4 except fluvastatin, rosuvastatin and pravastatin.
- Fluvastatin and rosuvastatin are metabolized by CYP2C9, whereas **pravastatin is excreted unchanged in urine.**
- All statins after metabolism are excreted in bile, i.e. finally with feces, except pravastatin which is excreted in urine.

103. Ans. (c) α_2, β_1, δ and ε

(Ref: Goodman Gilman 13th E/P177)

- Nicotinic acetylcholine receptors are pentameric structures made up of 5 protein subunits.
- These are 2 alpha, 1 beta, 1 delta and 1 gamma or epsilon.

104. Ans. (b) Macrolides

(Ref: Goodman Gilman 13th E/P1053)

- Macrolides inhibit production of proinflammatory cytokines and hence produce anti-inflammatory and immunomodulatory effect.
- This effect improves pulmonary function and decreases airway infection and hence macrolides are sometimes used post lung transplantation.
- Because of this anti-inflammatory effect macrolides might be effective in inflammatory disorders like sinusitis, asthma and rheumatoid arthritis.

105. Ans. (d) Hallucinations

(Ref: Goodman Gilman 13th E/P1017)

- Neurological side-effects like headache and dizziness are common but hallucinations, delirium and seizures are rare.
- Most common side-effect are related to GIT i.e. nausea, vomiting and abdominal discomfort.
- Hypoglycemia is a common side-effect that can be seen with fluoroquinolones due to release of insulin by block of ATP sensitive potassium channels.
- QT prolongation can be commonly seen with fluoroquinolones; risk is maximum with moxifloxacin and minimum with ciprofloxacin among the available drugs.

106. Ans. (c) Atorvastatin + Itraconazole

(Ref: Katzung 13th E/P62)

- Atorvastatin is metabolized by CYP3A4 and itraconazole is an inhibitor of CYP3A4.
- Hence itraconazole can block metabolism of atorvastatin and hence increase its toxicity.
- Carbamazepine and phenytoin both are enzyme inducers and hence decrease each other's plasma concentration.

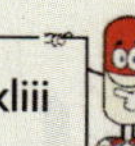

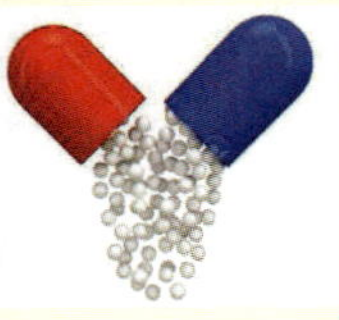

- Phenytoin and rifampicin are enzyme inducers and hence decrease each other's plasma concentration.
- Cimetidine is an enzyme inhibitor of CYP 1A2/2C9/2D6 and not 3A4 and hence won't block metabolism of amiodarone as it is metabolized by CYP3A4.

107. Ans. (c) Sotalol

- Defibrillation threshold is the amount of electrical energy required to produce a desirable effect on the myocardium.
- Shock applied during defibrillation depolarizes the myocardial cells and increases the refractory period of cells.
- Thus sodium channel blockers like lidocaine will increase the electrical energy required for depolarization i.e. increase defibrillation threshold.
- Whereas potassium channel blockers like sotalol or ibutilide will delay repolarization and increase refractoriness. Hence these drugs decrease the electrical energy required to make cells refractory i.e. decrease defibrillation threshold.
- Amiodarone though a potassium channel blocker, is also a sodium channel blocker and hence can increase defibrillation threshold.

108. Ans. (b) Acts through blocking cytoplasmic proteins

(Ref: Goodman Gilman 13th E/P1096)

- Isavuconazonium or isavuconazole is an azole which acts by blocking ergosterol synthesis.
- It has been approved by FDA in 2015 for treatment of invasive aspergillosis and mucormycosis.

109. Ans. (b) Apixaban

(Ref: Goodman Gilman 13th E/P595)

- Out of the given drugs apixaban is least excreted unchanged by urine and hence is relatively contraindicated in chronic kidney disease.
- Dabigatran (80%) > Edoxaban (50%) > Rivaroxaban (33%) > Apixaban (27%) are excreted unchanged by urine.

110. Ans. (a) Antihistamines

(Ref: Katzung 13th E/P1056)

- Antihistamines i.e. H2 blocker cimetidine can block androgen receptors, inhibit metabolism of estradiol and increase prolactin.
- Hence in males it can cause impotence and gynecomastia and in females it can cause galactorrhea.

111. Ans. (a) 40-year-old with Barrett's esophagus

(Ref: Goodman Gilman 13th E/P912)

- PPIs are given lifelong in patients of **Barrett's esophagus**, as it is a precancerous lesion.
- PPIs can be stopped in other disorders e.g. after healing of gastric ulcer.

112. Ans. (a) 7 days

(Ref: Goodman Gilman 13th E/P647)

- There are two anti-CD 25 monoclonal antibodies i.e. basiliximab and daclizumab.
- Basiliximab has a half-life of 7 days and daclizumab of 20 days.

113. Ans. (b) Serratia and (d) Burkholderia

(Ref: Goodman Gilman 13th E/P1058)

- Colistin is not active against both serratia and burkholderia.
- However, in KDT only serratia is mentioned and hence can be chosen as the best answer for the question.
- But remember it is an incorrect question with two right options.

114. Ans. (b) Has long half-life

(Ref: Goodman Gilman 13th E/P973)

- Artemisinin group drugs have a very short half-life and hence are never used as monotherapy for treatment or for prophylaxis of malaria.
- No dose adjustment is required as such in hepatic or renal failure.
- Oral bioavailability is around 30%.
- Artemisinin and artemether can induce enzymes CYP 2B6/3A4 which metabolize them and hence can increase their own metabolism (autoinduction).

115. Ans. (d) Tisagenlecleucel

(Ref: Goodman Gilman 13th E/P1224)

- Tisagenlecleucel is a CAR-T cell (Chimeric Antigen Receptor-T cell) which is approved for treatment of refractory B cell ALL.
- CAR is made up of antigen binding domain of monoclonal antibody that recognizes the tumor antigen, which is coupled with intracellular domains that activate T cells.
- When these CAR is attached to T cell, then T cell is activated against the tumor cells.

116. Ans. (b) SSRIs

(Ref: Goodman Gilman 13th E/P268)

- SSRIs are very effective class of drugs for treatment of major depression.
- Out of all anti-depressant SSRIs are the safest as well, as they are devoid of side-effects associated with TCAs, due to block of muscarinic, Alpha1, serotonin and H1 receptors.
- They are also devoid of a myriad of drug interactions that can be seen with MAO inhibitors.

117. Ans. (c) Diltiazem

(Ref: Goodman Gilman 13th E/P742)

- Nuclear Factor-KappaB (NF-Kb) is a transcription factor that plays a key role in embryonic/neuronal development, immune response to infections, inflammation and cell proliferation.
- Hence block of this factor has therapeutic implications for treatment of neoplasia and inflammatory disorders.
- Examples of drugs blocking NF-Kb are sunitinib, emetine, bortezomib, bithionol, lestaurtinib, olmesartan and iguratimod.
- Iguratimod is used in Japan and China for treatment of rheumatoid arthritis.

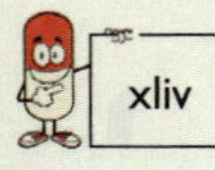

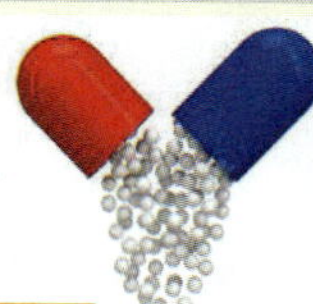

118. **Ans. (d) Bisoprolol**

(Ref: Goodman Gilman 13th E/P217)

- **Nebivolol is most cardioselective beta blocker followed by bisoprolol.**

119. **Ans. (a) Alemtuzumab**

(Ref: Goodman Gilman 13th E/P652)

- Alemtuzumab is an ant-CD 52 monoclonal antibody.
- Anti-TNF drugs in current use are infliximab, adalimumab, etanercept, golimumab, certolizumab.
- These are approved for treatment of rheumatoid arthritis, Crohn's disease, ulcerative colitis, ankylosing spondylitis, plaque psoriasis and psoriatic arthritis.

120. **Ans. (c) Osteoporosis**

(Ref: Goodman Gilman 13th E/P661)

- Denosumab is an anti-RANK ligand monoclonal antibody approved for treatment of postmenopausal osteoporosis in females with high risk of fractures in patients who are not able to tolerate bisphosphonates.

PGI MAY 2019

121. **Ans. (a) Bioavailability of an orally administered drug is calculated by comparing the area under curve after oral and IV drug administration, (b) Studies in zero phase of clinical trials, (c) Can be determined by plasma level and urinary excretion**

(Ref: Goodman Gilman 13th E/P24)

- Bioavailability of an orally administered drug is calculated by comparing the area under curve after oral and IV drug administration.
- Bioavailability is calculated in phase 0 and 1.
- It can be calculated by multiplying clearance with steady state plasma concentration and then diving it by dosing rate.
- Low oral bioavailability can be due to low absorption or high fist pass metabolism.
- It is the fraction of unchanged drug that reaches systemic circulation.

122. **Ans. (a) Verapamil, (d) Mibefradil, (e) Ethosuximide**

(Ref: Goodman Gilman 13th E/P315)

T type calcium channel blocker	T and L type calcium channel blocker	L type calcium channel blocker
Valproate	**Verapamil**	Diltiazem
Ethosuximide	**Mibefradil**	Nifedipine
Zonisamide	Nimodipine	Clevidipine
Lamotrigine	Nicardipine	Isardipine
	Amlodipine	

123. **Ans. (a) Rate of elimination is directly proportional to drug concentration, (b) Plasma half-life is independent of drug concentration, (d) Constant fraction of drug is eliminated over time**

(Ref: Goodman Gilman 13th E/P20)

124. **Ans. (a) Vegetables of Brassica family, (b) Perchlorates**

(Ref: Goodman Gilman 13th E/P797)

- Thiocyanate, perchlorate and fluoborate inhibit iodide trapping by blocking sodium iodide symporter.
- Vegetables of brassica family like cabbage, have thiocyanate and hence can produce same effect.

125. **Ans. (b) Omeprazole, (c) Calcium channel blockers, (d) Penicillamine, (e) Amiodarone**

(Ref: CMDT 2018/1206)

Drugs causing gynecomastia
Gy – GnRH Agonists
N – **Nifedipine**
E – Estrogen
C – Cimetidine, Copper chelating agent (Penicillamine)
O – **Omeprazole**
M – Metoclopramide
A – **Amiodarone**
S – Spironolactone
T – Testosterone
I – Isoniazid
A – Alcohol

126. **Ans. (e) Verapamil**

(Ref: Goodman Gilman 13th E/P554)

- **All calcium channel blockers are racemic mixture of enantiomers except diltiazem and nifedipine.**

127. **Ans. (b) Beta-blocker: Bradycardia, (e) Deafness from aminoglycoside overdose**

(Ref: Goodman Gilman 13th E/P57, 58)

- **Kindly go through text in chapter 2 i.e. clinical pharmacology for details of ADR types.**

128. **Ans. (a) Also called Acetyl cholinesterase**

(Ref: Goodman Gilman 13th E/P128)

- ***Pseudocholinesterase is also known as plasma cholinesterase* or butyrylcholinesterase.**
- ***It is synthesized by liver and is present in plasma, where it metabolizes drugs like succinylcholine, esmolol, clevidipine, remifentanil, mivacurium etc.***
- ***Acetyl cholinesterase or true cholinesterase is synthesized in synapse or RBC.***

129. **Ans. (a) Neurotoxicity, (b) Nephrotoxicity, (c) Ototoxicity, (d) Neuropathy, (e) Cardiac toxicity**

(Ref: Goodman Gilman 13th E/P1177)

- Cisplatin can cause nephrotoxicity, ototoxicity, neurotoxicity (peripheral neuropathy), cardiotoxicity and severe nausea and vomiting.

130. **Ans. (a) Ustekinumab**

(Ref: Goodman Gilman 13th E/P648)

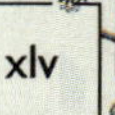

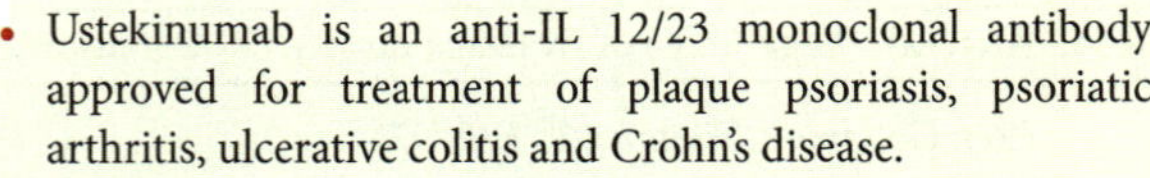

- Ustekinumab is an anti-IL 12/23 monoclonal antibody approved for treatment of plaque psoriasis, psoriatic arthritis, ulcerative colitis and Crohn's disease.

131. Ans. (b) Lead to decrease in absorption of sodium and chloride in Distal tubule

(Ref: Goodman Gilman 13th E/P455)

- Thiazides block Na/Cl cotransporter in the distal convoluted tubule and thus decrease absorption of sodium and chloride.
- Effectiveness of thiazides decreases with decreasing GFR.
- Thiazides cause hyperglycemia by decreasing insulin release.

132. Ans. (b) Ivacaftor

(Ref: Goodman Gilman 13th E/P66)

133. Ans. (b) Atomoxetine, (d) Pentazocine, (e) Clonidine

(Ref: Goodman Gilman 13th E/P205)

- *Methylphenidate and amphetamine are CNS stimulant and hence are used for treatment of narcolepsy.*
- *For same reason they have abuse potential as well.*

134. Ans. (a) Eptifibatide, (b) Tirofiban, (c) Abciximab

(Ref: Goodman Gilman 13th E/P599)

- Abciximab, Eptifibatide and tirofiban are inhibitors of alpha IIb beta 3-integrin.
- Rivaroxaban is a factor Xa inhibitor.
- Ticagrelor is an ADP inhibitor.

135. Ans. (a) Macrolides, (c) Vancomycin, (d) Linezolid, (e) β-lactams

(Ref: Katzung 13th E/P879)

- **For the list of antibiotics with TDK and CDK please go through the topic of antimicrobial drugs.**

136. Ans. (a) Verapamil, (b) Amiodarone, (c) Statins, (d) Cyclosporine

(Ref: Katzung 13th E/P62)

- For the list of drugs metabolized by CYP3A4 please go through the topic of general pharmacology.

137. Ans. (a) Daratumumab, (c) Lenalidomide, (d) Bortezomib, (e) Bendamustine

(Ref: Goodman Gilman 13th E/P1125-28)

- Drugs used for treatment of multiple myeloma are bortezomib, lenalidomide, dexamethasone, Panobinostat, daratumumab and bendamustine.

138. Ans. (a) Metformin, (e) Pioglitazone

(Ref: Goodman Gilman 13th E/P807)

- Hypoglycemia is a side effect caused by insulin or drugs that act by increasing insulin release (sulfonylureas, meglitinides and GLP1 related drugs).
- GLP1 related drugs are GLP1 agonists like exenatide and DPP-4 inhibitors like sitagliptin.

139. Ans. (a) Synthetic opioid, (b) 100 times more potent than morphine, (c) Acts on dorsal horn cells, (d) Metabolized into inactive metabolite norfentanyl (e) μ agonist

(Ref: Goodman Gilman 13th E/P373-74)

- **Fentanyl is a purely synthetic opioid, which is mu receptor agonist and is 100 times more potent than morphine.**
- **It acts on the dorsal horn of spinal cord.**
- **It is metabolized in to inactive metabolite norfentanyl.**

Recently Changed AIIMS Pattern Questions Review 2019

ASSERTION REASON TYPE QUESTIONS

1. **Assertion: Antibiotics can cause OCP failure.**
   Reason: Antibiotic use causes gut sterilization.
   a. Both Assertion and Reason are independently true statements and the Reason is correct explanation for the Assertion
   b. Both Assertion and Reason are independently true statements, but the Reason is not the correct explanation for the Assertion
   c. Assertion is independently true statement, but reason is independently a false statement
   d. Assertion is independently false statement, but reason is independently a true statement
   e. Both Assertion and Reason are independently false statements

Ans. (a) Both Assertion and Reason are independently true statements and the Reason is correct explanation for the Assertion

- Estrogen is metabolized by glucuronidation and converted in to water soluble form. But in the gut bacteria produce glucuronidase which deconjugates estrogen and makes it lipid soluble. Thus, estrogen is reabsorbed in colon; this being called as enterohepatic circulation.
- Antibiotics by killing the bacteria in gut can prevent this enterohepatic circulation, which leads to OCP failure.

2. **Assertion: Nitroglycerine is administered by sublingual route.**
   Reason: In acute attack of angina sublingual route is best.
   a. Both Assertion and Reason are independently true statements and the Reason is correct explanation for the Assertion.
   b. Both Assertion and Reason are independently true statements, but the Reason is not the correct explanation for the Assertion
   c. Assertion is independently true statement, but reason is independently a false statement
   d. Assertion is independently false statement, but reason is independently a true statement
   e. Both Assertion and Reason are independently false statements

Ans. (b) Both Assertion and Reason are independently true statements, but the Reason is not the correct explanation for the Assertion

- Nitroglycerine is given by sublingual route because of high first pass metabolism.
- Sublingual route produces rapid effect and hence is best in an acute attack of angina.
- Hence both Assertion and Reason are correct, but the Reason is not a correct explanation of the Assertion.

3. **Assertion: Digoxin has high volume of distribution.**
   Reason: Highly lipid soluble drugs get sequestered in fat tissue.
   a. Both Assertion and Reason are independently true statements and the Reason is correct explanation for the Assertion
   b. Both Assertion and Reason are independently true statements, but the Reason is not the correct explanation for the Assertion
   c. Assertion is independently true statement, but reason is independently a false statement
   d. Assertion is independently false statement, but reason is independently a true statement
   e. Both Assertion and Reason are independently false statements

Ans. (b) Both Assertion and Reason are independently true statements, but the Reason is not the correct explanation for the Assertion

- Digoxin has a high volume of distribution due to binding to Na/K ATPase channels in skeletal muscles and not because of high lipid solubility.

4. **Assertion: Sulfonamides can cause kernicterus in newborns.**
   Reason: Drugs with low plasma protein binding can cause hemolysis.
   a. Both Assertion and Reason are independently true statements and the Reason is correct explanation for the Assertion
   b. Both Assertion and Reason are independently true statements, but the Reason is not the correct explanation for the Assertion
   c. Assertion is independently true statement, but reason is independently a false statement
   d. Assertion is independently false statement, but reason is independently a true statement
   e. Both Assertion and Reason are independently false statements

Ans. (c) Assertion is independently true statement, but reason is independently a false statement.

- Sulfonamides have a high plasma protein binding and hence can displace bilirubin from albumin and cause kernicterus in newborns.

5. **Assertion: Partial agonist can never behave as an antagonist.**
   Reason: A partial agonist behaves as an inverse agonist in presence of a full agonist.
   a. Both Assertion and Reason are independently true statements and the Reason is correct explanation for the Assertion
   b. Both Assertion and Reason are independently true statements, but the Reason is not the correct explanation for the Assertion
   c. Assertion is independently true statement, but reason is independently a false statement
   d. Assertion is independently false statement, but reason is independently a true statement
   e. Both Assertion and Reason are independently false statements

Ans. (e) Both Assertion and Reason are independently false statements

- A partial agonist behaves as an antagonist in the presence of a full agonist.

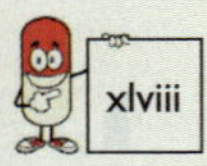

6. Assertion: Pralidoxime is most specific drug for organophosphate poisoning.
Reason: Organophosphates block ACHE enzyme.

a. Both Assertion and Reason are independently true statements and the Reason is correct explanation for the Assertion
b. Both Assertion and Reason are independently true statements, but the Reason is not the correct explanation for the Assertion
c. Assertion is independently true statement, but reason is independently a false statement
d. Assertion is independently false statement, but reason is independently a true statement
e. Both Assertion and Reason are independently false statements

Ans. (a) Both Assertion and Reason are independently true statements and the Reason is correct explanation for the Assertion

- Most specific drugs are drugs that act on the cause. It is to be noted here that most specific drugs do not mean drug of choice.
- Organophosphates block ACHE enzyme and pralidoxime reactivates ACHE enzyme.
- Hence pralidoxime is the most specific drug for organophosphate poisoning. But the drug of choice for organophosphate poisoning is atropine.

7. Assertion: Edrophonium is used for diagnosis of myasthenia gravis.
Reason: Tertiary amines can cross blood brain barrier.

a. Both Assertion and Reason are independently true statements and the Reason is correct explanation for the Assertion
b. Both Assertion and Reason are independently true statements, but the Reason is not the correct explanation for the Assertion
c. Assertion is independently true statement, but reason is independently a false statement
d. Assertion is independently false statement, but reason is independently a true statement
e. Both Assertion and Reason are independently false statements

Ans. (b) Both Assertion and Reason are independently true statements, but the Reason is not the correct explanation for the Assertion

- Edrophonium is used in diagnosis of myasthenia gravis because it is shortest acting ACHE inhibitor and being a quaternary amine, it does not have central side-effects.
- Tertiary amines like physostigmine can cross blood brain barrier.

8. Assertion: Quinidine can cause QT prolongation.
Reason: Class Ia drugs have maximum sodium channel blocking effect.

a. Both Assertion and Reason are independently true statements and the Reason is correct explanation for the Assertion
b. Both Assertion and Reason are independently true statements, but the Reason is not the correct explanation for the Assertion
c. Assertion is independently true statement, but reason is independently a false statement
d. Assertion is independently false statement, but reason is independently a true statement
e. Both Assertion and Reason are independently false statements

Ans. (c) Assertion is independently true statement, but reason is independently a false statement.

- Quinidine causes QT prolongation because of significant delay in repolarization due to potassium channel block.
- Maximum sodium channel block is caused by Class Ic drugs and not Ia.

9. Assertion: Sacubitril is contraindicated with ACE inhibitors.
Reason: Neutral endopeptidase is inhibited by sacubitril.

a. Both Assertion and Reason are independently true statements and the Reason is correct explanation for the Assertion
b. Both Assertion and Reason are independently true statements, but the Reason is not the correct explanation for the Assertion
c. Assertion is independently true statement, but reason is independently a false statement
d. Assertion is independently false statement, but reason is independently a true statement
e. Both Assertion and Reason are independently false statements

Ans. (b) Both Assertion and Reason are independently true statements, but the Reason is not the correct explanation for the Assertion

- Sacubitril is contraindicated with ACE inhibitors due to increased risk of angioedema.
- Sacubitril is a neutral endopeptidase inhibitor.

10. Assertion: Acetazolamide is used in treatment of motion sickness.
Reason: Cerebral edema is responsible for motion sickness.

a. Both Assertion and Reason are independently true statements and the Reason is correct explanation for the Assertion
b. Both Assertion and Reason are independently true statements, but the Reason is not the correct explanation for the Assertion
c. Assertion is independently true statement, but reason is independently a false statement
d. Assertion is independently false statement, but reason is independently a true statement
e. Both Assertion and Reason are independently false statements

Ans. (a) Both Assertion and Reason are independently true statements and the Reason is correct explanation for the Assertion

- Carbonic anhydrase inhibitors like acetazolamide decrease CSF production and decrease cerebral edema.
- Since cerebral edema is implicated in motion sickness, acetazolamide is used for same.

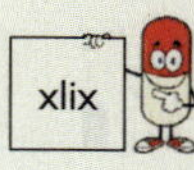

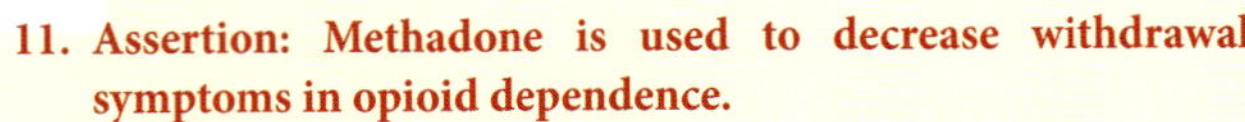

11. Assertion: Methadone is used to decrease withdrawal symptoms in opioid dependence.
Reason: Short acting drugs do not produce withdrawal symptoms.

a. Both Assertion and Reason are independently true statements and the Reason is correct explanation for the Assertion
b. Both Assertion and Reason are independently true statements, but the Reason is not the correct explanation for the Assertion
c. Assertion is independently true statement, but reason is independently a false statement
d. Assertion is independently false statement, but reason is independently a true statement
e. Both Assertion and Reason are independently false statements

Ans. (b) Assertion is independently true statement, but reason is independently a false statement

- Methadone is used to decrease withdrawal symptoms in opioid dependence because it is sequestered in tissues and slowly released.
- Long acting drugs do not produce withdrawal symptoms.

12. Assertion: Rufinamide is most preferred drug for treatment of Lennox Gastaut syndrome.
Reason: Lennox Gastaut syndrome is mixed seizure syndrome of elderly.

a. Both Assertion and Reason are independently true statements and the Reason is correct explanation for the Assertion
b. Both Assertion and Reason are independently true statements, but the Reason is not the correct explanation for the Assertion
c. Assertion is independently true statement, but reason is independently a false statement
d. Assertion is independently false statement, but reason is independently a true statement
e. Both Assertion and Reason are independently false statements

Ans. (e) Both Assertion and Reason are independently false statements

- Valproate is the drug of choice for treatment of Lennox Gastaut syndrome.
- Lennox Gastaut syndrome is a mixed seizure syndrome seen in children.

13. Assertion: Vancomycin is not effective against gram negative organisms.
Reason: Drugs with huge size can not pass through porins of gram negatives.

a. Both Assertion and Reason are independently true statements and the Reason is correct explanation for the Assertion
b. Both Assertion and Reason are independently true statements, but the Reason is not the correct explanation for the Assertion
c. Assertion is independently true statement, but reason is independently a false statement
d. Assertion is independently false statement, but reason is independently a true statement
e. Both Assertion and Reason are independently false statements

Ans. (a) Both Assertion and Reason are independently true statements and the Reason is correct explanation for the Assertion

- Vancomycin is a large molecule and hence can not pass through small porins of gram negatives.

14. Assertion: Cotrimoxazole is a bactericidal drug.
Reason: The ratio of trimethoprim to sulfamethoxazole in cotrimoxazole is 1:5 in plasma.

a. Both Assertion and Reason are independently true statements and the Reason is correct explanation for the Assertion
b. Both Assertion and Reason are independently true statements, but the Reason is not the correct explanation for the Assertion
c. Assertion is independently true statement, but reason is independently a false statement
d. Assertion is independently false statement, but reason is independently a true statement
e. Both Assertion and Reason are independently false statements

Ans. (c) Assertion is independently true statement, but reason is independently a false statement.

- Cotrimoxazole is a bactericidal drug because of sequential block of dihydropteroate synthase and dihydrofolate reductase by sulfamethoxazole and trimethoprim respectively.
- The ratio if trimethoprim to sulfamethoxazole in a table is 1:5, but in plasma is 1:20 due to high volume of distribution of trimethoprim.

15. Assertion: Bedaquiline is used along with clofazimine in XDR TB.
Reason: Two drugs acting on same target can antagonize each other.

a. Both Assertion and Reason are independently true statements and the Reason is correct explanation for the Assertion.
b. Both Assertion and Reason are independently true statements, but the Reason is not the correct explanation for the Assertion.
c. Assertion is independently true statement, but reason is independently a false statement.
d. Assertion is independently false statement, but reason is independently a true statement.
e. Both Assertion and Reason are independently false statements

Ans. (d) Assertion is independently false statement, but reason is independently a true statement.

- Bedaquiline is not used with clofazimine due to risk of cross tolerance.
- Two drugs acting on same target can compete with each other and hence antagonize.

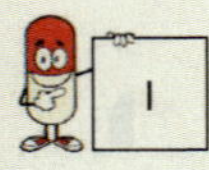

16. **Assertion: The number of drugs used in multibacillary and paucibacillary leprosy are different, but duration of treatment is same.**

Reason: Clofazimine is most effective anti-leprosy drug.

a. Both Assertion and Reason are independently true statements and the Reason is correct explanation for the Assertion
b. Both Assertion and Reason are independently true statements, but the Reason is not the correct explanation for the Assertion
c. Assertion is independently true statement, but reason is independently a false statement
d. Assertion is independently false statement, but reason is independently a true statement
e. Both Assertion and Reason are independently false statements

Ans. (e) Both Assertion and Reason are independently false statements

- The duration of multibacillary therapy is 12 months and paucibacillary therapy is 6 months. However, the number of drugs used are same because some time by mistake multibacillary is treated as paucibacillary.
- Rifampicin is the most effective anti-leprosy drug.

17. **Assertion: Amphotericin B is a fungicidal drug.**

Reason: Sequestration of ergosterol breaks the cell membrane.

a. Both Assertion and Reason are independently true statements and the Reason is correct explanation for the Assertion.
b. Both Assertion and Reason are independently true statements, but the Reason is not the correct explanation for the Assertion.
c. Assertion is independently true statement, but reason is independently a false statement.
d. Assertion is independently false statement, but reason is independently a true statement.
e. Both Assertion and Reason are independently false statements

Ans. (a) Both Assertion and Reason are independently true statements and the Reason is correct explanation for the Assertion

- Amphotericin B is a fungicidal drug because it sequesters ergosterol in the cell membrane and breaks it.
- The old mechanism is formation of pores in the cell membrane.

18. **Assertion: Dextrose is administered along with Amphotericin B.**

Reason: Amphotericin B is a nephrotoxic drug.

a. Both Assertion and Reason are independently true statements and the Reason is correct explanation for the Assertion
b. Both Assertion and Reason are independently true statements, but the Reason is not the correct explanation for the Assertion
c. Assertion is independently true statement, but reason is independently a false statement
d. Assertion is independently false statement, but reason is independently a true statement
e. Both Assertion and Reason are independently false statements

Ans. (b) Both Assertion and Reason are independently true statements, but the Reason is not the correct explanation for the Assertion

- Dextrose is a carrier for amphotericin B; it has nothing to do with nephrotoxicity.
- To decrease nephrotoxicity of amphotericin B, normal saline is administered.

19. **Assertion: Bleomycin can cause pulmonary fibrosis.**

Reason: Type II pneumocyte damage results in type I pneumocyte hyperplasia.

a. Both Assertion and Reason are independently true statements and the Reason is correct explanation for the Assertion
b. Both Assertion and Reason are independently true statements, but the Reason is not the correct explanation for the Assertion
c. Assertion is independently true statement, but reason is independently a false statement
d. Assertion is independently false statement, but reason is independently a true statement
e. Both Assertion and Reason are independently false statements

Ans. (c) Assertion is independently true statement, but reason is independently a false statement

- Bleomycin causes pulmonary fibrosis is a correct statement.
- The reason statement is not correct because bleomycin induced type I pneumocyte damage results in type II pneumocyte hyperplasia.

20. **Assertion: Normal saline preloading is done prior to cisplatin administration.**

Reason: Chloride inactivates cisplatin.

a. Both Assertion and Reason are independently true statements and the Reason is correct explanation for the Assertion
b. Both Assertion and Reason are independently true statements, but the Reason is not the correct explanation for the Assertion
c. Assertion is independently true statement, but reason is independently a false statement
d. Assertion is independently false statement, but reason is independently a true statement
e. Both Assertion and Reason are independently false statements

Ans. (a) Both Assertion and Reason are independently true statements and the Reason is correct explanation for the Assertion

- Cisplatin is a potent nephrotoxic drug and hence normal saline is preloaded prior to cisplatin administration.
- Cisplatin is inactivated by chloride. Mannitol is also administered which causes forced diuresis and removes inactivated cisplatin.

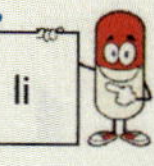

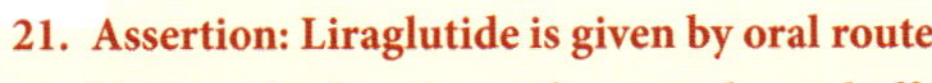

21. Assertion: Liraglutide is given by oral route.

Reason: Oral route produces prolonged effect.

a. Both Assertion and Reason are independently true statements and the Reason is correct explanation for the Assertion
b. Both Assertion and Reason are independently true statements, but the Reason is not the correct explanation for the Assertion
c. Assertion is independently true statement, but reason is independently a false statement
d. Assertion is independently false statement, but reason is independently a true statement
e. Both Assertion and Reason are independently false statements

Ans. (e) Both Assertion and Reason are independently false statements

- Liraglutide is given by subcutaneous route because it is a peptide which can not be given by oral route.
- Oral route has nothing to do with duration of action.

22. Assertion: Teriparatide is not given for more than 2 years.

Reason: Teriparatide can cause osteosarcoma.

a. Both Assertion and Reason are independently true statements and the Reason is correct explanation for the Assertion
b. Both Assertion and Reason are independently true statements, but the Reason is not the correct explanation for the Assertion
c. Assertion is independently true statement, but reason is independently a false statement
d. Assertion is independently false statement, but reason is independently a true statement
e. Both Assertion and Reason are independently false statements

Ans. (a) Both Assertion and Reason are independently true statements and the Reason is correct explanation for the Assertion

- Teriparatide is not given for more than 2 years due to risk of osteosarcoma.

23. Assertion: Allopurinol can cause acute gout.

Reason: Inhibition of uric acid synthesis mobilizes tissue store of uric acid in to plasma.

a. Both Assertion and Reason are independently true statements and the Reason is correct explanation for the Assertion
b. Both Assertion and Reason are independently true statements, but the Reason is not the correct explanation for the Assertion
c. Assertion is independently true statement, but reason is independently a false statement
d. Assertion is independently false statement, but reason is independently a true statement
e. Both Assertion and Reason are independently false statements

Ans. (a) Both Assertion and Reason are independently true statements and the Reason is correct explanation for the Assertion

- Allopurinol can cause acute gout in the first 2 weeks of therapy due to mobilization of uric acid from stores of body to plasma.
- Hence NSAID or colchicine is always given along with allopurinol for first 2 weeks.

24. Assertion: Azathioprine dose is decreased with allopurinol.

Reason: Azathioprine and allopurinol cause bone marrow suppression.

a. Both Assertion and Reason are independently true statements and the Reason is correct explanation for the Assertion
b. Both Assertion and Reason are independently true statements, but the Reason is not the correct explanation for the Assertion
c. Assertion is independently true statement, but reason is independently a false statement
d. Assertion is independently false statement, but reason is independently a true statement
e. Both Assertion and Reason are independently false statements

Ans. (c) Assertion is independently true statement, but reason is independently a false statement

- Azathioprine dose is decreased with allopurinol as allopurinol is a xanthine oxidase inhibitor and azathioprine is metabolized by xanthine oxidase. Hence allopurinol can precipitate azathioprine toxicity.

25. Assertion: Ciclesonide is an ICS with lesser systemic side-effects.

Reason: Soft steroids are metabolized in the airway.

a. Both Assertion and Reason are independently true statements and the Reason is correct explanation for the Assertion.
b. Both Assertion and Reason are independently true statements, but the Reason is not the correct explanation for the Assertion
c. Assertion is independently true statement, but reason is independently a false statement
d. Assertion is independently false statement, but reason is independently a true statement
e. Both Assertion and Reason are independently false statements

Ans. (a) Both Assertion and Reason are independently true statements and the Reason is correct explanation for the Assertion

- Ciclesonide and beclomethasone are metabolized in airway and associated with lesser side-effects and hence are known as soft steroids.

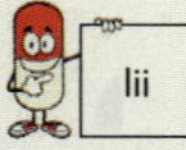

EXTENDED MATCHING QUESTIONS

26. Theme and focus: Basic terminology in pharmacology

Answer option list:

a. PKa b. Pharmacogenomics
c. Bioavailability d. Pharmacogenetics
e. Enzyme induction f. Drug clearance
g. Enzyme inhibition h. Area under the curve

Lead in question: For each of the following description find the appropriate term from the list given above.

1. Study of interindividual variability in genes governing drug response.
2. pH at which a drug is 50% ionized and 50% unionized.
3. Fraction of unchanged drug that reaches the systemic circulation.
4. A definite ml of plasma becomes drug free per hour.
5. Rifampicin can cause OCP failure.

Ans. 1-d, 2-a, 3-c, 4-f, 5-e

- Study of interindividual variability in genes governing drug response is called as pharmacogenetics. Application of pharmacogenetics to individualize drug therapy in a patient is called as pharmacogenomics.
- pH at which a drug is 50% ionized and 50% unionized is called as pKa.
- Fraction of unchanged drug that reaches the systemic circulation is called a bioavailability. Area under the curve in a concentration time curve is used to calculate bioavailability.
- Amount of plasma cleared off the drug per unit time is called as drug clearance.
- Rifampicin is an enzyme inducer and hence can cause OCP failure.

27. Theme and focus: Pharmacokinetics

Answer option list:

a. Amiodarone b. Captopril
c. Levodopa d. Vancomycin
e. Prazosin f. Lithium
g. Bendroflumethiazide h. Sulfadoxine

Lead in question: For each of the following pharmacokinetic parameter find the appropriate drug in the list above.

1. Oral absorption is negligible.
2. Half-life is several days.
3. Undergoes active tubular reabsorption
4. Is a prodrug which needs to be activated
5. Has a very high plasma protein binding

Ans. 1-d, 2-a, 3-f, 4-c, 5-h

- Vancomycin has a large size because of which it has poor oral absorption.
- Amiodarone is the longest acting antiarrhythmic and has a half-life of 53 days.
- Lithium is similar in structure to sodium and hence is reabsorbed in the collecting duct by ENaC.
- Levodopa is a prodrug which is activated by dopa decarboxylase in to dopamine.
- Sulfonamides have a high plasma protein binding and hence can displace bilirubin from albumin and cause kernicterus.

28. Theme and focus: Absorption and route of administration

Answer option list:

a. Cisplatin b. Levodopa
c. Erythromycin d. Rectal diazepam
e. Minocycline f. Octreotide
g. Nifedipine h. Methotrexate

Lead in question: Find the appropriate drug from the list above for the statements below.

1. Undergoes 50% first pass metabolism
2. 100% bioavailability
3. Sublingual administration prevents first pass metabolism
4. Poorly crosses blood brain barrier and hence given by intrathecal route for CNS use
5. Never administer with aluminum equipments

Ans. 1-d, 2-e, 3-g, 4-h and 5-a

- By rectal route of drug administration 50% of drug is absorbed vial portal vein and 50% of drug is absorbed directly in to inferior vena cava. Hence by rectal route only 50% of administered drug undergoes first pass metabolism.
- Minocycline has maximum bioavailability among tetracyclines which is 100%.
- Nifedipine among the given options can be given by sublingual route.
- Methotrexate poorly crosses blood brain barrier and hence is given by intrathecal route for treatment of CNS leukemia.
- Cisplatin is inactivated by aluminum and hence should never be administered with equipments made up of aluminum.

29. Theme and focus: Pharmacodynamics

Answer option list:

a. Quantal DRC b. Graded DRC
c. Vitamins d. Unparallel DRC
e. Competitive antagonism f. Parallel DRC
g. Noncompetitive antagonism
h. Full agonist

Lead in question: For each of the following statement find the appropriate parameter given in the options above.

1. A decrease in slope of DRC is seen.
2. Affinity of two drugs cannot be compared.
3. DRC shifts to right side.
4. DRC plotted for a population.
5. U shaped DRC can be seen.

Ans. 1-e, 2-d, 3-e, 4-a, 5-c

- In competitive antagonism there is a right shift in DRC, whereas in noncompetitive antagonism there is a decrease in slope of DRC.
- Affinity of two drugs can be compared if they act on same target. For drugs with unparallel DRC, their targets are different and hence affinity can not be compared.
- In graded DRC is plotted for an individual, whereas quantal DRC is plotted for a population.
- U shaped DRC can be seen with vitamins.

30. Theme and focus: Sympathetic agonists and antagonists

Answer option list:

a. Isoprenaline b. Adrenaline
c. Noradrenaline d. Tamsulosin
e. Clonidine f. Phenoxybenzamine
g. Phentolamine h. Carvedilol

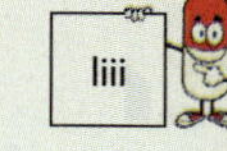

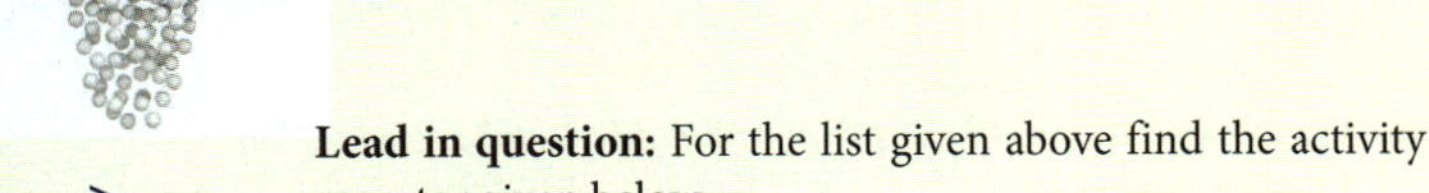

Lead in question: For the list given above find the activity at receptor given below.

1. Agonist at alpha 1, alpha 2, beta 1 and beta 2
2. Antagonist at alpha 1, beta 1 and beta 2
3. Agonist at beta 1 and beta 2
4. Agonist at alpha 1, alpha 2 and beta 1
5. Irreversible antagonist at alpha 1a

Ans. 1-b, 2-h, 3-a, 4-c, 5-f

- Adrenaline is an agonist at alpha 1, alpha 2, beta 1 and beta 2, whereas noradrenaline is an agonist at alpha 1, alpha 2 and beta 1.
- Carvedilol is a nonselective beta blocker (antagonist at beta 1 and beta 2) with antagonism at alpha 1 receptors.
- Isoprenaline is an agonist at beta 1 and beta 2 receptors.
- Phenoxybenzamine is an irreversible alpha 1 blocker including alpha 1a.

31. Theme and focus: Parasympathetic agonists and antagonists

Answer option list:

a. Atropine
b. Scopolamine
c. Pilocarpine
d. Donepezil
e. Edrophonium
f. Pyridostigmine
g. Methacholine
h. Revefenacin

Lead in question: For the list given above find the appropriate use given below.

1. Used in diagnosis of bronchial asthma.
2. Used in treatment of COPD.
3. Used in differential diagnosis of myasthenia gravis and cholinergic crisis.
4. Used in nicotinic poisoning.
5. Used in motion sickness.

Ans. 1-g, 2-h, 3-e, 4-a, 5-b

- Methacholine is used in bronchial challenge test for diagnosis of bronchial asthma.
- Revefenacin is a latest anticholinergic approved by FDA for treatment of COPD.
- Edrophonium is used for differential diagnosis of myasthenia gravis from cholinergic crisis.
- Atropine can be used in nicotinic poisoning for treatment of associated cholinergic symptoms.
- Scopolamine is the drug of choice for treatment of motion sickness.

32. Theme and focus: Uses of antiarrhythmic drugs

Answer option list:

a. Lidocaine
b. Verapamil
c. Atropine
d. Propranolol
e. Amiodarone
f. Digoxin
g. Mexiletine
h. Flecainide

Lead in the question: For the list of antiarrhythmic drugs mentioned above find the appropriate use given below.

1. Antiarrhythmic used for treatment of diabetic neuropathy
2. Antiarrhythmic preferred for long term management of congenital long QT syndrome
3. Antiarrhythmic used in ACLS
4. Antiarrhythmic used in inferior wall MI

Ans. 1-g, 2-d, 3-e and 4-c

- Mexiletine is an oral derivative of lidocaine used for treatment of diabetic neuropathy.
- Beta blockers are preferred for long term management of congenital long QT syndrome.
- Amiodarone is the preferred antiarrhythmic in ACLS guidelines.
- Inferior wall MI causes MI due to irritation of vagus and hence atropine is used.

33. Theme and focus: Drugs used in CHF

Answer options list:

a. Milrinone
b. Levosimendan
c. Carvedilol
d. Nesiritide
e. Sacubitril
f. Digoxin
g. Dobutamine
h. Enalapril

Lead in the question: For the drugs used in CHF given above find the appropriate statement below.

1. Inotrope of choice in acute CHF
2. Inotrope with calcium channel sensitizing effect
3. Drug which can cause maximum decrease in mortality in chronic CHF
4. Drug which is used with valsartan for chronic CHF

Ans. 1-g, 2-b, 3-c and 4-e

- Dobutamine is the inotrope of choice in acute CHF.
- Levosimendan inhibits PDE-3, sensitizes myocardium to calcium and opens potassium channels.
- Beta blockers cause maximum decrease in mortality in chronic CHF.
- Sacubitril is used along with valsartan to decrease mortality in chronic CHF.

34. Theme and focus: Diuretics

Answer option list:

a. Acetazolamide
b. Chlorthalidone
c. Spironolactone
d. Furosemide
e. Amiloride
f. Mannitol
g. Chlorothiazide
h. Eplerenone

Lead in the question: For the features of diuretics given below find the appropriate drug from the list given above.

1. Decreases both positive and negative free water clearance
2. Can cause both hyponatremia and hypernatremia as side-effect
3. Never used in a patient of liver cirrhosis

Ans. 1-d, 2-f and 3-a

- Loop diuretics decrease both positive and negative free water clearance, thiazides decrease positive free water clearance and carbonic anhydrase inhibitor increase positive free water clearance.
- Mannitol can cause both hyponatremia and hypernatremia as side-effects.
- Carbonic anhydrase inhibitors like acetazolamide cause hyperammonemia and hence never used in patients of liver cirrhosis, as hyperammonemia increases risk of hepatic encephalopathy.

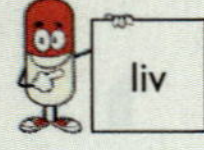

35. Theme and focus: Antiepileptics

Answer option list:

a. Lamotrigine b. Valproate
c. Rufinamide d. Carbamazepine
e. Phenytoin f. Ethosuximide
g. Topiramate h. ACTH

Lead in the question: For the given clinical presentation, find the drug of choice from the list given above.

1. A patient who has seizures shortly after awakening and is often precipitated by sleep deprivation.
2. A child with multiple seizure types and mental retardation.
3. A patient has twitching on the neck, head turning and lip smacking along with crawling sensation on the skin.
4. A 7 month old child with stiffness of muscle in the limbs and bending of head in forward direction during a seizure episode.

Ans. 1-b, 2-b, 3-d and 4-h

- The first one is a classical case of juvenile myoclonic epilepsy for which valproate is the drug of choice.
- Child with multiple seizure type and mental retardation is Lennox Gastaut syndrome, for which drug of choice is valproate.
- The third one is a classical case of partial seizure for which drug of choice is carbamazepine.
- The fourth one is infantile spasm for which ACTH is drug of choice.

36. Theme and focus: Opioids

Answer option list:

a. Methadone b. Morphine
c. Dezocine d. Buprenorphine
e. Codeine f. Pentazocine
g. Pethidine h. Fentanyl

Lead in the question: For the effect on the opioid receptors given below, find the appropriate opioid from the list given above.

1. Partial agonist at μ and antagonist at kappa
2. Partial agonist at μ and full agonist at kappa
3. Antagonist at μ and full agonist at kappa

Ans. 1-d, 2-f and 3-c

Mixed agonist antagonist opioids:

Buprenorphine	Partial agonist at μ and antagonist at kappa
Pentazocine	Partial agonist at μ and full agonist at kappa
Dezocine Nalbuphine Butorphanol	Antagonist at μ and full agonist at kappa

37. Theme and focus: Antibiotic use

Answer option list:

a. Ampicillin b. Ceftazidime
c. Vancomycin d. Meropenem
e. Metronidazole f. Ceftriaxone
g. Penicillin G h. Doxycycline

Lead in the question: For each of the infectious disease symptoms described below, find the appropriate drug of choice from the list mentioned above.

1. An admitted patient with prolonged therapy with ceftriaxone develops fever, diarrhoea with blood in stool and pain abdomen.
2. A patient with rashes, headache, neck stiffness, vomiting and light sensitivity.
3. A female with symptoms of dysuria and green colored discharge.

Ans. 1-c, 2-f and 3-e

- The first case is pseudomembranous enterocolitis, for which oral vancomycin is the current drug of choice.
- The second case is meningococcal meningitis for which ceftriaxone is the drug of choice.
- The third case is trichomoniasis for which metronidazole is drug of choice.

38. Theme and focus: Spectrum of antifungal drugs

Answer option list:

a. Amphotericin B b. Terbinafine
c. Tavaborole d. Natamycin
e. Fluconazole f. Griseofulvin
g. Sulfadiazine h. Caspofungin

Lead in the question: For the spectrum of antifungal drugs described below find the appropriate drug mentioned in the list above.

1. Most wide spectrum drug covers candida, dermatophytes, cryptococcus and endemic mycoses
2. Topical drug of choice for treatment of fungal corneal ulcers
3. Drug of choice for systemic fungal infections and mucormycosis
4. Used for treatment of dermatophytes and is drug of choice for kerion

Ans. 1-e, 2-d, 3-a and 4-f

- Azoles like fluconazole are most wide spectrum antifungals.
- Natamycin is a topical drug and is drug of choice for treatment of fungal corneal ulcer.
- Amphotericin B is the drug of choice for treatment of systemic fungal infections, mucormycosis and cryptococcal meningitis.
- Griseofulvin is used for treatment of dermatophytes and is drug of choice for T. capitis which causes kerion or boggy swelling. The drug of choice for dermatophytes is terbinafine though.

39. Theme and focus: Anticancer drug mechanism of action

Answer option list:

a. Cisplatin b. Paclitaxel
c. Vincristine d. Pentostatin
e. Cyclophosphamide f. Belinostat
g. Bleomycin h. Palbociclib

Lead in question: For each of the mechanism of action of anticancer drugs given below, find the appropriate anticancer drug from the list above.

1. Alkylates DNA at N7 position of guanine
2. Inhibits DNA synthesis by inhibiting adenosine deaminase
3. Inhibits S phase of cell cycle by inhibiting histone deacetylase

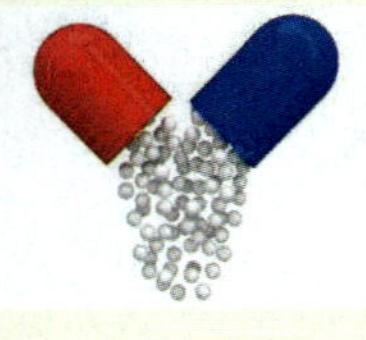

4. Inhibits M phase of cell cycle by increasing polymerization of microtubules

Ans. 1-e, 2-d, 3-f and 4-b

- Alkylating agents like cyclophosphamide alkylate DNA at N7 position of guanine.
- Pentostatin inhibits DNA synthesis by inhibiting adenosine deaminase.
- Belinostat is a histone deacetylase inhibitor, which inhibits S phase of cell proliferation.
- Paclitaxel inhibits M phase by increasing polymerization of microtubules, whereas vincristine inhibits M phase by decreasing polymerization of microtubules.

40. Theme and focus: Antidiabetic drugs

Answer option list:

a. Metformin b. Glibenclamide
c. Pioglitazone d. Acarbose
e. Pramlintide f. Sitagliptin
g. Semaglutide h. Canagliflozin

Lead in question: For the mechanism of action mentioned below, find the appropriate drug from the list given above.

1. Inhibition of metabolism of complex carbohydrates
2. Inhibition of hepatic glucose production
3. A decrease in insulin resistance

Ans. 1-d, 2-a and 3-c

- Acarbose inhibits alpha glucosidase enzyme which metabolizes complex carbohydrates like starch and disaccharides in to glucose.
- The primary mechanism of action of metformin is a decreased hepatic glucose production.
- Pioglitazone acts by stimulating PPAR gamma which leads to a decreased insulin resistance.

41. Theme and focus: Drugs acting on reproductive system

Answer option list:

a. Toremifene b. Ospemifene
c. Raloxifene d. Tamoxifen
e. Ulipristal f. Clomiphene
g. Fluvestrant h. Exemestane

Lead in question: For the drugs described below, find the appropriate drug from the list mentioned above.

1. Drug of choice for treatment of premenopausal ER positive breast cancer
2. Drug of choice for postmenopausal ER positive breast cancer
3. SPRM used in emergency contraception
4. SERM used in postmenopausal dyspareunia

Ans. 1-d, 2-h, 3-e and 4-b

- Tamoxifen is drug of choice for treatment of ER positive premenopausal breast cancer, whereas exemestane is the drug of choice for postmenopausal ER positive breast cancer.
- Ulipristal is an SPRM used for emergency contraception.
- Ospemifene is an SERM specifically approved for treatment of postmenopausal dyspareunia.

42. Theme and focus: Drugs acting on serotonin receptors

Answer option list:

a. Ondansetron b. Cyproheptadine
c. Locaserin d. Methysergide
e. Alosetron f. Buspirone
g. Sumatriptan h. Cisapride

Lead in question: For a description of drug acting on serotonin receptors find the appropriate drug from the list above.

1. A serotonin receptor agonist used for treatment of obesity
2. A serotonin receptor antagonist used in treatment of IBS associated with diarrhoea
3. A serotonin receptor agonist used as anxiolytic

Ans. 1-c, 2-e and 3-f

- Locaserin is a 5HT2 agonist used for treatment of obesity.
- Alosetron is a 5HT-3 antagonist used for treatment of IBS associated with diarrhoea.
- Buspirone is a 5HT1A agonist used as an anxiolytic.

43. Theme and focus: Immunomodulators

Answer option list:

a. Basiliximab b. Belatacept
c. Muromonab d. Leflunomide
e. Azathioprine f. Tacrolimus
g. Sirolimus h. Mycophenolate mofetil

Lead in question: For the mechanism of action mentioned below, find the appropriate immunomodulator from the list given above.

1. Decreases transcription of IL 2
2. Inhibits S phase of lymphocyte proliferation
3. Inhibits T cell costimulation

Ans. 1-f, 2-e and 3-b

- Tacrolimus and cyclosporine inhibit calcineurin, which leads to a decrease in transcription factors for production of IL 2.
- Azathioprine inhibits DNA synthesis i.e. S phase of lymphocyte proliferation.
- Belatacept is an inhibitor of T cell costimulation.

44. Theme and focus: Treatment of bronchial asthma

Answer option list:

a. Theophylline b. Fluticasone
c. Prednisolone d. Hydrocortisone
e. Salbutamol f. Salmeterol
g. Cromolyn h. Zileuton

Lead in question: For a particular clinical scenario of bronchial asthma, find the appropriate drug for treatment mentioned in the list above.

1. A patient of bronchial asthma who needs SABA more than 2 times in a week for symptom relief.
2. In acute attack of bronchial asthma, a steroid is to be administered.
3. A patient develops symptoms of asthma only during exercise.

Ans. 1-b, 2-d and 3-b

- The first case is persistent bronchial asthma, for which ICS like fluticasone is the drug of choice.
- In acute attack of bronchial asthma the steroid of choice is intravenous hydrocortisone.
- The third case is exercise induced asthma, for which ICS like fluticasone is drug of choice.

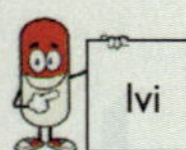

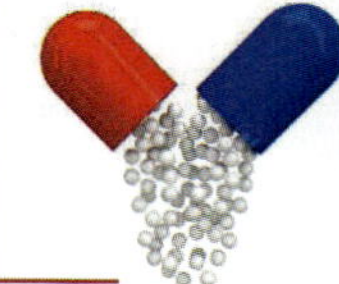

45. Theme and focus: Anticoagulant monitoring

Answer option list:

a. Lepirudin
b. Argatroban
c. Edoxaban
d. Dabigatran
e. Warfarin
f. Enoxaparin
g. Fondaparinux

Lead in question: For the monitoring parameter given below, find the appropriate drugs from the options above.

1. PT/INR
2. aPTT
3. PT and aPTT

Ans. 1-e, 3-a and 4-b

Anticoagulant drugs requiring monitoring are given below.

Unfractionated Heparin Parenteral direct thrombin inhibitors except argatroban	aPTT
Argatroban	aPTT and PT
Warfarin	PT/INR

46. Theme and focus: ASA physical status classification

Answer option list:

a. Class I
b. Class II
c. Class III
d. Class IV
e. Class V
f. Class VI

Lead in question: For the described physical status below, find the appropriate class mentioned in options above.

1. Patients with severe systemic disease that is a constant threat to life
2. Patient with mild systemic disease

Ans. 1-d and 2-b

American Society of Anaesthesiologists (ASA) Physical Status Classification

Class	Physical status
I	Normal healthy patient
II	Patients with mild systemic disease
III	Patients with severe systemic disease
IV	Patients with severe systemic disease that is a constant threat to life
V	Moribund patients who are not expected to survive without the operation
VI	A declared brain-dead patient whose organs are being removed for donor purposes

47. Theme and focus: Cylinder color

Answer option list:

a. Nitrous oxide
b. Carbon dioxide
c. Entonox
d. Air
e. Oxygen
f. Cyclopropane

Lead in question: For the colors described below, find the appropriate anesthetic agents from the options above.

1. Blue body with blue and white shoulders
2. Black with white shoulders
3. Gray body with black and white shoulders

Ans. 1-c, 2-e and 3-d

Cylinder color and pin index (Mnemonic: At ONCE)

Gas	Pin Index	Forms of Physical Content	Cylinder Color
At: Air	1, 5	Gas	Gray body with black and white shoulders
O: Oxygen	2, 5	Gas or Liquid	Black with white shoulders
N: Nitrous oxide	3, 5	Liquid	Blue
C: $CO_2 \geq 7.5\%$ $CO_2 < 7.5\%$ Cyclopropane	1, 6 2, 6 3, 6	Liquid Liquid	Grey Orange
Entonox	7	Liquid	Blue body with blue and white shoulder

Note: The color of helium cylinder is brown

48. Theme and focus: Anesthetic agent properties

Answer option list:

a. Thiopentone
b. Propofol
c. Enflurane
d. Desflurane
e. Ketamine
f. Etomidate
g. Halothane
h. Isoflurane

Lead in question: For the property described below find the appropriate anesthetic agent from the list above.

1. Intravenous agent that causes maximum nausea/vomiting
2. Intravenous agent that causes maximum pain on injection
3. Inhalational agent that causes maximum increase in intracranial pressure
4. Inhalational agent that maintains cardiac output

Ans. 1-f, 2-b, 3-g, 4-h

- Etomidate causes maximum nausea vomiting, whereas propofol has antiemetic effect.
- Maximum pain on injection (intravenous) is seen with propofol, whereas pain on accidental intraarterial injection is seen with thiopentone.
- Inhalational agent with maximum increase in ICP is halothane, whereas least increase in ICP is sevoflurane.
- Inhalational agent that maintains cardiac output is isoflurane.

49. Theme and focus: Use of local anesthetics

Answer option list:

a. Tetracaine
b. Chlorprocaine
c. Benzocaine
d. Bupivacaine
e. Dibucaine
f. Cocaine

Lead in question: For the property of local anesthetic mentioned below, find the appropriate drug from the list above.

1. Not used in Bier's block due to cardiotoxicity
2. Contraindicated in spinal anesthesia due to neurotoxicity'
3. Causes vasoconstriction and is contraindicated with epinephrine

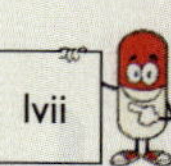

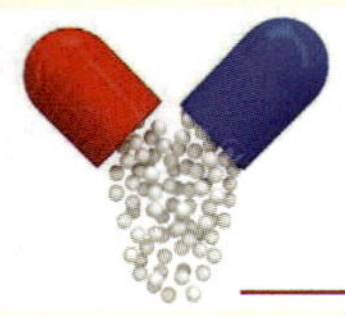

Ans. 1-d, 2-b, 3-f

- Bupivacaine is a cardiotoxic anesthetic agent and hence is contraindicated in Bier's block.
- Chlorprocaine is neurotoxic and hence is contraindicated in spinal anesthesia.
- Cocaine cause vasoconstriction and hence is contraindicated with epinephrine.

MATCH THE FOLLOWING TYPE

50. Match the appropriate enzyme in column A that metabolizes drug in column B.

Column A	Column B
1. Monoamine oxidase	a. Atazanavir
2. UGT1A1	b. Clozapine
3. Thiopurine methyl transferase	c. Azathioprine
	d. Propranolol
4. CYP2C9	e. Isoniazid
	f. Paracetamol
	g. Phenytoin
	h. Phenylephrine

Ans. 1-h, 2-a, 3-c and 4-g

- Monoamine oxidase metabolizes monoamines like norepinephrine, dopamine and serotonin. It also metabolizes drugs like phenylephrine.
- UGT1A1 metabolizes drugs like atazanavir, irinotecan, statins, benzodiazepines and estrogen.
- Thiopurine methyl transferase metabolizes immunomodulator azathioprine.
- CYP2C9 metabolizes drugs like phenytoin and warfarin.

51. Match the appropriate gene in column A, whose polymorphism can affect metabolism of drugs in column B.

Column A	Column B
1. CYP2D6	a. Clopidogrel
2. N acetyl transferase	b. Aspirin
3. CYP2C19	c. Digoxin
4. Butyryl choline esterase	d. Warfarin
	e. Succinylcholine
	f. Isoniazid
	g. Sildenafil
	h. Tramadol

Ans. 1-h, 2-f, 3-a and 4-e

- CYP2D6 enzyme metabolizes drugs like tramadol, antipsychotics, antidepressants and beta blockers. Hence polymorphism in CYP2D6 gene can affect metabolism of these drugs.
- N acetyl transferase metabolizes drugs like sulfonamides, dapsone, isoniazid, hydralazine and procainamide. Hence polymorphism in N acetyl transferase gene can affect their metabolism.
- Butyryl choline esterase metabolizes succinyl choline and hence polymorphism of butyryl choline esterase gene can affect metabolism.

52. Match the appropriate name of a phase of clinical trial in column A to the phases given in column B.

Column A	Column B
1. Phase 0	a. Therapeutic confirmatory trial
2. Phase II	b. Pharmacovigilance
3. Phase IV	c. Pharmacoepidemiology
4. Phase V	d. Microdosing
	e. Preclinical trial
	f. Post marketing surveillance
	g. Therapeutic exploratory trial
	h. Human pharmacology and toxicity study

Ans. 1-d, 2-g, 3-f and 4-c

Names of different phases of clinical trial	
Phase 0	Microdosing
Phase I	Human pharmacology and toxicity study
Phase II	Therapeutic exploratory trial
Phase III	Therapeutic confirmatory trial
Phase IV	Post marketing surveillance
Phase V	Pharmacoepidemiology

53. Match the route of drug administration in column A to the drugs in column B.

Column A	Column B
1. Sublingual	a. Nicardipine
2. Transdermal	b. Scopolamine
3. Intrathecal	c. Levodopa
4. Intranasal	d. Baclofen
	e. Nesiritide
	f. Fentanyl
	g. Buprenorphine
	h. Lorazepam

Ans. 1-g, 2-b, 3-d and 4-f

Kindly refer to the chapter of general pharmacology for examples of drugs given by different routes.

54. Match the drug class in column A with the appropriate drug in column B.

Column A	Column B
1. Ganglionic blocker	a. Atropine
2. Nicotinic agonist	b. Edrophonium
3. Carbamate	c. Acetylcholine
4. Direct cholinergic	d. Varenicline
	e. Reserpine
	f. Trimethaphan

Ans. 1-f, 2-d, 3-b, 4-c

- Trimethaphan is a ganglionic blocker used for treatment of hypertension.
- Varenicline is a nicotinic agonist used in smoking dependence.

- Edrophonium is the shortest acting carbamate used for diagnosis of myasthenia gravis.
- Acetylcholine is a direct cholinergic used as a miotic agent in ocular surgery.

55. Match the antiglaucoma drugs in column A to their side-effects in column B.

Column A	Column B
1. Latanoprost	a. Iris cysts
2. Brimonidine	b. Nasolacrimal duct obstruction
3. Epinephrine	c. Accommodative spasm
4. Timolol	d. Apnea in neonates
	e. Conjunctival pigmentation
	f. Trichomegaly

Ans. 1-f, 2-d, 3-e and 4-b

- Latanoprost can cause trichomegaly i.e. overgrowth of eye lashes.
- Brimonidine can cross blood brain barrier and cause apnea in neonates and drowsiness.
- Epinephrine can cause black pigmentation of conjunctiva.
- Timolol can cause nasolacrimal duct stenosis causing obstruction.

56. Match the antiarrhythmic drug class mentioned in column A to the appropriate drug in column B.

Column A	Column B
1. Class Ia	a. Adenosine
2. Class Ic	b. Verapamil
3. Class II	c. Amiodarone
4. Class V	d. Disopyramide
	e. Propranolol
	f. Lidocaine
	g. Moricizine
	h. Sotalol

Ans. 1-d, 2-g, 3-e and 4-a

Kindly refer to the text on antiarrhythmic drugs in chapter of CVS for details on classification of antiarrhythmics.

57. Match the mechanism of action of antianginal drugs in column A to the appropriate drug in column B.

Column A	Column B
1. Rho kinase inhibitor	a. Metoprolol
2. PFOX inhibitor	b. Nitroglycerine
3. Funny channel inhibitor	c. Trimetazidine
4. Sodium channel blocker	d. Ranolazine
	e. Nicorandil
	f. Fasudil
	g. Ivabradine
	h. Amlodipine

Ans. 1-f, 2-c, 3-g and 4-d

- Fasudil is a vasodilator which acts by inhibition of rho kinase and can be used in stable angina.
- Trimetazidine is a PFOX inhibitor that can be used in stable angina.
- Ivabradine is an inhibitor of funny channel and used in stable angina and chronic CHF.
- Ranolazine primarily acts by inhibition of sodium channel. Though it can inhibit PFOX, it is not the primary mechanism of action.

58. Match the diuretics in column A to their appropriate uses in column B.

Column A	Column B
1. Furosemide	a. Gynecomastia
2. Spironolactone	b. Mild to moderate hypertension
3. Mannitol	c. Cerebral edema
4. Chlorthalidone	d. Metabolic acidosis
	e. Hypertensive emergency
	f. Cirrhotic edema
	g. Hyperuricemia
	h. Angina

Ans. 1-e, 2-f, 3-c and 4-b

- Furosemide is used for treatment of hypertensive emergency. Furosemide and chlorthalidone can cause hyperuricemia as a side-effect.
- Spironolactone is drug of choice for cirrhotic edema. It can cause gynecomastia as a side-effect.
- Mannitol is drug of choice for cerebral edema.
- Chlorthalidone is the thiazide of choice for treatment of mild to moderate hypertension.

59. Match the side-effect of antiepileptic drugs given in column A to the appropriate drugs in column B.

Column A	Column B
1. Blue pigmentation of skin and nails	a. Phenytoin
2. Tremor	b. Carbamazepine
3. Metabolic acidosis	c. Lamotrigine
4. SIADH	d. Valproate
	e. Topiramate
	f. Ezogabine
	g. Gabapentin
	h. Cannabidiol

Ans. 1-f, 2-d, 3-e and 4-b

- Ezogabine is a potassium channel opener which can cause blue pigmentation of skin and nails.
- Valproate can cause tremor.
- Topiramate and Zonisamide can block carbonic anhydrase and hence cause metabolic acidosis, nephrolithiasis and hypohidrosis.
- Carbamazepine can cause SIADH, which can lead to dilutional hyponatremia.

60. Match the dependence disorder in column A to the FDA approved drug for treatment in column B.

Column A	Column B
1. Opioid dependence	a. Diazepam
2. Cocaine dependence	b. Bupropion
3. Alcohol dependence	c. Clonidine
4. Smoking dependence	d. Morphine
	e. Acamprosate
	f. Baclofen
	g. Bromocriptine
	h. Methadone

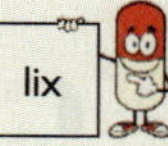

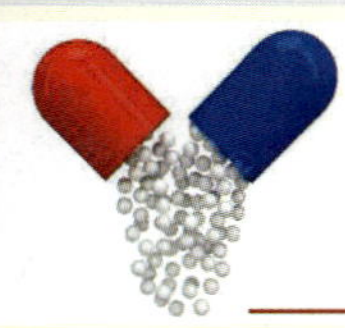

Ans 1-h, 2-g, 3-e and 4-b

- In opioid dependence methadone and buprenorphine are used to decrease withdrawal symptoms, whereas naltrexone is used to prevent relapse.
- In cocaine dependence bromocriptine and desipramine can be used.
- In alcohol dependence naltrexone, acamprosate and disulfiram are the only FDA approved drugs.
- In smoking dependence bupropion and varenicline can be used.

61. Match the drugs of choice in column A with the microbes/ infections in column B.

Column A	Column B
1. Ceftazidime	a. Typhoid
2. Linezolid	b. Traveler's diarrhoea
3. Clindamycin	c. Meningococcal meningitis case
4. Ciprofloxacin	d. Toxic shock syndrome
	e. Febrile neutropenia
	f. Pseudomembranous enterocolitis
	g. VRSA pneumonia
	h. MRSA

Ans. 1-e, 2-g, 3-d and 4-b

- Ceftazidime is drug of choice for treatment of febrile neutropenia, melioidosis and pseudomonas.
- Linezolid is drug of choice for treatment of VRSA pneumonia and VRE.
- Clindamycin inhibits toxin synthesis in staphylococcus and streptococcus and hence is drug of choice for treatment of toxic shock syndrome.
- Ciprofloxacin is drug of choice for traveler's diarrhoea.

62. Match the mechanism of action of antifungal drugs in column A to the appropriate drug in column B.

Column A	Column B
1. Sequesters ergosterol	a. Fluconazole
2. Blocks beta glucan synthase	b. Flucytosine
3. Blocks DNA synthesis	c. Griseofulvin
4. Blocks RNA synthase	d. Terbinafine
	e. Tavaborole
	f. Caspofungin
	g. Amphotericin B

Ans. 1-g, 2-f, 3-b and 4-e

- Amphotericin B sequesters ergosterol in the cell membrane is the updated mechanism. It forms pores in the cell membranes is the old mechanism.
- Echinocandins like caspofungin inhibit beta glucan synthase.
- Flucytosine is a prodrug of anticancer drug 5-FU which acts by inhibiting DNA synthesis.
- Tavaborole is a topical antifungal solution for fungal toe nail infection, which acts by inhibiting fungal RNA synthase.

63. Match the helminths in column A to the drugs of choice in column B.

Column A	Column B
1. Strongyloides	a. Metrifonate
2. Fasciola hepatica	b. Albendazole
3. Trichinella spiralis	c. DEC
4. Schistosoma	d. Metronidazole
	e. Ivermectin
	f. Praziquantel
	g. Pyrantel pamoate
	h. Triclabendazole

Ans. 1-e, 2-h, 3-b and 4-f

- Ivermectin is the drug of choice for thread worm or Strongyloides.
- Triclabendazole is drug of choice for Fasciola hepatica.
- Albendazole is drug of choice for Trichinella spiralis.
- Praziquantel is drug of choice for Schistosoma.

64. Match the anticancer drugs mentioned in column A to their appropriate side-effects in column B.

Column A	Column B
1. Bleomycin	a. Peripheral neuropathy
2. Capecitabine	b. Interstitial pneumonitis
3. Cytarabine	c. SIADH
4. Fludarabine	d. Hemolytic uremic syndrome
	e. Hand and foot syndrome
	f. Flagellate dermatitis
	g. Hemorrhagic cystitis
	h. Dementia

Ans. 1-f, 2-e, 3-h and 4-b

- Bleomycin causes flagellate dermatitis and pulmonary fibrosis.
- Capecitabine and 5-FU cause hand and foot syndrome.
- Cytarabine causes cerebellar and cerebral toxicity. Cerebral toxicity can present as dementia and seizures.
- Fludarabine can cause interstitial pneumonitis.

65. Match the drug used to decrease toxicity of anticancer drug mentioned in column A to the appropriate anticancer drug in column B.

Column A	Column B
1. Leucovorin + Vitamin B12	a. Cisplatin
2. Vitamin B6	b. Bleomycin
3. Loperamide	c. Methotrexate
4. Mannitol	d. Pemetrexed
	e. 5 fluorouracil
	f. Vincristine
	g. Irinotecan
	h. Cyclophosphamide

Ans. 1-d, 2-e, 3-g and 4-a

- Methotrexate and pemetrexed can cause bone marrow suppression. To prevent it, leucovorin or folic acid is used along with methotrexate. But pemetrexed causes more severe bone marrow suppression and hence leucovorin or folic acid plus vitamin B12 is used.

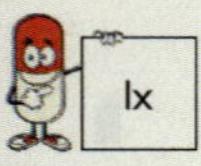

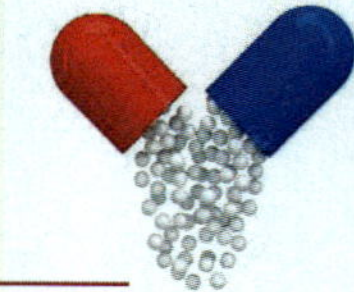

- 5 fluorouracil and capecitabine can cause hand and foot syndrome which can be prevented by vitamin B6.
- Irinotecan can cause nonsecretory diarrhoea which can be treated by loperamide.
- Cisplatin is a very potent nephrotoxic drug which can be prevented by normal saline (chloride diuresis) and mannitol.

66. Match the side-effects of antidiabetic drugs in column A to the appropriate drug in column B.

Column A	Column B
1. Vaginal pruritus	a. Metformin
2. Flatulence	b. Glimepiride
3. Congestive heart failure	c. Acarbose
4. Lung cancer	d. Sitagliptin
	e. Insulin
	f. Canagliflozin
	g. Saxagliptin
	h. Colesevelam

Ans. 1-f, 2-c, 3-g and 4-e

- SGLT-2 inhibitors like canagliflozin can cause UTI and vaginal pruritus as most common side-effect.
- Alpha glucosidase inhibitors like acarbose cause flatulence as most common side-effect.
- DPP-4 inhibitor saxagliptin and PPAR gamma agonist like pioglitazone can cause congestive heart failure.
- Inhalational insulin afrezza can cause lung cancer and hence is contraindicated in smokers.

67. Match the property of a steroid in column A to the appropriate drug in column B.

1. Most potent glucocorticoid	a. Aldosterone
2. Least potent glucocorticoid	b. Dexamethasone
3. Most potent mineralocorticoid	c. Prednisolone
4. Soft steroid	d. Triamcinolone
	e. Hydrocortisone
	f. Ciclesonide
	g. Fludrocortisone
	h. DOCA

Ans. 1-b, 2-e, 3-a and 4-f

- Dexamethasone and betamethasone are most potent glucocorticoid, whereas hydrocortisone is least potent glucocorticoid.
- Aldosterone is the most potent mineralocorticoid.
- Ciclesonide is metabolized by esterase in airway and hence is known as soft steroid.

68. Match the mechanism of action in column A to the appropriate DMARD in column B.

Column A	Column B
1. IL-6 inhibitor	a. Cyclosporine
2. TNF alpha inhibitor	b. Anakinra
3. Inhibitor of dihydroorotate dehydrogenase	c. Leflunomide
4. JAK inhibitor	d. Abatacept
	e. Adalimumab
	f. Rituximab
	g. Tofacitinib
	h. Tocilizumab

Ans. 1-h, 2-e, 3-c and 4-g

IL 6 inhibitor	Tocilizumab
TNF alpha inhibitors	Adalimumab Infliximab Etanercept Golimumab
Inhibitor of dihydroorotate dehydrogenase	Leflunomide
JAK inhibitors	Tofacitinib Baricitinib

69. Match the mechanism of action of antiasthmatic drugs in column A with the appropriate drug in column B.

Column A	Column B
1. IL5 inhibitor	a. Magnesium sulphate
2. Decreased leukotriene production	b. Salbutamol
3. Increased beta 2 receptor density	c. Reslizumab
4. Potassium channel opener	d. Omalizumab
	e. Hydrocortisone
	f. Zileuton
	g. Monteleukast
	h. Cromakalim

Ans. 1-c, 2-f, 3-e and 4-h

- Reslizumab is an IL5 inhibitor approved for treatment of severe eosinophilic asthma.
- Zileuton inhibits 5-LOX and thus decreases synthesis of leukotrienes.
- Steroids like hydrocortisone increase transcription of beta-2 receptors and increase effectiveness of beta2 agonists in bronchial asthma.
- Cromakalim is a potassium channel opener which can cause bronchodilation and can be used in acute attack of bronchial asthma.

70. Match the mechanism of action of laxative in column A with appropriate drug in column B.

Column A	Column B
1. Decreases surface tension of stool	a. Senna
2. Stimulates chloride channels	b. Bisacodyl
3. Promotes beneficial microbe growth in gut	c. Lubiprostone
4. Stimulates CFTR	d. Psyllium husk
	e. Polyethylene glycol
	f. Plecanatide
	g. Lactobacillus
	h. Docusate sodium

Ans. 1-h, 2-c, 3-d and 4-f

- Docusate sodium and calcium are surfactants that decrease surface tension of stool.
- Lubiprostone stimulates type II chloride channels in the intestine.
- Psyllium husk is dietary fiber that promotes growth of beneficial microbes in gut. Lactobacillus in itself is a beneficial microbe.
- Plecanatide and linaclotide stimulate CFTR.

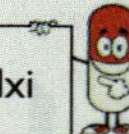

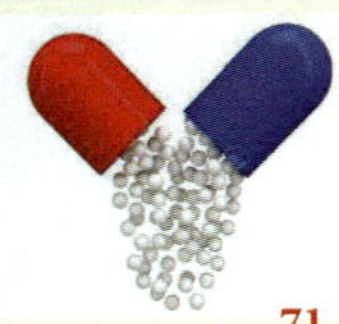

71. Match the mechanism of action of drug in column A to the appropriate drug in column B.

Column A	Column B
1. Reversible ADP inhibitor	a. Filgrastim
2. Plasmin inhibitor	b. Sargamostim
3. Oral direct thrombin inhibitor	c. Tranexamic acid
4. G-CSF analog	d. Edoxaban
	e. Clopidogrel
	f. Ticagrelor
	g. Dabigatran
	h. Lepirudin

Ans. 1-f, 2-c, 3-g and 4-a

- Ticagrelor and cangrelor are reversible ADP inhibitors, whereas clopidogrel, prasugrel and ticlopidine are irreversible ADP inhibitors.
- EACA and tranexamic acid are plasmin inhibitors used for treatment of fibrinolytic induced bleeding.
- Dabigatran and Ximelagatran are oral direct thrombin inhibitors.
- Filgrastim is a G-CSF analog, whereas sargamostim is a G-CSF analog.

72. Match the anesthetic agent in column A with the colour of vaporizer in column B.

Column A	Column B
1. Desflurane	a. Purple
2. Isoflurane	b. Black
3. Sevoflurane	c. Yellow
4. Enflurane	d. Red
	e. Orange
	f. Blue

Ans. 1-f, 2-a, 3-c and 4-e

Color coding for different vaporizers

Volatile anesthetic agent	Vaporizer color
Desflurane	Blue
Halothane	Red
Isoflurane	Purple
Sevoflurane	Yellow
Enflurane	Orange

73. Match the properties of nondepolarizing muscle relaxants in column A to the appropriate drug in column B.

Column A	Column B
1. Fastest acting	a. Mivacurium
2. Longest acting	b. Atracurium
3. Spontaneous metabolism	c. Pipecuronium
4. Shortest acting	d. Rocuronium
	e. Rapacuronium
	f. Vecuronium
	g. Doxacurium

Ans. 1-d, 2-g, 3-b, 4-e

- Rocuronium is fastest acting NDMR and hence is NDMR of choice in intubation. Overall the muscle relaxant of choice in intubation is succinyl choline.
- Doxacurium is the longest acting and most potent NDMR.
- Atracurium undergoes spontaneous metabolism called as Hoffman's elimination.
- Rapacuronium is shortest acting NDMR.

74. Match the safe dose of local anesthetic in column A to the appropriate drug in column B.

Column A	Column B
1. 1 mg/kg	a. Bupivacaine
2. 2 mg/kg	b. Prilocaine
3. 3 mg/kg	c. Dibucaine
4. 4 mg/kg	d. Etidocaine
	e. Procaine
	f. Chlorprocaine
	g. Tetracaine

Ans. 1-c, 2-a, 3-g and 4-d

Safe dose of local anesthetics	
Lidocaine	Without adrenaline: 3 mg/kg or 200 mg With adrenaline: 7 mg/kg or 500 mg
Bupivacaine	2 mg/kg
Chlorprocaine Procaine	12 mg/kg or 1000 mg
Tetracaine	3 mg/kg
Prilocaine	8 mg/kg
Mepivacaine	4.5 mg/kg
Etidocaine	4 mg/kg
Dibucaine	1 mg/kg

MULTIPLE COMPLETION TYPE QUESTIONS

75. GPCR among the options include

a. Glucocorticoid receptor
b. Alpha adrenoreceptor
c. Nicotinic receptor
d. $GABA_B$ receptor

1. a, b and c are correct
2. a and c are correct
3. b and d are correct
4. All four options are correct

Ans. 3 i.e. b and d are correct

- Alpha adrenoreceptor and $GABA_B$ receptor are GPCR.
- Glucocorticoid receptors are nuclear receptors.
- Nicotinic receptors are ion channel receptors.

76. Dialysis is ineffective in case of toxicity of

a. Digoxin
b. Benzodiazepines
c. Opioids
d. Aspirin

1. a, b and c are correct
2. a and c are correct
3. b and d are correct
4. All four options are correct

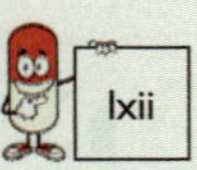

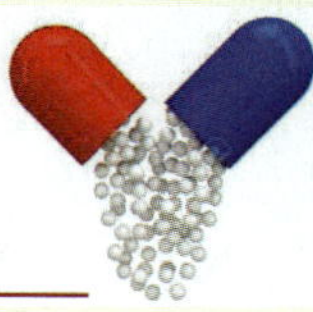

Ans. 1 i.e. a, b and c are correct

Drugs against which dialysis is ineffective
B: Benzodiazepines, Beta blockers
A: Amphetamines
D, D: Digoxin
O: Organophosphates, Opioids
C: Calcium channel blockers

77. Enzyme inducers among the following are

a. Rifampicin b. Fluoxetine
c. DDT d. Grapefruit juice

1. a, b and c are correct 2. a and c are correct
3. b and d are correct 4. All four options are correct

Ans. 2 i.e. a and c are correct

- Among the given options rifampicin and DDT are enzyme inducers.
- Fluoxetine and grapefruit juice are enzyme inhibitors.

78. Volume of distribution of a drug depends on

a. Lipid solubility b. Plasma protein binding
c. Body fat content d. PKa

1. a, b and c are correct 2. a and c are correct
3. b and d are correct 4. All four options are correct

Ans. 4 i.e. All four options are correct

Please refer to the text on volume of distribution in the topic of general pharmacology for details.

79. Drugs following zero order kinetics are

a. Alcohol b. Carbamazepine
c. Phenytoin d. Pioglitazone

1. a, b and c are correct 2. a and c are correct
3. b and d are correct 4. All four options are correct

Ans. 2 i.e. a and c are correct

- Among the given options only alcohol and phenytoin follow zero order kinetics.
- Other drugs following zero order kinetics are theophylline, tolbutamide, heparin, warfarin and methanol.

80. True statements regarding mechanism of action of drugs acting on autonomic nervous system are

a. Valbenazine inhibits dopamine beta hydroxylase enzyme
b. Cocaine inhibits reuptake of norepinephrine
c. Botulinum toxin inhibits release of norepinephrine
d. Reserpine inhibits VMAT2

1. a, b and c are correct 2. a and c are correct
3. b and d are correct 4. All four options are correct

Ans. 3 i.e. b and d are correct

- Reserpine, Valbenazine and tetrabenazine are inhibitors of VMAT2.
- Cocaine inhibits reuptake of norepinephrine.
- Botulinum toxin inhibits release of acetylcholine.

81. Cardioselective beta blockers are

a. Esmolol b. Labetalol
c. Nebivolol d. Timolol

1. a, b and c are correct 2. a and c are correct
3. b and d are correct 4. All four options are correct

Ans. 2 i.e. and c are correct

- Esmolol and nebivolol are cardioselective beta blockers.
- Labetalol is nonselective beta blocker with alpha blocking effect.
- Timolol is nonselective beta blocker.

82. True statements regarding antianginal drugs

a. Ranolazine inhibits sodium channels
b. Nicorandil is a potassium channel opener
c. Nitroglycerine produces effect by decreasing preload in stable angina
d. Nitroglycerine produces effect by coronary vasodilation in variant angina

1. a, b and c are correct 2. a and c are correct
3. b and d are correct 4. All four options are correct

Ans. 4 i.e. All four options are correct

- Ranolazine is a sodium channel blocker used in stable angina.
- Nicorandil is a potassium channel opener used in stable angina.
- Nitroglycerine primarily produces effect in stable angina by decreasing preload and in variant angina by coronary vasodilation.

83. Antihypertensive drugs causing postural hypotension

a. Enalapril b. Minoxidil
c. Prazosin d. Nifedipine

1. a, b and c are correct 2. a and c are correct
3. b and d are correct 4. All four options are correct

Ans. 2 i.e. a and c are correct

- For postural hypotension as a side-effect venodilation is required.
- RAAS inhibitors, alpha blockers, nitrates and nitroprusside can cause venodilation and postural hypotension.
- Minoxidil and nifedipine are arterial dilators and hence will not cause postural hypotension.

84. Diuretics decreasing positive free water clearance

a. Acetazolamide b. Furosemide
c. Spironolactone d. Chlorothiazide

1. a, b and c are correct 2. a and c are correct
3. b and d are correct 4. All four options are correct

Ans. 3 i.e. b and d are correct

- Loop diuretics decrease both positive and negative free water clearance, thiazides decrease positive free water clearance and carbonic anhydrase inhibitor increase positive free water clearance.

85. Antiepileptics causing hepatotoxicity are

a. Topiramate b. Valproate
c. Zonisamide d. Cannabidiol

1. a, b and c are correct 2. a and c are correct
3. b and d are correct 4. All four options are correct

Ans. 3 i.e. b and d are correct

- Valproate and cannabidiol are hepatotoxic antiepileptic drugs.

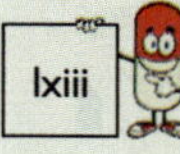

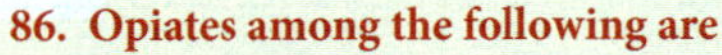

86. Opiates among the following are

a. Morphine b. Codeine
c. Papaverine d. Buprenorphine

1. a, b and c are correct 2. a and c are correct
3. b and d are correct 4. All four options are correct

Ans. 1 i.e. a, b and c are correct

- Opiate is the term used for natural opioid derived from the plant Papaver somniferum.
- Morphine, codeine, noscapine, thebaine and papaverine are natural opioids.

87. True regarding mechanism of action of antihelminthic drugs

a. Pyrantel pamoate causes flaccid paralysis
b. Piperazine causes flaccid paralysis
c. Praziquantel causes flaccid paralysis
d. Metrifonate causes spastic paralysis

1. a, b and c are correct 2. a and c are correct
3. b and d are correct 4. All four options are correct

Ans. 3 i.e. b and d are correct

Spastic paralysis	Flaccid paralysis
Praziquantel	Ivermectin
Metrifonate	Moxidectin
Pyrantel pamoate	Piperazine

88. True statements regarding anti-leprosy drugs

a. Rifampicin is most cidal drug
b. Clofazimine is cidal drug
c. Dapsone is static drug
d. Ofloxacin is static drug

1. a, b and c are correct 2. a and c are correct
3. b and d are correct 4. All four options are correct

Ans. 2 i.e. a and c are correct

- Rifampicin is most cidal anti-leprosy as well as antitubercular drug.
- Clofazimine is cidal against mycobacterium tuberculosis but static against mycobacterium leprae. Since this question is about anti-leprosy drugs this option is not correct.
- Dapsone is a static drug.
- Ofloxacin being a DNA gyrase inhibitor is a cidal drug.

89. Fluoroquinolones that can be safely given in renal impairment

a. Ciprofloxacin b. Pefloxacin
c. Ofloxacin d. Moxifloxacin

1. a, b and c are correct 2. a and c are correct
3. b and d are correct 4. All four options are correct

Ans. 3 i.e. b and d are correct

- Pefloxacin and moxifloxacin are excreted by liver and hence are safe in renal impairment.

90. Antibiotics that are bacteriostatic

a. Cotrimoxazole b. Sulfamethoxazole
c. Daptomycin d. Linezolid

1. a, b and c are correct 2. a and c are correct
3. b and d are correct 4. All four options are correct

Ans. 3 i.e. b and d are correct

- Sulfamethoxazole and linezolid are bacteriostatic drugs.
- Cotrimoxazole and daptomycin are bactericidal drugs.

91. M phase specific drugs among the following are

a. Methotrexate b. Vincristine
c. Bleomycin d. Eribulin

1. a, b and c are correct 2. a and c are correct
3. b and d are correct 4. All four options are correct

Ans. 3 i.e. b and d are correct

- Vincristine and eribulin act on microtubules and are specific for M phase.
- Methotrexate is specific for S phase.
- Bleomycin is specific for G1-S phase.

92. Cardiotoxic anticancer drugs are

a. Doxorubicin b. Cyclophosphamide
c. Trastuzumab d. 6 Mercaptopurine

1. a, b and c are correct 2. a and c are correct
3. b and d are correct 4. All four options are correct

Ans. 1 i.e. a, b and c are correct

- Doxorubicin, daunorubicin, trastuzumab and cyclophosphamide are cardiotoxic drugs.

93. Bone marrow suppression is not seen with

a. Methotrexate b. Cisplatin
c. Cyclophosphamide d. Vincristine

1. a, b and c are correct 2. a and c are correct
3. b and d are correct 4. All four options are correct

Ans. 3 i.e. b and d are correct

- Bone marrow suppression is not seen with cisplatin, vincristine and bleomycin.

94. Pure glucocorticoids are

a. Dexamethasone b. Triamcinolone
c. Betamethasone d. Prednisolone

1. a, b and c are correct 2. a and c are correct
3. b and d are correct 4. All four options are correct

Ans. 1 i.e. a, b and c are correct

- Dexamethasone, betamethasone and triamcinolone are pure glucocorticoids i.e. glucocorticoids without any mineralocorticoid effect.

95. Hypoglycemia as a side-effect is seen with

a. Repaglinide b. Metformin
c. Sitagliptin d. Pramlintide

1. a, b and c are correct 2. a and c are correct
3. b and d are correct 4. All four options are correct

Ans. 2 i.e. a and c are correct

- Hypoglycemia as a side-effect is caused by insulin or drugs which release insulin like sulfonylureas, meglitinides (repaglinide), GLP1 agonists and DPP-4 inhibitors (Sitagliptin).

96. Hepatotoxic NSAIDs are

a. Acetaminophen b. Diclofenac
c. Lumiracoxib d. Nimesulide

1. a, b and c are correct 2. a and c are correct
3. b and d are correct 4. All four options are correct

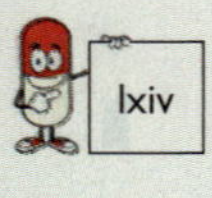

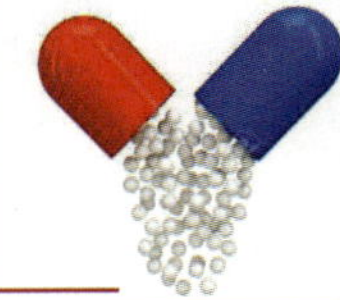

Ans. 4 i.e. All four options are correct

- All the NSAIDs mentioned in the options are hepatotoxic drugs.

97. Cyclosporine causes

a. Hirsutism
b. Hypokalemia
c. Hyperplasia of gums
d. Bone marrow suppression

1. a, b and c are correct
2. a and c are correct
3. b and d are correct
4. All four options are correct

Ans. 2 i.e. a and c are correct

- Cyclosporine causes hirsutism and hyperplasia of gums from the given options.

98. Mechanism of action of theophylline is

a. Phosphodiesterase inhibition
b. Adenosine receptor antagonism
c. Histone deacetylase stimulation
d. Release of IL10

1. a, b and c are correct
2. a and c are correct
3. b and d are correct
4. All four options are correct

Ans. 4 i.e. All four options are correct

- All the options mentioned in the question are mechanism of action of theophylline.

99. True statements regarding proton pump inhibitors

a. Lansoprazole is safest PPI in pregnancy
b. Esomeprazole is shorter acting then omeprazole
c. Rabeprazole is most potent PPI
d. Pantoprazole is most potent enzyme inhibitor

1. a, b and c are correct
2. a and c are correct
3. b and d are correct
4. All four options are correct

Ans. 2 i.e. a and c are correct

- PPI are contraindicated in pregnancy, but lansoprazole is the safest PPI in pregnancy.
- S isomer of omeprazole is slowly eliminated and hence esomeprazole is longer acting than omeprazole.
- Rabeprazole is most potent and longest acting PPI.
- Omeprazole is the most potent enzyme inhibitor, whereas pantoprazole is the least potent enzyme inhibitor.

MULTIPLE TRUE FALSE TYPE QUESTIONS

100. The following statements are true/false regarding volume of distribution of drugs.

a. Drugs with high volume of distribution are primarily located in the intravascular compartment.
b. Volume of distribution is important in calculating loading dose of a drug.
c. A drug with high plasms protein binding has high volume of distribution.
d. Dialysis is effective mode of treatment for toxicity if a drug with high volume of distribution.
e. Unit of volume of distribution is liters.

Ans. True: b and e, False: a, c and d

- Drugs with volume of distribution are located in tissues and not in intravascular compartment.
- Volume of distribution multiplied by plasma concentration gives loading dose.
- A drug with high plasma protein binding is located primarily in intravascular compartment and has a low volume of distribution.
- Dialysis is not effective for drugs with high volume of distribution, high plasma protein binding and irreversible binding with targets.
- The unit of volume of distribution is liters.

101. The following statements are true/false regarding kinetics of drug elimination.

a. In zero order a constant proportion of drug is eliminated
b. In zero order half-life is constant
c. In first order clearance is constant
d. Most drugs follow first order
e. In first order a constant amount of drug is eliminated

Ans. True: c and d, False: a, b and e

- In zero order a constant amount of drug is eliminated whereas in first order a constant proportion of drug is eliminated.
- In zero order as dose increases half life increases and clearance decreases.
- In first order half-life and clearance are constant.
- Most drugs follow first and only few drugs follow zero order.

102. The following statements are true/false regarding GPCRs.

a. Beta is the most important subunit of a GPCR
b. GPCRs are the most common receptor targeted by drugs
c. Cyclic AMP is a secondary messenger in Gq subtype of GPCR
d. GPCRs are also known as heptahelical receptors
e. Go subtype of GPCR produces effect via beta-gamma subunits

Ans. True: b, d and e, False: a and c

- Alpha is the most important subunit in a GPCR.
- GPCR is the most common target of drugs.
- Cyclic AMP is a secondary messenger of Gs subtype of GPCR, whereas IP3 is a secondary messenger of Gq subtype of GPCR.
- GPCRs are also known as heptahelical/serpentine/7 transmembrane/metabotropic receptor.
- All GPCRs produce effect by alpha subunit except Go subunit, which produces effect by beta-gamma subunit.

103. The following statements are true/false regarding mechanisms of drug absorption.

a. Active transport is the most common mechanism of drug absorption
b. ATP is not required in diffusion
c. Active transport can happen against concentration gradient
d. Insulin is absorbed by passive diffusion after subcutaneous injection
e. Facilitated diffusion does not require a carrier for absorption

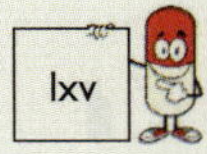

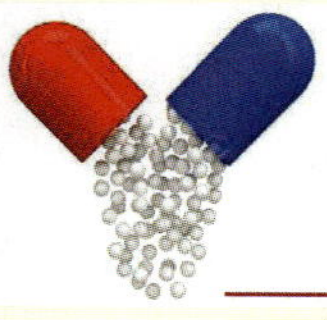

Ans. True: b and c, False: a, d and e

- Passive diffusion is the most common mechanism of drug absorption.
- ATP is not required in diffusion and filtration but absolutely required in active transport.
- Active transport happens against concentration gradient but diffusion happens with concentration gradient.
- Insulin is absorbed by filtration after a subcutaneous injection.
- Facilitated diffusion and active transport are carrier mediated drug absorption mechanisms.

104. The following statements are true/false regarding drug trials.

a. Patients are first introduced in phase II trial
b. In phase I trial toxicity is studied in patients
c. Maximum number of patients are studied in phase III trial
d. Efficacy is confirmed in phase II trial
e. Phase IV is done before releasing the drug in to the market

Ans. True: a and c, False: b, d and e

- In phase I normal healthy volunteers are taken and in phase II patients are taken for the first time in the trial.
- In phase I toxicity is studied but in normal healthy volunteers and not patients.
- Maximum number of patients i.e. 500-3000 are taken in phase III.
- Efficacy is determined in phase II, whereas confirmed in phase III.
- Phase IV which is known as post marketing surveillance is done after releasing drug in to the market.

105. The following statements are true/false regarding drugs used in urinary incontinence

a. Tolterodine is preferred in stress incontinence
b. Darifenacin is most selective drug for bladder among anticholinergics
c. Mirabegron is a beta 3 agonist used in stress incontinence
d. Duloxetine is an SNRI used in urge incontinence
e. Trospium does not have central side-effects

Ans. True: b and e, False: a, c and d

- Anticholinergics like tolterodine are used in treatment of urge incontinence.
- Darifenacin is most selective for M3 receptors (bladder) among all anticholinergics used in urge incontinence.
- Mirabegron is a beta 3 agonist used in urge incontinence.
- Duloxetine is an SNRI used in stress incontinence.
- Trospium is the only quaternary amine anticholinergic used in urge incontinence. It is lipid insoluble and hence does not cross blood brain barrier and does not produce central side-effects.

106. The following statements are true/false regarding effects of catecholamines on heart rate and blood pressure

a. Epinephrine has a biphasic effect on blood pressure
b. Norepinephrine decreases heart rate in presence of atropine
c. Isoprenaline causes bradycardia
d. Norepinephrine increases mean blood pressure
e. Epinephrine causes tachycardia

Ans. True: a, d and e

- Epinephrine first increases blood pressure due to alpha 1 receptor and then decreases due to beta 2 receptor; this effect is known as biphasic response of blood pressure.
- Norepinephrine decreases heart rate but in presence of atropine it increases heart rate.
- Isoprenaline causes significant tachycardia.
- Norepinephrine significantly increases mean blood pressure.
- Epinephrine causes tachycardia but lesser than isoprenaline.

107. The following statements are true/false regarding side-effects of antiarrhythmic drugs

a. Lidocaine can cause QT prolongation
b. Quinidine can cause diarrhoea
c. Procainamide can cause hypotension
d. Amiodarone can cause ceruloderma
e. Flecainide has least proarrhythmic effect

Ans. True: b, c and d; False: a and e

- QT prolongation as a side-effect is seen with Class Ia drugs and class III drugs; lidocaine rather causes QT shortening.
- Quinidine causes diarrhoea and procainamide causes hypotension.
- Amiodarone causes blue pigmentation of skin known as ceruloderma.
- Class Ic drugs like procainamide are most proarrhythmic drugs.

108. The following statements are true/false regarding antihypertensive drugs

a. Beta blockers are preferred in old age hypertension
b. Thiazides are preferred in young age hypertension
c. Spironolactone is reserved for treatment of resistant hypertension
d. Nicardipine is preferred for treatment of high blood pressure associated with end organ damage
e. Antihypertensive drug associated with maximum erectile dysfunction are thiazides

Ans. True: c, d and e; False: a and b

- ACE inhibitors/ARBs and beta blockers are preferred in young age hypertension, whereas thiazides and calcium channel blockers are preferred in old age hypertension.
- Spironolactone is drug of choice for treatment of resistant hypertension.
- Nicardipine is drug of choice for treatment of hypertensive emergency i.e. high blood pressure with endo organ damage.
- Thiazides > beta blockers cause maximum erectile dysfunction among antihypertensives.

109. The following statements are true/false regarding loop diuretics

a. Furosemide is most commonly used
b. Loop diuretics cause irreversible ototoxicity
c. Ethacrynic acid is most ototoxic
d. Bumetanide is most potent
e. Torsemide is longest acting

Ans. True: a, c, d and e; False: b

- Loop diuretics cause reversible ototoxicity.
- Other options are correct.

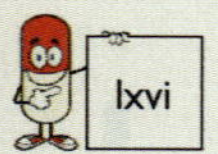

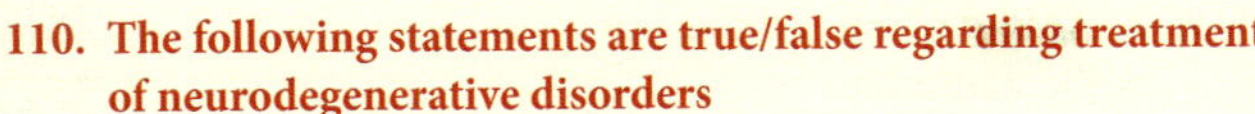

110. The following statements are true/false regarding treatment of neurodegenerative disorders

a. Levodopa is used in early onset Parkinson's disease
b. Edaravone is a recent drug approved for treatment of Huntington's chorea
c. Baclofen is used for treatment of ALS
d. Memantine is the most preferred drug for Alzheimer's disease
e. Apomorphine is used for treatment of on-off phenomena

Ans. True: c and e; False: a, b and d

- MAO inhibitors are preferred for treatment of early onset Parkinson's disease. Levodopa is not preferred in early onset type as there is risk of dyskinesia.
- Edaravone is a recent drug approved for treatment of ALS.
- Baclofen is used in ALS for treatment of muscle spasticity.
- Donepezil is the most preferred drug in Alzheimer's disease.
- Apomorphine is used as rescue therapy in on-off phenomena.

111. The following statements are true/false regarding sedative hypnotics

a. Barbiturates have both GABA facilitatory and mimetic action
b. Benzodiazepines have only GABA facilitatory action
c. Ramelteon is more effective than zolpidem in insomnia
d. Zolpidem has more addiction potential than ramelteon
e. Triazolam is the preferred benzodiazepine in insomnia

Ans. True: a, b and e; False: c and d

- Barbiturates at normal doses have GABA facilitatory effect, but at high doses have GABA mimetic effect.
- Benzodiazepines have only GABA mimetic effect.
- Benzodiazepines and Z compounds like zolpidem are more effective in insomnia and have higher addiction potential as compared to ramelteon.

112. The following statements are true/false regarding antiretroviral drugs

a. Nevirapine is effective against both HIV 1 and 2
b. Zidovudine is a first line drug in adults
c. Tenofovir is contraindicated in renal failure patients
d. Protease inhibitors are more effective than NNRTI in children < 3 years
e. Zidovudine should not be used in patients of anemia

Ans. True: c, d and e; False: a and b

- NNRTI class drugs like nevirapine is effective only against HIV 1.
- Zidovudine is a first line drug in children but not in adults.
- Tenofovir is a nephrotoxic drug and hence not used in renal failure patients.
- Children < 3 years on protease inhibitors have better survival than children on NNRTI.
- Zidovudine causes anemia and hence is not used in patients with hemoglobin < 9 gm%.

113. The following statements are true/false regarding antimalarial drugs

a. Tafenoquine is an erythrocytic schizontocidal drug approved for falciparum malaria
b. Primaquine is contraindicated in pregnancy
c. Artemisinin group drugs are fastest acting erythrocytic schizontocidal drugs
d. Quinine is the drug of choice for severe falciparum malaria
e. Chloroquine is drug of choice for falciparum malaria

Ans. True: b, c and d; False: a and e

- Tafenoquine is a hypnozoite cidal drug approved for radical cure of malaria in vivax and ovale like primaquine. The difference is primaquine is given for 14 days where as tafenoquine is given only once on second day.
- Primaquine is contraindicated in pregnancy and hence should be used only in postpartum period.
- Artemisinin group drugs are fastest acting and most potent schizontocidal drugs and hence are drug of choice for severe falciparum malaria.
- Falciparum is universally resistant to chloroquine and hence artemisinin group drugs are the drug of choice.

114. The following statements are true/false regarding monoclonal antibodies

a. Phlebitis is the most common side-effect
b. Only parenteral route is possible
c. Humanized monoclonal antibodies are completely derived from humans
d. Most monoclonal antibodies are excreted unchanged by kidney
e. Monoclonal antibodies are produced by hybridoma technique

Ans. True: b and e; False: a, c and d

- Acute infusion reaction like fever and rash is the most common side-effect of monoclonal antibodies.
- Monoclonal antibodies have poor oral absorption and hence only parenteral route is possible.
- Human monoclonal antibodies are completely derived from humans, whereas humanized monoclonal antibodies are derived from both human and mouse.
- Most monoclonal antibodies are eliminated by receptor mediated endocytosis and cellular metabolism.
- Monoclonal antibodies are produced by hybridoma technique.

115. The following statements are true/false regarding antidiabetic drugs

a. Pramlintide is used in only type II diabetes mellitus
b. Acarbose is FDA approved for both type I and II diabetes mellitus
c. Canagliflozin is used only in type I diabetes mellitus
d. Insulin is used only in type I diabetes mellitus
e. Sitagliptin is used only in type II diabetes mellitus

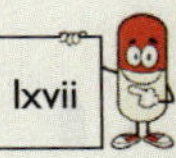

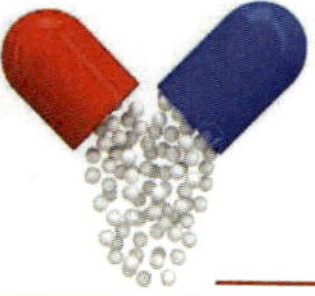

Ans. True: e, False: a, b, c and d

- Insulin and pramlintide are the only drugs that are used in both type I and II diabetes mellitus.
- All other drugs are used only in type II diabetes mellitus.

116. The following statements are true/false regarding drugs used in osteoporosis

a. Teriparatide inhibits bone resorption
b. Denosumab stimulates bone formation
c. Strontium ranelate inhibits bone resorption and stimulates bone formation
d. Alendronate stimulates bone formation
e. Raloxifene inhibits bone resorption

Ans. True: c and e; False: a, b and d

- Teriparatide stimulates bone formation. Strontium ranelate stimulates bone formation and inhibits bone resorption.
- All other drugs act by inhibiting bone resorption.

117. The following statements are true/false regarding antithyroid drugs

a. Methimazole is fastest acting antithyroid drug
b. Propylthiouracil is preferred to methimazole in thyroid storm
c. Propranolol inhibits sodium iodide symporter
d. Methimazole is longer acting than propylthiouracil
e. I^{123} is used in thyroid cancer treatment

Ans. True: b and d; False: a, c and e

- Potassium iodide is the fastest acting antithyroid drug that acts by inhibiting release of thyroid hormones.
- Propylthiouracil inhibits peripheral conversion of T4 to T3 and hence is preferred in thyroid storm.
- Propranolol inhibits peripheral conversion of T4 to T3.
- Methimazole is long acting drug given by once a day dosing, whereas propylthiouracil is a short acting drug given by QID dosing.

118. The following statements are true/false regarding gout treatment

a. Allopurinol can cause acute gout
b. Benzbromarone is effective in renal failure
c. Colchicine inhibits microtubules
d. Aspirin is the NSAID of choice in acute gout
e. Pegloticase is given by oral route

Ans. True: a, b and c; False: d and e

- Allopurinol can cause acute gout in the first 2 weeks of therapy due to mobilization of uric acid from stores of body to plasma. Hence NSAID or colchicine is always given along with allopurinol for first 2 weeks.
- Uricosuric agents are not effective in renal failure except benzbromarone.
- Colchicine inhibits microtubules in leucocytes, which leads to inhibition of chemotaxis.
- Indomethacin is the NSAID of choice in acute gout.
- Rasburicase and pegloticase are enzymes and hence can not be given by oral route; intravenous route is preferred.

119. The following statements are true/false regarding antihistaminics

a. Desloratadine is a third generation antihistaminic
b. Chlorpheniramine is preferred for day time use
c. Cetirizine is least sedating antihistaminic
d. Azelastine is a topical antihistaminic
e. Promethazine has local anesthetic effect

Ans. True: a, b, d and e; False: c

- Desloratadine, levocetirizine and fexofenadine being derivatives of second generation drugs are considered as third generation antihistaminics.
- Chlorpheniramine being least sedating first generation drug is preferred for day time use.
- Cetirizine is the most sedating second generation drug, whereas fexofenadine overall is the least sedating antihistaminic.
- Azelastine, alcaftadine, olopatadine and levocarbastine are topical antihistaminics.
- Promethazine and diphenhydramine have local anesthetic effect.

120. The following statements are true/false regarding immunomodulators

a. Mycophenolate mofetil is a neurotoxic drug
b. Cyclosporine is more toxic than tacrolimus
c. Sirolimus can cause hyperkalemia
d. Azathioprine is a hepatotoxic drug
e. Leflunomide causes bone marrow suppression

Ans. True: d and e; False: a, b and c

- Mycophenolate mofetil causes only GIT upset as side-effect.
- Nephrotoxicity, hepatotoxicity, neurotoxicity is seen with tacrolimus > cyclosporine.
- Sirolimus causes hypokalemia, whereas tacrolimus causes hyperkalemia.
- Leflunomide and azathioprine can cause bone marrow suppression and hepatotoxicity.

121. The following statements are true/false regarding drugs used in bronchial asthma

a. Vilanterol can be used in asthma and COPD
b. Palpitation is the most common side-effect of salbutamol
c. Terbutaline is a long acting beta2 agonist
d. Nedocromil is a hepatotoxic drug
e. Ketotifen is a mast cell stabilizer

Ans. True: e; False: a, b, c and d

- Vilanterol is a VLABA approved only for treatment of COPD.
- Tremor is the most common side-effect of beta2 agonists like salbutamol
- Terbutaline is a short acting beta2 agonist.
- Nedocromil and cromolyn sodium are safest antiasthmatic drugs and are not associated with hepatotoxicity.
- Ketotifen has mast cell stabilizing effect, H1 blocking effect and increases release of NO.

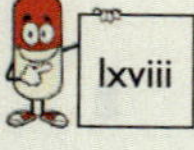

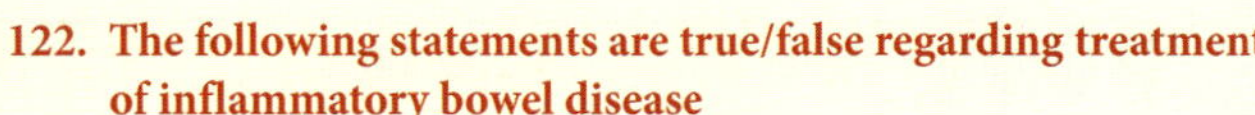

122. The following statements are true/false regarding treatment of inflammatory bowel disease

a. Steroids are used in long term management of ulcerative colitis
b. For Crohn's disease with fistula Infliximab is drug of choice
c. Sulfasalazine is more preferred than mesalamine in ulcerative colitis
d. Prednisolone is the steroid of choice in inflammatory bowel disease
e. In steroid resistant cases of ulcerative colitis azathioprine is drug of choice

Ans. True: b, False: a, c, d and e

- Steroids are used only in acute attack of ulcerative colitis or Crohn's disease
- For a mild to moderate case of Crohn's disease steroids are used, whereas for severe cases i.e. with fistula, infliximab is used.
- Mesalamine is more preferred than sulfasalazine as, mesalamine is less toxic.
- The steroid of choice in inflammatory bowel disease is budesonide.
- In steroid resistant cases of ulcerative colitis cyclosporine is drug of choice, whereas in steroid dependent cases azathioprine is drug of choice.

123. The following statements are true/false regarding antiaggregant drugs

a. Aspirin should be stopped 7 days before surgery
b. Clopidogrel need not be stopped before surgery
c. Vorapaxar is contraindicated in stroke
d. Ticlopidine is most toxic ADP inhibitor
e. Prasugrel is most effective ADP inhibitor

Ans. True: c, d and e; False: a and b

- Aspirin can be continued and need not be stopped before surgery, but clopidogrel nshould be stopped 7 days before surgery.
- Vorapaxar is associated with an increased risk of intracranial bleeding and hence contraindicated in patients of stroke.
- Ticlopidine is most toxic ADP inhibitor and can cause agranulocytosis, GIT upset and TTP-HUS.
- Prasugrel is most effective ADP inhibitor and has high risk of bleeding. Hence it is not used in patients with cerebrovascular disorders.

124. The following statements are true/false regarding intravenous anesthetic agents.

a. Fospropofol causes pain on injection
b. Thiopentone has cerebroprotective effect
c. Ketamine is contraindicated in bronchospastic disorders
d. Etomidate is a hemodynamically stable agent
e. Methohexital is used in ECT

Ans. True: b, d and e; False: a and c

- Fospropofol is a water soluble form of propofol, which does not require oily medium and hence does not cause pain on injection.
- Thiopentone decreases cerebral oxygen demand and metabolism and hence has cerebroprotective effect.
- Ketamine causes bronchodilation and hence is preferred in bronchospastic disorders.
- Etomidate is a hemodynamically stable agent and hence preferred in old patients and cardiovascular disorders.
- Methohexital causes seizure and hence is preferred in ECT.

SEQUENTIAL ARRANGEMENT TYPE QUESTIONS

125. Arrange the following drugs in decreasing order of volume of distribution i.e. drug with highest volume of distribution first and drug with least volume of distribution last.

a. Digoxin
b. Fluoxetine
c. Chloroquine
d. Nortriptyline

Ans. (c) Chloroquine, (b) Fluoxetine, (a) Digoxin, (d) Nortriptyline

Volume of distribution of some drugs with very high volume of distribution is given below.

Drug	Volume of distribution in liters
Chloroquine	13,000
Fluoxetine	2500
Imipramine	1600
Nortriptyline	1300
Labetalol	660
Digoxin	500
Verapamil	350
Meperidine	310

126. Arrange the following drugs in decreasing order of their half-life i.e. drug with longest half-life first and shortest half-life last.

a. Midazolam
b. Amiodarone
c. Chloroquine
d. Adenosine

Ans. (b) Amiodarone, (c) Chloroquine, (a) Midazolam, (d) Adenosine

Drug	Half-life
Amiodarone	53 days
Chloroquine	214 hours
Midazolam	1.9 hours
Adenosine	1-5 seconds

127. Arrange the sequence of events after stimulation of a Gs subtype of GPCR from beginning till end in descending order.

a. Stimulation of protein kinase
b. Increase in cyclic AMP
c. Stimulation of adenylate cyclase
d. Synthesis of α_s-GTP

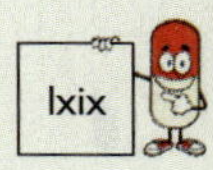

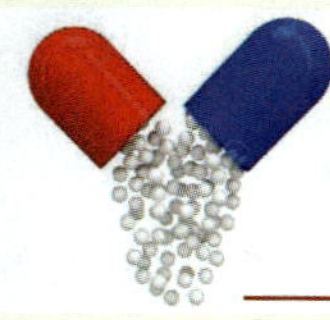

Ans. (d) Synthesis of α_s-GTP, (c) Stimulation of adenylate cyclase, (b) Increase in cyclic AMP, (a) Stimulation of protein kinase

- When a Gs subtype of GPCR is stimulated there is an increase in αs-GTP.
- α_s-GTP stimulates an enzyme called as adenylate cyclase, which increases production of cyclic AMP.
- Cyclic AMP stimulates an enzyme called as protein kinase, which phosphorylates different proteins.

128. Arrange bioavailability of the following drugs in increasing order i.e. drug with lowest bioavailability first and drug with highest bioavailability last.

a. Lithium   b. Ramelteon
c. Digoxin   d. Propranolol

Ans. (b) Ramelteon, (d) Propranolol, (c) Digoxin, (a) Lithium

Drug	Bioavailability (%)
Ramelteon	2
Propranolol	30
Digoxin	70
Lithium	100

129. Arrange the sequence of passage of ADR information in pharmacovigilance from the option given below i.e. at first who receives information and at last who receives information.

a. Indian pharmacopoeia commission
b. Uppsala monitoring center
c. CDSCO
d. Hospitals

Ans. (d) Hospitals, (a) Indian pharmacopoeia commission, (c) CDSCO, (b) Uppsala monitoring center

Kindly refer to the topic of pharmacovigilance in the chapter of clinical pharmacology for the detailed flow chart.

130. Arrange the enzymes responsible for synthesis/metabolism of catecholamines in sequence i.e. enzyme with which starts and enzyme with which ends.

a. Dopa decarboxylase   b. Monoamine oxidase
c. Tyrosine hydroxylase   d. Dopamine beta hydroxylase

Ans. (c) Tyrosine hydroxylase, (a) Dopa decarboxylase, (d) Dopamine beta hydroxylase, (b) Monoamine oxidase

Kindly refer to the text on synthesis of catecholamines in the topic of autonomic nervous system.

131. Arrange dilutions of epinephrine used by a particular route or use given below in decreasing order i.e. route which uses maximum dilution first and route which uses minimum dilution last.

a. Subcutaneous   b. Intraosseous
c. With local anesthetics   d. As a local vasoconstrictor

Ans. (c) With local anesthetics, (d) As a local vasoconstrictor, (b) Intraosseous, (a) Subcutaneous

The dilutions of epinephrine used for the options is given below.

With local anesthetics	1:200,000
As a local vasoconstrictor	1:100,000
Intraosseous	1:10,000
Subcutaneous	1:1000

132. Arrange the drugs used in chronic CHF in order as they are used i.e. first the drug with which treatment is started followed by other drugs.

a. Spironolactone   b. Ivabradine
c. Enalapril   d. Carvedilol

Ans. (c) Enalapril, (d) Carvedilol, (a) Spironolactone, (b) Carvedilol

Kindly refer to the topic of CVS for the flowchart of drug use in chronic CHF.

133. Arrange the following antiarrhythmics in order of classification i.e. class I first and Class IV last.

a. Esmolol   b. Lidocaine
c. Verapamil   d. Sotalol

Ans. (b) Lidocaine, (a) Esmolol (d) Sotalol, (c) Verapamil

Lidocaine	Class Ib
Esmolol	Class II
Sotalol	Class III
Verapamil	Class IV

134. Arrange the diuretics in order of sequence they act on the nephron i.e. first that acts on PCT and last that acts on collecting duct.

a. Furosemide
b. Chlorthalidone
c. Acetazolamide
d. Spironolactone

Ans. (c) Acetazolamide, (a) Furosemide, (b) Chlorthalidone, (d) Spironolactone

Acetazolamide	PCT
Furosemide	TAL
Chlorthalidone	DCT
Spironolactone	Collecting duct

135. Arrange the antiepileptics in order of their use in status epilepticus i.e. begin with the drug used first.

a. Phenytoin
b. Lorazepam
c. Phenobarbital
d. Propofol

Ans. (b) Lorazepam, (a) Phenytoin, (c) Phenobarbital, (d) Propofol

- The first drug used in status epilepticus is lorazepam followed by phenytoin infusion.
- If patient does not respond, then phenobarbital is used. If patient still does not respond then anesthetic agent propofol is used.

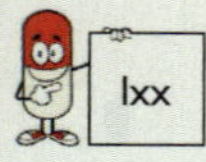

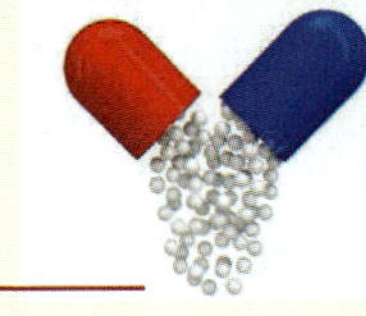

136. Arrange the following drugs for prophylaxis of pneumocystis in decreasing order of preference i.e. most preferred drug first and least preferred drug last.

a. Atovaquone b. Cotrimoxazole
c. Dapsone d. Pentamidine

Ans. (b) Cotrimoxazole, (c) Dapsone, (a) Atovaquone, (d) Pentamidine

Drugs used in prophylaxis of pneumocystis in descending order of their preference
1. Cotrimoxazole
2. Dapsone
3. Atovaquone
4. Pentamidine

137. Arrange the following penicillins in decreasing order of their spectrum i.e. extended spectrum first and narrow spectrum last.

a. Ampicillin b. Penicillin G
c. Oxacillin d. Piperacillin

Ans. (d) Piperacillin, (a) Ampicillin, (b) Penicillin G, (c) Oxacillin

Piperacillin	Extended spectrum
Ampicillin	Broad spectrum
Penicillin G	Intermediate spectrum
Oxacillin	Narrow spectrum

138. Arrange the following antibiotics in order of which resistance was developed with respect to time in staphylococcus i.e. first the one to which resistance developed first and last the one to which resistance developed last.

a. Vancomycin b. Oxacillin
c. Penicillin G d. Daptomycin

Ans. (c) Penicillin G, (b) Oxacillin, (a) Vancomycin, (d) Daptomycin

- First penicillin G was effective and used against staphylococcus, but resistance developed due to penicillinase production.
- Then penicillinase resistance penicillins like oxacillin was produced. But even in this case resistance developed due to alteration of penicillin binding protein and these strains were named as MRSA.
- Then for MRSA, vancomycin was used for treatment but even to vancomycin resistance developed and then these strains were termed as VRSA.
- The current drug of choice for VRSA is daptomycin.

139. Arrange the following antiretroviral drugs in order of their action on life cycle of viral replication i.e. first the drug which acts on first step of replication and last the drug which acts on last step of replication.

a. Elvitegravir
b. Abacavir
c. Ritonavir
d. Ibalizumab

Ans. (d) Ibalizumab, (b) Abacavir, (a) Elvitegravir, (c) Ritonavir

- The first step is viral entry in to CD4 cells which is blocked by anti CD4 monoclonal antibody ibalizumab.
- The second step is synthesis of DNA from RNA by reverse transcriptase which is blocked by drugs like Abacavir.
- The third step is integration of viral DNA to human DNA by integrase which is blocked by elvitegravir.
- The last step is assembly and maturation of virus mediated by enzyme protease, which is blocked by drugs like ritonavir.

140. Arrange the anticancer drug in order of their use for treatment of CML i.e. the drug of choice first and the drug for resistant cases last.

a. Dasatinib b. Omacetaxine
c. Imatinib d. Ponatinib

Ans. (c) Imatinib, (a) Dasatinib, (d) Ponatinib, (b) Omacetaxine

- Imatinib a first generation bcr-abl tyrosine kinase inhibitor is the drug of choice for treatment of CML.
- In case of imatinib resistance second generation drug like bosutinib is used.
- In case of bosutinib resistance a third-generation drug ponatinib is used.
- In case of resistance to multiple tyrosine kinase inhibitors omacetaxine is used.

141. Arrange the steps of monoclonal antibody production in a normal sequence i.e. first step in the beginning and last step at end.

a. HAT medium is added
b. Antigen injected to mouse
c. Fused cells divide and produce monoclonal antibodies
d. Cell suspension from mice spleen is mixed with polyethylene glycol and myeloma cells

Ans. (b) Antigen injected to mouse, (d) Cell suspension from mice spleen is mixed with polyethylene glycol and myeloma cells, (a) HAT medium is added, (c) Fused cells divide and produce monoclonal antibodies

- First the antigen of interest is injected in to mouse and then the cell suspension from mouse spleen is mixed with polyethylene glycol and myeloma cells. Polyethylene glycol fuses 1% of myeloma cells.
- HAT medium is added which inhibits de novo nucleotide synthesis.
- Non fused cells die as salvage pathway is absent. But fused cells divide due to presence of salvage pathway and produce monoclonal antibodies.

142. Arrange the site of insulin injection in decreasing order of preference i.e. most preferred site first and least preferred site last.

a. Upper arm b. Buttock
c. Abdomen d. Thigh

Ans. (c) Abdomen, (d) Thigh, (b) Buttock, (a) Upper arm

- The preference of insulin injection site is abdomen > anterior thigh > upper buttock > upper arm.

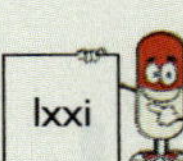

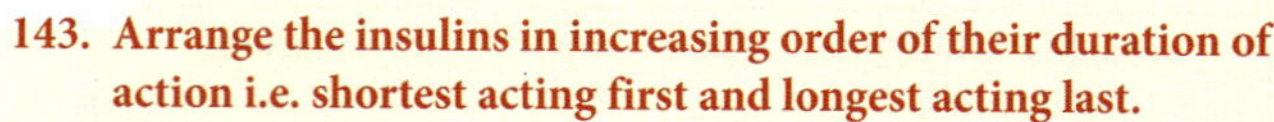

143. Arrange the insulins in increasing order of their duration of action i.e. shortest acting first and longest acting last.

a. NPH b. Glargine
c. Detemir d. Degludec

Ans. (a) NPH, (c) Detemir, (b) Glargine, (d) Degludec

- The duration of action of given insulins is NPH < Detemir < Glargine < Degludec.

144. Arrange the given glucocorticoids in decreasing order of potency i.e. most potent first and least potent last.

a. Triamcinolone b. Hydrocortisone
c. Dexamethasone d. Prednisolone

Ans. (c) Dexamethasone, (a) Triamcinolone, (d) Prednisolone, (b) Hydrocortisone

- Least potent glucocorticoid is hydrocortisone.
- Prednisolone is 4 times more potent, triamcinolone is 5 times more potent and dexamethasone is 30 times more potent as compared to hydrocortisone.

145. Arrange the following drugs in decreasing order of antiaggregant potency i.e. most potent drug first and least potent drug last.

a. Clopidogrel b. Aspirin
c. Abciximab d. Prasugrel

Ans. (c) Abciximab, (d) Prasugrel, (a) Clopidogrel, (b) Aspirin

- The order of potency of antiaggregant in option is abciximab > prasugrel > clopidogrel > aspirin.

146. Arrange the structure visible in increasing order of Mallampati score i.e. first structure visible in Class I and last structure visible in class IV.

a. Soft palate b. Only hard palate
c. Soft palate, uvula and faucial pillars
d. Soft palate and uvula

Ans. (c) Soft palate, uvula and faucial pillars, (d) Soft palate and uvula, (a) Soft palate, (b) Only hard palate

Mallampati Score

Classes	Structures visible
Class I	S: Soft Palate U: Uvula F: Faucial Pillars
Class II	S: Soft Palate U: Uvula
Class III	S: Soft Palate
Class IV	Only hard palate visible

147. Arrange the masks in decreasing order of percentage of oxygen delivered i.e. first which delivers maximum and last which delivers minimum.

a. Venturi mask b. Rebreathing mask
c. Nasal cannula d. Nonrebreathing mask

Ans. (b) Rebreathing mask, (d) Nonrebreathing mask, (a) Venturi mask, (c) Nasal cannula

Percentage of oxygen delivered from the oxygen delivery devices

Oxygen delivery devices	Percentage of oxygen delivered
Venturi mask	60%
Oxygen mask	60%
Rebreathing mask	100%
Nonrebreathing mask	80%
Nonrebreathing mask with reservoir	95%
Nasal cannula	44%
Face mask with reservoir connected to Ambu bag	100%

148. Arrange the steps of Allen's test in sequence i.e. first step first and last step last.

a. Radial artery released
b. Ask patient to raise hand for 30 seconds
c. Ask patient to clench fist
d. Occlude radial and ulnar artery

Ans. (c) Ask patient to clench fist, (d) Occlude radial and ulnar artery, (b) Ask patient to raise hand for 30 seconds, (a) Radial artery released

Steps in Allen's Test

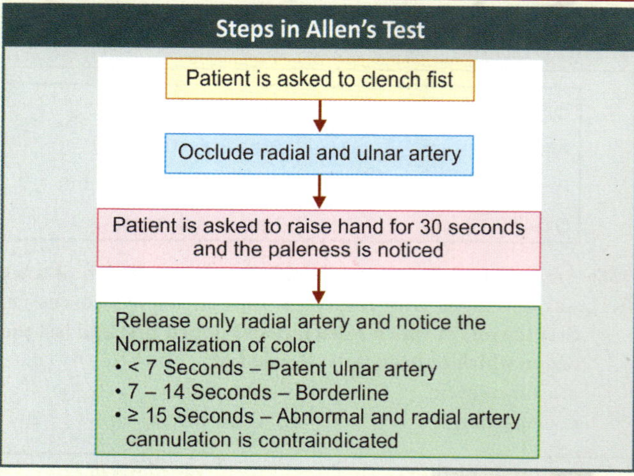
Patient is asked to clench fist
Occlude radial and ulnar artery
Patient is asked to raise hand for 30 seconds and the paleness is noticed
Release only radial artery and notice the Normalization of color
• < 7 Seconds – Patent ulnar artery
• 7 – 14 Seconds – Borderline
• ≥ 15 Seconds – Abnormal and radial artery cannulation is contraindicated

149. Arrange the following inhalational anesthetic agents in decreasing order of MAC i.e. agent with maximum MAC first and agent with minimum MAC last.

a. Enflurane b. Isoflurane
c. Nitrous oxide d. Methoxyflurane

Ans. (c) Nitrous oxide, (a) Enflurane, (b) Isoflurane, (d) Methoxyflurane

Inhalational Anesthetic Agent Properties

Inhalational agent	Mac	Blood gas partition coefficient	Odor
Nitrous oxide	104	0.47	Nil
Halothane	0.75	2.5	Sweet
Enflurane	1.58	1.9	Nil
Isoflurane	1.28	1.4	Irritant
Desflurane	6.0	0.45	Pungent
Sevoflurane	2.05	0.65	Nil
Methoxyflurane	0.2	12	Nil
Xenon	71	0.14	Nil

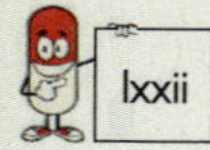

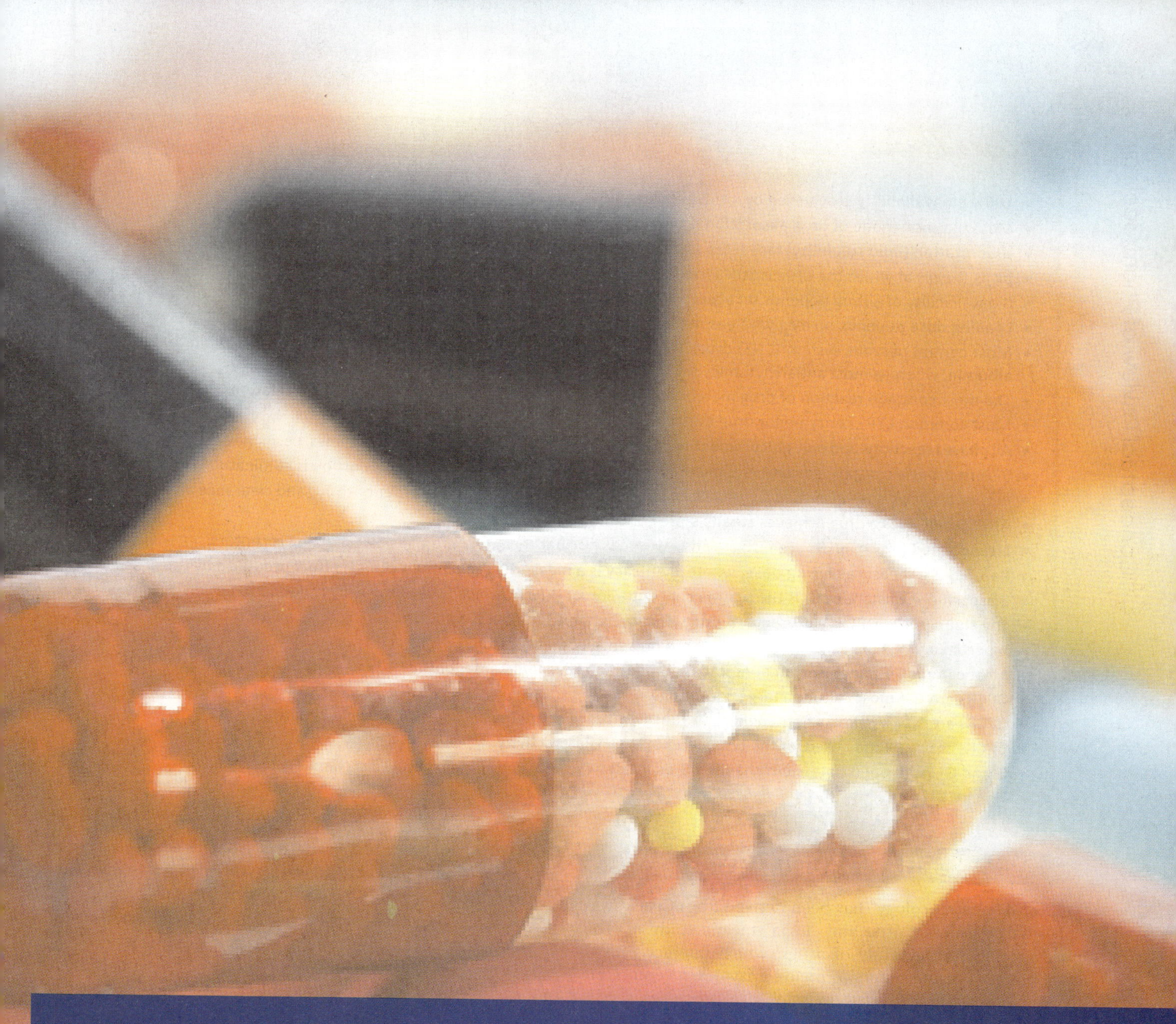

General Pharmacology

One Liners

- **100% bioavailability** is achieved by intravenous route.
- Most common mode of drug absorption is by **passive diffusion**.
- **Unionization (lipid solubility)** facilitates absorption whereas **ionization (water solubility)** facilitates excretion of drug.
- **pK_a** is the pH at which the drug is 50% ionized and 50% unionized.
- Bioavailability of a drug depends on **absorption** and **first-pass metabolism**.
- **Loading dose** depends on **aV_d**, whereas **maintenance dose** depends on **clearance**.
- Most central nervous system (CNS) drugs [except tricyclic antidepressants (TCA) and opioids] and antibiotics are bound to **albumin**, whereas most antiarrhythmics are bound to **alpha 1 acid glycoprotein**.
- The most common reaction of drug metabolism in phase I is **oxidation** and phase II is **glucuronidation**.
- Most common CYP_{450} enzyme for drug metabolism is **CYP3A4**.
- All **phase I reactions** and only **glucuronidation in phase II** are reactions by microsomal enzymes, i.e. in the sarcoplasmic reticulum.
- In **zero order** a constant amount is eliminated, whereas in **first order** a constant proportion is eliminated per unit time.
- In zero order as dose increases $T_{1/2}$ increases but clearance decreases. In first order both $T_{1/2}$ and clearance are constant.
- After **5 half-lives** a drug achieves **steady state concentration**.
- **Ligand gated ion channels** are fastest acting whereas **nuclear receptors** are the slowest acting receptors.
- **Potency** is a measure of drug **dose**, whereas **efficacy** is a measure of **maximum clinical effect** produced by the drug.
- Dissociation constant or K_D is the plasma concentration of drug at which 50% of the drug is bound to target.
- The **slope of the DRC** is a measure of **drug efficacy**, whereas the position of **DRC on log dose axis indicates potency.**
- A **partial agonist** behaves as an antagonist in presence of an agonist.
- Most common antagonism encountered is **competitive reversible antagonism**.
- **GPCRs** are the most common targets for drugs.
- GPCRs are also known as **heptahelical**, **7 transmembrane spanning** and **metabotropic** receptors.
- GPCRs are classified based on the type of α having **GTPase activity**.
- **G_i** and **G_o**, both open potassium channel; **G_i** decreases CycAMP and **G_i** inhibits calcium channel.

PHARMACOLOGY

The word "pharmacology" has been derived from **Greek** words "pharmakon" means drug and "logia" means study of. Thus, pharmacology is the study of drugs, which interact with the components of living system (proteins, enzymes, receptors, etc.) to attenuate or inhibit the pathophysiological processes.

DRUG

- World Health Organization (WHO) defines drug as a chemical agent, which alters the biochemical and physiological processes of tissues or organisms.
- A drug can be a chemical derived from living sources (plants, animals and microorganisms), synthetic and semisynthetic chemical or product of genetic engineering.
- Drug also includes psychoactive substances (alcohol, nicotine and caffeine) and poisons.
- Drug does not include nutrients and essential dietary ingredients required by the living system.

ROUTES OF DRUG ADMINISTRATION

Drugs can be administered by local routes like topical (mucosal, ocular and cutaneous), intrathecal, intra-articular and Intra-arterial or systemic routes like oral, sublingual, rectal, parenteral (IV, IM and SC), pulmonary, transdermal and intranasal.

Table 1: Local Routes of Drug Administration

Routes	Comments	Drugs
Topical	For local effect	• Cutaneous: Steroids • Ocular: Antiglaucoma drugs, steroids • Mucosal: Anticancer drugs in bladder cancer
Intrathecal	Preferred, If rapid or local effect in CNS is required or the drug poorly crosses blood brain barrier (e.g. Aminoglycosides)	• Methotrexate in childhood leukemia • Anesthetic agents like bupivacaine • Baclofen in muscle spastic disorders • Aminoglycosides in CNS infections
Intra-articular	For local effect	• Steroids in rheumatoid arthritis

Contd...

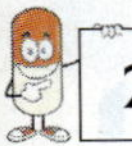

Routes	Comments	Drugs
Intra-arterial	For local effect on a particular organ supplied by an artery. Limited exposure decreases toxicity and there is lesser first pass metabolism as well	• Anticancer drugs in hepatocellular and Head and neck cancer

Table 2: Systemic Routes of Drug Administration

Routes	Benefits	Drawbacks	Drugs
Oral	Cheapest Convenient Safest	First pass metabolism **Most variable absorption** due to various factors like lipid solubility, food intake, digestive enzymes, etc.	Most drugs Remember: A drug with suffix tide or ase (e.g. Octreotide, Nesiritide, Asparginase etc) are peptides. Hence, these are broken down in GIT and never given by oral route.
Sublingual	No first pass metabolism and faster effect as drug is absorbed directly into SVC Drug can be spitted out after desirable effect	Tooth discoloration and decay Cardiac side effects	Nitroglycerine IDN Nifedipine Ephedrine Ergotamine Buprenorphine
Rectal	50% lesser first pass metabolism as from rectum 50% blood directly drains into IVC bypassing liver **Unpleasant and irritant drugs can be given**	Unreliable absorption	Diazepam for febrile seizures in children
Intravenous	100% bioavailability Fastest acting (Preferred in emergency) Irritants can be given Large volume can be given Peptides with high molecular weight are given	Increased chances of acute toxicity Drugs in oily medium cause hemolysis and hence are contraindicated	IV Drugs of choice Nicardipine: Hypertensive emergency Furosemide: Pulmonary edema Adenosine: PSVT Lorazepam: Status epilepticus
Intramuscular	Drugs in oily medium and irritants can be given Self-administration possible	Drugs in oily medium cause pain on injection NE is contraindicated as it can cause muscle necrosis due to potent vasoconstriction	IM Drugs of choice Adrenaline: Anaphylactic shock
Subcutaneous	Prolonged duration of action due to slow absorption	Irritants cannot be given as pain and necrosis can be seen	Insulin Contraceptives Adrenaline
Pulmonary	Faster effect due to rapid absorption by huge capillary network No first pass metabolism Local effect possible as in BA or COPD	Irritants can precipitate bronchospasm	Insulin (Exubera) Zanamivir Tobramycin SABA in BA Anticholinergics in COPD ICS
Transdermal	Longer duration of effect	Only lipid soluble drugs can be given	Nitroglycerine Fentanyl Scopolamine Nicotine Contraceptives HRT Clonidine
Intranasal	Rapid absorption and faster effect Ease of administration Preferred for peptides	Possible only for potent drugs Variable absorption	**Desmopressin** GnRH agonists Calcitonin Fentanyl

METHODS TO DELAY DRUG ACTION

By delaying drug action, the **number of doses required considerably decreases** and hence **compliance increases.** Apart from this there is a gradual rise in drug plasma concentration that is maintained throughout the day, thus **avoiding peaks of high** and **troughs of low plasma concentration.**

Delaying Absorption

Oral Drugs

- For oral route **extended release formulations** are made, which can be **sustained release** or **controlled release** preparation.
- Sustained release (SR) preparations cause a prolonged release of drug thereby prolonging plasma concentration. SR formulations are made by combining drugs with polymers such as hydroxypropyl methyl cellulose. When drug is ingested, first these polymers absorb water and then the drug is dissolved and released for absorption. SR drugs if taken with food, more amount of drug can be released **(dose dumping)** due to mechanical pressure, which can cause toxicity.
- Controlled release (CR) preparations have a true control on drug release rate. CR formulations are made by coating the drug with permeable membrane. This membrane allows water into the core and dissolution and release of drug is controlled by the parameters of membrane like its thickness, number of pores, etc.
- These preparations are suitable for drugs with **half-life lesser than 4 hours**.

Parenteral Drugs

Mechanism of increase in duration of action	Drugs
Addition of chemicals to make insoluble salts so that they are slowly absorbed from the site of injection	Procaine penicillin G Benzathine penicillin G
Esterification of drugs increases lipid solubility and on injection in oily medium, drugs are slowly absorbed from site of injection	Medroxyprogesterone acetate Testosterone propionate Fluphenazine decanoate
Addition of a vasoconstrictor delays absorption	Adrenaline with local anesthetics
Subcutaneous implants slowly release drugs	Estradiol

Transdermal

Polymers and adhesives are used to administer drug by transdermal route, which give a prolonged effect due to slow absorption.

Limiting Drug Metabolism

Inhibitors of drug metabolizing enzymes boost the half-life of drugs.

Inhibitors of enzymes	Drugs
Ritonavir and cobicistat inhibit CYP3A4	Protease inhibitors
Cilastatin inhibits dihydropeptidase	Imipenem

Limiting Drug Excretion

Drug excretion can be limited by adding a substrate that competitively inhibits drug excretion, e.g. Probenecid penicillin G.

Increasing Plasma Protein Binding

Plasma protein binding can be increased by combining drugs with insulin (Detemir = insulin + albumin) or by making drug which can avidly bind to plasma proteins sulfadoxine.

INTRODUCTION TO PHARMACOKINETICS AND PHARMACODYNAMICS

- Whenever a drug is given by oral route it undergoes **absorption** into the systemic circulation, following which a certain amount diffuses into various organs and tissues, a process known as **drug distribution**. After this the remaining drug in plasma attains a plasma concentration and is the source of a target to produce effect in the body. A definite amount of drug is continuously moving through liver depending upon hepatic blood flow, where it undergoes **metabolism**, i.e. inactivated

Conceptual Box-1

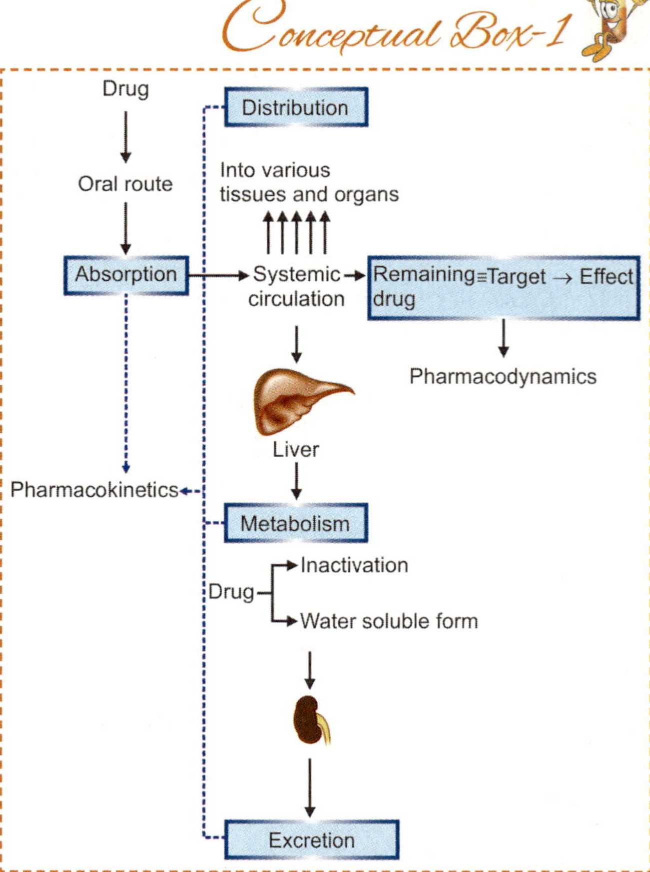

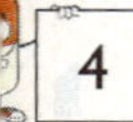

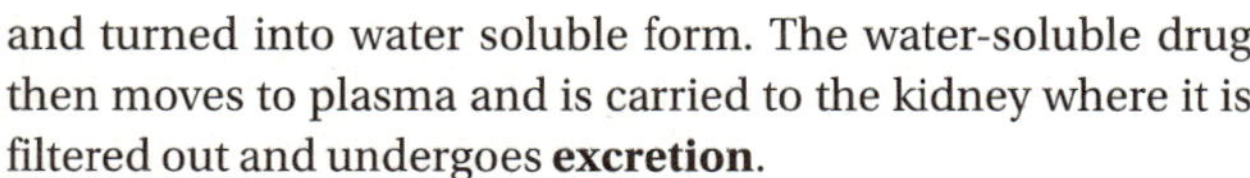

and turned into water soluble form. The water-soluble drug then moves to plasma and is carried to the kidney where it is filtered out and undergoes **excretion**.

- **Pharmacokinetics** is a word derived from Greek words "pharmakon" meaning drug and "kinesis" meaning movement. In this process, the phases involved with drug movement are described, i.e. absorption, distribution, metabolism and excretion are called as **pharmacokinetics**. In other words, this is what the body does to the drug.
- **Pharmacodynamics** is a word derived from Greek words "pharmakon" meaning drug and "dynamos" meaning change. The phase where drug is not moving when it is attached to the target and produces effect in the form of a change in the body, is known as **pharmacodynamics**. In other words, this is what the drug does to the body.

PHARMACOKINETICS

Absorption

In simple words, absorption of a drug by oral route means crossing over of the drug from the intestinal lumen to the blood vessel lumen. What lies in between these two lumens are the epithelial and endothelial membranes, which are made up of lipids and proteins. The proteins are ion channels, carriers, transporters, etc. The various ways of drug absorption are passive transport, carrier-mediated transport and pinocytosis.

Drug absorption in GIT is affected by drug **ionization/unionization**, **food**, **gastric emptying**, **size of drug particles** and **expression of P-glycoprotein pumps** for a drug.

Conceptual Box-2

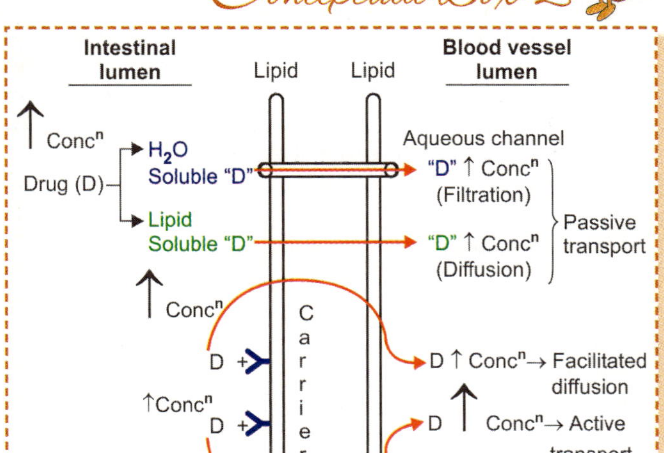

Lipinski Rule of Five

Lipinski rule of five give us criteria for drug absorption. A drug has poor absorption if

- Molecular weight >500 Dalton
- Log pH >5
- >5 hydrogen bond donors
- >5 hydrogen bond acceptors

Passive Transport

- Passive transport of drugs can take place through aqueous channels by filtration and through lipid membrane by passive diffusion.
- The drug present in the GIT can be in lipid and water soluble form. The amount of both depends on the pH of the drug (acidic or basic) and the medium (e.g. acidic pH in stomach and basic pH in intestine) in which it is located. If the pH is equal the drug is unionized, but if they are unequal then drug is ionized.
- The charge on the proteins in lipid barrier will not allow ionized drug to pass through lipid and hence the drug is called lipid insoluble or water soluble. In this form the drug can be absorbed through **aqueous channels (filtration)**.
- When the drug is unionized it can easily cross the lipid barrier and get absorbed by passive diffusion and hence is called as lipid soluble. **Most common process of drug absorption is passive diffusion** through lipid barrier and hence it is generalized that a drug is absorbed when it is in lipid soluble form.
- For passive transport a **concentration gradient** is mandatory, i.e. the drug is absorbed till the concentration is more in intestinal lumen as compared to blood vessel lumen. Passive transport can be compared to swimming in a river with the stream of water, where you do not have to spend energy; similarly here **ATP is not required**.

Table 3: Effect of pH on Drug Ionization and Unionization

- The effect of pH on drug ionization and unionization can be calculated for acidic and basic drug by Hasselbach equations given below:

  Basic drug: $\dfrac{\text{Log}_{10}\text{ (Ionized drug)}}{\text{(Unionized drug)}} = pK_a - pH$

  Acidic drug: $\dfrac{\text{Log}_{10}\text{ (Unionized drug)}}{\text{(Ionized drug)}} = pK_a - pH$

- What is pK_a?

  If the ionized drug = unionized drug, i.e. 50% each, then the equation becomes,

  $\text{Log}_{10} 1 = pK_a - pH$

  Or, $0 = pK_a - pH$

  Or, $pK_a = pH$

  Hence, pK_a is the pH at which the drug is 50% ionized and 50% unionized.

- Let us take an example of an acidic drug with pK_a 4. What would be the percentage of ionized and unionized drug in stomach and duodenum?
- **Stomach:** The drug has a pK_a 4 and Ph in stomach is 2 and using these values in the equation we get,

  $\dfrac{\text{Log}_{10}\text{ (Ionized drug)}}{\text{(Unionized drug)}} = 4 - 2 = 2$

  Or $\dfrac{\text{Unionized}}{\text{Ionized}} = 100$ (As Log_{10} 100 or $10^2 = 2$)

Contd...

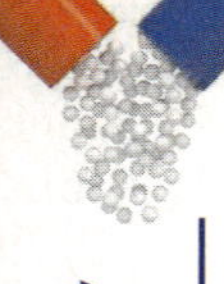

Thus, unionized drug is 100 times more than ionized drug or the ionized drug is approximately 99% and unionized drug is 1% in stomach. This proves that an acidic drug is more unionized in an acidic medium.

- **Duodenum:** The drug has a pK_a 4 and Ph in duodenum is 8 and using these values in the equation we get,

$$\frac{\text{Log}_{10}\text{ (Ionized drug)}}{\text{(Ionized drug)}} = 4 - 8 = -4$$

$$\text{Or, } \frac{\text{Unionized}}{\text{Ionized}} = 1/10{,}000 \text{ (As Log}_{10}\text{ } 1/10{,}000 \text{ or } 10^{-4} = -4)$$

Thus, ionized drug is 10,000 times more than unionized drug or the unionized drug is approximately 0.0001% and ionized drug is 99.9% in duodenum. This proves that an acidic drug is more ionized in a basic medium.

Table 4: Application of pH on Drug Absorption and Excretion

- **Absorption:** If the pH of the drug and the medium are same then drug is unionized and absorbed. Thus, an acidic drug is maximum unionized in acidic medium, i.e. stomach and basic drug in basic medium, i.e. small intestine. Thus, basic drug is maximum absorbed from small intestine. Stomach has a thick mucosal covering and small surface area, hence **maximum unionized acidic drug is also absorbed from small intestine.** Acidic or basic, the most common site for drug absorption is small intestine.
- **Excretion:** If the pH of the drug and the medium are different, then drug is ionized or water soluble and can be excreted. Hence in case of **weak acidic** or **weak basic** drug toxicity, the pH of urine can be changed into basic or acidic respectively to facilitate drug excretion. Most of the drugs are basic and few are acidic. Some examples of acidic drugs are given below.

Acidic Drugs

Mnemonics

Weak ACID

Weak : Warfarin
A : Antiepileptic (Phenobarbital and Phenytoin), Antifolate (Methotrexate and Sulfamethoxazole)
C : Chlorothiazide
I : Ibuprofen and Aspirin
D : Dopamine prodrug (Levodopa)

Carrier-Mediated Transport

Absorption of a drug can take place by carrier on epithelial membrane of intestine which has affinity to bind to drug and then propagate it into blood vessel lumen. Based on the type of transport absorption can be by facilitated diffusion or active transport.

- **Facilitated diffusion:** The carrier involved functions till there is a **concentration gradient**, i.e. it is also diffusion. But as this diffusion is facilitated by a carrier, it is known as facilitated diffusion. Just like passive diffusion, **no ATP is required**.
- **Active transport:** The carrier involved can function even **against the concentration gradient**, i.e. drug is absorbed even if the concentration of drug is more in blood vessel lumen than intestinal lumen. This can be compared with swimming against the stream of water, where you have to spend your energy. Hence, **ATP is absolutely required** for active transport.

Pinocytosis

Pinocytosis is acquiring drugs into vesicles and then releasing into systemic circulation by exocytosis. Proteins and large molecules like insulin cross the blood brain barrier via pinocytosis.

Table 5: Summary of Drug Absorption Modes

Passive diffusion	Facilitated diffusion	Active transport	Pinocytosis
No ATP required with concentration gradient	No ATP required with concentration gradient	ATP required against concentration gradient	No ATP required gradient not important
Most common mode of drug absorption	Requires carrier	Requires carrier	Absorbed by vesicle formation followed by exocytosis

Bioavailability and Bioequivalence

- When a drug is given by oral route, a particular amount is absorbed from the small intestine into portal circulation. The drug further has to pass through liver and then via hepatic vein into IVC. This is the road map for the drug to reach systemic circulation by oral route.
- While passing through liver, for the very first time some amount undergoes metabolism and is known as **first pass metabolism**. Though the enzymes (CYP3A4) and **efflux pump (P-glycoprotein pumps)** present in **intestinal epithelial cells** also contribute to first pass metabolism.
- After absorption and first pass metabolism, the fraction of unchanged drug that reaches the systemic circulation is known as **bioavailability**. In other words, it is the extent of absorption, which **depends on drug absorption and first pass metabolism**.
- The clinical effect depends not only on bioavailability or extent of absorption, but also on rate of absorption, i.e. time required to achieve that bioavailability. When both are taken into consideration. concept of **bioequivalence** comes into picture.
- **Bioavailability** can be calculated by dividing the **AUC** of a drug by oral route to IV route. Suppose the AUC_{oral} is 50 and AUC_{IV} is 500, then by using the formulae given below, bioavailability is 50/500 × 100 = 10%. Thus, bioavailability is 10% or 0.1. This is the fraction of drug reaching systemic circulation and hence bioavailability is also denoted as F.

$$\text{Bioavailability} = AUC_{oral}/AUC_{IV} \times 100$$

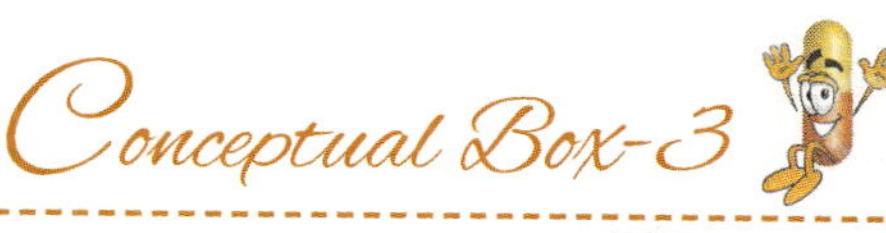

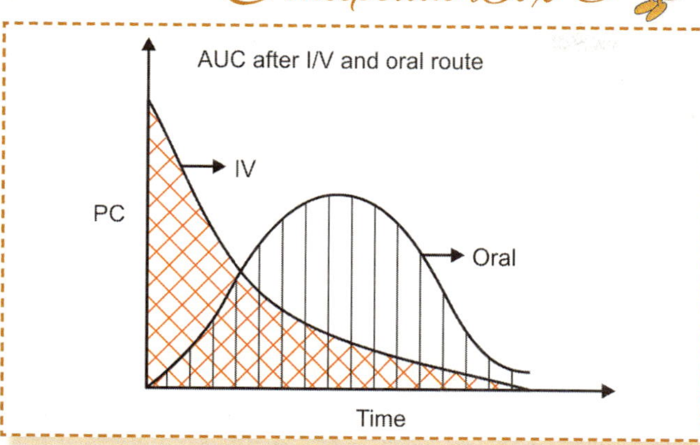

Table 6: Concept of Bioequivalence

- To understand the concept of bioequivalence let us take example of 2 drug companies, i.e. Dr Reddy and Cipla. Suppose Dr Reddy drug company invented drug X, for which it will get a **patent for exclusive right for 20 years.**
- After 20 years any company like Cipla can copy drug X and it is called as a generic drug. Cipla has to prove that its drug is as good as Dr Reddy drug for approval by FDA and this is done by proving that not only bioavailability, i.e. extent of absorption, but the rate of absorption of Cipla's drug is similar to Dr Reddy's drug X.
- **Thus, a generic drug is bioequivalent to branded drug, if the rate and extent of absorption are similar.**
- Since bioequivalence cannot be exactly same, an acceptable range of 20% is given, i.e. the generic drug (Cipla's) with a bioequivalence of 20% more or less than branded drug (Dr Reddy's) is approved by FDA.

P-glycoprotein Pumps (PgP)

- PgP are active transporters present in epithelial cell of intestine. When a drug is absorbed into the epithelial cell by various methods, it is actively pumped back into intestinal lumen by PgP. This is partly responsible for first pass effect that happens in intestine.
- Tumor cells can express these pumps to develop resistance by drug efflux. Inducers and inhibitors of these PgP can cause drug failure and toxicity respectively.
- Most of the drugs metabolized by CYP3A4 like protease inhibitors like benzodiazepines, etc. are substrates for PgP. Hence, the inducers and inhibitors of CYP3A4 also affect PgP.
- The enzyme inducers like rifampicin, etc. are also inducers of PgP, whereas the list of PgP inhibitors is different and given below:

Mnemonics

PgP Inhibitors

V: Verapamil, Valbenazine
A: Amiodarone
C: Cyclosporine
I: Itraconazole
N: Nifedipine
E: Erythromycin

Recent Advances

As PgP and MRP are responsible for drug efflux and resistance to anticancer drugs, several PgP inhibitors are currently under development. These are drugs like **zosuquidar, elacridar. Biriocodar** and **Timcodar** are dual PgP as well as MRP inhibitors for same purpose.

Distribution

- After a drug is absorbed into the systemic circulation, its diffusion into various organs and tissues is known as drug distribution. Then the remaining drug in plasma is source for target to produce effect.
- Hence, at same doses a drug with high volume of distribution will produce lesser plasma concentration and drug inefficacy and a drug with low volume of distribution will produce higher plasma concentration and toxicity.
- Thus, it is important to determine a drug's distribution. Distribution cannot be directly calculated and hence a hypothetical parameter called as **apparent volume of distribution (aV_d)** is used.
- **Apparent volume of distribution (aV_d) is the amount of plasma required to accommodate administered drug in the whole body at concentration that is achieved in plasma.**

Factors Determining aV_d

Apparent volume of distribution (aV_d) depends on factors like **lipid solubility (pKa), plasma protein binding, body fat and water content, tissue protein/receptor binding and accumulation in tissues with poor blood flow**.

- **Higher is lipid solubility,** more drug diffuses into compartments and **more is aV_d**, whereas **more is protein binding** drug is confined to plasma and **lesser is aV_d**.
- More fat content in body means **more aV_d** as seen in **obesity** and less fat content means **less aV_d as seen in athletes. Females have higher volume of distribution than males** due to higher fat content.
- The water content of body decreases with age and hence more plasma would be required to dilute the drug into body to plasma concentration; hence **with age aV_d increases.**
- Drugs with higher affinity for tissue proteins/receptors have higher aV_d, as is the case with digoxin due to high binding to Na/K ATPase pump in skeletal muscles.

Concept of aV_d and Loading Dose

Let us take an example of a drug "D" mg with high aV_d, given by IV route achieves an initial plasma concentration "C_0" mg/mL. To calculate aV_d, we have to determine the amount of plasma required to accommodate D mg in the whole body at concentration equal to "C" mg/mL.

Derivation of formula:

Amount of plasma required for C_0 mg = 1 mL
Amount of plasma required for D mg = D/C_0 mL
Hence the formula for aV_d is,

Contd...

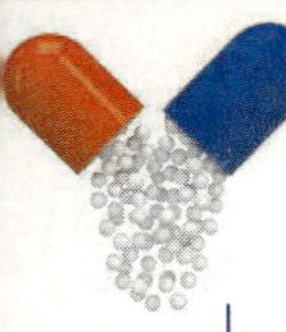

$$aV_d = D/C_0$$

D = Amount of administered drug by IV route

C_0 = Initial plasma concentration before elimination has begun

Loading dose:

To achieve a particular concentration C_p faster as in case of emergency, a loading dose might be required. The formula for aV_d for the particular plasma concentration will be:

$$aV_d = D/C_p$$

or,

$$D = aV_d \times C_p$$

The plasma concentration must be specific for a particular clinical effect. If drug has a high volume of distribution, then to maintain a specific plasma concentration, in the equation above we must increase the dose "D" of the drug. This increased dose of drug for drugs with high aV_d to maintain a specific plasma concentration is known as loading dose. Thus, **loading dose depends on aV_d** and the formula for calculation for drug given by IV route is,

$$\textbf{Loading dose (LD)} = aV_d \times C_p$$

If a drug is given by a route other than IV, then bioavailability plays an important role and hence in this case amount of drug in systemic circulation can be calculated by multiplying administered dose (D) with fraction of bioavailability (F). Hence our equation for aV_d becomes,

$$aV_d = D \times F/C_p$$

or,

$$D \times F = aV_d \times C_p$$

Thus, the loading dose in this case, i.e. $D = aV_d \times C_0/F$ and the formula for loading dose by oral route can be written as below:

$$\text{Loading dose (LD)} = \frac{aV_d \times C_p}{F}$$

Relation of Body Water to Volume of Distribution

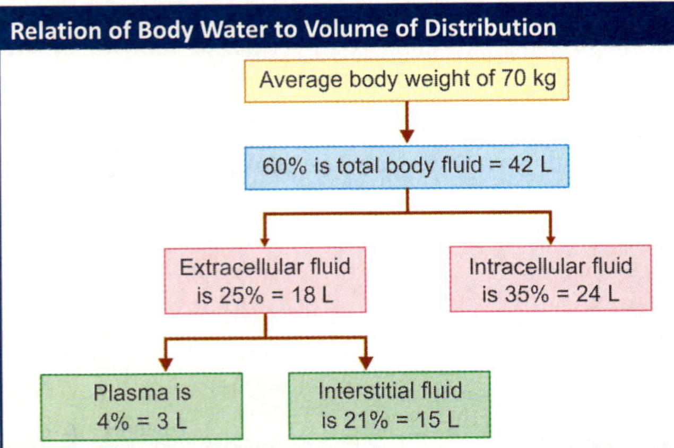

Thus, if a drug has a aV_d of 14–15 L, it is primarily distributed into interstitial fluid, whereas if aV_d is 40–42 L the drug is distributed into total body fluid. If a drug has aV_d more than 42 L, it is distributed into tissues as well.

Dialysis and Volume of Distribution

- Drugs with high aV_d are lesser in plasma and hence **dialysis is not effective** for treatment of toxicity. Some drugs with very high volume of distribution are chloroquine, calcium channel blockers, amphetamine, benzodiazepines, digoxin and opioids.
- Dialysis is not effective in case of **irreversible binders** of targetS like organophosphates and carbamates, as drug does not come back to plasma. Dialysis is not effective for drugs with a high plasma protein binding like beta blockers. The list of drugs against which dialysis is not effective is given below:

Mnemonics

BAD DOC

B: Benzodiazepines, Beta blockers

A: Amphetamine

D: ⎤
D: ⎦→Digoxin

O: Opioids, Organophosphates

C: CCBs, Chloroquine

Plasma Protein Binding

- Plasma protein binding is an important factor that determines apparent volume of distribution as only free drug is distributed to tissues.
- Acidic drugs bind to albumin and basic drugs to alpha1 acid glycoprotein.
- A decrease in plasma albumin is seen in conditions like nephrotic syndrome and cirrhosis can lead to freer acidic drugs in plasma and toxicity.
- Inflammatory disorders like rheumatoid arthritis and inflammatory bowel disease can increase alpha1 acid glycoprotein and decrease free basic drugs and their effect.
- For drugs with high plasma protein binding and narrow therapeutic index like phenytoin, unbound plasma drug concentration is more helpful clinically than total plasma drug concentration.
- A **highly plasma protein bound drug is primarily located in plasma** and by displacing other drugs with same feature can precipitate toxicity. These drugs can also displace bilirubin from albumin and precipitate kernicterus in a newborn.

Table 7: Drugs with High Plasma Protein Binding

High albumin bound drugs	High alpha 1 Acid glycoprotein bound drugs
CNS drugs: Barbiturates, Benzodiazepines, Phenytoin, valproate **Antibiotics:** Penicillin, Tetracyclines, Sulfonamides Warfarin NSAIDs	**Antiarrhythmics:** Verapamil, Lidocaine, Disopyramide, Beta blockers, Quinidine **CNS drugs:** Opioids, TCA Prazosin Bupivacaine

Note: Most **CNS drugs** are high albumin bound except TCA and opioids. Most **antiarrhythmics** are alpha 1 acid glycoprotein bound drugs.

Redistribution

- After binding to a target and producing effect, drug comes back to plasma. For drugs with very **high lipid solubility**

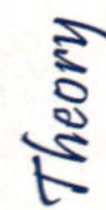

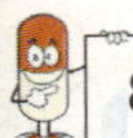

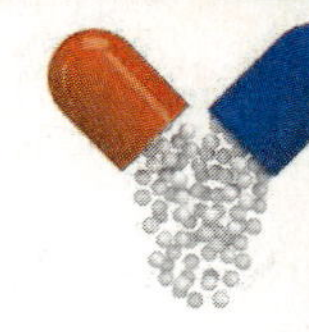

they GET immediately distributed into tissues again and this phenomenon is known as redistribution.

- Because of this rapid movement of drug into tissues, drugs with high redistribution are **short acting**. Thiopentone has a long $T_{1/2}$ life, but is short acting due to redistribution.
- Drugs which undergo significant redistribution are **thiopentone**, **propofol** and **diazepam**.

Metabolism

- Since drug metabolizing enzymes are maximum in the liver, it is the primary site of drug metabolism. These enzymes are present in the endoplasmic reticulum (microsomal) and cytoplasm (nonmicrosomal). The enzymes of endoplasmic reticulum are also called as microsomal enzymes, as centrifugation of endoplasmic reticulum precipitates its broken fragments in the microsomal fraction; the remaining cytoplasmic ones are called nonmicrosomal enzymes.
- Metabolism of drug happens in two phases, i.e. phase I and II, the **first one being slower** and hence determines the time required for drug clearance. Phase I metabolism **inactivates the drug** by breaking it down and then adds or exposes a functional group to the drug known as functionalization. The functional group partially increases the water solubility of drug. Some drugs which are inactive (prodrugs) are rather activated in phase I.
- In phase II a polar conjugate is attached to the functional group exposed or attached in phase I, which makes the drug **polar or water soluble** and facilitates its excretion.

Phase I

- In phase I the drugs are metabolized by reactions carried out by CYP_{450} enzymes, which are present in the **endoplasmic reticulum (microsomal) of cells in liver and intestinal epithelium**.
- The most common reaction of drug metabolism in phase I is **oxidation**.
- In a CYP_{450} enzyme **CY** denotes cytochrome, **P** denotes pigment which absorbs light at a wavelength of **450** nm. Cytochrome is a **hem protein** which accepts oxygen for drug metabolism.
- In a particular CYP_{450} enzyme like CYP1A2, the first number denotes family (1), alphabet denotes subfamily (A) and last number denotes chromosome number (2) for location of gene for the enzyme.
- Most common CYP_{450} enzyme for drug metabolism is **CYP3A4** followed by others (CYP3A4> CYP2D6> CYP2C9> CYP1A2> CYP2B6> CYP2C19).
- Apart from drugs these enzymes also metabolize various exogenous chemicals that come from environment, food etc and together with drugs these are known as xenobiotics. CYP_{450} enzymes also synthesize endogenous products like **steroids** and **bile acids**.

Reactions of Drug Metabolism in Phase I and II

Mnemonics

Phase I: ORCHAD

O: Oxidation
R: Reduction
C: Cyclization
H: Hydrolysis
A: Aliphatic and aromatic hydroxylation
D: Deamination

Phase II: GAMS

G: Glucuronidation, Glutathionylation, Glycation
A: Acetylation
M: Methylation
S: Sulfation

In phase I grow fruits in an ORCHAD and then in phase II make fruit GAMS.

Table 8: Drugs Metabolized by CYP_{450} Enzymes

CYP_{450} enzymes	Substrate drugs
CYP1A2	Paracetamol Tacrine Theophylline Tamoxifen
CYP2B6	Cyclophosphamide Methadone Efavirenz Artemisinin
CYP2C9	Phenytoin Warfarin Glipizide Losartan
CYP2C19	PPIs Clopidogrel is activated Propranolol
CYP2D6	Beta blockers except propranolol Drugs of psychiatry (TCA, SSRI, Antipsychotics)
CYP2E1	Enflurane, Paracetamol Ethanol
CYP3A4	C : CCBs, Cyclosporine H : H mg CoA reductase inhibitors (Statins) A : Anti arrhythmics (Lidocaine, Mexiletine, Quinidine) R: Rapamycin L: Long acting benzodiazepines, e.g. diazepam I : Inhibitors of protease E : Erythromycin, Estrogen, Progesterone and its antagonist **Mifepristone**

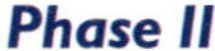

Phase II

- The conjugation reactions of phase II take place in cytoplasm (non-microsomal) except glucuronidation, which takes place in endoplasmic reticulum (microsomal).
- The most common drug metabolizing reaction in phase II is glucuronidation. In **Crigler-Najjar** syndrome there is decrease or absence of glucuronyl transferase and hence metabolism of drugs by glucuronidation is compromised and toxicity can be seen. Drugs with established incidence of toxicity are **irinotecan** and **atazanavir**.

Table 9: Drugs Metabolized by Conjugation

Conjugation reaction	Drug substrate
Glucuronidation	Irinotecan Atazanavir Estrogen Statins Benzodiazepines
Glutathionation	Fosfomycin Doxorubicin Bleomycin Ethacrynic acid
Glycination	Salicylic acid Nicotinic acid
Acetylation	D: Dapsone I : Isoniazid
	N: Nitrazepam C: Clonazepam H: Hydralazine A: Acebutolol, Amantadine, Amrinone K: K(c)affeine Sexy: Sulphonamides Padosan: Procainamide, Phenelzine
Methylation	Methyldopa Mercaptopurine
Sulfation	Steroids

Drug Interaction

- Drug interaction can take place as some drugs can inhibit or induce the microsomal enzymes thereby increasing chances of drug toxicity or failure respectively.
- Rifampicin is an inducer of CYP3A4 (metabolizes estrogen, protease inhibitors) and by increasing power of CYP3A4 rifampicin can induce metabolism of estrogen and protease inhibitors resulting in OCP and ART failure.
- Terfenadine can cause cardiac arrhythmia which can be fatal if combined with enzyme inhibitors like ketoconazole.
- Drugs like estrogen are metabolized by glucuronidation in phase II and estrogen attached to glucuronic acid becomes water soluble and is excreted with bile into intestine. In the colon bacteria produce enzyme glucuronidase which breaks glucuronic acid and renders estrogen free and lipid soluble, so that it is reabsorbed back (enterohepatic circulation). **Antibiotics** by killing bacteria in colon **(gut sterilization)** prevent this enterohepatic circulation of estrogen and can cause **OCP failure**.

Mnemonics

GRAB DJ Priyanka Chopra and invite her for QuICK VEG Dish.

Enzyme inducers	Enzyme inhibitors
G: Griseofulvin	**Qu:** Quinidine
R: Rifampicin	**I:** Isoniazid, Inhibitors of protease
A: Alcohol	**C:** Cimetidine, Chloramphenicol, Ciprofloxacin
B: Benzopyrene	**K:** Ketoconazole, Itraconazole, Fluconazole
D: DDT	**V:** Valproate
J: St. John's wort	**E:** Erythromycin
Priyanka: Phenytoin, Phenobarbital, Primidone	**G:** Grape juice
Chopra: Carbamazepine, Cigarette smoke	**Dish:** DEC, Delavirdine, Disulfiram

Note: **Omeprazole** is an inducer of **CYP1A2** and inhibitor of **CYP2C19**. **Acute alcohol** consumption causes **enzyme inhibition**, whereas **chronic alcohol** consumption causes **enzyme induction**.

Prodrugs

Prodrugs are inactive form of drugs which are activated in phase I of metabolism. Some prodrugs are deliberately made to increase lipid solubility for better oral absorption.

Table 10: Prodrugs List

- All ACEIs except captopril and lisinopril
- ARBs like olmesartan and candesartan
- Azathioprine
- Bitolterol
- Capecitabine
- Cyclophosphamide
- Carisoprodol
- Carbimazole
- Cortisone
- Dipivefrine
- 5FU
- Flucytosine
- Fluoxetine
- Levodopa
- Methyldopa
- 6 MP, 6 TG
- Mycophenolate mofetil
- Prednisone
- Proguanil
- Statins like lovastatin and simvastatin
- Sulfasalazine
- Sulindac
- Zidovudine

Excretion

For excretion of a drug by all organs it has to be water soluble except for lungs where it is excreted in lipid soluble form.

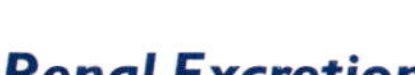

Renal Excretion

Renal excretion of drugs can be via glomerular filtration and tubular secretion. Since only 20% of plasma is filtered, rest 80% of drug in plasma is excreted via tubular secretion. A plasma protein bound drugs cannot be filtered but removed by tubular secretion. Penicillin G is highly plasma protein bound, but is short acting due to rapid tubular secretion.

Hepatic Excretion

Hepatic excretion is facilitated by transporters which secrete drug into bile. The glucuronidated polar drugs in the bile are deglucuronidated in the colon by glucuronidase enzyme produced by bacteria. This deglucuronidated non-polar or lipid soluble drug is reabsorbed into liver by enteric circulation and is known as enterohepatic circulation. This process of enterohepatic circulation of estrogen is inhibited by **antibiotics** and hence they can also cause **OCP failure** as discussed earlier.

Drugs that Undergo Enterohepatic Circulation

- Amphetamine
- Doxorubicin
- Estrogen
- Indomethacin
- Metronidazole
- Morphine
- Mefloquine
- Piroxicam
- Tetracycline

Extraction Ratio

Extraction ratio is the ability of an organ to remove the drug in a single pass. The value ranges from 0 to 1; 0 extraction ratio signifies THAT THE drug is not at all removed by organ and 1 signifies complete removal of drug by organ. Extraction ratio is affected by various factors like organ blood flow, plasma protein binding and intrinsic ability of organ to eliminate drug.

- **Organ blood flow:** For drugs with low extraction ratio (<0.3) venous and arterial concentration are same and ER is not affected by blood flow. For drugs with high extraction ratio (>0.7) drug eliminated is directly proportional to blood flow.
- **Plasma protein binding:** For low ER drugs only, free drug is eliminated but for high ER drugs both free and bound drugs are eliminated.
- **Intrinsic ability of organ:** For drugs with low ER, change in organ's ability to eliminate drug significantly affects ER, which is not the case with drugs having high ER.
- A drug propranolol which has a high extraction ratio of >0.9 is immediately removed by liver after absorption due to first pass metabolism. Hence, its oral dose is around 20 times more than IV dose.

Extraction Ratio Formula

$$E = C_A - C_V/C_A$$

E = Extraction ratio, C_A = Arterial drug concentration, C_V = Venous drug concentration

Rate of Drug Elimination

The rate at which a drug is eliminated can be calculated with the help of drug clearance and plasma concentration.

Table 11: Concept of RDE and MD

RDE

- Drug clearance (Cl) is the amount of plasma that is cleared off the drug per unit time (mL/hour).
- Plasma concentration (PC) is the amount of drug present in per unit of plasma (mg/mL).
- Let us multiply units of both parameters,
  mL/hour × mg/mL = mg/hour
  = Amount of drug eliminated per unit time
  = Rate of drug elimination (RDE)
- Hence, one formula for RDE is given below:

$$RDE = Cl \times PC$$

- If a drug is given by IV route the above formula also gives the infusion rate.

$$\text{Infusion rate} = Cl \times PC$$

- Derivation of another formula for RDE
  $aV_d = D/C$ or PC, or $PC = D/aV_d$
  $T_{1/2} = 0.693 \times aV_d/Cl$, or $Cl = 0.693 \times aV_d/T_{1/2}$
  Placing the above value of Cl and PC in formula of RDE we get,
  $RDE = D/aV_d \times 0.693 \times aV_d/T_{1/2} = 0.693 \times D/T_{1/2}$

$$RDE = 0.693 \times D/T_{1/2}$$

- The above formula derived are for drug given by IV route. If drug is given by any other route then bioavailability (F) is considered and one formula for RDE is:

$$RDE = \frac{0.693 \times D \times F}{T_{1/2}}$$

- Derivation of another formula for RDE when drug is given by route other than IV.
  $aV_d = D \times F/C$ or PC or $D = aV_d \times PC/F$
  $T_{1/2} = 0.693 \times aV_d/Cl$
  Placing the above value of D and $T_{1/2}$ in the formula for RDE by IV route we get

$$RDE = 0.693 \times D/T_{1/2} = 0.693 \times \frac{aV_d \times PC/F}{0.693 \times aV_d/Cl}$$

$$\frac{Cl \times PC}{F}$$

$$RDE = \frac{Cl \times PC}{F}$$

MD

- Maintenance dose is given after a certain period to maintain the plasma concentration within therapeutic window. The amount of drug given back after a period should be the amount lost in that period or time.
- Hence, MD can be calculated by first finding out the amount of drug eliminated per unit time (RDE) and then multiplying it with time. Thus, MD can be calculated for IV route by below given.

Contd...

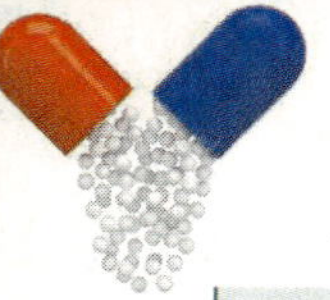

$$MD = Cl \times PC \times Time$$

- For routes other than oral bioavailability is taken into account and hence the formula for MD changes as given below:

$$MD = \frac{Cl \times PC \times Time}{F}$$

Note: In patients with renal or hepatic impairment the maintenance dose is reduced, whereas the loading dose does not change.

Kinetics of Drug Elimination

- The kinetics of drug elimination depends on the order of plasma concentration and based on THIS it can be either **zero order/saturation/linear kinetics** or **first order/ nonsaturation/non-linear kinetics**.
- Since the drug eliminating enzymes and pumps are usually in abundance and do not get saturated at normal doses (nonsaturation kinetics), most drugs follow first order kinetics. At high doses the drug eliminating mechanisms are saturated and all drugs follow zero order kinetics.
- Only few drugs, for which eliminating enzymes and pumps are saturated (saturation kinetics) at very low doses follow zero order kinetics at normal doses. Zero order is not true zero order as in the beginning till enzymes and pumps are saturated, first order persists and hence **zero order is also known as pseudo zero order kinetics**.

Drugs Following Zero Order Kinetics

Mnemonics

Zero **ATP H**as **M**ade **W**eaker
Zero
A : Aspirin, Alcohol
T : Theophylline, Tolbutamide
P : Phenytoin, Phenylbutazone
Has: Heparin
Made : Methanol
Weaker: Warfarin

Table 12: Concept of Zero and First Order Kinetics

Zero Order Kinetics

- Let us apply the formula of RDE to evaluate kinetics of drug elimination. Cl is constant for a drug at constant dose.

  RDE = PC × Cl (Constant)
- In zero order kinetics order of PC is 0 and hence the equation will be

  $RDE = [PC]^0 \times Constant$

  Or, RDE = 1 × Constant

  Or, amount of drug eliminated per unit time = Constant
- **Thus in zero order kinetics a constant amount of drug is eliminated per unit time.**

Contd...

First Order Kinetics

- In first order kinetics order of PC is 1 and hence the equation will be

  $RDE = [PC]^1 \times Constant$

  Or, RDE α PC

  Or, Amount of drug eliminated per unit time α PC
- **Thus is first order kinetics a constant proportion of drug is eliminated per unit time.**

Table 13: Relation of $T_{1/2}$ and Cl to dose in Elimination Kinetics

Zero Order Kinetics

- Let us take an example of a drug at a dose of 100 mg, which follows zero order and is removed at a rate of 20 mg/hour. What is the $T_{1/2}$?
- The time taken for 100 mg to 50 mg, i.e. $T_{1/2}$ is 2.5 hours.
- If the dose is increased to 200 mg, then now the time taken for 200 mg to become 100 mg is 5 hours.
- Thus, as the dose increases $T_{1/2}$ increases and Cl decreases (As $T_{1/2}$ $1/\alpha$ Cl) for drugs following zero order kinetics.

First Order Kinetics

- Let us take an example of a drug at a dose of 100 mg, which follows first order kinetics and is removed at a rate of 20%/hour. What is the $T_{1/2}$?
- The time taken for 100 mg to become 50 mg is approximately 3 hours.
- If dose is increased to 200 mg, then now the time taken for 200 mg to become 100 mg is again 3 hours.
- **Thus for drugs following first order kinetics $T_{1/2}$ and Cl, both are constant.**

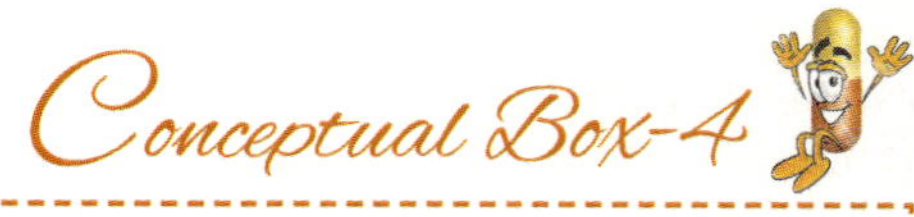

Zero and First Order Kinetics

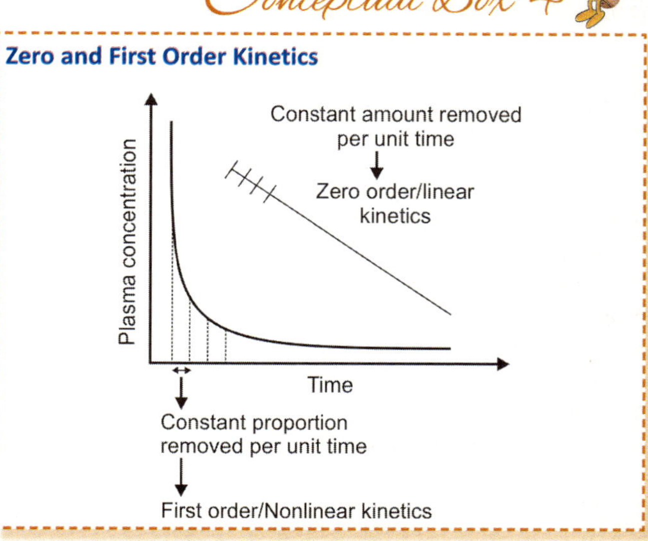

Half-life ($T_{1/2}$)

Half-life or $T_{1/2}$ is the time required for a drug's plasma concentration to be decreased by 50%. $T_{1/2}$ is directly proportional to aV_d as the more is drug distributed in tissues, more is time

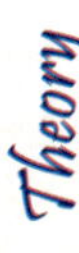

required for its metabolism and clearance. $T_{1/2}$ is inversely proportional to clearance. Faster is the clearance, lesser is the half-life. Hence the formula for half-life is -

$$T_{1/2} = 0.693 \times aV_d/Cl$$

Steady State Concentration

- In one half-life, the drug is decreased by 50%, in second by 75%, third by 87.25%, fourth by **93.75%** and fifth by **96.86%.**
- If a drug is given by continuous IV infusion, it takes approximately at least **5 half-lives** for the drug to disappear from plasma and here after the amount of drug administered is equal to drug removed. This plasma concentration at this state is called as **steady state concentration**.
- The knowledge of half-life and steady state concentration is important to decide about dosing of drug. If a drug has a very long half-life, e.g. Amiodarone has half-life OF 53 days; it will take 265 days to achieve a steady state concentration and hence a loading dose might be given to achieve quick steady state concentration in case of emergency.
- As all the drugs are not given by continuous infusion, this pattern can be mimicked by multiple dosing.

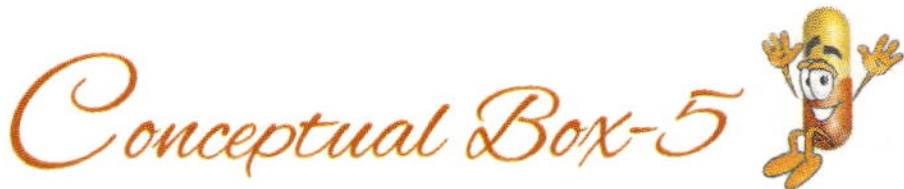

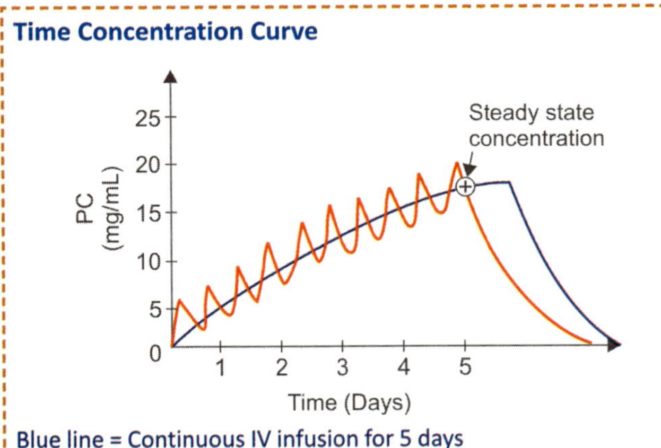

Blue line = Continuous IV infusion for 5 days

Red line = BD dosing for 5 days

Time-concentration curve for a drug with $T_{1/2}$ = 24 hours. Steady state concentration at continuous IV infusion and BD dosing, is achieved at same time, i.e. day 5 (after 5 $T_{1/2}$)

Summary of Pharmacokinetics

- As given in the conceptual box-6, when A drug is administered there is an absorption phase, at the end of which a maximum plasma concentration is achieved (C_{max}).
- The time taken to achieve absorption is denoted as $\mathbf{T_{max}}$, which determines **rate of drug absorption**.
- This is followed by a rapid decline in plasma concentration due to **drug distribution**, which is called as α phase. After distribution there is a slow decline in concentration of DRUG IN plasma due to **drug elimination** known as β phase.

Conceptual Box-6

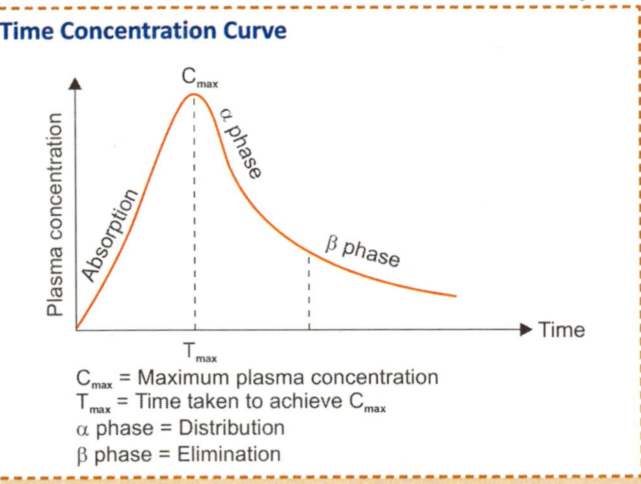

PHARMACODYNAMICS

As described earlier, pharmacodynamics (PD) is the part where the drug is not moving, i.e. attached to target and this is when a particular effect is produced. The target for a drug can be receptors, enzymes, transporters and ion channels.

In PD, there are two things in sequence, i.e. drug acting on target and the target giving an effect and it has been described below in conceptual box. The tendency of a drug to bind the target is **affinity**, whereas once drug is bound to target, the ability of drug to generate effect is known as **efficacy**.

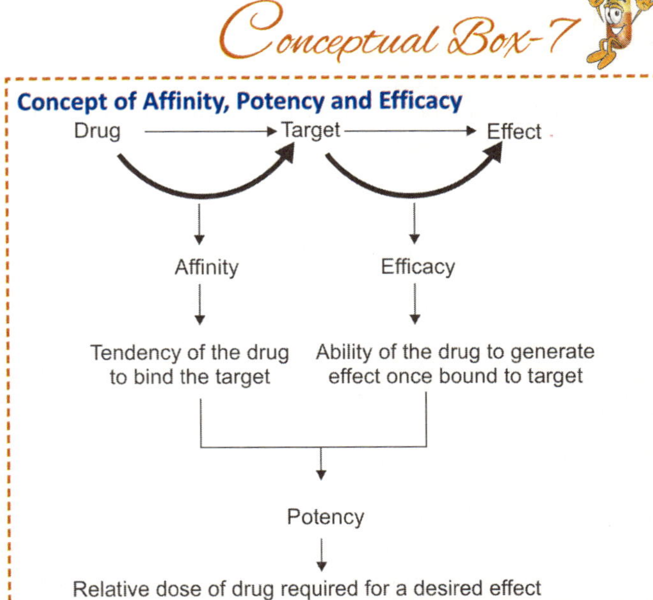

Affinity

Affinity of a drug is its tendency to bind to a particular target. Affinity of two drugs can be compared only if they act on the same target.

Efficacy

Efficacy is the ability of the drug to generate **maximum effect by acting on target**. It is the **most important parameter** of drug clinically. Quantification of efficacy is given in the section of drug receptor interaction.

Potency

Potency is the relative dose of a drug required for a desired effect. The dose of drug required for an effect depends both on affinity and efficacy. Potency of two drugs acting on different targets can also be compared. If lesser dose is required for a particular effect, higher is the potency and vice versa.

Dissociation Constant (K_D)

If drug is denoted by 'D', target by 'T' and effect by 'E', then in an equation we can write drug, receptor and effect as below.

$$D + T \rightleftharpoons DT = E$$

- Dissociation constant or K_D is the ratio of concentration of D and T separately to concentration of DR together. If affinity of D for T is lesser than D and T separately, more is K_D. Hence, K_D is inversely proportional to drug affinity and potency.

$$K_D = [D]\,[T]/[DT]$$

- If K_D is equal to concentration of drug [D], then the equation becomes:

$$K_D = [D]\,[T]/[DT]$$

Or, $K_D = K_D\,[T]/[DT]$

Or $[T]/[DT] = 1$

Or $[T] = [DT]$

If concentration of target is equal to concentration of drug bound to target, then 50% targets or receptors are bound to drug. Hence, **K_D is the concentration of drug at which 50% of drug is bound to target.**

- The affinity constant K_A is inverse of K_D. Hence, higher is K_A, higher is the affinity and potency of the drug.

$$K_A = 1/K_D$$

Dose-Response Curve

Dose-response curve (DRC) can be of two types, i.e. graded and quantal. Graded DRC is determined in an individual whereas quantal DRC is determined in a population.

Graded DRC

Graded DRC is the graph obtained by plotting the log of dose on X axis and the effect produced in an individual by each dose on Y axis. The **slope of the DRC** is a measure of **drug efficacy**, whereas the position of **DRC on log dose axis indicates potency**. More is the height of the slope, more is efficacy and more is the inclination of DRC towards left, lesser is dose and more is potency.

- If two DRCs are parallel then they act on same target and hence affinity can be compared along with potency and efficacy. When the drugs A and B are plotted to observe the DRC (conceptual Box no 8 A), it can be observed that drug A is more efficacious and potent and with more affinity.
- But if two DRCs are unparalleled, then though affinity can not be compared, potencies and efficacies can still be compared. About drugs C and D plotted in the DRC (conceptual Box no 8 B), it can be said that drug C is more efficacious and potent than drug D.

Conceptual Box-8

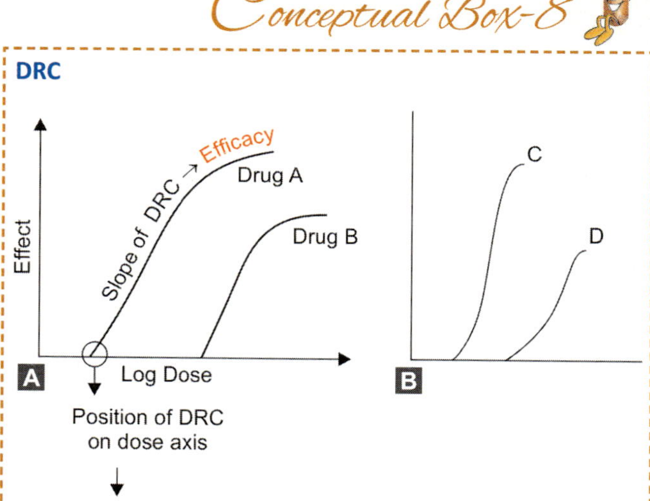

Quantal DRC

Quantal DRC is the graph obtained by plotting the log of dose in X axis and effect produced in the population by each dose on Y axis as all or none phenomenon (a drug produces either sedation or no sedation).

- In conceptual box 9 an example of a quantal DRC is given. The first graph shows the percentage of population responding at a particular dose.
- In the second graph the cumulative response is drawn and the dose at which 50% of the population responds is known as **median effective dose (ED_{50})**, which is a marker of **drug potency**. Similarly, dose at which 50% of population will have toxicity, i.e. **median toxic dose (TD_{50})** and dose at which 50% animals die, i.e. **median lethal dose (LD_{50})** can be calculated.

Conceptual Box-9

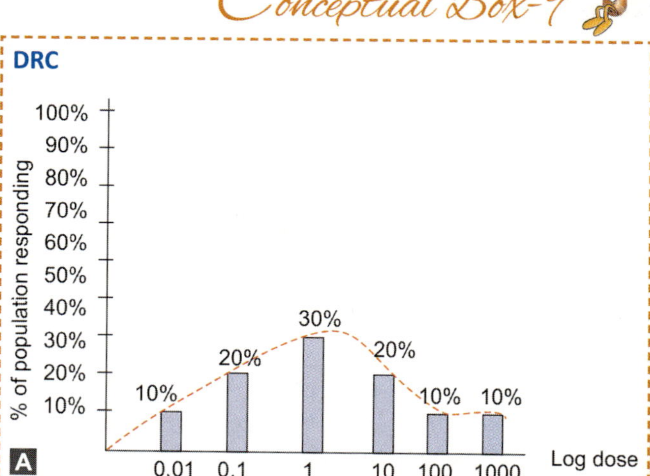

Contd...

Conceptual Box-9

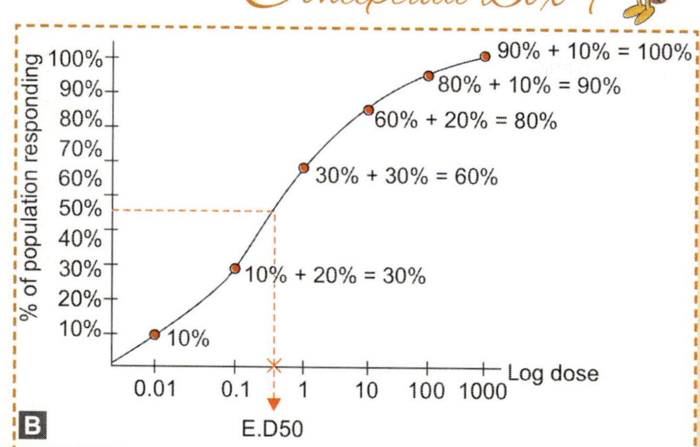

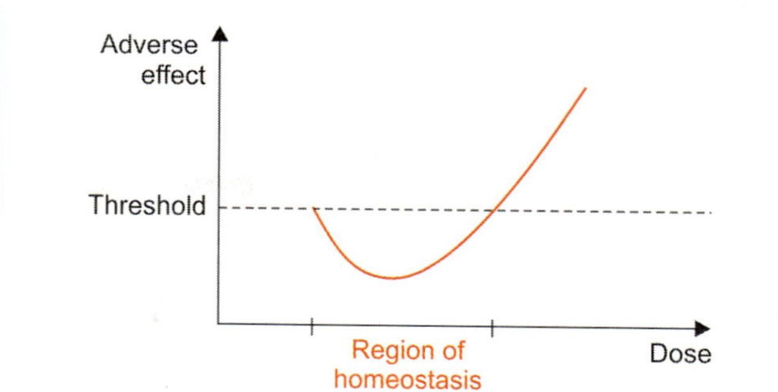

Contd...

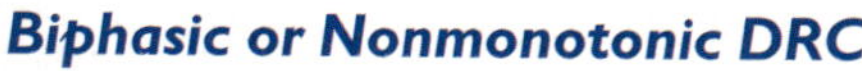

Biphasic or Nonmonotonic DRC

Some DRCs for certain drugs and chemicals do not follow the classical sigmoid shape, rather produce effect in two phases and are known as biphasic DRC.

- **Bell-shaped or inverted U-shaped DRC** is seen mostly with ligands and drugs that can downregulate receptors. At low doses adequate effect is seen but at high doses due to receptor downregulation, the effect decreases. It is mostly seen with hormones like estrogen.

Bell-shaped or inverted U-shaped DRC

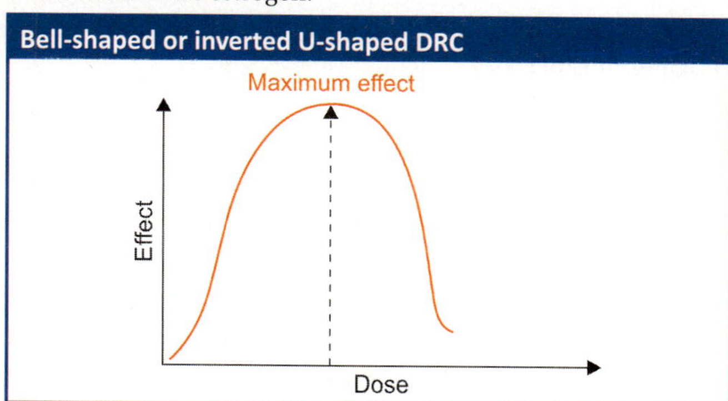

- **U shaped and J shaped DRC** is seen with vitamins and minerals, as both deficiency and excess of these can cause adverse reaction. Thus, there is a normal range of dose for vitamins and minerals to maintain region of homeostasis.

U- and J-shaped DRC

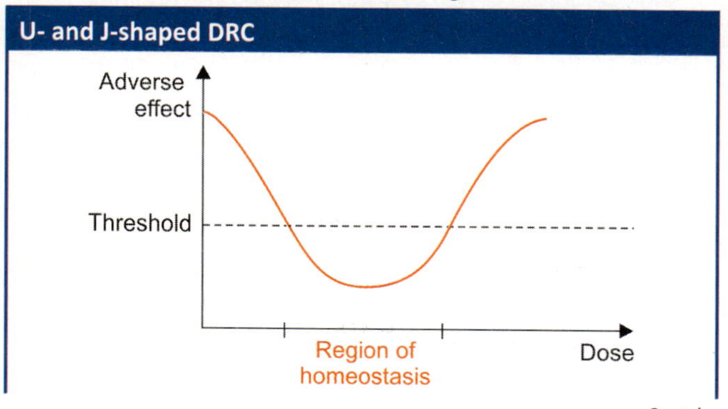

- **Hockey stick-shaped DRC** is the one in which adverse effects are seen only after breach of a particular threshold and then it follows a linear pattern. It is seen with toxic chemicals like formaldehyde.

Hockey stick-shaped DRC

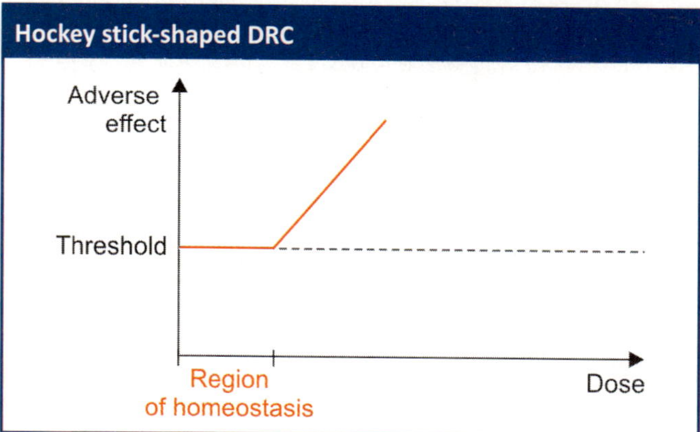

Drug Receptor Interaction

Drugs can interact with targets and produce various magnitudes of effect. Based on quantification of effects, drugs can be full agonist, partial agonist, antagonist or inverse agonist. The intrinsic efficacy of these drugs is shown in mathematical representation on a scale of +1 to –1.

- **Full agonist:** A full agonist is a drug that binds to target and produces **maximal effect** with an intrinsic efficacy of **+1**.
- **Partial agonist:** A partial agonist is a drug that binds to target and produces **submaximal effect** with an intrinsic efficacy value in between **+1 to 0**.
- **Antagonist:** An antagonist is a drug that binds to target and **doesn't produce any effect** and thus has an intrinsic efficacy **0**.
- **Inverse agonist:** An inverse agonist is a drug that binds to target and produces **opposite effect** with an intrinsic efficacy in between 0 to **–1**.

The maximal effect of an agonist can be compromised in the presence of a partial agonist and hence it can be said that a partial agonist behaves as an antagonist in presence of a full agonist.

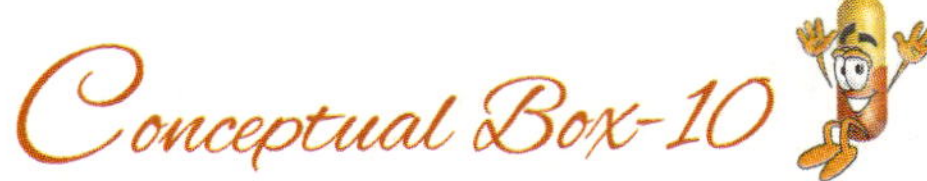

Suppose four drugs A, B, C and D are taken that can bind to β_1 receptors and change the normal heart rate of 70 beats/minute. Let us take the maximum and minimum drug induced increase and decrease in HR as 200 and 40 beats/minute respectively.

- Drug A increases the HR to maximum, i.e. 200 and is a full agonist with intrinsic efficacy of +1.
- Drug B increases HR but lesser than maximum, i.e. to 100 and hence is a partial agonist with intrinsic efficacy between 0 to +1.
- Drug C acts on receptor but doesn't change HR, i.e. no effect and hence is antagonist with 0 intrinsic efficacy.
- Drug D on the contrary decreases HR, i.e. no effect and hence is inverse agonist with intrinsic efficacy between 0 to –1.

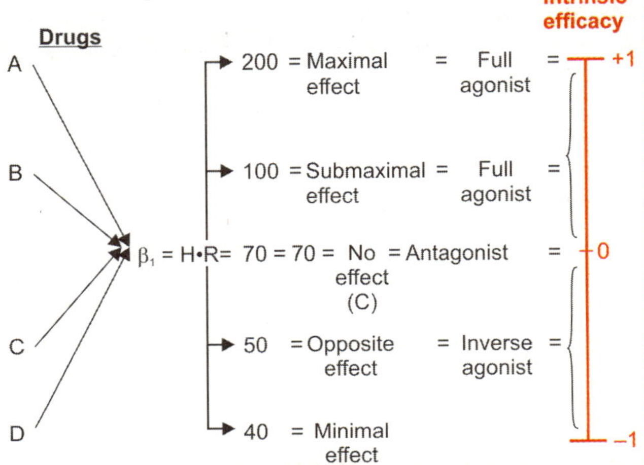

Conceptual Box-11

DRC of Agonists and Antagonists

Full agonist
Full agonist + partial agonist or antagonist
Partial agonist
Antagonist
Inverse agonist + antagonist
Inverse agonist
Response
20
15
10
5
0
–5
–10
–15
–20
Log dose

Types of Antagonism

In broad sense when one drug decreases or completely neutralizes effect of another drug, it is called as antagonism. Based on the different ways of preventing effects antagonism can be pharmacokinetic, chemical, physiological, pharmacological (competitive) and noncompetitive.

Pharmacokinetic Antagonism

One drug prevents another drug's action by acting on its pharmacokinetic parameters like absorption, metabolism, etc. Examples are given below

- Charcoal binds to alcohol and prevents its absorption.
- Enzyme inducers decrease the effect of drugs which are substrate for that enzyme.
- Probenecid inhibits excretion of penicillin-G.

Chemical Antagonism

One drug prevents another drug's action by chemically combining with it in a solution. Examples are given below:

- Binding of dimercaprol to heavy metals
- Binding of protamine sulfate to heparin
- Binding of monoclonal antibodies to protein targets

Physiological Antagonism

One drug prevents another drug's action by acting on a **different receptor**. Examples are given below:

- Bronchoconstriction caused by histamine on H_1 receptor IS prevented by bronchodilation caused by adrenaline on b_2 receptors.
- Hydrochloric acid production by histamine IS inhibited by proton pump inhibitors.
- Aggregant effect of TxA_2 is prevented by PgI_2.

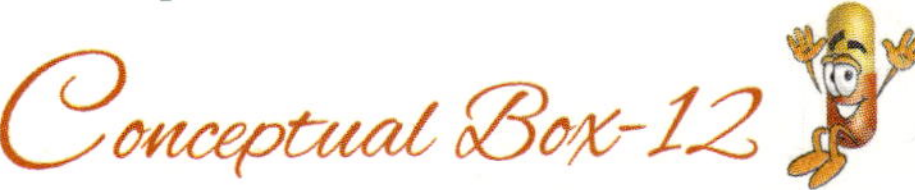

DRC in Competitive Reversible Antagonism

In competitive reversible antagonism the receptors captured by antagonist can be taken away by agonist if its concentration is increased and hence this antagonism is also known as surmountable. Thus, to retain a particular effect, the dose of agonist has to be increased and if dose increases the DRC shifts toward right side and potency decreases.

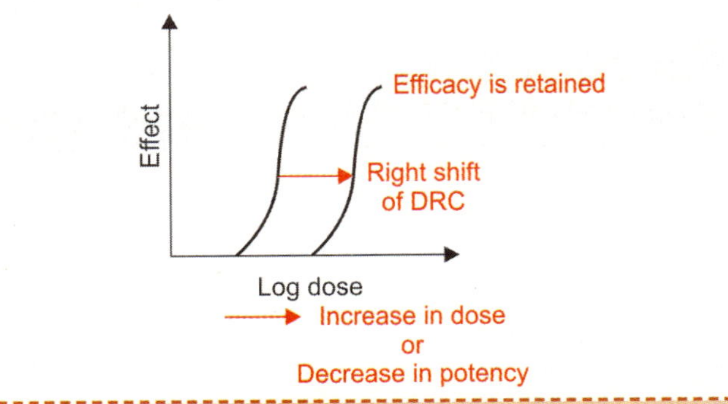

Pharmacological or Competitive Antagonism

One drug prevents another drug's action by acting on the same receptor. The antagonist can bind to receptors by forming ionic or covalent bonds. Since ionic bonds are weaker AND the

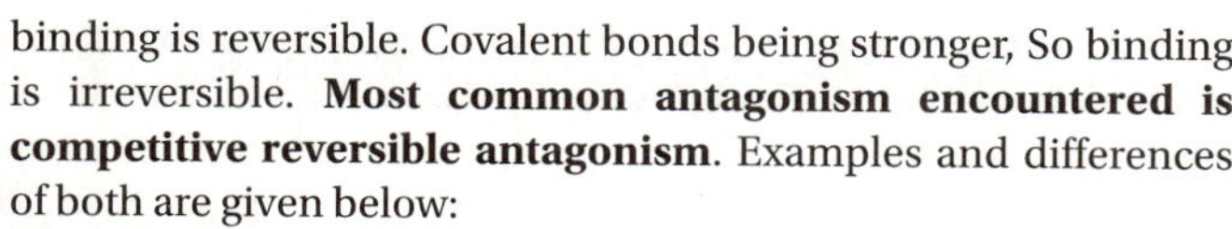

binding is reversible. Covalent bonds being stronger, So binding is irreversible. **Most common antagonism encountered is competitive reversible antagonism**. Examples and differences of both are given below:

- **Competitive reversible (equilibrium) antagonism:** Most antagonists are of this type and examples include beta blockers preventing effect of catecholamines on b_1 receptors, cimetidine inhibiting hydrochloric acid production by acting on H_2 receptors, etc.
- **Competitive irreversible (nonequilibrium) antagonism:** This type of antagonism is rare and examples are aspirin inhibiting TxA_2, PPIs inhibiting proton pumps, phenoxybenzamine inhibiting α receptors and MAO inhibitors. The change of DRC in this is similar to noncompetitive antagonism.

Noncompetitive Antagonism

One drug prevents another drug's action by acting on a site distal to the receptor for agonist, e.g. Verapamil blocks calcium channel and decreases intracellular calcium; acetylcholine induces muscle contraction by acting on nicotinic receptors, but at the end calcium is required for contraction. Hence, verapamil is a noncompetitive antagonist of acetylcholine.

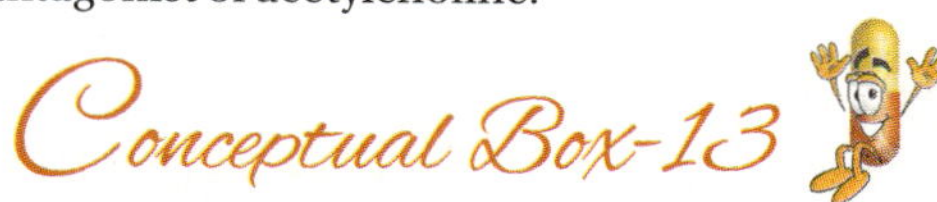

DRC in Noncompetitive Antagonism

In noncompetitive inhibition, since the site of action for antagonist is distal to the site of agonist, the receptors captured by antagonist can never be taken away by agonist. Hence, the effect has to decrease and the slope of DRC and efficacy decreases.

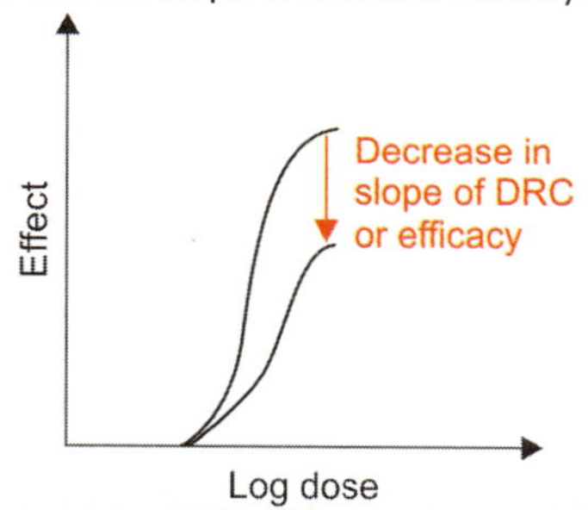

Competitive and noncompetitive antagonism of enzymes by drugs

we discussed the inhibition of receptors above. If enzymes are taken into consideration as targets, then inhibition can be competitive (reversible and irreversible) and noncompetitive. In competitive antagonism the site of drug and antagonist is same, whereas in noncompetitive the antagonist acts on allosteric site and hence this type is also known as **allosteric antagonism**.

Michaelis Menten Equation

- To understand enzyme antagonism, let us have a look at the **Michaelis Menten equation** which states:

$$V = V_{max} \times [D] / K_m + [D]$$

V = Velocity of reaction
V_{max} = Maximum velocity of reaction
[D] = Drug concentration

Contd...

K_m = Concentration of drug [D], required to achieve ½ of V_{max}

- If a graph is drawn taking V_{max} on Y axis and drug concentration on X axis, a hyperbolic curve is formed as given below:

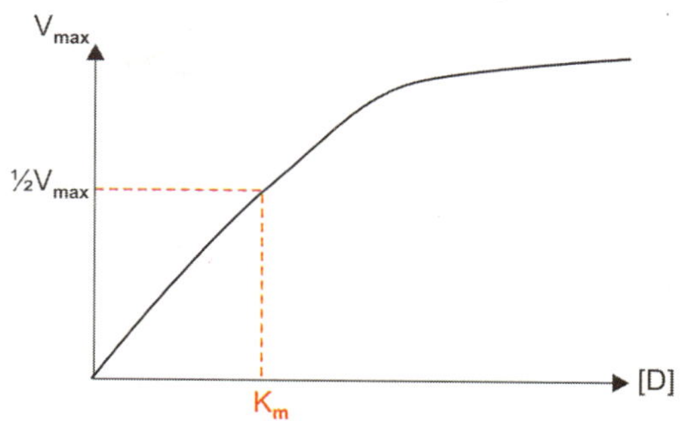

- The V_{max} or maximum velocity of reaction between drug and enzyme will produce maximum clinical effect and hence **V_{max} is directly proportional to efficacy**.
- K_m or Concentration of drug [D], required to achieve ½ of V_{max} represents drug dose. Since drug dose is inversely proportional to potency, **K_m is also inversely proportional to potency**.
- **Competitive reversible antagonism:** Potency decreases, and efficacy does not change and hence K_m increases, and V_{max} does not change.
- **Noncompetitive or allosteric antagonism:** Efficacy decreases but potency does not change and hence V_{max} decreases, and K_m does not change.
- The graphical representation of same is given below:

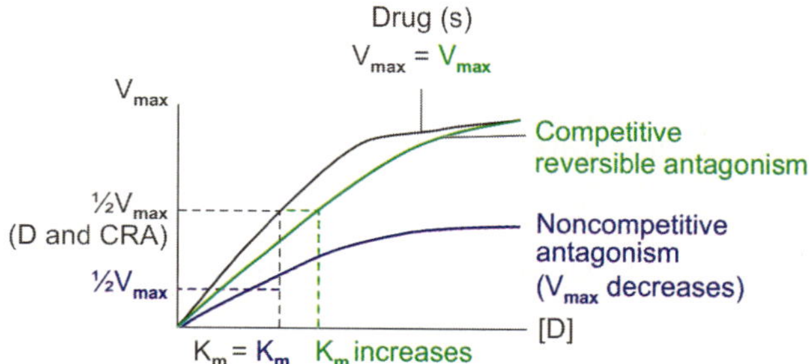

Double Reciprocal or Lineweaver Burk Plot

- Double reciprocal plot is a linear representation of Michael Menten equation, which can be achieved as given below:

$V = V_{max} \times [D] / K_m + [D]$

Or $1/V = K_m + [D] / V_{max} \times [D]$

Or $1/V = K_m / V_{max} \times 1 / [D] + 1 / V_{max}$

- Since for a particular drug K_m and V_{max} are constant, in the equation above 1/V and 1/[D] are variables. Out of these variables if 1/V is taken on Y axis and 1/[D] on X axis then a linear graph is achieved as given below:

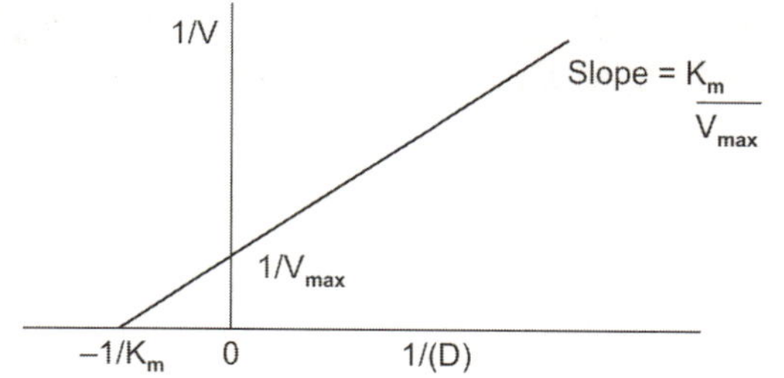

Contd...

- The changes in presence of a competitive reversible antagonist and irreversible antagonist are similar as described before and are represented as given below.

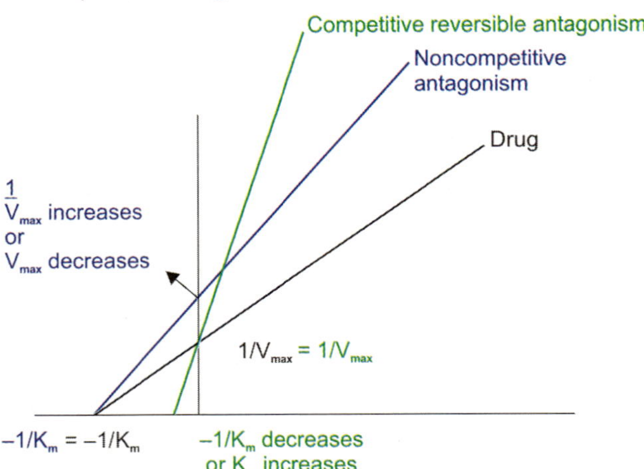

Dixon Plot

- A Dixon plot is again a linear graph like previous one. Here a graph is drawn by plotting I/V on Y axis and the antagonist concentration [A] on X axis at different drug concentration [D].
- The different lines derived at different concentration intersect with each other behind Y axis in case of a competitive antagonist and the perpendicular drawn from that point to X axis is the point which is K_A (affinity of the Antagonist for enzyme).
- In case of noncompetitive antagonist, the lines intersect on X axis and this point is K_A.
- The K_A value is calculated by graph is used to compare potencies of different antagonists.

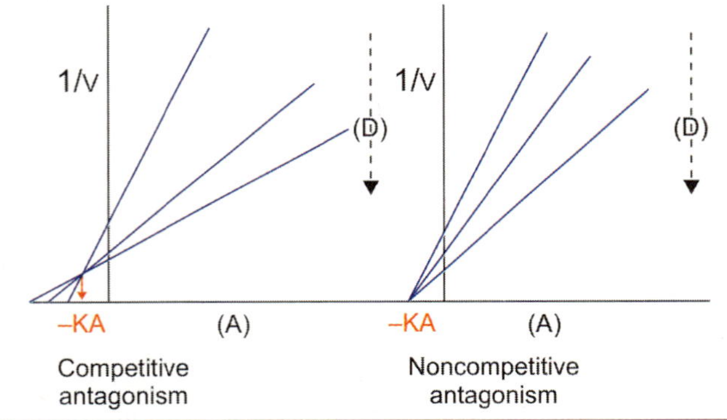

Table 14: Comparison between Competitive and Non-Competitive Antagonism

Competitive antagonism	Noncompetitive antagonism
At same site	At different sites
DRC shifts to right side	Slope of DRC decreases
Efficacy and V_{max} does not change	Efficacy and V_{max} decreases
Dose and K_m increases as potency decreases	Dose, potency and K_m does not change

RECEPTORS

Receptors are the most important targets for drugs and hence have been discussed in detail below. The various types of receptors are GPCRs, ion channel receptors, enzyme linked receptors and nuclear receptors.

G-PROTEIN COUPLED RECEPTORS (GPCRS)

- These are the most important ones as most of the drugs target GPCRs. Some examples of GPCRs are **muscarinic receptors**, beta adrenergic receptors, alpha adrenergic receptors, eicosanoid receptors, thrombin receptors (Protease Activated Receptors), serotonergic receptors (except 5HT3), **oxytocin receptor** and histaminergic receptors.
- G protein coupled receptors are located outside the cell membrane and while entering into cytoplasm they spin the cell membrane seven times. Hence, they are also called as **heptahelical or 7-transmembrane spanning receptors**. Another name for these is **metabotropic receptors**.
- After entering into the cytoplasm, receptor attaché S to G protein, which has 3 subunits α, β and γ; α subunit being attached to a molecule of GDP.
- When receptor is stimulated, GDP is phosphorylated to GTP, which pulls α subunit away from G protein, forming two active components, i.e. αGTP and βγ.
- αGTP has a short half-life, as α-GTPase activity **breaks down GTP into GDP** forming α–GDP; followed by reunion of α–GDP with βγ and receptor comes back to inactive state.
- The effect produced by αGTP depends on the subtype of α protein (s, q, i, o, 12/13) and based on this GPCRs are named as $G\alpha_s$, $G\alpha_q$, $G\alpha_i$, $G\alpha_o$, $G\alpha_{12/13}$. Hence α **is the most important subunit** of GPCR.

$G\alpha_s$ Subtype

- Its activation increases intracellular α_sGTP, which stimulates **adenylyl cyclase** to increase **cycAMP**.
- CycAMP stimulates **PKA (Protein Kinase A)** which results in phosphorylation of intracellular proteins and calcium channels.
- One example is beta-1 receptors which phosphorylate calcium channels and by increased calcium, contraction of myocardium increases. Another example is Beta-2 receptors which phosphorylate proteins in smooth muscles like mLCP (Myosin Light Chain Phosphorylase), which dephosphorylates myosin and relaxes smooth muscles.

$G\alpha_q$ Subtype

- Its activation increases intracellular α_qGTP, which stimulate **PLC (Phospholipase C)** to increase **PIP-2 (Phosphoinositol bisphosphonates-2)**.
- PIP-2 further degrades into terminal active products **IP-3 (Inositol triphosphate)** and **DAG (Diacylglycerol)**.
- IP-3 activates IP-3 receptors in sarcoplasmic reticulum and **releases calcium.** One example is α_1 adrenoreceptors which CAUSES vasoconstriction by this mechanism.
- DAG stimulates **PKC (Protein Kinase C)** present in cell membranes and phosphorylates ion channels, receptors, etc.

$G\alpha_i$ Subtype

- Its activation **decreases intracellular cycAMP** and **opens potassium channel**. They reverse the effects of previous two subtypes.
- One example is M2 muscarinic receptors in heart which decrease cycAMP and calcium, thus decreasing contraction, heart rate and conduction.
- The other examples of $G\alpha_i$ subtype of receptors are α_2 adrenergic, $5HT_1$, A_1/A_3 (Adenosine), H_3 and CB_1/CB_2 (Cannabinoid) receptors.

$G\alpha_o$ Subtype

- Its primary effect is seen by the βγ subunit, which **opens potassium channels** and **inhibits calcium channels**.
- The end effect is quite similar to $G\alpha_i$ subtype, i.e. relaxation.
- One example is analgesic effect of opioid receptors due to opening of potassium channels by βγ subunits.

$G\alpha_{12/13}$ Subtype

- Its activation phosphorylates Rho-GDP to Rho-GTP, which stimulates **Rho kinase**.
- Rho kinase is responsible for protein phosphorylation in smooth muscles, which causes **vasoconstriction** and is considered as a cause of pulmonary hypertension.
- Rho kinase has smooth muscle proliferative, angiogenic and synaptic remodelling effects.
- Hence, Rho kinase inhibitor **fasudil** has been developed for treatment of pulmonary problems, hypertension, angina and cerebral vasospasm.

Recent Advances

Netarsudil is a topical rho kinase inhibitor recently approved for treatment of open angle glaucoma. It acts by increasing aqueous outflow through trabecular meshwork.

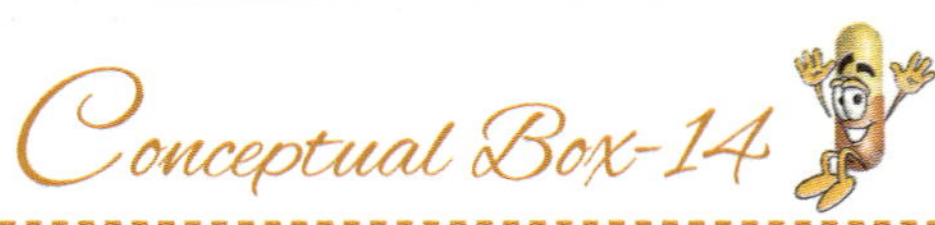

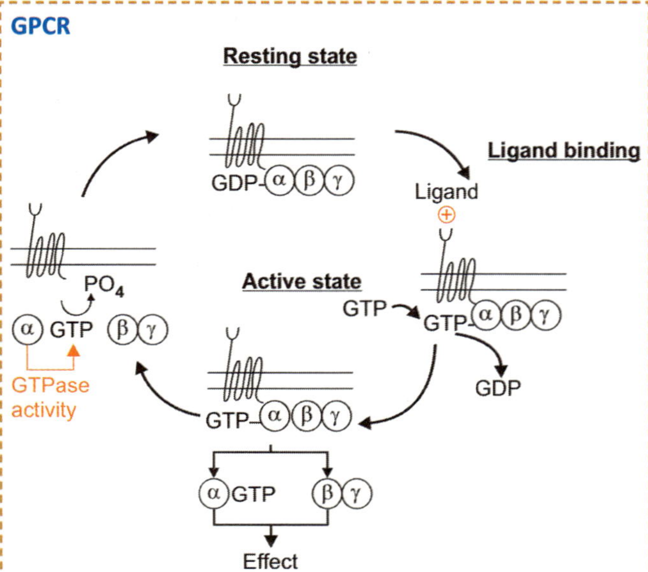

LIGAND GATED ION CHANNEL RECEPTORS

- The action of ligand on an ion channel receptor opens the ion channel, which conducts a specific ion and leads to depolarization (Na ion channels) or hyperpolarization (Cl ion channels).
- Since these effects are immediately seen after ligand's action, **ligand gated ion channel receptors are fastest acting receptors**.
- **$GABA_A$**, glutamate (AMPA, kainate and NMDA subtypes), nicotinic and **$5HT_3$** receptors are some examples of ligand gated ion channel receptors.

ENZYME LINKED RECEPTORS

An extracellular receptor is linked by a single helix to intracellular enzymes like tyrosine kinase, serine/threonine kinase, janus kinase and guanylyl cyclase. Activation of receptor leads to enzyme activation that causes intracellular effects.

Examples of enzyme linked receptors	
Tyrosine kinase receptors	EGFR, VEGFR, Her-2, Insulin, IGF1 and Toll like receptors
Serine/threonine kinase receptors	TGFR
Janus kinase	Cytokine receptors, growth hormone receptor, **prolactin receptor**
Guanylyl cyclase linked receptor	Receptor of ANP and BNP

NUCLEAR RECEPTORS

- The nuclear receptors are located both in cytoplasm and nucleus but are termed AS nuclear because on activation, the cytoplasmic receptors translocate to nucleus and regulate gene expression.
- The effect produced is delayed as changes in gene followed by transcription factors take time and hence nuclear receptors are the **slowest acting receptors**. Based on their location though receptors can be nuclear or cytoplasmic.

Nuclear receptors located in nucleus	Nuclear receptors located in cytoplasm
Vitamin D receptor Thyroid receptor Retinoic acid receptor PPAR (Peroxisome Proliferator Activated Receptor) Estrogen receptor Progesterone receptor	Mineralocorticoid receptor Glucocorticoid receptor Androgen receptor

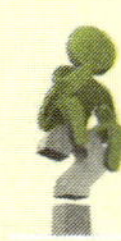

Image-based Questions

1. **The mode of drug absorption shown in the picture is:**

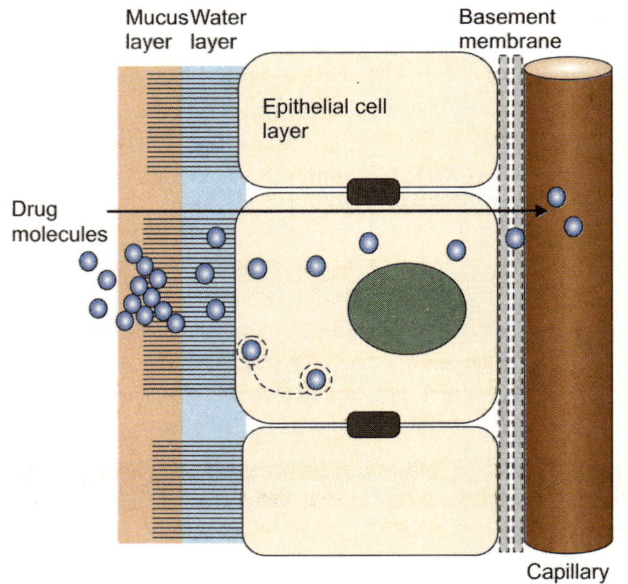

a. Passive diffusion
b. Active transport
c. Facilitated diffusion
d. Pinocytosis
e. Diffusion

2. **Which of the following is true regarding the graph given below:**

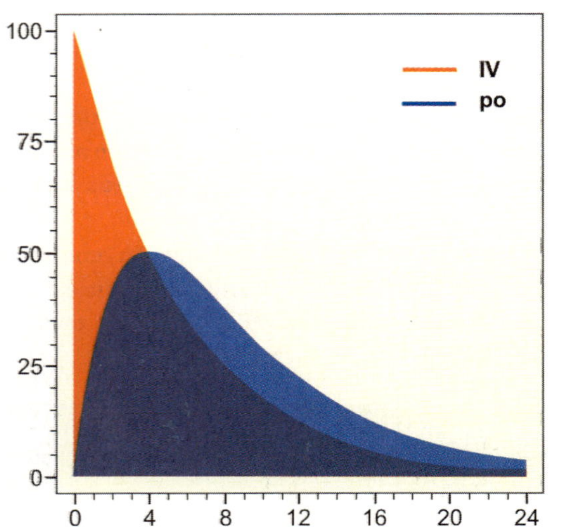

a. Area under red graph is bioavailability
b. Area under blue graph is bioavailability
c. Area under both red and blue graph is bioavailability
d. Area under blue graph by area under red graph is bioavailabilty

3. **A patient weighing 100 kg was given a drug at a dose of 2000 mg/kg by IV route. The plasma concentration at first hour to fifth hour is given in the picture below. What is the aV_d, for the drug?**

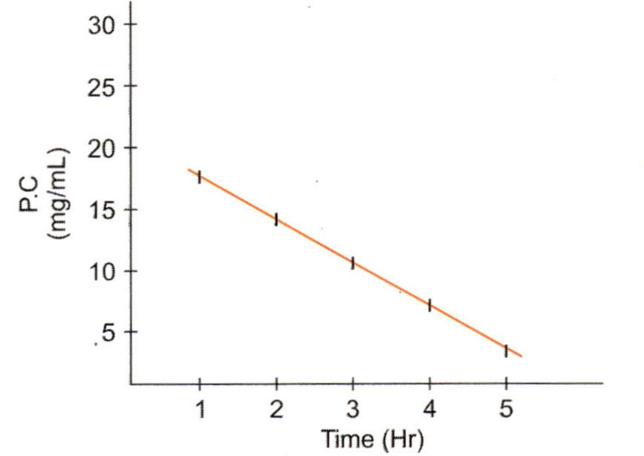

a. 2 L
b. 4 L
c. 8 L
d. 10 L
e. 20 L

4. **A drug has the following time concentration curve. What is the order of elimination?**

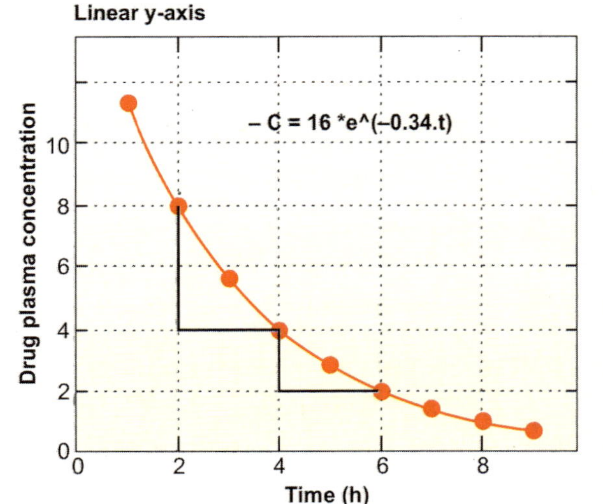

a. Zero order
b. First order
c. Second order
d. Pseudo zero order

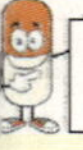

5. A drug has the following time concentration curve. Which of the following statement is correct regarding this drug?

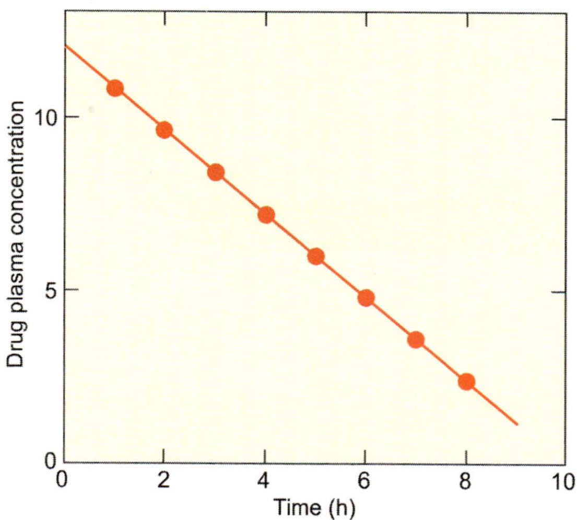

a. Most drug follow this pattern
b. As dose increases T1/2 of drug increases
c. As dose increases Cl of drug increases
d. P.C determines elimination

6. The DRC for three drugs A, B and C are given in the picture below. Which of the following statements is not correct.

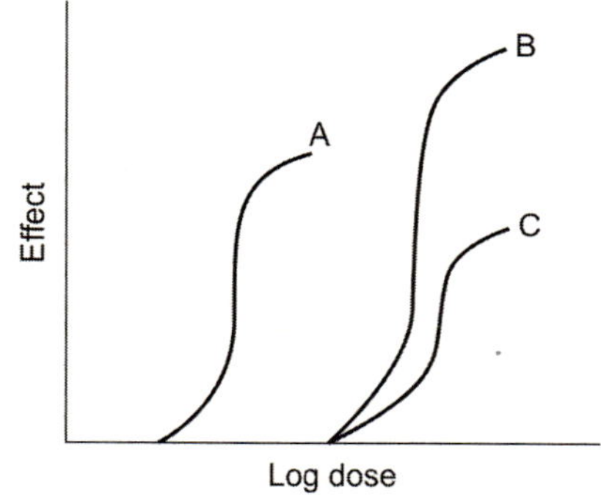

a. A and B act on same target
b. B and C act on different targets
c. B is more potent than C
d. A has more efficacy than C
e. Affinity of B and C cannot be compared

7. DRC of a drug is shown in the picture before and after administration of antagonist. What is the type of antagonism?

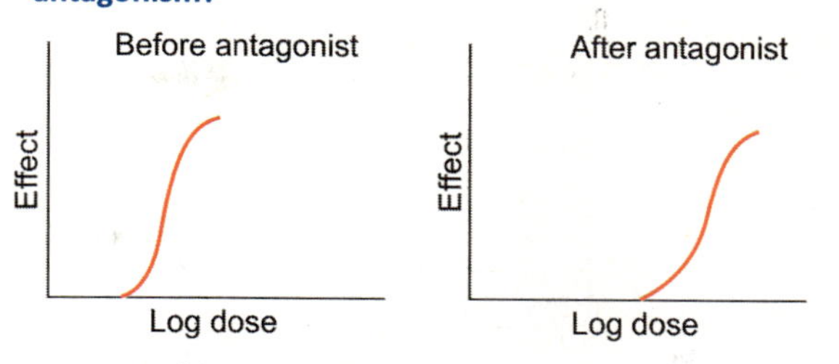

a. Reversible competitive
b. Irreversible competitive
c. Reversible noncompetitive
d. Irreversible noncompetitive
e. No antagonism

8. The receptor given in the picture is also known as:

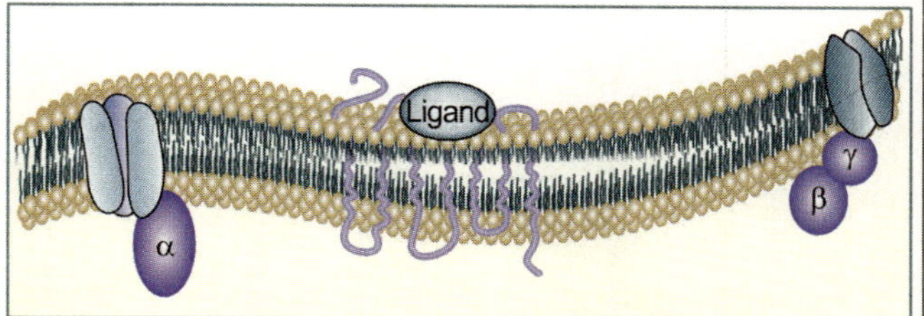

a. Metacentric
b. Metabolic
c. Metabotropic
d. Octahelixal

9. The drug given in the picture is

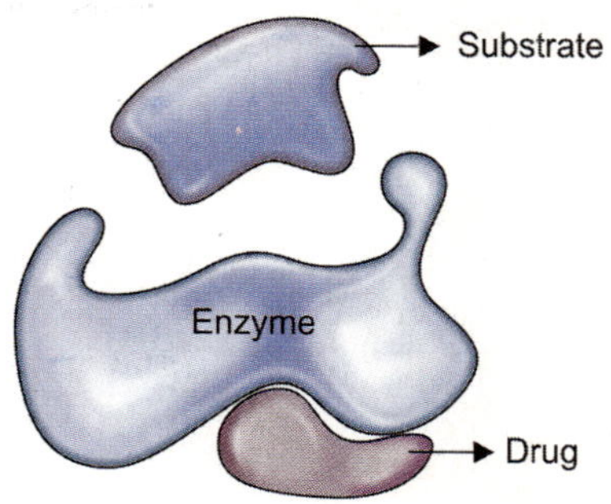

a. Reversible competitive inhibitor
b. Irreversible competitive inhibitor
c. Noncompetitive
d. Enzyme inhibitor
e. Allosteric inhibitor
f. Both c and e

10. **The drug in the delivery system given below is for:**

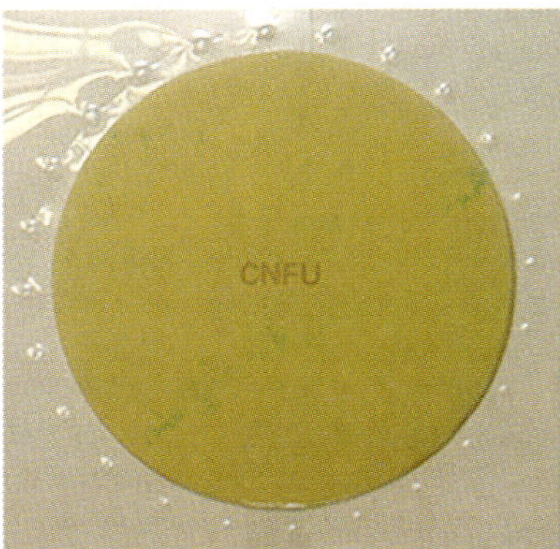

a. Topical use
b. Systemic use
c. Both topical and systemic use
d. None

11. **The drug given in the picture is given by which route:**

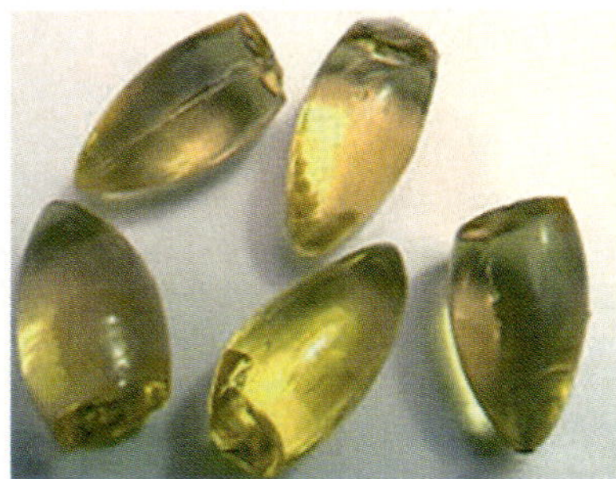

a. Oral
b. Sublingual
c. Ocular
d. Rectal

12. **The structure given in the picture is responsible for all, except:**

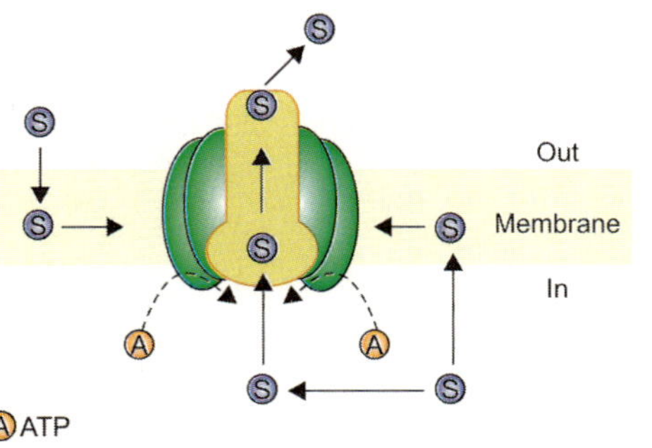

a. Drug absorption
b. Drug resistance
c. First pass metabolism
d. Drug efflux

13. **Which of the following statement is correct regarding the drug whose concentration time curve is given below?**

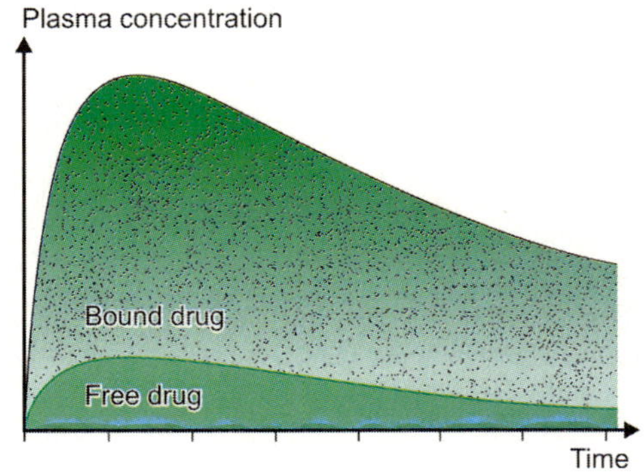

a. High volume of distribution
b. Possible drug interactions
c. High lipid solubility
d. Low lipid solubility

14. **The reaction of drug metabolism given below is:**

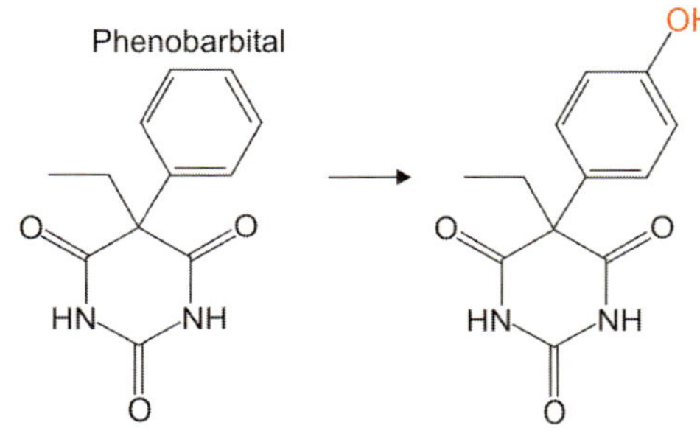

a. Phase II – Glucuronidation
b. Phase II – Hydroxylation
c. Phase I – Hydroxylation
d. Phase I – Glucuronidation

15. **What is the type of receptor given in the picture?**

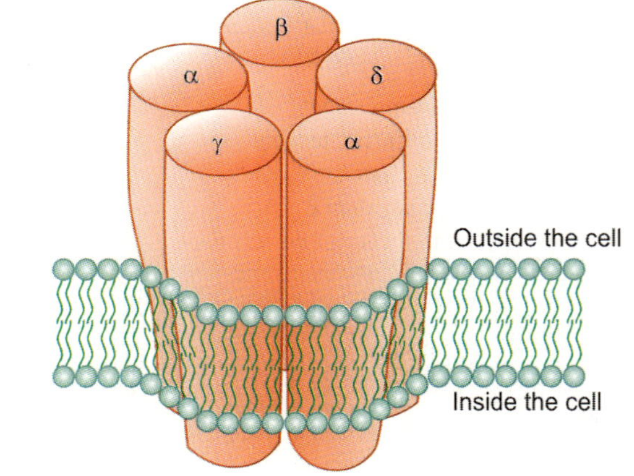

a. GPCR
b. Ion channel receptor
c. Enzyme linked receptor
d. Nuclear receptor

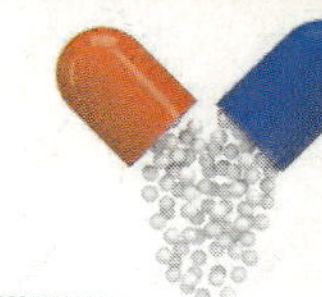

Answers with Explanations to Image-based Questions

1. Ans. (a) Passive diffusion

- The passage of drug through the epithelial membrane of intestine and endothelial membrane of blood vessels (lipid barrier) is known as passive diffusion.
- Passive diffusion is the most common mode of drug absorption.
- Since the drug has to be lipid soluble for passive diffusion, it is generalized that a drug is absorbed if it is lipid soluble.

2. Ans. (d) Area under blue graph by area under red graph is bioavailabilty

- The area under the red curve is for IV dose and blue graph is for oral dose.
- Bioavailability can be calculated by dividing the area under the curve for oral route by intravenous route and then multiplying with 100.

$$\text{Bioavailability} = AUC_{oral}/AUC_{IV} \times 100$$

3. Ans. (d) 10 L

- Dose of the drug given to the patient = 100 × 2000 = 200000 mg
- The plasma concentration in the beginning, if we extend the graph will be 20 mg/mL.
- Hence V_d = D/C = 200000/20 = 10000 mL = 10 L

4. Ans. (b) First order

- As it can be seen in the graph a constant proportion is eliminated per unit time and hence the given drug follows first order kinetics.

5. Ans. (b) As dose increases $T_{1/2}$ increases

As it can be seen in the graph, a constant amount of drug is eliminated per unit time and hence this drug follows zero order kinetics.

- Most drugs follow first order kinetics.
- In zero order as dose increases $T_{1/2}$ increases and Cl decreases.
- In zero order drug elimination is independent of P.C.

6. Ans. (c) B is more potent than C

- B and C are equipotent as potency is related to dose and position of DRC on dose axis, which is same for B and C.
- A and B are parallel DRC and hence act on same target, whereas B and C are not parallel and hence act on different targets.
- Affinity of B and C cannot be compared as they act on different targets.

7. Ans. (a) Reversible competitive

- The right shift in the DRC is suggestive of competitive antagonism, which is reversible.
- In reversible competitive antagonism if dose is increased the efficacy can be retained, as shown in tvhe DRC.
- DRC of irreversible competitive antagonism is similar to noncompetitive antagonism.

8. Ans. (c) Metabotropic

- The receptor given in the picture is a GPCR, which spins the cell membrane seven times and hence is also known as an heptahelical receptor or seven pass transmembrane receptor.
- The other synonyms of GPCR are metabotropic and serpentine receptor.

9. Ans. (f) Both c and e

- The drug in the picture is acting on the allosteric site of the enzyme and changes site of action for substrate.
- Hence increasing substrate concentration has no effect on drug.
- This type of inhibition is known as noncompetitive or allosteric inhibition.

10. Ans. (b) Systemic use

(Ref: Goodman Gilman 12th E/P22)

- This is a transdermal patch and this route is for systemic use of drugs.

11. Ans. (d) Rectal

(Ref: Goodman Gilman 12th E/P22)

- The drug in the picture are suppositories given by rectal route.

12. Ans. (a) Drug absorption

(Ref: Goodman Gilman 12th E/P97)

- The structure in the picture is an active transporter involved in drug efflux, i.e. P-glycoprotein.
- It is present in intestinal epithelial cells, where drug efflux partially contributes to first pass metabolism.
- In tumor cells its expression is one of the mechanism for drug resistance.

13. Ans. (b) Possible drug interactions

(Ref: Goodman Gilman 12th E/P24)

- The drug has a high plasma protein binding as given in the graph.
- For such drugs the volume of distribution is usually low.
- Drug interactions are possible as such drugs can displace other high plasma protein bound drugs and cause toxicity.

14. Ans. (c) Phase I – Hydroxylation

(Ref: Goodman Gilman 12th E/P131)

- The reaction is hydroxylation of phenobarbital, which is a phase I reaction of drug metabolism.

15. Ans. (b) Ion channel receptor

(Ref: Goodman Gilman 12th E/P59)

- The pentameric structure in the picture is a nicotinic receptor made up of 2 alpha, 1 beta and 1 delta subunit.
- Nicotinic receptor is a Na ion channel receptor.

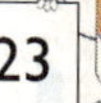

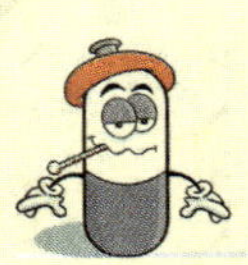

Annexures

Drugs whose Absorption is Increased by Fatty Food

Mnemonics

PLAGuE

- **P** : Posaconazol
- **L** : Lumeantrine
- **A** : Albendazole, Atovaquone
- **Gu** : Griseofulvin
- **E** : Efavirenz

Drugs with High First Pass Metabolism

Mnemonics

Very High **METABOLISM of NTG**

- **Very** : Verapamil
- **High** : Hydrocortisone
- **M** : Morphine
- **E** : Estrogen
- **T** : Testosterone, Trinitrate glycerine
- **A** : Antipsychotic (Chlorpromazine)
- **B** : Beta blockers (Propranolol and Carvedilol)
- **O** : Opioids (Morphine, Pethidine and Pentazocine)
- **L** : Levodopa, Lignocaine
- **I** : Isoprenaline
- **S** : Saquinavir, Salbutamol
- **M** : Midazolam
- Of
- **NTG** : Nitroglycerine

Extremes of Bioavailability

Drugs with 0% BA	Drugs with 100% BA
• Tubocurare • Aminoglycosides • Heparin	• Valproate • Lithium • Diazepam • Doxycycline, Minocycline • Linezolid • Indomethacin, Salicylic acid • Penbutalol, Pindolol

Drugs with Very Short Half-Life (<10 Minutes)

- Adenosine (1–5 seconds)
- Esmolol
- Dopamine
- Dobutamine
- Nitroprusside
- Alteplase
- 5-FU

Drugs with Very Long Half-Life (Days)

- Suramin
- Amiodarone
- Mefloquine
- Chloroquine
- Eratnacept
- Phenylbutazone
- Gold salts

Hit and Run Drugs

Drug whose terminal half-life is longer than biological half-life show this phenomenon. PPIs have a short half-life of 5–2 hours, but duration of action is 24–36 hours due to irreversible binding.

- **M** : MAO inhibitors
- **O** : Omeprazole
- **R** : Reserpine
- **Gue** : Guanethidine

Drugs Excreted in Saliva

- Lithium
- Rifampicin
- Heavy metals
- Clarithromycin
- Phenytoin
- Disulfiram
- Metoclopromide

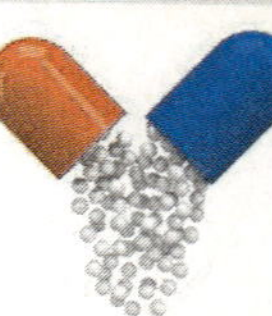

Multiple Choice Questions

PHARMACOKINETICS

1. **Among the following, maximum rate of drug absorption is indicated by:** ***(AIIMS May 2018)***
   a. Cmax b. AUC
   c. Tmax d. T 1/2
2. **Therapeutic index is a measure of:** ***(AIIMS May 2018)***
   a. Potency b. Efficacy
   c. Safety d. Toxicity
3. **From which of the following routes, bioavailability of the drug is likely to be 100 percent?** ***(AIIMS May 2018)***
   a. Intravenous b. Subcutaneous
   c. Intramuscular d. Intradermal
4. **Hepatic First pass metabolism will be encountered by which of the following routes of drug administration?** ***(AIIMS May 2018)***
   a. Oral b. Intravenous
   c. Sublingual d. Subcutaneous
5. **You have to give 180 mg of ceftriaxone to a patient in 2 mL syringe which has 10 divisions per mL. Concentration of this drug in vial is 500mg/5ml. How many divisions should be filled in 2 mL syringe to give 180 mg?** ***(AIIMS May 2018, Nov 2017)***
   a. 18 b. 1.8
   c. 2 d. 20
6. **Initial feature of storage of drug in tissues is:** ***(AIIMS May 2017)***
   a. Large apparent volume of distribution
   b. Less excretion in urine
   c. Small apparent volume of distribution
   d. High excretion of drug in urine
7. **A patient was administered 200 mg of a drug. 75 mg of the drug is eliminated in 90 minutes. If the drug follows first order kinetics how much drug will remain after 6 hours?** ***(AIIMS May 2017)***
   a. 6.25 mg b. 12.5 mg
   c. 25 mg d. 50 mg
8. **A drug x was given continuous IV 1.6mg/min and elimination rate of x was 640ml/min. With t1/2 of 1.8h, what would be the concentration of drug after achieving study state?** ***(AIIMS May 2017)***
   a. 2.88 mg/mL
   b. 0.004 mg/mL
   c. 0.002 mg/mL
   d. 3.25 mg/mL
9. **Which of the following is a P glycoprotein inducer:** ***(AIIMS May 2017)***
   a. Rifampicin
   b. Erythromycin
   c. Voriconazole
   d. Ketoconazole
10. **True about pKa is:** ***(Recent Question 2017)***
    a. pH at which ionized fraction of drug equals to unionized fraction
    b. pH at which ionized fraction of drug is more than unionized fraction
    c. pH at which ionized fraction of drug is less than unionized fraction
    d. pH at which ionized fraction of drug is twice unionized fraction
11. **Which of the following correctly represents the sequence of maximum absorption of a drug when applied topically?** ***(AIIMS Nov 2016)***
    a. Post auricular >scrotum>scalp>dorsum of arm>plantar area
    b. Scalp>scrotum>post auricular >dorsum of arm>plantar area
    c. Plantar area>dorsum of arm>scalp>scrotum>post auricular
    d. Scrotum> scalp > post auricular >dorsum of arm > plantar area
12. **Digoxin has a half-life of 40 hours, which helps in prescribing to determine:** ***(AIIMS Nov 2016)***
    a. Regimen for smooth discontinuation
    b. Need for loading dose in order to give immediate effect
    c. Regimen for maintenance dose
    d. Can be given once in 2 days
13. **An 80kg man is in shock. Vasopressor has to be started at 10microg/kg/min. One vial has 200 mg in 5 mL and 2 vials were diluted to 250ml. If 16 drops = 1ml, calculate drops per min required.** ***(AIIMS Nov 2016)***
    a. 4 b. 8
    c. 16 d. 24
14. **Low volume of distribution indicates:** ***(AIIMS Nov 2018, Nov 2015)***
    a. Low efficacy
    b. Decreased distribution in tissues and organ
    c. Short biological life
    d. Poor bioavailability
15. **Glyceryl trinitrate is used by sublingual route because it is** ***(AIIMS May 2015)***
    a. Nonionic and more lipid soluble
    b. Ionic and more lipid soluble
    c. Ionic and less lipid soluble
    d. Non Ionic and less lipid soluble
16. **Which of the following is not converted into an active metabolite?** ***(AIIMS May 2014)***
    a. Lisinopril b. Fluoxetine
    c. Cyclophosphamide d. Diazepam
17. **Ritonavir inhibits the action of all except:** ***(AIIMS May 2013)***
    a. Cisapride b. Phenytoin
    c. Amiodarone d. Midazolam

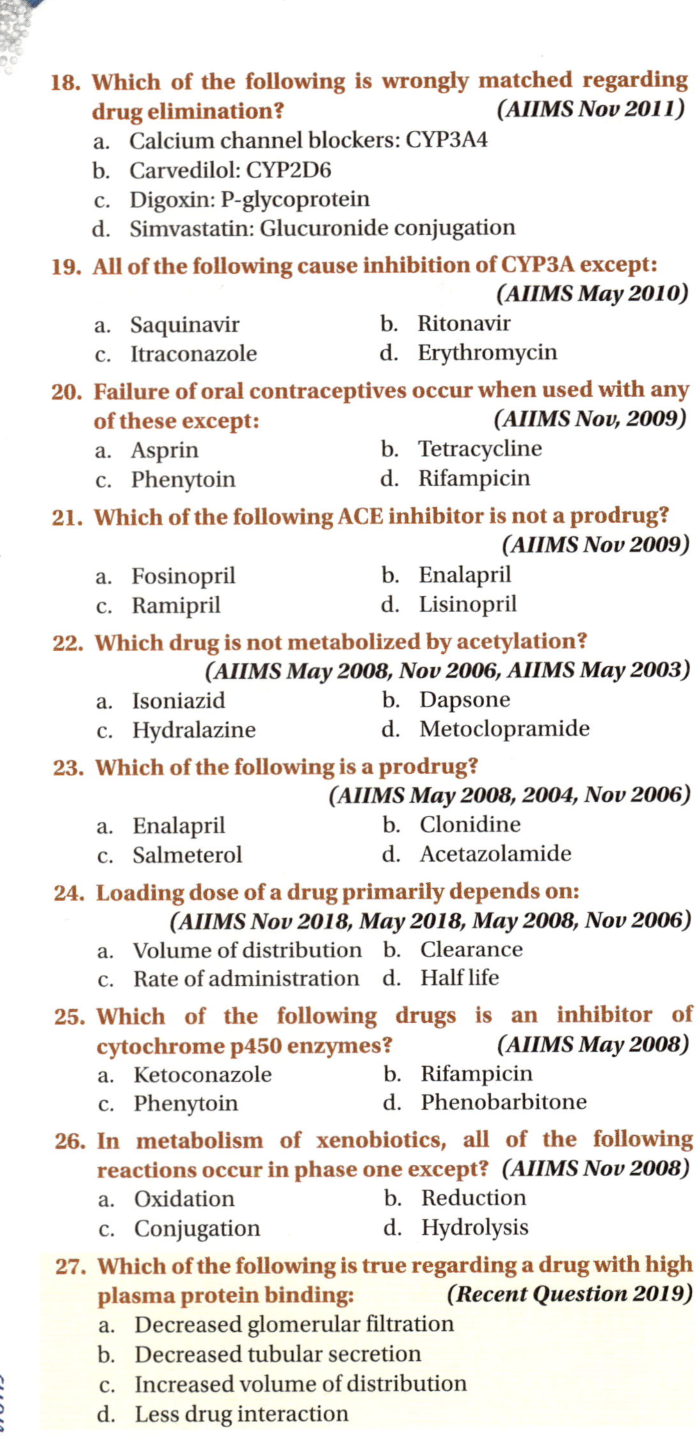

18. Which of the following is wrongly matched regarding drug elimination? ***(AIIMS Nov 2011)***

a. Calcium channel blockers: CYP3A4
b. Carvedilol: CYP2D6
c. Digoxin: P-glycoprotein
d. Simvastatin: Glucuronide conjugation

19. All of the following cause inhibition of CYP3A except: ***(AIIMS May 2010)***

a. Saquinavir b. Ritonavir
c. Itraconazole d. Erythromycin

20. Failure of oral contraceptives occur when used with any of these except: ***(AIIMS Nov, 2009)***

a. Asprin b. Tetracycline
c. Phenytoin d. Rifampicin

21. Which of the following ACE inhibitor is not a prodrug? ***(AIIMS Nov 2009)***

a. Fosinopril b. Enalapril
c. Ramipril d. Lisinopril

22. Which drug is not metabolized by acetylation? ***(AIIMS May 2008, Nov 2006, AIIMS May 2003)***

a. Isoniazid b. Dapsone
c. Hydralazine d. Metoclopramide

23. Which of the following is a prodrug? ***(AIIMS May 2008, 2004, Nov 2006)***

a. Enalapril b. Clonidine
c. Salmeterol d. Acetazolamide

24. Loading dose of a drug primarily depends on: ***(AIIMS Nov 2018, May 2018, May 2008, Nov 2006)***

a. Volume of distribution b. Clearance
c. Rate of administration d. Half life

25. Which of the following drugs is an inhibitor of cytochrome p450 enzymes? ***(AIIMS May 2008)***

a. Ketoconazole b. Rifampicin
c. Phenytoin d. Phenobarbitone

26. In metabolism of xenobiotics, all of the following reactions occur in phase one except? ***(AIIMS Nov 2008)***

a. Oxidation b. Reduction
c. Conjugation d. Hydrolysis

27. Which of the following is true regarding a drug with high plasma protein binding: ***(Recent Question 2019)***

a. Decreased glomerular filtration
b. Decreased tubular secretion
c. Increased volume of distribution
d. Less drug interaction

28. Beta phase of semilog of plasma concentration and time is due to drug ***(Recent Question Dec 2016)***

a. Metabolism b. Excretion
c. First Pass metabolism d. Distribution

29. Drug transport across the cell membrane mainly by: ***(Recent Question Dec 2016)***

a. Passive transport b. Active
c. Facilitated d. Pinocytosis

30. Drug inhibiting the P-glycoprotein is: ***(Recent Question Dec 2016)***

a. Chloramphenicol b. Ketoconazole
c. Tetracycline d. Erythromycin

31. Which of the following is a pro drug? ***(Recent Question 2016)***

a. Ampicillin b. Captopril
c. Levodopa d. Phenytoin

32. Zero order kinetics is shown by all except: ***(Recent Question 2016)***

a. High dose salicylates b. Phenytoin
c. Ethanol d. Methotrexate

33. Ciprofloxacin should not be given to an asthmatic using theophylline because: ***(Recent Question 2016)***

a. Ciprofloxacin inhibits theophylline metabolism
b. Theophylline inhibits ciprofloxacin metabolism
c. Ciprofloxacin decreases effect of theophylline
d. Theophylline induces metabolism of ciprofloxacin

34. Isoniazide is metabolized by ***(Recent Question 2016)***

a. Acetylation b. Oxidation
c. Reduction d. Hydrolysis

35. False regarding Cytochrome P 450 is: ***(Recent Question 2016)***

a. They are essential for the production of cholesterols, steroids, prostacyclins and thromboxane A2
b. They absorb light with 450nm wavelength
c. They occur predominantly in liver
d. They are non-heme proteins

36. Glucuronidation takes place in ***(Recent Question 2016)***

a. Liver b. RBC
c. Pancreas d. Thyroid

37. A drug having 40% absorption and hepatic extraction ratio of 0.6. What is the bioavailability of that drug? ***(Recent Question 2016)***

a. 16%
b. 24%
c. 20%
d. 28%

38. Maintainence dose is calculated by using value of: ***(Recent Question 2016)***

a. Clearance
b. Volume of distribution
c. Oral bioavailability
d. Daily dosage

39. Action of theophylline is reduced by: ***(Recent Question 2016)***

a. Smoking
b. Erythromycin
c. Cimetidine
d. Lithium

40. Xenobiotics are metabolized to: ***(Recent Question 2016)***

a. Increase water solubility b. Increase lipid solubility
c. Make them nonpolar d. None of the above

41. About rectal route true is: ***(Recent Question 2016)***

a. Used for irritant and unpleasant drugs
b. Cannot be used in unconscious patient
c. There is predictable absorption of drug
d. Diazepam cannot be given via rectal route of administration

42. Plasma protein bound drug distributed in which compartment: ***(Recent Question 2016)***

a. Extracellular b. Intravascular
c. Interstitial d. Extravascular

43. **Following are the advantages of sustained release preparation over the conventional preparations except:** *(Recent Question 2016)*
   a. Decreased frequency of administration
   b. Improved compliance
   c. Less incidence of high peak side effects
   d. Drugs with half-life > 4 hours are suitable

44. **Following drugs show zero order** *(Recent Question 2016)*
   a. Phenytoin b. Tolbutamide
   c. Alcohol d. Fomepizole

45. **Most variable absorption is seen with which route** *(Recent Question 2016)*
   a. Oral b. Intramscular
   c. Intravenous d. Per rectal

46. **Which of the following drug substrate combinations do not match- combinations do not match:** *(Recent Question 2016)*
   a. CYP 3A4/5 – simvastatin
   b. CYP 2D6 – SSRI
   c. CYP 2C8/9 – mifepristone
   d. CYP 2C19 - propranolol

47. **Which does not affect metabolism of oral contraceptive pill** *(Recent Question 2016)*
   a. Phenytoin b. Gresiofulvin
   c. Primidone d. Penicillin

48. **Most common mitochondrial enzyme for metabolism detoxification reaction is:** *(Recent Question 2016)*
   a. CYP 3A4 b. CYP 1A2
   c. CYP 2A6 d. CYP 2B6

49. **Alkaline dieresis is done for treatment of poisoning due to** *(Recent Question 2016)*
   a. Morphine b. Amphetamine
   c. Phenobarbitone d. Atropine

50. **Which of the following is a prodrug?** *(Recent Question 2016)*
   a. Enalapril b. Clonidine
   c. Salmeterol d. Acetazolamide

51. **Which of the following drugs should be removed by dialysis?** *(Recent Question 2016)*
   a. Digoxin b. Salicylates
   c. Benzodiazepines d. Organophosphates

52. **Urinary alkalinizing agents are administered in case of poisoning due to drugs which are:** *(Recent Question 2016)*
   a. Weak bases
   b. Weak acids
   c. Strong bases
   d. Strong acids

53. **Drug administered by intranasal route?** *(Recent Question 2016)*
   a. Adrenaline
   b. Desmopressin
   c. Ganirelix
   d. Insulin

54. **Major mechanism of transport of drugs across biological membranes is by** *(Recent Question 2016)*
   a. Passive diffusion b. Facilitated diffusion
   c. Active transport d. Endocytosis

55. **Induction of microsomal enzymes can result in:** *(Recent Question 2016)*
   a. Tolerance
   b. Dependence
   c. Super sensitivity to a drug
   d. Toxicity of a drug

56. **Thiopentone is used for induction of anesthesia. It shows marked redistribution which is a characteristic of:** *(Recent Question 2016)*
   a. Highly lipid soluble drugs
   b. Highly water soluble drugs
   c. Weak electrolytes
   d. Highly plasma protein bound drugs

57. **Most common phase II drug metabolizing reaction** *(Recent Question 2016)*
   a. Glucuronidation
   b. Acetylation
   c. Oxidation
   d. Glutathione conjugation

58. **Detoxification of drugs is controlled by** *(Recent Question 2016)*
   a. Cytochrome B
   b. Cytochrome p450
   c. Cytochrome C
   d. Cytochrome A

59. **Elimination after 4 half-life in first order kinetics** *(Recent Question 2016)*
   a. 84%
   b. 93%
   c. 80%
   d. 75%

60. **Drugs with high plasma protein binding have** *(Recent Question 2016)*
   a. Short duration of action
   b. Less drug interactions
   c. Lower volumes of distribution
   d. All of the above

61. **Drug not having active metabolite** *(Recent Question 2016)*
   a. Diazepam
   b. Propranolol
   c. Allopurinol
   d. Lisinopril

62. **First pass metabolism is seen in all except** *(Recent Question 2016)*
   a. Insulin b. Propranolol
   c. Lignocaine d. Isoprenaline

63. **Removal of acidic drugs from body is done by** *(Recent Question 2016)*
   a. Ammonium chloride
   b. Sodium bicarbonate
   c. Hydrochloric acid
   d. Citric acid

64. **The elimination of alcohol follows:** *(Recent Question 2016)*
   a. Zero order kinetics
   b. 1st order kinetics
   c. 2nd order kinetics
   d. 3rd order kinetics

65. **Which of the following is excreted in saliva?** *(Recent Question 2016)*
   a. Tetracyclines
   b. Ampicillin
   c. Lithium
   d. Chloramphenicol

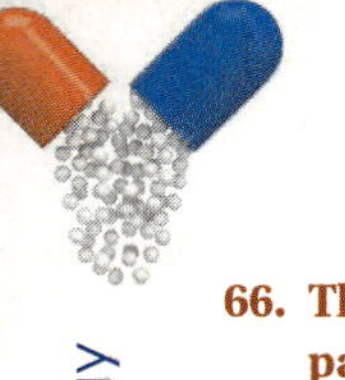

66. The pharmacokinetics change occurring in geriatric patients is decline in *(Recent Question 2016)*
a. Gastric absorption
b. Liver metabolism
c. Renal clearance
d. Hypersensitivity

67. Redistribution phenomenon is seen in *(Recent Question 2016)*
a. Halothane b. Ether
c. Thiopentone d. All

68. Which of the following is not a prodrug? *(Recent Question 2016)*
a. Enalapril b. Imipramine
c. Sulphasalazine d. Cyclophosphamide

69. Potential microsomal enzymes inhibitor drug is *(Recent Question 2016)*
a. Phenobarbitone b. Griseofulvin
c. Sodium valproate d. Phenytoin

70. Drug having the least oral bioavailability *(Recent Question 2016)*
a. d-tubocurarine b. Morphine
c. Ampicillin d. Phenytoin

71. Potent microsomal enzyme inducer drug is *(Recent Question 2016)*
a. Captopril b. Erythromycin
c. Rifampicin d. Cimetidine

72. True about zero order kinetics *(Recent Question 2016)*
a. Constant fraction of the drug is eliminated per unit time.
b. Dependent on plasma concentration
c. Constant amount of the drug is eliminated per unit time
d. Half-life is constant

73. Most common cytochrome associated with drug metabolism *(Recent Question 2016)*
a. CYP3A b. CYP2C
c. CYP2D6 d. CYPA1E

74. Inducer of cytochrome p-450 *(Recent Question 2016)*
a. Rifampicin b. Dicumarol
c. Disulfiram d. Penicillin

75. Inhibitor of cytochrome p-450 *(Recent Question 2016)*
a. Rifampicin
b. Phenytoin
c. Theophylline
d. Omeprazole

76. Volume of distribution V_d <5 indicates that the drug is *(Recent Question 2016)*
a. Inside the cell
b. Within vascular compartment
c. ECF
d. Interstitial fluid

77. Which of the following is an effect of grapefruit juice on drug metabolism? *(Recent Question 2016)*
a. Enzyme inducer
b. Enzyme inhibitor
c. Inhibits tubular secretion
d. Inhibits tubular reabsorption

78. Which of the following drug is highly albumin bound? *(Recent Question 2016)*
a. Propranolol b. Tricyclic anti-depressants
c. Barbiturate d. Quinidine

79. Zero order kinetics is independent of: *(Recent Question 2016)*
a. Plasma concentration b. Clearance
c. Volume of distribution d. Half-life

80. Which is true about a prodrug? *(Recent Question 2016)*
a. Drug which is active and is converted into an active metabolite
b. Drug that is given before an active drug to increase its action
c. Drug which is inactive and converted to active metabolite in body
d. Drug which is active and converted in inactive metabolite

81. Which amongst the following is a prodrug? *(Recent Question 2016)*
a. Candesartan b. Lisinopril
c. Ramiipril d. Telmisartan

82. Drug not metabolized by acetylation is *(Recent Question 2016)*
a. Salicylates b. PAS
c. Dapsone d. Procainamide

83. Drug not given sublingually is *(Recent Question 2016)*
a. Isosorbide dinitrate b. Buprenorphine
c. Ergotamine tartrate d. Isosobide-5-mononitrate

84. Kinetics of phenytoin *(Recent Question 2016)*
a. Zero order b. First order
c. Pseudo zero order d. All of the above

85. Drug maintenance dose is calculated by *(Recent Question 2016)*
a. Amount of drug eliminated/Time taken
b. Rate of elimination of a drug/Plasma concentration
c. C_L × Target plasma concentration
d. V_d × Target plasma concentration

86. Which of the following do not increase the action of warfarin? *(DS2'2012)*
a. Cimetidine b. Lsoniazid
c. Rifampicin d. Cotrimoxazole

87. All of the following increases effect of warfarin EXCEPT? *(DS2'2012)*
a. Cimetidine b. Disulfiram
c. Cotrimoxazole d. Griseofulvin

88. Zero order kinetics occurs in following drug? *(Recent Question 2003)*
a. Phenytoin and ethanol
b. Digoxin and propranolol
c. Amiloride and probenecid
d. Lithium and theophylline

89. The clearance of drug means? *(Recent Question 2002)*
a. Unit volume of plasma which is cleared off drug in unit of time
b. Amount of drug excreted in urine
c. Amount of drug metabolized in unit of time
d. All of the above

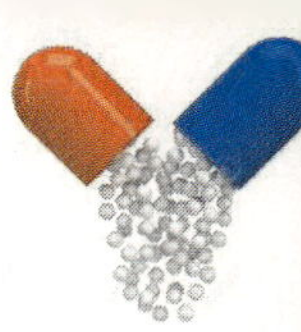

90. Theophyline levels in blood are increased by?
(Recent Question 2000)
a. Barbiturates
b. Methotrexate
c. Cimetidine
d. All of the above

91. Chloramphenicol does not increases the blood level of which drug? *(Recent Question 2008)*
a. Phenytoin
b. Tolbutamide
c. Phenylbutazone
d. Cyclophosphamide

92. Dialysis is contraindicated in? *(Recent Question 2000)*
a. Hyperkalemia
b. Hypercalcemia
c. Aspirin
d. Digitalis toxicity

93. All decrease effectiveness of OC pills except:
(Recent Question 2007)
a. Rifampicin
b. Phenytoin
c. Phenobarbitone
d. Ketoconazole

PHARMACODYNAMICS

94. Diamox is given for glaucoma, which is a noncompetitive antagonist of carbonic anhydrase. The effect is:
(AIIMS Nov 2018)
a. Increase in K_m and V_{max}
b. Decrease in K_m
c. Decrease in V_{max}
d. No change in V_{max}

95. Which of the following receptor is GPCR?
(AIIMS May 2018)
a. Muscarinic
b. Nicotinic
c. GABA
d. Insulin

96. Which of the following statement is correct regarding the given DRCs? *(AIIMS Nov 2016)*

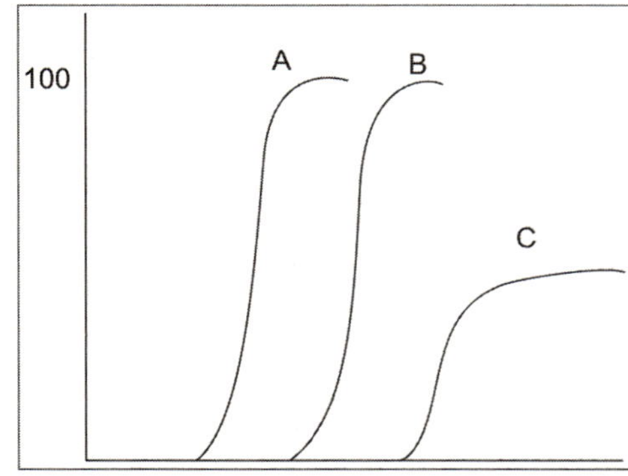

a. A and B are full agonists
b. C is noncompetitive antagonist
c. B more potent than A
d. A more efficacious than B

97. The neurotransmitters; noradrenaline, adrenaline and dopamine act through which of the following receptors?
(AIIMS Nov 2011)
a. Single pass transmembrane receptors
b. Four pass transmembrane receptors
c. Seven pass transmembrane receptors
d. Ligand gated receptors

98. True about G protein coupled receptors is:
(AIIMS May 2008)
a. G proteins bind to hormones on the cell surface
b. All the three subunits alpha, beta and gamma should bind to each other for G proteins to act
c. G proteins act as inhibitory and excitatory because of difference in alpha subunit
d. G protein is bound to GTP in resting state

99. All are second messengers except: *(AIIMS Nov 2008)*
a. Cyclic amp
b. Guanylyl cyclase
c. Diacylglycerol
d. Inositol triphosphate

100. Action of alpha subunit of G-protein is:
(AIIMS Nov 2008)
a. Binding of agonist
b. Conversion of GDP to GTP
c. Breakdown of GTP to GDP
d. Internalization of receptors

101. Quantal DRC, true is: *(Recent Question 2019)*
a. Response in population seen with increasing dose of drug
b. Efficacy calculated
c. Potency calculated
d. Affinity calculated

102. GABA B is which type of receptor?
(Recent Question 2018)
a. Ligand gated
b. Nuclear
c. GPCR
d. Enzymatic

103. When two drugs acting on different receptors have opposite action, it is known as:
(Recent Question Dec 2016)
a. Physiological antagonism
b. Competitive antagonism
c. Non-competitive antagonism
d. Chemical antagonism

104. Which of the following is a JAK receptor?
(Recent Question Dec 2016)
a. Prolactin
b. Estrogen
c. TSH
d. TRH

105. In competitive inhibition, true is:
(Recent Question Dec 2016)
a. K_m increased, V_{max} unchanged
b. K_m unchanged
c. Both K_m & V_{max} increase
d. V_{max} increases, K_m unchange

106. Which of the following terms best describes the antagonism of leukotriene's bronchoconstrictor effect (mediated at the leukotriene receptor) by terbutaline (acting at adrenoreceptors) in a patient with asthma?
(Recent Question 2016)
a. Pharmacologic antagonist
b. Partial agonist
c. Physiologic antagonist
d. Chemical antagonist

107. 1, 25 dihydrocholecalciferol acts on:
(Recent Question 2016)
a. Surface receptors
b. Cytosolic receptors
c. Intranuclear receptors
d. None of the above

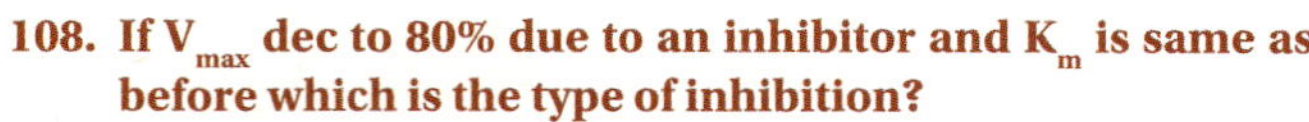

108. If V_{max} dec to 80% due to an inhibitor and K_m is same as before which is the type of inhibition? *(Recent Question 2016)*
a. Competitive Equilibrium type
b. Noncompetitive
c. Competitive Non Equilibrium type
d. None of the above

109. Agonist antagonist combination acting on the same receptor is *(Recent Question 2016)*
a. Isoprenaline and propranolol
b. Adrenaline and histamine
c. Salbutamol and leukotriene
d. Estrogen and tamoxifen

110. Which of the following property of the drug will enable it to be used in low concentration? *(Recent Question 2016)*
a. High affinity
b. High specificity
c. Low specificity
d. High stability

111. A partial agonist has *(Recent Question 2016)*
a. High affinity but low intrinsic activity
b. High affinity but no intrinsic activity
c. Low affinity but high intrinsic activity
d. Low affinity but low intrinsic activity

112. Which of the following drugs act through heptahelical (serpentine) receptors? *(Recent Question 2016)*
a. Insulin
b. Estrogen
c. Local anesthetics
d. Salbutamol

113. Antagonism between acetylcholine and atropine: *(Recent Question 2016)*
a. Competitive antagonism
b. Physiological antagonism
c. Noncompetitive antagonism
d. None

114. Agonist is having *(Recent Question 2016)*
a. Affinity with intrinsic activity is 1
b. Affinity with intrinsic activity is 0
c. Affinity with intrinsic activity is -1
d. None

115. Efficacy of a drug meas *(Recent Question 2016)*
a. Maximum absorption of a drug
b. Maximum metabolism of a drug
c. Maximum response that can be elicited by the drug
d. Maximum binding to its receptor

116. Heparin and protamine sulfate is an example of *(Recent Question 2016)*
a. Physical antagonism
b. Chemical antagonism
c. Competitive antagonism
d. Noncompetitive antagonism

117. Which of the following is an example of endogenous/ physiological antagonism? *(Recent Question 2016)*
a. Heparin-Protamine
b. Prostacyclin-Thromboxane
c. Adrenaline-Phenoxybenzamine
d. Physostigmine-Acetylcholine

118. When a drug binds to the receptor and causes action opposite to that of agonist this is called as? *(Recent Question 2016)*
a. Complete agonist
b. Inverse agonist
c. Partial agonist
d. Neutral antagonist

119. When a drug binds to the receptor and causes action submaximal to that of agonist this is called as: *(Recent Question 2016)*
a. Complete agonist
b. Partial agonist
c. Inverse agonist
d. Neutral antagonist

120. Potency of a drug is a measure of its: *(Recent Question 2016)*
a. Dose
b. Efficacy
c. Safety
d. Therapeutic index

121. U shaped dose response curve is seen in: *(Recent Question 2016)*
a. Vitamins
b. Anti-cancer drugs
c. Steroids
d. Chelators

122. Regarding 1st order drug kinetics, which of the following is true: *(PGI May 2018)*
a. Constant fraction of drug is eliminated per unit time
b. Rate of elimination has no correlation with concentration of drug
c. As concentration of drugs increases, rate of elimination increases
d. Elimination half-life is dose dependent
e. Clearance (CL) increases as drug concentration increases

123. True about 1st order kinetics: *(PGI Nov 2017)*
a. Variable t1/2
b. Fraction eliminated is constant
c. Amount eliminated is constant
d. Variable clearance

124. Competitive antagonist true is: *(PGI Nov 2017)*
a. Shift of the drug response curve parallel to right
b. Low efficacy
c. Low potency
d. Shift of drug response curve to left non-parallel

125. A drug has V_d = 70L, clearance = 350 mL/min. In case of renal failure where renal function is 50%, which of the following is true? *(PGI Nov 2017)*
a. High loading dose
b. Low maintenance dose
c. V_d will be same = 70 L
d. Clearance = 700 mL/min
e. t1/2 will be same

126. Which of the following is/are true about First order kinetics: *(PGI May 2017)*
a. Applied to majority of drugs
b. Rate of elimination is directly proportional to the drug concentration
c. Very few drug follow it
d. Clearance decreases with increase in concentration

127. Which of the following is/are true about pharmacodynamics of drugs: *(PGI NOV 2016)*
a. Affinity means how strongly drug binds to receptor
b. Efficacy means maximal effect by a drug
c. Irreversible antagonist mainly forms ionic bonds with receptor
d. Agonist potency depends on two parameters: affinity and efficacy
e. For antagonists, efficacy is zero

128. All are true about plasma protein binding except: ***(PGI Nov. 2016)***
a. Acidic drugs generally bind to plasma albumin and basic drugs to a1 acid glycoprotein
b. Plasma binding determines volume of distribution
c. More plasma protein binding means more storage in liver
d. More plasma protein binding means less penetration in vascular membrane
e. High degree of protein binding generally makes the drug long acting

129. First pass metabolism is significant problem in drug given through: ***(PGI Nov. 2016)***
a. Sublingual route
b. Rectal route
c. Intramuscular route
d. Directly into stomach
e. Directly into large intestine

130. Which of the following drug interact with Warfarin: ***(PGI Nov 2014/May 2014)***
a. ACE inhibitor b. Azithromycin
c. Fluconazole d. Aspirin
e. Benzodiazepine

131. Which of the following is/are true regarding plasma concentration time curve of a drug: ***(PGI Nov 2014/May 2014)***
a. Peak concentration determine bioavailability
b. Intramuscular administration have curve different from oral administration
c. Area under curve determine therapeutic response
d. Bioavailability of an orally administered drug can be calculated by comparing the area under curve after oral & after i.v. administration
e. Changes in the rate of absorption and extent of bioavailability can influence both the duration of action and the effectiveness of the same total dose of a drug administered in different formulations

132. Which of the following pair of G receptors is correctly matched with its action: ***(PGI May 2014)***
a. Gi- Activation of calcium channel
b. Gq- ↑ cytoplasmic calcium
c. Gs- Opening of calcium channel
d. Go- Opening of potassium channel
e. Gt- Activation of potassium channel

133. A person has given 0.175 g oral digoxin with bioavailability 70%. The amount of drug reaching in systemic circulation is: ***(PGI May 2014)***
a. 0.175 b. 0.175×0.7
c. 0.175/7 d. $0.175 + 0.7$
e. $0.175 + 1/0.7$

134. Which of the following is/are true about Zero Order kinetics: ***(PGI Nov 2013)***
a. Rate of elimination remains constant irrespective of drug concentration
b. Constant amount of drug is excreted
c. T1/2 decreases with dose
d. Clearance decreases with increase in concentration
e. Clearance remain constant

135. Drugs, which are enzyme inducers: ***(PGI Nov 2013)***
a. Rifampicin b. Ketoconazole
c. Phenytoin d. Griseofulvin

136. Isoniazid is metabolised in body by: ***(PGI May 2013)***
a. Acetylation b. Sulfation
c. Hydroxylation d. Methylation
e. First metabolized in liver and then excreted in urine

137. Regarding drug transport which of the following is/ are true except: ***(PGI May 2013)***
a. Active transport: it is energy dependent
b. Passive diffusion: Most common method of drug transport
c. Faciliated diffusion: not need energy
d. Faciliated diffusion: carrier mediated diffusion
e. Pinocytosis: transport by diffusion

138. KD constant of drug-receptor interactions is: ***(PGI May 2013)***
a. Concentration of drug at which half the receptors are bound
b. Concentration of drug at which maximal response is seen
c. Concentration at which antagonist is able to bind to half of the receptors
d. Concentration of drug at which half of the maximal response is seen

139. Repeated i.v bolus dose of a drug is given to a person. Correct statement regarding the drug is/are: ***(PGI Nov 2011)***
a. No significant change in T1/2 if drug follow zero order kinetics
b. Increase in T1/2 if drug follow first order kinetics
c. Steady state Plama concentration increases with linear relation on increasing dose rate in case of drug eliminated by first order kinetics
d. Steady state plama concentration increases with linear relation on increasing dose rate in case of drug eliminated by zero order kinetics
e. 87.5% of drug is eliminated in 3 T1/2

140. True statement about bioavailability of orally administered drug: ***(PGI Nov 2011)***
a. First pass metabolism occur in gut
b. First pass metabolism occur in liver
c. Bioavailability is 100%
d. Depends on extent of absorption
e. Enterohepatic circulation leads to reabsorption of some drugs like estrogen

141. Non-medicinal substance that causes enzyme induction: ***(PGI May 2011)***
a. Grape juice b. Ecstasy (MDMA)
c. Hyperforin d. DDT
e. St. John's wort

142. Which of the following drug will be more absorbed from stomach: ***(PGI May 2011)***
a. pKa 3.4 for weakly basic drug
b. pKa 3.4 for weakly acidic drug
c. pKa 6.4 for weakly basic drug
d. pKa 6.4 for weakly acidic drug
e. Not affected by pKa value

143. Which of the following is prodrug: *(PGI May 2011)*
a. Sulindac b. Scholine
c. Bitolterol d. Tyramine
e. Lisonopril

144. Theophylline toxicity level is increased by all except: *(PGI May 2010)*
a. Smoking b. Carbamazepine
c. Alcohol intake d. Rifampicin
e. Ciprofloxacin

145. Following are drugs except: *(PGI May 2010)*
a. Nutrients b. Blood component
c. Essential dietary ingredient
d. Poison

146. Volume of distribution depends on: *(PGI Nov 2009/June 2009)*
a. Protein binding b. Lipid solubility
c. Glomerular secretion d. Tissue affinity
e. pKa

147. True about active transport of the drug: *(PGI June 2009)*
a. Carrier mediated b. Requires ATP (energy)
c. Transport drugs along concentration gradient
d. Saturation occurs

148. CYP 3A inhibitors is/are: *(PGI June 2009)*
a. Ritonavir b. Amiodarone
c. Verapamil d. Rifampin
e. Barbiturates

149. True about competitive inhibition: *(PGI June 2009)*
a. Raise V_{max} & K_m
b. Inhibitors bind to substance binding site on enzyme
c. Example is malonate
d. Inhibitor resemble structurally to the substance

150. True about competitive antagonist: *(PGI June 2009)*
a. Maximum rate of reaction can be attained by increasing agonist concentration
b. ED50 remain same with or without antagonist
c. Binding site of agonist & antagonist are essentially same
d. Reversal of blockade by antagonist can be achieved by higher dose of agonist

151. Which of the following HIV drug inhibit drug metabolizing enzymes: *(PGI Nov 2008)*
a. Ritonavir b. Lamivudine
c. Nevirapine d. Delavirdine
e. Enfuvirtide

152. Which of the following statement (s) is/are true regarding drug transport mechanism: *(PGI Nov 2008)*
a. Facilitated diffusion require energy
b. Faciliated diffusion is carrier mediated
c. Active transport is carrier mediated
d. Passive diffusion is same as faciliated diffusion
e. Faciliated diffusion may transport against concentration gradient

153. Absorption of drug in gut is decreased by: *(PGI Nov 2008)*
a. Food b. Nonionised state
c. First pass metebolism d. Small size of particle
e. Increase expression of p-glycoprotein

154. A drug has Volume of distribution of 13.6 L/kg. Which of the following statement is/are true: *(PGI Nov 2008)*
a. It is present in plasma & interstitium
b. Confined to extracellular intravascular space
c. Hemodialysis is effective
d. Substance solubility is more
e. Less protein bound

155. Following are prodrug except: *(PGI June 2008)*
a. Enalapril b. Diazepam
c. Lisinopril d. Cyclophosphamide

156. True about first- pass metabolism: *(PGI June 2008)*
a. Only seen in orally taking drugs
b. High rectal administration, less first pass metabolism
c. Vomiting affect first pass metabolism
d. Affected by portal and gastrointestinal endothelium
e. Prodrug has low first- pass metabolism

157. Physiological antagonism found in: *(PGI Nov 2007)*
a. Isoprenaline & Salbutamol
b. Isoprenaline & Adrenalin
c. Isoprenaline & Propanolol
d. Adrenaline & Histamine

158. Which is a prodrug: *(PGI Nov 2007)*
a. Cyclophosphamide b. Lisinopril
c. Metochlorpramide d. Ranitidine
e. Eptifibatide

159. Which is a pro-drug: *(Recent Question 2016)*
a. Cyclophosphamide b. Lisinopril
c. Metochlorpramide d. Ranitidine
e. Eptifibatide

160. Narrow therapeutic index are seen in: *(Recent Question 2016)*
a. Metfomin b. Phenytoin
c. Cyclosporin d. Digitalis

161. Hemodialysis is *not* useful in: *(PGI June 2007)*
a. Benzodiazepines b. Methanol
c. Digitalis d. Theophylline
e. Salicylates

162. On I.V. drug administration, elimination of a drug depend on: *(PGI Nov 2006)*
a. Lipid solubility b. Volume of distribution
c. Clearance d. Drug concentration

163. IV drug duration of action depends on: *(PGI June 2006)*
a. Protein binding b. Clearance
c. Volume of distribution d. Lipid solubility

164. Drug transport mechanism include: *(PGI June 2006)*
a. Active transport b. Passive transport
c. Lipid solubility

165. Causes for less bioavailability: *(PGI June 2006)*
a. High first pass metabolism
b. Increased absorption
c. IV drug administration
d. High solubility

166. CYP 3A4 affected by *(PGI Nov 2005)*
a. Fexofenadine b. Phenytoin
c. Carbamazapine

167. Which of the following is not true ***(PGI Nov 2005)***
a. If drug administered rectally it follow '1' order kinetics
b. If drug administered I.M. it follows '0' order kinetics
c. If drug administered I.V. it follows '1' order kinetics
d. Bioavailability is lower after oral administration

168. CYP-450 inducers are: ***(PGI June 2005)***
a. Cimetidine b. Ketoconazole
c. Phenobarbitone d. DDT
e. Theophylline

169. Drug distribution is influenced by: ***(PGI June 2005)***
a. Drug binding b. Drug solubility
c. Degree of blood flow d. Age

170. Type of receptor of oxytocin? ***(JIPMER Nov 2018)***
a. Gq b. Cytoplasmic / nuclear
c. Cytokines mediated d. Tyrosine kinase

171. Phospholipase c acts via? ***(JIPMER Nov 2018)***
a. Gs b. Gq
c. Gi d. G12

172. IGF-1 acts on which type of receptor?
a. Tyrosine kinase ***(JIPMER Nov 2018)***
b. Nuclear/Cytoplasmic
c. JAK STAT
d. GPCR

173. False regarding volume of distribution is:
a. Proportional to T1/2 ***(JIPMER Nov 2018)***
b. Equal to the log of 2 multiplied with half-life
c. Skeletal muscle relaxants have low volume of distribution
d. High plasma protein bound drugs have low volume of distribution

174. IP3 increases intracellular: ***(JIPMER Nov 2018)***
a. Na b. Cl
c. Ca d. K

175. A patient comes 6 hours after consuming morphine and presents with pin point pupils and respiratory depression. T ½ of morphine is 3 hours and Volume of distribution (V_d) is 200 L. Plasma concentration is 0.5 microgram/ml. Calculate the initial morphine dose consumed. ***(JIPMER May 2018)***
a. 100 mg b. 400 mg
c. 10 mg d. 50 mg

176. Drug that does not cross transdermally is: ***(JIPMER 2017)***
a. Scopalamine b. Nitroglycerine
c. Clonidine d. Dexmeditomidine

177. Which of the following drugs does not bind to alpha-1 acid glycoprotein? ***(JIPMER 2017)***
a. Quinine b. Lidocaine
c. Propranolol d. Dipyridamole

178. The cause of OCP failure with ampicillin is:
a. Alteration of gut flora ***(JIPMER 2017)***
b. Enzyme induction
c. Enzyme inhibition
d. High plasma protein binding

179. True regarding loading dose are all except:
a. Achieves target levels fast ***(JIPMER 2014)***
b. Rapid activation of receptors
c. Depends on volume of distribution
d. Proportional to the half life of the drug

180. False regarding Cytochrome P450 is: ***(JIPMER 2013)***
a. Found only in bone marrow
b. CYP3A4 is the most common isoform
c. Participate in Phase 1 Xenobiotic reactions
d. They are present in Smooth Endoplasmic reticulum within cells

181. All are true regarding phase II biotransformation reaction except: ***(JIPMER 2013)***
a. Converts drug to lipid soluble
b. Introduces covalent bonds
c. Attachment of polar compounds
d. Produces large molecular weight product

182. Drug bound to alpha 1 acid glycoprotein are all except: ***(JIPMER 2012)***
a. Lignocaine b. Tolbutamide
c. Quinidine d. Propranolol

183. Which of the following is a Phase 1 reaction in Xenobiotics? ***(JIPMER 2011,2010)***
a. Hydroxylation b. Methylation
c. Conjugation d. Acetylation

184. All the following drugs inhibit cytochrome P-450 except: ***(JIPMER 2010)***
a. Alcohol b. Cyclophosphamide
c. Isoniazid d. Disulfiram

185. Carbamazepine toxicity is precipitated by:
a. Erythromycin b. Vitamin K ***(JIPMER 2007)***
c. Theophyllin d. Phenytoin

186. Which one of the following is not an NMDA receptor?
a. Kappa b. Kainite ***(JIPMER 2006)***
c. AMPA d. Glutamate

187. Rate of elimination of drug is: ***(JIPMER 2006)***
a. Clearance b. T1/2
c. Biotransformation d. Bioavailability

188. All have high hepatic clearance EXCEPT: ***(NIMHANS 2014)***
a. Labetalol b. Simvastatin
c. Morphine d. Paracetamol

189. All of the following are enzyme inducers of cytochrome EXCEPT ***(NIMHANS 2011)***
a. Phenytoin b. Rifampicin
c. Isoniazid d. Erythromycin

190. CYP_{450} is inhibited by ***(NIMHANS 2011)***
a. Ketoconazole b. Rifampin
c. Alcohol d. Phenytoin

191. Protein bound drug is ***(NIMHANS 2010)***
a. Propranolol b. Atenolol
c. Phenylbutazone d. Warfarin

192. Drug that does not follow nonlinear dose dependent saturation kinetics ***(NIMHANS 2009)***
a. Paracetamol b. Salicylates
c. Phenytoin d. Ethanol

Practice Questions & Answers from 193 to 224 are given at the end of the chapter.

Answers with Explanations to Multiple Choice Questions

1. Ans. (c) Tmax

(Ref: Goodman Gilman 13th E/P25)

- Tmax is the time required to achieve the maximum plasma concentration (Cmax) for a drug.
- Thus lesser is the Tmax, faster is absorption and vice versa. Hence Tmax tells us about the rate of drug absorption.

2. Ans. (c) Safety

(Ref: Goodman Gilman 13th E/P36)

3. Ans. (a) Intravenous

(Ref: Goodman Gilman 13th E/P17)

4. Ans. (a) Oral

(Ref: Goodman Gilman 13th E/P16)

- Hepatic first pass metabolism is encountered by oral and rectal routes of administration. The reason being by these routes drug is absorbed into enteric circulation and then it goes via portal vein into liver, which is responsible for first pass metabolism.
- Though by rectal route only 50% drug flows through portal vein and hence only 50% of drug undergoes first pass metabolism. Rest 50% is directly absorbed into inferior vena cava.

5. Ans. (a) 18

- 2 mL syringe has 10 divisions for each mL and hence each division measures = 2 mL/20 = .1 mL
- 500 mg of drug is in 5 mL and hence 100 mg is in 1 mL. Thus 180 mg is in 1.8 mL.
- So 0.1 mL in 1 division

1 mL in 1/.1 division

1.8 mL in 1/.1•1.8 = 18 divisions

6. Ans. (a) Large apparent volume of distribution

(Ref: Goodman Gilman 12th E/P24)

- Large volume of distribution indicates storage of drug in tissues.
- Small volume of distribution indicates presence of drug in plasma.

7. Ans. (d) 50 mg

First of all calculate the half life of drug:

Rate of drug elimination = 0.693 • Dose/T1/2

Here rate of drug elimination is 75/90 mg/min

Hence 75/90 = 0.693 • 200/T/1/2

Or T1/2 = 0.693•200• 90/75 = 166.32 minutes = approximately 3 hours.

So drug becomes 50% in 3 hours, i.e. 100 mg.

So in another 3 hours drug ll become 50% of 100 mg = 50 mg

8. Ans. (c) 0.002 mg/mL

The formula for infusion rate is similar to rate of drug elimination.

RDE = Infusion rate = PC at steady state • Cl

Or 1.6 = PC at steady state • 640

Or PC at steady state = 1.6/640 = 0.0025 mg/mL = 0.002 mg/mL

9. Ans. (a) Rifampicin

(Ref: Goodman Gilman 12th E/P91)

P glycoprotein inducers are similar to CYP3A4 enzyme inducers like

- Phenytoin
- Phenobarbital
- Rifampicin
- St. Johns wort
- Carbamazepine etc

10. Ans. (a) pH at which ionized fraction of drug equals to unionized fraction

(Ref: Goodman Gilman 12th E/P18)

pKa is the pH at which as drug is 50% ionized and 50% unionized, i.e. the fraction of ionized drug equals to the fraction of unionized drug.

11. Ans. (a) Post auricular >scrotum>scalp>dorsum of arm> plantar area

(Ref: Goodman Gilman 12th E/P1803)

- Permeability is inversely proportional to thickness of stratum corneum.
- Thickness of stratum corneum is least in postauricular area/face < Scrotum < Rest part < Palms/Soles

12. Ans. (b) Need for loading dose in order to give immediate effect

(Ref: Goodman Gilman 12th E/P37)

- Half-life tells us about the time we need to achieve steady state, i.e. 4–5 half lives.
- Thus for digoxin, it ll require 200 hours to achieve steady state.
- Hence to achieve steady state faster loading dose is given.

An 80 kg man is in shock. Vasopressor has to be started at 10microg/kg/min. One vial has 200 mg in 5 mL and 2 vials were diluted to 250 mL. If 16 drops = 1mL,

13. Ans. (b) 8

- Drug to be given per min = 80•10 = 800 mcg/min = 0.8 mg/min
- Total amount of drug given = 400 mg in 250 mL
- So in 1 mL we have = 400/250 mg

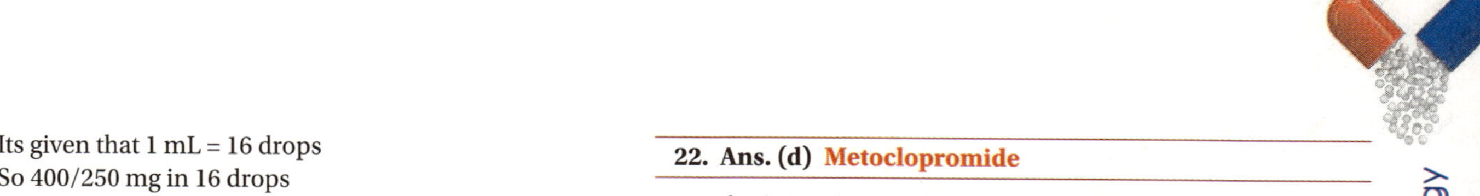

- Its given that 1 mL = 16 drops
- So 400/250 mg in 16 drops
- 0.8 mg is in 16•2500.8/400 = 8 drops
- **Thus to give 0.8 mg per min we have to give 8 drops/min.**

14. Ans. (b) Decreased distribution in tissues and organs

(Ref: Goodman Gilman 12th E/P31)

Low Volume of Distribution Means

- Decreased amount of drug in tissues and organs
- Increased amount of drug in plasma

15. Ans. (a) Nonionic and more lipid soluble

(Ref: Goodman Gilman 12th E/P18)

- Unionized drugs are lipid soluble which facilitates absorption.
- Ionized drugs are water soluble which facilitates excretion.

16. Ans. (a) Lisinopril

(Ref: Rang and Dale 6th E/P117)

- All ACEIs are prodrugs except captopril and lisinopril.

17. Ans. (b) Phenytoin

(Ref: Katzung 12th E/P58)

- Ritonavir is an enzyme inhibitor of CYP3A4 and hence inhibits metabolism of drugs which are substrate for CYP3A4.
- Phenytoin is not affected by ritonavir as phenytoin is metabolized primarily by CYP2C9.

18. Ans. (c) Digoxin: P-glycoprotein

(Ref: Katzung 12th E/P58)

- All drugs are metabolized by the CYP enzymes in the options.
- P-glycoprotein is an efflux pump and responsible for efflux of drug from the intestinal epithelium, which is a part of first pass effect. Thus it is a better answer.

19. Ans. (a) Saquinavir

(Ref: Katzung 12th E/P58)

- Though all drugs in the options are enzyme inhibitors, saquinavir is the least potent of all and is the best possible answer here.

20. Ans. (a) Aspirin

(Ref: Katzung 12th E/P58)

- Rifampicin and phenytoin being enzyme inducers can cause OCP failure by accelerating estrogen metabolism.
- Antibiotics like tetracycline can also cause OCP failure by inhibiting the enterohepatic circulation of estrogen.

21. Ans. (d) Lisinopril

(Ref: Rang and Dale 6th E/P117)

22. Ans. (d) Metoclopromide

(Ref: Goodman Gilman 12th E/P138)

Drugs Metabolized by Acetylation

D : Dapsone
I : Isoniazid
N : Nitrazepam
C : Clonazepam
H : Hydralazine
A : Acebutalol, Amantidine, Amrinone
K : K(c)affeine
Sexy : Sulfonamides
Padosan : Procainamide, Phenelezine

23. Ans. (a) Enalapril

(Ref: Rang and Dale 6th E/P117)

24. Ans. (a) Volume of distribution

(Ref: Goodman Gilman 12th E/P37)

Loading Dose

$$aV_d = D/C$$

or

$$D = aV_d \times C$$

The plasma concentration must be specific for a particular clinical effect. If drug has a high volume of distribution, then to maintain a specific plasma concentration, in the equation above we must increase the dose "D" of the drug. This increased dose of drug for drugs with high aV_d to maintain a specific plasma concentration is known as loading dose. Thus **loading dose depends on aV_d** and the formula for calculation is,

Loading dose (LD) = $aV_d \times C$

25. Ans. (a) Ketoconazole

(Ref: Katzung 12th E/P58)

26. Ans. (c) Conjugation

(Ref: Goodman Gilman 12th E/P138)

Reactions of Phase I and II

Mnemonics

Phase I: ORCHAD
O : Oxidation
R : Reduction
C: Cyclization
H : Hydrolysis
A : Aliphatic and aromatic hydroxylation
D : Deamination

Phase II: GAMS
G : Glucuronidation, Glutathionylation, Glycination
A : Acetylation
M : Methylation
S : Sulfation

In phase I grow fruits in an ORCHAD and then in phase II make fruit GAMS.

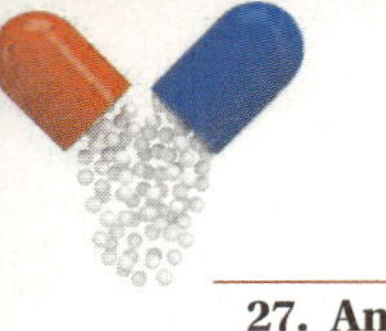

27. Ans. (a) Decreased glomerular filtration

(Ref: Goodman Gilman 13th E/P18)

- It is a basic concept in physiology that proteins can never get filtered out from a normal kidney as the glomerular bed is charged and proteins are also charged particles.
- Hence plasma protein bound drugs cannot undergo glomerular filtration.
- Though plasma protein bound drugs can undergo tubular secretion.

28. Ans. (b) Excretion

(Ref: Mark Tomlin's Pharmacology and Pharmacokinetics/P21)

In semilog of plasma concentration and time curve

- Alpha phase = Distribution
- Beta phase = Elimination

29. Ans. (a) Passive transport

(Ref: Goodman Gilma 12th E/P20)

Most common process of drug absorption is passive diffusion through lipid barrier and hence it is generalized that a drug is absorbed when it is in lipid soluble form.

30. Ans. (d) Erythromycin

(Ref: Harrison 19th E/P34)

Mnemonics

PgP Inhibitors

V : Verapamil
A : Amiodarone
C : Cyclosporine
I : Itraconazole
N : Nifedipine
E : Erythromycin

31. Ans. (c) Levodopa

(Ref: Rang and Dale 6th E/P117/KDT 7th E/P23)

Prodrugs List

- 5FU
- Capecitabine
- Cyclophosphamide
- 6 MP, 6 TG
- Flucytosine
- Mycophenolate mofetil
- All ACEIs except captopril and lisinopril
- ARBs like olmesartan and candesartan
- Statins like lovastatin and simvastatin
- **Levodopa**
- Methyldopa
- Carsioprodol
- Carbimazole
- Azathioprine
- Prednisone
- Cortisone
- Fluoxetine
- Proguanil
- Zidovudine

32. Ans. (d) Methotrexate

(Ref: Goodman Gilman 19th E/P 34)

Drugs Following Zero Order Kinetics

Mnemonics

Zero ATP Has Made Weaker

Zero

A : Aspirin, Alcohol
T : Theophylline, Tolbutamide
P : Phenytoin, Phenylbutazone
Has : Heparin
Made : Methanol
Weaker : Warfarin

33. Ans (a) Ciprofloxacin inhibits theophylline metabolism

(Ref: Goodman Gilman 19th E/P 130)

34. Ans. (a) Acetylation

(Ref: Goodman Gilman 12th E/P138)

35. Ans. (d) They are non-heme proteins

(Ref: Katzung 12th E/P55)

Drug Metabolism by CYP_{450} Enzymes

- In phase I the drugs are metabolized by reactions carried out by CYP_{450} enzymes, which are present in the endoplasmic reticulum (microsomal). Cytochrome is a **heme protein** which accepts oxygen for drug metabolism. In a CYP_{450} enzyme, e.g. CYP1A2, the first number denotes family (1), alphabet denotes subfamily (A) and last number denotes gene number (2). Most common CYP_{450} enzyme for drug metabolism is CYP3A4 followed by others.
- P3A4>CYP2D6>CYP2C9>CYP1A2>CYP2B6>CYP2C19).
- The number **450 denotes wavelength** as which they absorb light.
- Apart from drugs these enzymes also metabolize various exogenous chemicals that come from environment, food etc and together with drugs these are known as xenobiotics.
- CYP_{450} enzymes also synthesize endogenous products like **steroids** and **bile acids**.

36. Ans. (a) Liver

(Ref: Goodman Gilman 12th E/P129)

37. Ans. (a) 16%

(Ref: Goodman Gilman 12th E/P20)

- Suppose 100 mg of drugs was given to the patient.
- Since absorption is 40%, only 40 mg reaches to liver.
- Hepatic extraction ratio is 0.6, i.e. 60% is removed in liver (24 mg).
- Thus the drug that reaches the systemic circulation in unchanged form is 16 mg, which from 100 mg comes to 16%.
- Extraction ratio is the ability of an organ to remove the drug in a single pass. The value ranges from 0 to 1; 0 extraction ratio signifies drug is not at all removed by organ and 1signifies complete removal of drug by organ.

38. Ans. (a) Clearance

(Ref: Goodman Gilman 12th E/P34)

- Maintenance dose depends on clearance.
- Loading dose depends on volume of distribution.

39. Ans. (a) Smoking

(Ref: Katzung 12th E/P58)

- Cigarette smoke is an enzyme inducer and hence smoking can reduce the effect of theophylline.

40. Ans. (a) Increase water solubility

(Ref: Goodman Gilman 12th E/P139)

41. Ans. (a) Used for irritant and unpleasant drugs

(Ref: Goodman Gilman 12th E/P22)

Features of Rectal Route of Drug Administration

- 50% lesser first pass metabolism as from rectum 50% blood directly drains into IVC bypassing liver
- Unpleasant and irritant drugs can be given.
- Unreliable absorption and hence effect is unpredictable.
- Can be given in unconscious patients.
- Diazepam for febrile seizures in children when it is difficult to find an IV line.

42. Ans. (b) Intravascular

(Ref: Goodman Gilman 12th E/P24)

43. Ans. (d) Drugs with half-life > 4 hours are suitable

(Ref: Goodman Gilman 12th E/P21)

- By delaying drug action the **number of doses required considerably decreases** and hence **compliance increases.** Apart from this, there is a gradual rise in drug plasma concentration that is maintained throughout the day, thus **avoiding peaks of high** and **troughs of low plasma concentration.**
- For oral route **extended release formulations** are made, which can be **sustained release** or **controlled release** preparation. Sustained release (SR) preparations cause a prolonged release of drug thereby prolonging plasma concentration. SR formulations are made by combining drugs with polymers such as hydroxypropyl methyl cellulose. When drug is ingested first these polymers absorb water and then the drug is dissolved and released for absorption. SR drugs if taken with food, more amount of drug can be released **(dose dumping)**, which can cause toxicity.
- Controlled release (CR) preparations have a true control on drug release rate. CR formulations are made by coating the drug with permeable membrane. This membrane allows water into the core and dissolution and release of drug is controlled by the parameters of membrane like its thickness, number of pores, etc. These preparations are suitable for drugs with **half-life lesser than 4 hours**.

44. Ans. (d) Fomepizole

(Ref: Goodman Gilman 12th E/P34)

45. Ans. (a) Oral

(Ref: Goodman Gilman 12th E/P20)

Features of Oral Route

Benefits	Drawbacks	Drugs given
Cheapest Convenient Safest	First pass metabolism Most variable absorption due to various factors like lipid solubility, food intake, digestive enzymes, etc.	Most drugs Remember: A drug with suffix tide or ase (e.g. Octreotide, Nesiritide, Asparginase etc) are peptides. Hence these are broken down in GIT and never given by oral route.

46. Ans. (c) CYP 2C8/9 – mifepristone

(Ref: Katzung 12th E/P58)

- Mifepristone and statins are metabolized by CYP3A4 primarily.
- SSRI, TCA, antipsychotics and beta blockers (except propranolol by CYP2C19) are metabolized by CYP2D6.

47. Ans. (d) Penicillin

(Ref: Katzung 12th E/P58)

- The first three options are enzyme inducers and hence can cause OCP failure.
- Out of penicillins, amoxicillin and ampicillin are also associated with OCP failure by inhibition of enterohepatic circulation of estrogen.
- Thus here we don't have a correct answer, but if we have to go for one, penicillin is best answer as the specific penicillin has not been specified.

48. Ans. (a) CYP3A4

(Ref: Goodman Gilman 12th E/P129)

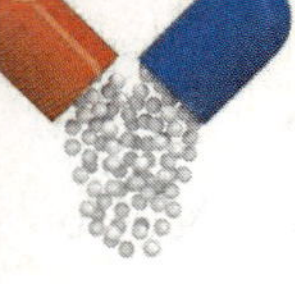

The sequence of CYP_{450} enzymes involvement in drug metabolism is CYP3A4>CYP2D6>CYP2C9>CYP1A2>CYP2B6>CYP2C19

49. Ans. (c) Phenobarbitone

(Ref: Goodman Gilman 12th E/P26)

Alkalinization of urine is done for toxicity of acidic drugs.

Acidic Drugs

Mnemonics

Weak ACID
- Weak : Warfarin
- A : Antiepileptic (Phenobarbital and Phenytoin), Anti-folate (Methotrexate and Sulphamethoxazole)
- C : Chlorthiazide
- I : Ibuprofen and Aspirin
- D : Dopamine prodrug (Levodopa)

50. Ans. (a) Enalapril

(Ref: Rang and Dale 6th E/P117, KDT 7th E/P23)

51. Ans. (b) Salicylates

(Ref: Goodman Gilman 12th E/P24)

Drugs with High Volume of Distribution

Drugs with high aV_d are lesser in plasma and hence **dialysis is not effective** for treatment of toxicity. Dialysis is also not effective in case of **irreversible binders** of target like organophosphates and carbamates, as drug does not come back to plasma.

Mnemonics

BAD DOC
- B : Benzodiazepines, Beta blockers
- A : Amphetamine
- D, D : Digoxin
- O : Opioids
- C : CCBs, Chloroquine

52. Ans. (b) Weak acids

(Ref: Goodman Gilman 12th E/P26)

53. Ans. (b) Desmopressin

(Ref: Rang and Dale 6th E/P107)

Drugs given by Intranasal Route

- Desmopressin
- GnRH agonists
- Calcitonin
- Fentanyl

54. Ans. (a) Passive diffusion

(Ref: Goodman Gilman 12th E/P18)

Characteristics of Passive Diffusion

- Most common method of drug absorption
- No ATP required
- Requires a concentration gradient

55. Ans. (a) Tolerance

(Ref: Goodman Gilman 12th E/P140)

- On enzyme induction the effect of the drug will be compromised or in other words we can say there will be induced tolerance.

56. Ans. (a) High lipid soluble drugs

(Ref: KDT 7th E/P18)

57. Ans. (a) Glucuronidation

(Ref: Goodman Gilman 12th E/P139)

Most common mechanism of drug metabolism in

- Phase I: CYP3A4
- Phase II: Glucuronidation

58. Ans. (b) Cytochrome P450

(Ref: Goodman Gilman 12th E/P129)

59. Ans. (b) 93%

(Ref: Goodman Gilman 12th E/P33)

Drug is decreased in

- One half-life : By 50%
- Two half-lives: By 75%
- Three half-lives: By 87.25%
- Four half-lives: By 93.75%
- Five half-lives: By 96.86%

60. Ans. (c) Low volume of distribution

(Ref: Goodman Gilman 12th E/P31)

Factors Determining aV_d

- **aV_d** depends on factors like **lipid solubility (pKa), plasma protein binding, age, sex and tissue protein/ receptor binding.**
- **Higher is lipid solubility,** more drug diffuses into compartments and **more is aV_d**, whereas **more is protein binding** drug is confined to plasma and **lesser is aV_d**.
- The water content of body decreases with age and hence more plasma would be required to dilute the drug into body to plasma concentration; hence **with age aV_d increases. Females** have lesser total body water than males and hence have a **higher aV_d** for similar reason.
- Drugs with higher affinity for tissue proteins/receptors have higher aV_d, as is the case with digoxin due to high binding to Na/K ATPase pump in skeletal muscles.

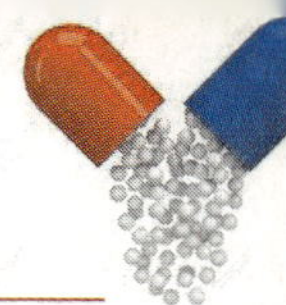

61. Ans. (d) Lisinopril

(Ref: Rang and Dale 6th E/P117, KDT 7th E/P23)

62. Ans. (a) Insulin

(Ref: KDT 7th E/P27)

Drugs with High First Pass Metabolism

Mnemonics

Very High METABOLISM

Very : Verapamil
High : Hydrocortisone
M : Morphine
E : Estrogen
T : Testosterone, Trinitrate glycerine
A : Antipsychotic (Chlorpromazine)
B : Beta blockers (Propranolol and Carvedilol)
O : Opioids (Morphine, Pethidine and Pentazocine)
L : Levodopa, Lignocaine
I : Isoprenaline
S : Saquinavir, Salbutamol
M : Midazolam

63. Ans. (b) Sodium bicarbonate

(Ref: Goodman Gilman 12th E/P26)

64. Ans. (a) Zero order kinetics

(Ref: Goodman Gilman 12th E/P34)

65. Ans. (c) Lithium

(Ref: KDT 7th E/P28)

Drugs Excreted in Saliva

- Lithium
- Rifampicin
- Heavy metals
- Clarithromycin
- Phenytoin
- Disulfiram
- Metoclopromide

66. Ans. (c) Renal clearance

(Ref: Goodman Gilman 12th E/P30)

67. Ans. (c) Thiopentone

(Ref: KDT 7th E/P18)

68. Ans. (b) Imipramine

(Ref: Rang and Dale 6th E/P117, KDT 7th E/P23)

69. Ans. (c) Sodium valproate

(Ref: Katzung 12th E/P58)

70. Ans. (a) d-tubocurarine

(Ref: Goodman Gilman 12th E/P

Drugs with 0% bioavailability
Tubocurare
Aminoglycosides
Heparin

71. Ans. (c) Rifampicin

(Ref: Katzung 12th E/P58)

72. Ans. (c) Constant amount of drug is eliminated per unit time

(Ref: Goodman Gilman 12th E/P34)

- Zero order: Constant amount eliminated per unit time.
- First order: Constant proportion eliminated per unit time.

73. Ans. (a) CYP3A

(Ref: Goodman Gilman 12th E/P129)

74. Ans. (a) Rifampicin

(Ref: Katzung 12th E/P58)

75. Ans. (d) Omeprazole

(Ref: Katzung 12th E/P58)

- Omeprazole is an inducer of CYP1A2 and inhibitor of CYP2C19.

76. Ans. (b) Within vascular compartment

(Ref: Goodman Gilman 12th E/P31)

Total plasma volume is 5 liters and if a drug has Vd

- >5 L – It is located in tissues and organs
- <5 L – It is located in plasma

77. Ans. (b) Enzyme inhibitor

(Ref: Katzung 12th E/P58)

78. Ans. (c) Barbiturate

(Ref: KDT 7th E/P19)

High albumin bound drugs	High alpha 1 acid glycoprotein bound drugs
cNS drugs: Barbiturates, Benzodiazepines, Phenytoin, valproate	**Antiarrhythmics:** Verapamil, Lidocaine, Disopyramide, Beta blockers, Quinidine
Antibiotics: Penicillins, Tetracyclines	**CNS drugs:** Opioids, TCA
Warfarin	Prazosin
NSAIDs	Bupivacaine

Note: Most CNS drugs are high albumin bound except TCA and opioids. Most antiarrhythmics are alpha 1 acid glycoprotein bound drugs.

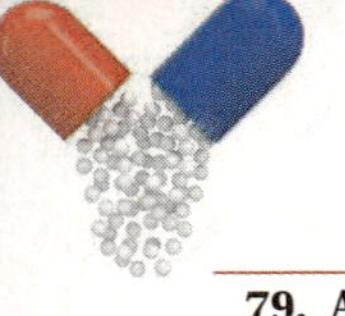

79. Ans. (a) Plasma concentration

(Ref: Goodman Gilman 12th E/P34)

80. Ans. (c) Drug which is inactive and converted to active metabolite

(Ref: Rang and Dale 6th E/P117, KDT 7th E/P23)

81. Ans. (a) Candesartan, (c) Ramipril

(Ref: Rang and Dale 6th E/P117, KDT 7th E/P23)

- Only ARBs which are prodrugs are olmesartan and candesartan.
- All ACEIs are prodrugs except captopril and lisinopril.

82. Ans. (a) Salicylates

(Ref: Goodman Gilman 12th E/P138)

83. Ans. (d) Isosorbide-5-mononitrate

(Ref: Goodman Gilman 12th E/P22)

Drugs given by Sublingual Route

- Nitroglycerine
- IDN
- Nifedipine
- Ephedrine
- Ergotamine
- Buprenorphine

84. Ans. (d) All of the above

(Ref: Goodman Gilman 12th E/P26)

- **Phenytoin follows zero order kinetics.**
- Zero order is not true zero order as in the beginning till enzymes and pumps are saturated, **first order persists** and hence **zero order is also known as pseudo zero order kinetics**.

85. Ans. (c) C_L × Target plasma concentration

(Ref: Goodman Gilman 12th E/P36)

86. Ans. (c) Rifampicin

(Ref: Katzung 12th E/P58)

- Rifampicin is an enzyme inducer and hence will decrease the effect of warfarin.
- Drugs in other options are enzyme inhibitors and will increase the effect of warfarin.

87. Ans. (d) Griseofulvin

(Ref: Katzung 12th E/P58)

88. Ans. (a) Phenytoin and ethanol

(Ref: Goodman Gilman 12th E/P26)

89. Ans. (a) Unit volume of plasma which is cleared off drug in unit time

(Ref: Goodman Gilman 12th E/P33)

90. Ans. (c) Cimetidine

(Ref: Katzung 12th E/P58)

91. Ans. (c) Phenylbutazone

(Ref: Katzung 12th E/P58)

- Phenylbutazone is metabolized by non-microsomal enzymes and hence enzyme inducers or inhibitors have no effect.

92. Ans. (d) Digitalis toxicity

(Ref: Goodman Gilman 12th E/P31)

93. Ans. (d) Ketoconazole

(Ref: Katzung 12th E/P58)

94. Ans. (c) Decrease in V_{max}

(Ref: Goodman Gilman 13th E/P36)

Competitive antagonism	Non-competitive antagonism
At same site	At different sites
DRC shifts to right side	Slope of DRC decreases
Efficacy and V_{max} does not change	Efficacy and **V_{max} decreases**
Dose and K_m increases as potency decreases	Dose, potency and K_m does not change

95. Ans. (a) Muscarinic

(Ref: Goodman Gilman 13th E/P40)

- Muscarinic receptors are GPCRs, whereas nicotinic receptors are ion channel receptors.
- M1, M3 and M5 are Gq subtype of GPCRs, whereas M2 and M4 are Gi subtype of CPCRs.
- Other examples of GPCRs are beta adrenergic, alpha adrenergic, eicosanoid receptors, thrombin receptors (Protease Activated Receptors), serotonergic receptors (except 5HT3), oxytocin receptor and histaminergic receptors.

96. Ans. (a) A and B are full agonists

(Ref: Goodman Gilman 12th E/P44)

- As A and B are producing maximum clinical effect they are full agonists.
- C is not a non competitive antagonist as potency is different.
- A and B have equal efficacy.
- A is more potent than B

97. Ans. (c) Seven pass transmembrane receptor

(Ref: Goodman Gilman 12th E/P55)

Examples of seven pass transmembrane/GPC/Metabotropic receptors

- Alpha and beta adrenergic receptors
- Muscarinic receptors
- 5HT receptors except 5HT3

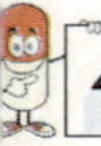

- Histamine receptors
- Dopamine receptors

98. Ans. (c) G proteins act as inhibitory and excitatory because of difference in alpha subunit

(Ref: Goodman Gilman 12th E/P55)

- G-proteins bind to receptors on cell surface not hormones.
- All three subunits of G protein are together, when the receptor is not activated.
- When receptor is activated alpha separates from beta and gamma subunits.
- The effect produced by αGTP depends on the subtype of α protein (s, q, i, o, 12/13), and based on this GPCRs are named as $G\alpha_s$, $G\alpha_q$, $G\alpha_i$, $G\alpha_o$, $G\alpha_{12/13}$.

99. Ans. (b) Guanylyl cyclase

(Ref: Goodman Gilman 12th E/P56)

Examples of Second Messengers

- Cyc AMP
- Cyc GMP
- IP3
- DAG
- Calcium

100. Ans. (b) Conversion of GDP to GTP

(Ref: Goodman Gilman 12th E/P56)

- α subunit has GTPase activity and hence it breaks GTP to GDP.
- This is why αGTP has a short half-life.

101. Ans. (c) Potency calculated

(Ref: Goodman Gilman 13th E/P36)

- Quantal DRC is calculated in a population by plotting log of dose on X axis to response on Y axis as all or none phenomenon (not graded response).
- ED50 is calculated in a quantal dose response curve, which represents potency of drug.

102. Ans. (c) GPCR

(Ref: Goodman Gilman 12th E/P251)

GABA Receptors

GABA A	GABA B
Chloride ion channel receptor	Gi subtype of GPCR

103. Ans. (a) Physiological antagonism

(Ref: Goodman Gilman 12th E/P46)

Physiological Antagonism

One drug prevents another drug's action by acting on a **different receptor**. Examples are given below.

- **Bronchoconstriction caused by histamine on H_1 receptor prevented by bronchodilation caused by adrenaline on β_2 receptors.**
- **Hcl production by histamine inhibited by PPIs.**
- **Aggregant effect of TxA_2 prevented by PgI_2.**

104. Ans. (a) Prolactin

(Ref: Goodman Gilman 12th E/P63)

Examples of enzyme linked receptors	
Tyrosine kinase receptors	EGFR, VEGFR, Her-2, Insulin and Toll like receptors
Serine/threonine kinase receptors	TGFR
Janus kinase	Cytokine receptors, Growth hormone receptor, **Prolactin receptor**
Guanylyl cyclase linked receptor	Receptor of ANP and BNP

105. Ans. (a) K_m increased, V_{max} unchanged

(Ref: Goodman Gilman 12th E/P46)

Competitive antagonism	Noncompetitive antagonism
At same site	At different sites
DRC shifts to right side	Slope of DRC decreases
Efficacy and V_{max} does not change	Efficacy and V_{max} decreases
Dose and K_m increases as potency decreases	Dose, potency and K_m does not change

106. Ans. (c) Physiological antagonist

(Ref: Goodman Gilman 12th E/P 42)

Physiological Antagonism

One drug prevents another drug's action by acting on a different receptor. Examples are given below.

- Bronchoconstriction caused by histamine on H_1 receptor prevented by bronchodilation caused by adrenaline on β_2 receptors.
- HCl production by histamine is inhibited by PPIs.
- Aggregant effect of TxA_2 is prevented by PgI_2.

107. Ans. (c) Intranuclear receptors

(Ref: Rang and Dale 6th E/P48)

Nuclear receptors	Cytoplasmic receptors
Vitamin D receptor Thyroid receptor Retinoic acid receptor	Mineralocorticoid receptor Glucocorticoid receptor
PPAR (Peroximal Proliferator of Activated Receptor) LXR (Liver Oxysterol Receptor) RXR (Retinoid X Receptor) FXR (Farnesoid X Receptor)	Estrogen receptor Progesterone receptor

108. Ans. (b) Noncompetitive

(Ref: Rang and Dale 6th E/P18)

Competitive antagonism	Noncompetitive antagonism
At same site	At different sites
DRC shifts to right side	Slope of DRC decreases
Efficacy and V_{max} does not change	Efficacy and $\mathbf{V_{max}}$ **decreases**
Dose and K_m increases as potency decreases	Dose, potency and $\mathbf{K_m}$ **does not change**

109. Ans. (a) Isoprenaline and propranolol

(Ref: Goodman Gilman 12th E/P46)

Pharmacological or Competitive Antagonism

One drug prevents another drug's action by acting on the same receptor. The antagonist can bind to receptors by forming ionic or covalent bonds. Since ionic bonds are weaker so the binding is reversible and covalent bonds being stronger, the binding is irreversible. Most common antagonism encountered is competitive reversible antagonism. Examples and differences of both are given below.

- Competitive reversible (equilibrium) antagonism: Most antagonists are of this type and examples include beta blockers preventing effect of catecholamines on β_1 receptors, cimetidine inhibiting Hcl production by acting on H_2 receptors, etc.
- Competitive irreversible (non-equilibrium) antagonism: This type of antagonism is rare and examples are aspirin inhibiting TxA_2, PPIs inhibiting proton pumps, phenoxybenzamine inhibiting α receptors, and MAO inhibitors. The change of DRC in this is similar to noncompetitive antagonism.

110. Ans. (a) High affinity

(Ref: Rang and Dale 6th E/P11)

- High affinity for the receptor means high potency and hence a drug can be used at lower dose.
- High specificity for a receptor means, drug acts lesser on other receptors and chances of side effects are lesser.

111. Ans. (a) High affinity but low intrinsic activity

(Ref: Rang and Dale 6th E/P11)

- Full agonist: High affinity with high intrinsic activity, i.e. +1
- Partial agonist: High affinity with low intrinsic activity, i.e. 0 to +1
- Antagonist: High affinity without intrinsic activity, i.e. 0
- Inverse agonist: High affinity with negative intrinsic activity, i.e. 0 to -1

112. Ans. (d) Salbutamol

(Ref: Rang and Dale 6th E/P33)

- All adrenergic receptors are GPCRs or heptahelical receptors.
- Salbutamol is a beta-2 agonist and hence acts on GPCR or heptahelical receptor.
- Estrogen acts on nuclear receptor.
- LA acts on Na channels.
- Insulin acts on TK linked receptor.

113. Ans. (a) Competitive antagonists

(Ref: Rang and Dale 6th E/P16)

- Ach and atropine act on same receptors, i.e. muscarinic and hence are pharmacological or competitive antagonists.

114. Ans. (a) Afinity with intrinsic activity 1

(Ref: Rang and Dale 6th E/P11)

115. Ans. (c) Maximum response that can be elicited by the drug

(Ref: Rang and Dale 6th E/P11)

- The tendency of the drug to activate the receptor and produce maximal effect is known as efficacy.
- Affinity of the drug to bind the receptor is called potency. In other words potency is the minimal dose required to produce a particular effect.

116. Ans. (b) Chemical antagonism

(Ref: Rang and Dale 6th E/P15)

Chemical Antagonism

One drug prevents another drug's action by chemically combining with it in a solution. Examples are given below.

- Binding of dimercaprol to heavy metals.
- Binding of protamine sulfate to heparin
- Binding of monoclonal antibodies to protein targets.

117. Ans. (b) Prostacyclin-Thromboxane

(Ref: Rang and Dale 6th E/P15)

Physiological/Functional Antagonism

One drug prevents another drug's action by acting on a different receptor. Examples are given below.

- Bronchoconstriction caused by histamine on H_1 receptor prevented by bronchodilation caused by adrenaline on β_2 receptors.
- HCl production by histamine is inhibited by PPIs.
- **Aggregant effect of TxA_2 is prevented by PgI_2**

118. Ans. (b) Inverse agonist

(Ref: Rang and Dale 6th E/P15)

Full agonist	Maximal effect
Partial agonist	Submaximal effect
Antagonist	No effect
Inverse agonist	Opposite effect

119. Ans. (b) Partial agonist

(Ref: Rang and Dale 6th E/P11)

120. Ans. (a) Dose

(Ref: Rang and Dale 6th E/P10)

Parameters Signifying a Particular Feature of Drug

Potency	Dose
Efficacy	Clinical effect
Therapeutic index	Safety

121. Ans. (a) Vitamins

(Ref: Goodman Gilman 12th E/P45)

- Drugs which cause stimulation of response at low dose and inhibition at high dose give a U shaped dose response curve.
- Examples are vitamins, minerals, prostaglandins, endothelin, serotonergic and purinergic drugs.
- As it can be seen in the diagram, at low doses adequate clinical effect is seen with vitamins and then at high doses the clinical effect might disappear and signs of toxicity appear.
- With anticancer drugs inverted U or J shape curve is seen.

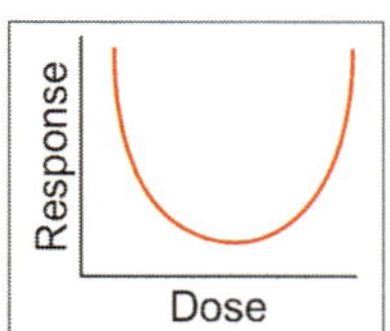

122. Ans. (a) 'b' and 'c' i.e. Constant fraction of drug is eliminated per unit time, (b) Rate of elimination has no correlation with concentration of drug, (c) As concentration of drugs increases, rate of elimination increases

(Ref: Goodman Gilman 13th E/P25)

123. Ans. (b) Fraction eliminated is constant

(Ref: Goodman Gilman 12th E/P28)

Zero order kinetics	First order kinetics
As dose increases t1/2 increases and clearance decreases	Both t1/2 and clearance are constant
A constant amount is eliminated per unit time	A constant fraction is eliminated per unit time

124. Ans.(a) Shift of the drug response curve parallel to right, (c) Low potency

(Ref: Goodman Gilman 12th E/P44)

Competitive antagonism	Noncompetitive antagonism
At same site	At different sites
DRC shifts to right side	Slope of DRC decreases
Efficacy and V_{max} does not change	Efficacy and V_{max} decreases
Dose and K_m increases as potency decreases	Dose, potency and K_m does not change

125. Ans. (b) Low maintenance dose and (c) V_d will be same = 70 L

(Ref: Goodman Gilman 12th E/P34)

- In Case of renal failure and a decrease in renal function by 50%, the renal clearance will decrease by 50% and hence becomes 350/2 = 175 mL/min.
- Since maintenance dose depends on clearance, a decrease in clearance will decrease maintenance dose.
- V_d does not depend on clearance and hence V_d will not change.
- Loading dose depends on V_d and since V_d does not change, loading dose will not change.
- T ½ is inversely proportional to clearance; since clearance decreases here, t ½ will increase.

126. Ans. (a) Applied to majority of drugs and (b) Rate of elimination is directly proportional to the drug concentration

(Ref: Goodman Gilman 12th E/P34)

- **Most of the drugs follow first order kinetics and only a few drugs follow zero order kinetics.**
- **In first order kinetics the rate of drug elimination is directly proportional to the plasma concentration of drug.**
- **Half-life and clearance is constant for drugs following first order kinetics.**

127. Ans. (a) Affinity means how strongly drug binds to receptor, (b) Efficacy means maximal effect by a drug, (d) Agonist potency depends on two parameters: affinity and efficacy, (e) For antagonists, efficacy is zero

(Ref: Goodman Gilman 12th E/P46)

Irreversible antagonist mainly forms covalent bonds with the receptors.

128. Ans. (c) More plasma protein binding means more storage in liver

(Ref: Goodman Gilman 12th E/P24)

More plasma protein binding means more drug remains in plasma and lesser in tissues.

129. Ans. (d) Directly into stomach, (e) Directly into large intestine

(Ref: Goodman Gilman 12t E/P20)

- By oral and large intestinal administration most of the drugs go into liver through portal circulation and hence there is significant first pass metabolism.

- By rectal route only 50% drug undergoes first pass metabolism as, rectal blood flow drains 50% via portal vein and 50% directly into inferior vena cava.

130. Ans. (c) Fluconazole, (d) Aspirin

(Ref: Katzung 12th E/P58)

- Fluconazole is an enzyme inhibitor and hence can increase effect of warfarin.
- Aspiring being an antiaggregant can cause excessive bleeding if given with anticoagulants like warfarin.

131. Ans. (b) Intramuscular administration have curve different from oral administration, (d) Bioavailability of an orally administered drug can be calculated by comparing the area under curve after oral & after i.v. administration, (e) Changes in the rate of absorption and extent of bioavailability can influence both the duration of action and the effectiveness of the same total dose of a drug administered in different formulations

(Ref: KDT 7th E/P16)

- Bioavailability is calculated by dividing the AUC by oral to IV route and then multiplying with 100.
- Different routes of administration have different AUC.
- Extent of absorption or bioavailability along with rate of absorption determine the therapeutic response.

132. Ans. (b) Gq- ↑ cytoplasmic calcium, (c) Gs- Opening of calcium channel, (d) Go- Opening of potassium channel

(Ref: Rang and Dale 6th E/P36)

Effect of GPCRs

Gs	Increase in CycAMP Calcium channel opening
Gq	Increase in calcium Stimulation of membrane protein kinase
Gi	Decrease in Cyc AMP Opening of K channel
Go	Opening o K channel Inhibition of calcium channel
G12/13	Rho kinase stimulation

133. Ans. (b) 0.175 × 0.7

(Ref: Goodman Gilman 12th E/P33)

Amount of drug reaching systemic circulation

= 70% of 0.175 gm

$$= 70/100 \times 0.175$$
$$= 0.7 \times 0.175$$

134. Ans. (a) Rate of elimination remains constant irrespective of drug concentration, (b) Constant amount of drug is excreted, (d) Clearance decreases with increase in concentration

(Ref: Goodman Gilman 12th E/P26)

135. Ans. (a) Rifampicin, (c) Phenytoin (d)Griseofulvin

(Ref: Katzung 12th E/P58)

136. Ans. (a) Acetylation, (e) First metabolized in liver then excreted in urine

(Ref: Goodman Gilman 12th E/P138)

137. Ans. (e) Pinocytosis: transport by diffusion

(Ref: Goodman Gilman 12th E/P18)

Features of Various Modes of Drug Absorption

Passive diffusion	Facilitated diffusion	Active transport	Pinocytosis
No ATP required With concentration gradient Most common mode of drug absorption	No ATP required With concentration gradient Requires carrier	ATP required Against concentration gradient Requires carrier	No ATP required Gradient not important Absorbed by vesicle formation followed by exocytosis

138. Ans. (a) Concentration of drug at which half of the receptors are bound, (c) Concentration at which antagonist is able to bind to half of the receptors

(Ref: Goodman Gilman 12th E/P45)

Potency and K_D

Potency of a drug is its affinity to bind the target and hence higher affinity means higher potency. Higher potency/affinity requires lesser dose of drug to bind same number of targets and hence lesser side effects are seen. If drug is denoted by 'D', target by 'T' and effect by 'E', then in an equation we can write drug, receptor and effect as below.

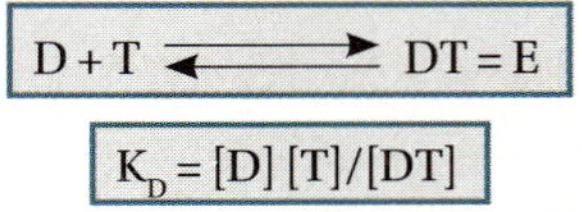

$$K_D = [D]\,[T]/[DT]$$

Dissociation constant or K_D is the ratio of concentration of D and T separately to concentration of DR together. If affinity of D for T is lesser then more are D and T separately and more is K_D. Hence K_D is inversely proportional to drug affinity and potency.

- If K_D is equal to concentration of drug [D], then the equation becomes,

$$K_D = [D]\,[T]/[DT]$$
or $$K_D = K_D\,[T]/[DT]$$
or $$[T]/[DT] = 1$$
or $$[T] = [DT]$$

If concentration of target is equal to concentration of drug bound to target, then 50% targets or receptors are bound to drug. Hence **K_D is the concentration of drug at which 50% of drug is bound to target**.

$$K_A = 1/K_D$$

The affinity constant K_A is inverse of K_D. Hence higher is K_A, higher is the affinity and potency of the drug.

139. Ans. (c) Steady state Plama concentration increases with linear relation on increasing dose rate in case of drug eliminated by first order kinetics, 87.5% of drug is eliminated in 3 T1/2

(Ref: Goodman Gilman 12th E/P26)

140. Ans. (a) First pass metabolism occur in gut, (b) First pass metabolism occur in liver, (d) Depends on extent of absorption, (e) Enterohepatic circulation leads to reabsorption of some drugs like estrogen

(Ref: Goodman Gilman 12th E/P20)

- Bioavailability is 100% by IV route.
- It depends on absorption and first pass metabolism, which takes place in liver as well as intestinal epithelial cells.
- Eneterohepatic circulation is primarily seen with drug metabolized in phase II by glucuronidation like estrogen.

141. Ans. (c) Hyperforin, (d) DDT, (e) St. John's wort

(Ref: Katzung 12th E/P58)

142. Ans. (b) pKa 3.4 for weakly acidic drug, (d) pKa 6.4 for weakly acidic drug

(Ref: Goodman Gilman 12th E/P18)

143. Ans. (a) Sulindac, (c) Bitolterol

(Ref: Rang and Dale 6th E/P117, KDT 7th E/P23)

Prodrugs List

- 5FU
- Capecitabine
- Cyclophosphamide
- 6 MP, 6 TG
- Flucytosine
- Mycophenolate mofetil
- All ACEIs except captopril and lisinopril
- ARBs like olmesartan and candesartan
- Statins like lovastatin and simvastatin
- Levodopa
- Methyldopa
- Carsioprodol
- Carbimazole
- Azathioprine
- Prednisone
- Cortisone
- Fluoxetine
- Proguanil
- Zidovudine
- Sulfasalazine
- Sulindac
- Dipivefrine
- Bitolterol

144. Ans. (a) Smoking, (b) Carbamazepine, (c) Alcohol intake, (d) Rifampicin

(Ref: Katzung 12th E/P58)

145. Ans. (a) Nutrients, (b) Blood component, (c) Essential dietary ingredients

(Ref: Rang and Dale 6th E/P3)

Drug

- WHO defines drug as a chemical agent which alters the biochemical and physiological processes of tissues or organisms.
- A drug can be a chemical derived from living sources (plants, animals, microorganisms), synthetic and semisynthetic chemicals or product of genetic engineering.
- Drug also includes psychoactive substances (alcohol, nicotine, caffeine) and poisons.
- Drug does not include nutrients and essential dietary ingredients required by the living system.

146. Ans. (a) Protein binding, (b) Lipid solubility, (d) Tissue affinity, (e) pKa

(Ref: Goodman Gilman 12th E/P31)

Factors Determining aV_d

- Lipid solubility (pKa)
- Plasma protein binding
- Age
- Sex
- Tissue protein/receptor binding

147. Ans. (a) Carrier mediated, (b) Requires ATP (energy), (d) Saturation occurs

(Ref: Goodman Gilman 12th E/P18)

148. Ans. (a) Ritonavir and (c) Verapamil

(Ref: Katzung 12th E/P58)

149. Ans. (b) Inhibitors bind to substance binding site on enzyme, (c) Example is malonate, (d) Inhibitor resemble structurally to the substance

(Rang and Dale 6th E/P16)

Competitive inhibition	Noncompetitive inhibition
At same site	At different sites
DRC shifts to right side	Slope of DRC decreases
Efficacy and V_{max} does not change	Efficacy and V_{max} decreases
Dose and K_m increases as potency decreases	Dose, potency and K_m does not change

150. Ans. (a) Maximum rate of reaction can be attained by increasing agonist concentration, (c) Binding site of agonist & antagonist are essentially same, (d) Reversal of blockade by antagonist can be achieved by higher dose of agonist

(Ref: Rang and Dale 6th E/P16)

151. Ans. (a) Ritonavir, (d) Delavirdine

(Ref: Katzung 12th E/P58)

152. Ans. (b) Faciliated diffusion is carrier mediated, (c) Active transport is carrier mediated

(Ref: Goodman Gilman 12th E/P18)

153. Ans. (a) Food, (e) Increase expression of p-glycoprotein

(Ref: Goodman Gilman 12th E/20)

Absorption of Drug in Gut is Decreased by

- Ionization
- Large size of particle
- P-glycoprotein pumps that can throw drug back to intestinal lumen
- Gastric emptying delay (Estrogen decreases)

154. Ans. (d) Substance solubility is more, (e) Less protein binding

(Ref: Goodman Gilman 12th E/P31)

155. Ans. (b) Diazepam, (c) Lisinopril

(Ref: Rang and Dale 6th E/P117, KDT 7th E/P23)

156. Ans. (d) Affected by portal and GI system, (e) Prodrug has low first - pass metabolism

157. Ans. (d) Adrenaline and Histamine

(Ref: Rang and Dale 6th E/P18)

158. Ans. (a) Cyclophosphamide

(Ref: Rang and Dale 6th E/P117, KDT 7th E/P23)

159. Ans. (a) Cyclophosphamide

160. Ans. (b) Phenytoin, (c) Cyclosporine, (d) Digitalis

161. Ans. (a) Benzodiazepines, (c) Digitalis

(Ref: Goodman Gilman 12th E/P31)

162. Ans. (a) Lipid solubility, (b) Volume of distribution, (c) Clearance, (d) Drug concentration

163. Ans. (a) Protein binding, (b) Clearance, (c) Volume of distribution, (d) Lipid solubility

(Ref: Goodman Gilman 12th E/P35)

164. Ans. (a) Active transport, (b) Passive transport

(Ref: Goodman Gilman 12th E/P18)

165. Ans. (a) High first pass metabolism

(Ref: Goodman Gilman 12th E/P20)

Lesser Bioavailabilty is seen in case of

- Decreased absorption
- Increased first pass metabolism

166. Ans. (b) Phenytoin, (c) Carbamazapine

(Ref: Katzung 12th E/P58)

167. Ans. (a) If drug administered rectally it follow '1' order kinetics, (b) If drug administered I.M. it follows '0' order kinetics, (c) If drug administered I.V. it follows '1' order kinetics

(Ref: Goodman Gilman 12th E/P26)

168. Ans. (c) Phenobarbitone, (d) DDT

(Ref: Katzung 12th E/P58)

169. Ans. (a) Drug binding, (b) Drug solubility, (c) Degree of blood flow, (d) Age

(Ref: Goodman Gilman 12th E/P31)

170. Ans.(a) Gq

(Ref: Goodman Gilman 13th E/P783)

- Oxytocin acts via a Gq/G11 subtype of GPCR.
- This leads to stimulation of phospholipase C, which increases inositol triphosphate (IP3). IP3 by acting on the sarcoplasmic reticulum releases calcium, which leads to contraction of uterus.
- Oxytocin also stimulates release of prostaglandin, which contracts uterus.

171. Ans. (b) Gq

(Ref: Goodman GILMAN 13th E/P43)

- Stimulation of Gq subtype of GPCR, increases alpha-q GTP which stimulates an enzyme called as phospholipase C.
- Phospholipase C activates phosphatidylinositol bisphosphonate (PIP2) which breaks down into inositol triphosphate (IP3) and diacyl glycerol (DAG).
- IP3 acts on the IP3 receptors present in endoplasmic reticulum and releases calcium.
- DAG activates protein kinase C, which phosphorylates proteins present in cell membrane.

172. Ans. (a) Tyrosine kinase

(Ref: Goodman Gilman 13th E/P774)

- GHRH acts on Gs subtype of GPCR in somatotroph cells of pituitary and increases release of growth hormone (GH).
- Growth hormone acts on growth hormone receptors, which are JAK-STAT subtype of receptors.
- Growth hormone increases IGF-1 which acts on IGF-1 receptors, which are like insulin receptors i.e. are tyrosine kinase receptors.

173. Ans. (b) Equal to the log of 2 multiplied with half life

(Ref: Goodman Gilman 13th E/P23)

- A drug with high volume of distribution takes longer time to get eliminated and hence V_d is directly proportional to half-life.
- Volume of distribution equals to dose of drug upon plasma concentration.
- Muscle relaxants have a low volume of distribution.
- High plasma protein bound drugs are restricted to intravascular compartment and thus have a low V_d.

174. Ans. (c) Ca

(Ref: Goodman GILMAN 13th E/P43)

175. Ans. (b) 400 mg

(Ref: Goodman Gilman 13th E/P28)

- Volume of distribution = 200 L
- Plasma concentration = 0.5 mcg/ml = 500 mcg/L
- Amount of drug present in plasma currently = V_d × PC = 200 × 500 = 100,000 mcg = 100 mg
- Since the half life of drug is 3 hours the amount of drug before 3 hours was 200 mg and similarly before 6 hours was 400 mg.

176. Ans. (d) Dexmeditomidine

(Ref: Goodman Gilman 12th E/P22)

Drugs given by transdermal route are

- Nitroglycerine
- Fentanyl
- Scopalamine
- Nicotine
- Contraceptives
- HRT
- Clonidine

177. Ans. (d) Dipyridamole

(Ref: Goodman Gilman 12th E/P24)

Drugs with High Plasma Protein Binding

High albumin bound drugs	High alpha 1 acid glycoprotein bound drugs
CNS drugs: Barbiturates, Benzodiazepines, Phenytoin, valproate Antibiotics: Penicillins, Tetracyclines, Sulfonamides Warfarin NSAIDs	Antiarrhythmics: Verapamil, Lidocaine, Disopyramide, Beta blockers, Quinidine CNS drugs: Opioids, TCA Prazosin Bupivacaine

Note: Most **CNS drugs** are high albumin bound except TCA and opioids. Most **antiarrhythmics** are alpha 1 acid glycoprotein bound drugs.

178. Ans. (a) Alteration of gut flora

(Ref: Goodman Gilman 12th E/P28)

- Drugs like estrogen are metabolized by glucuronidation in phase II and estrogen attached to glucuronic acid becomes water soluble and is excreted with bile into intestine.
- In the colon bacteria produce enzyme glucunoridase which breaks glucunoric acid and renders estrogen free and lipid soluble, so that it is reabsorbed back (enterohepatic circulation).
- Antibiotics by killing bacteria in colon (gut sterilization) prevent this enterohepatic circulation of estrogen and can cause OCP failure.

179. Ans. (d) Proportional to the half-life of drug

(Ref: Goodman Gilman 12th E/P37)

Loading Dose

aV_d = Drug dose/Concentration

or, Drug dose = aV_d × Concentration

- The plasma concentration must be specific for a particular clinical effect. If drug has a high volume of distribution, then to maintain a specific plasma concentration, in the equation above we must increase the dose "D" of the drug.
- This increased dose of drug for drugs with high aV_d to maintain a specific plasma concentration is known as loading dose. Thus loading dose depends on aV_d and the formula for calculation for drug given by IV route is,

Loading dose (LD) = aV_d × C

- Loading dose is used for drugs with long half-life to attain steady state concentration faster in emergency conditions.

180. Ans. (a) Found only in bone marrow

(Ref: Goodman Gilman 12th E/P127)

- In phase I the drugs are metabolized by reactions carried out by CYP_{450} enzymes, which are present in the endoplasmic reticulum (microsomal) of cells in liver and intestinal epithelium.
- The most common reaction of drug metabolism in phase I is oxidation. Cytochrome is a heme protein which accepts oxygen for drug metabolism. In a CYP_{450} enzyme, e.g. CYP1A2, the first number denotes family (1), alphabet denotes subfamily (A) and last number denotes gene number (2).
- Most common CYP_{450} enzyme for drug metabolism is CYP3A4.

181. Ans. (a) Converts drug to lipid soluble

(Ref: Goodman Gilman 12th E/P131)

- Metabolism of drug happens in two phases, i.e. phase I and II, the first one being slower and hence determines the time required for drug clearance. Phase I metabolism inactivates the drug by breaking it down and then adds or exposes a functional group to the drug known as functionalization.

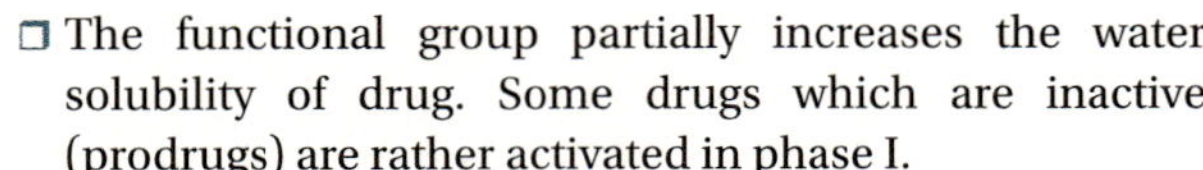

- The functional group partially increases the water solubility of drug. Some drugs which are inactive (prodrugs) are rather activated in phase I.
- In phase II a polar conjugate is attached to the functional group exposed or attached in phase I, which makes the drug polar or water soluble and facilitates its excretion.

182. Ans. (b) Tolbutamide

(Ref: Goodman Gilman 12th E/P24)

Drugs with High Plasma Protein Binding

High albumin bound drugs	High alpha 1 acid glycoprotein bound drugs
CNS drugs: Barbiturates, Benzodiazepines, Phenytoin, valproate Antibiotics: Penicillins, Tetracyclines, Sulfonamides Warfarin NSAIDs	Antiarrhythmics: Verapamil, **Lidocaine**, Disopyramide, Beta blockers, **Quinidine** CNS drugs: Opioids, TCA Prazosin **Propranolol** Bupivacaine

Note: Most **CNS drugs** are high albumin bound except TCA and opioids. Most **antiarrhythmics** are alpha 1 acid glycoprotein bound drugs.

183. Ans. (a) Hydroxylation

(Ref: Goodman Gilman 12th E/P131)

184. Ans. (b) Cyclophosphamide

(Ref: Harrison 19th E/P34)

185. Ans. (a) Erythromycin

(Ref: Harrison 19th E/P34)

Erythromycin being an enzyme inhibitor can cause toxicity of other drugs metabolized by microsomal enzymes like carbamazepine.

186. Ans. (a) Kappa

(Ref: Goodman Gilman 12th E/P55)

187. Ans. (a) Clearance

(Ref: Goodman Gilman 12th E/P29)

188. Ans. (d) Paracetamol

(Ref: Goodman Gilman 12th E/P30)

Drugs with High Hepatic Clearance

- Diltiazem
- Imipramine
- Lidocaine
- Morphine
- Propranolol
- Statins

189. Ans. (d) Erythromycin

(Ref: Harrison 19th E/P34)

190. Ans. (a) Ketoconazole

(Ref: Harrison 19th E/P34)

191. Ans. (d) Warfarin

(Ref: Goodman Gilman 12th E/P24)

192. Ans. (a) Paracetamol

(Ref: Goodman Gilman 12th E/P34)

Practice Questions

193. A patient was administered 500 mg by oral route, out of which 400 mg was absorbed and 200 mg was metabolized in liver. If the drug has a volume of distribution of 50 L and a plasma concentration of 10 mg/L, what is the loading dose of the drug.

a. 1.25 mg
b. 1.25 gm
c. 125 mg
d. 125 gm
e. 1250 gm

Ans. (b) 1.25 gm

- The total amount of drug that has reached systemic circulation = 500 – 300 = 200 mg (As 100 mg is not absorbed and 200 mg underwent first pass metabolism.
- Thus, the fraction of bioavailability (F) = 200/500 = 0.4
- Volume of distribution = 50 L and PC = 10 mg/L
- Now using the formula for loading dose

$$LD = \frac{aV_d \times PC}{F} = \frac{50 \times 10}{0.4} = 1250\text{ mg} = 1.25\text{ gm}$$

194. A patient was given a dose of 1000 mg, which has a bioavailability of 50% and its half-life is 20 hours. What is the maintenance dose of the drug by TDS dosing?

a. 1.4 gm
b. 1.4 mg
c. 14 gm
d. 14 mg
e. 140 gm
f. 140 mg

Ans. (f) 140 mg

- The fraction of bioavailability = 50% = 0.5
- Half-life = 20 hours and Time after which next dose is given = 8 hours
- Now using the formula for maintenance dose

$$MD = \frac{0.7 \times \text{Dose} \times F}{T_{1/2}} = \frac{0.7 \times 1000 \times 0.5}{200} = 140\text{ mg}$$

195. An anticancer drug is given by continuous intravenous infusion. If the plasma concentration at steady state is 10 mg/mL and clearance is 20 mL/hour, what would be the infusion rate if half-life is 2 minutes?

a. 200 mg/hour
b. 400 mg/hour
c. 800 mg/hour
d. 1600 mg/hour
e. 3200 mg/hour

Ans. (a) 200 mg/hour

- PC = 10 mg/mL and Cl = 20 mL/hour
- For an intravenous drug, the infusion rate is the rate of drug elimination, which can be calculated as, RDE or Infusion rate = PC × Cl
  = 20 × 10 mg/hour
  = 200 mg/hour

196. A drug following zero order kinetics was administered at a dose of 200 mg and the half-life calculated was 2 hours. If the dose is increased by 400 mg, what is the half-life?

a. 2 hours
b. 4 hours
c. 6 hours
d. 12 hours
e. 24 hours

Ans. (c) 6 hours

- For drugs following zero order kinetics, as dose increases half-life increases.
- In this case dose is increased by 400 mg, so total dos becomes 600 mg.
- The half-life for 200 mg is 2 hours and thus for 600 mg is 6 hours.

197. A drug following first order kinetics was administered at a dose of 300 mg and the half-life calculated was 3 hours. If the dose is increased by 600 mg, what is the half–life?

a. 3 hours
b. 6 hours
c. 9 hours
d. 18 hours
e. 36 hours

Ans. (a) 3 hours

- For a drug following first order kinetics the half-life is constant.
- Hence even after increasing the dose in this case half-life continues to be 3 hours.

198. The most common site of absorption of an acidic drug is:

a. Stomach
b. Duodenum
c. Jejunum
d. Ileum
e. Colon

Ans. (b) Duodenum

- An acidic drug is maximum unionized in an acidic medium, i.e. stomach, but is not absorbed maximally in stomach due to thick mucosal barrier and a smaller surface area.
- After the drug is turned into unionized form in stomach, it is dumped into small intestine, where it is maximum absorbed in the duodenum.

199. A patient was given 1000 mg of drug and following concentration at different time were achieved as given below. What is the volume of distribution of the drug?

Plasma concentration (mg/L)	Time after dose (hours)
100	2
67	4
45	6

a. 5 L
b. 6.7 L
c. 22.2 L
d. 10 L
e. 15 L

Ans. (b) 6.7 L

- Dose of drug = 1000 mg
- If percentage of drug eliminated is calculated it comes to 33%, as if 33% from 100 mg is removed 67 mg remains and 33% from 67 mg is removed 45 mg remains.
- To find out the C0, i.e. initial plasma concentration, we have to find out plasma concentration at zero hours, i.e. 2 hours before the plasma concentration was 100. Let's assume the C0 is A, then
  A = 100 + 33% of A (As after 33% was removed from A we got 100)
  Or A - 33% of A = 100
  Or A - 0.33A = 100
  Or 0.67 A = 100
  Or A = 100/0.67 = 150 approximately
- V_d = D/C0 = 1000/150 = 6.7 L

200. A patient was started on IV lidocaine for treatment of ventricular tachycardia. The very next day patient developed myocardial infarction. In this setting at the same dose of lidocaine the effect will be

a. Increased
b. Decreased
c. Unchanged
d. Variable
e. Cannot be said based on given information

Ans. (b) Decreased

- Lidocaine in plasma binds to alpha1-acid glycoprotein, which increases in case of myocardial infarction.
- Due to increased plasma protein binding the free lidocaine will decrease in plasma and hence effect will decrease.
- This is the reason why the dose of lidocaine is adjusted based on the ECG findings, i.e. a decrease or increase in arrhythmia and not based on plasma concentration.

201. A patient was given an alpha 2 agonist dexmedetomidine for sedation prior to surgery. The weight of dexmedetomidine is 200 Dalton. What is the most probable mechanism by which it crosses the blood brain barrier to produce sedation?

a. Filtration
b. Passive diffusion
c. Pinocytosis
d. Facilitated diffusion
e. Active transport

Ans. (b) Passive diffusion

- As it has been discussed in the theory for drug absorption the size should be less than 500 Dalton and the most common mode of drug absorption is passive diffusion.
- Similarly for blood brain barrier crossing the same criteria holds true and hence passive diffusion is the answer here.

202. A patient developed anaerobic infection for which clindamycin was prescribed. However after few days the patient's condition deteriorated and he presented with complaints of diarrhoea, fever, abdominal pain and pus in stool. He was started on vancomycin by oral route as it has a molecular weight of:

a. 100 Dalton
b. 200 Dalton
c. 300 Dalton
d. 400 Dalton
e. 1500 Dalton

Ans. (e) 1500 Dalton

203. A patient of gestational diabetes mellitus was started on subcutaneous insulin, which was injected on abdomen and thigh with alteration. Absorption of insulin from the site of injection to systemic circulation is via

a. Passive diffusion
b. Active transport
c. Facilitated diffusion
d. Pinocytosis
e. Filtration

Ans. (e) Filtration

- Insulin being a protein has a huge molecular weight and hence can't undergo passive diffusion.
- It is absorbed from the site of injection into capillaries through aqueous channels by a mechanism known as filtration.
- Insulin however crosses the blood brain barrier by facilitated diffusion.

204. A patient was given aspirin by oral route which has a pKa of 3.5. What would be the amount of unionized drug in the stomach at fasting state?

a. 1%
b. 10%
c. 100%
d. 50%
e. 99%

Ans. (d) 50%

- Taking the average gastric pH of 3 at fasting state, the pKa and pH of the drug are nearly equal.
- In such a case the amount of ionized and unionized drug are equal, i.e. 50% each.

205. A °patient was prescribed methotrexate for treatment of osteosarcoma following which crystallization lead to obstructive renal failure. Bicarbonate was administered to the patient for alkalinisation of urine and prevent nephrotoxicity. What could be the possible mechanism by which bicarbonate acts here?

a. Covalently binds to methotrexate
b. Inactivates methotrexate by metabolizing it
c. Ion trapping of methotrexate in renal tubules
d. Facilitates recrystallization of methotrexate
e. Facilitates reabsorption of methotrexate

Ans. (c) Ion trapping of methotrexate in renal tubules

- When the pH of drug and medium is different drug is ionized.
- Methotrexate is an acidic drug and when urine is alkalinized with bicarbonate, methotrexate becomes ionized or water soluble and hence excreted.
- This is known as ion trapping, which prevents methotrexate induced nephrotoxicity.

206. A patient of dyslipidemia was started on niacin. After a couple of days he developed flushing for which aspirin was given to the patient. Aspirin has a pKa of 3.5 and hence is maximum absorbed from

a. Stomach
b. Duodenum
c. Colon
d. Rectum
e. Oral cavity

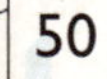

Ans. (b) Duodenum

- Acidic drugs are maximum unionized in stomach and basic drugs in small intestine.
- However both acidic and basic drugs are maximum absorbed in the small intestine due to its huge surface area.
- Drugs are poorly absorbed in stomach due to small surface area and a thick mucosal coating.

207. Pharmacology is a word derived from which language?

a. Latin b. English
c. Greek d. German

Ans. (c) Greek

(Ref: Rang and Dale 6th E/P3)

208. Which of the following is not a systemic route of drug administration?

a. Transdermal b. Intravenous
c. Subcutaneous d. Intra-arterial

Ans. (d) Intra-arterial

(Ref: Goodman Gilman 12th E/P23)

209. Which of the following is a drawback of extended release preparation?

a. Frequent high peak side effects
b. Decreased compliance
c. Increased cost
d. No dose dumping

Ans. (c) Increased cost

(Ref: Goodman Gilman 12th E/P21)

- Extender release drugs are associated with gradual rise in drug plasma concentration that is maintained throughout the day, thus avoiding peaks of high and troughs of low plasma concentration.
- By delaying drug action the number of doses required considerably decreases and hence compliance increases.
- Though the cost is higher than normal preparation drugs.
- Extended release drugs if taken with food, more amount of drug can be released (dose dumping), which can cause toxicity.

210. Lipinski rule of five is associated with drug

a. Absorption b. Toxicity
c. Metabolism d. Excretion

Ans. (a) Absorption

(Ref: Structure Based Drug Discovery by Hubbard/P143)

211. 1000 mg of a drug was given by oral route. 800 mg was absorbed following which enzymes in liver and intestine metabolized 200 mg of drug. The drug is also substrate for Pgp, which can effectively pump out 10% of administered dose. What is the bioavailability?

a. 520 b. 500
c. 720 d. 700

Ans. (b) 500

(Ref: Goodman Gilman 12th E/P20)

- Drug absorbed = 800 mg
- First pass metabolism = 200 + 10% of 1000 = 300 mg
- Hence bioavailability = 800 – 300 = 500 mg

212. P-glycoprotein pump is involved in

a. Active transport b. Facilitated transport
c. Passive transport d. Pinocytosis

Ans. (a) Active transport

(Ref: Goodman Gilman 12th E/P27)

- P-glycoprotein is an active transporter involved in drug efflux.

213. All of the following reactions take place in sarcoplasmic reticulum except

a. Oxidation b. Reduction
c. Glucuronidation d. Glutathionylation

Ans. (c) Glutathionylation

(Ref: Goodman Gilman 12th E/P125)

- All phase I reactions and only glucuronidation in phase II are reactions by microsomal enzymes, i.e. in the sarcoplasmic reticulum.

214. Which of the following drug toxicity can be seen in Crigler Najjar syndrome?

a. Tenofovir b. Zidovudine
c. Atazanavir d. Nevirapine

Ans. (c) Atazanavir

(Ref: Goodman Gilman 12th E/P133)

- Drugs with established toxicity in case of Crigler Najjar syndrome are irinitecan and atazanavir.
- These drugs are metabolized by glucuronidation,

215. A patient was given a drug at a dose of 1000 mg and it has a half-life of 5 hours. What is the TDS dose of the drug?

a. 100 mg b. 200 mg
c. 300 mg d. 400 mg

Ans. (a) 100 mg

(Ref: Goodman Gilman 12th E/P36)

- At TDS dosing, drug is to be given every 8 hours, so we have to calculate the maintenance dose after 8 hours.
- MD = 0.693 × D/T1/2 = 0.693 × 1000/5 = 111.68 mg
- Hence 100 is the best option here.

216. An acidic drug is maximally absorbed from

a. Stomach b. Small intestine
c. Large intestine d. Oral cavity

Ans. (b) Small intestine

(Ref: Goodman Gilman 12th E/P18)

- An acidic drug is maximally unionized in the stomach, but as it has thick mucosa and small surface area, maximum absorption takes place in small intestine.

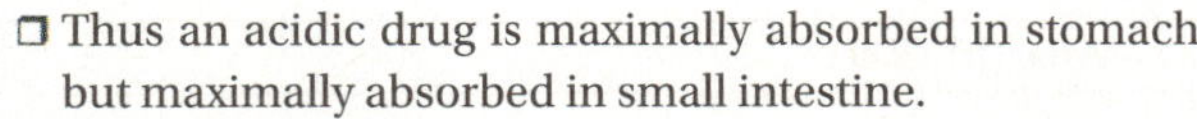

❒ Thus an acidic drug is maximally absorbed in stomach but maximally absorbed in small intestine.

217. K_D is a measure of drug

a. Efficacy b. Potency
c. Toxicity d. Safety

Ans. (b) Potency

(Ref: Goodman Gilman 12th E/P45)

218. Most common type of antagonism is

a. Reversible competitive
b. Reversible noncompetitive
c. Irreversibe competitive
d. Irreversible noncompetitive

Ans. (a) Reversible competitive

(Ref: Rang and Dale 6th E/P16)

219. Rifampicin and ritonavir are

a. Physical antagonist
b. Chemical antagonist
c. Pharmacokinetic antagonist
d. Competitive antagonist

Ans. (c) Pharmacokinetic antagonist

(Ref: Rang and Dale 6th E/P16)

220. Diazepam and bicuculine are

a. Physical antagonist
b. Competitive antagonist
c. Noncompetitive antagonist
d. Physiological antagonist

Ans. (c) Noncompetitive antagonist

(Ref: Rang and Dale 6th E/P18)

❒ Bicuculine acts on the GABA binding site on GABAA receptor, whereas the site of binding for benzodiazepines and barbiturates are different.

❒ Hence they are noncompetitive antagonists.

221. G_i and G_o subtype of GPCRs are located primarily on:

a. Postsynaptic membrane
b. Presynaptic membrane
c. Axons
d. Dendrites

Ans. (b) Presynaptic membranes

(Ref: Goodman Gilman 12th E/P55)

❒ Gi and Go subtype of GPCRs are presynaptic membranes where they control release of neurotransmitters.

❒ These presynaptic receptors are also known as auto receptors.

222. Which of the following is fastest acting receptor?

a. Beta 1 b. M2
c. GABAA d. Estrogen receptor

Ans. (c) GABAA

(Ref: Goodman Gilman 12th E/P60)

❒ Ligand gated ion channels are the fastest acting receptors.

❒ Out of the options, the only ion channel receptor is GABAA.

223. Which of the following is slowest acting receptor?

a. Beta 1
b. M2
c. Tyrosine kinase receptors
d. Mineralocorticoid receptor

Ans. (d) Mineralocorticoid receptor

(Ref: Goodman Gilman 12th E/P65)

❒ Nuclear receptors are the slowest acting receptors.

❒ The only nuclear receptor in the options is mineralocorticoid receptors.

224. Which of the following is not a tyrosine kinase receptor

a. TLR b. Insulin receptor
c. EGFR d. ANP receptor

Ans. (d) ANP receptor

(Ref: Rang and Dale 6th E/P43)

Examples of enzyme linked receptors	
Tyrosine kinase receptors	EGFR, VEGFR, Her-2, Insulin and Toll like receptors
Serine/threonine kinase receptors	TGFR
Janus kinase	Cytokine receptors
Guanylyl cyclase linked receptor	Receptor of ANP and BNP

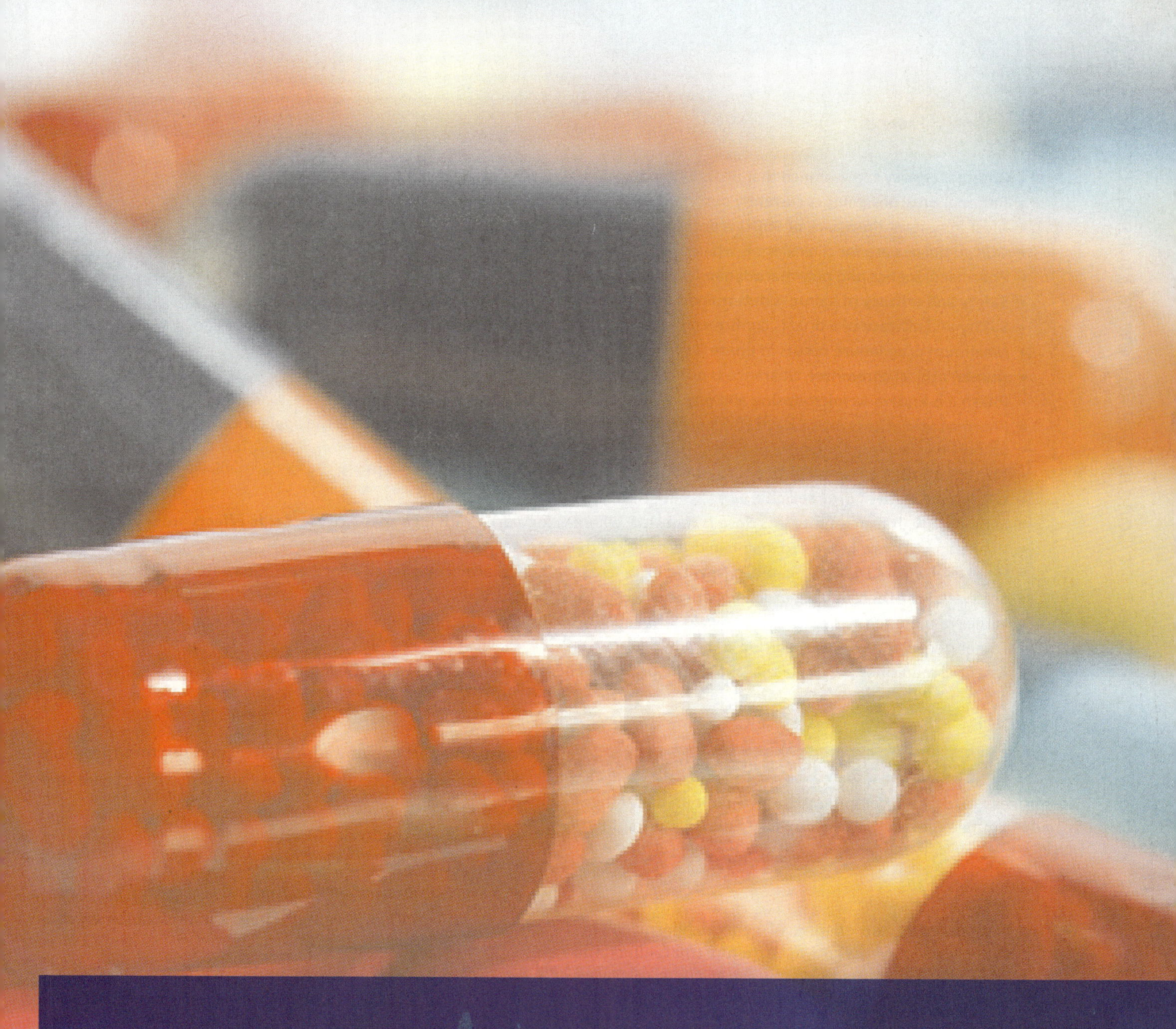

Clinical Pharmacology

One Liners

- **Pharmacognosy** is the branch that deals with natural sources of drug, i.e. plants, animals and microorganisms.
- **Rational drug designing** is currently best method as understanding structure of receptor enhances better target.
- Most important **drawback of SBDD** is decreased interaction of the drug with target proteins.
- **GCP** guidelines are for clinical trials whereas **CPCSEA** guidelines are for preclinical trials.
- **Pharmacokinetics** and **pharmacodynamics** of a drug can be determined in phase 0 and phase I clinical trial.
- **Safety** and **efficacy** of a drug is **determined in phase II** as compared to a placebo or a standard drug.
- **Safety** and **efficacy** of a drug is **confirmed in phase III** as compared to a placebo or a standard drug.
- **Maximum drug failure occurs in phase II** of clinical trial due to poor efficacy of drugs.
- **Human ethical committee clearance** is not required in phase IV clinical trials.
- **Phase 0 is known as microdosing and phase V is known as pharmacoepidemiology.**
- **Pharmacogenetics** is the study of effect of genes on drugs whereas pharmacogenomics is the application of pharmacogenetics to individualize drug therapy.
- **Therapeutic index** is a measure of drug **safety** and is calculated by dividing LD_{50} with ED_{50}.
- LD_{50} is a measure of **drug toxicity**, whereas ED_{50} is a measure of **drug potency**.
- For a drug with **high affinity less dose is required**, whereas for a drug with **high specificity less side effects are seen**.
- **Pharmacovigilance** is done to maintain drug safety in the society.
- Head quarter of **CDSCO** is located in **New Delhi**, whereas **NCC of pharmacovigilance** is located in **Ghaziabad (UP).**
- **Software for ADR reporting** used in pharmacovigilance is known as **vigiflow**.
- Father of modern pharmacology is Oswald Schmiedberg, whereas father of Indian pharmacology is **Sir. Ram Nath Chopra**.
- Father of evidence-based medicine is **David Sackett**.
- Essential medicines are those that **satisfy the priority of health care needs of majority of population**.

DRUG DEVELOPMENT

The process of drug development is very tedious and ranges from designing a molecule till testing it in animals and humans in trials.

DRUG DESIGNING

As it was discussed in the chapter of general pharmacology, a drug is a chemical with known structure that alters the pathophysiology for therapeutic gain. These chemicals were initially discovered from the pre-existing chemicals in the nature from plants, animals or microorganisms. The branch that deals with these sources is called **pharmacognosy**. But due to its limitation the drug development process has moved with invention of latest technologies into **"Rational drug designing"**.

CONVENTIONAL DRUG DISCOVERY

- The concept of drug discovery was laid down in 18th century, only after a new branch called as **medicinal chemistry** came into existence.
- Medicinal chemistry dealt with mere isolation of active components of plants, which were then screened in isolated organs followed by screening in whole animals. This gave an idea about the clinical effect that the component can bring about as a whole without any knowledge of molecular mechanism of action.
- If any desired effect was produced, then drug toxicity studies were carried out in animals followed by clinical trials. However, no change was made in the active component.
- Most drugs in use nowadays have been discovered by this conventional technique, which is also known as **"trial and error method"**.
- The drawbacks of this methods are
  - **It is a time consuming method**
  - **Larger amount of new compound is required for study**
  - **No information is gained about the molecular mechanism of drug**
- Examples of drugs discovered by this method

Morphine	*Papaver somniferum*
Atropa	*Atropa belladonna*
Quinine and quinidine	*Cinchona succirubra*
Ephedrine	*Ephedra sinica*
Theophylline	*Theobroma cacao*
Pentoxiphylline	*Camellia sinensis*
Glycosides	*Digitalis lanata*

SERENDIPITOUS DRUG DISCOVERY

- The word serendipity itself means a "happy accident" or a "pleasant surprise". These are drugs which were developed for one indication, but later were found to be effective in some other disorder.

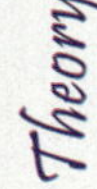

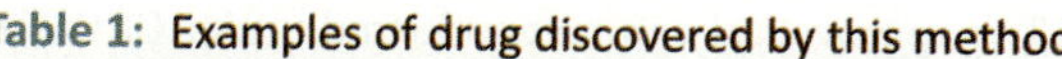

Table 1: Examples of drug discovered by this method

Drug	Initial use	New use
Sildenafil	Pulmonary hypertension	Erectile dysfunction
Sulfonylureas	Antibacterial	Oral hypoglycemic agent
Allopurinol	Antineoplastic	Antigout
Atomoxetine	Antidepressant	ADHD
Carbamazepine	Antipsychotic	Antiepileptic
Imipramine	Sedative	Antidepressant
Chlorpromazine	Antihelminthic	Antipsychotic
Disulfiram	Antihelminthic	Alcohol dependence
Raloxifene	Contraceptive	Osteoporosis
Gabapentin	Antiepileptic	Peripheral neuropathy
Bremelanotide	Tanning cream	Erectile dysfunction

RATIONAL DRUG DESIGNING

- Rational drug design came into existence in the 20th century when radio-ligand binding assay gave enormous information about various ligands and receptors. Further the structure of receptors, enzymes and ligands were extensively studied with the invention of NMR Spectroscopy and X-RAY crystallography.
- This is the best method of drug development because, **understanding the structure of receptor enhances better target**.
- This followed the development of a new procedure for chemical production called as **combinational chemistry**. These specialists combined different chemical entities to create a chemical with definite structure which is composite to the structure of an enzyme or a receptor (e.g. ACE inhibitor for enzyme ACE).
- Rational drug discovery based on this concept can be classified into:
  1. Structure-based drug designing
  2. Ligand-based drug designing
  3. In silico drug designing
  4. Homology modeling

- **Structure-based drug designing**
  - Structure-based drug designing (SBDD) is applied when the target is a protein or an enzyme in the pathway.
  - The disease of interest is studied and based on the pathophysiology, targets of interest are identified. For example, one would study hypertension and find RAAS system, where ACE or angiotensin receptor could be a potential target.
  - Based on the 3D structure of the target, e.g. ACE, desired complementary compounds (Let's say 100,000) are suggested by chemists, e.g. future ACE inhibitors.
  - These collections of compounds are called drug library (100,000 chemicals) which is further subjected to screening on living system for drug discovery.
- **Ligand-based drug designing (LBDD)**
  - Similarly, disease of interest is studied and the target of interest is identified, e.g. angiotensin.
  - Then 3D structure of ligand-receptor interaction is determined, e.g. angiotensin with angiotensin receptor, which helps in detection of the active part of ligand which binds to target.
  - This active part of ligand which is minimum necessary structural characteristic of a ligand and is necessary to bind to a receptor is called **"pharmacophore".**
  - Based on the structure of pharmacophore, chemist can synthesize desired compounds (Let's say 100,000) that can bind to angiotensin receptor.
  - These collections of compounds are again called **drug library** (100,000 chemicals) which is further subjected to screening on living system for drug discovery.
- **In silico drug designing (ISDD)**
  - "In silico" is an expression used to mean performed on computer.
  - The structure of the target of interest, i.e. receptor or enzyme (e.g. ACE) that is obtained by NMR spectroscopy or X-ray crystallography is plotted in a computer.
  - Different computational algorithms are used to produce various virtual compounds (in millions) which can bind to virtual receptors and these virtual chemicals form a virtual drug library.
  - This virtual library is screened on the virtual receptor by software tools, which gives us the drugs that can best interact with target (Let's say 10,000).
  - These 10,000 chemicals when synthesized, form the real drug library and then can be used for drug screening for drug discovery.
- **Homology modeling (HM)**
  - This refers to construction of an atomic resolution model of the target protein from its amino acid sequence and an experimental 3D structure of a related homologous protein.
  - This 3D structure can be used for screening of various drug libraries.

Screening in RDD

- Once a drug library is formed the next thing required for drug discovery is an assay. The different types of screening are high throughput screening and ultra high throughput screening.
- After drug library is screened in an assay, some of the chemicals from drug library produce desired effect which can be detected by radiolabelling, luminescence and fluorescent techniques. Very less chemicals from drug library usually produce effect, let's say only 100 out of 100,00.
- These chemicals from drug library which produce effect in a bioassay or living system is called as a "HIT" (100). One thing that is not known yet is if these HITs are producing effect by acting on target of interest.

Hit to Lead

- Once the "HIT" is found, the structure of HIT with target is determined and we get the HITs producing effect by acting

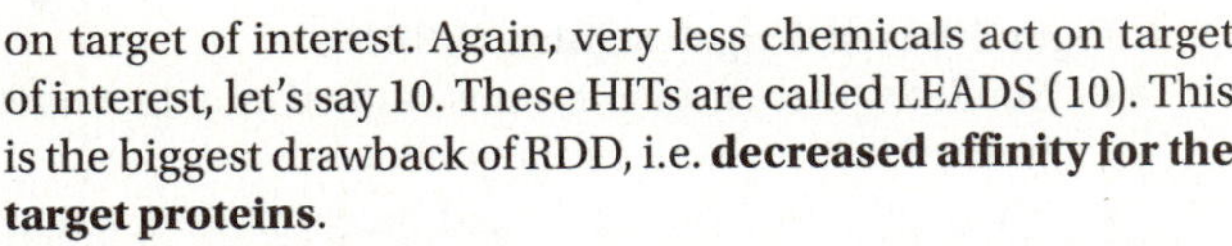

on target of interest. Again, very less chemicals act on target of interest, let's say 10. These HITs are called LEADS (10). This is the biggest drawback of RDD, i.e. **decreased affinity for the target proteins**.

- The leads generated still need some modification for better outcome as a drug and this is called lead optimization. Parameters requiring optimization are their affinity for target, agonist/antagonist activity, permeability across cell membranes and ADMET.
- These optimized leads are now ready for entering the preclinical trial in animals followed by clinical trials in humans. The most potent lead first enters into preclinical trial and is called "LEAD COMPOUND". If the first compound fails at any level, then we can start with the second most potent lead.

Conceptual Box-1

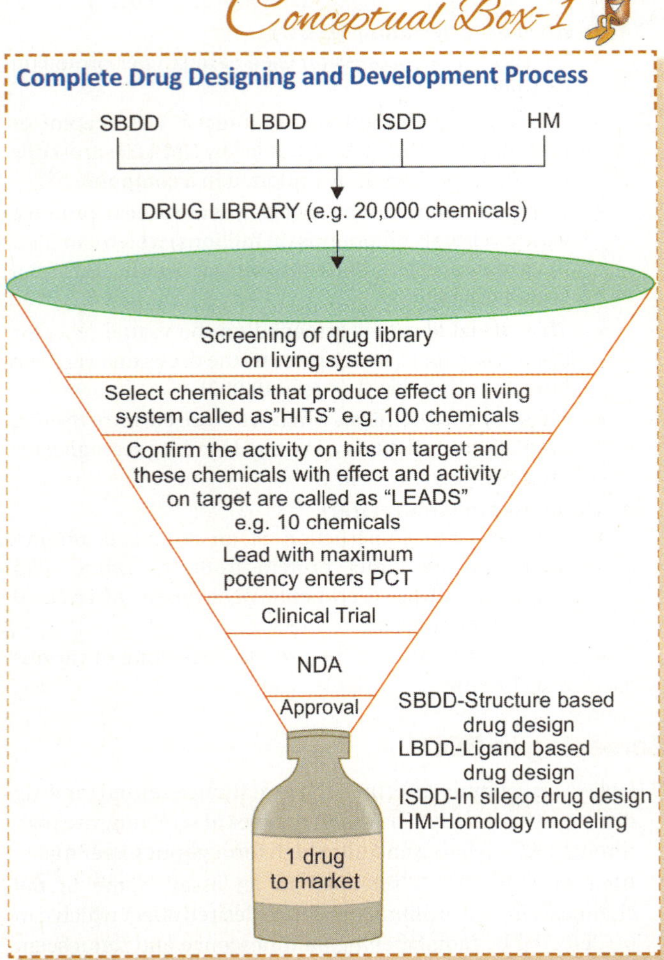

PRECLINICAL TRIAL (PCT)

Before the drug is given in humans, it is administered in animals to confirm the efficacy, toxicity, teratogenicity and other effects of drugs.

- To begin with a protocol is made that is a document, which states about the process of trial, e.g. animals to be used, doses of drug to be given, samples to be taken, analysis to be done, etc.
- This protocol is submitted to the animal ethical committee, which takes a final decision on approval of the PCT.
- Once PCT is approved, it can be conducted under **CPCSEA** (Committee for the purpose of control and supervision of experiments in animals) guidelines.

CLINICAL TRIAL (CT)

A clinical trial is one type of bioassay done to compare the efficacy of a drug with an existing drug or placebo.

Concept of Bioassay

Bioassay is the procedure to evaluate a drug or endogenous substance potency or concentration by correlating it to the biological response produced. Bioassays are designed to check the pharmacological activity/efficacy of a new drug (clinical trial), to find the role of endogenous ligands and to find drug toxicity.

There are four mandatory phases of clinical trial I to III for approval of a drug and the fourth (phase IV) mandatory phase follows drug approval. Similar to preclinical trial a protocol is made, which in this case is submitted to the human ethical committee. Once it is approved the clinical trial can be started from phase I under GCP (Good Clinical Practice guidelines).

Phase I–Human Pharmacology and Toxicity Study

- Phase I, trial is carried out in 20–100 **healthy volunteers**, as they can better tolerate toxicity than a patient. However healthy volunteers cannot be taken, if the drug belongs to a highly toxic class like anticancer drugs and hence patients are directly included in phase I. The trials are open label with placebo as control.
- The aim of the first phase is to determine the **safety**, **toxicity** and **maximum tolerated dose (MTD) of drug** in healthy volunteers, which helps to determine the dose range for Patients in phase II.
- The second aim is to determine the **pharmacokinetics** (supports formulation development) and **pharmacodynamics** (indicator of potency and efficacy that guides dosage and regimens) of drugs.

Phase II–Therapeutic Exploratory Trial

- Phase II, trials are carried out in 100–500 patients at few centers (2–4) and the study time is for 1 to 2 years. Randomized controlled trials are done and **placebo** or a **standard drug** may be used as control.
- The aim of this phase is to find the **dose range of drug** (phase IIa) and **determine safety** and **efficacy** (phase IIb) of the drug in comparison to a placebo or standard drug in patients.
- This phase is known for **maximum drug failure**, i.e. around 75%.

Placebo

A placebo is an **unreal drug that has no active substance** but is administered to the patient in a trial who believes it to be a real drug. Some patients get therapeutic effect from a placebo and is known as placebo effect, e.g. Intake of placebo can stimulate endorphin release that can have analgesic effect. In a clinical trial in phase II and III it is always advisable to take standard drug as control than placebo, as it is not advised to give placebo to a patient for a disease, if an established treatment option is available. However, in phase I placebo is universally taken as a control.

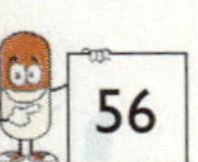

Phase III–Therapeutic Confirmatory Trial

- Phase III, trials are carried out in 500–3000 patients for 3–5 years in many centers (multicentric). Phase III can be **randomized controlled trials (RCT)** or **randomized uncontrolled trials** and **placebo or a standard drug may** be used as control.
- This phase is a replica of phase II and the aim is to **confirm the safety and efficacy** in a larger group of patients (As in a study the subjects increase, error decreases) as compared to placebo or standard drug. Thus, safety and efficacy of a drug in a patient is best determined in phase IIIa.
- Phase IIIb can be done after NDA submission and before approval to support the drug approval. **Pharmacoeconomic analysis** is done in this phase, which weighs the economic benefit to the patient from new drug as compared to available drugs.
- After this phase the documents are collected from the first day of drug designing till last day of phase III trial and a New Drug Application (NDA) is filed with the FDA. Once FDA gives permission for marketing, the drug is available to patients throughout the country.

Phase IV–Post-Marketing Surveillance

- There is no definite time period for the phase IV trials and these are open label trials. Since no active trial is being done here, permission is not required from the human ethical committee.
- **Safety (long-term and rare ADR)**, drug effectiveness, new therapeutic indications (beta blockers in CHF), drug-drug interaction, use in other age group population, alternative routes of administration, change in dosing (phenytoin from TDS to OD dosing), **comparison with existing treatment** and new formulations, etc. are explored in this phase.
- The company is bound to submit Periodic Safety Update Report (PSUR) regarding the drug to the CDSCO 6 monthly for first two years, followed by yearly.

Recent Advances

Clinical Trial

There are two more phases included in clinical trial namely "Phase 0" and "Phase V", which are nonmandatory.

Phase 0–Microdosing

- In this phase healthy volunteers are administered drug at doses of **100 micrograms or 1/100th** of normal dose whichever is lesser.
- At such low doses volunteers are not exposed to drug toxicity, but still drug effect can be determined because the drug used is bound to a radioligand, which makes detection of even traces, possible by powerful detection techniques like AMS (Accelerated Mass Spectrometry).
- Samples are drawn and pharmacokinetics and pharmacodynamics of the drug is studied. If any discrepancy is found that indicates at drug inefficacy or toxicity that may be seen in Phase I or II, the trial is aborted at Phase 0 itself.

Contd...

Recent Advances

- Thus not only the volunteers are not exposed to toxic drugs, the company saves money and time by avoiding such drugs in early phase of trial.

Phase V – Pharmacoepidemiology

- The main aim of this phase is to supplement the findings of Phase IV trial or pharmacovigilence. If inconclusive ADR reports are found in phase IV then this phase can be helpful in confirming those signals.
- The study designs used are like case reports, case control studies, cohort studies and active surveillance.

E.g. if only few cases are found with ADR related to a drug, we can do a case control study and find if other patients exposed to that drug ever developed that particular ADR or design a cohort study and follow patients to find if they develop that ADR.

PHARMACOGENETICS AND PHARMACOGENOMICS

Pharmacogenetics is the study of effects of genes on drug fate. Genes are responsible for production of targets (enzymes and receptors) for drugs, drug metabolizing enzymes and drug transporters. A decrease, increase or absence in production of these can cause either drug inefficacy or toxicity. Genetic variations can be due to single nucleotide polymorphisms (most common), insertion, deletion or duplication of DNA sequence.

If one knows about the genetic defect present in a patient, then the drug dose can be modified to prevent drug failure or toxicity. This individualization of drug therapy based on pharmacogenetics is called as **pharmacogenomics**.

GENETIC POLYMORPHISM OF DRUG TARGET

VKORC1 Polymorphism

Vitamin K is activated by an enzyme vitamin K epoxide reductase (VKORC1) which is target for anticoagulant warfarin. Mutation of VKOR gene can **decrease the effect of warfarin**.

Ryanodine Receptor Gene Polymorphism

Increased activity of genes increases ryanodine receptors, which are present is sarcoplasmic reticulum and release calcium. Drugs like **halothane**, **lidocaine** and **Sch** which act on this receptor increases excessive release of calcium (passive), which is then taken up by sarcoplasmic reticulum (active). This depletes a huge number of ATP, generating heat energy and leads to malignant hyperthermia.

ACE Polymorphism

ACE polymorphism with homozygous deletion genotypes poorly respond to ACE inhibitors.

β_2 Receptor Polymorphism

Poor response to beta-2 agonists in bronchial asthma.

HMG Co-A Polymorphism

Poor response to statin therapy in dyslipidemia.

GENETIC POLYMORPHISM OF DRUG METABOLIZING AND OTHER ENZYMES

CYP450 Polymorphmism

- **CYP2D6 polymorphism:** CYP2D6 activates **tamoxifen to its active product endoxifen**, which inhibits ER, metabolizes drugs used in psychiatry (antidepressants and antipsychotics). Hence decreased CYP2D6 can cause failure of tamoxifen and toxicity of beta blockers and psychiatry drugs.
- **CYP2C19 polymorphism:** CYP2C19 metabolizes PPI and activates clopidogrel. Hence decreased expression of CYP2C19 causes decreased activation of **clopidogrel** and decreased metabolism of PPI. Decreased activation of clopidogrel can compromise clinical effect and hence a **black box warning** has been issued by FDA against it.
- **CYP2C9 Polymorphism:** Decreased CYP2C9 can decrease warfarin metabolism and increase its toxicity. **VKORC1** and **CYP2C9** gene polymorphism together account for variation of dose in **25% of patients**.

Thiopurine Methyl Transferase (TMT) Polymorphism

This enzyme metabolizes 6MP, GTG and azathioprine and hence in its absence toxicity can be seen.

Butyryl Cholinesterase Polymorphism

A variant allele codes for an **atypical butyryl choline esterase** or **pseudocholinesterase**, which poorly metabolizes Sch and hence prolonged apnea is seen.

N-acetyl Transferase Polymorphism

People with NAT1 gene are fast acetylators and hence can cause drug failure, whereas people with NAT2 gene are slow acetylators and can cause drug toxicity for drugs metabolized by **acetylation**. Isoniazid is metabolized by acetylation, which causes neuropathy in slow acetylators and hepatotoxicity in fast acetylators.

UDP Glucunoryl Transferase Polymorphism

A decrease in this enzyme can enhance toxicity of drugs metabolized by glucuronidation like **irinotecan**. Hence FDA recommends genotyping prior to irinotecan therapy.

G6PD Polymorphism

G6PD deficiency can cause hemolysis by certain drugs due to oxidative stress. Drugs with definite risk of hemolysis are given below:

Mnemonics

New Delhi ChAMPS

New : Nalidixic acid, Nitrofurantoin, Niridazole, Naphthalene
Delhi : Dapsone
Ch : Chlorproguanil, Cotrimoxazole
A : Acetanilide
M : Methylene blue
P : Primaquine > Chloroquine, Phenazopyridine
S : Sulphamethoxazole

ALA Polymorphism

ALA polymorphism can lead to increased porphyrin synthesis. If enzyme inducers like thiopental sodium and phenobarbital are used in these patients, AIP can be seen.

GENETIC POLYMORPHISM OF DRUG TRANSPORTERS

- **P-glycoprotein** polymorphism can have effect on plasma concentration of drugs which are substrate for it like, digoxin.
- **Breast cancer resistance protein (BRCP)** polymorphism can cause toxicity of diflomotecan (absorbed by BRCP) and increased effect of rosuvastatin (excreted by BRCP).
- **Organic anionic transporter (OATP)** polymorphism can increase plasma concentration of drugs like pravastatin and repaglinide, which are cleared from plasma by this transporter.

MISCELLANEOUS

- Apo-E4 positive patients poorly respond to cholinergics in Alzheimer's disease.
- HLA polymorphism can cause increased risk of hypersensitivity with abacavir and carbamazepine.

Mnemonics

PHARMACOGEN

P : Pseudocholinesterase causing apnea with Sch
H : HMG Co-A reductase polymorphism, HLA polymorphism
A : ACE polymorphism
R : Rosuvastatin increased effect in BRCP polymorphism
M : Malignant hyperthermia with RyR gene polymorphism
A : Anticoagulant warfarin associated VKOR polymorphism
C : CYP450 polymorphism
O : OATP polymorphism
G : G6PD deficiency associated hemolysis
E : ApoE-4 A positive patients
N : N-acetyl transferase polymorphism

THERAPEUTIC INDEX AND WINDOW

THERAPEUTIC INDEX

Therapeutic index is calculated by dividing **LD_{50}** to **ED_{50}**. LD_{50} is the minimum dose required to kill 50% of animals and hence is a measure of drug toxicity. ED_{50} is the minimum dose required to produce clinical effect in 50% of population and hence is a measure of drug potency (Lower dose required to produce effect, higher potency and vice a versa). Potency as discussed in general pharmacology is a measure of drug dose.

$$TI = LD_{50}/ED_{50}$$

Hence on dividing drug toxicity by drug dose, we get a range of dose at which drug use is safe and thus **TI is a measure of drug safety**. For drugs with low TI, TDM is done to maintain the plasma concentration within safe range and is discussed below.

THERAPEUTIC WINDOW

TI is a crude measure for drug safety and is of little clinical usefulness. Hence a better measure of drug's clinical usefulness called as therapeutic window (TW) is used. TW is a range of plasma concentration ranging from minimum effective concentration to minimum toxic concentration. The drug produces adequate clinical effect without sign of toxicity within this range.

Some drugs like **TCA**, **clonidine** and **glipizide** have a distinct type of TW, as they are effective only between the MEC and MTC. The clinical effect seems to wean off below and above both these concentrations respectively.

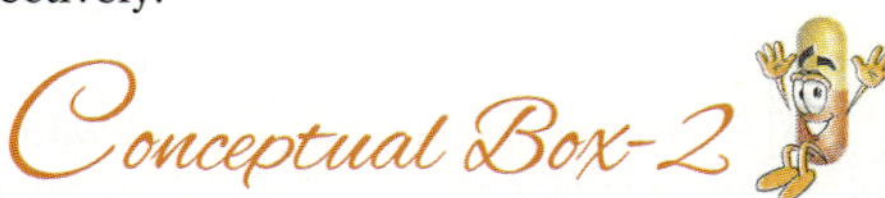

Therapeutic Window

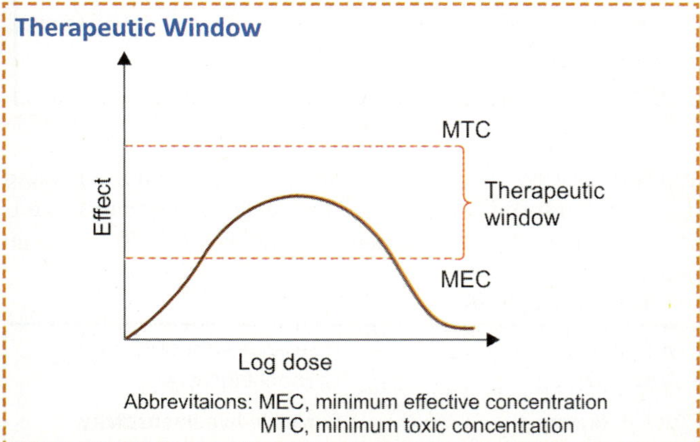

Abbrevitaions: MEC, minimum effective concentration
MTC, minimum toxic concentration

THERAPEUTIC DRUG MONITORING

Therapeutic drug monitoring (TDM) is based on the principle that for some drugs there is a good correlation between the serum plasma concentration and clinical effect/side effect. Based on the plasma concentration, accordingly dose can be adjusted. The best time for sampling is **just before the maintenance dose**, however for drugs with ling $T_{1/2}$ like phenytoin at least 4-5 half-lives must have elapsed before TDM to attain steady state concentration. The various indications for TDM are given below.

Calculation of dose by TDM

New dose = Old dose × Desired drug concentration/Old drug concentration

Drugs with Poorly Defined Clinical end Points

If the clinical effect of drug cannot be easily quantified, e.g. one cannot measure epilepsy, TDM is done. This means, if clinical effect can be easily quantified, TDM is not required. Examples of such drugs for which in place of TDM, the clinical effect can be measured are:

- Beta blocker - Blood pressure
- OHA–RBS
- Warfarin–INR

TDM is not done also for hit and run drugs, irreversible binders and drugs activated in body like levodopa.

Drugs with Low Therapeutic Index

These drugs can cause toxicity even with slight fluctuation of plasma concentration. Example of such drugs with low therapeutic index is given below.

Mnemonics

A Low Therapeutic Drug Causes Toxicity

- **A** : Antiepileptics, Aminoglycosides, Antiarrhythmics
- **Low** : Lithium, Lidocaine
- **Therapeutic** : Theophylline
- **Drug** : Digoxin
- **Causes** : Cyclosporine/Tacrolimus
- **Toxicity** : TCA

Noncompliance of Patients

Compliance is a problem specifically with **antipsychotics**, for which TDM is done.

Therapeutic Failure

TDM can be done to find the reason of therapeutic failure. One of the best examples is that of antiepileptic drug **phenytoin**. In case of a break through seizure for a patient on phenytoin, serum levels are measured; if it's normal the drug is changed and if decreased then dose is increased.

Drugs with Variation in Metabolism in Population

Variable metabolism can be seen in population due to **pharmacogenetic conditions** like acetyl transferase polymorphism. So TDM can be done for drugs metabolized by acetylation like sulfonamides, procainamide, hydralazine, dapsone, etc.

To Prevent Organ or Fetal Toxicity

- A patient with resistant pseudomonas and renal impairment, aminoglycosides can be given with TDM.
- A pregnant female of JME on valproate, is **continued on valproate with TDM** as stopping or changing the drug might cause a break through seizure.

ADVERSE DRUG REACTION

Adverse drug reaction (ADR) is an appreciably harmful or unpleasant reaction resulting from an intervention related to the use of a medicinal product, which predicts hazard from future use and requires withdrawal of drug or alteration of dosage along with treatment of ADR. **Drug specificity is inversely proportional to ADR**, as the drug is more specific for a receptor, lesser is the interaction with other receptors and lesser is side effect. The various types of ADRs are mentioned below in detail.

SIDE EFFECT

Side effect is an undesired effect, which is other than therapeutic one. It may be dose dependent like anticholinergic side effect of TCA and dose independent like anaphylaxis seen with penicillin.

TOXIC EFFECT

Toxic effect is an exaggeration of desired therapeutic effect seen at high doses or on long term therapy. It is always dose related like headache with calcium channel blockers due to meningeal artery dilation and hypoglycemia with sulfonylureas.

SERIOUS ADR

Any ADR which is associated with following features is labeled as serious,

- Death
- Requires hospitalization
- Prolongation of existing hospital stay
- Results in disability
- Life threatening

ALLERGIC REACTION

Allergic reaction is an ADR in which prior sensitization of the immune system by drugs leads to immunogenic reaction on subsequent use. There are four types of allergic reactions.

Conceptual Box-3

Types of Allergic Reactions

Type I: Anaphylatic reaction	Type II: Cytolytic reaction	Type III: Arthus reaction/ serum sickness	Type IV: Delayed hypersensitivity reaction
IgE induced release of mediators like histamine, leukotrienes, prostaglandins, etc.	Ig G and Ig M induced cell damage	Ig G induced damage to blood vessels	T lymphocytes and macrophages induced damage to skin and other organs
• Penicillin • Streptokinase • Heparin • Vaccines	• Hemolytic anemia with penicillin • Thrombocytopenia with quinine and heparin • Agranulocytosis with sulfonamides • Hepatic necrosis with halothane	• SLE with procainamide and hydralazine • Antibiotics-induced serum sickness	• SJS with carbamazepine and lamotrigine

IDIOSYNCRATIC REACTION

Idiosyncratic reaction is an ADR that is seen in a **particular patient** due to absence/decrease/increase in an enzyme or receptor for that drug, which can be caused by genetic polymorphism. Isoniazid causes more peripheral neuropathy in slow acetylators, hemolysis caused by drugs due to G6PD deficiency, etc. are examples of idiosyncrasy.

TERATOGENICITY

Teratogenicity is the ability of a drug to induce gross structural malformation during fetal development. Thus, drugs have been categorized (A, B, C, D and X) based upon their safety of use during pregnancy. Some examples of drugs associated with teratogenicity and pregnancy drug category is given in the annexure.

MUTAGENICITY

Drug (primary carcinogens) or reactive metabolites of drug (secondary carcinogens) induced direct damage to DNA can cause mutagenesis, the latter being more common. Examples are anticancer drugs (alkylating agents, platinum compounds and etoposide) induced secondary leukemia. Epigenetic carcinogens are agents that promote and assist in carcinogenesis, like estrogen dependent breast cancer.

Classification of ADR

Type	Example
Type A: Augmented (Dose related)	Headache with calcium channel blockers
Type B: Bizarre (Non-dose related)	Penicillin hypersensitivity
Type C: Chronic (Dose and Time Related)	HPA suppression by steroids
Type D: Delayed (Time related)	Tardive dyskinesia with antipsychotics, Teratogenicity, Carcinogenesis
Type E: End of use (Withdrawal)	• Opioid withdrawal syndrome • Clonidine withdrawal hypertension
Type F: Failure (Unexpected failure of therapy)	Rifampicin causes OCP failure

PHARMACOVIGILANCE

- Pharmacovigilance is a continuous post marketing monitoring system to detect the rare and long term side effects of drugs to **maintain drug safety**.
- Sources of information for pharmacovigilance are
  - ADR reporting system
  - Medical literature published worldwide
  - Action taken by drug regulatory authorities in other countries
- The pharmacovigilance program was initiated in the year **2010**, by the government of India at AIIMS as National Coordinating center (NCC) but shifted to **Indian Pharmacopoeia Commission (IPC) building, Ghaziabad (U.P)** in the year 2011, which is the current NCC.
- Pharmacovigilance is conducted by **CDSCO (Center for Drug Standard Control Organization)**, Delhi and coordinated by IPC.
- Any ADR detected throughout India in hospitals and medical colleges is reported to the NCC through a software **VIGIFLOW**. When a statistically significant and conclusive ADR is found, NCC reports it to CDSCO. CDSCO does the needful by informing the patients to stop taking the drug, doctors to stop prescribing the drug and drug companies to withdraw the drug from the market.
- Thus, the aim is to maintain **drug safety** in the society.

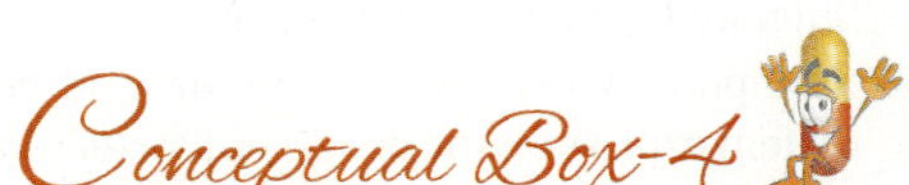

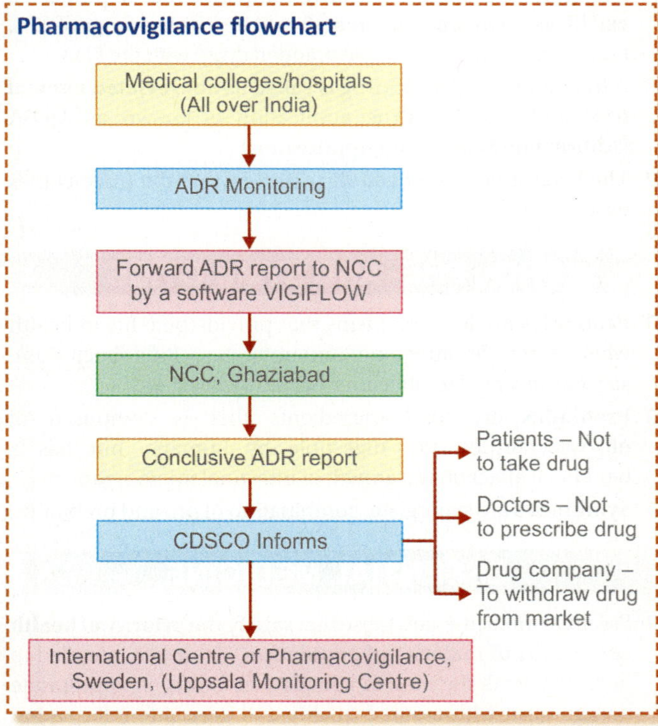

Note: VIGIBASE – worldwide drug safety database of pharmacovigilance.

BIOVIGILANCE AND HEMOVIGILANCE

- The aim of the programs is to track adverse reactions and events associated with blood and blood product transfusion, tissue, organ or cell therapy transplantation.
- It was launched in the year **2012** under pharmacovigilance program of India with following control mechanism, i.e. **NIB (National Institute of Biologics)** as the coordinating center (Conducts) and CDSCO (Controls) as headquarter.

ADVERSE EFFECTS FOLLOWING IMMUNIZATION (AEFI)

- Since majority of the vaccines are administered to a vulnerable population, i.e. children, it is essential to monitor safety.
- AEFI is defined as a medical event that takes place after immunization, causes concern and is believed to be caused by immunization.
- In India safety of vaccines is monitored by division of **AEFI (MOHFW)** through the pharmacovigilance program of India.

DRUG TOLERANCE

Tolerance is defined as requirement of higher than earlier doses of drug for same response production.

INNATE TOLERANCE

Innate tolerance is genetically determined lack of sensitivity to drugs, as it happens in case of pharmacogenetics. It does not take time and is observed the first time drug is administered.

ACQUIRED TOLERANCE

Acquired tolerance is usually seen after some doses of drug have been administered. Various types of acquired tolerance are given below.

- **Pharmacokinetic tolerance:** Changes in pharmacokinetic parameters on repeated drug administration, e.g. enzyme induction by barbiturates increases its own metabolism and higher doses are required.
- **Pharmacodynamic tolerance:** Adaptive changes in the system due to drug exposure. It can be due to change in receptor density or changes in the signaling pathways. Most drugs develop tolerance due to this mechanism like opioids, alcohol, etc.
- **Learned tolerance:** A reduction in effect of drug due to compensatory mechanisms acquired from past experience. E.g. gradually learning to walk in a straight line after alcohol intoxication.
- **Reverse tolerance:** Increase in response with use of same dose of drug again, as seen with cocaine and amphetamine.
- **Cross tolerance:** Repeated administration of drug confers tolerance to other drugs with similar structure or mechanism of action. E.g. diminished effects of sedatives in alcoholics.
- **Acute tolerance or tachyphylaxis:** Rapid development of tolerance after few doses of drug. E.g. **ephedrine**, **methylphenidate**, **amphetamine**, **tyramine**, etc.

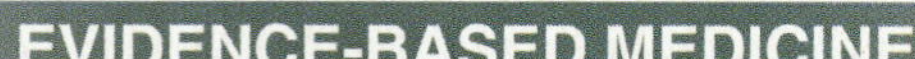

EVIDENCE-BASED MEDICINE

- The concept of evidence-based medicine (EBM) was laid down by **David Sackett** and hence is known as father of EBM.
- Process of developing evidence
  - Formulate a question – e.g. what is the DOC for HTN with CHF?
  - Search literature, e.g. metanalysis, RCT, etc. pertaining to the question.
  - Evaluate the evidence gathered and apply statistics to find the answer to question. E.g. Maximum decrease in mortality is found to be with thiazides and hence is the DOC for HTN with CHF.
- Grades of evidence
  - Systemic reviews and metanalysis are best quality evidence.
  - Professional opinion is poorest quality opinion.

SPURIOUS, ADULTERATED AND MISBRANDED DRUGS

The terms spurious, adulterated and misbranded have been described in the "Drugs and Cosmetics Act, 1940" as given below.

SPURIOUS DRUGS

In India the term spurious drug is used whereas world wide the term counterfeit drug is more accepted. A drug is considered as spurious drug if

- It has been substituted completely or partially by another drug or substance
- It is manufactured under a name which belongs to another drug
- Its label has name of a company which is fictitious or does not exist
- It purports to be the product of a manufacturer of whom it is not truly a product
- It is an imitation or substitute for another drug in a manner likely to deceive

ADULTERATED DRUG

A drug is considered as adulterated if

- It contains any filthy, putrid or decomposed substance
- It has been prepared, packed or stored in insanitary conditions which can cause contamination
- Its container is composed of poisonous or deleterious substance which can make the drug hazardous
- It contains a color other than prescribed one
- It contains harmful or toxic substance
- It has been mixed with any substance to decrease its quality or strength

MISBRANDED DRUG

A drug is considered misbranded if

- It is colored, coated, polished or powdered to conceal damage or to make it appear of more therapeutic value than it really is
- It is not labelled in a prescribed manner
- Its label or container bears any statement that is false or misleading

REVERSE PHARMACOLOGY

- The concept of reverse pharmacology is to find drugs or herbal products in current use with collateral effects (e.g. statins improve cognition) and take them back into lab and conduct trial for any other indication (e.g. Statins for Alzheimer's disease).
- This concept was laid down by **Gnanath Sen** and is known as Father of Reverse Pharmacology.

PARADOXICAL PHARMACOLOGY

- This term was coined by **Richard Bond**, who reported intriguing observations that "Chronic use of some drug types have the opposite effect to those following acute administration of those".
- Examples of paradoxical pharmacology
  - Beta blockers are contraindicated in acute heart failure but decrease mortality in chronic compensated heart failure.
  - Stimulants methylphenidate and amphetamines used in ADHD.
  - Skin irritants like retinoic acid used to treat acne.

GENERIC DRUG

- A generic drug is a product (Company X) that is comparable to a branded drug (Company Y) in dosage form, strength, route of administration, quality and performance characteristics, intended use and bioequivalence.
- Company X can legally copy drug of company Y after the patent expires for the drug, i.e. after 20 years.
- For approval of the generic drug company X has to produce a **certificate of bioequivalence** (should be within a range of 20%, i.e. 20% more or less from the branded drug) with the FDA.
- A trial done for generic drug is called as **abbreviated clinical trial** and the new drug application is known as **ANDA (Abbreviated New Drug Application)**.
- The biggest benefit of generic drugs is, that the price comes down considerably.

PRO-, PRE- AND SYMBIOTICS

- **Probiotics** are live organisms that provide benefits to health when taken at adequate amounts. E.g. Bifidobacterium, saccharomyces, lactobacillus, bacillus calusii, etc.
- **Prebiotics** are food ingredients that is composed of oligosaccharides, not digestible by humans, but has a beneficial effect on the growth of intestinal microorganisms.
- **Symbiotics** are synergistic combination of pro and prebiotics.

ESSENTIAL MEDICINE

- Essential medicines are those that **satisfy the priority of health care needs of majority of population**. These are intended to be available all the time in adequate amounts, in appropriate dosage form with assured quality and adequate information and at a price the individuals and community can afford.
- The concept was introduced by WHO in **1977** and then adopted by many countries.

- The list of essential medicine should be country specific addressing the disease burden of the nation and the commonly used drug at all levels of health care.
- Indian National List of Essential Medicine (NLEM) contains **348 drugs**.

ME TOO DRUGS

"Me too drugs" are structurally similar with only minor changes to the already existing drugs. These drugs have their own share of benefits (better efficacy, new uses, etc.) and drawbacks (deliberate production of "Me too" drugs to increase price). Examples of some me too drugs are given below.

Old drug	Me too drug
Omeprazole	Esomeprazole
Loratadine	Desloratadine
Citalopram	Escitalopram
Zopiclone	Eszopiclone

DRUG SYNERGISM

When two drugs are given in combination, the total effect can be

- **Antagonistic:** Neutralization of effect
- **Sub additive:** Combined effect lesser than sum of individual effect
- **Additive:** Combined effect = sum of individual effect
- **Synergistic:** Combined effect > sum of individual effect

MECHANISMS OF DRUG SYNERGISM

- **Inhibition of drug metabolizing enzyme:** Ritonavir with other protease inhibitors, penicillin with beta lactamase inhibitors, levodopa with carbidopa and imipenem with cilastatin.
- **Sequential blocking of enzyme:** Sulfamethoxazole with trimethoprim, sulfadiazine with pyrimethamine block DHFR and DHPS.
- **Efflux pump inhibitor:** Penicillin G with probenecid.
- **Multiple drugs for same target:** ATT drug combination.

EVERGREENING OF DRUG

Ever greening refers to different ways by which drug companies take undue advantage and manipulate law to extend patent of drug.

The various routes taken by companies for these are:

- Me too drug production
- Prescription to OTC switch
- Exclusive partnership with the cream generic companies

NUTRACEUTICALS

Nutraceuticals are food or food ingredients that may provide health benefits beyond the traditional nutrition that it contains. Common examples are beta carotene in carrot, **lycopene** intomatoes, flavonoids in onions, caffeic and ferulic acid in fruits, **coenzyme Q**, **tryptophan**, ginseng, ginkgo biloba, etc.

FDA approved nutraceuticals

Neutraceutical	Approved for
Soy protein	CHD
Calcium	Osteoporosis
Fibres containing fruits and vegetables	Cancer
Folic acid	NTD

EXCLUSION LIST FOR NEUTRACEUTICALS

- Allopathic, ayurvedic, siddha and yunani drugs defined in section 3 of drugs and cosmetics act.
- Product does not claim to mitigate any specific disease or disorder.
- Does not contain a narcotic or psychotropic substance.

DRUG ADVERTISEMENT GUIDELINES IN INDIA

The required information for pharmaceutical advertising are given by the OPPI (Organization of Pharmaceutical Products of India). All printed promotional materials must be legible and include:

- The 'name' of the product (normally the brand name).
- The 'active ingredients', using approved names where they exist.
- The 'name and address' of the pharmaceutical company or its agent responsible for marketing the product.
- The 'date of production' of the advertisement.
- The 'abbreviated prescribing information' which should include an approved indication or indications for use together with the dosage and method of use; and a succinct statement of the contraindications, precautions and side effects.

DRUG DESENSITIZATION

Drug desensitization is the development of a temporary state of tolerance within hours to days to hypersensitivity caused by a particular drug. Desensitization is done if no better drug is available for a condition and the benefit of drug outweighs the risk. The most commonly studied drug for desensitization is **penicillin**, followed by others like rifampicin, isoniazid, allopurinol, insulin, aspirin, platinum compounds, taxanes, rituximab and trastuzumab. The various principles of drug desensitization are given below.

- No better alternative is available for the condition, e.g. penicillin for syphilis in pregnancy, allopurinol in chronic gout, cisplatin in recurrent ovarian cancer, etc.
- Drug used for the condition is superior to alternative, e.g. rifampicin and isoniazid in TB.
- The hypersensitivity reaction should not be life threatening like SJS and TEN for desensitization to be done.
- Starting dose is $1/1,000,000^{th}$ to $1/100^{th}$ of normal dose in desensitization depending upon severity of hypersensitivity.
- Dose escalations are doubled at 15–30 minutes interval for immediate reactions and up to 24 hours for delayed reactions.

- CPR facility should be readily available.
- Premedication with steroids and antihistaminics are not given.
- Drug is continued daily to maintaintolerance as there can be breakthrough hypersensitivity if skipped.

DESIGNER DRUGS

Designer drugs are made illegally by altering the chemical structure of legal drugs like pethidine to increase their potency several times which have addiction potential. These drugs are also known as club drugs. The examples of designer drugs are **methamphetamine**, ecstasy, GHB, rohypnol, ketamine and various analgesic analogs.

PHOTOPHARMACOLOGY

- A **photo switch** is a molecule that gets activated by a wavelength of light.
- This photo switch molecule can be attached to a drug molecule and thus by a wavelength of light the drug can be selectively activated in a particular organ or tissue of interest.
- This is a step to reduce adverse drug reactions associated with action of drug on undesirable tissues.
- Let's take an example: Ciprofloxacin used for prostatitis causes tendinitis as side effect. If a photo switch is attached with ciprofloxacin and a wavelength is directed to prostate tissue ciprofloxacin will act only on prostate. And hence there will be no tendinitis.
- Some examples of drugs being developed with photo switches
  - Insulin with incretin switch
  - Ciprofloxacin
  - Sulfonylureas 4th gen
  - Histone deacetylase inhibitors
  - Proteasome inhibitors

FIXED DOSE COMBINATIONS (FDC)

- Fixed dose combinations are two or more drugs in a single formulation. FDC are acceptable only if the combination has a proved advantage over single compounds given separately in terms of efficacy or safety.
- There are benefits and drawbacks of FDC as mentioned below in the table.

Benefits	Drawbacks
• Better compliance • Decreased cost • Increased efficacy (Trimethoprim sulfamethoxazole) • Decreased side effect (Spironolactone prevents thiazide induced hyperkalemia) • Decreased resistance (ATT)	• Individual drug dose titration is not possible • Difficulty in finding cause of ADR • Limited use as one drug's contraindication limits other drug's use

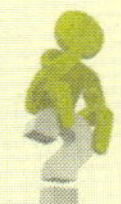

Image-based Questions

1. **The person shown in the picture is:**

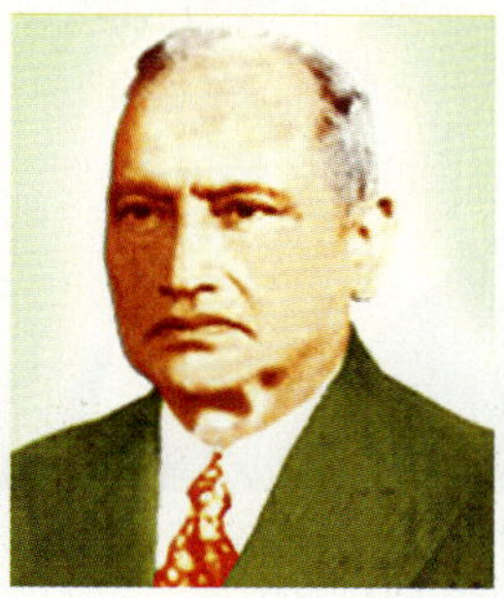

a. Gnanath Sen b. Sir. Ram Nath Chopra
c. Prem Chopra d. Milap Nahata

2. **The person in the picture is known as Father of:**

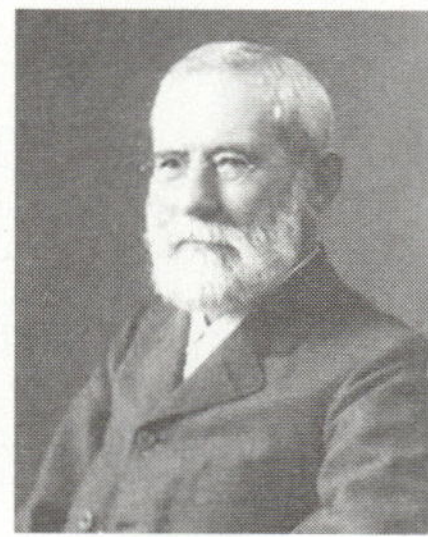

a. Paradoxical pharmacology
b. Reverse pharmacology
c. Chronopharmacology
d. Modern pharmacology

3. **The ultrasonographic finding is consistent with teratogenic effect of**

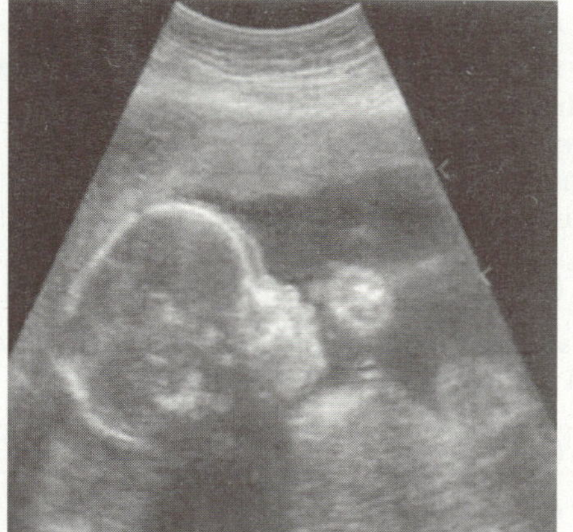

a. Valproate b. Phenytoin
c. Thalidomide d. Warfarin

4. **The picture shown below is suggestive of teratogenic effect due to:**

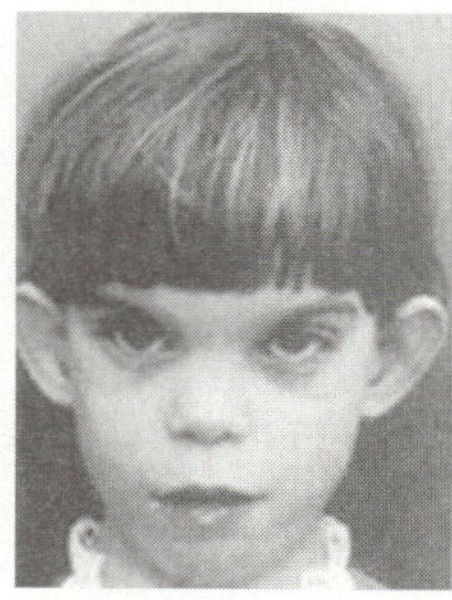
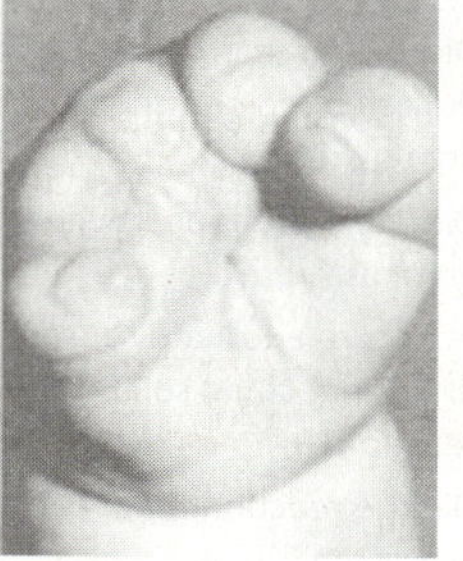

a. Phenytoin b. Valproate
c. Thalidomide d. Warfarin

5. **The baby shown in the picture was born after exposure of**

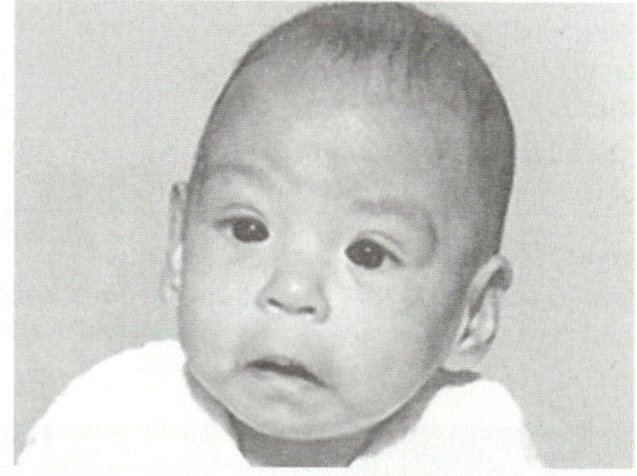

a. Valproate b. Phenytoin
c. Warfarin d. Alcohol

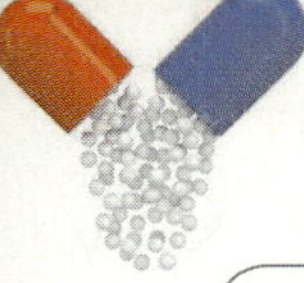

6. The scale given in the picture is known as

	Question	Yes	No	Don't know
1	Are there previous conclusion reports on this reaction?	+1	0	0
2	Did the adverse event appear after the suspect drug was administered?	+2	−1	0
3	Did the AR improve when the drug was discontinued or a specific antagonist was administered?	+1	0	0
4	Did the AR reappear when drug was re-administered?	+2	−1	0
5	Are there alternate causes [other than the drug] that could solely have caused the reaction?	−1	−2	0
6	Did the reaction reappear when a placebo was given?	−1	−1	0
7	Was the drug detected in the blood [or other fluids] in a concentration known to be toxic?	+1	0	0
8	Was the reaction more severe when the dose was increased, or less severe when the dose was decreased?	+1	0	0
9	Did the patient have a similar reaction to the same or similar drug in any previous exposure?	+1	0	0
10	Was the adverse event confirmed by objective evidence?	+1	0	0

a. Langley scale
b. ADR scale
c. Naranjo scale
d. Pharmacovigilance scale

7. The person in the picture is known as father of:

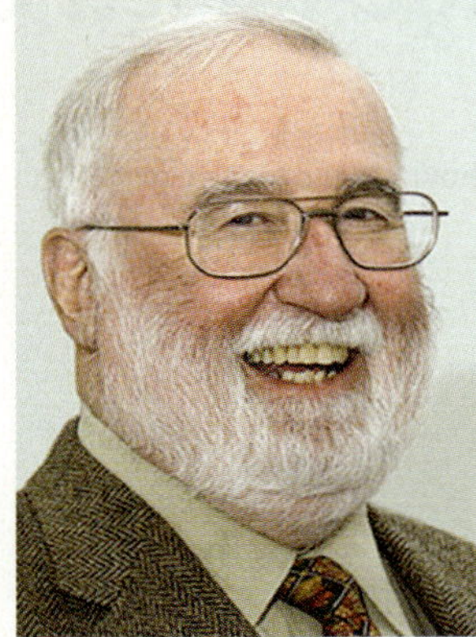

a. Modern Pharmacology
b. Reverse Pharmacology
c. Evidence based medicine
d. Clinical Pharmacology

Answers with Explanations to Image-based Questions

1. Ans. (b) Sir. Ram Nath Chopra

- The person in the picture is Sir. Ram Nath Chopra, who is known as the father of Indian Pharmacology.
- He established the first pharmacology institute in India in Calcutta.

2. Ans. (d) Modern Pharmacology

(Ref: KDT 7th E/P1)

- The person in the picture is Oswald Schmiedberg, who is known as father of modern pharmacology.
- He established the first pharmacology institute ever in this world.

3. Ans. (d) Warfarin

(Ref: Rang and Dale 6th E/P759)

- The finding of nasal hypoplasia in USG of fetus is confirmatory of warfarin fetopathy.

4. Ans. (a) Phenytoin

(Ref: Rang and Dale 6th E/P759)

The features of the child suggestive of fetal hydantoin syndrome are

- Facial cleft
- Microcephaly

5. Ans. (d) Alcohol

(Ref: Rang and Dale 6th E/P759)

The features of the baby suggestive of fetal alcohol syndrome are

- Small palpebral fissures
- Thin vermilion border
- Smooth philtrum

6. Ans. (c) Naranjo scale

The scale given in the picture is called as Naranjo scale used for detection of ADR causality.

7. Ans. (c) Evidence based medicine

(Ref: KDT 7th E/P73)

- The person in the picture is David Sackett, who is known as the father of evidence based medicine.

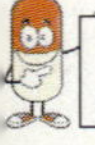

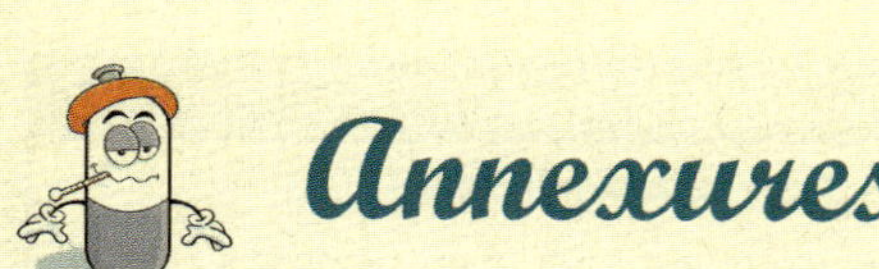

Annexures

Drug Storage Temperature

Condition	Temperature
Freezer	–20 –10°C
Refrigerator	2–8°C
Cold	Temperature not exceeding 8°C
Cool	8–15°C
Room temperature	15–30°C
Warm	30–40°C
Excessive heat	Above 40°C

Drugs Banned and Withdrawn

Drugs	Reason for ban or withdrawal
Astemizole Terfenadine Cisapride Tegaserod	QT prolongation
Fenfluramine	Cardiac valve defects Pulmonary hypertension
Gatifloxacin	Hyperglycemia
Letrozole banned in pregnancy	Teratogenicity Bone malformation Cardiac stenosis
Phenylpropanolamine	Stroke
Phenformin	Lactic acidosis
Nimesulide banned in children < 12 years	Hepatotoxicity
Refecoxib Valdecoxib	Myocardial infarction Stroke
Rimonabant	Depression Suicidal tendency
Rosiglitazone	Myocardial infarction Stroke
Sibutramine	Myocardial infarction Stroke
Troglitazone	Hepatic necrosis

Important Drug Schedules in India

Schedule G	List of drugs that don't need prescription but requires a mandatory text on label "Caution: It is dangerous to take this preparation, except under medical supervision". E.g. antihistaminics.
Schedule H	List of drugs that can be sold only when a prescription is produced. Most drugs belong to this category.
Schedule P	It is about drug expiry period, i.e. maximum period till which drug can be used with intact potency.
Schedule W	List of drugs marketed under generic names only.
Schedule X	List of psychotropic drugs which need special license for manufacture and sale.
Schedule Y	Guidelines on clinical trials, import and manufacture of new drugs.

Note:
- OTC (Over the counter) drugs don't require a prescription and are drugs which don't belong to schedule H and X.
- Drugs under schedule G, H and X cannot be directly advertised to the patient.

Important Drug Schedules in USA

Schedule I	Drugs with high abuse potential, which cannot be prescribed. E.g. Heroin, LSD, Flunitrazepam.
Schedule II	Drugs with high abuse potential but can be prescribed. E.g. Morphine, Codeine, Methylphenidate, Amphetamines.
Schedule III	Drugs associated with moderate abuse potential. E.g. Buprenorphine, Phenobarbital.
Schedule IV	Drugs associated with low abuse potential. E.g. Benzodiazepines.
Schedule V	Drugs associated with least abuse potential. Most of these are OTC (Over the counter) drugs.

Contributors to Pharmacology

Oswald Scmiedberg	Father of modern pharmacology
Rudolf Buchheim	Founded first pharmacology institute
Sir Ram Nath Chopra	Father of Indian pharmacology
Gnanath Sen	Father of reverse pharmacology
James black	Discovered beta-2 and H2 receptors followed by their blockers
Freidrich Seruner	Purified morphine from opium
Paul Ehrlich	Used arsenical compounds for syphilis
Gerhard Domagk	Discovered first antibiotics, i.e. sulfonamides
Chain and Florey	Developed penicillin based on Fleming's work
Langley	Gave receptor theory
James Gregory	Introduced allopathy
Hahnemann	Introduced homeopathy
Richard bond	Coined term paradoxical pharmacology

Drugs and Teratogenicity

Drug	Teratogenic effect
Alcohol	**Fetal Alcohol Syndrome** • Dysmorphic facial features (all 3 are required) ▪ Small palpebral fissures ▪ Thin vermilion border ▪ Smooth philtrum • Prenatal and/or postnatal growth impairment • Central nervous system abnormalities (1 required) ▪ Structural: head size < 10th percentile, significant brain abnormality on imaging ▪ Neurological ▪ Functional: global cognitive or intellectual deficits ▪ Functional deficits in at least three domains
Fluconazole	• Oral clefts • Abnormal facies • Cardiac abnormalities • Skull, long-bone, and joint abnormalities
ACE inhibitors	• **Fetal RAAS inhibition** followed by hypotension and reduced perfusion causes fetal-growth restriction and calvarium maldevelopment • Oligohydramnios causes pulmonary hypoplasia and limb contractures.
Leflunomide	• Hydrocephalus • Eye anomalies • Skeletal abnormalities

Contd...

Drug	Teratogenic effect
Chloramphenicol	• Grey baby syndrome
Nitrofurantoin	• Hypoplastic left heart syndrome • Microphthalmia/anophthalmia • Facial clefts • Atrial septal defects
Sulfonamides	• Anencephaly • Left ventricular outflow tract obstruction • Choanal atresia • Diaphragmatic hernia
Tetracycline	• Yellow discoloration of deciduous teeth • Bone growth abnormality
Fluoroquinolones	Cartilage growth defect
Cyclophosphamide	• Skeletal abnormalities • Limb defects • Cleft palate • Eye abnormalities
Methotrexate	Fetal methotrexate aminopterin syndrome • Craniosynostosis with "clover-leaf" skull • Wide nasal bridge • Low-set ears • Micrognathia • Limb abnormalities
Trastuzumab	• Pulmonary hypoplasia • Skeletal abnormalities
Diethylsilbestrol	Vaginal adenosis, vaginal and cervical cancer in female fetus after 20+ years
Corticosteroids	Facial clefts
Lithium	Ebstein's anomaly
Isotretinoin	• Bilateral microtia • Anotia with stenosis of external ear canal • Flat, depressed nasal bridge and ocular hypertelorism • Cleft lip and palate
Thalidomide	• Phocomelia • Cranial nerve defects • Anorectal stenosis • Cardiac defects
Warfarin	• Stippling of the vertebrae and femoral epiphyses • Nasal hypoplasia with depression of the nasal bridge (saddle nose)
Valproate	• Neural tube defect • Cardiovascular defect
Phenytoin	**Fetal hydantoin syndrome** • Facial cleft • Microcephaly • IUGR • Hypertelorism • Triphalangeal thumb
Penicillamine	Loose skin

Pregnancy Drug Categories

Categories	Significance	Examples
Category A	No risk to fetus in human studies	• Levothyroxine • Potassium • Supplementation • $MgSO_4$
Category B	• Animal studies show no risk • Human studies are lacking	• Penicillin • Cephalosporin • Macrolides • Brimonidine
Category C	• Animal studies show positive teratogenic risk • Human studies are not available	• Albuterol • Zidovudine • CCB • Morphine • Atropine
Category D	• Human and animal studies show positive teratogenic risk • Can be used in pregnancy because of benefits greater than risk might be acceptable	• Corticosteroids • Azathioprine • Carbamazepine • Valproate • Methotrexate • Lithium
Category X	• Human and animal studies show positive teratogenic risk • Absolutely contraindicated in pregnancy because of risk greater than benefits	• Thalidomide • Isotretinoin • Fluoroquinolones • Tetracyclines • Chloramphenicol • Warfarin • ACE inhibitors

Drug-Induced Ion Abnormalities

Hypokalemia	Hyperkalemia

• Beta 2 agonists
• Alpha blockers
• Insulin
• Theophylline/Caffeine
• B12/Folic acid
• Amphotericin B
• Diuretics except K sparing ones
  ▪ CA inhibitors
  ▪ Loops
  ▪ Thiazides
  ▪ Osmotic diuretics
• Penicillin
• Fludrocortisone
	• Beta blockers (Non-selective)
	• Digoxin
	• Succinyl choline
	• RAAS inhibitors
	  ▪ ACEI
	  ▪ ARB
	  ▪ Renin inhibitors
	  ▪ Aldosterone antagonists
	• Amiloride/Triamterene
	• Trimethoprim
	• Pentamidine
	• NSAIDS
	• Cyclosporine/Tacrolimus
	• Heparin

Hypomagnesemia	Hypermagnesemia

• PPI
• Ethanol
• Diuretics
  ▪ Loops
  ▪ Thiazides
  ▪ Osmotic
• Pentamidine
• Foscarnet
• Cyclosporine
• Aminoglycosides
• Amphotericin B
• Cetuximab
	• Cathartics
	• Urologic irrigants
	• Antacids
	• Enemas
	• Laxatives
	• Lithium
	• Theophylline

Hyponatremia	**Hypernatremia**
• Chlorpropamide • Vincristine • Cyclophosphamide • Nicotine • Clofibrate • SSRI • NSAIDS • Oxytocin • TCA • Nicotine	• Bicarbonate • Steroids • Androgens • Estrogen • Lithium • Demeclocycline • Foscarnet • Expired tetracycline
Hypocalcemia	**Hypercalcemia**
• Bisphosphonates • Cisplatin • Foscarnet • Calcitonin • Loops • Glucocorticoids • Antiepileptics • PPI • PTU • Colchicine toxicity	• Thiazides • Lithium • Vitamin D • Vitamin A intoxication • Aluminium intoxication • Theophylline • Estrogen • Tamoxifen

Multiple Choice Questions

1. **Manufacturer of a drug company labels the drug contains 500 mg paracetamol. On government analysis, it was found to contain only 200 mg of drug. Which type of drug it is known as?** ***(AIIMS May 2018)***
   a. Unethical drug
   b. Spurious drug
   c. Adulterant drug
   d. Unbranded drug
2. **Which one is a placebo:** ***(AIIMS Nov 2017)***
   a. Herbal medication with no effect known
   b. Physiotherapy
   c. Sham surgery
   d. Cognitive behavioural therapy
3. **What instruction do you give to a mother who is lactating for drug use?** ***(AIIMS Nov 2017)***
   a. No advice as most of drug are not present in breast milk
   b. Give longer half-life drugs
   c. Tell the mother to feed when it is least efficacious
   d. Just before the next dose, when the plasma concentration of the drug would be the least
4. **Drug advertisement literature which tells the efficacy and indications of drugs need not mention:** ***(AIIMS Nov 2016)***
   a. Common side effects but nonserious
   b. Rare side effects but serious
   c. Expiry date of drugs
   d. Should quote for reference for all inference regarding the drug
5. **What is the weight of rabbit used for ocular experiment of miotics and mydriatics?** ***(AIIMS Nov 2016)***
   a. 0.5–1 kg
   b. 1.5–2.5 kg
   c. 4–6 kg
   d. 6–8 kg
6. **Which of the following drugs might have produced the effect in the picture?** ***(AIIMS Nov 2016)***

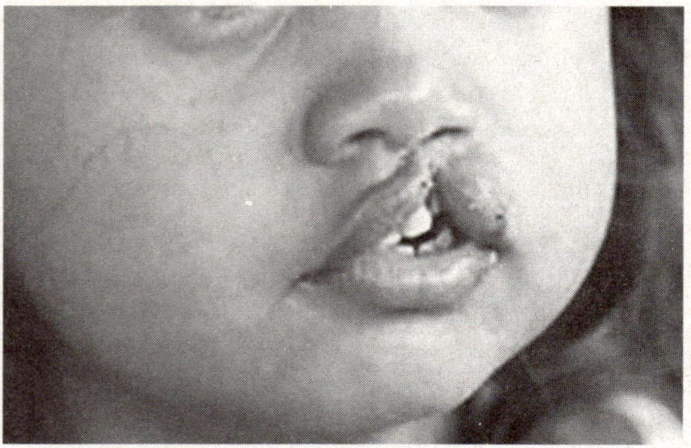

   a. Nicotinic acid
   b. Retinoic acid
   c. Folic acid
   d. Pantothenic acid
7. **Which of the following phase of clinical trials is carried out after a new drug is marketed:** ***(AIIMS May 2016)***
   a. Phase 1
   b. Phase 2
   c. Phase 4
   d. Phase 0
8. **Pigmentation of nail can be seen with all except:** ***(AIIMS Nov 2016)***
   a. Chloroquine
   b. Cyclophosphamide
   c. Chlorpromazine
   d. Amiodarone
9. **Store a drug in a cool place refers to:** ***(AIIMS Nov 2018, NOV 2015)***
   a. Below freezing pt of water
   b. 0 degree
   c. 2–4 degree
   d. 8 to 15 degree
10. **Phase 1 clinical trial is for?** ***(AIIMS, Nov 2018, Nov 2015)***
   a. Pharmacokinetics
   b. Dose
   c. Safety
   d. Efficacy
11. **Schedule of drug to be sold only on prescription?** ***(AIIMS MAY, 2018, Nov 2015)***
   a. H
   b. P
   c. G
   d. X
12. **Which of the following drug is considered as category B in pregnancy?** ***(AIIMS Nov 2014)***
   a. Latanoprost
   b. Pilocarpine
   c. Brimonidine
   d. Dorazolamide
13. **Father of evidence-based medicine is:** ***(AIIMS May 2014)***
   a. David Sackett
   b. Oswald Schmeidberg
   c. Arachibald Cochrane
   d. Gananath Sen
14. **Maximum tolerated dose of a new drug is evaluated in:** ***(AIIMS May 2013)***
   a. Phase 1 trial
   b. Phase 2 RCT
   c. Phase 4 RCT
   d. Case Control
15. **True about orphan drugs:** ***(AIIMS May 2013)***
   a. Drug for rare diseases
   b. Developed for orphans
   c. Rare drug for common diseases
   d. Rarely using drugs
16. **Comparison of efficacy of a drug with placebo is confirmed in which phase of clinical trials?** ***(AIIMS May 2013)***
   a. Phase 1
   b. Phase 2
   c. Phase 3
   d. Phase 4
17. **In new drug designing, problem arises in:** ***(AIIMS Nov 2012)***
   a. Decreasing interaction of drug with target proteins
   b. Increasing drug interaction with nontarget proteins
   c. Decreasing potency of drugs
   d. Increased binding with target protein
18. **Unfavorable interaction of drug and substrate in human beings are all except:** ***(AIIMS Nov 2012)***
   a. Omeprazole reduces stomach acid secretion
   b. Methotrexate inhibiting folate
   c. Barbiturates decreases B_{12} absorption
   d. Retinoic acid inhibits vitamin E

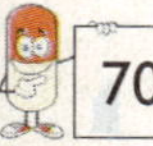

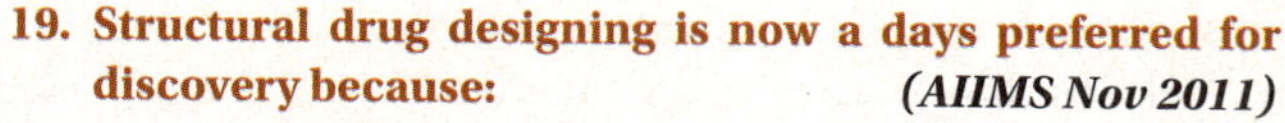

19. **Structural drug designing is now a days preferred for discovery because:** ***(AIIMS Nov 2011)***
    a. It avoids the need to develop a lead compound
    b. It makes the use of drug library redundant
    c. Understanding the structure of the receptor can enhance better target
    d. It is very easy and less time consuming
20. **Evidence-based medicine all are true except:** ***(AIIMS Nov 2011)***
    a. It is based on clinical model and decision analysis
    b. The research paper is investigated by the tools quoted in the research paper itself to check validity
    c. The opinions of medical professionals and researchers is given least importance
    d. Evidence is formed from weak and poor studies
21. **Pharmacovigilance means:** ***(AIIMS May 2010)***
    a. Monitoring of drug safety
    b. Monitoring of unethical trade of drugs
    c. Monitoring pharma students
    d. Monitoring drug efficacy
22. **Pharmacovigilance is used:** ***(AIIMS May 2009)***
    a. To monitor drug toxicity
    b. To monitor unauthorized drug manufacture
    c. For monitoring of students
    d. To check costs
23. **Therapeutic drug monitoring is required in all except:** ***(AIIMS Nov 2007)***
    a. Phenytoin   b. Metformin
    c. Tacrolimus   d. Cyclosporin
24. **Good clinical practice (GCP) is not required in:** ***(AIIMS Nov 2007)***
    a. Preclinical phase   b. Phase I trial
    c. Phase II studies   d. Phase IV studies
25. **Which of the following property of the drug will enable it to be used in low concentration?** ***(AIIMS Nov 2005)***
    a. High affinity
    b. High specificity
    c. Low specificity
    d. High stability
26. **Side effects of a drug arise due to interactions of the drug to molecules other than the target. These effects of the drug can be minimized by its high:** ***(AIIMS Nov 2005)***
    a. Specificity   b. Solubility
    c. Affinity   d. Hydrophobicity
27. **Which of the following is correct regarding clinical trials?** ***(Recent Question 2019)***
    a. Phase 3 is RCT
    b. Phase 1 is for safety and efficacy
    c. Phase 4 is done in animals
    d. Phase 2 is done for toxicity
28. **Fixed dose combinations benefits** ***(Recent Question 2019)***
    a. Hepatic status affects both components equally
    b. Dose of individual components can be adjusted
    c. Adverse effect of one overcome by other
    d. Easy to find cause of ADR
29. **Which is most common drug studied for desensitization?** ***(Recent Question Dec 2016)***
    a. Penicillin   b. Allopurinol
    c. Isoniazid   d. Insulin
30. **Which of the following drug is contraindicated in G6PD deficiency?** ***(Recent Question Dec 2016)***
    a. Quinine   b. Nitrofurantoin
    c. Hydralazine   d. Methotrexate
31. **A patient developed porphyria while on thiopentone. This can be studied under:** ***(Recent Question Dec 2016)***
    a. Pharmacogenetic   b. Pharmacogenomics
    c. Pharmacognosy   d. Pharmacopoeia
32. **Phase 3 trials are for whom?** ***(Recent Question Dec 2016)***
    a. Normal subjects
    b. Few patients
    c. Hundreds of patients
    d. Thousands of patients
33. **Human ethical committee permission is not necessary for?** ***(Recent Question Dec 2016)***
    a. Phase 1   b. Phase 2
    c. Phase 3   d. Phase 4
34. **Which of the following drug doesn't come under Category C in pregnancy?** ***(Recent Question Dec 2016)***
    a. Adenosine   b. Metoprolol
    c. Amiodarone   d. Diltiazem
35. **Which of the following is a designer drug?** ***(Recent Question Dec 2016)***
    a. Cocaine   b. Heroin
    c. Methamphetamine   d. Cannabis
36. **Therapeutic drug monitoring must be done for:** ***(Recent Question 2016)***
    a. Penicillin   b. Lithium
    c. Erythromycin   d. Lignocaine
37. **Therapeutic drug monitoring is used in:** ***(Recent Question 2016)***
    a. Diuretic
    b. Metformin
    c. Levodopa
    d. Digoxin
38. **Pharmacovigilance is used for:** ***(Recent Question 2016)***
    a. To monitor drug toxicity
    b. To monitor unauthorize d. Drug manufacture
    c. Monitoring of students d. Check costs
39. **Branch that deals with medicinal drugs obtained from plants and other natural resources:** ***(Recent Question 2016)***
    a. Pharmacognosy   b. Pharmacogenetics
    c. Pharmacogenomics   d. Pharmacopia
40. **Counterfeit drug is:** ***(Recent Question 2016)***
    a. Fake medicine
    b. Contains the wrong ingredient
    c. They have active ingredient in wrong dose
    d. All the above
41. **Approximate dose of drug in a 5 years old child:** ***(Recent Question 2016)***
    a. Same as adult dose   b. 1/2 of adult dose
    c. 1/3 of adult dose   d. 1/4 of adult dose

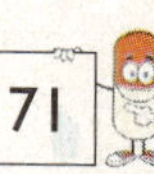

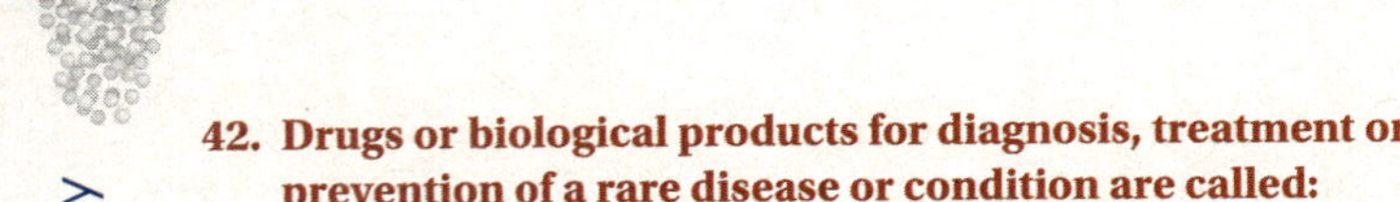

42. Drugs or biological products for diagnosis, treatment or prevention of a rare disease or condition are called: ***(Recent Question 2016)***

a. Orphan drugs b. Rare drugs
c. Extinct drugs d. Essential drugs

43. Essential drugs: ***(Recent Question 2016)***

a. Included in national pharmacopoeia
b. Should always be present at PHC
c. Those that satisfy the primary health care needs of the population
d. Life saving medications

44. Father of pharmacology: ***(Recent Question 2016)***

a. Radolf buchheim b. Oswald schmiedeberg
c. J langley d. P ehrilich

45. Therapeutic monitoring of plasma level of drug is done for all except: ***(Recent Question 2016)***

a. Warfarin b. Gentamicin
c. Cyclosporine d. Phenytoin

46. Therapeutic index is a measure of: ***(Recent Question 2016)***

a. Safety b. Potency
c. Efficacy d. Selectivity

47. In which of the following phases of clinical trial of drugs, ethical clearance is not required? ***(Recent Question 2016)***

a. Phase I b. Phase II
c. Phase III d. Phase IV

48. All the following drugs can cross placenta except: ***(Recent Question 2016)***

a. Phenytoin b. Diazepam
c. Morphine d. Heparin

49. Which of the following is most likely due to a pharmacogenetic condition? ***(Recent Question 2016)***

a. Hypoglycemia by insulin
b. Tachycardia by albuterol
c. Metoclopramide induced muscle dystonia
d. Primaquine-induced hemolytic anemia

50. Drug requiring serum level monitoring: ***(Recent Question 2016)***

a. Lorazepam b. Lithium
c. Amitryptylline d. Haloperidol

51. In which of the following phases of clinical trials, healthy normal human volunteers participate: ***(Recent Question 2016)***

a. Phase-I b. Phase-II
c. Phase-III d. Phase-IV

52. The aim of post marketing studies is:

a. Efficacy of the drug ***(Recent Question 2016)***
b. Dosage of the drug
c. Deals with alteration of the drug includes absorption, distribution, binding/storage
d. Safety and comparisons with other medicines

53. ED50 is used for determining: ***(Recent Question 2016)***

a. Potency
b. Efficacy
c. Safety
d. Toxicity

54. Stage IV clinical trial is also called as:

a. Human pharmacology and safety
b. Postmarketing surveillance ***(Recent Question 2016)***
c. Therapeutic exploration and does ranging
d. Therapeutic confirmation

55. As per 'Drugs and cosmetic act' prescription drugs are included in: ***(Recent Question 2016)***

a. Schedule C b. Schedule H
c. Schedule J d. Schedule I

56. Phase IV of clinical trials collect information specifically about: ***(Recent Question 2016)***

a. Drug efficacy
b. Drug potency
c. Drug shelf life
d. Other possible uses of the drug

57. The study of how variations in the human genome affect the response to medications is known as: ***(Recent Question 2016)***

a. Pharmacogenomics b. Pharmacokinetics
c. Pharmacotherapeutics d. Pharmacovigilance

58. Idiosyncrasy is: ***(Recent Question 2016)***

a. Unpredictable reaction to a drug
b. Predictable effect of a drug at normal concentration
c. Predictable effect of a drug at high concentration
d. Non of the above

59. Drug which causes tachyphylaxis: ***(Recent Question 2016)***

a. Adrenaline b. Amoxicillin
c. Amphetamine d. Atropine

60. Pharmacognosy is: ***(Recent Question 2016)***

a. Study of animal extracts
b. Study of genetic polymorphisms due to drug effect
c. Study of drugs from plants
d. Study and development of sustained release drugs

61. The study of adverse effects, toxicity and appropriate corrections of drugs is: ***(Recent Question 2016)***

a. Pharmacovigilance b. Pharmacodynamics
c. Pharmacokinetics d. Pharmacogenomics

62. LD 50/ED 50 is a measure for: ***(Recent Question 2016)***

a. Affinity b. Potency
c. Therapeutic index d. Toxicity

63. Drug withdrawn in india is? ***(Recent Question 2016)***

a. Levofloxacin b. Gatifloxacin
c. Moxifloxacin d. Ofloxacin

64. Phocomelia is best described as:*(Recent Question 2016)*

a. Defect in development of long bones
b. Defect in development of flat bones
c. Defect in intramembranous ossification
d. Defect in cartilage replacement by bones

65. Which amongst the following is contraindicated in pregnancy? ***(Recent Question 2016)***

a. ACE inhibitors b. Indomethacin
c. Carbamezapine d. All of the above

66. Drug contraindicated in pregnancy are all, except: ***(Recent Question 2016)***

a. Phenytoin b. Methyl dopa
c. Lithium d. Methotrexate

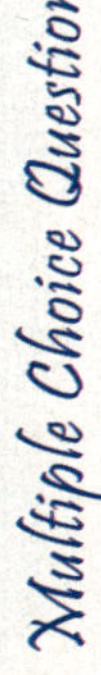

67. Hemolysis in G6PD deficiency is precipitated by following, except: *(Recent Question 2016)*
a. Dapsone b. Cotrimoxazole
c. Quinine d. Penicillin

68. Which antimalarial drug can be safely administered in a baby with glucose-6 phosphate dehydrogenase' deficiency (2002)? *(Recent Question 2016)*
a. Chloroquine b. Quinine
c. Dapsone d. Primaquine

69. True about Placebo: *(PGI May 2014)*
a. It works only in psychiatric person
b. Response is both objective & subjective
c. Effect also seen in normal person
d. It is an inert substance

70. True statement about essential medicines: *(PGI May 2013)*
a. Emergency medicine
b. Costly but necessary
c. Drug listed in pharmacopoeia
d. Need for society
e. Should be available at all times

71. Which of the following are neutraceuticals: *(PGI May 2010)*
a. Coq10 b. Tryptophan
c. β-carotene d. Lycopene

72. True statement regarding Bioassay: *(PGI May 2010)*
a. Done to know activity of endogenous substance
b. To know toxicity & efficacy of drug

73. Therapeutic drug monitoring (TDM) involves monitoring of plasma concentration of the drug when there is similar relation b/w plasma drug concentration & its effect. TDM has widely used to guide therapy with which of the following group of drugs: *(PGI June 2009)*
a. Antiarrhythmics b. Anticoagulants
c. Antihypertensive agents d. Hypoglycemic agents
e. Antidepressants

74. Compliance of drug increased by: *(PGI Nov 2008)*
a. ↑ no. of dose
b. ↑ duration of treatment
c. Past history of unpleasant events like myocardial infarction
d. Less frequent dose
e. Involvement of family member

75. Narrow therapeutic index are seen in: *(PGI Nov 2007)*
a. Metfomin
b. Phenytoin
c. Cyclosporin
d. Digitalis

76. Advantages of fixed drug combinations: *(PGI Nov 2007)*
a. ↓ Cost
b. ↑ Efficacy
c. ↑ Compliance
d. ↓ Resistance
e. Dose titration can be done

77. In G6PD deficiency, drugs contraindicated are: *(PGI Nov 2007)*
a. Primaquine b. Chloroquine
c. Hydralazine d. Losartan

78. True about tachyphylaxis: *(PGI Nov 2006)*
a. Direct sympathemimetic involved
b. Mechanism clearly understood
c. Ephedrine tachyphylaxis reversed with noradrenline
d. Indirect sympathomimetics involved
e. It is an anaphylaxis reaction

79. Pharmacogenetics is associated with: *(PGI Nov 2005)*
a. Variability of enzyme action
b. Environmental influence
c. Individual variability in oral absorption
d. Different mechanism of actions in different individuals
e. Different DRC in different individual.

80. Which of the following is not a cat C drug? *(JIPMER 2017)*
a. Amiodarone b. Nifedipine
c. Salbutamol d. Atropine

81. Entry of new drug into the market: *(JIPMER 2012)*
a. Phase 1
b. Phase 2
c. Phase 3
d. Phase 4

82. All are true about Phase II trials except: *(JIPMER 2006)*
a. Safety and efficacy
b. Done in healthy human volunteers
c. Therapeutic exploratory trial
d. Positive evidence in Phase I is a prerequisite

Practice Questions & Answers from 83 to 92 are given at the end of the chapter.

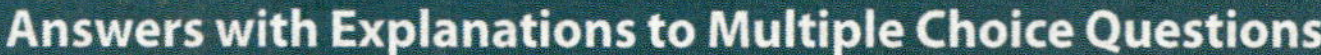

Answers with Explanations to Multiple Choice Questions

1. Ans. (b) Spurious drug

(Ref: Drugs and Cosmetic ACT 1940)

- This is a case where there is a decreased dose of active ingredient and hence is a counterfeit or spurious drug. Please refer to text for details on spurious drugs.

2. Ans. (c) Sham surgery

(Ref: Tsui's Pain Medicine/P87)

Examples of placebo are:
- Inactive tablets (Sugar pills)
- Vehicle infusion
- Sham surgery: A fake surgery that mimics the real procedure.

3. Ans. (d) Just before the next dose, when the plasma concentration of the drug would be the least

(Ref: Katzung 12th E/P1047)

- The drugs are present in breast milk in variable amount but lesser than in plasma of mother.
- Breast feeding is advised 3–4 hours after drug intake so that plasma concentration is lesser and so is drug less in breast milk of mother.

4. Ans. (c) Expiry date of drugs

(Ref: OPPI Guidelines)

Drug Advertisement Guidelines in India

The required information for pharmaceutical advertising are given by the **OPPI (Organization of Pharmaceutical Products of India)**. All printed promotional materials must be legible and include
- The 'name' of the product (normally the brand name).
- The 'active ingredients', using approved names where they exist.
- The 'name and address' of the pharmaceutical company or its agent responsible for marketing the product.
- The 'date of production' of the advertisement.
- The 'abbreviated prescribing information' which should include an approved indication or indications for use together with the dosage and method of use; and a succinct statement of the contraindications, precautions and side effects.

5. Ans. (b) 1.5–2.5 kg

(Ref: Bikas Medhi Experimental and Clinical Pharmacology/P231)

6. Ans. (b) Retinoic acid

(Ref: Goodman Gilman 12th E/P1812)

Teratogenic effects of retinoic acid
- Bilateral microtia
- Anotia with stenosis of external ear canal
- Flat, depressed nasal bridge and ocular hypertelorism
- Cleft lip and palate

7. Ans. (c) Phase 4

(Ref: Goodman Gilman 12th E/P79)

8. Ans. (d) Amiodarone

(Ref: Tracey's Dermatological Manifestation/P402)

Drugs causing pigmentation of nails
- Melphalan
- Hydroxyurea
- Doxorubicin
- Busulfan
- 5-FU
- Methotrexate
- Cyclophosphamide
- Bleomycin
- Tetracyclines
- Antimalarials
- Sulfonamides
- Phenothiazines
- Mercury
- Gold
- Phenytoin
- Timolol

9. Ans. (d) 8 to 15 degree

(Ref: Vogel Drug Discovery/P235)

Drug Storage Temperature

Condition	Temperature
Freezer	–20–10°C
Refrigerator	2–8°C
Cold	Temperature not exceeding 8°C
Cool	8–15°C
Room temperature	15–30°C
Warm	30–40°C
Excessive heat	Above 40°C

10. Ans. (a) Pharmacokinetics

(Ref: Goodman Gilman 12th E/P8)

- Pharmacokinetics is a better answer as it is determined only in phase I, whereas safety is determined in all phases.

Clinical Trial	Purpose
Phase I	Safety and toxicity in healthy volunteers Maximum tolerable dose **Pharmacokinetics** Pharmacodynamics
Phase II	Efficacy and **safety** determined in patients in comparison to placebo or standard drug Determine dose range

Contd...

Clinical Trial	Purpose
Phase III	Efficacy and **safety** confirmed in patients in comparison to placebo or standard drug
Phase IV	**Safety** (Rare and long term ADR) Comparison with existing treatment Drug effectiveness New uses New formulations and routes of drug Drug-drug interaction Use in extremes of age group

11. Ans. (a) H

(Ref: Drug and Cosmetics act 1940)

Schedule G	List of drugs that don't need prescription but requires a mandatory text on label "Caution: It is dangerous to take this preparation, except under medical supervision". E.g. antihistaminics
Schedule H	List of drugs that can be sold only when a prescription is produced. Most drugs belong to this category
Schedule P	It is about drug expiry period, i.e. maximum period till which drug can be used with intact potency
Schedule W	List of drugs marketed under generic names only
Schedule X	List of psychotropic drugs which need special license for manufacture and sale
Schedule Y	Guidelines on clinical trials, import and manufacture of new drugs

12. Ans. (c) Brimonidine

(Ref: Goodman Gilman 12th E/P1846)

Pregnancy Drug Categories

Categories	Significance	Examples
Category A	No risk to fetus in human studies	• Levothyroxine • Potassium • Supplementation • MgSO4
Category B	• Animal studies show no risk • Human studies are lacking	• Penicillin • Cephalosporin • Macrolides • Brimonidine
Category C	• Animal studies show positive teratogenic risk • Human studies are not available	• Albuterol • Zidovudine • CCB • Morphine • Atropine
Category D	• Human and animal studies show positive teratogenic risk • Can be used in pregnancy because of benefits greater than risk might be acceptable	• Corticosteroids • Azathioprine • Carbamazepine • Valproate • Methotrexate • Lithium
Category X	• Human and animal studies show positive teratogenic risk • Absolutely contraindicated in pregnancy because of risk greater than benefits	• Thalidomide • Isotretinoin • Fluoroquinolones • Tetracyclines • Chloramphenicol • Warfarin • ACE inhibitors

Contd...

13. Ans. (a) David Sackett

(Rang and Dale 6th E/P92)

Evidence-Based Medicine

- The concept of EBM was laid down by David Sackett and hence is known as father of EBM.
- Process of developing evidence
  - Formulate a question, e.g. what is the DOC for HTN with CHF?
  - Search literature, e.g.meta-analysis, RCT, etc. pertaining to the question.
  - Evaluate the evidence gathered and apply statistics to find the answer to question. E.g. maximum decrease in mortality is found to be with thiazides and hence is the DOC for HTN with CHF.
- **Grades of evidence**

Grade I	Systemic reviews Meta-analysis	Best quality evidence
Grade II	Randomized control trials	Good evidence but may require support from similar studies
Grade III	Open label trials Pilot studies Observational studies (Case control, cohort studies)	Less reliable evidence
Grade IV	Case reports Professional opinion Anecdotal reports	Poorest quality evidence

14. Ans. (a) Phase 1 trial

(Ref: Goodman Gilman 12th E/P8)

15. Ans. (a) Drug for rare disease

(Ref: KDT 7th E/P5)

- An orphan drug is a drug used for treatment of a rare disease.
- An orphan receptor is a receptor without any known ligand.

16. Ans. (c) Phase 3

(Ref: Goodman Gilman 12th E/P8)

- Efficacy of a drug is determined in comparison to placebo in phase II.
- Efficacy of a drug is confirmed in comparison to placebo in phase III.

Clinical Trial	Purpose
Phase I	Safety and toxicity in healthy volunteers Maximum tolerable dose Pharmacokinetics Pharmacodynamics
Phase II	**Efficacy** and safety **determined** in patients in comparison to **placebo** or standard drug Determine dose range
Phase III	**Efficacy** and safety **confirmed** in patients in comparison to **placebo** or standard drug
Phase IV	Rare and long term ADR Drug effectiveness New uses New formulations and routes of drug Drug-drug interaction Use in extremes of age group

17. Ans. (a) Decreasing interaction of the drug with target protein

(Ref: Vogel Drug Discovery/P12)

- There is a decreased interaction of drugs with target protein and increased interaction with non-target proteins.
- However out of these two more important drawback is that, the drug has a poor interaction with target protein.

18. Ans. (a) Omeprazole reduces stomach acid secretion

(Ref: KDT 7th E/P84)

- Omeprazole reducing stomach acid secretion is the therapeutic effect.
- Other options are unfavorable effects that leads to side effects.

19. Ans. (c) Understanding the structure of the receptor can enhance better target

(Ref: Vogel Drug Discovery/P12)

Rational Drug Designing

- Rational drug design came into existence in the 20th century when radio-ligand binding assay gave enormous information about various ligands and receptors. Further the structure of receptors, enzymes and ligands were extensively studied with the invention of NMR Spectroscopy and X-ray crystallography.
- This is the best method of drug development because, **understanding the structure of receptor enhances better target**.
- This followed the development a new procedure for chemical production called as combinational chemistry. These specialists combine different chemical entities to create a chemical with definite structure which is composite to the structure of an enzyme or receptor (e.g. ACE inhibitor for enzyme ACE).
- Rational drug discovery based on this concept can be classified into
  - Structure based drug designing
  - Ligand based drug designing
  - In silico drug designing
  - Homology modeling

20. Ans. (d) Evidence is formed from weak and poor studies

(Ref: Rang and Dale 6th E/P92)

- Evidence is formed from stronger possible studies like meta-analysis and RCT.
- Opinion of medical professionals and researchers is a weakest form of evidence.

21. Ans. (a) Monitoring of drug safety

(Ref: KDT 7th E/P82)

Pharmacovigilance

- Pharmacovigilance is a continuous post marketing monitoring system to detect the rare and long term side effects of drugs to maintain drug safety.
- Sources of information for pharmacovigilance are
  - ADR reporting system
  - Medical literature published worldwide
  - Action taken by drug regulatory authorities in other countries
- The pharmacovigilance program was initiated in the year 2010, by the government of India at AIIMS as National Coordinating center (NCC), but shifted to Indian Pharmacopoeia Commission (IPC) building, Ghaziabad (U.P.) in the year 2011, which is the current NCC.
- Pharmacovigilance is conducted by CDSCO (Center for Drug Standard Control Organization), Delhi and coordinated by IPC.

22. Ans. (a) To monitor drug toxicity

(Ref: KDT 7th E/P82)

23. Ans. (b) Metformin

(Ref: Goodman Gilman 12th E/P38)

If the clinical effect of drug cannot be easily quantified, e.g. one cannot measure epilepsy, TDM is done. This means, if clinical effect can be easily quantified, TDM is not required. Example of such drugs for which in place of TDM, the clinical effect can be measured are

- Beta blocker—Blood pressure
- OHA—RBS
- Warfarin—INR

24. Ans. (a) Preclinical phase

(Ref: Goodman Gilman 12th E/P8)

Guidelines in Trials

- Preclinical trial: CPCSEA guidelines
- Clinical trial: GCP guidelines

25. Ans. (a) High affinity

(Ref: Rang and Dale 6th E/P10)

- Higher is the affinity of the drug for target, higher is the potency and hence lesser dose is required.
- Higher is the specificity of the drug for a target, lesser are chances it will bind to other receptors and hence lesser are side effects.

26. Ans. (a) Specificity

(Ref: Rang and Dale 6th E/P10)

27. Ans. (a) Phase 3 is RCT

(Ref: Goodman Gilman 13th E/P6)

- Phase 3 is randomized controlled (RCT) or uncontrolled trial, whereas phase 2 is always RCT.
- Phase 1 is done for determination of toxicity, maximum tolerable dose, pharmacokinetics and pharmacodynamics of drugs.
- Phase 4 is post marketing surveillance done in patients.
- Phase 2 is done for safety and efficacy in patients.

28. Ans. (c) Adverse effect of one overcome by other

(Ref: KDT 7th E/P62)

Fixed dose combinations are two or more drugs in a single formulation. There are benefits and drawbacks of FDC, mentioned below.

Benefits	Drawbacks
• Better compliance • Decreased cost • Increased efficacy (Trimethoprim sulfamethoxazole) • Decreased side effect (Spironolactone prevents thiazide induced hyperkalemia) • Decreased resistance (ATT)	• Individual drug dose titration is not possible • Difficulty in finding cause of ADR • Limited use as one drug's contraindication limits other drug's use

29. Ans. (a) Penicillin

(Ref: Rang and Dale 6th E/P761)

30. Ans. (b) Nitrofurantoin

(Ref: Goodman Gilman 12th E/P

31. Ans. (a) Pharmacogenetics

(Ref: Goodman Gilman 12th E/P145)

32. Ans. (d) Thousands of patients

(Ref: Goodman Gilman 12th E/P8)

33. Ans. (d) Phase 4

(Ref: Goodman Gilman 12th E/P8)

34. Ans. (d) Diltiazem

(Ref: Litt's drug eruption 19th E/P130)

35. Ans. (c) Methamphetamine

(Ref: Foster's Designer drugs/P8)

Designer Drugs

Designer drugs are made illegally by altering the chemical structure of legal drugs like pethidine to increase their potency several times which have addiction potential. These drugs are also known as club drugs. The examples of designer drugs are **methamphetamine**, ecstasy, GHB, rohypnol, ketamine and various analgesic analogs.

36. Ans. (b) Lithium

(Ref: Goodman Gilman 19th E/P 37-38)

Drugs with Low Therapeutic Index

These drugs can cause toxicity even with slight fluctuation of plasma concentration. Example of such drugs with low therapeutic index for which TDM is done are

Drugs with Low Therapeutic Index

Mnemonics

A Low Therapeutic Drug Causes Toxicity

A : Antiepileptics, Aminoglycosides, Antiarrhythmics
Low : Lithium, Lidocaine
Therapeutic : Theophylline
Drug : Digoxin
Causes : Cyclosporine/Tacrolimus
Toxicity : TCA

37. Ans. (d) Digoxin

(Ref: Goodman Gilman 12th E/P38)

38. Ans. (a) To monitor drug toxicity

(Ref: KDT 7th E/P82)

39. Ans. (a) Pharmacognosy

(Ref: Eugenia Pharmacology/P23)

40. Ans. (d) All of the above

(Ref: Satoskar 24th E/P54)

Types of Counterfeit Drugs

- Counterfeit drug containing
  - Same dose of the active ingredient
  - Incorrect dose of active ingredient
  - Potentially harmful substance
  - Unlisted active ingredient
- Counterfeit drug without active ingredient
- Mislabeled drugs

41. Ans. (c) 1/3 of adult dose

(Ref: Bob Handbook of Pediatrics/P47)

Prescribing Drug Dose in Children

Age	Part of Adult Dose Given
0–1 month	1/18
1–6 months	1/14
6–12 months	1/7
1–2 years	1/5
2–4 years	1/4
4–6 years	1/3
6–9 years	2/5
9–14 years	1/2

Calculation of Dose in Child

Child BSA/Adult BSA × Adult dose of drug = Child dose

42. Ans. (a) Orphan drugs

(Ref: KDT 7th E/P5)

43. Ans. (c) Those that satisfy the primary health care needs of the population

(Ref: KDT 7th E/P4)

Essential Medicine

- Essential medicines are those that **satisfy the priority of health care needs of majority of population**. These are intended to be available all the time in adequate amounts, in appropriate dosage form with assured quality and adequate information and at a price the individuals and community can afford.
- The concept was introduced by WHO in 1977 and then adopted by many countries.
- The list of essential medicine should be country specific addressing the disease burden of the nation and the commonly used drug at all levels of health care.
- Indian National List of Essential Medicine (NLEM) contains 348 drugs.

44. Ans. (b) Oswald schmiedberg

(Ref: KDT 7th E/P1)

Oswald Scmiedberg	Father of modern pharmacology
Rudolf Buchheim	Founded first pharmacology institute
Sir Ram Nath Chopra	Father of Indian pharmacology
Gananath Sen	Father of reverse pharmacology
James black	Discovered beta-2 and H2 receptors followed by their blockers

45. Ans. (a) Warfarin

(Ref: Goodman Gilman 12th E/P38)

46. Ans. (a) Safety

(Ref: Rang and Dale 6th E/P95)

Therapeutic Index

- Therapeutic index is calculated by dividing LD_{50} to ED_{50}. LD_{50} is the minimum dose required to kill 50% of animals and hence is a measure of drug toxicity. ED50 is the minimum dose required to produce clinical effect in 50% of population and hence is a measure of drug potency (Lower dose required to produce effect, higher potency and vice a versa. Potency as discussed in general pharmacology is a measure of drug dose.

$$TI = LD_{50}/ED_{50}$$

Hence by dividing drug toxicity by drug dose, we get a range of dose with which drug use is safe and thus **TI is a measure of drug safety**. For drugs with low TI, TDM is done to maintain the plasma concentration within safe range and is discussed below.

47. Ans. (d) Phase IV

(Ref: Goodman Gilman 12th E/P8)

- Ethical clearance is not required in phase IV, as it is done post approval of drug by FDA.

48. Ans. (d) Heparin

(Ref: Goodman Gilman 12th E/P26)

- **Heparin is a large molecule that does not cross placenta.**

49. Ans. (d) Primaquine-induced hemolytic anemia

(Ref: Rang and Dale 6th E/P52)

Pharmacogenetic Conditions

Mnemonics

PHARMACOGEN

- **P:** Pseudocholinesterase causing apnea with Sch
- **H:** HMG Co-A reductase polymorphism, HLA polymorphism
- **A:** ACE polymorphism
- **R:** Rosuvastatin increased effect in BRCP polymorphism
- **M:** Malignant hyperthermia with RyR gene polymorphism
- **A:** Anticoagulant warfarin associated VKOR polymorphism
- **C:** CYP450 polymorphism
- **O:** OATP polymorphism
- **G:** G6PD deficiency associated hemolysis
- **E:** ApoE-4 A positive patients
- **N:** N-acetyl transferase polymorphism

50. Ans. (b) Lithium

(Ref: Goodman Gilman 12th E/P38)

51. Ans. (a) Phase-I

(Ref: Goodman Gilman 12th E/P8)

Participants in Trial

- Phase I – Normal healthy volunteers
- Phase II, III and IV – Patients

52. Ans. (d) Safety and comparisons with other medicines

(Ref: Goodman Gilman 12th E/P8)

Clinical trial	Purpose
Phase I	Safety and toxicity in healthy volunteers Maximum tolerable dose Pharmacokinetics Pharmacodynamics
Phase II	Efficacy and safety determined in patients in comparison to placebo or standard drug Determine dose range
Phase III	Efficacy and safety confirmed in patients in comparison to placebo or standard drug
Phase IV	Safety (Rare and long term ADR) Comparison with existing treatment Drug effectiveness New uses New formulations and routes of drug Drug-drug interaction Use in extremes of age group

53. Ans. (a) Potency

(Ref: Rang and Dale 6th E/P96)

- ED50 is a measure of drug potency
- LD50 is a measure of drug toxicity.

54. Ans. (b) Postmarketing surveillance

(Ref: Goodman Gilman 12th E/P8)

Name of Clinical Trials

Phase I	Human pharmacology and toxicity study
Phase II	Therapeutic exploratory trial
Phase III	Therapeutic confirmatory trial
Phase IV	Post marketing surveillance

55. Ans. (b) Schedule H

(Ref: Drug and Cosmetics act 1940)

56. Ans. (d) Other possible uses of drug

(Ref: Goodman Gilman 12th E/P8)

Clinical trial	Purpose
Phase I	Safety and toxicity in healthy volunteers Maximum tolerable dose Pharmacokinetics Pharmacodynamics
Phase II	Efficacy and safety determined in patients in comparison to placebo or standard drug Determine dose range
Phase III	Efficacy and safety confirmed in patients in comparison to placebo or standard drug
Phase IV	Safety (Rare and long term ADR) Comparison with existing treatment Drug effectiveness New uses New formulations and routes of drug Drug-drug interaction Use in extremes of age group

57. Ans. (a) Pharmacogenomics

(Ref: Rang and Dale 6th E/P742)

- The best answer to the MCQ is pharmacogenetics, but as it is not in the option the best possible answer is pharmacogenomics, which is application of pharmacogenetics.

58. Ans. (a) Unpredictable reaction to a drug

(Ref: Rang and Dale 6th E/P744)

59. Ans. (c) Amphetamine

(Ref: KDT 7th E/P70)

Acute tolerance or tachyphylaxis: Rapid development of tolerance after few doses of drug. e.g. ephedrine, methyl phenidate, amphetamine, tyramine, etc.

60. Ans. (c) Study of drugs from plants

(Ref: Eugenia Pharmacology/P23)

61. Ans. (a) Pharmacovigilance

(Ref: KDT 7th E/P82)

62. Ans. (c) Therapeutic index

(Ref: Rang and Dale 6th E/P95)

63. Ans. (b) Gatifloxacin

(Ref: KDT 9th E/P969)

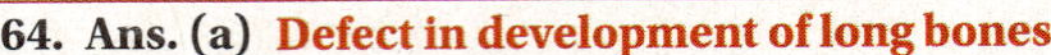

64. Ans. (a) Defect in development of long bones

(Ref: Rang and Dale 6th E/P760)

Drugs and Teratogenicity

Drug	Teratogenic effect

Alcohol	**Fetal Alcohol Syndrome**
	• Dysmorphic facial features (all 3 are required)
	  ▪ Small palpebral fissures
	  ▪ Thin vermilion border
	  ▪ Smooth philtrum
	• Prenatal and/or postnatal growth impairment
	• Central nervous system abnormalities (1 required)
	  ▪ Structural: head size < 10th percentile, significant brain abnormality on imaging
	  ▪ Neurological
	  ▪ **Functional:** Global cognitive or intellectual deficits functional deficits in at least three domains

Fluconazole	• Oral clefts • Abnormal facies • Cardiac abnormalities • Skull, long-bone, and joint abnormalities
ACE inhibitors	• Fetal RAAS inhibition followed by hypotension and reduced perfusion causes fetal-growth restriction and calvarium maldevelopment • Oligohydramnios causes pulmonary hypoplasia and limb contractures
Leflunomide	• Hydrocephalus • Eye anomalies • Skeletal abnormalities
Chloramphenicol	• Gray baby syndrome
Nitrofurantoin	• Hypoplastic left heart syndrome • Microphthalmia/anophthalmia • Facial clefts • Atrial septal defects
Sulfonamides	• Anencephaly • Left ventricular outflow tract obstruction, • Choanal atresia • Diaphragmatic hernia
Tetracycline	• Yellow discoloration of deciduous teeth • Bone growth abnormality
Fluoroquinolones	Cartilage growth defect
Cyclophosphamide	• Skeletal abnormalities • Limb defects • Cleft palate • Eye abnormalities
Methotrexate	Fetal methotrexate aminopterin syndrome • Craniosynostosis with "clover-leaf" skull • Wide nasal bridge • Low-set ears • Micrognathia • Limb abnormalities
Trastuzumab	• Pulmonary hypoplasia • Skeletal abnormalities
Diethylsilbestrol	Vaginal adenosis, vaginal and cervical cancer in female fetus after 20+ years
Corticosteroids	Facial clefts
Lithium	Ebstein's anomaly
Isotretinoin	• Bilateral microtia • Anotia with stenosis of external ear canal • Flat, depressed nasal bridge and ocular hypertelorism
Thalidomide	• Phocomelia • Cranial nerve defects • Anorectal stenosis • Cardiac defects
Warfarin	• Stippling of the vertebrae and femoral epiphyses • Nasal hypoplasia with depression of the nasal bridge (saddle nose)
Valproate	• Neural tube defect • Cardiovascular defect
Phenytoin	**Fetal hydantoin syndrome** • Facial cleft • Microcephaly • IUGR • Hypertelorism • Triphalangeal thumb
Penicillamine	Loose skin

Contd...

65. Ans. (d) All of the above

(Ref: Rang and Dale 6th E/P760)

66. Ans. (b) Methyl dopa

(Ref: Rang and Dale 6th E/P760)

67. Ans. (d) Penicillin

(Ref: Rang and Dale 7th E/P742)

68. Ans. (b) Quinine

(Ref: Rang and Dale 7th E/P742)

Hemolysis in G6PD Deficiency with Antimalarials

Primaquine—Definite
Chloroquine—Probable
Quinine—Doubtful

69. Ans. (b) Response is both objective & subjective, (c) Effect also seen in normal person, (d) It is an inert substance

(Ref: Rang and Dale 6th E/P95)

- A placebo is an unreal drug that has no active substance, but is administered to the patient in a trial who believes it to be a real drug.
- Some patients get therapeutic effect from a placebo and is known as placebo effect.

70. Ans. (d) Need for society and (e) Should be available at all times

(Ref: KDT 7th E/P4)

71. Ans. (a) Coq10, (b) Tryptophan, (c) β-carotene, (d) Lycopene

(Ref: Ritter's Clinical Pharmacology 5th E/P97)

Neutraceuticals

Neutraceuticals are food or food ingredients that may provide health benefits beyond the traditional nutrition that it contains. Common examples are beta carotene in carrot, lycopene intomatoes, flavonoids in onions, caffeic and ferrulic acid in fruits, coenzyme Q, tryptophan, ginseng, ginkgo biloba, etc.

72. Ans. (a) Done to know activity of endogenous substance, (b) To know toxicity & efficacy of drug

(Ref: Rang and Dale 6th E/P90)

73. Ans. (a) Antiarrhythmics, (e) Antidepressants

(Ref: KDT 7th E/P34)

74. Ans. (d) Less frequent dose, (e) Involvement of family member

(Ref: KDT 7th E/P34)

75. Ans. (b) Phenytion, (c) Cyclosporine, (d) Digitalis

(Ref: KDT 7th E/P34)

76. Ans. (a) ↓ Cost, (b) ↑ Efficacy, (c) ↑ Compliance, (d) ↓ Resistance

(Ref: KDT 7th E/P62)

Fixed dose combinations are two or more drugs in a single formulation. There are benefits and drawbacks of FDC, mentioned below.

Benefits	Drawbacks
• Better compliance • Decreased cost • Increased efficacy (Trimethoprim sulfamethoxazole) • Decreased side effect (Spironolactone prevents thiazide induced hyperkalemia) • Decreased resistance (ATT)	• Individual drug dose titration is not possible • Difficulty in finding cause of ADR • Limited use as one drug's contraindication limits other drug's use

77. Ans. (a) Primaquine, (b) Chloroquine

(Ref: Rang and Dale 7th E/P742)

78. Ans. (b) Mechanism clearly understood, (d) Indirect sympathomimetics involved

(Ref: KDT 7th E/P70)

79. Ans. (a) Variability of enzyme action, (c) Individual variability in oral absorption, (e) Different DRC in different individual

(Ref: Rang and Dale 7th E/P742)

80. Ans. (a) Amiodarone

(Ref: Goodman Gilman 12th E/P1846)

Amiodarone is a pregnancy category D drug. Other drugs in the option belong to pregnancy category C.

81. Ans. (d) Phase 4

(Ref: Goodman Gilman 12th E/P8)

82. Ans. (b) Done in healthy volunteers .

(Ref: Goodman Gilman 12th E/P8)

Practice Questions

83. All of the following are rational drug designing methods except
a. Structure based drug designing
b. In silico drug designing
c. Homology modeling
d. Trial and error designing

Ans. (d) Trial and error designing

(Ref: Vogel Drug Discovery/P12)

84. A drug library is a
a. Collection of drugs in pharmacy
b. Collection of drugs in hospitals
c. Collection of chemicals for drug discovery
d. Collection of chemicals for drug toxicity

Ans. (c) Collection of chemicals for drug discovery

(Ref: Vogel Drug Discovery/P14)

85. Which of the following is fastest method of drug designing?
a. SBDD b. LBDD
c. In silico d. Homology modeling

Ans. (c) In silico

(Ref: Vogel Drug Discovery/P27)

❒ In silico drug designing is computer based drug designing, which is the fastest method.

86. CPCSEA guidelines are for
a. Phase I clinical trial
b. Preclinical trial
c. Phase 0 clinical trial
d. Phase IV clinical trial

Ans. (b) Preclinical trial

(Ref: Rang and Dale 6th E/92)

87. Most common reason for drug failure in clinical trials is
a. Toxicity
b. Inefficacy
c. Inadequate potency
d. Pharmacokinetic incompatibility

Ans. (b) Inefficacy

(Ref: Goodman Gilman 12th E/P8)

❒ Maximum drug failure occurs in phase II due to poor efficacy of drugs.

88. Maximum drug failure occurs in which phase of clinical trial
a. Phase I b. Phase II
c. Phase III d. Phase IV

Ans. (b) Phase II

(Ref: Goodman Gilman 12th E/P8)

89. Long-term side effect of a drug is determined in which phase of clinical trial
a. Phase I b. Phase II
c. Phase III d. Phase IV

Ans. (d) Phase IV

(Ref: Goodman Gilman 12th E/P8)

90. Phase 0 clinical trial is known as
a. Primitive trial b. Pharmacoepidemiology
c. Microdosing d. Nanodosing

Ans. (c) Microdosing

(Ref: Goodman Gilman 12th E/P8)

91. A patient with slow acetylator genotype is given decreased doses of isoniazid. This is known as
a. Pharmacogenetics b. Pharmacogenomics
c. Pharmacoepidemiology d. Pharmacoeconomics

Ans. (b) Pharmacogenomics

(Ref: Rang And Dale 6th E/P642)

92. Pharmacovigilance program of India was started in the year
a. 1990 b. 1980
c. 2010 d. 2012

Ans. (c) 2010

(Ref: KDT 7th E/P83)

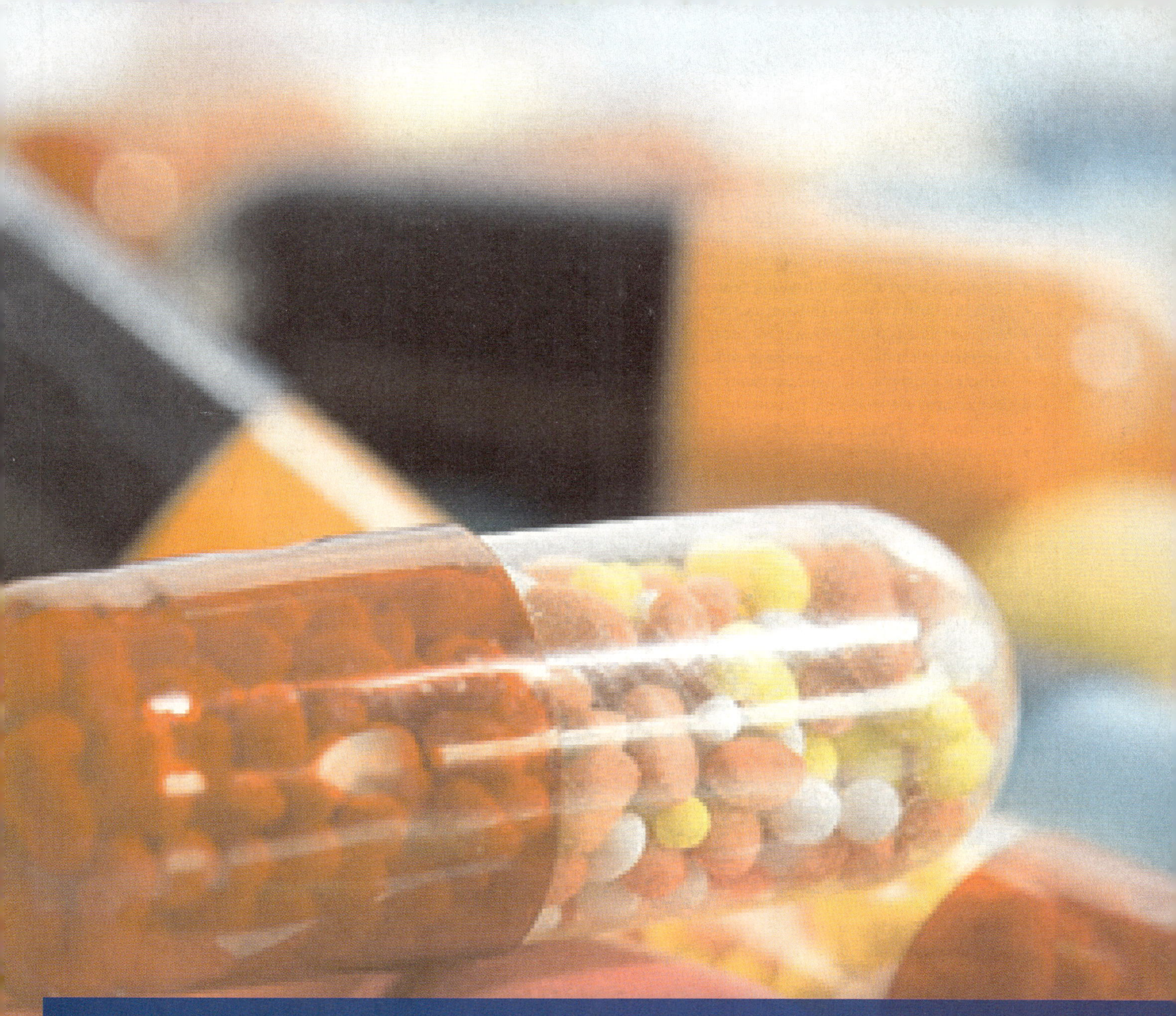

Autonomic Nervous System

One Liners

- Rate limiting step of acetylcholine synthesis is **choline transport from synaptic cleft** to presynaptic neuron.
- Rate limiting step for NE synthesis is conversion of tyrosine to dopa by **tyrosine hydroxylase (RLE).**
- The neurotransmitter in ganglion is acetylcholine, postganglionic parasympathetic axon is **acetylcholine** and postganglionic sympathetic axon is norepinephrine.
- Botulinum toxin acts by **inhibiting release of acetylcholine** from presynaptic neuron.
- **M_3** is the most common muscarinic receptor in the body.
- Methacholine is most active at **M_2** receptors.
- **Varenicline** is a nicotinic agonist used for smoking dependence.
- **Atropine** is used in **nicotinic poisoning** for treatment of cholinergic effect.
- **Carbamates** are reversible (pseudo irreversible) inhibitors, whereas **organophosphates** are irreversible inhibitors of ACHE.
- **Atropine** is the **drug of choice** for organophosphate poisoning, whereas **oximes** are the **most specific drugs**.
- **Pralidoxime** is the most commonly used oxime for organophosphate poisoning.
- **Physostigmine** is the drug of choice for treatment of **atropine or belladonna poisoning**.
- **Donepezil** is the drug of choice for treatment of **Alzheimer's disease.**
- **Edrophonium** is **shortest acting** ACHE inhibitor as it inhibits only **anionic site**.
- **Edrophonium** is the drug of choice for diagnosis of myasthenia gravis in **Tensilon's test**.
- **Pyridostigmine** is the drug of choice for **treatment of myasthenia gravis**.
- **Prostaglandin analogs** are drug of choice for **open angle and normal tension glaucoma**.
- **Acetazolamide** is the drug of choice for **closed angle glaucoma**.
- **Atropine** is the most effective in inhibiting the **salivary glands secretions**.
- **Scopolamine** is the drug of choice for **motion sickness**.
- **Tropicamide** is **shortest and fastest acting** cycloplegic and mydriatic; preferred in adults.
- **Atropine** is **longest acting and most potent** mydriatic and cycloplegic; preferred in children.
- **Glycopyrrolate is a quaternary amine (lipid insoluble)** used as preanesthetic medication.
- **Tiotropium** is the drug of choice for treatment of **COPD**.
- **Darifenacin** is the drug of choice for **overactive bladder, detrusor instability or urge incontinence**.
- **Tetrabenazine** is the drug of choice for treatment of **Huntington's chorea**.
- **Anticholinergics** are the drug of choice for **EPS** like acute dystonia, parkensomism and oculogyric crisis.
- Methylphenidate is the drug of choice for treatment of **ADHD**.
- **Atomoxetine** is the drug of choice for treatment of **ADHD associated with Tensilon's syndrome**.
- **Norephedrine (phenylpropanolamine)** has been banned due to risk of **cerebral hemorrhage**.
- **Modafinil** is the drug of choice for treatment of **narcolepsy, shift worker disease and excessive sleepiness associated with OSA.**
- **Bromocriptine** is the drug of choice for treatment of **cocaine dependence**.
- **Epinephrine** increases systolic blood pressure and has a variable effect on heart rate and diastolic blood pressure.
- **Norepinephrine** increases both systolic and diastolic blood pressure but **decreases heart rate**.
- **Epinephrine** is the drug of choice for treatment of **brittle asthma**.
- **Epinephrine** is the drug of choice in **anaphylactic shock** and the preferred route is **intramuscular** at **1:1000 dilution**.
- **Norepinephrine** is the drug of choice for treatment of **vasodilatory shock e.g. septic shock**.
- **Dopamine** is the drug of choice for treatment of **CHF with oliguria and cardiogenic shock.**
- **Dobutamine** is the inotrope of choice in **acute CHF**.
- **Phenylephrine** is the drug of choice or treatment of **anesthetic agent induced hypotension**.
- **Clonidine** is the drug of choice for **hypertensive urgency and tics associated with Tourette's syndrome.**
- **SABA** are the drug of choice for an **acute attack of asthma** and **LABA** for **prophylaxis of asthma**.
- **Terazosin and doxazosin** are drug of choice for treatment of hypertension associated with BPH or dyslipidemia.
- **Tamsulosin and silodosin** are drug of choice for treatment of **BPH.**
- **Yohimbine** is an **α_2 blocker** that can be used for treatment of **erectile dysfunction**.
- **Phentolamine** is the drug of choice for treatment of **cheese reaction** and **clonidine withdrawal hypertension.**
- **Pheochromocytoma** is treated by an **alpha blocker followed by a beta blocker.**
- β blockers are contraindicated in **variant angina**.
- **Nadolol** is **longest acting** whereas **esmolol** is **shortest acting** beta blocker, as it is metabolized by **esterase in plasma**.
- **Butaxamine** is a **β_2 antagonist** used as an experimental drug.
- **Nonselective beta blockers** have unfavorable effect (increase LDL and triglycerides and decrease HDL) on lipid profile and increase insulin resistance.
- **Vasodilating beta blockers** like **bucindolol** have favorable effect on lipid profile (decrease LDL and triglycerides and increase HDL) and decrease insulin resistance.

INTRODUCTION

Nervous system is divided into central and peripheral parts. The central nervous system is made up of cortex, cerebellum, diencephalon, brain stem and spinal cord. The peripheral nervous system is classified into autonomic nervous system and, sensory and somatic nervous system. The peripheral nervous system relays information to the CNS, which processes the information and sends it back that leads to an appropriate response. The sensory and somatic nervous system are responsible for voluntary movements whereas the autonomic nervous system is responsible for effects on smooth muscles, glands, etc. i.e. involuntary response. This autonomous nature gives the name **autonomic nervous system (ANS)**.

Conceptual Box-1

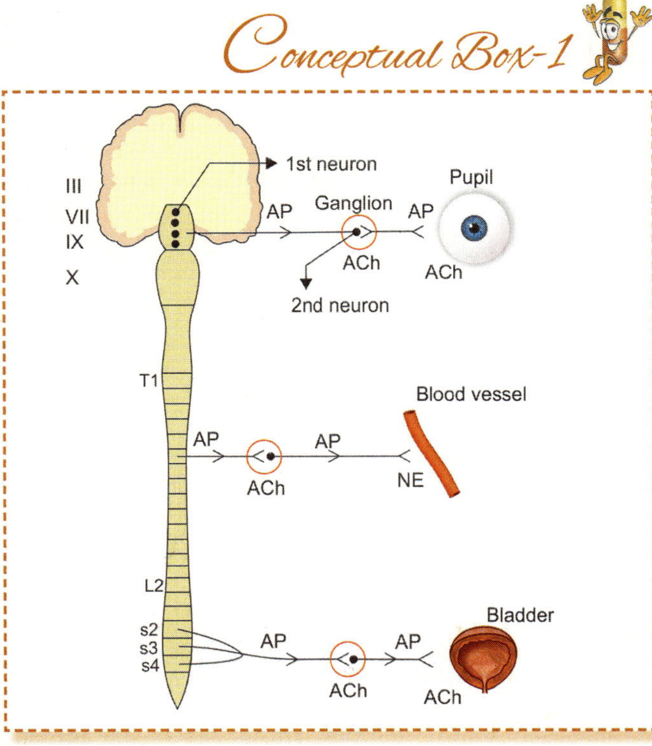

Note: ACH = acetylcholine; AP = Action potential; Nonepinephrine

- ANS is broadly classified into sympathetic, parasympathetic and enteric nervous system. The sympathetic nervous system bears its origin from the **T_1 to L_2 segment** of spinal cord and hence is also called thoracolumbar segment. The parasympathetic nervous system originates from brain stem, i.e. **cranial nerve nuclei III, VII, IX and X** and the **sacral segments, i.e. S_2 to S_4**.
- The ANS functions with two neurons - the first one is located in the brain stem or spinal cord and the second one is located in a ganglion. The first neuron propagates the command in the form of action potential (AP) to the ganglionic neuron, which further propagates it to particular organs.
- For example, the III cranial nerve nuclei propagate action potential via a ganglion to pupil, which gets depolarized and contracts. Similarly in sympathetic nervous system the action potential is propagated via ganglion to blood vessels, which leads to vasoconstriction.
- Thus propagation of action potential is the most crucial aspect in ANS, which requires two things. One is a **neurotransmitter (NT)** present in the presynaptic neuron and another is a **receptor** in the postsynaptic membrane. As the action potential depolarizes presynaptic neuron, it releases NT into the synapse which acts on postsynaptic receptors and causes depolarization or generation of action potential.
- The neurotransmitter in a ganglion is always acetylcholine (ACH) as the receptors are N_N subtype. In parasympathetic nervous system, the neurotransmitter, both in preganglionic and postganglionic axons is acetylcholine. In sympathetic preganglionic axons the neurotransmitter is **acetylcholine**, whereas in postganglionic axons, it is **norepinephrine**. The exceptions are **adrenal glands (ACH)**, **renal blood vessels (Dopamine)** and **sweat glands (ACH)**.

Conceptual Box-2

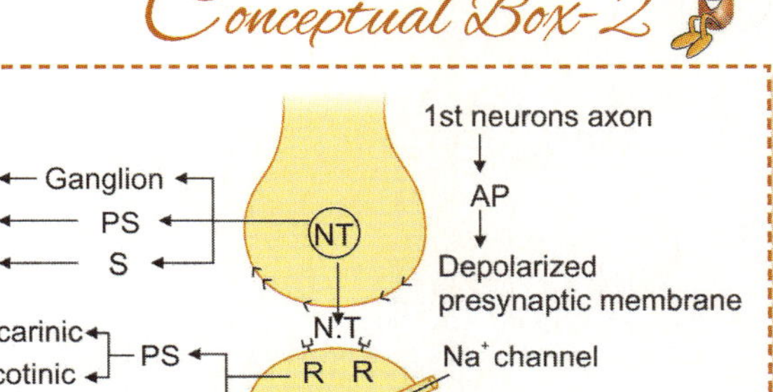

Note: ACH = acetylcholine; AP = Action potential; NE = Non-epinephrine; PS = Parasympathetic; S = Sympathetic

PARASYMPATHETIC NERVOUS SYSTEM

NEUROTRANSMITTER

- As discussed earlier, the universal neurotransmitter in the parasympathetic nervous system is acetylcholine. Acetylcholine is synthesized in the presynaptic neuron from two substances, i.e. **Acetyl CoA** and **choline**, with the help of enzyme **choline acetyltransferase (CAT)**.
- Acetyl CoA is produced by metabolism of glucose and fat in our body, whereas we are dependent on exogenous source for choline as it cannot be synthesized. Choline is also recycled from the synapse after breakdown of acetylcholine in the synapse and this being the most important source of choline, is the **rate limiting step in acetylcholine synthesis**.
- After synthesis, acetylcholine enters into a vesicle by H^+-Ach ATPase. The vesicle has a protein attached called SVP (synaptic vesicular protein).
- Once the action potential strikes the presynaptic membrane, it is depolarized, and this results in opening of calcium channels. Rise in intracellular calcium stimulates vesicle movement until it fuses with presynaptic membrane and acetylcholine is outpoured into the synaptic cleft.

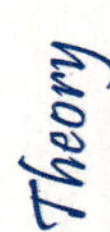

- The duration of acetylcholine action in the synaptic cleft is only for milliseconds, as it is immediately metabolized by ACHE (Acetyl Choline Esterase) into choline and acetate. Choline is recycled into presynaptic neuron for synthesis of acetylcholine and this is the rate limiting step of acetylcholine synthesis.

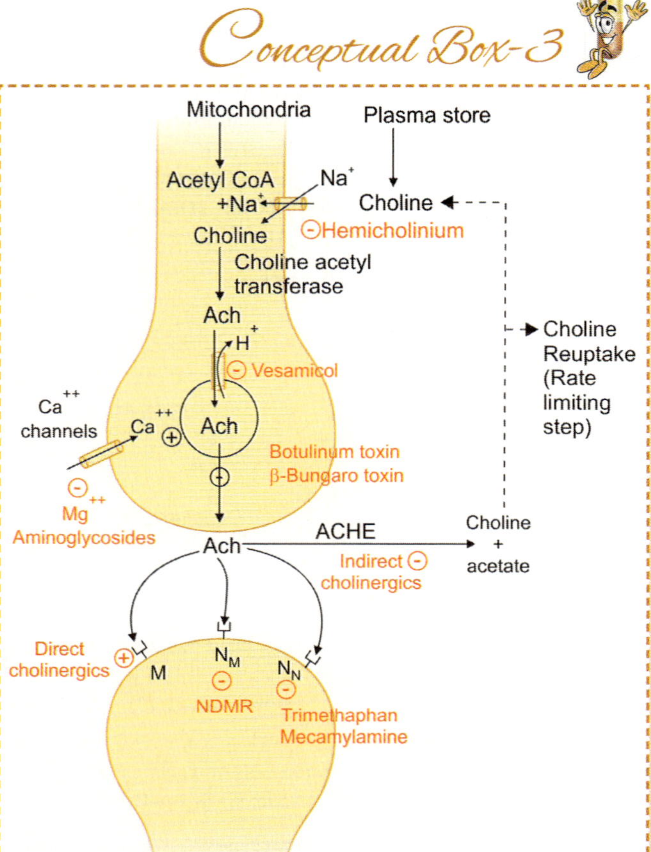

Drugs Acting on Acetylcholine Synthesis, Storage and Release

- **Hemicholinium** blocks the choline Na^+ cotransporter and decreases availability of choline for acetylcholine synthesis. **Vesamicol** inhibits the Ach-H^+ antiporter and decreases acetylcholine entry into vesicles. Both these drugs are not used clinically, rather utilized in research.

- **Botulinum toxin prevents release of acetylcholine** into the synaptic cleft, which decreases stimulation of N_M receptors and muscle contraction. Hence its primary use is in conditions with increased muscle tone like hemifacial spasm, achalasia, torticollis, strabismus and blepharospasm. It is also used in cosmetology for removal of wrinkles and for treatment of various headache. The only problem with this toxin is its temporariness of effect.

RECEPTORS

The receptors in parasympathetic nervous system are of two types, i.e. **muscarinic (M)** and **nicotinic (N)**. Nicotinic receptors are ligand gated Na^+ ion channels, whereas muscarinic receptors are GPCRs.

Nicotinic Receptors

- Nicotinic receptors are pentameric structures made up of four protein subunits i.e. α (2), β, ε and δ. There are two sites for binding of acetylcholine on α subunit, which opens the ion channel and conducts Na^+ and Ca^{++} into the cells causing depolarization.

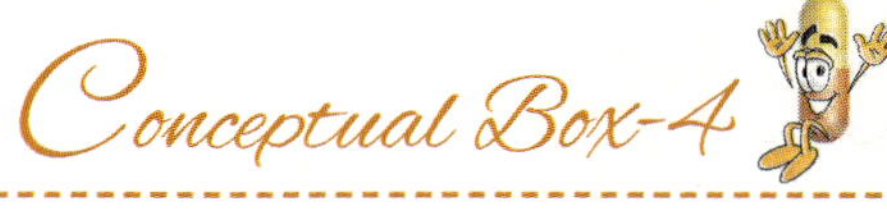

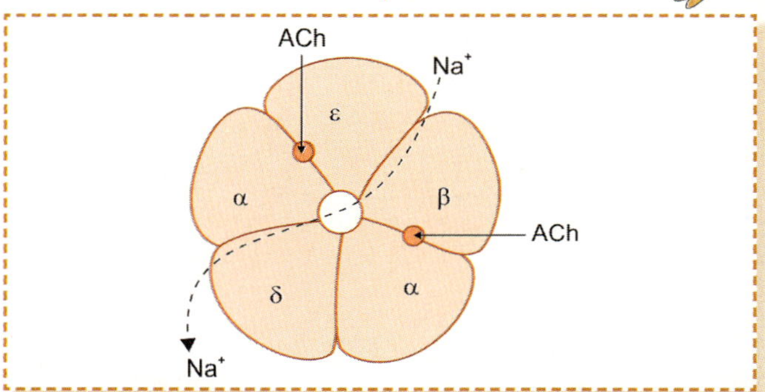

- Nicotinic receptors are of two subtypes, i.e. **muscular (N_M)** and **neuronal (N_N)**. The N_M subtypes are located in **neuromuscular junction**, where they cause muscle contraction. The N_N subtypes are located in the **adrenal medulla** depolarize the cells, which release norepinephrine and is subsequently converted into epinephrine and then released into blood. N_N receptors in the **ganglions** generate action potential that is propagated in the postganglionic axons. N_N receptors in **CNS** cause stimulation (arousal and attention) and analgesia.

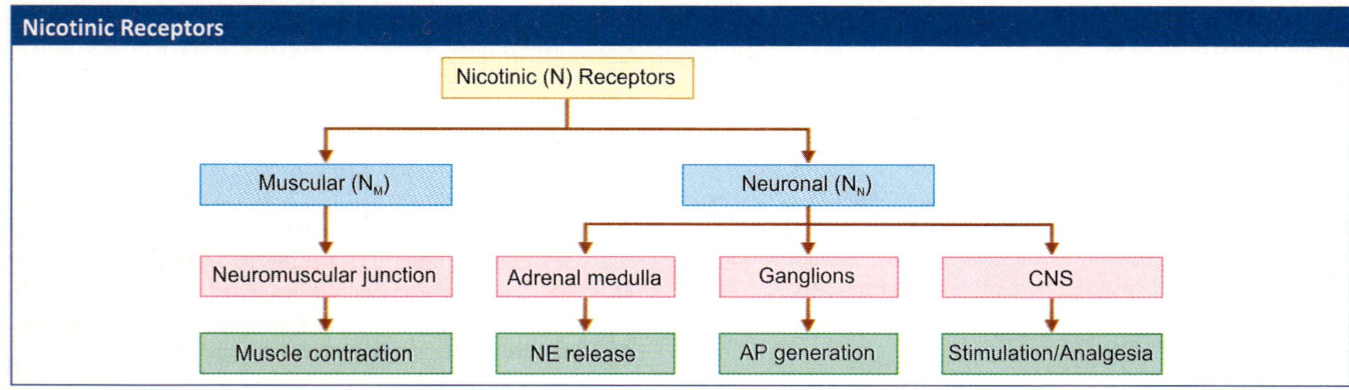

Muscarinic Receptors

- Muscarinic receptors are of five subtypes and all of them are **GPCRs**. The odd ones are **M_1, M_3 and M_5 are G_q subtypes,** which on stimulation increases calcium. The even ones, i.e. **M_2 and M_4 are G_i subtypes** and on stimulation decreases cyclic AMP and **open K^+ channel**. Overall **M_3 subtype** has the widest distribution and is the **most common muscarinic receptor**.
- Thus, wherever the odd ones are present, they will produce an effect corresponding to increase in calcium and the even ones will produce an effect corresponding to decrease in cyclic AMP and opening of K^+ channels, which causes relaxation.

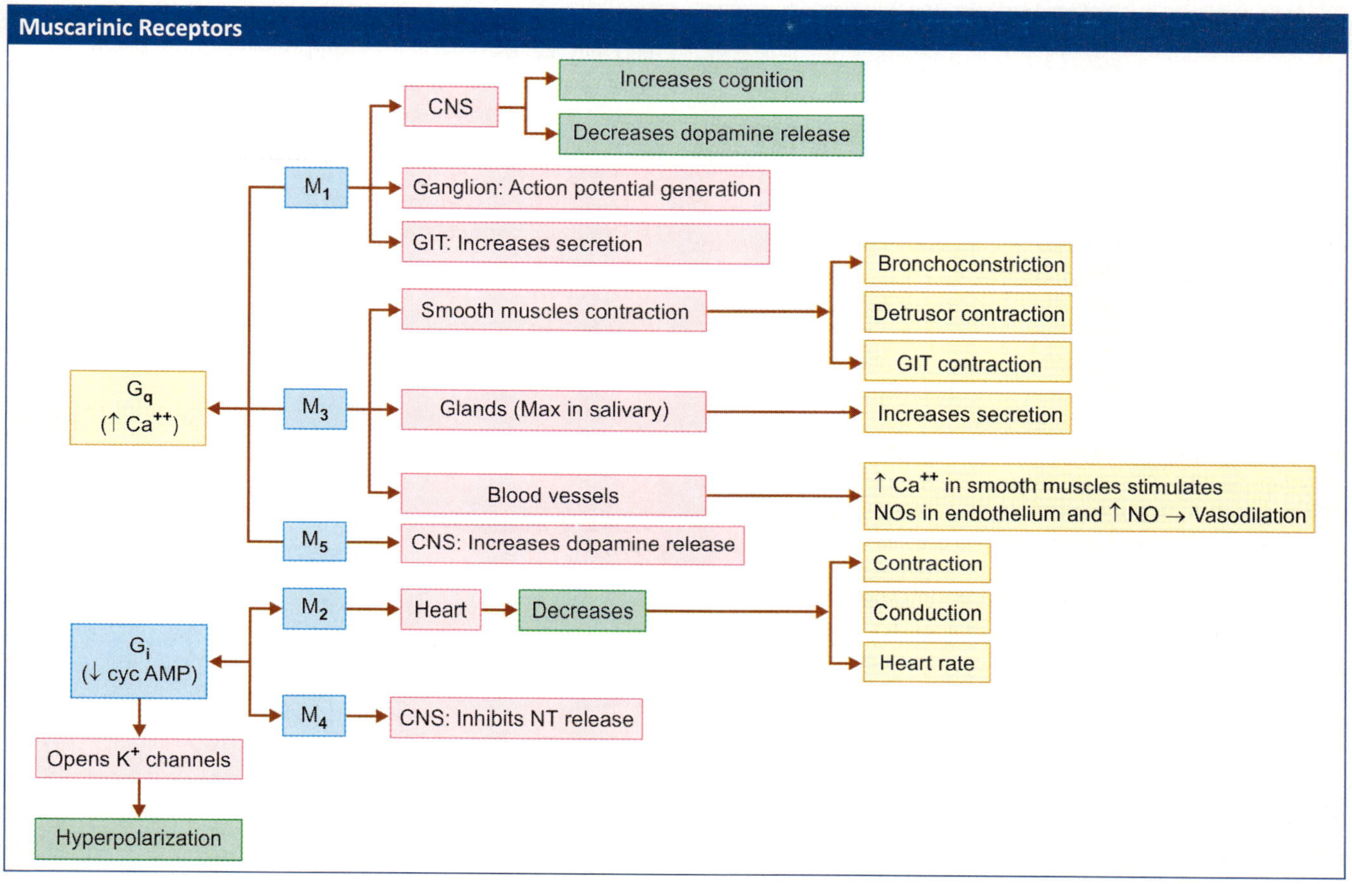

Muscarinic Receptors
Gq
(↑ Ca++)
M1
CNS
Increases cognition
Decreases dopamine release
Ganglion: Action potential generation
GIT: Increases secretion
M3
Smooth muscles contraction
Bronchoconstriction
Detrusor contraction
GIT contraction
Glands (Max in salivary)
Increases secretion
Blood vessels
↑ Ca++ in smooth muscles stimulates NOs in endothelium and ↑ NO → Vasodilation
M5
CNS: Increases dopamine release
Gi
(↓ cyc AMP)
M2
Heart
Decreases
Contraction
Conduction
Heart rate
M4
CNS: Inhibits NT release
Opens K+ channels
Hyperpolarization

CHOLINERGIC (PARASYMPATHOMIMETIC) DRUGS

Cholinergic effect can be achieved by directly stimulating muscarinic receptors (Direct Cholinergics) with agonists or by inhibiting ACHE which leads to decreased metabolism of ACH (Indirect Cholinergics).

Direct Cholinergics

Direct cholinergics are drugs that are agonist at the receptors of parasympathetic nervous system. Hence they can be classified as muscarinic and nicotinic agonists.

Muscarinic Agonists

Muscarinic agonists can be broadly classified into **alkaloids** and **choline esters**.

Muscarinic Agonists
Muscarinic Agonists
Alkaloids
Choline Esters
• Pilocarpine
• Cevimeline
• Aricoline
• Muscarine
• Ach
• Methacholine
• Carbachol
• Bethanechol

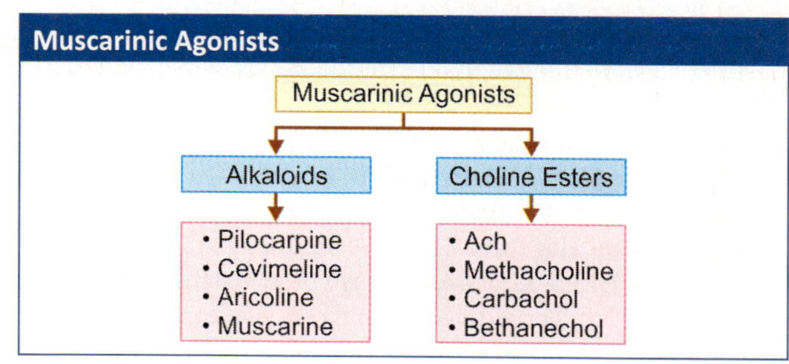

Alkaloids

Alkaloids like pilocarpine, cevimeline and arecoline are **tertiary amines**, whereas muscarine is a quaternary amine. **Tertiary amines are lipid-soluble compounds** and hence can **cross blood brain barrier** and **biological membranes like cornea** and **have central cholinergic side effects**.

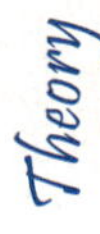

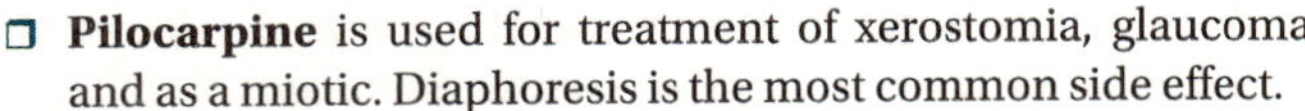

- **Pilocarpine** is used for treatment of xerostomia, glaucoma and as a miotic. Diaphoresis is the most common side effect.
- **Cevimeline** is more selective at M_3 receptors and hence is more effective and less toxic than pilocarpine. It is the **drug of choice for xerostomia**.

Choline Esters

All choline esters are **quaternary amines**. Quaternary amines are lipid insoluble and hence don't cross blood brain barrier and are devoid of central cholinergic side effects. Thus are preferred for **peripheral use**. **Acetyl choline** is immediately metabolized by **plasma esterases** (ACHE and butyryl choline esterase) and hence is **very short acting**. Thus, esterase resistant derivatives of acetylcholine methacholine, bethanechol and carbachol were synthesized. **Methacholine** is resistant only to **butyryl choline esterase**, whereas **carbachol** and **bethanechol** are **resistant to both ACHE and butyryl choline esterase**. These drugs are longer acting than acetylcholine, but overall are still short acting due to rapid excretion by kidney.

- **Acetylcholine** is not used by systemic route because of its short duration of action and non-selectivity. It is rather used as a miotic agent in ocular surgery.
- **Methacholine** is most active at the **M_2 receptors**, though it is not used for this vagomimetic effect on heart. It is used in bronchial challenge test for diagnosis of bronchial asthma.
- **Bethanechol** is a pure muscarinic drug as it does not have any nicotinic action and hence preferred for systemic use. Its maximum effect is on M_1 (GIT) and M_3 (bladder). Hence it is used for treatment of atonic bladder, gastroparesis and paralytic ileus.
- **Carbachol** is used as a miotic agent in ocular surgery and in glaucoma. It has **maximum nicotinic action**, because of which it is not used by systemic route. Its muscarinic effect is least antagonized by **atropine**.

Nicotinic Agonists

Nicotinic receptors are stimulated by natural alkaloids like nicotine and lobeline and synthetic drug like varenicline.

- **Varenicline** is a partial agonist at $\alpha_4\beta_2$ subtype and full agonist at α_7 subtype of nicotinic receptor and is used for treatment of **smoking dependence**. Its use has been associated with mood changes.
- **Nicotine** is a nonselective agonist, but is more potent at N_N as compared to N_M receptors. It is also used for **smoking dependence** in the form of transdermal, gum, nasal spray and vapor inhaler form. Nicotine stimulates the ganglion at low doses, which increases release of acetylcholine and NE in the postganglionic fibers leading to vasoconstriction and tachycardia. However at high doses, it has inhibitory effect on the ganglions due to receptor downregulation, which causes hypotension, reflex tachycardia, vomiting, seizures and **death from respiratory paralysis**. The fatal dose of nicotine is around 60 mg. Treatment aims at symptomatic management with **ventilation** and **antiepileptics** and **atropine** to inhibit cholinergic activity.
- **Tetramethylammonium (TMA) and 1,1-dimethyl-4-phenyl piperazinium iodide (DMPP)** are more selective nicotinic agonists at the ganglion. The drugs after stimulation do not cause ganglion block like, nicotine.

Indirect Cholinergics or ACHE Inhibitors

ACHE is an enzyme with two primary sites for acetylcholine metabolism, i.e. **anionic** and **esteratic site**. An anionic site (negatively charged) binds to the positively charged choline molecule of acetylcholine. Then the acetyl group is transferred to esteratic site. In this process both choline and acetate are liberated due to metabolism of acetylcholine. ACHE inhibitors can compete with acetylcholine for binding to these sites and then they are liberated like acetylcholine but more slowly.

- **Carbamates** bind to both anionic and esteratic site, following which they carbamylate the esteratic site and slowly dissociate as compared to acetylcholine. Hence though they are longer acting, their **binding is reversible**; because they bind for longer period, it is also termed as **pseudo irreversible**.
- **Organophosphates** bind only to the esteratic site and phosphorylate it; further this phosphate bond is replaced after few hours with more strong bonds and this process is known as **aging**. After aging, the effects can be reversed only after new ACHE enzymes are synthesized and hence these are termed as **irreversible inhibitors of ACHE**.

Conceptual Box-5

ACH degradation by ACHE

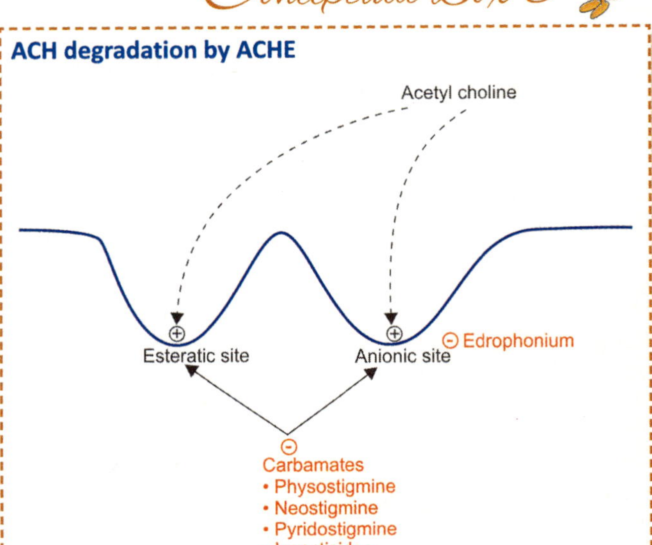

Carbamates

Carbamates, which are reversible ACHE inhibitors can be broadly classified based on their chemical structures into **tertiary amines** and **quaternary amines**. Carbamates are also used as insecticides, herbicides and fungicides as given in the box below.

Tertiary Amines

As discussed earlier, tertiary amines are lipid soluble and can cross blood brain barrier and hence have CNS use as well as side effects.

- **Physostigmine** is the drug of choice for treatment of **atropine or belladonna poisoning** because atropine is also a tertiary amine that can cross blood brain barrier. It is also used for treatment of glaucoma (like pilocarpine) and ataxia. Physostigmine is the **only natural drug** in this class derived from a plant called **Physostigma venenosum**.

- **Tacrine, donepezil, rivastigmine and galantamine** are other tertiary amines that can cross blood brain barrier and hence used for treatment of **mild to moderate Alzheimer's disease**. **Donepezil** is also approved for severe Alzheimer's disease and hence is the **drug of choice**. It has 100% bioavailability and is the longest acting in this class. **Rivastigmine** is approved for treatment of **dementia associated with Parkinson's disease**. **Tacrine** is not preferred due to **hepatotoxicity**.

Carbamates

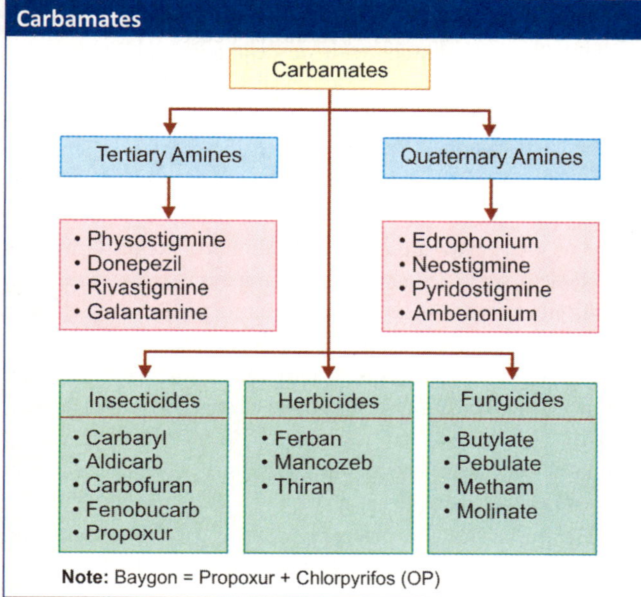

Note: Baygon = Propoxur + Chlorpyrifos (OP)

Quaternary Amines

Quaternary amines are lipid insoluble and hence don't cross blood brain barrier and have poor oral absorption. These are devoid of central side effects and hence preferred for peripheral use like **myasthenia gravis**. In myasthenia gravis, anti N_M antibodies are produced which are competitive inhibitors of acetylcholine. Thus, by increasing acetylcholine in the synapse this competitive inhibition can be reversed.

- **Edrophonium** inhibits only anionic site in the ACHE enzyme by an ionic bond and hence is **shortest acting**. Ionic bond being weaker, it binds for a small interval. It is drug of choice for diagnosis of **myasthenia gravis in Tensilon test**, due to its faster and shorter action; **neostigmine** is used in case if more time is required for diagnosis. A dose of 2 mg of edrophonium is given by rapid intravenous route. An improvement in muscle strength confirms myasthenia gravis, whereas worsening indicates towards **cholinergic crisis**. Cholinergic crisis is caused by persistent depolarization of postsynaptic membrane due to acetylcholine excess. Edrophonium can be used for treatment of an acute attack of **PSVT** as well.
- **Pyridostigmine**, **neostigmine** and **Ambenonium** can be used for treatment of myasthenia gravis, with **pyridostigmine** being preferred as it is **longest acting**. Pyridostigmine is also used for prophylaxis of biological warfare ACHE inhibitors like soman.
- **Neostigmine** is also used for treatment of **paralytic ileus**, **abdominal distention** and **detrusor atony,** however it is contraindicated in these cases if obstruction is present. Neostigmine is preferred for **reversal of NDMR** effect after surgery and **cobra bite**.

Insecticides, Fungicides and Herbicides

- The carbamates used as insecticides, fungicides and herbicides are mention in the box.
- Apart from this these carbamates are also relevant for **cholinergic poisoning** associated with suicidal or homicidal attempts. The symptoms and treatment of the same are discussed in the section of organophosphates.

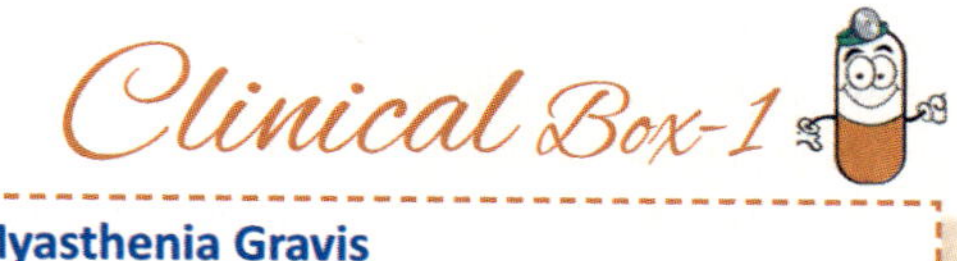

Treatment of Myasthenia Gravis

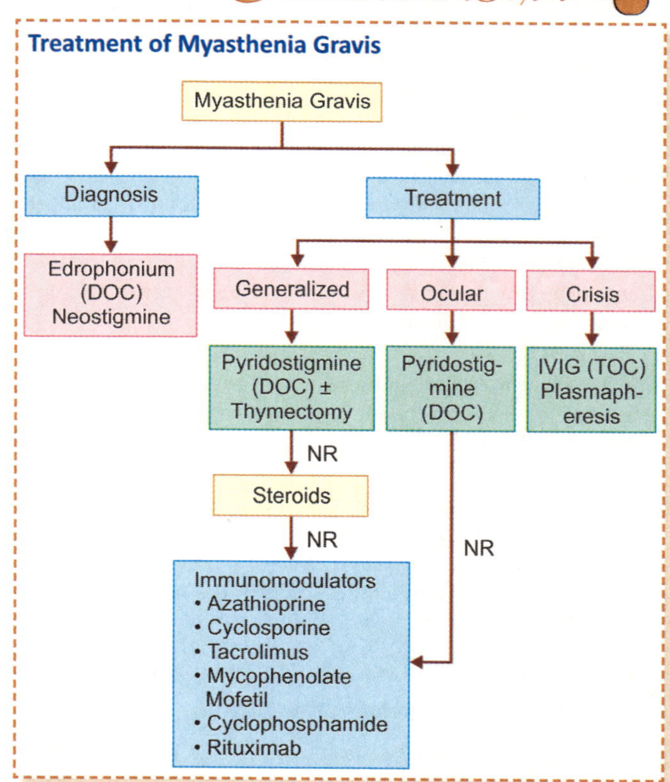

Organophosphates

Organophosphates which are the only irreversible ACHE inhibitors due to the chemical process called as aging discussed before.

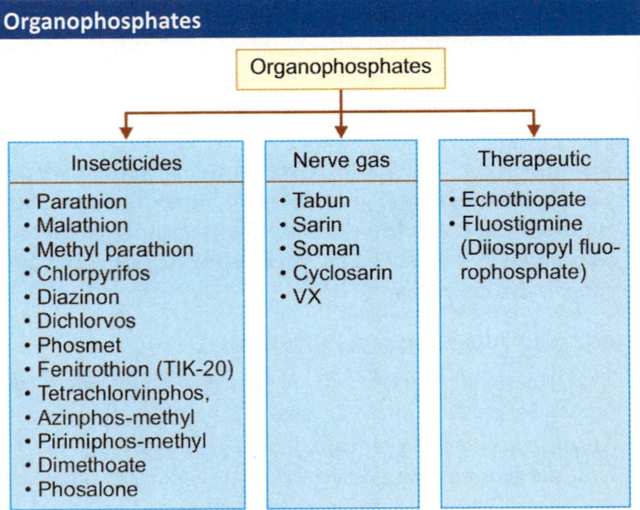

Organophosphates
Organophosphates
Insecticides
• Parathion
• Malathion
• Methyl parathion
• Chlorpyrifos
• Diazinon
• Dichlorvos
• Phosmet
• Fenitrothion (TIK-20)
• Tetrachlorvinphos,
• Azinphos-methyl
• Pirimiphos-methyl
• Dimethoate
• Phosalone
Nerve gas
• Tabun
• Sarin
• Soman
• Cyclosarin
• VX
Therapeutic
• Echothiopate
• Fluostigmine (Diiospropyl fluorophosphate)

- **Organophosphates** were primarily synthesized as **insecticides** and **nerve gas poison**, which is a biological warfare agent. These chemicals list is given in the box.
- Some of them have clinical indications as well. **Echothiophate** and **fluostigmine** can be used for treatment of **glaucoma** and **esotropia**, whereas **Malathion** can be used for treatment of **pediculosis**.
- Organophosphates and carbamates are abused for suicidal and homicidal attempts and these patients present to the medical emergency with muscarinic symptoms like **miosis (pin point pupil)**, brow ache, increased secretions, confusion, ataxia, nausea and vomiting, diarrhea, etc. The latter GIT symptoms are first to be seen. Nicotinic symptoms like weakness, fasciculation and respiratory paralysis are associated. **Respiratory paralysis is the most common cause of death.**
- The drug of choice for organophosphate and carbamate poisoning is **atropine** that reverses the muscarinic symptoms but has no effect on nicotinic ones. **Atropine** is given to the patient until the cholinergic symptoms subside and the **pupil size is used as a marker**.
- Nicotinic symptoms are reversed by ACHE reactivators like pralidoxime, obidoxime and diacetyl mono-oxime. **Pralidoxime is most commonly used and at dose of 1-2 mg over less than 5 minutes**. These compounds bind to the anionic site and remove the phosphate group from the esteratic site thereby dephosphorylating and activating ACHE. Since carbamates bind to both esteratic and anionic sites, **ACHE reactivators are ineffective in carbamate poisoning**.

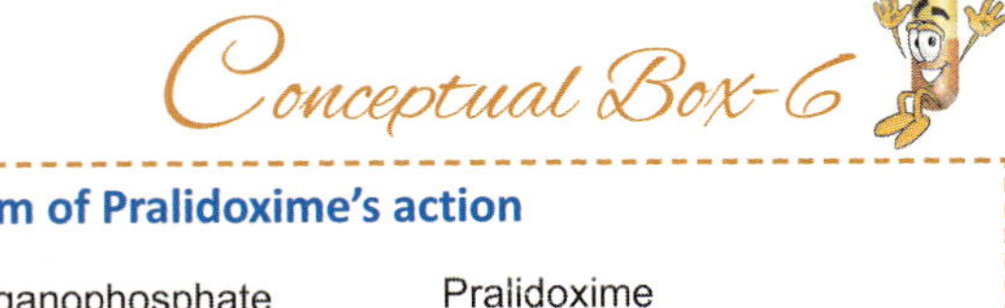

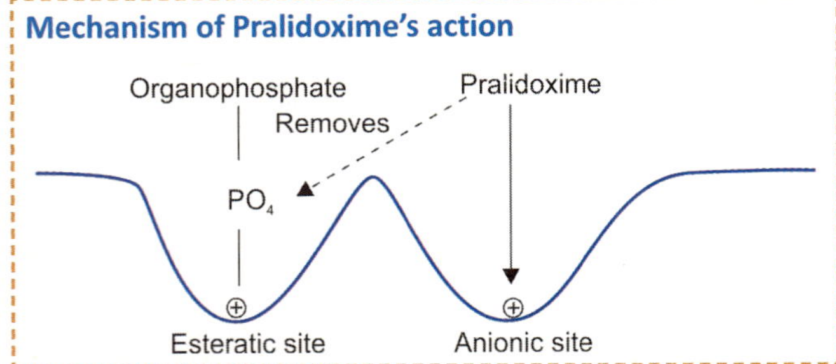

Glaucoma Treatment

- Glaucoma was considered as an increase in IOP more than 21 mm Hg, but since it has been seen that symptoms of glaucoma can be seen even with normal IOP (normal tension glaucoma), this definition is obsolete. Glaucoma can be broadly classified into primary angle closure glaucoma (PACG) and primary open angle glaucoma (POAG).
- In case of an acute attack of PACG (acute congestive glaucoma) IV mannitol (DOC) and/or oral acetazolamide can be used. Once IOP begins to fall topical pilocarpine can be used to open the angle and continued till iridectomy.
- POAG with a gradual increase in IOP and the management is initially medical along with surgical, followed by definitive surgical procedure in drug resistant cases, as given in conceptual box. Treatment of normal tension glaucoma is identical to open angle glaucoma.

Miotic Agents

- Pilocarpine, physostigmine, carbachol and echothiopate are applied topically in acute closed angle glaucoma and open angle glaucoma. These drugs by causing pupil constriction **to increase the trabecular aqueous outflow**.
- These drugs can cause **ciliary body (accommodative) spasm**, induced myopia, brow ache, corneal edema and retinal detachment.
- Echothiopate can cause iris cysts and nasolacrimal duct obstruction also due to stenosis.
- ACHE inhibitors like physostigmine and echothiopate can cause cataract and hence not used in phakic patients.

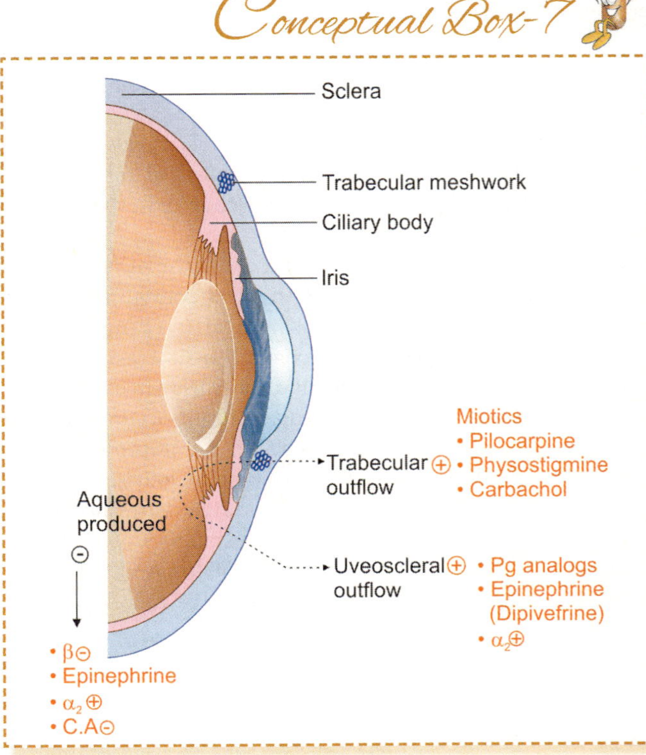

Prostaglandin Analogs

- Latanoprost, travoprost and bimatoprost **OD at night** are drug of choice for open angle and normal tension glaucoma. **Bimatoprost** has been approved for treatment of **hypotrichosis**, e.g. in chemotherapy-induced loss of eye lashes.
- They decrease IOP by increasing **uveoscleral outflow** of aqueous.
- An increase in tyrosinase activity in melanocytes increases melanin content which can lead to **pigmentation of iris (heterochromia iridis), periocular skin** and **eyebrow**. Other side effects seen are **trichomegaly, dry (sandy) eyes, cystoid macular edema** and periorbital fat depletion.
- These drugs are contraindicated in patients with **uveitis** and **herpetic keratitis**.

Beta Blockers

- Topical non-selective beta blockers like timolol, levobunolol, metipranolol, carteolol and **selective beta$_1$ blocker** like **betaxolol** are second line drugs for treatment of open angle and normal tension glaucoma. Timolol is the most potent, whereas betaxolol is the longest acting topical beta blocker.
- Beta blockers have **retinal neuroprotective effect, that is maximum with betaxolol**. They decrease IOP by **decreasing aqueous production**.
- Topical beta blockers can cause systemic side effects and hence are **contraindicated with systemic beta blockers**. Systemic side effects are more common with nonselective beta blockers than selective one like betaxolol. They can also cause dyspnea and apnea in young children.
- Timolol can cause **nasolacrimal duct obstruction** and **ocular cicatricial pemphigoid**. Metipranolol can cause granulomatous anterior uveitis characterized by mutton fat keratic precipitates.
- **Nonselective beta blockers** can block beta-2 receptors and cause bronchospasm; hence are contraindicated in patient of **asthma** and **COPD**.

Sympathomimetics

- **Epinephrine** and its prodrug **dipivefrine** are less preferred nowadays for treatment of glaucoma.
- α_2 agonists like **brimonidine** is third line drugs in open angle and normal tension glaucoma. **Apraclonidine** is primarily used for treatment of transient rise in IOP seen after anterior segment laser procedures.
- These drugs act primarily by **decreasing aqueous production** and contributed by an increase in uveoscleral outflow.
- Common side effect associated with this class is **ocular allergy**. Epinephrine and dipivefrine can cause **black pigmentation of the conjunctiva**.
- **Apraclonidine** being non-selective stimulates alpha 1 receptor and that can cause **lid retraction, mydriasis and conjunctival blanching**. Brimonidine being selective for alpha 2 is devoid of these side effects.
- **Brimonidine** is lipid soluble drug and hence can cross blood brain barrier and cause **drowsiness**/fatigue (sedation), dry mouth, hypotension and **apnea in young children** due to central sympatholytic effect. Apraclonidine being lipid insoluble is devoid of these side effects.

Carbonic Anhydrase Inhibitors

- Acetazolamide (oral) is used in both closed and open angle glaucoma as given in clinical box.
- Topical brinzolamide and dorzolamide are also third line drugs for treatment of open angle and normal tension glaucoma. These drugs act by **decreasing aqueous production**.
- Transient myopia, corneal edema and periorbital dermatitis can be seen with topical drugs. Systemic side effects like hypersensitivity (sulfonamide group in these drugs), paresthesia, metabolic acidosis, hyperammonemia, hyperkalemia etc. can be seen with these drugs.

Recent Advances

Netarsudil: It is rho kinase inhibitor recently approved for treatment of open angle glaucoma, which acts by increasing aqueous out flow via trabecular meshwork.

Antiglaucoma drugs	Mechanism of action
Prostaglandin analogs	Increase uveoscleral outflow
Miotics	Increase trabecular outflow
β blockers and CA Inhibitors	Decrease aqueous production
Sympathomimetics	Decrease aqueous production > Increase uveoscleral outflow

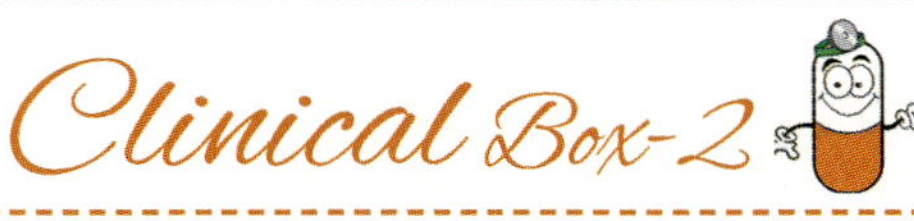

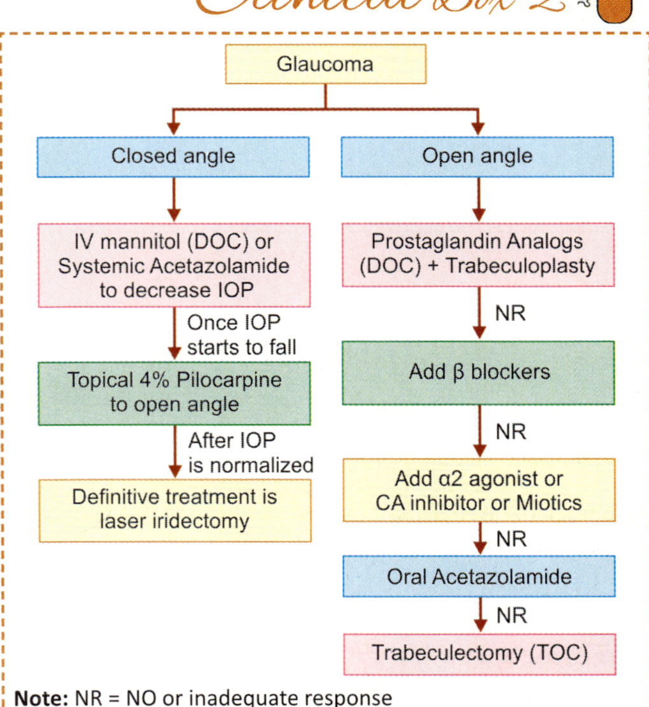

Mushroom Poisoning

- Mushrooms are an important part of diet in most of the tribal people and hence cases of toxicity can be seen. Clinically mushroom toxicity can be broadly classified as early onset and late onset.

- Early onset symptoms are seen within 30 to 120 minutes whereas late onset symptoms are seen only after 6 to 12 hours of mushroom intake.
- The symptoms can range from nausea and vomiting to liver or renal failure depending on the type of mushroom and hence managed accordingly. The **most fatal among the mushrooms is amanita phalloides** and death is usually seen due to massive liver necrosis. The toxin **amanitin inhibits RNA polymerase II**, which decreases protein synthesis and cell death.
- The different types of mushroom poisoning, symptoms and management is given below in the form of a table.

Early onset of mushroom poisoning			
Mushroom type	**Toxin**	**Symptoms**	**Treatment**
Inocybe Clitocybe	Muscarine	Cholinergic	Atropine
Amanita muscaria	Muscimol and ibotenic acid	Anticholinergic	Physostigmine Note: Muscarine content is less and hence atropine is not used.
Coprinus	Coprine	Disulfiram like reaction	Avoid alcohol for 72 hours
Psilocybe Panaeolus	Psilocybin Psilocin	Hallucinations	Supportive care
Late onset mushroom poisoning			
Amanita phalloides **(Death Cap)**	Amanitin	Renal failure Hepatic failure Gastroenteritis	**More effective** • Charcoal • **IV silymarin (silibinin)** • N acetyl cysteine **Less effective** • Thioctic acid • Penicillin-G • **Steroids**
Gyromitra	Mono-methylhydrazine	Gastroenteritis Seizures Renal and hepatic failure	IV Pyridoxine for seizures
Cortinarius	Orellanine	GIT upset Renal failure	Supportive care

ANTICHOLINERGIC (PARASYMPATHOLYTIC) DRUGS

Anticholinergic drugs are antagonists at the muscarinic and nicotinic receptors and hence can be broadly classified as muscarinic and nicotinic antagonists.

Muscarinic Antagonists

Muscarinic antagonists have an inhibitory effect on all parts of body except heart, where they have stimulatory effect.

CNS Effects and Uses

- Muscarinic antagonist used for CNS effects are **tertiary amines**, as lipid solubility is important to cross the **blood brain barrier**.
- Muscarinic antagonists in CNS decrease cognition without causing retrograde amnesia. Hence **scopolamine (hyoscine)** is used in **narco analysis** and is known as truth serum. **Scopolamine** is the **drug of choice for motion sickness** by transdermal route. It has to be given at least 4 hours before journey and thereafter every 72 hours if journey continues.
- Muscarinic antagonists by acting on M_1 receptors increase dopamine release in CNS and hence are beneficial in **Parkinson's disease** and treatment of **EPS** like **acute dystonia, parkinsonism, akathisia and oculogyric crisis associated with antipsychotics**. The tertiary amines (lipid soluble) preferred are **benztropine, biperiden and trihexyphenidyl**.

Ocular Effects and Uses

- Muscarinic antagonists decrease pupil contraction (mydriasis) and accommodation (cycloplegia), whereas sympathomimetics like phenylephrine cause only mydriasis. The drugs used for these effects are **atropine**, scopolamine, tropicamide, cyclopentolate and homatropine.
- **Mydriasis** makes them useful for visualization and examination of retina and optic disc. They are combined with miotics to prevent **synechiae formation in iridocyclitis** and **fungal corneal ulcer** and in case synechiae is formed, they are combined with sympathomimetics like phenylephrine to increase mydriatic effect that breaks the synechiae.

- Cycloplegia is essential to cancel the accommodation for accurate **refractive error testing**. Cycloplegic doses are higher than mydriatic doses. In **adults tropicamide** is preferred as it is **shortest** and **fastest** acting and hence side effect like photophobia due to mydriasis is short lived; adults can resume work faster. In **children 1% atropine ointment** is preferred as children have a powerful accommodation and **atropine** is the **most potent cycloplegic**. Cycloplegic effect is also beneficial to decrease pain associated with **anterior uveitis**.
- Due to mydriatic effect any anticholinergic or a drug with anticholinergic side effects (TCA, antihistaminics, typical and atypical antipsychotics) can **precipitate an acute attack of closed angle glaucoma**.

Effects on Secretions and Uses

- Muscarinic antagonists decrease secretions from oropharyngeal cavity, bronchi, lacrimal gland, sweat gland, nasal cavity and sinuses.
- **Glycopyrrolate** being a **quaternary amine (lipid insoluble) does not cross blood brain barrier** and hence used as a **preanesthetic medication** to decrease oropharyngeal and bronchial secretions to prevent aspiration.
- Methscopolamine is a quaternary amine derivative of scopolamine used for treatment of allergic rhinitis and sinusitis. Ipratropium is also used in rhinitis to decrease secretions. Because of anticholinergic effect, antihistaminics are also beneficial in rhinitis.

Effect on Bronchial Smooth Muscles and Uses

- Bronchial smooth muscle contraction is decreased by muscarinic antagonists and hence causes bronchodilation. Bronchodilatory effect makes these drugs useful in treatment of **COPD** and bronchial asthma.
- Since cholinergic effect mediated bronchoconstriction is the only reversible component in COPD, these are the **drug of choice in COPD**. In bronchial asthma major cause of bronchoconstriction are mediators like histamine and leukotrienes; cholinergic effect plays a minor role and hence these drugs though used in bronchial asthma are not as effective as β_2 agonists.
- The drugs in this class like **ipratropium, tiotropium, oxitropium and** umeclidinium are **quaternary amine** derivatives of atropine. **Tiotropium being the longest acting and most effective is the drug of choice for COPD**.

Effects on Heart and Uses

- Muscarinic antagonists by acting on M_2 receptors **increase cardiac contraction and conduction and heart rate**.
- **Atropine** is used for treatment of **bradyarrhythmia** like sinus bradycardia and sinus arrest. It is also used for reversal of **AV block**.
- Bradyarrhythmia usually seen with inferior wall MI and AV block caused by digitalis respond well to atropine.

Effects on GIT and Uterus and Uses

- Muscarinic antagonists decrease contraction of GIT and uterus makes these drugs useful as **antispasmodic agents** and is useful in GIT spasm, diarrhea associated with IBS and in dysmenorrhea. The drugs preferred are **dicyclomine, scopolamine, atropine and glycopyrrolate**. Glycopyrrolate being a quaternary amine (lipid insoluble) does not cause central side effects and is more preferred.
- Muscarinic antagonists decrease hydrochloric acid secretion by parietal cells and makes them useful in **peptic ulcer disease**. **Pirenzepine and telenzepine** are M_1 antagonists that decrease acetylcholine release in intramural gastric ganglion. This interrupts acetylcholine release into the synapse of parietal cells containing M_3 receptors and thus decreases hydrochloric acid secretion by parietal cells.

Effects on Bladder and Uses

- A **decrease in detrusor contraction** makes them beneficial in a condition with increased/spontaneous detrusor contraction called as **overactive bladder or detrusor instability**, which leads to **urge incontinence**. These drugs are also useful in **enuresis** in children.
- The drugs used for this indication can be classified as nonselective and selective M_3 antagonists. Nonselective class contains drugs like **flavoxate, fesoterodine, oxybutynin, tolterodine** and **trospium**. Selective M_3 antagonists are **darifenacin** and **solifenacin**; **darifenacin is more M_3 selective than solifenacin**.
- Trospium, darifenacin and solefenacin do not cause central side effects like drowsiness, dizziness, confusion and decrease in cognition; as **trospium being a quaternary amine** does not cross blood brain barrier and darifenacin and solifenacin have no effect on central M_1 receptors. Most common side effect causing incompliance is xerostomia.
- Flavoxate and fesoterodine are not used nowadays due to toxicity. Among the remaining drugs the order of preference based on toxicity profile is **darifenacin** > **solifenacin** > **trospium** > **tolterodine** > **oxybutynin**. Since among the drugs currently used oxybutynin is the most toxic, transdermal formulations in the form of patch and gel are available.

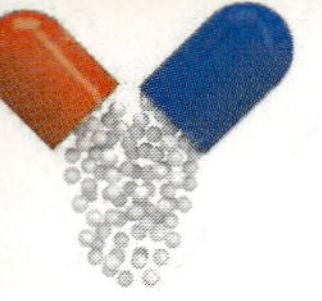

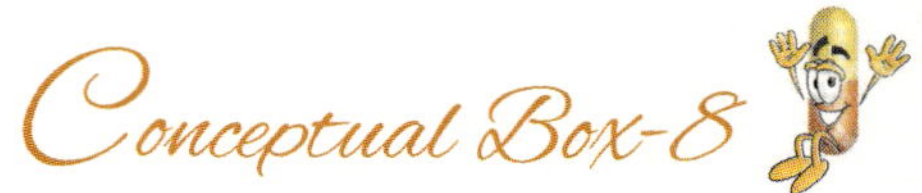

(↓DC) ↓Detrusor contraction ← (↑Cyc← G_s) Amp ← β_3

(↑DC) ↑Detrusor contraction ← (G_q→↑Ca^{++}) ← M_3

Detrusor

Trigone

Sphincter α1(G_q →↑Ca^{++}) → ↑Sphincter contraction (↑SC)

Sympathetic NS

β_3⊕ → Effect →↓DC → Indication→↑DC OAB/DI → Urge incontinence → Drug → Mirabegron

α1⊕ → Effect →↑SC → Indication→↓SC → Stress incontinence → Drug → Duloxetine →↑NE→⊕α1

Parasympathetic NS

⊕ Cholinergics → Effect →↑DC → Indication→↓DC Detrusoritony → Overflow incontinence → Drug → Bethanechol, Neostigmine

⊖ Anticholinergics → Effect →↓DC → Indication→↑DC OAB/DI → Urge incontinence → Drug

- Nonselective
  - Fesoterodine
  - Flavoxate
  - Oxybutynin
  - Tolterodine
  - Trospium
- Selective M3⊖
  - Darifenacin
  - Solifenacin

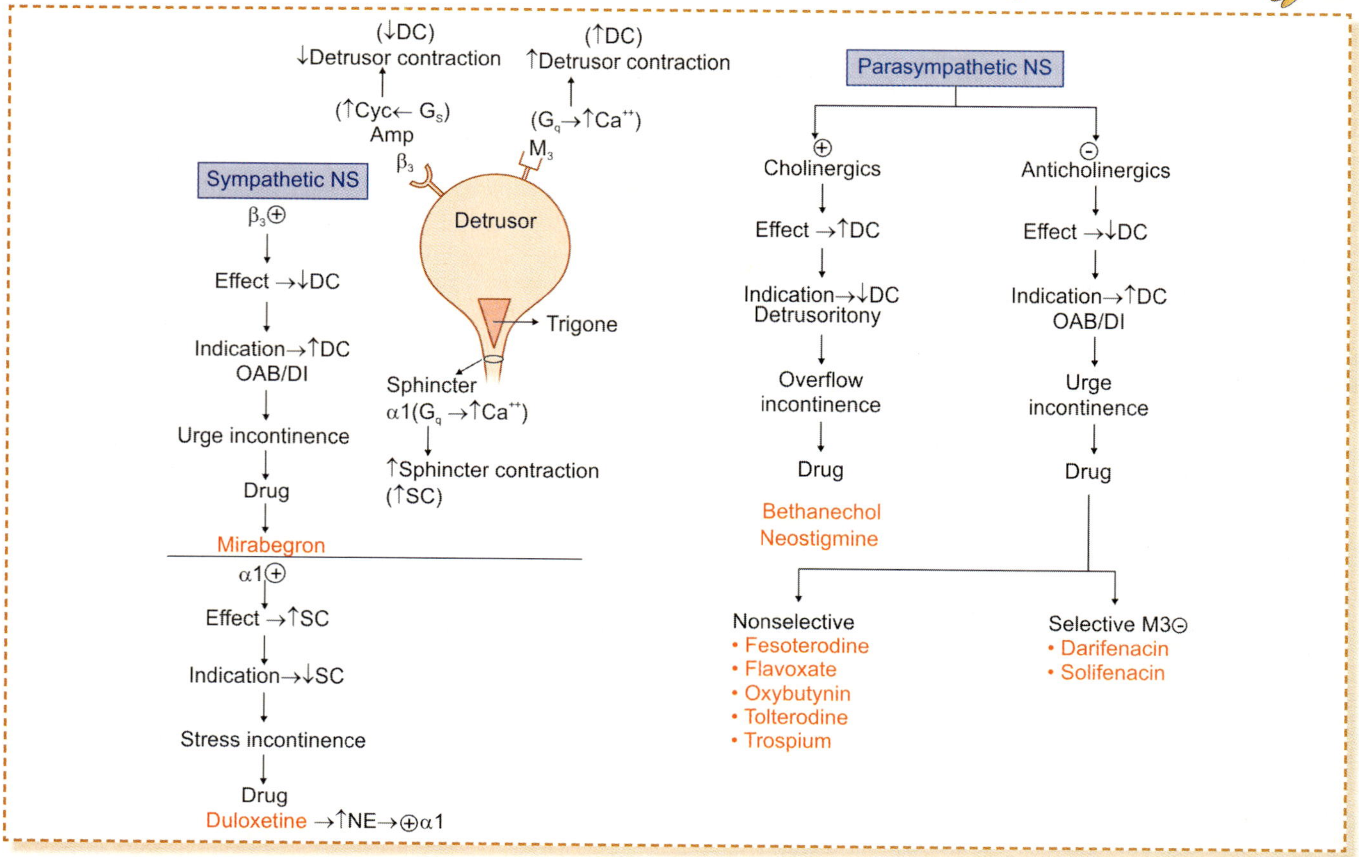

Nicotinic Antagonists

Nicotinic antagonists are drugs that inhibit the N_M and N_N subtype of nicotinic receptors.

N_M Receptor Antagonists

These drugs inhibit transmission at the neuromuscular junction and cause muscle relaxation. Thus, this class of drug is used as **muscle relaxant** in anesthesia. Muscle relaxants can be depolarizing ones like succinylcholine or nondepolarizing ones (NDMR) like tubocurare.

N_N Receptor Antagonists

- These are targeted at the ganglionic site which leads to inhibition of norepinephrine and acetylcholine release in the postganglionic fibers. Hence the effect that can be seen are vasodilation and mild reflex tachycardia associated with anticholinergic effects like dry mouth, constipation, urine retention etc.
- **Tetraethylammonium (TEA)**, **trimethaphan, hexamethonium and mecamylamine** are the drugs in this class, also known as **ganglionic blockers** were the first class of drug to be used in hypertension. Though nowadays less preferred due to associated side effects.
- Mecamylamine an oral drug, is also used for treatment of Tourette syndrome and as an adjunct to nicotine patch in smoking dependence.
- Trimethaphan is used by intravenous route for treatment of hypertensive emergency.
- **Tetraethylammonium** is currently used as a research agent that selectively **blocks potassium channel**.

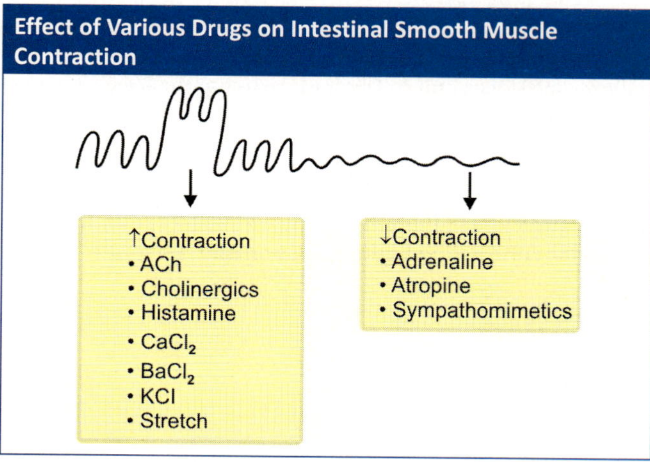

Effect of Various Drugs on Intestinal Smooth Muscle Contraction
↑Contraction
• ACh
• Cholinergics
• Histamine
• $CaCl_2$
• $BaCl_2$
• KCl
• Stretch
↓Contraction
• Adrenaline
• Atropine
• Sympathomimetics

SYMPATHETIC NERVOUS SYSTEM

NEUROTRANSMITTER

- The precursor for norepinephrine synthesis is amino acid **tyrosine**, which is taken up into presynaptic neurons by aromatic amino acid transporter. Tyrosine is converted into dopa by the rate limiting enzyme **tyrosine hydroxylase**.
- Dopa is further converted into dopamine by dopa decarboxylase and then dopamine is taken up into vesicles by vesicular monoamine transporters (VMAT). Inside vesicle, dopamine is converted into NE by an enzyme called dopamine-β-hydroxylase.
- In the adrenal gland cells, norepinephrine is **methylated** into epinephrine by phenyl ethanolamine-N-methyltransferase, which is activated by cortisol.
- After the action potential strikes the presynaptic membrane, calcium channels open and rise in intracellular calcium causes movement of vesicle and release of norepinephrine into the synaptic cleft.
- Norepinephrine acts on α and β receptors following which **90% of undergoes reuptake** into presynaptic neuron by NET (Norepinephrine Transporter). The remaining 10% is either metabolized by enzymes like COMT and MAO into **vanillylmandelic acid (VMA)** or simply diffuses out of the synaptic cleft.

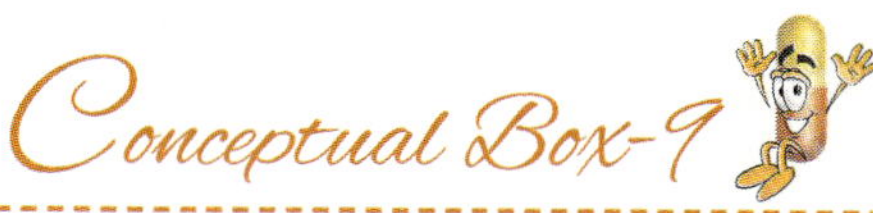

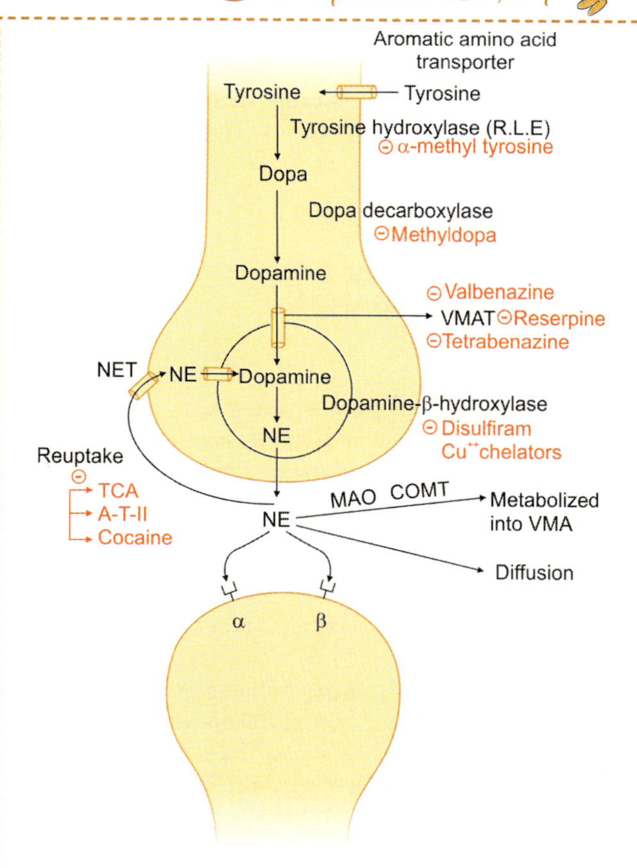

Drugs Acting on NE Synthesis

Methyl tyrosine is an analog of tyrosine and hence competitively inhibits the rate limiting enzyme of NE synthesis, i.e. tyrosine hydroxylase. It is used along with phenoxybenzamine for treatment and preoperative preparation **pheochromocytoma**. It is also used in **malignant pheochromocytoma** for long term management of hypertension. Crystalluria is a specific side effect that is associated.

Drugs Acting on NE Storage

VMAT-2 Inhibitors

VMAT-2 inhibitors act by inhibiting uptake of catecholamines like norepinephrine, dopamine and serotonin by the vesicles.

- **Reserpine** is a natural **alkaloid** derived from a plant called ***Rauwolfia serpentina***. It irreversibly blocks VMAT-2 and is used for treatment of **hypertension** along with diuretics in elderly patients and in **tardive dyskinesia** caused by antipsychotics. Overall it is rarely used nowadays due to toxicity.
- **Tetrabenazine** is a reversible inhibitor of VMAT-2 which is more selectively located in dopaminergic neurons It is also a weak D_2 antagonist. Since it is reversible inhibitor, it is shorter acting than reserpine and is less toxic. It is the current **drug of choice for Huntington's chorea** and is also used for treatment of tics associated with **Tourette syndrome**. It is also useful in other movement disorders like tardive dyskinesia, hemiballismus and dystonia. Side effects associated are sedation, depression, parkinsonism, etc.
- Side effects of these drugs are related to depletion of catecholamines as given below.

Decreased catecholamines	Side effect
Norepinephrine Serotonin	Depression with suicidal tendency Sedation
Norepinephrine	Hypotension
Dopamine	Parkinsonism

Recent Advances

- **Valbenazine** and **deutetrabenazine** are derivatives of tetrabenazine which also act by inhibiting VMAT-2 and have been recently approved for treatment of **tardive dyskinesia** associated with antipsychotics, whereas deutetrabenazine is also approved for treatment of **Huntington's chorea** as well. These drugs have similar side effect as tetrabenazine.
- **Deutetrabenazine** is synthesized by adding deuterium (heavy hydrogen, an isotope of regular hydrogen) in place of normal hydrogen in tetrabenazine molecule. The deuterium bond is difficult to break and hence slowly metabolized by liver; deutetrabenazine is longer acting than tetrabenazine. This effect of adding an isotope of hydrogen is called **primary kinetic isotope effect**.

False Neurotransmitters

False neurotransmitters are taken up into the vesicles which displace NE into the synaptic cleft and produce sympathomimetic effect. On repeated dosing though, the NE gets depleted and after some doses only false neurotransmitter is released; in the absence of norepinephrine sympatholytic effect is seen. Thus at intermittent doses these drugs cause sympathomimetic effect and at continuous doses cause sympatholytic effect. The effect is seen at initial doses and then disappears after few doses, this phenomenon is called as **tachyphylaxis**.

Tyramine

- It is a dietary amine present in red wine and cheese. Tyramine is metabolized in the GIT and liver by MAO.
- Earlier, when MAO inhibitors were a popular class of antidepressant drug, consumption of cheese and red wine along with inhibited metabolism of tyramine. This tyramine released NE from vesicles into synapse and an acute surge in blood pressure resulted in many cases of hypertensive crisis.
- This reaction was classically known as **cheese reaction**, for which α blocker, **phentolamine is the drug of choice**.

Guanethidine and Guanadrel

- These drugs at continuous doses can decrease NE in the synapse and hence are beneficial in hypertension. Initial release of NE can worsen pheochromocytoma and hence are contraindicated in same.
- Postural hypotension is a persistent side effect seen due to sympathetic blockade even on chronic administration.

Amphetamine

- Apart displacing NE, it is also an inhibitor of DAT (dopamine transporter) and VMAT-2.
- Amphetamine can be used for treatment of **ADHD, obesity** and **narcolepsy**. **Dextroamphetamine** is more specific for central action and hence preferred to amphetamine. **Lis dexamphetamine** is a prodrug of amphetamine used for treatment of **ADHD**.
- **Methamphetamine or crystal meth (crank)** is a drug of abuse and is known as **designer drug**. When a drug banned by the narcotic act is produced with slight modification to avoid law is known as **designer drug**, e.g. **methamphetamine from amphetamine**.
- Amphetamine toxicity can be treated by **urine acidification** with aluminum hydrochloride, as it is a basic drug. Consumption in pregnancy can cause teratogenic effects like **IUGR, cardiac defects, cleft lip and biliary atresia**.

Methylphenidate

- It is an analog of amphetamine and is the **drug of choice for treatment of ADHD**.
- Stimulants like methylphenidate and amphetamine worsen tics of Tourette syndrome and have potential for abuse. Hence in case of **ADHD with Tourette syndrome or family history of drug abuse, atomoxetine is drug of choice**.

Ephedrine

- Ephedrine not only displaces norepinephrine but also stimulates alpha and beta receptors. Hence it is known as a **mixed acting sympathomimetic**.
- Ephedrine is drug of choice for treatment of **hypotension in pregnancy and hypotension with anesthetic agents**. It is given by oral route, has a **longer duration of action (6 hours) as compared to catecholamines**.
- **Norephedrine (phenylpropanolamine)** was used as nasal decongestant and as anorexic agent but has been banned due to risk of **cerebral hemorrhage**.
- **Pseudoephedrine** an isomer of ephedrine. Both ephedrine and pseudoephedrine are used as nasal decongestant**.**

Modafinil

- Modafinil is the drug of choice for **narcolepsy, shift worker disease** and **sleepiness in patients of OSA (Obstructive Sleep Apnea)**. Armodafinil, the R enantiomer is longer acting.
- It acts by inhibiting DAT, which leads to an increase in dopamine in CNS.

Drugs Acting on NE Reuptake

- **TCA** are nonselective inhibitors of all monoamines, i.e. NE, dopamine and serotonin, whereas SNRI inhibits reuptake of only NE and serotonin. An increase in these monoamines has antidepressant effect; thus methyltyrosine and reserpine by depleting these amines cause depression. These drugs are discussed in detail in the chapter of CNS.
- **Cocaine** inhibits reuptake of monoamines; dopamine by acting on D_2 receptors in CNS gives kick and hence is a substance of abuse. For **cocaine dependence** D_2 agonist **bromocriptine is the drug of choice**, whereas TCA desipramine can also be used.

RECEPTORS

The adrenergic receptors are broadly classified into α and β receptors; both subtypes are GPCRs.

α Receptors

α receptors are of two subtypes, i.e. α_1 and α_2.

- α_1 **receptors** are G_q subtype of GPCR, located on postsynaptic membranes. Stimulation of three subtypes, i.e. α_{1A}, α_{1B} **and** α_{1D} increases intracellular calcium which causes contraction of blood vessels, bronchi, uterus, prostatic urethra, bladder sphincter and radial muscles of iris (mydriasis). Calcium dependent K^+ channels open in GIT, which causes relaxation. In the liver α_1 receptors induce glycogenolysis and gluconeogenesis.
- α_2 **receptors** being G_i subtype decrease cyclic AMP, inhibit calcium channels and open K^+ channels, which causes relaxation. Their primary site of location is presynaptic membrane where they **decrease NE release**. Postsynaptic α_2 receptors can cause vasoconstriction, GIT relaxation and a decrease in insulin release.

α_1 Receptors		α_2 Receptors	
α_{1A}	Prostatic urethra and bladder sphincter contraction, glycogenolysis and gluconeogenesis in liver	α_{2A}	Decrease in NE release in synapse Vasoconstriction
α_{1B}	Vasoconstriction	α_{2B}	Vasoconstriction
α_{1D}	Vasoconstriction and prostatic urethra and bladder contraction	α_{2C}	Inhibits dopamine release in CNS and catecholamine release from adrenals
Note: Cardiac hypertrophy is caused by both α_{1A} and α_{1B}		Note: Insulin release is decreased by both α_{2A} and α_{2B}	

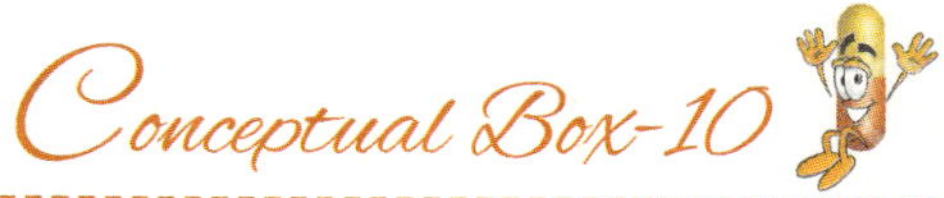

Control of NE Release

NE release is controlled by **presynaptic α_2 and β_2 receptors**. When NE is released into the synapse it can act these two receptors, but the selectivity depends on amount of NE in synapse.

- Threshold concentration of NE for β receptor activation is lesser than α receptor activation. Hence at low NE concentration in synapse, β receptors are predominantly stimulated. Thus in the beginning when NE is lesser in synapse, NE stimulates β receptors, which are G_s subtype and stimulate NE release.
- At high NE concentration though α receptors are predominantly stimulated. After some time when there is excess of NE in synapse, α_2 is predominantly stimulated which inhibits NE release. Because of this automatic control of NE release these receptors are also called as **autoreceptors**.

β Receptors

- β receptors are classified into three subtypes, i.e. β_1, β_2 **and** β_3; all are G_s subtype and act by increasing cyclic AMP.
- β_1 receptors are predominantly located in the **heart**, where raised cyclic AMP stimulates Ca^{++} channels that leads to **increase in cardiac contraction and conduction, heart rate**. In the kidney β_1 receptors are present in **JG cells** where they stimulate renin release.
- β_2 receptors have a differential action based upon location. In **cardiac and skeletal muscles** they act by β_1 pathway and hence **increase contraction**. In **smooth muscles** β_2 receptors induced increase in cyclic AMP, stimulates myosin light chain phosphorylase, inhibits myosin light chain kinase and opens K^+ channels, which collectively cause **relaxation**. The effect seen are bronchodilation, vasodilation and uterine relaxation. β_2 receptors in liver and muscle induce gluconeogenesis and glycogenolysis (hyperglycemia +++), and in beta islet cells of pancreas increase insulin release (hypoglycemia -). The overall effect is **hyperglycemia (++)**. Initially opening of K^+ channel causes **hyperkalemia (transient)**, which is followed by **hypokalemia** (persistent) due to insulin release.
- β_3 receptors present in **adipocytes** increase cyclic AMP, which increases production of hormone-sensitive lipase and induces **lipolysis**. These are also present in detrusor where they facilitate relaxation.

β Receptors	Location and effect
β_1	Heart = Increased contraction, conduction and HR Kidney (JG Cells) = Renin release
β_2	Heart = Increased contraction, conduction and HR Skeletal muscles = Increased Contraction Blood vessels = Dilation Bronchi = Dilation Uterus = Relaxation Liver = Glycogenolysis and gluconeogenesis Pancreas = Insulin release
β_3	Adipocytes = Lipolysis Detrusor = Relaxation

SYMPATHOMIMETICS (ADRENERGICS)

Sympathomimetics can be broadly classified into **catecholamines, noncatecholamines** and **miscellaneous**. The miscellaneous class contains drugs which are false neurotransmitters and have been discussed earlier.

Catecholamines

Catecholamines are either endogenous products like NE, epinephrine and dopamine or exogenous synthetic chemicals like dobutamine, isoprenaline, dopexamine, fenoldopam and droxidopa.

Endogenous Catecholamines

Epinephrine (Adrenaline)

- Epinephrine is a nonselective agonist at **all subtypes of α and β receptors**. As discussed earlier the effect on α and β receptors depends on the dose of epinephrine. At low/physiological doses β receptors are predominantly stimulated, that causes vasodilation, whereas at high doses α_1 receptor stimulation causes vasoconstriction.

Dale's Phenomenon

Epinephrine when administered initially raises blood pressure due to α_1 followed by a decrease in blood pressure due to β_2; this **biphasic pattern** of blood pressure is called as Dale's phenomenon. If patient is given epinephrine being on α blocker, then only vasodilation is seen due to β_2; this effect is known as vasomotor reversal of dale.

- The effect of epinephrine on heart rate and blood pressure is given in the conceptual box below.
- Epinephrine is the drug of choice for **prophylaxis and treatment of anaphylactic shock** because of both α_1 (vasoconstriction) and β_2 (bronchodilation) effects. The **preferred route of administration is intramuscular**, though intravenous route is used in case patient does not respond. It is also drug of choice for treatment of **brittle asthma** and for treatment of **bradycardia in infants and children**. It is used along with local anesthetics as a vasoconstrictor to increase

duration of action and decrease toxicity. It can also be used in cardiac arrest (1 mg IV), parainfluenza virus associated ARDS, GIT bleeding, scombroid sea food poisoning and mastocytosis.

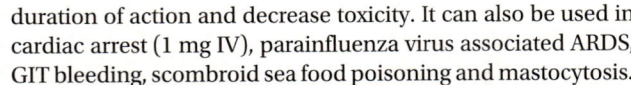

- Epinephrine is available at various dilutions with doses e.g. 1 mg/mL at **1:1000** dilution for subcutaneous and intramuscular use and 0.1 mg/mL or **1:10,000** dilutions for intravenous and topical use.

Table 1: Epinephrine Dilutions Used

Route of administration	Epinephrine dilution used
Intramuscular Subcutaneous Endotracheal	1:1000
Intravenous Intraosseous Intracardiac	1:10,000
Local injection to decrease blood loss	1:100,000
With local anesthetics	1:200,000

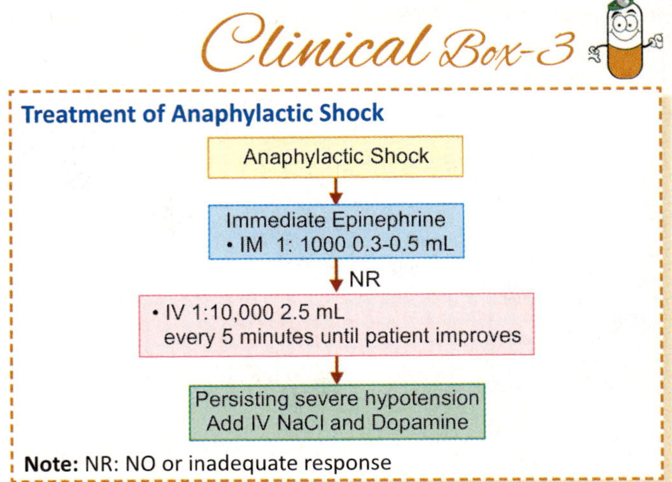

Norepinephrine (Noradrenaline)

- Norepinephrine is a nonselective **agonist at α subtype but more selective at β_1 receptors**. Because of this NE is a more potent vasoconstrictor than epinephrine and hence is contraindicated by intramuscular route as it can cause muscle necrosis. Vasoconstriction causes an increase in diastolic BP but a reflex decrease in HR (- - -) due to vagus. NE is a less potent cardiac stimulator as compared to epinephrine and hence increases heart rate directly (++) and systolic BP, but lesser than epinephrine. The overall effect is an **increase in both diastolic and systolic BP but a decrease in HR (-)**. If the patient has a **transplanted heart or is on anticholinergic like atropine**, the effect of vagus is missing and hence NE in such cases causes an **increase in HR (++)**.
- A high dose of epinephrine has an effect similar to that of norepinephrine, which can be differentiated by use of an α_1 blocker to decrease blood pressure. In case of epinephrine α_1 block causes a greater decrease in blood pressure to β_2 action.

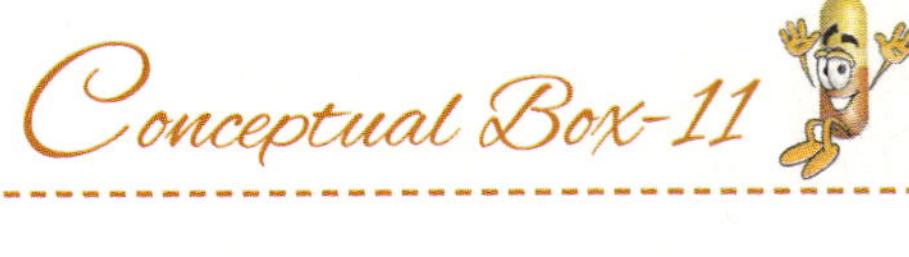

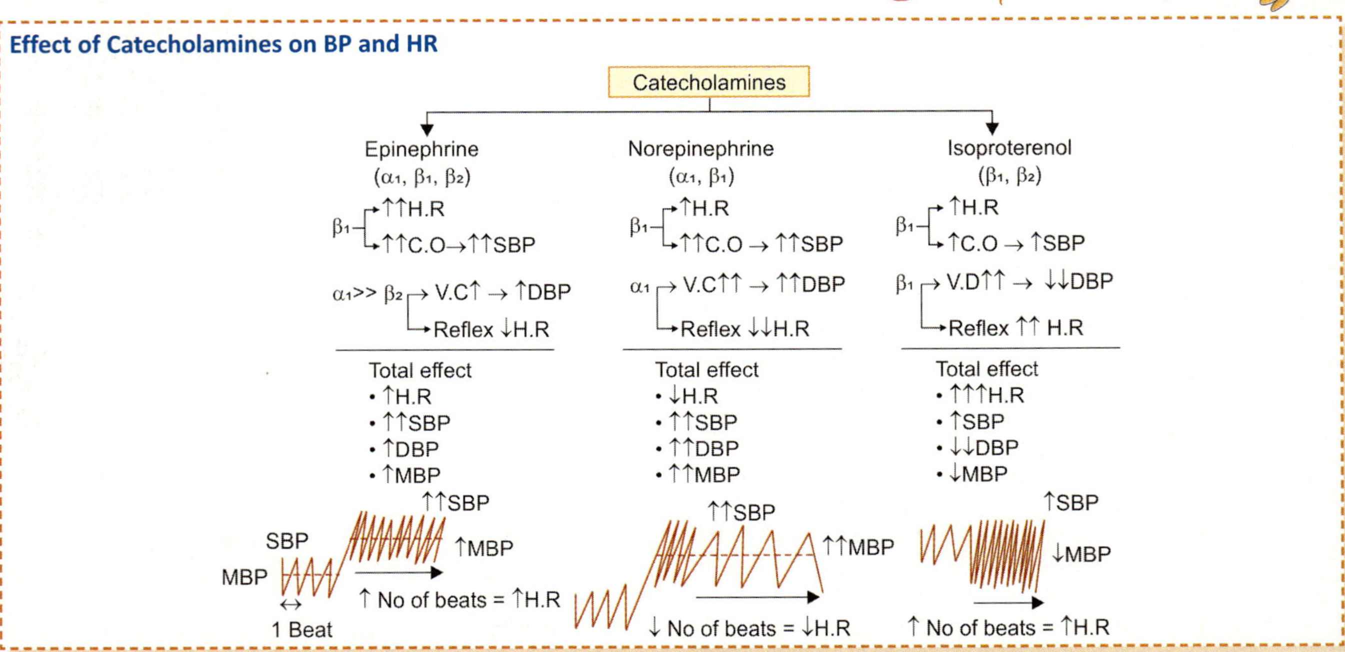

Note: HR = Heart Rate, SBP = Systolic Blood Pressure, DBP = Diastolic Blood Pressure, MBP = Mean Blood Pressure

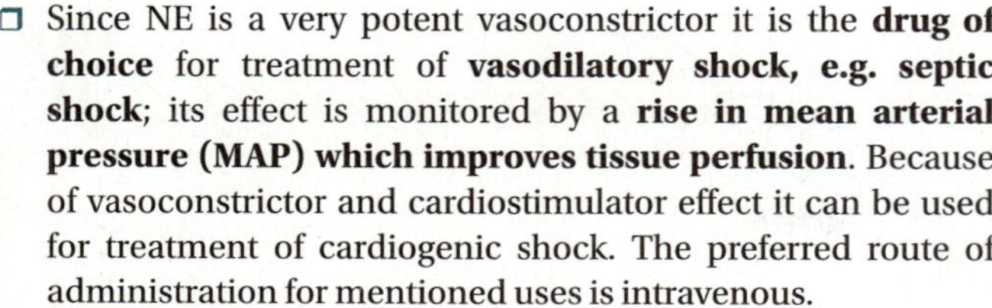

- Since NE is a very potent vasoconstrictor it is the **drug of choice** for treatment of **vasodilatory shock, e.g. septic shock**; its effect is monitored by a **rise in mean arterial pressure (MAP) which improves tissue perfusion**. Because of vasoconstrictor and cardiostimulator effect it can be used for treatment of cardiogenic shock. The preferred route of administration for mentioned uses is intravenous.

Dopamine

- Dopamine has a dose dependent action as mentioned below.

Dose (continuous IV infusion)	Target receptor/organ affected	Therapeutic indication
<2 μg/kg/min	D_1 receptors in renal blood vessels = **Renal vasodilatation** = Diuresis	Oliguria
2-10 μg/kg/min	β_1 receptors in heart = Inotropic effect	CHF
> 10 μg/kg/min	α_1 receptors in blood vessels = Vasoconstriction	Shock

- Dopamine is the drug of choice for treatment of **cardiogenic shock**, **CHF with oliguria** and **hypotension associated with hypothermia**. It differs from other sympathomimetics in causing **renal vasodilation** and preserving renal function in **shock**.
- The route of administration is intravenous, preferably into large veins to prevent extravasation as it causes necrosis of tissue.

Sympathomimetics	Target receptors
Epinephrine	$\alpha_1\ \alpha_2\ \beta_1\ \beta_2$
Norepinephrine	$\alpha_1\ \alpha_2\ \beta_1$
Dopamine (Dose dependent action)	$D_1\ \beta_1\ \alpha_1$
Fenoldopam	$D_1\ \alpha_2$
Dopexamine	$D_1\ \beta_2$
Isoprenaline (Isoproterenol)	$\beta_1\ \beta_2$

Exogenous Catecholamines

- **Dobutamine** is an agonist at **β1 and** β2 receptors and increase cardiac output more than heart rate, and also causes vasodilation. Hence it is used for treatment of cardiogenic shock and is the inotrope of choice in case of acute CHF as it reduces PCWP. Dobutamine is also used as a pharmacological stressor in PET/SPECT myocardial perfusion testing and echocardiography. D isomer of dobutamine is α1 antagonist, whereas L isomer is α1 agonist; the net effect on α1 remains unchanged as they cancel each other effect. It is given by continuous IV infusion owing to its short half-life of 2 minutes.
- **Isoproterenol** is a nonselective β receptor agonist. Because of its β_1 effect on heart it can be used for treatment of AV block and bradycardia and β_2 mediated bronchodilation makes it useful in bronchial asthma.
- **Droxidopa** is a recently approved drug in 2014 for treatment of **neurogenic hypotension**. It is a prodrug of NE.
- **Dopexamine** is an agonist at β_2 and D1 receptor, whereas fenoldopam is an agonist as α_2 and D_1. The overall effect is a significant decrease in blood pressure, which makes these drugs useful in **hypertensive emergency**.

Dopexamine and Fenoldopam	D_1 agonism = Diuresis = Decrease in BP
Dopexamine	β_2 agonism = Vasodilation = Decrease in BP
Fenoldopam	α_2 agonism = decrease in NE release = Decrease in BP

Noncatecholamines

Noncatecholamines are agonists at α and β adrenergic receptors. α agonists can be further subclassified as α_1 and α_2 agonists and β agonists as β_2 and β_3 agonists.

α_1 Agonists

- **Phenylephrine** can be used for treatment of anesthetic agent induced hypotension and can be used as adjunct in shock. It is also approved for treatment of nasal congestion and as a mydriatic.
- **Midodrine is the vasopressor of choice for treatment of orthostatic hypotension**; the drug of choice if fludrocortisone. **Metaraminol** and **mephenteramine** can also be used for treatment of hypotension associated with spinal anesthesia and cardiac arrhythmia respectively. **Mephenteramine** like ephedrine also releases NE, which stimulates heart.
- **Methoxamine** can be used for treatment of shock by systemic route.
- **Oxymetazoline** and **tetrahydrozoline** are used by topical route for treatment of nasal congestion.

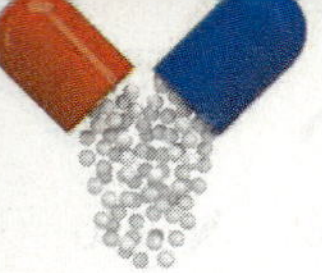

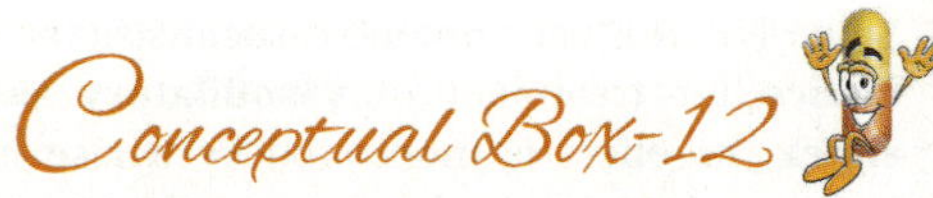

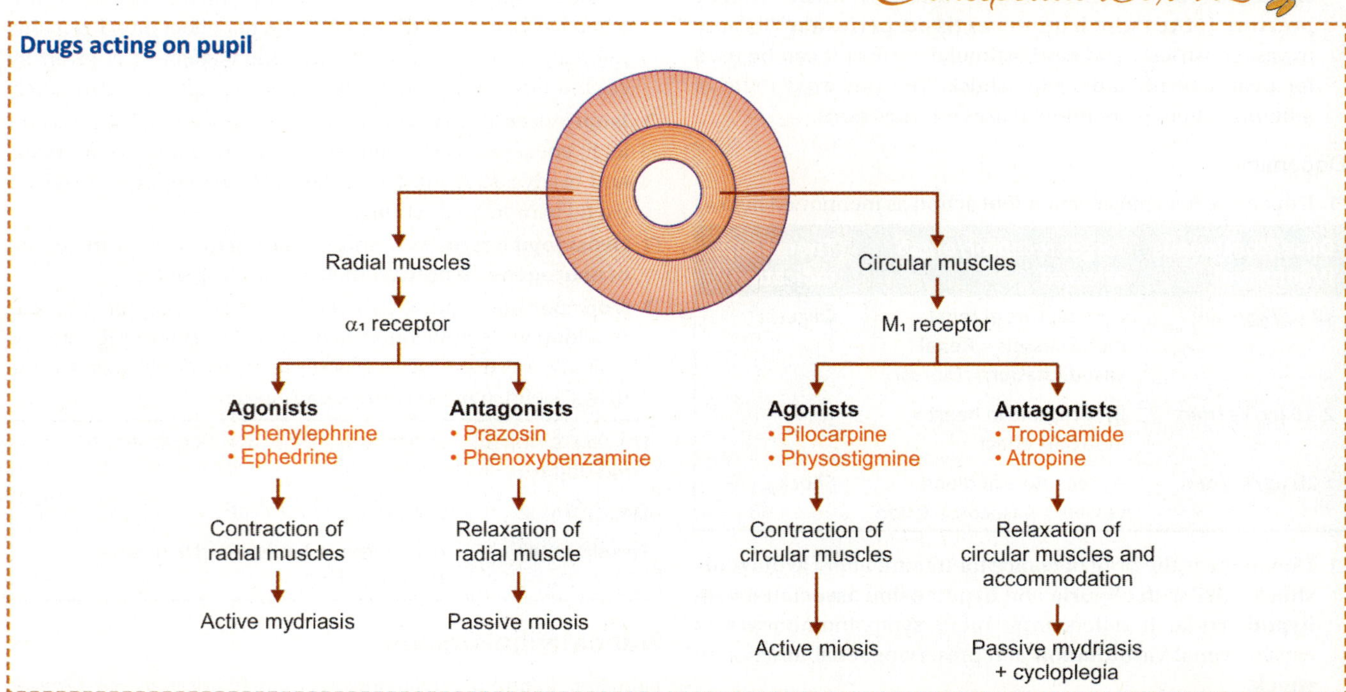

α_2 *Agonists*

α_2 agonists decrease NE release in the CVS center in CNS and thus are known as **central sympatholytics**. A decrease in NE release in presynaptic CNS neuron is seen specifically due to **α_{2A} subtype**.

- **Clonidine** is primarily used as a second line drug for treatment of hypertension. Oral clonidine is the **drug of choice for treatment of hypertensive urgency** and **tics associated with Tourette's syndrome**. Clonidine has found new uses in due course of time like diarrhea associated with DM (decreases Cl and water secretion), prophylaxis of migraine, ADHD (NE decrease decreases CNS stimulation), dependence (alcohol, smoking, opioid), postmenopausal hot flashes (transdermal route), preanesthetic medication and conscious sedation in ICU (NE is a stimulant and if decreased, sedation is seen), analgesic in cancer patients and diagnosis of pheochromocytoma. Clonidine in hypertension significantly decreases NE, which does not happen in pheochromocytoma. Side effects associated are **dry mouth, impotence and withdrawal hypertension**.

Mnemonics

Uses of Clonidine

C : Cl^- absorption treats diarrhea of DM
H : Hypertension
A : Analgesic in terminal cancer patients
M: Menopausal hot flashes, Migraine prophylaxis
A : ADHD
T : Tics associated with Tourette's syndrome
K : Kills dependence on alcohol, smoking and opioids
A : Atrial fibrillation
R : Restless leg syndrome

- **Dexmedetomidine** is also a **central α_2 agonist** used as preanesthetic medication like **clonidine**. The beneficial effect for surgery are seen are sedation, anxiolysis, **analgesia** and decreased secretions.
- **Apraclonidine** and **brimonidine** are used for treatment of **glaucoma** and have been discussed earlier in the section of glaucoma.
- **Methyldopa** is a prodrug converted into active compound α methyl NE, which not only an α_2 agonist, but also a false neurotransmitter that depletes vesicular NE. It has limited use in treatment of hypertension and is preferred in pregnancy induced hypertension. The current drug of choice for same is oral labetalol.
- **Guanfacine** and **guanabenz** can be used for treatment of ADHD. Guanfacine is also indicated for treatment of tics associated with Tourette's syndrome like clonidine.
- **Moxonidine** is an agonist at both alpha2 and imidazole receptors. It is used for treatment of resistant hypertension in elderly and for neuropathic pain. Another drug with similar properties is **rilmenidine**.
- **Tizanidine** is primarily used as a muscle relaxant in muscle spastic disorders like **amyotrophic lateral sclerosis (ALS)**.

β_2 *Agonists*

β_2 agonists are functional antagonists of histamine and leukotrienes and hence are **best bronchodilators in bronchial asthma**. Their use in COPD is limited and are preferred only if the patient does not respond to anticholinergics. Since these drugs can cause hypokalemia, they are also used for treatment of hyperkalemia.

- **Short acting β_2 agonists (SABA)** like salbutamol and terbutaline are the drug of choice for an acute attack of asthma.
- **Long acting β_2 agonists (LABA)** like salmeterol, formoterol and arformoterol are used for prophylaxis of bronchial asthma, exercise induced asthma, nocturnal asthma and along with ICS for management of persistent bronchial asthma.

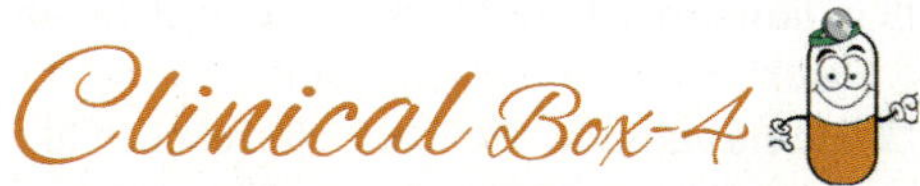

Treatment of Tourette's Syndrome Associated Tics and Huntington's Chorea

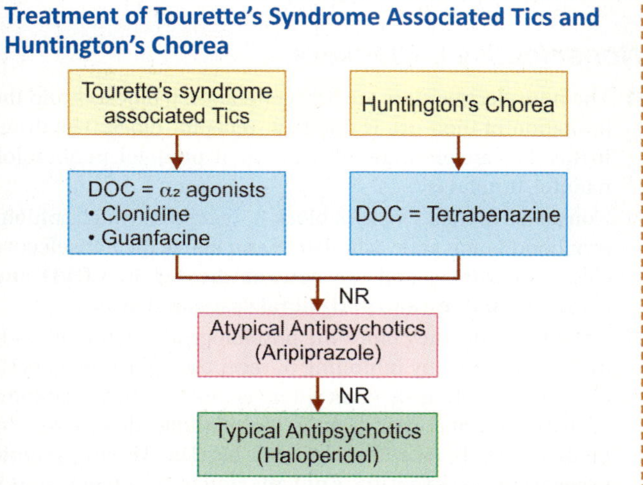

Other drugs effective for tics are clonazepam, verapamil, nifedipine, tetrabenazine, botulinum toxin, risperidone, pimozide and fluphenazine.

Note: NR = No or inadequate response

- **Very long acting β_2 agonists (VLABA)** carmoterol, indacaterol, olodaterol and vilanterol can be used for only COPD. These are not advised for treatment of asthma.
- Ritodrine is used as a tocolytic to halt premature labor.

Other details of this class have been covered in the chapter of respiratory system.

β_3 Agonist

- The only β_3 agonist approved by FDA is **mirabegron** for treatment of **urge incontinence** associated with detrusor instability or overactive bladder.
- Mirabegron is currently under trial for treatment of chronic **CHF**.
- Side effects associated are raised blood pressure, headache and urinary tract infection.

SYMPATHOLYTICS (ANTIADRENERGICS)

Sympatholytics are drugs which are antagonists at α and β receptors and are known as α and β blockers.

α Blockers

α blockers can be broadly classified into selective α blockers and nonselective α blockers. Selective α_1 blockers are more commonly used and have replaced the nonselective drugs for most of the indications.

Selective α Blockers

The selective α blockers can be further subclassified as selective α_1 **blockers**, α_2 **blockers** and more selective α_{1a} blockers.

Selective α_1 Blockers

This class effect is vasodilation due to block of α_{1b} and α_{1d} subtypes and prostatic urethra dilation due to block of α_{1a} subtype. Vasodilation is nonselective and venodilation is responsible for associated **postural hypotension**. To prevent postural hypotension related symptoms, these drugs should be **given at bed time**. Apart from this, this class also **increases HDL and decreases LDL**.

- **Prazosin, terazosin and doxazosin** are used in **essential hypertension** and are the **drug of choice for hypertension associated with dyslipidemia and hypertension associated with BPH**. Terazosin and doxazosin are **longer acting** and additionally induce apoptosis of smooth muscles in prostate. Though used in CHF to decrease preload and afterload, long term use does not decrease mortality.

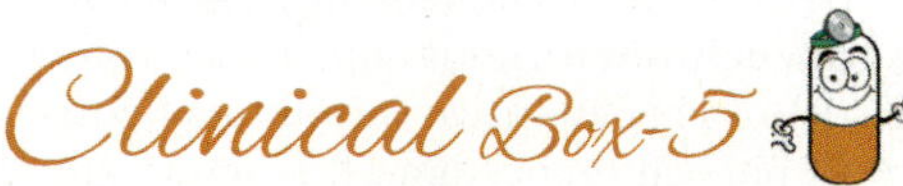

Treatment of Scorpion Sting

- Continuous **IV midazolam** for sedative effect.
- Vasodilators like **prazosin**, nitroprusside, nifedipine and hydralazine for treatment of hypertension and pulmonary edema.
- Atropine is used for treatment of life threatening bradyarrhythmia.

- Alfuzosin is used only for treatment of BPH.
- Indoramin, urapidil and bunazosin are used for treatment of hypertension in some parts of world.

Selective α_{1A} Blockers

- **Tamsulosin and silodosin** being **selective at α_{1a}** receptors are devoid of side effects like postural hypotension related to α_{1B} and α_{1D} receptors. Hence these are **drug of choice for treatment of BPH**.
- Though being more selective at α_{1A} receptors, the side effects related to these receptors are more commonly seen with tamsulosin and silodosin as compared to previous class. α_{1A} receptor block in iris can cause **flaccid or floppy iris** and prostatic urethra can cause **ejaculation abnormality**.

Selective α_2 Blocker

- **Yohimbine** is a selective α_2 blocker and hence increases central NE release. It is derived from root of Rauwolfia serpentine and hence is structurally similar to reserpine. Though not approved by FDA, but is used for treatment of **erectile dysfunction**, diabetic neuropathy and postural hypotension.

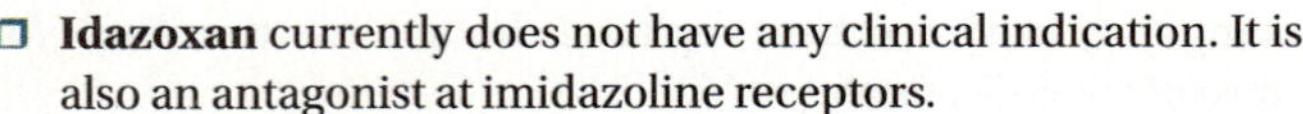

- **Idazoxan** currently does not have any clinical indication. It is also an antagonist at imidazoline receptors.

Nonselective α Blockers

Nonselective α blockers are antagonists at **both** α_1 **and** α_2 **receptor** subtypes. The primary effect that translates into therapeutic gain is vasodilation. Phentolamine and tolazoline are reversible competitive inhibitors, whereas phenoxybenzamine is an irreversible nonselective α blocker.

- **Phentolamine** is primarily used for treatment of erectile dysfunction, pheochromocytoma (short term management of hypertension, intraoperative hypertension), **withdrawal hypertension with clonidine and methyldopa, cheese reaction** and for dermal necrosis caused by epinephrine extravasation.
- **Tolazoline** primarily causes vasodilatation in the peripheral blood vessels and hence used in peripheral vascular disease like **Raynaud's disease**. It is also used as a **vasodilator to enhance angiography of peripheral blood vessels**.
- **Phenoxybenzamine** is an alkylating agent that covalently (strongest bond) binds with α receptors and hence acts for 3–4 days and effect is termed as **irreversible**. It can be used for treatment of hypertensive episode seen with **pheochromocytoma** and also used preoperatively to decrease risk of a hypertensive episode in pheochromocytoma surgery. In pheochromocytoma β blockers are also given to inhibit the effects of catecholamines on heart. **First α blockers are given followed by β blockers**, or else β blockers can block β_2 mediated vasodilation and worsen the condition.

β Blockers

β blockers primary use is by inhibition of β_1 receptors in the **heart,** which causes a decrease in cardiac contraction and conduction and heart rate. Inhibition of β_1 receptors in the **JG cells of kidney** decreases renin production, which causes a decrease in blood pressure. Thus beta blockers can be associated with side effects like bradycardia, conduction block (contraindicated with verapamil) and hypotension. Lipid soluble drugs can cross blood brain barrier and cause central side effects like insomnia, nightmares, seizures and depression.

Uses of β Blockers

- **Hypertension:** β blockers produce antihypertensive effect primarily by decreasing renin production and hence are more effective in hyperreninemic conditions. These are second line drugs for treatment of hypertension and also beneficial in hypertensive emergency.
- **HOCM** and **aortic dissection:** β blockers are drug of choice for treatment of both these conditions. By decreasing force and rate of contraction the left outflow tract obstruction decreases in HOCM; in aortic dissection this decreases chances of aneurysm formation and its rupture.
- **CHF** and **MI:** In both these conditions β blockers decrease mortality.
- **Angina:** Beta blockers are drug of choice for long term prophylaxis of stable angina.
- **Hyperthyroidism, essential tremor, anxiety with somatic presentation, variceal bleeding prophylaxis in portal hypertension, prophylaxis of migraine:** Propranolol is the preferred beta blocker for the mentioned conditions. Propranolol is the drug of choice for prophylaxis of migraine and essential tremors.
- **Glaucoma:** Beta blocker use in glaucoma is covered in the previous section of glaucoma.
- **Hemangioma:** Topical beta blocker like **timolol** is used to restrict growth of hemangiomas.

Nonselective β Blockers

- The nonselective class are first generation β blockers and the limitation of their use is due to β_2 receptor block. The drugs in this class are propranolol, oxprenolol, pindolol, penbutolol, nadolol, timolol etc.
- Nonselective beta blockers block β_2 receptors which inhibits bronchodilation and vasodilation and hence the nonselective class can worsen and are **contraindicated in COPD and bronchial asthma and peripheral vascular disease.**
- Apart from this they block the physiological reaction of body to hypoglycemia by inhibiting β_2 receptors; gluconeogenesis and glycogenolysis by β_2 receptors is blocked and symptoms of hypoglycemia like tremor, palpitation, dizziness, etc. mediated by β_2 receptors are also blocked **(hypoglycemic unawareness). Sweating is not affected** by beta blockers as it is mediated by acetylcholine.
- Nonselective β blockers due to β_2 receptor block increases **insulin resistance (hyperglycemia)** and have unfavorable effect on lipid profile (Increase LDL and triglyceride/Decrease HDL).
- Block of β_2 mediated vasodilation can precipitate vasospasm and hence this class is **contraindicated in variant angina**.
- Block of β_2 mediated vasodilation and glycogenolysis in muscles can dampen exercising ability.
- Hence selective β_1 blockers are more appropriate in the conditions mentioned above.

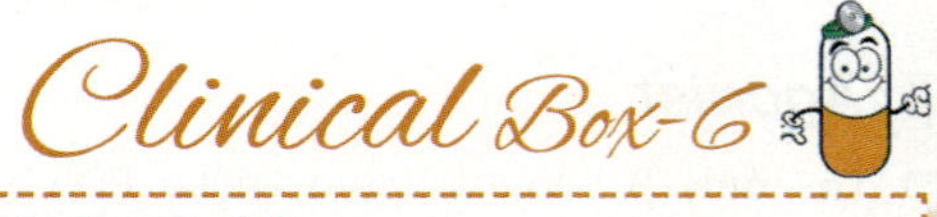

Treatment of β Blocker Toxicity

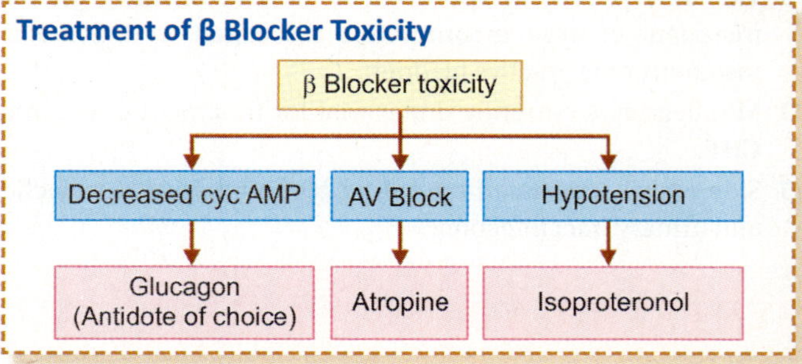

Selective β_1 Blockers (Cardioselective)

- Cardioselective class contains drugs of second generation like acebutolol, atenolol, metoprolol, esmolol and bisoprolol and some third-generation drugs like nebivolol, betaxolol and celiprolol. **Nebivolol** is most cardioselective beta blocker followed by **bisoprolol**.

- These drugs have negligible effect on the metabolic profile. Since they do not block beta 2 receptors, these are safe in diabetes mellitus, asthma, COPD and peripheral vascular disease.

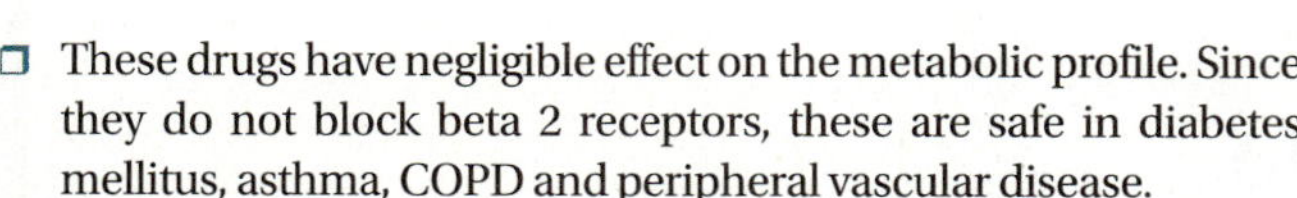

Mnemonics

Selective β_1 Blockers

My : Metoprolol
B : Betaxolol, Bisoprolol
E **t**: Esmolol
T : aTenolol
A : Acebutalol
O **N** : NebivOlol
Ce : Celiprolol

- Esmolol is the **shortest acting** β blocker because it is rapidly **metabolized by esterases** in erythrocytes. Thus **esmolol** is preferred in **surgery** for **prophylaxis and treatment of tachycardia** and for treatment of supraventricular tachycardia.

Beta Blockers with Vasodilatory Effect

- These are third generation beta blockers with vasodilatory effect due to various mechanisms mentioned below. β_1 block decreases **systolic blood pressure** and vasodilation decreases **diastolic blood pressure**.
- Unlike other classes of beta blockers these drugs have favorable effect on lipid profile (increase HDL and decrease LDL and triglycerides) and they also **decrease insulin resistance**.
- **Carvedilol** and **nebivolol** from this class have **antioxidant** effect as well.
- Carvedilol has also anti-inflammatory effect, **prevents LDL oxidation** and at high doses has calcium channel blocking effect. Since it has cardioprotective effect it is preferred in patients of **CAD** (stable angina and MI) and chronic CHF to decrease mortality.
- **Nebivolol** is a racemic mixture of enantiomers; **D isomer causes beta block** whereas L isomer causes NO release.

Mechanism of vasodilation	Beta blockers
β_2 agonism	**B: B**opindolol **C: C**eliprolol, **C**arteolol
NO release	**N: N**ipradilol, **N**ebivolol + **B:** Bopindolol **C:** Celiprolol, Carteolol
Calcium Channel block	**Be: Be**taxolol **Be: Be**vantolol **C: C**arvedilol
α_1 **block**	**Be: Be**vantolol **C: C**arvedilol + Bucindolol Labetalol Nipradilol
Po**T**assium Channel Block	**T**ilisolol

Beta Blockers with Additional Properties

- Beta blockers with partial agonist activity are least likely to cause bradycardia because of stimulatory effect and they have negligible effect on metabolic profile. These are not effective in prophylaxis of migraine as partial agonistic effect on beta 2 produces vasodilation. In myocardial infarction prophylaxis also, these are not used because of partial agonistic effect on beta 1.
- Beta blockers with membrane stabilizing effect are not used as topical agents in glaucoma, as anesthetic effect on cornea can lead to corneal damage.
- Beta blocker with maximum intrinsic agonistic effect is pindolol and beta blockers with maximum membrane stabilizing effect are carvedilol and propranolol.

Beta blockers with intrinsic sympathomimetic or partial agonistic effect	Beta blockers with membrane stabilizing or local anaesthetic effect
C: Carteolol, Celiprolol L: Labetalol A: **Acebutolol** P: Pindolol, Penbutolol	Can : Carvedilol Blow: Betaxolol L : Labetalol A : **Acebutolol** M : Metoprolol P : Propranolol and Pindolol

Selective Properties of Beta Blockers

Properties	Beta blockers
High lipid solubility	Penbutolol Propranolol
High water solubility	B: Bisoprolol E: Esmolol A: Acebutolol, Atenolol S: Sotalol T: Timolol
Longest acting	Nadolol
Shortest acting	Esmolol
Maximum bioavailability (100%)	Penbutolol Pindolol
Minimum bioavailability (30%)	Propranolol Carvedilol
Maximum plasma protein binding	Carvedilol
Minimum plasma protein binding	Celiprolol
Favorable effect on metabolic profile i.e. increased HDL, decreased LDL, triglycerides and insulin resistance	3rd generation drugs
Unfavorable effect on metabolic profile, i.e. decreased HDL, increased LDL, triglycerides and insulin resistance	1st generation drugs

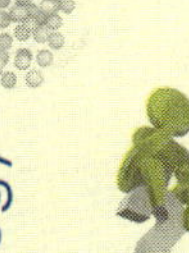

Image-based Questions

1. **Which of the following drug is used for the test given in the picture?**

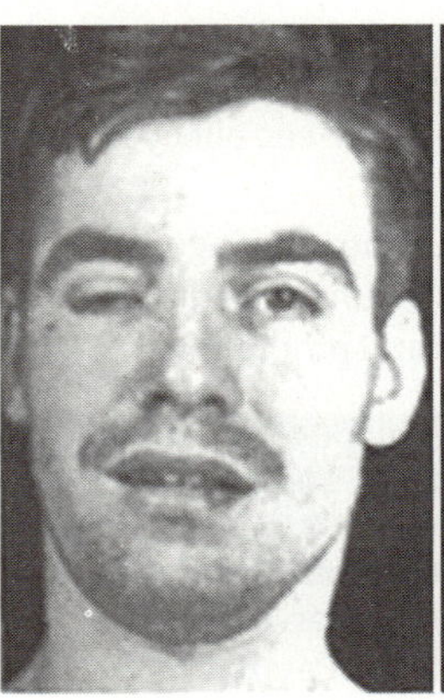
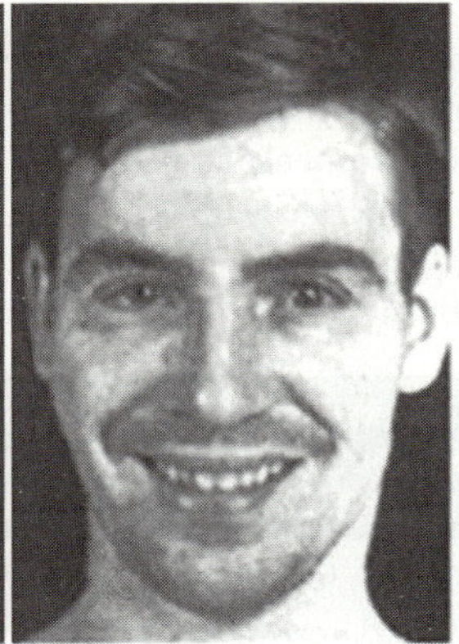

a. Atropine
b. Neostigmine
c. Edrophonium
d. Cyclopentolate

2. **The plant in the given picture is a source for:**

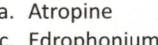

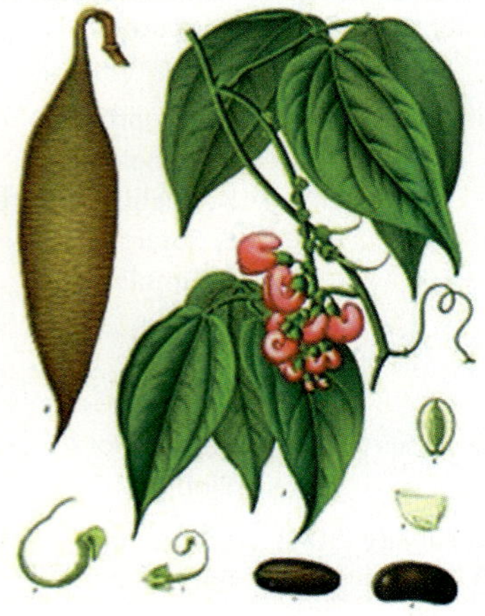

a. Neostigmine
b. Physostigmine
c. Edrophonium
d. Organophosphates

3. **Which of the following antiglaucoma drug can cause the side effect given in the picture?**

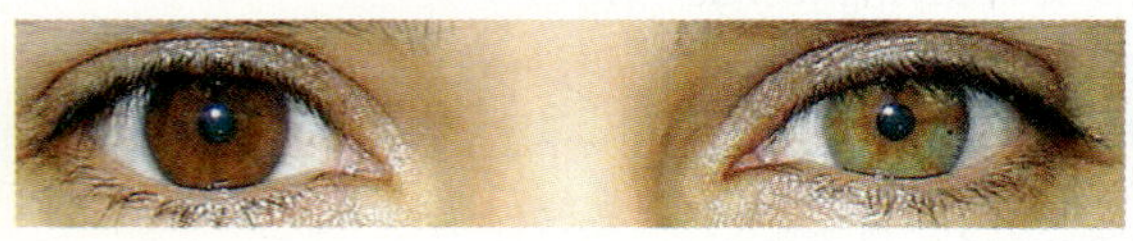

a. Dipivefrin
b. Pilocarpine
c. Latanoprost
d. Timolol

4. **A child accidentally consumed a fruit shown in the picture? Which of the following drug is used for management?**

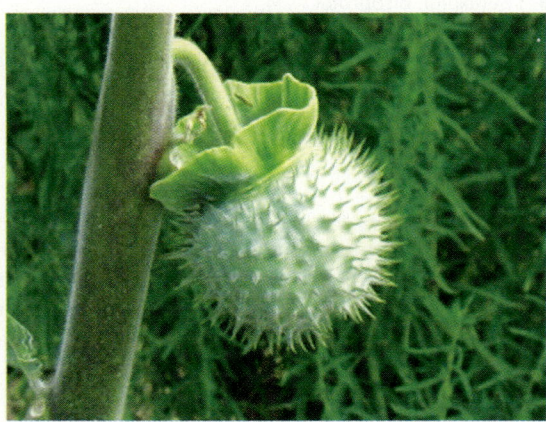

a. Atropine
b. Neostigmine
c. Pyridostigmine
d. Physostigmine

5. **After addition of a compound at point x in a graph of intestinal smooth muscle contraction, the amplitude of contraction decreases, what is added at point x?**

(AIIMS Nov 2015)

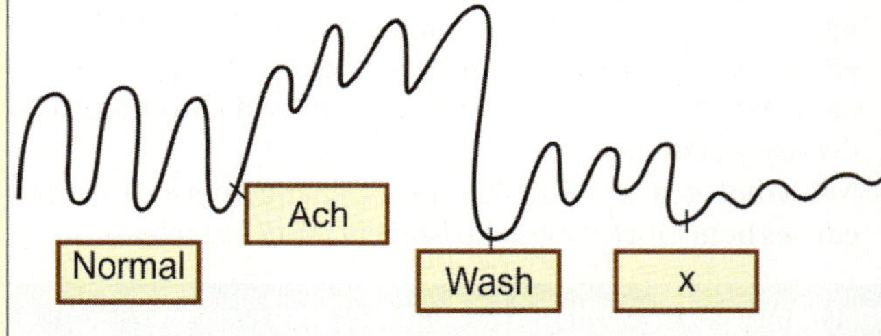

a. Adrenaline
b. Acetylcholine
c. KCl
d. Bacl2

6. **The drug given in the picture is used for treatment of**

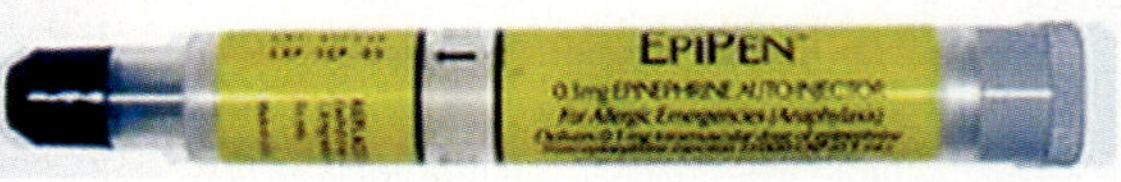

a. Cobra bite
b. Scorpion bite
c. Bee sting
d. Dog bite

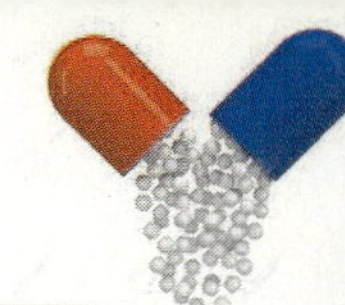

7. Which of the following drug is used for the procedure given in the picture?

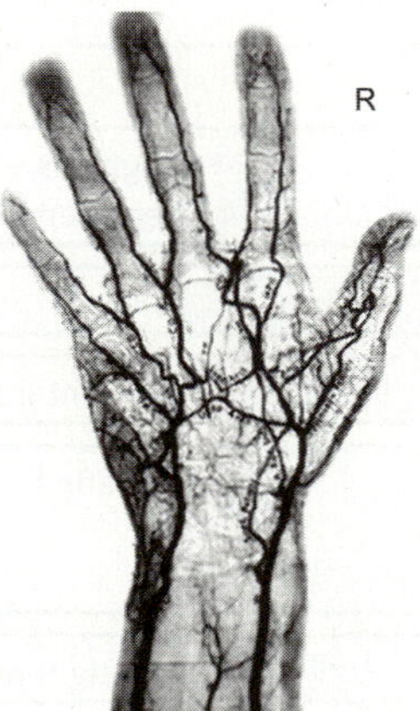

a. Phenoxybenzamine
b. Propranolol
c. Tolazoline
d. Nitrates

8. A patient after consumption of the mushroom given in picture presented with increased secretions, bradycardia, dry mouth and constipation. Which of the following drugs should be used? *(AIIMS Nov 2015)*

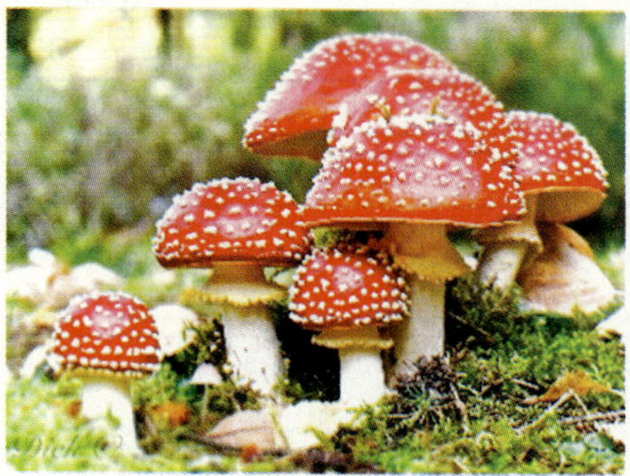

a. Atropine
b. Physostigmine
c. Silymarin
d. Pyridoxine

Answers with Explanations to Image-based Questions

1. Ans. (c) Edrophonium

(Ref: Goodman Gilman 12th E/P251)

- The given picture depicts improvement of ptosis and is suggestive of Tensilon test for diagnosis of myasthenia gravis.
- Though neostigmine can be used, the preferred drug for diagnosis is edrophonium due to its rapid and fast action.

2. Ans. (b) Physostigmine

(Ref: Goodman Gilman 12th E/P 242)

Physostigmine is a natural drug derived from calabar beans of the plant called as *physostigma venenosum* in the picture.

3. Ans. (c) Latanoprost

(Ref: Goodman Gilman 12th E/P1788)

The change of iris color given in the picture is called as heterochromia iridis, which is seen with prostaglandin analogs like latanoprost.

4. Ans. (d) Physostigmine

(Ref: Goodman Gilman 12th E/P309)

- The plant in the picture is Datura Stramonium, which contains atropine.
- The child thus has anticholinergic toxicity, for which physostigmine is the drug of choice.

5. Ans. (a) Adrenaline

(Ref: Goodman Gilman 12th E/P285)

- As shown in the graph, the contraction increases after Ach and comes back to normal. Then it decreases at point X. Among the given options only adrenaline decreases contraction of intestinal smooth muscles.

6. Ans. (c) Bee sting

(Ref: Goodman Gilman 12th E/P282)

- The device in the picture epipen contains epinephrine for emergency self-administration.
- It can be used in anaphylaxis; in bee sting it's use as anaphylactic can be seen.
- In cobra bite neostigmine is used.
- In scorpion bite vasodilators like prazosin are used.

7. Ans. (c) Tolazoline

(Ref: Goodman Gilman 12th E/P306)

Tolazoline, a nonselective alpha blocker is used as a vasodilator in digital angiography for proper visualization of blood vessels.

8. Ans. (b) Physostigmine

(Ref: Goodman Gilman 12th E/P225)

- The mushroom in the picture is Amanita Muscaria, which causes anticholinergic poisoning.
- The signs of poisoning are anticholinergic and hence physostigmine is used.

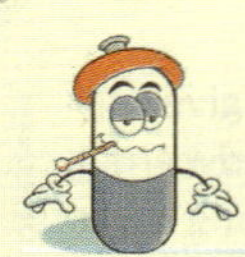

Annexures

Drug of Choice

ADHD	Methylphenidate
ADHD with Tourette syndrome	Atomoxetine
Alzheimer's disease	Mild to moderate – Donepezil Severe – Memantine
Aortic dissection HOCM Migraine prophylaxis	Beta blockers
Atropine or belladonna poisoning	Physostigmine
BPH	Tamsulosin
BPH with hypertension	Terazosin
Brittle asthma	Epinephrine
Bronchial challenge test	Methacholine
Cheese reaction Clonidine withdrawal hypertension Intraoperative hypertension in pheochromocytoma	Phentolamine
COPD	Tiotropium
Cycloplegia	Adult – Tropicamide Children – Atropine
CHF with oliguria Hypotension caused by hypothermia	Dopamine
Glaucoma	Closed angle – Acetazolamide Open angle – Latanoprost Normal tension – Latanoprost
Hutington's Chorea	Tetrabenazine
Hypotension in pregnancy Hypotension with anesthetic agents	Ephedrine
Motion sickness	Scopolamine
Myasthenia gravis	Diagnosis – Edrophonium Treatment – Pyridostigmine
Myasthenia crisis	IVIG
Narcoanalysis	Thiopental sodium
Narcolepsy Shift worker disease Sleepiness in OSA	Modafinil
NDMR reversal	Neostigmine
Nicotine toxicity	Atropine
Orthostatic hypotension	Fludrocortisone
Organophosphate poisoning	Atropine
Scorpion bite	Prazosin
Shock	Anaphylactic – Epinephrine Septic – Norepinephrine Cardiogenic – Dopamine
Stress ECHO	Dobutamine
Stress incontinence	Duloxetine
Tics associated with Tourette syndrome	Clonidine
Urge incontinence	Darifenacin
Xerostomia	Cevimeline

New Drugs

New drugs	Mechanism of action	Uses
Deutetrabenazine	VMAT 2 inhibitor	Huntington's chorea Tardive dyskinesia
Valbenazine	VMAT 2 inhibitor	Tardive dyskinesia
Mirabegron	Beta 3 agonist	Urge incontinence

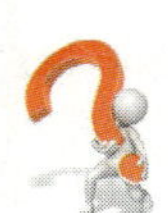

Multiple Choice Questions

PARASYMPATHETIC NERVOUS SYSTEM

1. **Mechanism by which Ach decreases heart rate is by** *(AIIMS Nov 2018)*
   a. Delayed diastolic depolarization
   b. Increase in plateau
   c. Decrease preload
   d. Increase afterload
2. **A Male with insulin dependent diabetes having macular edema develops glaucoma. Which drug should be used as the least resort to treat?** *(AIIMS Nov 2018)*
   a. Alpha agonist b. Prostaglandin analogue
   c. Pilocarpine d. Beta blocker
3. **Drug that is used as an adjuvant in fungal corneal ulcer?** *(AIIMS May 2018)*
   a. Dexamethasone b. Pilocarpine
   c. Atropine d. Lignocaine
4. **Atropine is not given in which of the following case of poisoning:** *(AIIMS Nov 2017)*
   a. Baygon b. Parathion
   c. Endrin d. TIK 20
5. **Treatment for motion sickness for a trip next morning:**
   a. Scopolamine patch a night before *(AIIMS Nov 2017)*
   b. Tab. Ranitidine one night before and then before the trip
   c. Dimenhydrinate 1 hour before
   d. Omeprazole
6. **Pirenzepine is used in:** *(Recent Question 2017)*
   a. Peptic ulcer disease b. Bronchial asthma
   c. Rheumatoid arthritis d. Motion sickness
7. **Methacholine is an agonist at** *(AIIMS May 2015, May 2014)*
   a. M2 b. M1
   c. M4 d. M3
8. **Which of one the following anticholinergics is not a tertiary amines?** *(AIIMS Nov 2014)*
   a. Atropine b. Glycopyrrolate
   c. Dicyclomine d. Scopolamine
9. **In which of the following condition, cholinomimetics are not used?** *(AIIMS Nov-2014, Nov 2012)*
   a. Glaucoma b. Postsurgical ileus/atony
   c. Myasthenia gravis d. Bradycardia
10. **What is the probable diagnosis in a patient with a dilated pupil not responsive to 1% pilocarpine?** *(AIIMS Nov 2011)*
    a. Diabetic 3rd nerve palsy b. Adie's tonic pupil
    c. Uncal herniation d. Pharmacological block
11. **Which of the following drug is used for overactive bladder?** *(AIIMS Nov 2010)*
    a. Duloxetine b. Darifenacin
    c. Oxybutynin d. Flavoxate
12. **A patient presented in emergency with tachycardia, hyperthermia, bronchial dilatation and constipation. The person is likely to be suffering from overdose of:**
    a. Atropine *(AIIMS Nov 2010)*
    b. Organophosphorus compound
    c. Mushroom d. Paracetamol
13. **A child presented with history of ingestion of some unknown plant and developed mydriasis, tachycardia, dry mouth, warm skin and delirium. Which of the following group of drugs is likely to be responsible for the symptoms of this child?** *(AIIMS May 2010)*
    a. Anticholinergic b. Sympathomimetic
    c. Opioid d. Benzodiazepine
14. **Vagal stimulation of heart causes?** *(AIIMS Nov 2008)*
    a. Increased heart rate
    b. Increased RR interval in ECG
    c. Increased cardiac output
    d. Increased force of contraction
15. **Ocular hypotensive drug causing apnea in young children is** *(Recent Question 2019)*
    a. Brimonidine b. Brinzolamide
    c. Latanoprost d. Pilocarpine
16. **A patient came to casualty with acute attack of asthma after starting treatment of glaucoma. The causative drug is** *(Recent Question 2019)*
    a. Timolol b. Betaxolol
    c. Clonidine d. Acetazolamide
17. **Drug used to differentiate between myasthenia gravis and cholinergic crisis is** *(Recent Question 2019)*
    a. Neostigmine b. Edrophonium
    c. Methacholine d. Bethanechol
18. **Post cardiac surgery delirium symptoms are worsened by** *(Recent Question 2018)*
    a. Antipsychotics b. Anticholinergics
    c. BZD d. Antihistaminics
19. **Pilocarpine is an** *(Recent Question 2018)*
    a. Active miotic b. Passive miotic
    c. Active Mydriatic d. Passive Mydriatic
20. **Tolterodine used in overactive bladder acts by which receptor** *(Recent Question 2018)*
    a. M1 b. M2
    c. M3 d. M4
21. **Sand eyes are due to which antiglaucoma drug?** *(Recent Question Dec 2016)*
    a. Apraclonidine b. Latanoprost
    c. Pilocarpine d. Timolol
22. **True about pilocarpine** *(Recent Question Dec 2016)*
    a. Sympathomimetic
    b. Decreases aqueous production
    c. Mainstay in glaucoma treatment
    d. Causes accommodative spasm

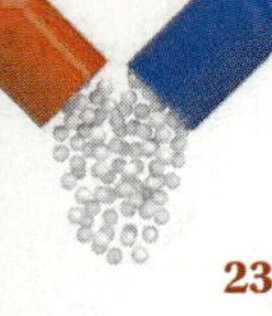

23. A 28-year-old woman has been treated with several autonomic drugs for about a month. Which of the following signs would distinguish between an overdose of muscarinic blocker and a ganglionic blocker? *(Recent Question 2016)*

a. Blurred vision
b. Dry mouth and constipation
c. Mydriasis
d. Postural hypotension

24. Which for the following is an antimuscarinic drug *(Recent Question 2016)*

a. Duloxetine b. Oxybutynin
c. Ephedrine d. Pilocarpine

25. Which of the following is drug of choice for belladonna poisoning *(Recent Question 2016)*

a. Physostigmine b. Neostigmine
c. Pyridostigmine d. Pralidoxime

26. The most preferred drug for diagnosis of myasthenia gravis is *(Recent Question 2016)*

a. Neostigmine b. Edrophonium
c. Pyridostigmine d. Physostigmine

27. Most effective agent to prevent motion sickness is *(Recent Question 2016)*

a. Ephedrine b. Nedocromil
c. Cyproheptadine d. Hyoscine

28. Most commonly used cholinesterase regenerator at NM junction is *(Recent Question 2016)*

a. Pralidoxime b. Obidoxime
c. Diacetyl monoxime d. Edrophonium

29. Cholinergic drug which acts of in levels of cAMP and due to opening of K+ channels is *(Recent Question 2016)*

a. Methacholine b. Oxotremorine
c. Bethanechol d. DMPP

30. Rivastigmine is used in *(Recent Question 2016)*

a. Dementia b. Dissociation
c. Depression d. Delusions

31. Neostigmine is used in the following except *(Recent Question 2016)*

a. Myasthenia gravis b. Cobra bite
c. Atony of bladder d. Glaucoma

32. Function of M2 receptor in heart *(Recent Question 2016)*

a. SA node hyperpolarisation
b. AV node increased velocity of conduction
c. Increased contractility of ventricles
d. Increased Ach release from cholinergic nerve endings

33. Pralidoxime acts by *(Recent Question 2016)*

a. Reactivating cholinesterase enzyme
b. Promoting synthesis of cholinesterase
c. Promoting synthesis of acetylcholine
d. Direct action on cholinergic receptors

34. Which of the following is a parasympatholytic agent? *(Recent Question 2016)*

a. Atropine
b. Neostigmine
c. Pyridostigmine
d. Acetylcholine

35. Regarding neostigmine, all the following are correct except

a. A quaternary ammonium compound
b. Shorter acting than edrophonium
c. Poorly absorbed orally *(Recent Question 2016)*
d. Does not cross the blood brain barrier

36. Latanoprost (PGF2 alpha is used in *(Recent Question 2016)*

a. Maintenance of ductus arteriosus
b. Pulmonary hypertension
c. Gastric mucosal protection
d. Glaucoma

37. Atropine is used in all except *(Recent Question 2016)*

a. Glaucoma b. Mydriatic
c. Cycloplegic d. Preanaesthetic medication

38. Atropine is most sensitive to *(Recent Question 2016)*

a. Mucous and pharyngeal secretions
b. Heart
c. Pupil
d. Gl tract motility

39. Which is not an effect of atropine? *(Recent Question 2016)*

a. Rise of body temperature
b. Decreased salivary secretion
c. Bradycardia
d. Increased A-V conduction

40. True about latanoprost are all except

a. PG inhibitor *(Recent Question 2016)*
b. Decrease IOP by increasing UV scleral outflow
c. Conjunctivitis is long-term complication
d. Used once a day

41. Anticholinergic drug to be given in over activity of detrusor muscle *(Recent Question 2016)*

a. Atropine b. Pirenzepine
c. Tolterodine d. Cyclopentolate

42. Treatment of amanita poisoning is *(Recent Question 2016)*

a. Adrenaline b. Dopamine
c. Atropine d. Hydrocortisone

43. Mechanism of action of carbamates

a. Reversible carbamylation *(Recent Question 2016)*
b. Reversible phosphorylation
c. Irreversible carbamylation
d. Irreversible phosphorylation

44. Anticholinesterases are used in *(Recent Question 2016)*

a. Myasthenia gravis b. Parkinsonism
c. Prostatic hypertrophy d. Cardiogenic shock

45. Oximes are contraindicated n which poisoning *(Recent Question 2016)*

a. Baygon b. Parathion
c. Malathion d. TIK-20

46. Fastest acting mydriatic *(Recent Question 2016)*

a. Atropine
b. Homatropine
c. Scopolamine
d. Tropicamide

47. **Synaptic transmission in the autonomic ganglion is usually** ***(Recent Question 2016)***
   a. Adrenergic b. Peptidergic
   c. Cholinergic d. Mediated by substance P
48. **Botulinum toxin produces skeletal muscle paralysis by** ***(Recent Question 2016)***
   a. Enhancing release of norepinephrine
   b. Inhibiting release of acetylcholine
   c. Direct damage to nerve endings
   d. Producing hemolysis
49. **All are seen with cholinergic muscarinic receptor stimulation except** ***(Recent Question 2016)***
   a. Sweating b. Rise in blood pressure
   c. Bradycardia d. Urination
50. **Which of the following properties make pyridostigmine different from neostigmine?** ***(Recent Question 2016)***
   a. It is more potent orally
   b. It is longer acting
   c. It produces less muscarinic side effect
   d. It does not have any direct action on NM receptors
51. **The neurotransmitter agent that is normally released in the SA node of the heart in response to increased blood pressure is** ***(Recent Question 2016)***
   a. Acetylcholine b. Dopamine
   c. Adrenaline d. Noradrenaline
52. **Dangerous effect of belladonna in children** ***(Recent Question 2016)***
   a. Dehydration b. Hallucination
   c. Hypertension d. Hyperthermia
53. **Drug of choice for treatment of acute organophosphate poisoning is** ***(Recent Question 2016)***
   a. Atropine b. Pralidoxime
   c. Neostigmine d. d-Tubocurare
54. **All are cholinergic agents except** ***(Recent Question 2016)***
   a. Galantamine b. Donepezil
   c. Tacrine d. Memantine
55. **Which drug is not used now in Alzheimer's disease?** ***(Recent Question 2016)***
   a. Tacrine b. Galantamine
   c. Donepezil d. Rivastigmine
56. **Drug used in ameliorative test for myasthenia gravis is** ***(Recent Question 2016)***
   a. Physostigmine b. Edrophonium
   c. Tacrine d. Pyridostigmine
57. **Treatment of atropine toxicity is** ***(Recent Question 2016)***
   a. 2-pralidoxime b. Naloxone
   c. Flumazenil d. Physostigmine
58. **Short acting mydriatic used in fundoscopy is** ***(Recent Question 2016)***
   a. Atropine b. Homatropine
   c. Cyclopentolate d. Tropicamide
59. **Anti-cholinesterases are ineffective against** ***(Recent Question 2016)***
   a. Belladonna poisoning b. Carbamate poisoning
   c. Postoperative ileus d. Cobra bite
60. **Which one of the following acts commonly both on parasympathetic and sympathetic division?** ***(Recent Question 2016)***
   a. Atropine b. Pilocarpine
   c. Acetylcholine d. Adrenaline
61. **The short acting anticholinesterase drug is** ***(Recent Question 2016)***
   a. Edrophonium b. Demecarium
   c. Dyflos d. Echtothiophate
62. **Which of the following drugs has no cycloplegic action?** ***(Recent Question 2016)***
   a. Atropine b. Cyclopentolate
   c. Tropicamide d. Phenylephrine
63. **The main mechanism of hyperpyrexia induced by atropine includes** ***(Recent Question 2016)***
   a. Vasodilation
   b. Inhibition of sweating
   c. Through central actions
   d. Increase in basal metabolic rate
64. **Antismoking drug** ***(Recent Question 2016)***
   a. Varenicline b. Veratridine
   c. Azelastine d. Fexofenadine
65. **The drug which acts on both muscarinic and nicotinic receptors** ***(Recent Question 2016)***
   a. Benzoylcholine b. Butyrylcholine
   c. Carbachol d. Methacholine
66. **Uroselective anti-cholinergic drug is** ***(Recent Question 2016)***
   a. Darifenacin b. Solifenacin
   c. Tolterodine d. Trospium chloride
67. **Drugs used in parkinsonism like symptom** ***(Recent Question 2016)***
   a. Benztropine b. Levodopa and carbidopa
   c. Ropinirole d. Selegiline
68. **Atropine causes all except** ***(Recent Question 2016)***
   a. Hypothermia b. Fever
   c. Coma d. Mydriasis
69. **All are tertiary amines except** ***(Recent Question 2016)***
   a. Hyoscine b. Atropine
   c. Scopolamine d. Glycopyrrolate
70. **Central anticholinergics are used in treatment of all except** ***(Recent Question 2016)***
   a. Akathisia
   b. Parkinsonism
   c. Acute dystonia
   d. Neuroleptic malignant syndrome
71. **All are true about neostigmine except** ***(Recent Question 2016)***
   a. Tertiary ammonium compound
   b. Given to reduce effect of depolarizing muscle relaxation
   c. Given to reduce post-operative paralytic ileus
   d. Help in urinary retention
72. **Galantamine is used in?** ***(Recent Question 2016)***
   a. Alzheimer's disease b. Parkinson's disease
   c. Emesis d. Chorea

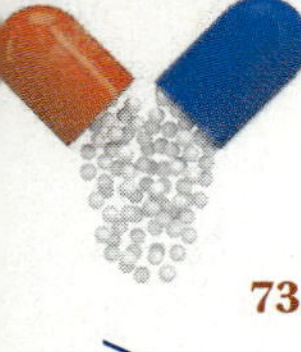

73. In organophosphorus (OP) poisoning OP compound binds to acetyl cholinesterase in which manner? ***(Recent Question 2016)***

a. Uncompetitively b. Non competitively
c. Irreversibly d. None of the above

74. Drugs given in Alzheimer's disease are?

a. Rivastigmine and donepezil ***(Recent Question 2016)***
b. Levodopa and carbidopa
c. Benzhexol and levodopa
d. Tacrine and benztropine

SYMPATHETIC NERVOUS SYSTEM

75. Side effects of salbutamol are all except ***(AIIMS Nov 2018, May 2018)***

a. Hypokalemia b. Hypoglycemia
c. Tremor d. Tachycardia

76. A placebo therapy given to one patient and new drug given to another patient. On comparing: ***(AIIMS Nov 2017)***

- **Heart rate in Placebo (72), Drug (86)**
- **SBP in Placebo (110), Drug (150)**
- **DBP in Placebo (80), Drug (68)**
- **Cardiac output in Placebo (5), Drug (6)**

Action of new drug best related to

a. Alpha 1 antagonist and beta 1 agonist
b. M2 agonist and M3 agonist
c. Alpha 1 agonist and beta 1 agonist
d. Beta 1 agonist and beta 2 agonist

77. During resuscitation of septic shock norepinephrine was given to the patient. Its response is checked by seeing.

a. Increased heart rate ***(AIIMS Nov 2017)***
b. Decreased heart rate
c. Increased MAP
d. Decreased renal perfusion and reduced urine output

78. What will you give in anaphylactic shock?

a. Adrenaline 0.5 mg 1/1000 IM ***(AIIMS Nov 2017)***
b. Adrenaline 1 mg 1/10000 IV
c. Atropine 3 mg
d. Adenosine 6 mg followed by 12 mg IV

79. In an animal model how will u show vasomotor reversal of dale ***(AIIMS May 2017)***

a. Beta 2 stimulation by low epinephrine and thereafter beta 1 stimulation
b. Stimulation of beta 1 followed by block of beta 2
c. Stimulation of beta 1 receptor followed by block of beta 2 receptor
d. Beta 2 stimulation by norepinephrine followed by beta 1 stimulation

80. Which of the following muscle relaxant is centrally acting alpha-2 agonist? ***(Recent Question 2017)***

a. Tizanidine
b. Baclofen
c. Diazepam
d. Dexmedetomidine

81. An alternative vasoconstrictor to epinephrine in advanced cardiac life support is: ***(Recent Question 2017)***

a. Vasopressin b. Atropine
c. Low dose dopamine d. Norepinephrine

82. Which of the following statements is correct regarding the graphs given? ***(AIIMS Nov 2016)***

a. Drug in graph A is epinephrine
b. The effect on HR in graph A can be overcome by anti-muscarinic
c. Drug acting in graph C is nor- epinephrine
d. Drug acting on graph B is isoproterenol

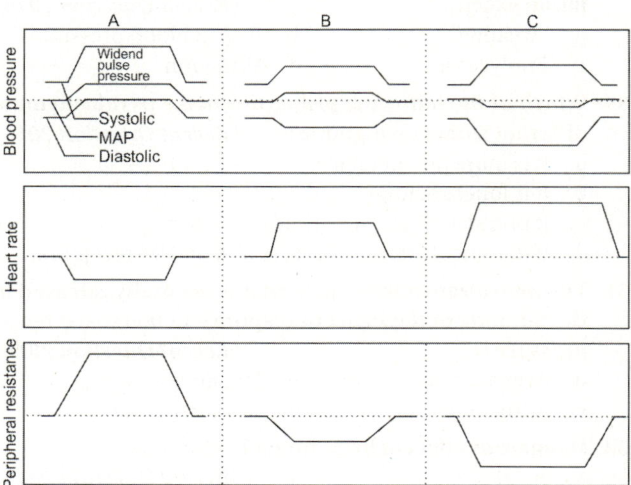

83. Which of the following does not contribute to the therapeutic levels of IV dopamine ***(AIIMS May 2016)***

a. Stimulation of cardiac beta receptor
b. Stimulation of vasomotor center
c. Stimulation of renal dopaminergic receptor
d. Stimulation of vasomotor alpha center

84. Black deposits on the conjunctiva are noted with use of one of the following drugs used in glaucoma

a. Prostaglandins ***(AIIMS May 2016)***
b. Adrenergic agonists
c. Beta blockers
d. Carbonic anhydrase inhibitors

85. One of the following is pharmacological effects of adrenaline which does not play a role in its anaphylaxis ***(AIIMS May 2016)***

a. Stimulation of vascular alpha receptors
b. Stimulation of pre-synaptic alpha receptors
c. Stimulation of beta 1 receptors in heart
d. Stimulation of beta two receptors on bronchial smooth muscles

86. Dopamine in dose concentration at 3-5mcg/kg/min acts predominantly on? ***(AIIMS Nov 2015)***

a. $\beta 1$ b. D1
c. $\alpha 1$ d. $\alpha 2$

87. Lipolysis in adipocyte is through which receptors- ***(AIIMS May 2015)***

a. Beta-1 b. Beta-2
c. Beta-3 d. Beta-4

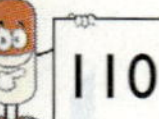

88. Dexmedetomidine is a *(AIIMS Nov 2014)*
a. Central alpha 2 agonist
b. Peripheral alpha 2 agonist
c. Central alpha 2 antagonist
d. Peripheral alpha 2 antagonist

89. α2 agonist cause all of the following except *(AIIMS May 2014)*
a. Analgesia b. Hyperalgesia
c. Sedation d. Anxiolysis

90. Which of the following is a mixed alpha and beta agonist? *(AIIMS May 2014)*
a. Dobutamine b. Fenoldopam
c. Epinephrine d. Phenylephrine

91. Drug which is correctly matched with MOA: *(AIIMS May 2013)*
a. Brimonidine-decreases aqueous production
b. Pilocarpine-increases UV outflow (drainage)
c. Latanoprost-carbonic anhydrase inhibitor
d. Betaxolol-decreases trabecular outflow

92. Which of the following drugs can be given by subcutaneous route? *(AIIMS May 2013)*
a. Terbutaline b. Albuterol
c. Fenoterol d. Metaproterenol

93. A patient with glaucoma is being treated with systemic beta blocker. All of the following can be given to the patient except? *(AIIMS Nov 2012)*
a. Brimonidine b. Dorzolamide
c. Levobunolol d. Prostaglandin

94. Lid retraction is caused by: *(AIIMS Nov 2011)*
a. Bimatoprost b. Latanoprost
c. Brimonidine d. Apraclonidine

95. Which of the following drug is a long acting beta-2 agonist? *(AIIMS May 2008, Nov 2006)*
a. Albuterol b. Salmeterol
c. Pirbuterol d. Orciprenaline

96. Tolazoline is used as: *(AIIMS May 2009)*
a. A thrombin inhibitor in peripheral angiography
b. A vasodilator in treating coronary artery stenosis during angio procedures
c. A vasoconstrictor in treatment of varices
d. An antispasmodic during biliary spasm

97. Drug used to perform stress ECHO is: *(AIIMS May 2008)*
a. Thallium b. Dobutamine
c. Adrenaline d. Adenosine

98. Which is not an endogenous catecholamine? *(AIIMS May, 2007)*
a. Dopamine b. Dobutamine
c. Adrenaline d. Noradrenaline

99. Which of the following is an alpha-2 agonist *(Recent Question 2019)*
a. Apraclonidine b. Latanoprost
c. Timolol d. Pilocarpine

100. Hypertension and pulmonary edema caused by scorpion poisoning treated by *(Recent Question 2019)*
a. Prazosin b. Furosemide
c. Enalaprilat d. Nitroglycerine

101. Metyrosine given in *(Recent Question 2018)*
a. Malignant pheochromocytoma
b. Addison's disease
c. Depression
d. Hypertensive emergency

102. Tizanidine has action on? *(Recent Question 2018)*
a. Alpha adrenergic b. GABA A action
c. Gaba B action d. Beta adrenergic

103. Which beta blocker is used to prevent and treat tachycardia intraoperatively? *(Recent Question Dec 2016)*
a. Carvedilol b. Metoprolol
c. Esmolol d. Nadolol

104. Beta blocker used in CAD is *(Recent Question Dec 2016)*
a. Carvedilol b. Bucindolol
c. Labetalol d. Metoprolol

105. Beta-Blocker used in which condition given below *(Recent Question Dec 2016)*
a. Icthyosis b. Hemangioma
c. Melanoma d. Photosensitivity

106. Crystal meth means *(Recent Question Dec 2016)*
a. Amphetamine b. Heroin
c. Cocaine d. Cannabis

107. Drug which acts at dopamine receptors, α-receptors, β1 but not β2 receptor is *(Recent Question Dec 2016)*
a. Dopamine b. Dobutamine
c. Epinephrine d. Norepinephrine

108. Beta blockers with intrinsic sympathomimetic activity and local anaesthetic property is: *(Recent Question 2016)*
a. Propranolol b. Metoprolol
c. Carvedilol d. Acebutolol

109. The oral bioavailability of propranolol is: *(Recent Question 2016)*
a. 26% b. 74%
c. 50% d. 26%

110. Drug used in Benign Prostatic Hypertrophy is? *(Recent Question 2016)*
a. Alpha 1 agonist b. Alpha 1 antagonist
c. Alpha 2 agonist d. Alpha 2 antagonist

111. sympathomimetic amine which increases the force of contraction but reduces heart rate *(Recent Question 2016)*
a. Epinephrine b. Norepinephrine
c. Phenylephrine d. Isoproteronol

112. Intravenous administration of NE in a patient already taking an effective dose of atropine will *(Recent Question 2016)*
a. Increase heart rate
b. Decrease total peripheral resistance
c. Decrease pupil size
d. Has no effect on cardiovascular system

113. Beta blocker that decreases both systolic and diastolic blood pressure is *(Recent Question 2016)*
a. Propranolol b. Sotalol
c. Atenolol d. Nebivolol

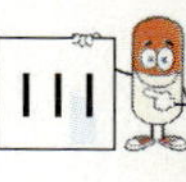

114. Which of the following is true regarding management of pheochromocytoma? ***(Recent Question 2016)***
a. Alpha blocker followed by beta blocker
b. Salt restriction
c. ACE inhibitors
d. Beta blocker followed by alpha blocker

115. Latest drug approved for urge incontinence is ***(Recent Question 2016)***
a. Darifenacin b. Oxybutynin
c. Mirabegron d. Duloxetine

116. Alpha 1a blocker ***(Recent Question 2016)***
a. Tamsulosin b. Prazosin
c. Terazosin d. Clonidine

117. Amphetamine causes which of the following ***(Recent Question 2016)***
a. IUGR b. Cardiac anomaly
c. Cleft lip d. All the above

118. Selective beta 2 blocker is ***(Recent Question 2016)***
a. Butoxamine b. Betaxolol
c. Esmolol d. Bisoprolol

119. Beta blocker with membrane stabilizing property are all except ***(Recent Question 2016)***
a. Acebutolol b. Betaxolol
c. Carvedilol d. Bevantolol

120. The shortest acting beta blocker ***(Recent Question 2016)***
a. Esmolol b. Nadolol
c. Acebutolol d. Sotalol

121. The longest acting beta blocker is ***(Recent Question 2016)***
a. Nadolol b. Esmolol
c. Carvedilol d. Atebnolol

122. Alpha 2 agonist used in glaucoma is ***(Recent Question 2016)***
a. Brimonidine b. Timolol
c. Phenylephrine d. Reserpine

123. Dopamine at 1-2 Microgram/Kg/min produces ***(Recent Question 2016)***
a. Renal vasodilatation
b. Positive ionotropic effect
c. Mesenteric vasoconstriction
d. Generalised vasoconstriction

124. Atomoxetine is used for ***(Recent Question 2016)***
a. Nocturnal enuresis b. ADHD
c. Temper tantrums d. Patent ductus arteriosus

125. Beta blocker with d isomer responsible for beta blocker action is ***(Recent Question 2016)***
a. Nebivolol b. Timolol
c. Esmolol d. Propranolol

126. Mechanism of action of timolol is ***(Recent Question 2016)***
a. Nonselective beta blocker
b. Nonselective alpha blocker
c. Selective beta 1 blocker
d. Selective beta 2 blocker

127. Treatment of choice for cheese reaction ***(Recent Question 2016)***
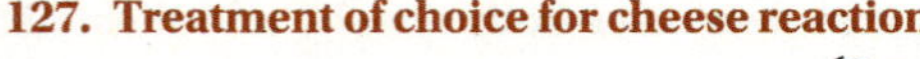
a. Prazosin b. Pentazocin
c. Phentolamine d. Phenoxybenzamine

128. Nonselective beta-adrenergic antagonist is ***(Recent Question 2016)***
a. Nadolol b. Atenolol
c. Bisoprolol d. Esmolol

129. Beta blockers mask all effects of hypoglycemia except ***(Recent Question 2016)***
a. Sweating b. Palpitations
c. Dizziness d. Tremors

130. Selective alpha-2 antagonist ***(Recent Question 2016)***
a. Prazosin b. Labetalol
c. Yohimbine d. Butaxamine

131. Alpha blocker useful in BPH is ***(Recent Question 2016)***
a. Phentolamine b. Prazosin
c. Tolazoline d. Phenoxybenzamine

132. M/C used drug for prophylaxis of migraine is ***(Recent Question 2016)***
a. Sumatriptan b. Propranolol
c. Valproate d. Flunarizine

133. Beta blocker with alpha blocking capacity is ***(Recent Question 2016)***
a. Atenolol b. Labetalol
c. Propranolol d. Metoprolol

134. Glaucoma drug which is selective beta 1 blockers is ***(Recent Question 2016)***
a. Timolol b. Levobunolol
c. Carteolol d. Betaxolol

135. Drug used for common cold that can cause stroke ***(Recent Question 2016)***
a. Phenylpropanolamine b. Oxymetazoline
c. Phenylephrine d. None of the above

136. Modafinil is use as an adjunct in treatment of ***(Recent Question 2016)***
a. Sleep apnea syndrome b. Narcolepsy
c. ADHD d. Somnolescence

137. Alpha 1a antagonist giving symptomatic relief in BPH ***(Recent Question 2016)***
a. Tamsulosin b. Prazosin
c. Doxazosin d. Tolazoline

138. Alpha-1 blocker without any effect on blood pressure is ***(Recent Question 2016)***
a. Tamsulosin b. Prazosin
c. Doxazosin d. Terazosin

139. Beta blockers are contraindicated in ***(Recent Question 2016)***
a. Decompensated CCF b. Asthma
c. Atherosclerosis d. All of the above

140. Not true for noradrenaline ***(Recent Question 2016)***
a. Increases heart rate b. Decreases heart rate
c. Increases systolic BP d. Increases diastolic BP

141. D1 receptors increase renal flow when given in ***(Recent Question 2016)***
a. Low dose b. Moderate dose
c. High dose d. At all doses

142. True for β1 receptors is ***(Recent Question 2016)***
a. Present of heart b. Present of JG cells in kidney
c. Present in adipose tissue d. Both A and B

143. In anaphylactic shock epinephrine given by which route *(Recent Question 2016)*
a. Intravenous b. Oral
c. Subcutaneous d. Intramuscular

144. Beta blocker with beta-2 agonism *(Recent Question 2016)*
a. Labetalol b. Carvedilol
c. Celiprolol d. Tilisolol

145. Sympathomimetic drug used in the treatment of anaphylactic shock is *(Recent Question 2016)*
a. Adrenaline b. Dopamine
c. Dobutamine d. Isoprenaline

146. Adrenergic blocker among the following *(Recent Question 2016)*
a. Prazosin b. Atropine
c. Hyoscine d. Salmeterol

147. β2 agonist action results in *(Recent Question 2016)*
a. Dilatation of bronchiolesb. Bronchoconstriction
c. Diuresis d. Vasoconstriction

148. Dobutamine acts on *(Recent Question 2016)*
a. β1 receptors b. β2 receptors
c. D1 receptors d. D2 receptors

149. Not a nonselective beta blocker *(Recent Question 2016)*
a. Esmolol b. Pindolol
c. Propranolol d. Sotalol

150. Beta agonist used to stop preterm labor *(Recent Question 2016)*
a. Ritodrine b. Salbutamol
c. Propranolol d. Salmeterol

151. The most important action of beta-blockers in glaucoma is *(Recent Question 2016)*
a. Membrane stabilizing effect
b. Retinal neuron protecting effect
c. Decrease in the production of aqueous humor
d. Pupillary constriction

152. A patient came to the casualty with acute bronchial asthma after treatment for glaucoma. The probable drug maybe *(Recent Question 2016)*
a. Timolol b. Betaxolol
c. Latanoprost d. Anticholinesterase

153. Vasopressor of choice in pregnancy is *(Recent Question 2016)*
a. Ephedrine b. Phenylephrine
c. Methoxamine d. Mephentermine

154. Longest acting ocular beta blocker *(Recent Question 2016)*
a. Timolol b. Betaxolol
c. Carteolol d. Metoprolol

155. The alpha-adrenergic blocker that paradoxically produces vasoconstriction is *(Recent Question 2016)*
a. Phenoxybenzamine b. Ergotamine
c. Prazosin d. Tolazoline

156. B2 selective agonists are often effective in
a. Angina due to coronary insufficiency
b. Asthma *(Recent Question 2016)*
c. Delayed labor d. All the above

157. Third generation beta-blocker is *(Recent Question 2016)*
a. Propranolol b. Timolol
c. Nadolol d. Nebivolol

158. Beta blocker without local anesthetic effects is *(Recent Question 2016)*
a. Metoprolol b. Pindolol
c. Propranolol d. Timolol

159. Dopamine is preferred in treatment of shock because of
a. Renal vasodilatory effect *(Recent Question 2016)*
b. Increased cardiac output
c. Peripheral vasoconstriction
d. Prolonged action

160. Which of the following increases systolic and diastolic BP for prolonged period? *(Recent Question 2016)*
a. Epinephrine b. Dopamine
c. Ephedrine d. All of these

161. Drug used for treatment of scorpion sting is *(Recent Question 2016)*
a. Adrenaline b. Morphine
c. Captopril d. Prazosin

162. Propranolol can be used in all except *(Recent Question 2016)*
a. Thyrotoxicosis b. Variant angina
c. Migraine d. Hypertension

163. Half-life of dobutamine is *(Recent Question 2016)*
a. 120 seconds b. 200 seconds
c. 20 seconds d. 20 minutes

164. Timolol is contraindicated in *(Recent Question 2016)*
a. Hypertension b. Glaucoma
c. COPD d. Aphakia

165. Biphasic reaction on blood pressure is seen with the administration of *(Recent Question 2016)*
a. Adrenaline b. Nor adrenaline
c. Dopamine d. Dobutamine

166. Major metabolite of noradrenaline in urine is *(Recent Question 2016)*
a. VMA b. HVA
c. Normetanephrine d. Metanephrine

167. Conversion of norepinephrine to epinephrine occur by *(Recent Question 2016)*
a. Methylation b. Decarboxylation
c. Oxidation d. Sulfation

168. Betaxolol is a *(Recent Question 2016)*
a. Alpha blocker b. Beta blocker
c. Calcium channel blockerd. Potassium channel opener

169. Beta blocker having both alpha and beta blocking property is *(Recent Question 2016)*
a. Carvedilol b. Sotalol
c. Nadolol d. Pindolol

170. Clonidine is used for *(Recent Question 2016)*
a. Migraine
b. Opioid withdrawal syndrome
c. To decrease anesthetic requirement
d. All of the above

171. **β blocker with intrinsic sympathomimetic activity** ***(Recent Question 2016)***
   a. Propranolol b. Atenolol
   c. Sotalol d. Pindolol

172. **Non-catecholamine sympathomimetic drug** ***(Recent Question 2016)***
   a. Ephedrine b. Dopamine
   c. Isoproterenol d. Dobutamine

173. **Dobutamine increases** ***(Recent Question 2016)***
   a. Heart rate b. Cardiac output
   c. Blood pressure d. Plasma volume

174. **Drug that acts on D1, D2, β1 and not on β2 receptors is** ***(Recent Question 2016)***
   a. Dobutamine b. Dopamine
   c. Noradrenaline d. Phenylephrine

175. **Drug of choice for beta blocker poisoning** ***(Recent Question 2016)***
   a. Calcium b. Glucagon
   c. Insulin d. Salbutamol

176. **Dexmedetomidine is** ***(Recent Question 2016)***
   a. Centrally acting α_{2a} agonist
   b. Centrally acting α_2 agonist
   c. Peripherally acting α_2 agonist
   d. Peripherally acting α_2 agonist

177. **Drug used for sexual arousal is** ***(Recent Question 2016)***
   a. SSRI b. Beta blocker
   c. Alpha 2 antagonist d. Alpha 1 antagonist

178. **Beta blockers are contraindicated in** ***(Recent Question 2016)***
   a. Acute aortic dissection b. Angina pectoris
   c. Post MI d. Sick sinus syndrome

179. **If dopamine is given at rate of 8μg/kg /min which of the following actions are seen:** ***(PGI May 2018)***
   a. Increased stroke volume
   b. Decreased systemic vascular resistance
   c. Increased systemic vascular resistance
   d. Renal vasodilation
   e. Increased heart rate

180. **Long acting β agonist(s) which is/are used as once a day drug:** ***(PGI May 2017)***
   a. Salmeterol b. Formoterol
   c. Olodaterol d. Vilanterol
   e. Indacaterol

181. **Adrenaline can be used in:** ***(PGI May 2017)***
   a. Bronchial asthma b. Allergic disorder
   c. Cardio-pulmonary resuscitation
   d. Anaphylaxis
   e. As anti-analgesic medicine

182. **Which of the following is/are true regarding muscarinic action except:** ***(PGI June 2015)***
   a. Miosis
   b. Detrusor muscle contraction
   c. Dicyclomine is antimuscarinic drug used for smooth muscle relaxation
   d. Cardiac muscarinic receptors are predominantly M 3 type
   e. ↓salivary gland secretion

183. **Common action(s) of epinephrine and norepinephrine includes:** ***(PGI Nov 2014)***
   a. Skin vasodilation
   b. Bronchial muscle contraction
   c. Increase systolic BP
   d. Increase HR
   e. Renal vasoconstriction

184. **Which of the following is function of muscarinic receptor:**
   a. Increase in conduction velocity of A-V node and His-purkinje fibres ***(PGI May 2014)***
   b. Eye-mydriasis
   c. Ciliary muscle contraction
   d. Contraction of circular muscle of iris
   e. Detrusor muscle contraction

185. **Which of the following is/are true about dobutamine:**
   a. Selective β 2 receptor agonist ***(PGI May 2014)***
   b. ↑ ventricular filling pressure
   c. Half-life is about 2 min
   d. Dopamine receptor agonist

186. **Acetylcholine esterase inhibitors are:** ***(PGI Nov 2013)***
   a. Neostigmine b. Atropine
   c. Edrophonium d. Methacholine
   e. Malathion

187. **Beta blocker with no α_1 antagonistic property:**
   a. Labetalol b. Carvedilol***(PGI May 2013)***
   c. Atenolol d. Nebivolol
   e. Betaxolol

188. **Adrenergic receptor effects includes:** ***(PGI May 2013)***
   a. Piloerection b. Urine retention
   c. Diarrhea d. Pupillary dilation
   e. Bronchodilation

189. **Which beta blockers have partial agonistic activity:** ***(PGI Nov 2012)***
   a. Atenolol b. Nadolol
   c. Propanolol d. Celiprolol
   e. Acebutolol

190. **Precursor of Adrenaline is:** ***(PGI Nov 2011)***
   a. Noradrenaline b. Phenylalanine
   c. Tryptophan d. Dobutamine
   e. Tyrosine

191. **True about Hyoscine:** ***(PGI Nov 2010)***
   a. Penetrate cornea
   b. Obtained from atropa belladonna
   c. Shorter duration of action than atropine
   d. Cross Brain-blood barrier
   e. Used in motion sickness

192. **Which of the following are β1selective antagonist:** ***(PGI May 2010)***
   a. Propranolol b. Atenolol
   c. Metoprolol d. Pindolol

193. **Use of α2 agonist:** ***(PGI Nov 2009)***
   a. Relief of spasticity/muscular spasm
   b. Erectile dysfunction
   c. Terminal cancer pain
   d. Conscious sedation in intubated ICU patients
   e. Postherpetic neuropathy

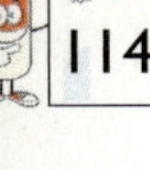

194. Correct about β blocker: *(PGI June 2009)*
a. Membrane stability
b. Used in glaucoma
c. Esmolol metabolize by kidney
d. Nadolol metabolize by liver
e. Have intrinsic sympathomimetic activity

195. Which of the following drug (s) is/are used in β-blocker overdose: *(PGI Nov 2008)*
a. Atropine
b. Acetylcholine
c. Glucagon
d. Octreotide
e. Isoprenaline

196. Drug(s) used in incontinence of urine is/are: *(PGI Nov 2008)*
a. Oxybutynin
b. Tolterodine
c. Tiotropium
d. Solifenacin
e. Imipramine

197. What is/are true about Terazosin w.r.t. phenoxybenzamine: *(PGI Nov 2008)*
a. More α1 selective
b. Less S/E
c. Longer acting
d. Once daily dosing

198. β-Blocker used in: *(PGI Nov 2007)*
a. Portal hypertension
b. Alcohol withdrawal
c. Anxiety
d. HOCM

199. Both alpha and beta blocker are:
a. Labetalol
b. Carvedilol
c. Prazosin
d. Tamsulosin
e. Milrinone

200. True about esmolol: *(PGI June 2006)*
a. Alpha Blocker
b. Long half life
c. Not cardioselective
d. Used in LV decompensation
e. Cause bradycardia

201. Uses of α2 agonist except *(PGI Dec 2005)*
a. Sedation
b. HTN
c. Glaucoma
d. BPH
e. Ischaemia

202. Which of the following is paired incorrectly *(PGI Dec 2005)*
a. Hemicholinium: prevents the release of Ach, from storage vesicle
b. Botulinum, increase the Ach release
c. Pralidoxime reactivates acetylcholine esterase
d. Vesamicol inhibit the uptake of choline
e. Organophosphorus inhibits acetylcholinesterase

203. Contraindications of B-blockers. *(PGI Dec 2005)*
a. Asthma
b. Heart block
c. HTN
d. Arrhythmias
e. CHF

204. Combined α and β blockers are A/E: *(PGI June 2005)*
a. Pindolol
b. Levobunolol
c. Carvedilol
d. Labetalol
e. Acebutolol

205. Mirabegron is a *(JIPMER Nov 2018)*
a. Beta 3 agonist
b. Beta 3 antagonist
c. Beta 1 agonist
d. Beta 1 antagonist

206. In a diabetic patient with autonomic neuropathy early morning hypotension and dizziness is seen; the drug of choice is: *(JIPMER Nov 2018)*
a. Dobutamine
b. Isoproterenol
c. Clonidine
d. Midodrine

207. Beta blocker which increases HDL: *(JIPMER May 2018)*
a. Celiprolol
b. Nebivolol
c. Carvedilol
d. Bucindolol

208. A child comes to you with ADHD. He has a family h/o drug addiction. Which is the DOC in this patient? *(JIPMER May 2018)*
a. Methylphenidate
b. Atomoxetine
c. Amphetamine
d. Clonidine

209. Tetraethylammonium blocks *(JIPMER 2017)*
a. Na channel
b. K channel
c. Cl channel
d. Ca channel

210. Which of the following is a new drug for treatment of tardive dyskinesia *(JIPMER 2017)*
a. Valbenazine
b. Deutetrabenazine
c. Tetrabenazine
d. Ropinirole

211. Mechanism of action of tetrabenazine is *(JIPMER 2017)*
a. Inhibits VMAT
b. Inhibits NE reuptake
c. Inhibits NE metabolism
d. Stimulates NE synthesis

212. Which of the following drugs is not used in Tourette syndrome *(JIPMER 2017)*
a. Clonidine
b. Carbamazepine
c. Haloperidol
d. Verapamil

213. Which of the following is a cardioselective beta blocker with antioxidant property? *(JIPMER 2017)*
a. Nebivolol
b. Sotalol
c. Betaxolol
d. Carvedilol

214. Antidote for metoprolol toxicity is *(JIPMER 2017)*
a. Glucagon
b. Atropine
c. Calcium gluconate
d. Naloxone

215. Which beta blocker has membrane stabilizing property? *(JIPMER 2014)*
a. Metoprolol
b. Atenolol
c. Propranolol
d. Esmolol

216. Which of the following drugs does not penetrate blood brain barrier and cause central effects? *(JIPMER 2014)*
a. Glycopyrrolate
b. Hyoscine hydrobromide
c. Hyoscine butylbromide
d. Atropine

217. Which beta blocker has antioxidant property? *(JIPMER 2014)*
a. Celiprolol
b. Carvedilol
c. Betaxolol
d. Propranolol

218. Drug used in the treatment of overactive bladder causing xerostomia is: *(JIPMER 2013)*
a. Serfanacin
b. Oxybutynin
c. Trospium
d. Darifenacin

219. Drug used in Narcoanalysis is: *(JIPMER 2013)*
a. Cocaine
b. Pethidine
c. Atropine
d. Scopolamine

220. True about beta blockers all except: *(JIPMER 2013)*
a. Postural hypotension
b. Bradycardia
c. Glucagon used for toxicity
d. Lipid soluble drug (cause bad dreams)

221. Glucagon hydrochloride is used in poisoning of: ***(JIPMER 2013)***
   a. Beta blocker
   b. Calcium channel blocker
   c. Tricyclic antidepressants
   d. SSRI

222. A patient is on propranolol. Adverse effects of beta blocker are all except: ***(JIPMER 2012)***
   a. Seizures
   b. Rebound tachycardia
   c. Hypotension
   d. Poor response to hypoglycemia

223. Which alpha 2 agonist is used to relieve spasticity in amyotrophic lateral sclerosis? ***(JIPMER 2011)***
   a. Clonidine
   b. Brimonidine
   c. Apraclonidine
   d. Tizanidine

224. All the following are beta-blockers except: ***(JIPMER 2009)***
   a. Esmolol
   b. Sotalol
   c. Celiprolol
   d. Formoterol

225. Which of the following is not an alpha-2 stimulant? ***(JIPMER 2009)***
   a. Guanabenz
   b. Guanadrel
   c. Clonidine
   d. Alpha methyl dopa

226. The neurotransmitter secreted by postganglionic sympathetic fibres innervating sweat glands is: ***(JIPMER 2008)***
   a. Nor epinephrine
   b. Epinephrine
   c. Acetylcholine
   d. Dopamine

227. Which of the following is the most beta-1 selective antagonist? ***(JIPMER 2007)***
   a. Acebutolol
   b. Atenolol
   c. Metoprolol
   d. Bisoprolol

228. Atropine is added with diphenoxylate to: ***(JIPMER 2007)***
   a. Increase effects
   b. Decrease side effects
   c. Decrease abuse potential
   d. Enhance absorption

229. Clonidine acts on: ***(JIPMER 2011)***
   a. Vasomotor center
   b. Sympathetic nerve
   c. Autonomic ganglia
   d. Vascular smooth muscle

230. A drug which is an alpha agonist and orally used prodrug for autonomic insufficiency and postural hypotension is: ***(JIPMER 2010)***
   a. Methamphetamine
   b. Midodrine
   c. Phenylephrine
   d. Metaraminol

231. Dexmedetomidine is a new drug used in: ***(JIPMER 2006)***
   a. General anaesthesia
   b. Treatment of VRSA
   c. Hypertension
   d. Multiple sclerosis

232. The indicated Dose of Pralidoxime with Atropine in Organophosphorus Poisoning is ***(NIMHANS 2013)***
   a. 500 mg
   b. 800 mg
   c. 1 gm
   d. 5 gm

233. All of the following stimulate Peristalsis except ***(NIMHANS 2010)***
   a. Neostigmine
   b. Bethanechol
   c. Metoclopramide
   d. Atropine

234. Clonidine mechanism of action is ***(NIMHANS 2010)***
   a. α-blockade
   b. β-blockade
   c. α 1-agonist
   d. α 2-agonist

235. Dales vasomotor reversal ***(NIMHANS 2007)***
   a. Stimulation of alpha-1 receptors
   b. Stimulation of alpha-2 receptors
   c. Stimulation of beta-1 receptors
   d. Stimulation of beta-2 receptors

Practice Questions & Answers from 236 to 245 are given at the end of the chapter.

Answers with Explanations to Multiple Choice Questions

1. Ans. (a) Delayed diastolic depolarization

- Acetyl choline decreases heart rate primarily by inhibiting the spontaneous depolarization of cells in SA node; also known as diastolic depolarization. This is achieved by inhibition of the funny current in the SA node.

Effect of acetylcholine on cardiovascular system	
Heart rate decreases	Ach inhibits funny current generation in the pacemaker cells of SA node
AV conduction decreases	Ach blocks L type calcium channels in the AV node
Atrial contraction decreases > ventricular contraction	Atrium is supplied by cholinergic fibers more than the ventricles. Ach opens potassium channels and decreases cyclic AMP in the myocardial cells
Vasodilation	Ach increases calcium in endothelial cells, which stimulates calcium dependent ENOS and releases NO which causes vasodilation

2. Ans. (b) Prostaglandin analogue

(Ref: Meyler's side effects of Endocrine and Metabolic drugs/ P124)

- Prostaglandin analogues like latanoprost can disrupt the blood aqueous barrier and cause macular edema. Hence this class should be used as a last resort in patients with macular edema.
- Beta blockers can mask the symptoms of hypoglycemia and hence can be problematic in patients of diabetes, specifically on insulin. But this can be tackled by regular monitoring of blood glucose level and hence is not an absolute contraindication.
- Other options are safe in patients of diabetes as well as macular edema.

3. Ans. (c) Atropine

(Ref: Goodman Gilman 13th E/P1261)

- Atropine 1% ointment is used as an adjuvant in fungal corneal ulcer to prevent synechiae formation.

4. Ans. (c) Endrin

(Ref: Goodman Gilman 12th E/P244)

- Endrin is an organochloride pesticide which causes neurotoxicity. There is no antidote available and hence only symptomatic treatment is done.
- Parathion and TIK-20 are organophosphates, and Baygon is a combination of organophosphate and carbamate; for all of these atropine is the drug of choice for poisoning.

5. Ans. (a) Scopolamine patch a night before

(Ref: Goodman Gilman 12th E/P233)

- Scopolamine is the most effective drug and hence drug of choice in motion sickness. It has to be given at least 4 hours before journey and thereafter every 72 hours if journey continues.
- Antihistaminics like dimenhydrinate, cyclizine and diphenhydramine are least effective and required to be given before one hour of travel and then every 4-6 hours during travel.

6. Ans. (a) Peptic ulcer disease

(Ref: Goodman Gilman 12th E/P1316)

7. Ans. (a) M2

(Ref: Goodman Gilman 12th E/P223)

Direct cholinergics	Muscarinic receptor activity maximum at	Nicotinic receptor activity
Methacholine	M_2	Low
Bethanechol	M_1 and M_3	Absent
Carbachol	M_1 and M_3	Maximum
Pilocarpine	M_1 and M_3	Absent
Ach	M_1, M_2 and M_3	Intermediate

8. Ans. (b) Glycopyrrolate

(Ref: Goodman and Gilman 12th E/P 226-27)

Anticholinergics

Tertiary amines	Quaternary amines
Atropine	Glycopyrrolate
Scopolamine	Trospium
Hyoscine	Ipratropium
Dicyclomine	Tiotropium
Benztropine	Oxitropium
Biperiden	

9. Ans. (d) Bradycardia

(Ref: Goodman and Gilman 12th E/P 221)

- **Cholinomimetics decrease heart rate and hence cannot be used in bradycardia.**
- **Anticholinergics like atropine is used for treatment of bradycardia.**

10. Ans. (d) Pharmacological block

(Ref: Goodman and Gilman 12th E/P 221)

- **If pilocarpine is not able to reverse mydriasis by acting on M_3 receptors, it means the receptors is blocked.**
- **When antagonism is because of same site, it is called as competitive or pharmacological antagonism.**

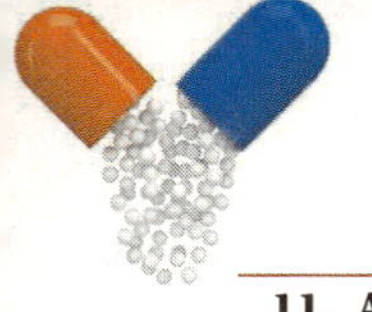

11. Ans. (b) Darifenacin

(Ref: Goodman and Gilman 12th E/P 231)

- **Though options b, c and d all can be used in overactive bladder, the best answer is option b i.e. darifenacin.**
- **Flavoxate is rarely used nowadays due to toxicity.**
- **Oxybutynin is the most toxic of available drugs in this class and hence it is used by transdermal formulation.**
- **Darifenacin and solifenacin being M_3 selective cause lesser toxicity and are more preferable.**

12. Ans. (a) Atropine

(Ref: Goodman and Gilman 12th E/P 234)

13. Ans. (a) Anticholinergic

(Ref: Goodman and Gilman 12th E/P 234)

14. Ans. (b) Increased RR interval in ECG

(Ref: Goodman and Gilman 12th E/P 221)

- Vagal stimulation of heart decreases conduction, heart rate and contraction.
- A decrease in heart rate manifests in ECG as increased RR interval and decreased conduction through AV node as a prolonged PR interval.

15. Ans. (a) Brimonidine

(Ref: Goodman Gilman 13th E/P203)

- Brimonidine is a lipid soluble drug and hence crosses blood brain barrier, which leads to side effects like hypotension, sedation and apnea in young children specifically.
- Apnea as a side effect can be seen with beta blockers like timolol both in young children.

16. Ans. (a) Timolol

(Ref: Goodman Gilman 13th E/P1291)

- Nonselective beta blockers like timolol, metipranolol, carteolol and levobunolol can block beta 2 receptors and hence precipitate bronchospasm.
- Cardioselective beta blockers like betaxolol is devoid of such effect.

17. Ans. (b) Edrophonium

(Ref: Goodman Gilman 13th E/P172)

- Edrophonium is the drug of choice for diagnosis of myasthenia gravis. As soon as it is given there is an improvement in muscle weakness.
- Cholinergic crisis is due to excessive Ach in the synapse (ACHE inhibitor overdosing), which downregulates the postsynaptic NM receptors and causes muscle weakness. If edrophonium is given in this case there will be further worsening of muscle weakness due to increase in Ach.

18. Ans. (b) Anticholinergics

(Ref: Goodman Gilman 13th E/P156)

- Delirium is an acute change in cognition and attention characterized by alteration in consciousness and disorganized thinking.
- Since anticholinergics decrease cognition, delirium can be worsened by anticholinergics.
- Postoperative delirium is decreased by drugs like
  - Antipsychotics: Haloperidol
  - Dexmedetomidine
  - Benzodiazepines: Midazolam

19. Ans. (a) Active miotic

(Ref: Goodman Gilman 13th E/P1259)

- Miosis: Contraction of pupil can be seen due to contraction of circular muscles (active miosis), due to M3 stimulation or it can be seen due to relaxation of radial muscles (passive miosis), due to $\alpha 1$ receptors block. Relaxation of radial muscles can cause miosis due to unopposed action of circular muscles. Thus, cholinergics like pilocarpine and physostigmine are active miotics, whereas alpha blockers like phentolamine and phenoxybenzamine are passive miotics.
- Mydriasis: Relaxation of pupil can be seen due to contraction of radial muscles (active mydriasis) due to $\alpha 1$ receptors stimulation or due to relaxation of circular muscles (passive mydriasis) due to M3 blockers. Relaxation of circular muscles cause mydriasis due to unopposed action of radial muscles. Thus, sympathomimetics like phenylephrine and ephedrine are active mydriatics, whereas anticholinergics like atropine, tropicamide and cyclopentolate are passive mydriatics.

Miotics		Mydriatics	
Active	Passive	Active	Passive
Pilocarpine	Phentolamine	Phenylephrine	Atropine
Physostigmine	Phenoxyben-zamine	Ephedrine	Tropicamide

20. Ans. (c) M3

(Ref: Goodman Gilman 13th E/P157)

- M3 are Gq subtype of GPCR, which increase calcium and that causes contraction of detrusor. In case of overactive bladder inhibition of M3 is crucial for treatment by anticholinergics like tolterodine.

21. Ans. (b) Latanoprost

(Ref: Katzung 11th E/P328)

Side effects of Topical Prostaglandin Analogs

- Pigmentation of iris (heterochromia iridis) and eyebrow
- Trichomegaly
- Dry (sandy) eyes
- Periorbital fat depletion

22. Ans. (d) Causes accommodative spasm

(Ref: Goodman Gilman 12th E/P1788)

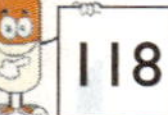

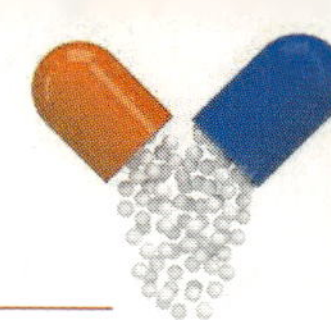

23. Ans. (d) Postural hypotension

(Ref: Goodman Gilman 12th E/P 273)

- Ganglionic blockers decrease release of both Ach and NE in the post ganglionic axons and hence will have inhibitory effect on both sympathetic and parasympathetic nervous system.
- Muscarinic blocker antagonizes only parasympathetic nervous system.
- Hence the common symptoms in both toxicities will be anticholinergic ones like blurred vision, mydriasis dry mouth, constipation, urine retention etc.
- The differential symptoms in ganglionic blockers will be because of decrease in NE, which will cause **postural hypotension**.

24. Ans. (b) Oxybutynin

(Ref: Goodman Gilman 12th E/P 231)

25. Ans. (a) Physostigmine

(Ref: Goodman Gilman 12th E/P 234)

- Physostigmine is the drug of choice for treatment of **atropine or belladonna poisoning** because atropine is also a tertiary amine that can cross blood brain barrier.

26. Ans. (b) Edrophonium

(Ref: Goodman Gilman 12th E/P 251)

- Edrophonium is preferred drug for diagnosis of myasthenia gravis due to its shorter duration of action and faster action.
- For diagnosis it is used in the test called as Tensilon's test.

27. Ans. (d) Hyoscine

(Ref: Goodman Gilman 12th E/P 233)

- **Hyoscine (scopolamine) is the drug of choice for treatment of motion sickness.**
- **Alternatively antihistaminics with good anticholinergic effect like promethazine and diphenhydramine can also be used.**

28. Ans. (a) Pralidoxime

(Ref: Goodman Gilman 12th E/P 249)

29. Ans. (a) Methacholine

(Ref: Goodman Gilman 12th E/P 223)

- Methacholine primarily acts on M_2 receptors in the heart, which are G_i subtype of receptors.
- Stimulation results in a decrease in cyc AMP and opening of K^+ channels and hyperpolarization of cells in the heart i.e. SA node, AV node and myocardium.
- Bethanechol and carbachol primarily act on M_1 and M_3, which are G_q subtypes of receptors and stimulation increases Ca^{++}.

30. Ans. (a) Dementia

(Ref: Goodman Gilman 12th E/P 253)

Cholinergics Used in Dementia

- Donepezil
- Rivastigmine
- Galantamine
- Tacrine

31. Ans. (d) Glaucoma

(Ref: Goodman Gilman 12th E/P 250, 251)

32. Ans. (a) SA node hyperpolarization

(Ref: Goodman Gilman 12th E/P 220, 221)

33. Ans. (a) Reactivating cholinesterase enzyme

(Ref: Goodman Gilman 12th E/P 249)

34. Ans. (a) Atropine

(Ref: Goodman Gilman 12th E/P 227)

35. Ans. (b) Shorter acting than edrophonium

(Ref: Goodman Gilman 12th E/P 250)

- Neostigmine being a quaternary amine is lipid insoluble and hence does not cross the blood brain barrier and has poor oral absorption.
- It is longer acting than edrophonium.

36. Ans. (d) Glaucoma

(Ref: Goodman Gilman 12th E/P1787)

- Prostaglandin analogs like latanoprost and bimatoprost are the drug of choice for treatment of open angle glaucoma.

37. Ans. (a) Glaucoma

(Ref: Goodman Gilman 12th E/P 233)

- Anticholinergics like atropine can cause mydriasis and precipitate an acute attack of glaucoma.
- Cholinergics like pilocarpine are used in glaucoma.

38. Ans. (a) Mucous and pharyngeal secretions

(Ref: Goodman Gilman 12th E/P 228)

39. Ans. (c) Bradycardia

(Ref: Goodman Gilman 12th E/P 228)

40. Ans. (a) PG inhibitor

(Ref: Goodman Gilman 12th E/P1787)

41. Ans. (c) Tolterodine

(Ref: Goodman Gilman 12th E/P 231)

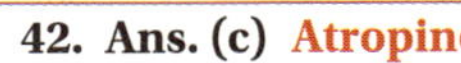

42. Ans. (c) Atropine

(Ref: Goodman Gilman 12th E/P 225)

Mushroom poisoning	Symptoms	Treatment
Inocybe Clitocybe	Cholinergic	Atropine
Amanita muscaria (Muscarine predominant)	Cholinergic	**Atropine**
Amanita muscaria (Atropine like compound predominant)	Anticholinergic	Physostigmine
Amanita phalloides	Renal failure Hepatic failure Gastroenteritis	Charcoal IV silymarin (Antidote of choice)
Psilocybe Panaeolus	Hallucinations	Supportive care
Cortinarius	GIT upset Renal failure	Supportive care
Gyromitra	Gastroenteritis Seizures Renal and hepatic failure	IV Pyridoxine for seizures

43. Ans. (a) Reversible carbamylation

(Ref: Goodman Gilman 12th E/P242)

- Carbamylation in itself is a reversible reaction and hence carbamates bind reversibly to ACHE.
- The binding to esteratic site though is longer than Ach and hence these are called as pseudoirreversible, as well.

44. Ans. (a) Myasthenia gravis

(Ref: Goodman Gilman 12th E/P251)

45. Ans. (a) Baygon

(Ref: Goodman Gilman 12th E/P249)

- Baygon contains carbamate propoxur and organophosphate chlorpyrifos. Oximes cannot reverse carbamate poisoning as the anionic site is bound.
- Other options are organophosphates, in which oximes are useful as their binding site i.e. anionic site is free.

46. Ans. (d) Tropicamide

(Ref: Goodman Gilman 12th E/P233)

- Tropicamide is shortest and fastest acting mydriatics.
- Atropine is longest acting and most potent mydriatic.

47. Ans. (c) Cholinergic

(Ref: Goodman Gilman 12th E/P189)

Organ	Neurotransmitter
Ganglion	Ach
Postganglionic parasympathetic	Ach
Postganglionic sympathetics	NE Exception: Sweat glands–Ach Adrenals–Ach Renal blood vessels–Dopamine

48. Ans. (b) Inhibiting release of acetylcholine

(Ref: Goodman Gilman 12th E/P186)

49. Ans. (b) Rise in blood pressure

(Ref: Goodman Gilman 12th E/P192-3)

50. Ans. (b) It is longer acting

(Ref: Goodman Gilman 12th E/P251)

51. Ans. (a) Acetylcholine

(Ref: Goodman Gilman 12th E/P219)

- Increase in blood pressure causes reflex activation of vagus, which releases Ach in heart.
- Ach by acting on M_2 receptors decrease cyc AMP and open potassium channel that causes hyperpolarization of cells of SA node, AV node and myocardium.

52. Ans. (d) Hyperthermia

(Ref: Goodman Gilman 12th E/P242)

- Belladonna or atropine can decrease generalized sweating and hence children are at risk of hyperthermia.

53. Ans. (a) Atropine

(Ref: Goodman Gilman 12th E/P249)

54. Ans. (d) Memantine

(Ref: Goodman Gilman 12th E/P252, 253)

- Memantine is an NMDA antagonist approved for treatment of Alzheimer's disease.

55. Ans. (a) Tacrine

(Ref: Goodman Gilman 12th E/P252)

- Tacrine has been abandoned due to risk of hepatotoxicity.

56. Ans. (b) Edrophonium

(Ref: Goodman Gilman 12th E/P251)

57. Ans. (d) Physostigmine

(Ref: Goodman Gilman 12th E/P252)

- Physostigmine being a tertiary amine is preferred for treatment of a tertiary amine like atropine's toxicity.

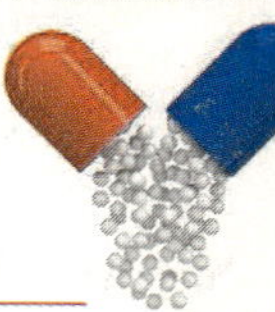

58. Ans. (d) Tropicamide

(Ref: Goodman Gilman 12th E/P233)

59. Ans. (b) Carbamate poisoning

(Ref: Goodman Gilman 12th E/P249)

- Carbamate itself is an anti-cholinesterase implicated in cholinergic toxicity.

60. Ans. (c) Acetylcholine

(Ref: Goodman Gilman 12th E/P189)

Organ	Neurotransmitter
Ganglion	Ach
Postganglionic parasympathetic	Ach
Postganglionic sympathetics	NE Exception: Sweat glands–Ach Adrenals–Ach Renal blood vessels–Dopamine

61. Ans. (a) Edrophonium

(Ref: Goodman Gilman 12th E/P251)

62. Ans. (d) Phenylephrine

(Ref: Goodman Gilman 12th E/P233)

- Anticholinergics are mydriatics as well as cycloplegics.
- Sympathomimetics are only mydriatics.

63. Ans. (b) Inhibition of sweating

(Ref: Goodman Gilman 12th E/P179)

64. Ans. (a) Varenicline

(Ref: Goodman Gilman 12th E/P272)

65. Ans. (c) Carbachol

(Ref: Goodman Gilman 12th E/P223)

66. Ans. (a) Darifenacin

(Ref: Goodman Gilman 12th E/P232)

- Darifenacin and Solifenacin are both selective M_3 antagonist and hence are known as uroselective.
- Since darifenacin is more M_3 selective it is a better answer.

67. Ans. (a) Benztropine

(Ref: Goodman Gilman 12th E/P234)

- Benztropin, biperiden and trihexphenydil are anticholinergics used for treatment of EPS spectrum side effects like parkinsonism, acute dystonia, akathisia and oculogyric crisis seen with antipsychotics.

68. Ans. (a) Hypothermia

(Ref: Goodman Gilman 12th E/P179)

- Atropine can inhibit generalized sweating and hence causes hyperthermia.

69. Ans. (d) Glycopyrrolate

(Ref: Goodman Gilman 12th E/P234)

70. Ans. (d) Neuroleptic malignant syndrome

(Ref: Goodman Gilman 12th E/P234)

- Benztropin, biperiden and trihexphenydil are anticholinergics used for treatment of EPS spectrum side effects like parkinsonism, acute dystonia, akathisia and oculogyric crisis seen with antipsychotics.
- In NMS there is already hyperthermia which can be worsened by anticholinergics by inhibition of sweating.

71. Ans. (a) Tertiary ammonium compound

(Ref: Goodman Gilman 12th E/P242)

72. Ans. (a) Alzheimer's disease

(Ref: Goodman Gilman 12th E/P253)

73. Ans. (c) Irreversibly

(Ref: Goodman Gilman 12th E/P249)

74. Ans. (a) Rivastigmine and donepezil

(Ref: Goodman Gilman 12th E/P253)

75. Ans. (b) Hypoglycemia

(Ref: Goodman Gilman 13th E/P201)

- Beta-2 agonists like salbutamol stimulate glycogenolysis and gluconeogenesis and increase plasma glucose (+++++++); they also increase insulin release and decrease plasma glucose (- -). However, the first effect is more predominant, and this leads to **hyperglycemia**.
- An increase in insulin release can cause **hypokalemia**.
- Stimulation of beta-2 receptors in skeletal muscles causes **tremor**.
- Stimulation of beta-2 receptors in heart causes **tachycardia**; beta-2 mediated vasodilation can also cause reflex **tachycardia**.

76. Ans. (a) Alpha 1 antagonist and beta 1 agonist

(Ref: Goodman Gilman 12th E/P178)

- Option 2 can be ruled out as M2 agonism causes bradycardia.
- Option 3 can be ruled out as alpha 1 agonism will cause vasoconstriction and increase diastolic BP.
- Option 4 beta 1 and 2 agonism will cause significant tachycardia which isn't in the case.
- Option a, alpha 1 antagonism will decrease diastolic BP and beta1 agonism will increase systolic BP and heart rate. This is the case here and hence option a is the best answer.

77. Ans. (c) Increased MAP

(Ref: CMDT 2017/P496)

- Septic shock is a vasodilatory shock; vasodilation is caused by the inflammatory mediator.
- The effect of NE that is beneficial in septic shock is an increase in MAP, as MAP increase is required for improvement in tissue perfusion. The aim is to maintain MAP at 65 mmHg or above. Infusion of NE is started at dose of 2-4 mcg/min; dose can be increased to a maximum of 30 mcg/min in case of no response.
- If patient does not respond to NE another vasopressor i.e. vasopressin can be combined.
- Phenylephrine is another vasopressor that can be used in place of NE, in case there is vasodilation but high cardiac output or presence of tachyarrhythmia.

78. Ans. (a) Adrenaline 0.5 mg 1/1000 IM

(Ref: Katzung 12th E/P145)

- Adrenaline 0.5 mg 1/1000 by intramuscular route (IM) is the drug of choice for treatment of anaphylactic shock. Hence it is the answer here.
- In case the patient develops life threatening condition, adrenaline 0.25 mg IV is given.

79. Ans. (a) Beta 2 stimulation by low epinephrine and thereafter beta 1 stimulation

(Ref: Goodman Gilman 12th E/P189)

Dale's Phenomenon:

When epinephrine is administered to a living system there is an initial rise in BP due to stimulation of alpha1 followed fall in blood pressure due to stimulation of beta 2.

Vasomotor Reversal of Dale:

When epinephrine is administered to a living system with an alpha blocker, there is only fall in blood pressure mediated by beta 2 stimulation.
Hence among the given option a is the best answer.

80. Ans. (a) Tizanidine

(Ref: Goodman Gilman 12th E/P297)

Tizanidine is a central alpha-2 agonist used as a muscle relaxant in spastic disorders like amyotrophic lateral sclerosis.

81. Ans. (c) Low dose dopamine

(Ref: ACLS 2017 guidelines)

- According to older guidelines vasopressin 40 units by intravenous route was used as an alternative to epinephrine as a vasoconstrictor in advanced cardiac life support. However currently vasopressin is not indicated in ACLS guidelines.
- Currently vasopressors used other than epinephrine are dopamine (2-10 mcg/kg) and norepinephrine.

82. Ans. (b) The effect on HR in graph A can be overcome by anti-muscarinic

(Ref: Goodman Gilman 12th E/P289)

- Graph A is NE, as there is an increase in both systolic and diastolic BP but decrease in HR. Decrease in **HR can be counteracted by antimuscarinics**.
- Graph B is epinephrine due to minor increase in systolic and decrease in diastolic BP and an increase in HR
- Graph C is isoprenaline as there is an instant and rapid increase in HR and a minor increase in systolic but major decrease in diastolic BP.

83. Ans. (d) Stimulation of vasomotor center

(Ref: Godman Gilman 12th E/P288)

- Dopamine has a dose dependent action as mentioned below.

Dose (continuous IV infusion)	Target receptor/organ affected
<2 μg/kg/min	D_1 receptors in renal blood vessels = **Renal vasodilatation** = Diuresis
2-10 μg/kg/min	β_1 receptors in heart = Inotropic effect
> 10 μg/kg/min	α_1 receptors in blood vessels = Vasoconstriction

84. Ans. (b) Adrenergic agonists

(Ref: Goodman Gilman 12th E/P1787)

- The precursor for adrenergic agonist like epinephrine is amino acid tyrosine.
- Hence topical administration can cause synthesis of melanin and can lead to black coloured pigmentation of conjunctiva.

85. Ans. (b) Stimulation of pre-synaptic alpha rectors

(Ref: Goodman Gilman 12th E/P282-83)

86. Ans. (a) β1

(Ref: Goodman Gilman 12th E/P288)

Dopamine's Action

Dose (continuous IV infusion)	Target receptor/ organ affected	Therapeutic indication
<2 μg/kg/min	D_1 receptors in renal blood vessels = Renal vasodilatation = Diuresis	Oliguria
2-10 μg/kg/min	β_1 receptors in heart = Inotropic effect	CHF
> 10 μg/kg/min	α_1 receptors in blood vessels = Vasoconstriction	Shock

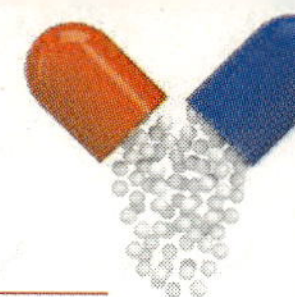

87. Ans. (c) Beta-3

(Ref: Goodman Gilman 12th E/P204)

88. Ans. (a) Central alpha 2 agonist

(Ref: Goodman and Gilman 12th E/P 297-99)

Central Alpha-2 Agonists

- Clonidine
- **Dexmedetomidine**
- Apraclonidine
- Brimonidine
- Guanfacine
- Guanabenz
- Tizanidine
- Methyldopa

89. Ans. (b) Hyperalgesia

(Ref: Goodman and Gilman 12th E/P 296)

Effects of α_2 Agonists

- **Analgesia**
- **Sedation**
- **Anxiolysis**
- **Decreased secretions**

90. Ans. (c) Epinephrine

(Ref: Goodman Gilman 12th E/P282)

Sympathomimetics	Target receptors
Epinephrine	α_1 α_2 β_1 β_2
Norepinephrine	α_1 α_2 β_1
Dopamine	D_1 β_1 α_1 (Dose dependent action)
Fenodolpam	$D_1\alpha_2$
Dopexamine	D_1 β_2
Isoprenaline (Isoproterenol)	β_1 β_2

91. Ans. (a) Brimonidine-decreases aqueous production

(Ref: Goodman Gilman 12th E/P1787)

Antiglaucoma drugs	Mechanism of action
Prostaglandin analogs	Increase uveoscleral outflow
Miotics	Increase trabecular outflow
β blockers and CA Inhibitors	Decrease aqueous production
Sympathomimetics	Decrease aqueous production > Increase uveoscleral outfloe

92. Ans. (a) Terbutaline

(Ref: Goodman Gilman 12th E/P293)

93. Ans. (c) Levobunolol

(Ref: Goodman Gilman 12th E/P1787)

- Topical beta blockers are contraindicated with systemic beta blockers due to risk of severe cardio suppression,

94. Ans. (d) Apraclonidine

(Ref: Goodman Gilman 12th E/P1787)

Side effects of Antiglaucoma Drugs

Drugs	Side effects
Prostaglandin analogs	Darkening of iris (heterochromia iridis) and eyebrow Trichomegaly Periorbital fat depletion
Miotics	Brow ache Corneal edema Retinal detachment
Timolol	Nasolacrimal duct stenosis (obstruction)
Sympathomimetics	Ocular allergy
Apraclonidine	Lid retraction
Apraclonidine Brimonidine	Drowsiness

95. Ans. (b) Salmeterol

(Ref: Goodman Gilman 12th E/293)

96. Ans. (b) A vasodilator in treating coronary artery stenosis during angio procedures

(Ref: Goodman Gilman 12th E/306)

97. Ans. (b) Dobutamine

(Ref: Harrison 19th E/P 270e-3)

- Dobutamine is used as a pharmacological stressor in myocardial perfusion testing and echocardiography.
- The pharmacological stressors of choice are coronary vasodilators like dipyridamole, adenosine and regadenson.

98. Ans. (b) Dobutamine

(Ref: Goodman Gilman 12th E/290)

Endogenous catecholamines	Exogenous catecholamines
Epinephrine Norepinephrine Dopamine	Dobutamine Isoprenaline Dopexamine Fenoldopam Droxidopa

99. Ans. (a) Apraclonidine

(Ref: Goodman Gilman 13th E/P203)

100. Ans. (a) Prazosin

(Ref: Harrison 19th E/P2748)

Treatment of Scorpion Sting

- Continuous IV midazolam for sedative effect.
- Vasodilators like prazosin, nitroprusside, nifedipine and hydralazine for treatment of hypertension and pulmonary edema.
- Atropine is used for treatment of life threatening bradya-rrhythmia.

101. Ans. (a) Malignant pheochromocytoma

(Ref: Goodman Gilman 13th E/P141)

- Metyrosine competitively inhibits tyrosine hydroxylase, thereby decreasing norepinephrine synthesis in the neurons.
- It is used for treatment of hypertension in patients with pheochromocytoma prior to surgery along with phenoxybenzamine, which is the drug of choice.
- It is also used in malignant pheochromocytoma for long term management.

102. Ans. (a) Alpha adrenergic

(Ref: Goodman Gilman 13th E/P203)

103. Ans. (c) Esmolol

(Ref: Goodman Gilman 12th E/P327)

Esmolol is shortest and fast acting, hence is preferred in surgery for

- Prophylaxis and treatment of tachycardia
- Treatment of SVT

104. Ans. (a) Carvedilol

(Ref: Goodman Gilman 12th E/P329)

105. Ans. (b) Hemangioma

(Ref: Peter Mattel's Pediatric Surgery/P885)

106. Ans. (a) Amphetamine

(Ref: Goodman Gilman 12th E/P663)

107. Ans. (a) Dopamine

(Ref: Goodman Gilman 12th E/P288)

108. Ans. (d) Acebutolol

(Ref: Goodman Gilman 12th E/P 311-12)

109. Ans. (d) 26%

(Ref: Goodman Gilman 12th E/P 313)

Beta blockers with maximum bioavailability = 100%	Penbutolol Pindolol
Beta blockers with minimum bioavailability = 30%	Carvedilol Propranolol

110. Ans. (b) Alpha1 antagonist

(Ref: Goodman Gilman 12th E/P 305)

Drug of choice for BPH	Alpha-1a antagonists Tamsulosin Silodosin
Drug of choice for BPH with HTN	Alpha-1 antagonists Terazosin Doxazocin

111. Ans. (b) Norepinephrine

(Ref: Goodman Gilman 12th E/P 283)

- NE stimulates beta-1 receptors and increases heart rate (++).
- NE also causes potent vasoconstriction due to alpha-1 receptors stimulation, which stimulates baroreceptors and causes reflex decrease in heart rate (- - -) due to vagus.
- The combined effect is a decrease in heart rate (–).
- If the patient is on atropine it will inhibit vagus action and there is an increase in heart rate.

112. Ans. (a) Increase heart rate

(Ref: Goodman Gilman 12th E/P 283)

113. Ans. (d) Nebivolol

(Ref: Goodman Gilman 12th E/P 313, 315)

Nebivolol decreases systolic blood pressure by beta-1 receptor block and decreases diastolic blood pressure due to vasodilation caused by NO release.

114. Ans. (d) Beta blocker followed by alpha blocker

(Ref: Goodman Gilman 12th E/P 314)

115. Ans. (c) Mirabegron

(Ref: CMDT 2015/P 66)

Mirabegron is a latest beta-3 receptor agonist approved for treatment of urge incontinence.

116. Ans. (a) Tamsulosin

(Ref: Goodman Gilman 12th E/P307)

117. Ans. (d) All of the above

(Ref: Goodman Gilman 12th E/P298)

Teratogenic Effects of Amphetamines

- **IUGR**
- **Cardiac anomaly**
- **Cleft lip**
- **Biliary atresia**

118. Ans. (a) Butoxamine

(Ref: Budhiraja 4th E/P182)

- Butoxamine is a β_2 antagonist used in experimental pharmacology.

119. Ans. (d) Bevantolol

(Ref: Goodman Gilman 12th E/P311)

Beta blockers with membrane stabilizing effect
Can : **Carvedilol**
Blow : **Betaxolol**
L : Labetalol
A : **Acebutolol**
M : Metoprolol
P : Propranolol and Pindolol

120. Ans. (a) Esmolol

(Ref: Goodman Gilman 12th E/P313)

- Esmolol is metabolized by esterases in erythrocytes and hence is short acting (8 minutes); it is fast acting as well.

121. Ans. (a) Nadolol

(Ref: Goodman Gilman 12th E/P313)

122. Ans. (a) Brimonidine

(Ref: Goodman Gilman 12th E/P1787)

Alpha-2 Agonists Used in Glaucoma are

- Apraclonidine
- Brimonidine

123. Ans. (a) Renal vasodilation

(Ref: Goodman Gilman 12th E/P288)

124. Ans. (b) ADHD

(Ref: Goodman Gilman 12th E/P288, E/P402)

- Atomoxetine is the drug of choice for ADHD associated with Tourette's syndrome.

125. Ans. (a) Nebivolol

(Ref: Goodman Gilman 12th E/P330)

126. Ans. (a) Nonselective beta blocker

(Ref: Goodman Gilman 12th E/P313)

127. Ans. (c) Phentolamine

(Ref: Goodman Gilman 12th E/P309, 310)

128. Ans. (a) Nadolol

(Ref: Goodman Gilman 12th E/P313)

129. Ans. (a) Sweating

(Ref: Goodman Gilman 12th E/P179)

- Localized sweating e.g. in the palms is caused by α_1 receptors and hence beta blockers cannot mask sweating.

130. Ans. (c) Yohimbine

(Ref: Goodman Gilman 12th E/P313)

131. Ans. (b) Prazosin

(Ref: Goodman Gilman 12th E/P307)

132. Ans. (b) Propranolol

(Ref: Goodman Gilman 12th E/P320)

133. Ans. (b) Labetalol

(Ref: Goodman Gilman 12th E/P315)

Beta blockers with alpha blocking effect

- Bucindolol
- Bevantolol
- Labetalol
- Nipradilol
- Carvedilol

134. Ans. (d) Betaxolol

(Ref: Goodman Gilman 12th E/P313)

135. Ans. (a) Phenylpropanolamine

(Ref: Goodman Gilman 12th E/P300)

- **Norephedrine (phenylpropanolamine)** was used as nasal decongestant and as anorexic agent, but has been banned due to risk of **cerebral hemorrhage**.

136. Ans. (b) Narcolepsy

(Ref: Goodman Gilman 12th E/P300)

- Modafinil is the drug of choice for **narcolepsy, shift worker disease** and **sleepiness in patients of OSA (Obstructive Sleep Apnea)**.
- Armodafinil the R enantiomer is longer acting.
- It acts by inhibiting DAT, which leads to an increase in dopamine in CNS.

137. Ans. (a) Tamsulosin

(Ref: Goodman Gilman 12th E/P307)

138. Ans. (a) Tamsulosin

(Ref: Goodman Gilman 12th E/P307)

139. Ans. (d) All of the above

(Ref: Goodman Gilman 12th E/P316)

140. Ans. (a) Increases heart rate

(Ref: Goodman Gilman 12th E/P287)

141. Ans. (a) Low dose

(Ref: Goodman Gilman 12th E/P288)

142. Ans. (d) Both A and B

(Ref: Goodman Gilman 12th E/P203)

β receptors	Location and effect
β_1	Heart = Increased contraction, conduction and HR Kidney (JG Cells) = Renin release
β_2	Heart = Increased contraction, conduction and HR Skeletal muscles = Increased Contraction Blood vessels = Dilation Bronchi = Dilation Uterus = Relaxation Liver = Glycogenolysis and gluconeogenesis Pancreas = Insulin release
β_3	Adipocytes = Lipolysis Detrusor = Relaxation

143. Ans. (c) Subcutaneous

(Ref: Goodman Gilman 12th E/P286)

- Though epinephrine can be given by subcutaneous, intramuscular and intravenous route for anaphylactic shock, the preferred route is **subcutaneous**.

144. Ans. (c) Celiprolol

(Ref: Goodman Gilman 12th E/P315)

Beta blocker with beta-2 agonism
B : Bopindolol **C :** Celiprolol, Carteolol

145. Ans. (a) Adrenaline

(Ref: Goodman Gilman 12th E/P287)

146. Ans. (a) Prazosin

(Ref: Goodman Gilman 12th E/P307)

147. Ans. (a) Dilation of bronchioles

(Ref: Goodman Gilman 12th E/P291)

148. Ans. (a) β1 receptors

(Ref: Goodman Gilman 12th E/P290)

149. Ans. (a) Esmolol

(Ref: Goodman Gilman 12th E/P313)

Mnemonics

Selective β_1 Blockers

My : Metoprolol
B : Betaxolol, Bisoprolol
E : Esmolol
T : aTenolol
A : Acebutalol
O, N : NebivOlol
Ce : Celiprolol

150. Ans. (a) Ritodrine

(Ref: Goodman Gilman 12th E/P294)

151. Ans. (c) Decrease in the production of aqueous humor

(Ref: Goodman Gilman 12th E/P1787)

152. Ans. (a) Timolol

(Ref: Goodman Gilman 12th E/P1787)

- Beta blocker like timolol by blocking beta 2 receptors can precipitate bronchial asthma.

153. Ans. (a) Ephedrine

(Ref: Goodman Gilman 12th E/P300)

154. Ans. (b) Betaxolol

(Ref: Goodman Gilman 12th E/P 313)

155. Ans. (b) Ergotamine

(Ref: Goodman Gilman 12th E/P348)

- Ergotamine at low doses produce α agonistic and at high doses α antagonistic effect.
- Hence it can cause both vasoconstriction and vasodilation depending on the dose.

156. Ans. (b) Asthma

(Ref: Goodman Gilman 12th E/P293)

157. Ans. (d) Nebivolol

(Ref: Goodman Gilman 12th E/P304)

158. Ans. (d) Timolol

(Ref: Goodman Gilman 12th E/P313)

Beta blockers with membrane stabilizing or local anaesthetic effect
Can : Carvedilol Blow : Betaxolol L : Labetalol A : Acebutalol M : Metoprolol P : Propranolol and Pindolol

159. Ans. (a) Renal vasodilatory effect

(Ref: Goodman Gilman 12th E/P301)

- Though dopamine has all actions mentioned in options a, b and c, it is more preferred in CHF and shock because of its vasodilatory effect due to D_1 agonism that preserves the renal function.

160. Ans. (c) Ephedrine

(Ref: Goodman Gilman 12th E/P300)

- Ephedrine is given by oral route, has a longer duration of action (6 hours). By increasing NE release, it increases both systolic and diastolic blood pressure.
- Epinephrine and dopamine have very short half-lives i.e. in minutes.

161. Ans. (d) Prazosin

(Ref: Harrison 19th E/P2748)

Treatment of Scorpion Sting

- Continuous IV midazolam for sedative effect
- Vasodilators like prazosin, nitroprusside, nifedipine and hydralazine for hypertension and pulmonary edema

162. Ans. (b) Variant angina

(Ref: Goodman Gilman 12th E/P316)

- Nonselective beta blockers like propranolol inhibit beta-2 mediated vasodilation and can cause vasospasm.
- Hence this class is contraindicated in variant angina.

163. Ans. (a) 120 seconds

(Ref: Goodman Gilman 12th E/P290)

164. Ans. (c) COPD

(Ref: Goodman Gilman 12th E/P316)

165. Ans. (a) Adrenaline

(Ref: Goodman Gilman 12th E/P283)

166. Ans. (a) VMA

(Ref: Goodman Gilman 12th E/P286)

167. Ans. (a) Methylation

(Ref: Goodman Gilman 12th E/P286)

In the adrenal gland cells, NE is **methylated** into epinephrine by phenylethanolamine-N-methyltranserase, which is activated by cortisol.

168. Ans. (b) Beta blocker

(Ref: Goodman Gilman 12th E/P313)

169. Ans. (a) Carvedilol

(Ref: Goodman Gilman 12th E/P315)

170. Ans. (d) All of the above

(Ref: Goodman Gilman 12th E/P296)

171. Ans. (d) Pindolol

(Ref: Goodman Gilman 12th E/P313)

Beta blockers with intrinsic agonistic effect
C : Carteolol, Celiprolol
L : Labetalol
A : Acebutolol
P : Pindolol, Penbutolol

172. Ans. (a) Ephedrine

(Ref: Goodman Gilman 12th E/P300)

173. Ans. (b) Cardiac output

(Ref: Goodman Gilman 12th E/P290)

174. Ans. (b) Dopamine

(Ref: Goodman Gilman 12th E/P288)

175. Ans. (b) Glucagon

(Ref: Goodman Gilman 12th E/P317)

176. Ans. (a) Centrally acting α_{2a} agonist

(Ref: Goodman Gilman 12th E/P201)

- Dexmedetomidine is an α_2 agonist which causes sedation by acting primarily on the α_{2a} subtype.

177. Ans. (c) Alpha 2 antagonist

(Ref: Goodman Gilman 12th E/P309)

178. Ans. (d) Sick sinus syndrome

(Ref: Goodman Gilman 12th E/P309)

179. Ans. (a) Increased stroke volume, (d) Renal vasodilation and (e) Increased heart rate

(Ref: Goodman Gilman 13th E/P198)

- At doses >0 to 2 mcg/kg D1 receptor stimulation causes renal vasodilation.
- At doses >2 to 10 mcg/kg beta 1 receptor stimulation increases stroke volume and heart rate.
- At doses >10 mcg/kg alpha1 stimulation causes vasoconstriction.

180. Ans. (c) Olodaterol, (d) Vilanterol and (e) Indacaterol

(Ref: Katzung 13th E/P148)

Ultralong acting Beta 2 agonists:

- Carmoterol
- Indacaterol
- Vilanterol
- Olodaterol

181. Ans. (a) Bronchial asthma, (b) Allergic disorder, (c) Cardio-pulmonary resuscitation, (d) Anaphylaxis

(Ref: Goodman Gilman 12th E/P287)

Uses of adrenaline

- Bronchial asthma
- Allergic reaction including anaphylaxis
- Cardiopulmonary resuscitation: In cardiac arrest
- Vasoconstrictor: Topical hemostatic agent and along with local anesthetics
- Post intubation and infectious croup
- Glaucoma

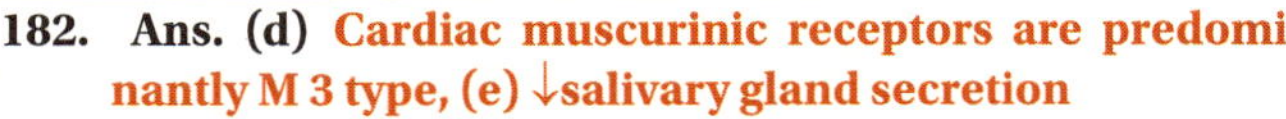

182. Ans. (d) Cardiac muscurinic receptors are predominantly M 3 type, (e) ↓salivary gland secretion

(Ref: Goodman Gilman 12th E/P178-79)

183. Ans. (c) Increase systolic BP, (e) Renal vasoconstriction

(Ref: Goodman Gilman 12th E/P283,287)

184. Ans. (c) Ciliary muscle contraction, (d) Contraction of circular muscle of iris, (e) Detrusor muscle contraction

(Ref: Goodman Gilman 12th E/178-79)

185. Ans. (c) Half-life is about 2 min

(Ref: Goodman Gilman 12th E/P290)

- Dobutamine has a half-life of 2 minutes, hence it is given by continuous IV infusion.
- It is is an agonist at β_1 and β_2 receptors.
- β_2 mediated vasodilation causes a decrease in ventricular filling pressure.

186. Ans. (a) Neostigmine, (c) Edrophonium, (e) Malathion

(Ref: Goodman Gilman 12th E/P242)

187. Ans. (c) Atenolol, (d) Nebivolol, (e) Betaxolol

(Ref: Goodman Gilman 12th E/P313)

188. Ans. (a) Piloerection, (b) Urine retention, (d) Pupillary dilation, (e) Bronchodilation

(Ref: Goodman Gilman 12th E/P178,179)

189. Ans. (d) Celiprolol, (e) Acebutolol

(Ref: Goodman Gilman 12th E/P313)

190. Ans. (e) Tyrosine

(Ref: Goodman Gilman 12th E/P194)

191. Ans. (a) Penetrate cornea, (c) Shorter duration of action than atropine, (d) Cross Brain-blood barrier, (e) Used in motion sickness

(Ref: Goodman Gilman 12th E/P194)

- Scopolamine is a tertiary amine i.e. lipid soluble and hence can cross blood brain barrier or biological membranes like cornea.
- It is derived form a plant called as Hyoscyamus niger.
- It is the drug of choice for motion sickness.
- Atropine is longest acting anticholinergics, scopolamine is shorter acting.

192. Ans. (b) Atenolol, (c) Metoprolol

(Ref: Goodman Gilman 12th E/P313)

193. Ans. (a) Relief of spasticity/muscular spasm, (c) Terminal cancer pain, (d) Conscious sedation in intubated ICU patients

(Ref: Goodman Gilman 12th E/P296)

Mnemonics

Uses of Clonidine

- **C :** Cl^- absorption treats diarrhoea of DM
- **H :** Hypertension
- **A :** Analgesic in terminal cancer patients
- **M :** Menopausal hot flashes, Migraine prophylaxis
- **A :** ADHD
- **T :** Tics associated with Tourette's syndrome
- **K :** Kills dependence on alcohol, smoking and opioids
- **A :** Atrial fibrillation
- **R :** Restless leg syndrome

194. Ans. (a) Membrane stability, (b) Used in glaucoma, (e) Have intrinsic sympathomimetic effect,

(Ref: Goodman Gilman 12th E/P313)

195. Ans. (a) Atropine, (c) Glucagon, (e) Isoprenaline

(Ref: Goodman Gilman 12th E/P313)

Treatment of β blocker toxicity

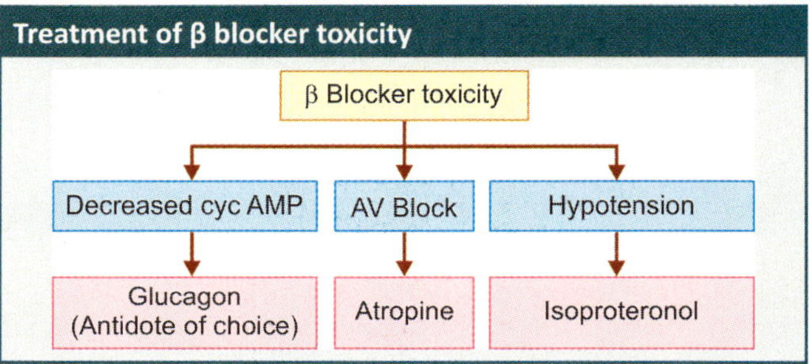

196. Ans. (a) Oxybutynin, (b) Tolterodine, (d) Solifenacin, (e) Imipramine

(Ref: Goodman Gilman 12th E/P231)

197. Ans. (a) More α_1 selective, (b) Less S/E, (d) Once daily dosing

(Ref: Goodman Gilman 12th E/P309)

198. Ans. (a) Portal hypertension, (c) Anxiety, (d) HOCM

(Ref: Goodman Gilman 12th E/P317-319)

199. Ans. (a) Labetalol, (b) Carvedilol

(Ref: Goodman Gilman 12th E/P313)

200. Ans. (e) Causes bradycardia

(Ref: Goodman Gilman 12th E/P313)

201. Ans. (d) BPH

(Ref: Goodman Gilman 12th E/P296)

- **Clonidine can improve cardiac ischemia associated with MI as well.**

202. Ans. (a) Hemicholinium: prevents the release of Ach, from storage vesicle, (b) Botulinum, increase the Ach release, (d) Vesamicol inhibit the uptake of choline

(Ref: Goodman Gilman 12th E/P309)

203. Ans. (a) Asthma, (b) Heart block

(Ref: Goodman Gilman 12th E/P319)

204. Ans. (a) Pindolol, (e) Acebutolol

(Ref: Goodman Gilman 12th E/P313)

205. Ans. (a) Beta 3 agonist

(Ref: Goodman Gilman 13th E/P202)

- Mirabegron is a beta 3 agonist approved for treatment of urge incontinence (detrusor instability or overactive bladder).
- Anticholinergics are the drug of choice for same and mirabegron is used as an addon drug.
- Side effects associated are headache, hypertension and urinary tract infection.
- It is an enzyme inhibitor (CYP2D6) and hence can inhibit metabolism of drugs like beta blockers, anti-depressants (SSRI, TCA), digoxin and opioids.

206. Ans. (d) Midodrine

(Ref: Goodman Gilman 13th E/P202)

- Hypotension in early morning period i.e. when patient gets up from bed indicates towards postural hypotension.
- Midodrine and alpha 1 agonist is the vasopressor of choice for treatment of postural hypotension.
- The drug preferred for long term management however is fludrocortisone and is the drug of choice for same.

207. Ans. (d) Bucindolol

(Ref: Goodman Gilman 13th E/P218)

208. Ans. (b) Atomoxetine

(Ref: Katzung 13th E/P149)

- Stimulants like amphetamine and methylphenidate have potential for abuse and patients of ADHD are at increased risk of substance abuse. Hence both should not be used in patients of ADHD with a family history of ADHD.
- Thus in these patients atomoxetine is preferred.

209. Ans. (b) K channel

(Ref: Katzung 12th E/P124)

Tetraethylammonium is a ganglionic blocking agent which is currently used only as a research agent that selectively blocks potassium channel.

210. Ans. (a) Valbenazine

(Ref: Goodman Gilman 13th E/P291, CMDT 2018/P1082)

- Valbenazine is a VMAT 2 (Vesicular Monoamine Transporter 2) inhibitor, which acts by inhibiting release of catecholamines into the synapse.
- It has been approved in 2017 for treatment of tardive dyskinesia in adults.

211. Ans. (a) Inhibits VMAT

(Ref: Goodman Gilman 12th E/P436)

Inhibitors of VMAT

- Reserpine
- Tetrabenazine
- Deutetrabenazine
- Valbenazine

212. Ans. (b) Carbamazepine

(Ref: CMDT 2018/P1027)

- Clonidine and guanfacine are the current drug of choice for treatment of tics associated with Tourette syndrome. Guanfacine is more preferred due to once daily dosing and lesser sedation.
- Atypical antipsychotics like risperidone can be tried in patients not responding to clonidine and guanfacine.
- Finally if above drugs are not effective or it is a case of severe tics then the drug of choice becomes typical antipsychotics like haloperidol, pimozide and fluphenazine.
- Other drugs that can be used are clonazepam, verapamil, nifedipine, tetrabenazine and botulinum toxin.
- Carbamazepine worsens tics associated with Tourette syndrome.

213. Ans. (a) Nebivolol

(Ref: Goodman Gilman 12th E/P330)

Antioxidant Effect is seen with:

- Cardioselective beta blocker: Nebivolol
- Nonselective beta blocker: Carvedilol

214. Ans. (a) Glucagon

(Ref: Goodman Gilman 12th E/P86)

- Beta blocker decrease cyclic AMP and glucagon being a source for cyclic AMP is used as an antidote for treatment of beta blocker toxicity.

215. Ans. (c) Propranolol

(Ref: Goodman Gilman 12th E/P320)

216. Ans. (a) Glycopyrrolate

(Ref: Goodman Gilman 12th E/P234)

217. Ans. (b) Carvedilol

(Ref: Goodman Gilman 12th E/P329)

Antioxidant effect is seen with beta-blockers like

- Carvedilol
- Nebivolol

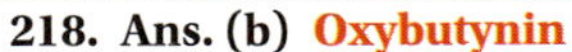

218. Ans. (b) Oxybutynin

(Ref: Goodman Gilman 12th E/P232)

- Flavoxate and fesoterodine are not used nowadays due to toxicity.
- Among the remaining drugs the order of preference based on toxicity profile is darifenacin > solifenacin > trospium > tolterodine > oxybutynin.
- Since among the drugs currently used oxybutynin is most toxic, transdermal formulations in the form of patch and gel are available.

219. Ans. (d) Scopolamine

(Ref: Goodman Gilman 12th E/P233)

- Scopolamine is used for narcoanalysis and is also known as truth serum.
- The drug of choice for narcoanalysis is thiopental sodium though.

220. Ans. (a) Postural hypotension

(Ref: Goodman Gilman 12th E/P316)

Postural hypotension is caused by drugs which can dilate veins i.e. with venodilators and mixed dilators like nitrates, nitroprusside, ACE inhibitors, ARBs and DRIs.

221. Ans. (a) Beta blocker

(Ref: Goodman Gilman 12th E/P316)

222. Ans. (b) Rebound tachycardia

(Ref: Goodman Gilman 12th E/P316)

223. Ans. (d) Tizanidine

(Ref: Goodman Gilman 12th E/P297)

224. Ans. (d) Formoterol

(Ref: Goodman Gilman 12th E/P321-33)

225. Ans. (b) Guanadrel

(Ref: Goodman Gilman 12th E/P299)

- Guanethidine and guanadrel are NE depletors and hence at continuous doses can decrease NE in the synapse and hence are beneficial in hypertension.
- Initial release of NE can worsen pheochromocytoma and hence are contraindicated in same. Postural hypotension is a persistent side effect seen due to sympathetic blockade even on chronic administration.

226. Ans. (c) Acetylcholine

(Ref: Goodman Gilman 12th E/P191)

The neurotransmitter in postganglionic sympathetic fibers is NE, except in:

- Adrenal glands - Ach
- Sweat glands - Ach
- Renal blood vessels - Dopamine

227. Ans. (d) Bisoprolol

(Ref: Goodman Gilman 12th E/P328)

Most cardioselective beta blocker is nebivolol > bisoprolol.

228. Ans. (c) Decrease abuse potential

(Ref: Goodman Gilman 12th E/P1338)

- Diphenoxylate is an opioid used for treatment of nonsecretory diarrhea.
- Atropine is combined with it to prevent abuse.

229. Ans. (a) Vasomotor center

(Ref: Goodman Gilman 12th E/P295)

230. Ans. (b) Midodrine

(Ref: Goodman Gilman 12th E/P295)

231. Ans. (a) General anesthesia

(Ref: Goodman Gilman 12th E/P296)

- Dexmedetomidine is also a central α_2 agonist used as preanesthetic medication like clonidine.
- The beneficial effect for surgery are sedation, anxiolysis, analgesia and decreased secretions.

232. Ans. (c) 1 gm

(Ref: Goodman Gilman 12th E/P248)

- For treatment of nicotinic symptoms pralidoxime is used at dose of 1–2 mg by IV route in less than 5 minutes time.
- If symptoms don't improve in 20-60 minutes, the dose is repeated.

233. Ans. (d) Atropine

(Ref: Goodman Gilman 12th E/P232)

234. Ans. (d) α2-agonist

(Ref: Goodman Gilman 12th E/P295)

235. Ans. (d) Stimulation of beta-2 receptors

(Ref: Goodman Gilman 12th E/P189)

Dale's Phenomenon

Epinephrine when administered initially raises blood pressure due to α_1 followed by a decrease in blood pressure due to β_2; this **biphasic pattern** of blood pressure is called as Dale's phenomenon. If patient is given epinephrine being on α blocker, then only vasodilation is seen due to β_2; this effect is known as vasomotor reversal of dale.

Practice Questions

236. A patient was given a placebo and a drug, which produced effects as given in the picture. The drug is

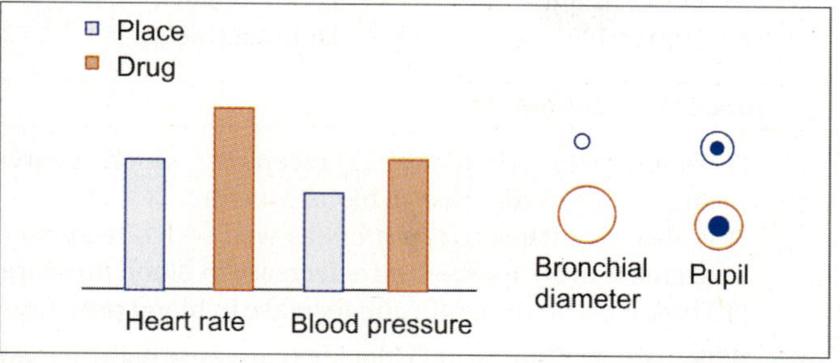

a. Isoproterenol b. Atropine
c. Epinephrine d. Norepinephrine

Ans. (c) Epinephrine

- The drug causes an increase in heart rate and hence it cannot be norepinephrine, which causes a decrease in heart rate.
- The drug causes a significant increase in blood pressure which cannot be seen with atropine.
- The drug causes mydriasis, which cannot be seen with isoproterenol.
- Hence the drug is atropine which has all the effects mentioned in the picture.

237. At high doses epinephrine's effect is similar to

a. Isoproterenol b. Dobutamine
c. Dopamine d. Norepinephrine

Ans (d) Norepinephrine

- At high doses epinephrine is more active at alpha-1 receptors and hence cause more vasoconstriction like norepinephrine and reflex bradycardia.

238. The heart rate and blood pressure tracing of two drugs A and B are given in the picture below. The drugs A and B are respectively

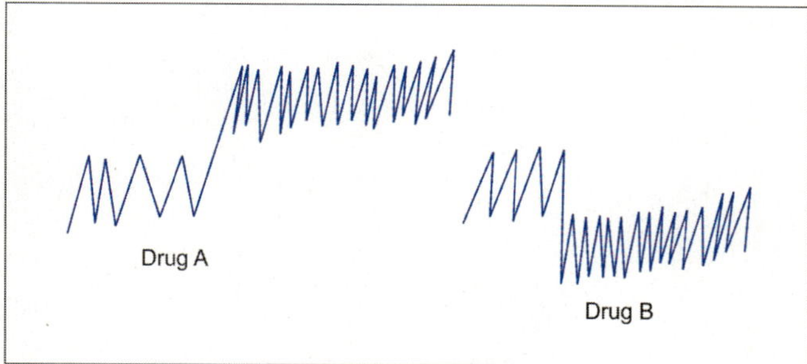

a. Epinephrine and Norepinephrine
b. Dobutamine and Epinephrine
c. Epinephrine and Isoproterenol
d. Norepinephrine and Epinephrine

Ans. (c) Epinephrine and Isoproterenol

- In the case of drug A there is an increase in blood pressure as the graph shifted up from baseline and there is an increase in heart rate as the tracings have come closer. Thus, there is an increase in blood pressure and heart rate. This can be seen with epinephrine but not norepinephrine as it causes bradycardia.
- In case of drug B similarly there is a decrease in blood pressure but an increase in heart rate, which can be seen with isoproterenol. Both epinephrine and norepinephrine will not cause a decrease in blood pressure.
- Hence the answer is epinephrine and isoproterenol.

239. The drug A given in the picture has the following effect on blood pressure and heart rate as given in the tracing below. The drug is

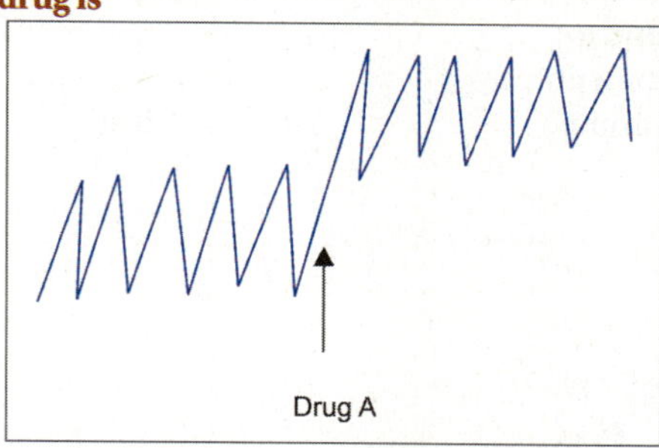

a. Isoproterenol b. Epinephrine
c. Phenylephrine d. Norepinephrine

Ans. (c) Phenylephrine

- In the tracing given in the picture there is an increase in blood pressure as it has shifted up from the base line.
- There is no change in heart rate as the distance between tracings remain same.
- Hence this drug A which causes only an increase in blood pressure is phenylephrine.

240. The beta blocker with anti-inflammatory effect is

a. Labetalol b. Carvedilol
c. Metoprolol d. Nebivolol

Ans. (b) Carvedilol

241. A new drug effect was compared as compared to placebo in phase I trial in healthy volunteers. The effect of the new drug is predominantly on which receptors

	Placebo	New
BP	120/80	100/50
HR	70/mm	110/mm

a. α_1 and α_2
b. β_1 and β_2
c. α_1, α_2 and β_1
d. α_2 and β_2

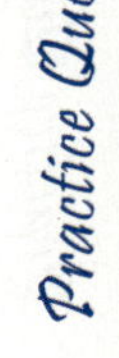

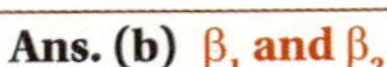

Ans. (b) β_1 **and** β_2

- The new drug is causing a greater decrease in diastolic blood pressure as compared to systolic blood pressure. This is because of vasodilation by β2 receptors decreasing diastolic blood pressure. Systolic blood pressure is maintained by β_1 effect.
- There is a significant increase in heart rate, which is seen both because of direct effect on β_1 and reflex tachycardia due to vasodilation by β_2.

242. Which of the following drug can cause mydriasis without any effect on accommodation?

a. Atropine
b. Tropicamide
c. Ephedrine
d. Pilocarpine

Ans. (c) Ephedrine

- Mydriasis can be caused by both sympathomimetics and parasympatholytics but cycloplegia is caused by only parasympatholytics.
- Hence, ephedrine being a sympathomimetic is the answer among the options.

243. A patient with denervation of radial muscle will not respond to

a. Epinephrine
b. Phenylephrine
c. Atropine
d. Ephedrine

Ans. (d) Ephedrine

- Denervated radial muscles do not respond to indirectly acting sympathomimetics like ephedrine and amphetamine.

244. A drug is administered to a patient which decreases blood pressure significantly due to its action on D_1 **and** α_2 **receptors. The drug is**

a. Dopexamine
b. Fenoldopam
c. Dopamine
d. Dobutamine

Ans. (b) Fenoldopam

- Fenoldopam stimulates D_1 receptors which causes diuresis and a decrease in blood pressure.
- It also stimulates α_2 receptors as well which leads to a decrease in NE release and a decrease in blood pressure.
- Thus, it causes a significant decrease in blood pressure.

245. Which of the following beta blockers can cause nightmares?

a. Sotalol
b. Pindolol
c. Nadolol
d. Betaxolol

Ans. (b) Pindolol

Pindolol being a lipid soluble drug can cross blood brain barrier and cause central side effects like nightmares and seizures.

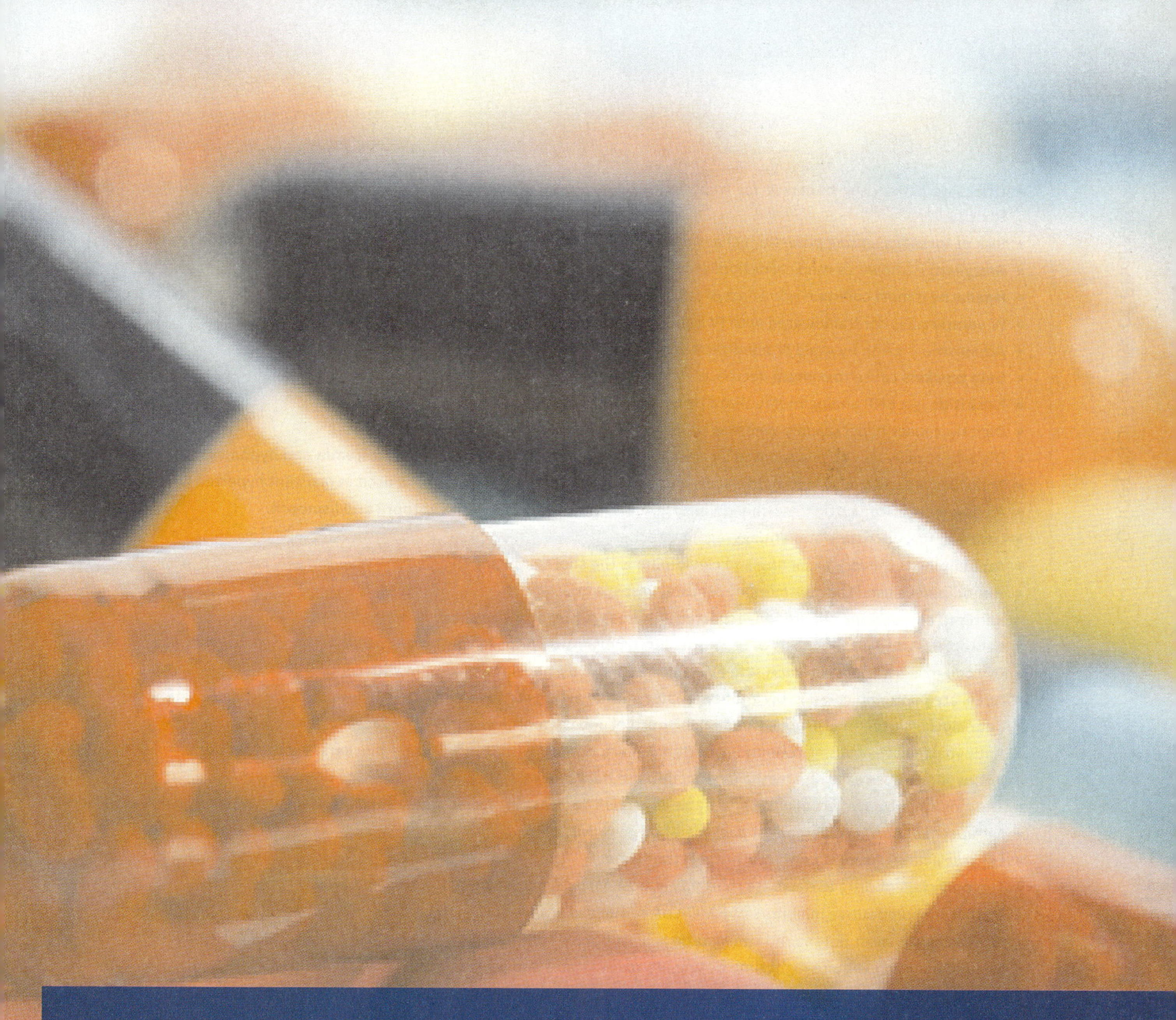

Cardiovascular System

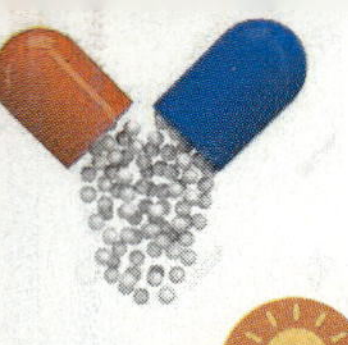

One Liners

- **Lidocaine** is the drug of choice for treatment of **ventricular arrhythmia** caused by myocardial infarction **(MI)** and **digitalis toxicity**.
- Risk of **torsades** among potassium channel blockers is **maximum with ibutilide** and **minimum with amiodarone**.
- **Bretylium** is known as medical defibrillator.
- **Headache** is most common side effect of calcium channel blockers (**CCBs**), followed by ankle edema and constipation (verapamil).
- **IV verapamil** is contraindicated with **IV beta blockers** due to risk of **conduction block**.
- **Adenosine** is given by rapid IV administration.
- **Beta blockers** cause maximum decrease in mortality in patients of congestive heart failure (CHF).
- **Nesiritide** is a BNP analog metabolized by **neutral endopeptidase**.
- Digitalis causes hyperkalemia whereas hypokalemia causes digitalis toxicity.
- Digitalis toxicity can be precipitated by **myocardial ischemia**, **hypokalemia**, **hypercalcemia** and **hypomagnesemia.**
- **Thiazides** are used in mild to moderate hypertension whereas spironolactone is used in resistant hypertension.
- All angiotensin-converting enzyme inhibitors (ACEIs) are prodrugs except **captopril** and **lisinopril**.
- **Losartan** has **uricosuric** and **antiaggregant** effect.
- **Amlodipine** is the longest acting and **clevidipine** is the shortest acting DHP.
- **Nimodipine** is used for treatment of **cerebral vasospasm**.
- **Ramipril and perindopril are longest acting** whereas **captropil** is the **shortest acting** ACEI.
- **Captopril** is used for **diagnosis of renovascular hypertension** prior to confirmation with renal angiography.
- **Dry cough** is the most common side effect of ACEIs and **dysgeusia** is maximum with **captopril**.
- **ACEIs** are contraindicated in **pregnancy**, **bilateral renal artery stenosis** and **single kidney with renal artery stenosis**.
- Beta blockers used in CHF are **carvedilol**, **bisoprolol** and **metoprolol**.
- Antihypertensives causing rebound hypertension are **clonidine** (maximum), **beta blockers** and **methyl dopa**.
- Antihypertensives causing **erectile dysfunction** are **beta blockers**, **thiazides** and **methyl dopa**.
- The most important effect of nitrates in stable angina is a **decrease in cardiac preload** and in variant angina is coronary vasodilation.
- Nitrate that doesn't undergo first pass metabolism is **IMN**.
- Longest acting nitrate is **pentaerythritol tetranitrate**.
- The only class of drug to decrease mortality in post MI patients are **beta blockers** and ACEI.
- Statins are competitive inhibitors of **HMG-CoA reductase**.
- **Pitavastatin** is most potent and **simvastatin** is least potent statin.
- Statins that don't require night time dosing are **rosuvastatin** and **atorvastatin**.
- HMG-CoA reductase is indirectly stimulated by **bile acid binding resins**.
- **Niacin** causes a maximum increase in **HDL** and is the only drug to decrease **lipoprotein(a)**.
- Fibrates stimulate **PPAR alpha** receptors and increase **lipoprotein lipase synthesis**.
- **Ezetimibe** inhibits **cholesterol absorption** by inhibiting **NPC1L1 (Niemann Pick C1 Like 1) protein** in the intestine.

ANTIARRHYTHMIC DRUGS

PHYSIOLOGY OF CARDIAC ACTION POTENTIAL

The resting membrane potential in a myocardial cell is -90 mV. The depolarization begins with opening of sodium channel and the rise of action potential is phase 0, followed by phase 1 notch caused by opening of potassium channels (early outward rectifiers). In phase 2 inward calcium channels open which maintain depolarization and give rise to plateau phase. As calcium channels closes and potassium channels open, again (delayed outward rectifier), phase 3 begins giving rise to repolarization, which brings the cell to resting membrane potential in phase 4.

The SA and AV nodes are significantly different as the resting membrane potential is -60 mV and depolarization is primarily by calcium and not sodium. Immediately after hyperpolarization an inward Na/K channel is activated termed as h (since it is after hyperpolarization) or of (funny because of its nature) channel. This initiates depolarization which is continued and completed by opening of calcium channels.

Conceptual Box-1

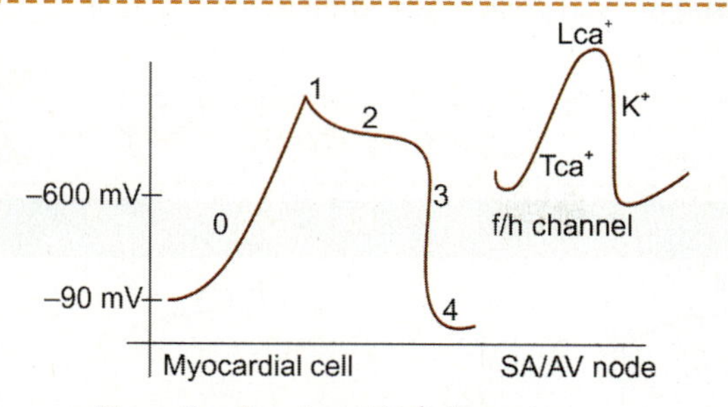

Phase 0 = Opening of Na^+ channels
Phase 1 = Opening of K^+ channels
Phase 2 = Opening of ca^{++} channels
Phase 3 = Opening of K^+ channels
Phase 4 = Return to resting membrane potential

CONCEPT OF ARRHYTHMIA TREATMENT

Conceptual Box-2

A patient of tachyarrhythmia with a heart rate of 200 beats/minute was advised for an ECG. A definite length of ECG paper having four graphs was taken.

ECG-1

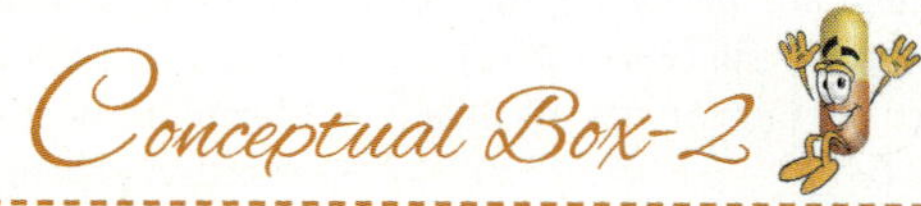

After treating the patient, the heart rate came down to 100 beats/minute and then again, an ECG was advised. Now if we take the same length of ECG paper, how many graphs will we be having? The answer is two. So, what we need to understand is how to make two graphs out of four or one out of two. That is explained in the graph below.

Contd...

Conceptual Box-2

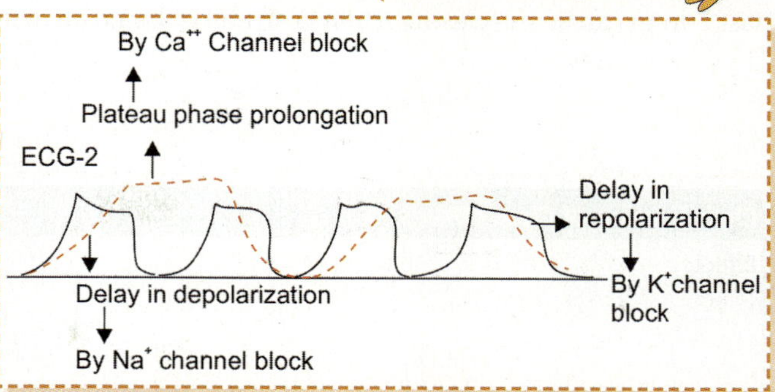

CLASSIFICATION OF ANTIARRHYTHMIC DRUGS

As it was derived in the conceptual box, antiarrhythmic effect can be obtained by blocking sodium, potassium and calcium channels and beta one receptors. These four classes of drugs fall under Vaughan William's classification of antiarrhythmic drugs. Apart from these miscellaneous classes includes drugs like adenosine, magnesium sulphate and digoxin.

Conceptual Box-3

Tip to remember class of antiarrhythmic drugs: Correlate with physiological location of ions and beta one receptor.

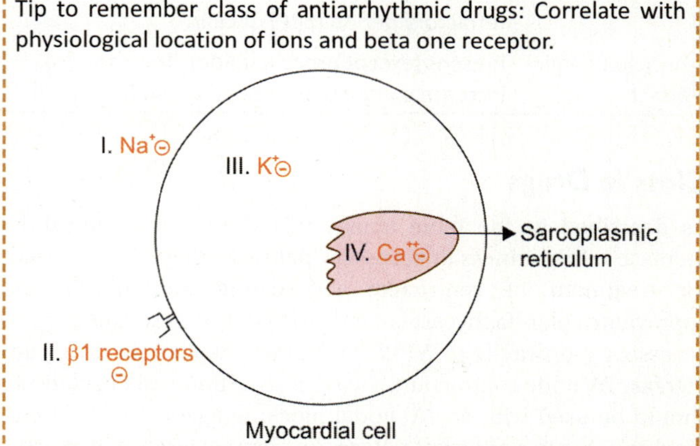

Classification of Antiarrhythmic Drugs

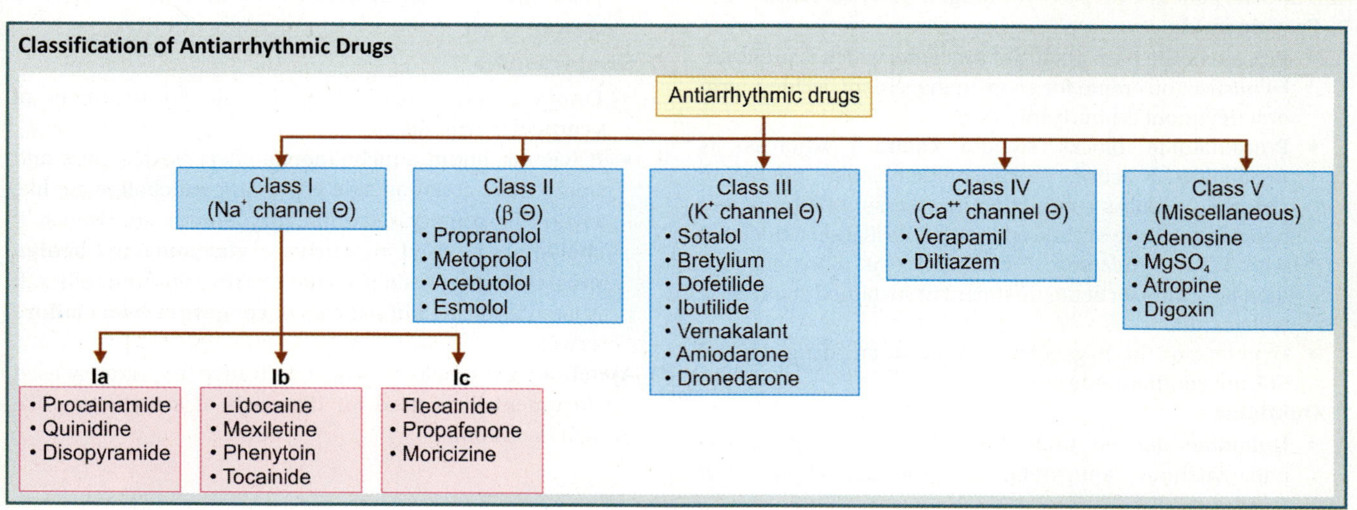

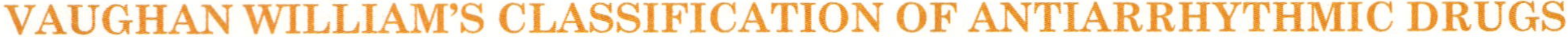

VAUGHAN WILLIAM'S CLASSIFICATION OF ANTIARRHYTHMIC DRUGS

Class I: Sodium Channel Blockers

Class I drugs can be sub classified into Ia, Ib and Ic, based on their effect on sodium and potassium channels.

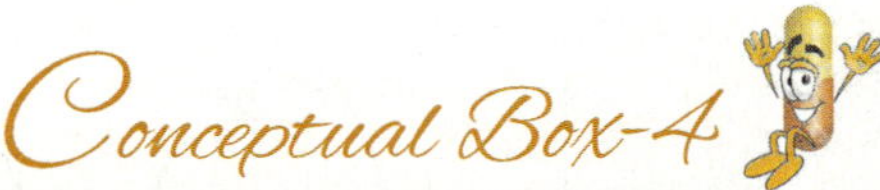

Classification of Class I Drugs			
Effects	Ia QT ↑ ed	Ib QT ↓ ed	Ic QT normal
Na channel	Blocked in **open state** for intermediate duration, as recovery time is 1–10 sec. Thus, the effects seen are: • Inhibition of conduction in normal cells and accessory pathways and increases effective refractory period (ERP) of cells. • Intermediate decrease in rate of rise of action potential (V_{max}). • Increase in AV node conduction due to anticholinergic effect	Blocked in **closed state** for minimum duration, as recovery time is <1 sec. Thus, the effects seen are: • Inhibition of conduction in tissue with slow conduction, i.e. in ischemic tissue (cells are partly depolarized and channels are in closed state). • No effect on rate of rise of action potential (V_{max}). • No effect on AV node conduction	Blocked in **open state** for maximum duration, as recovery time is >10 sec. Thus, the effects seen are: • Maximum inhibition of conduction in normal cells and accessory pathways and increases effective refractory period (ERP) of cells. • Maximum decrease in rate of rise of action potential (V_{max}). • Decrease in AV node conduction
K channel	Blocked: This increases action potential duration (APD) and increases effective refractory period (ERP) of cells.	Opened: This decreases APD	Negligible effect
Anticholinergic Effect	Present (except procainamide): This can increase conduction through AV node	Nil	Nil

Class Ia Drugs

As described in the table above, this class can significantly increase refractoriness in accessory pathway, they are indicated for treatment of ventricular tachycardia and fibrillation, supraventricular tachycardia and arrhythmia associated with accessory pathway (e.g. WPW syndrome). As class Ia drug can increase AV node conduction, if used in atrial flutter or fibrillation, should be used with an AV nodal blocking agent (CCB or beta blocker). Due to significant potassium channel block it increases APD and the patient is at risk of **prolonged QT syndrome**.

- **Procainamide**
  - Procainamide is an analog of procaine, which is preferred by intravenous route for acute management, as long-term oral treatment is poorly tolerated.
  - Procainamide blocks sodium channel, whereas its metabolite N-acetyl procainamide blocks potassium channel. It blocks conduction in accessory pathway and hence is the drug of choice for atrial fibrillation associated with **WPW syndrome**. Procainamide is more effective than lidocaine for acute treatment of sustained ventricular tachycardia.
  - Hypotension due to ganglionic blockade and drug induced SLE are common side effects.
- **Quinidine**
  - Quinidine derived from bark of cinchona plant has antiarrhythmic, antipyretic and antimalarial effect. It is used to maintain sinus rhythm in atrial flutter and fibrillation.
  - Most common side effect seen is **diarrhoea**, whereas most specific side effect is **cinchonism**, which is dose dependent as it improves with decrease in dose. High doses of quinidine can precipitate **ventricular tachycardia**. Hypotension can be seen due to alpha receptor blockade. It can also cause thrombocytopenia.
  - Unlike other drugs of this class, quinidine can cause **QT prolongation even at therapeutic and subtherapeutic doses**.
- **Disopyramide:**
  - Disopyramide is used by oral route for treatment of ventricular arrhythmia.
  - It has maximum anticholinergic effect in this class and hence most common side effects are anticholinergic like mydriasis, urinary retention, dry mouth etc. Hence it should not be used in patients of **glaucoma** and **benign prostate hyperplasia**. As it has negative inotropic effect, it is contraindicated in patients of **congestive heart failure** as well.
- **Ajmaline:** Ajmaline is rauwolfia derivative that is rarely used for treatment. It is used for diagnosis of arrhythmias like Brugada syndrome.

Class Ib Drugs

The class Ib drugs which block sodium channels mostly in closed state, that is seen in case of ischemia and digitalis toxicity and hence are preferred for treatment of **ventricular arrhythmia associated with myocardial infarction** and **digitalis induced arrhythmia**. This class has no effect on atrial cells (atrial cells have short action potential and channels remain in closed state for a very short period) and on accessory pathways. Since these drugs cause early opening of potassium channel, short QT interval can be seen.

- **Lidocaine**
  - Lidocaine undergoes a **high first pass metabolism** and hence for systemic use it is given by intravenous route. The **volume of distribution is high** and hence a loading dose is administered.
  - Lidocaine is the drug of choice for treatment of **digitalis and MI induced ventricular tachyarrhythmia**. It is **not effective in supraventricular arrhythmias** as it has no effect on atrial cells.
  - Higher dose of lidocaine is required in patients of myocardial infarction due to increased alpha-1 acid glycoproteinto which lidocaine binds. Dose is decreased in case of CHF and hepatic disorder due to decreased volume of distribution and clearance respectively.
  - Dose dependent neurological side effects are most commonly seen e.g. paresthesia, seizures, tremor, delirium, stupor, nystagmus (earliest sign of toxicity). Malignant hyperthermia can also be seen but on rare occasions. For treatment of seizures phenytoin is not used, rather benzodiazepines like diazepam is preferred.
- **Mexiletine**
  - Mexiletine is an analog of lidocaine developed to have lesser first pass metabolism. Hence, it is used by oral route for treatment of ventricular tachycardia. Other off label uses of mexiletine are for treatment of painful **sensory neuropathy** and myotonia.
  - Commonly associated side effects are nausea and tremor, which can be reduced with drug intake with food.
- **Phenytoin:** Phenytoin is an antiepileptic which is effective for treatment of **digitalis induced atrial and ventricular arrhythmia**, as the cells are in closed state due to depolarization. It is less effective for arrhythmia associated with ischemic tissue.
- **Tocainide:** Tocainide is also an analog of lidocaine, which is less preferred because of serious side effects like agranulocytosis, pulmonary fibrosis and conversion of ventricular tachycardia to fibrillation.

Class Ic Drugs

This class causes a maximum increase in refractoriness in normal cells and accessory pathway along with a delay in AV node conduction. Hence, these drugs are preferred for treatment of life threatening ventricular arrhythmia (tachycardia and fibrillation) and refractory supraventricular tachycardia. These drugs are contraindicated in patients with structural heart disease and myocardial infarction due to risk of proarrhythmic effect.

- **Flecainide:** Flecainide though can be used for treatment of arrhythmia mentioned above, its use is limited by its proarrhythmic effect that can worsen ventricular arrhythmia or induce a new ventricular arrhythmia. It can be used for diagnosis of Brugada syndrome, as it can cause ST elevation in V_1 leads characteristic of same. It can worsen congestive heart failure and can also cause blurring of vision.
- **Propafenone:** Propafenone apart from blocking sodium channel is also a weak beta blocker and calcium channel blocker. The uses are again same as mentioned above.
- **Moricizine:** Moricizine is less preferred nowadays due to its less effectiveness and high mortality rate associated with its proarrhythmic effect.

Class II: Beta Blockers

- Beta blockers inhibit catecholamines mediated if current induced action potential by F or H channels, which constitutes the phase 4 depolarization in SA and AV nodes.
- The primary use of beta blockers is for treatment of SVT and PSVT as it induces AV block due to above mentioned effect. They are the drugs of choice for **rate control in atrial fibrillation**, where the aim is to maintain the ventricular rate below 100 beats/minute; **metoprolol** (stable patient) and **esmolol** (unstable patient) are the preferred agents.
- Other agents used for rate control are verapamil and digoxin; if patient does not respond to any of these then it is resistant atrial fibrillation that can be treated by **catheter ablation or pulmonary vein isolation**.
- Beta blockers are also drug of choice for **idiopathic ventricular tachycardia and ventricular premature beats.** Beta blockers are also used for treatment of arrhythmias associated with adrenergic excess (pheochromocytoma, exercise, emotion and cocaine) and anesthetic agents (cyclopropane and halothane).

Class III: Potassium Channel Blockers

Potassium channel blockers delay repolarization and hence increase action potential duration (APD) and cell refractoriness. Thus, these drugs are primarily used to make cells and accessory pathways refractory to stimulation in high rate life threatening arrhythmias of atrium and ventricles like atrial and ventricular fibrillation, atrial flutter and WPW syndrome. Prolongation of APD leads to a common side effect seen with this class i.e. **QT prolongation**, however torsades de pointes is rarely seen with **amiodarone** and most commonly seen with **ibutilide**.

Mnemonics

Potassium-Channel Blockers

Sundar : Sotalol
Black : Bretylium
D : Dofetilide, Dronedarone
I : Ibutilide
V : Vernakalant
A : Amiodarone

Amiodarone

- Amiodarone has high lipid solubility, which is responsible for its **high volume of distribution** (5000 liters) and hence

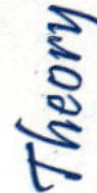

a loading dose of 800–1600 mg/day is given for many weeks to achieve steady state concentration. For same reason its concentration is 20 times more in heart and 300 times more in fat as compared to plasma. The average half-life is around 53 days and hence is the **longest acting antiarrhythmic**.

- Apart from blocking potassium channels, it also blocks sodium channels (in closed state), beta and alpha receptors and calcium channels. Hence, it is the antiarrhythmic with **most wide spectrum activity**. It is because of this wide spectrum effect that it is least associated with torsades de pointes.
- Oral route is preferred for treatment of recurrent ventricular tachycardia and fibrillation resistant to other antiarrhythmics and to maintain sinus rhythm in atrial fibrillation. Intravenous administration is reserved for termination of an acute attack of ventricular tachycardia or fibrillation. It is the preferred antiarrhythmic in **ACLS guidelines** for management of **cardiac arrest**.
- Being an analog of thyroid hormone, it has iodine which can cause thyroid related disorders. If it is given to patients living in euthyroid region, iodine inhibits release of thyroid hormones and causes hypothyroidism. However, if it is given to patients living in endemic iodine deficiency region, the iodine is taken up by thyroid and accelerated production of thyroid hormones causes hyperthyroidism. Since most patients live in euthyroid region, **hypothyroidism is more common than hyperthyroidism**.
- **Pulmonary fibrosis** is the most dangerous side effect which is common in case of associated lung disease, recent attack of pneumonia, oxygen therapy, male sex and a dose more than 400 mg/day. A decrease in DLCO is the earliest finding. Pathological study demonstrates destruction of **type II pneumocytes**.
- Hypotension is usually seen with IV administration (acute high dose toxicity) because of **myocardial suppression** and alpha block induced vasodilation.
- **Whorl like corneal microdeposits** (cornea verticillata) associated with amiodarone are usually **asymptomatic and reversible** on dose decrease or discontinuation of drug. The incidence is around 100% after six months of drug use.
- **Hepatotoxicity, peripheral neuropathy, photosensitivity,** bluish skin discoloration, and myocarditis can also be seen.

Mnemonics

Side Effects of Amiodarone

Potassium : Pulmonary fibrosis
Channel : Corneal microdeposits
Blocker : Blue colored skin
Makes : Myocarditis
Liver : Liver toxicity
Nerve : Neuropathy
And : Alpha receptor block causes hypotension
Skin : Photosensitivity
Toxic : Thyroid (Hypothyroidism > Hyperthyroidism)

Dronedarone

- Dronedarone is a derivative of amiodarone, which lacks the iodine molecule and hence is less toxic as compared to amiodarone. It is not only **less toxic** but also **less efficacious** than amiodarone. It is **shorter acting** than amiodarone and has a half-life of 24 hours.
- FDA has approved dronedarone for maintaining sinus rhythm and facilitate cardioversion in atrial fibrillation and flutter by oral route. **Food increases its absorption** and hence patient is advised to take dronedarone with food.
- It is absolutely contraindicated in pregnancy and breast feeding (as it is a **category X drug**) and **heart failure** (**black box warning**).

Recent Advances

Celivarone: It is a dronedarone derivative under trial for prevention of ventricular tachycardia.

Ibutilide

- Ibutilide has a high volume of distribution and high first pass metabolism (used by intravenous route only). Apart from blocking potassium channel, it **also activates an inward sodium current**, which contributes to refractoriness of cells.
- It is the drug of choice for treatment of an **acute attack of atrial fibrillation or flutter**. The treatment of choice is though **cardioversion** and ibutilide is used in case of unresponsiveness, as it significantly increases chances of a successful cardioversion. It is more effective in atrial flutter than fibrillation.
- Though QT prolongation is seen with all drugs of this class, the chances of **torsades de pointes is maximum with ibutilide**.

Clinical Box-1

Treatment and Prophylaxis of Atrial Fibrillation and Flutter

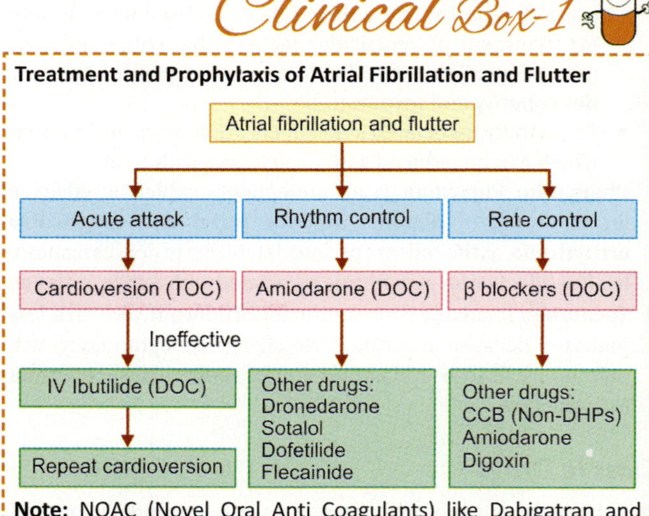

Note: NOAC (Novel Oral Anti Coagulants) like Dabigatran and Apixaban are the drugs of choice to prevent thrombosis in patients of atrial fibrillation.

Dofetilide

Dofetilide is used for treatment of acute attack as well as prophylaxis of atrial fibrillation and flutter by oral route. Since it is only potassium channel blocker, extra cardiac side effects are not seen. It has a bioavailability of 100%.

Sotalol

Sotalol is a racemic mixture, with both D and L isomers having potassium channel blocking effect, whereas only L isomer has beta blocking effect. It is an **orphan drug** approved for treatment of ventricular (tachycardia and fibrillation) and supraventricular arrhythmias (fibrillation and flutter).

Vernakalant

- Vernakalant is not only a potassium channel blocker, but also sodium and calcium channel blocker. These effects are predominantly seen in atrium with sparing of ventricles and hence QT prolongation is not seen with this drug.
- It is approved in many countries for treatment of an acute attack of atrial fibrillation. It is not approved by FDA as the trial was suspended in US, due to a case of cardiogenic shock in volunteer.

Bretylium

Bretylium is a quaternary amine with potassium channel blocking and sympatholytic effect (inhibits release of NE). It was used for treatment of life-threatening ventricular arrhythmias by intravenous route and was known as **medical defibrillator**. Most common presentation of toxicity is hypotension, which can be treated by **norepinephrine**.

Class IV: Calcium Channel Blockers

- All calcium channel blockers (CCB) are racemic mixtures of enantiomers except diltiazem and nifedipine. They act by inhibiting the $\alpha 1$ subunit of slow (L type) calcium channels and are broadly classified as dihydropyridines and non-dihydropyridines (verapamil and diltiazem).

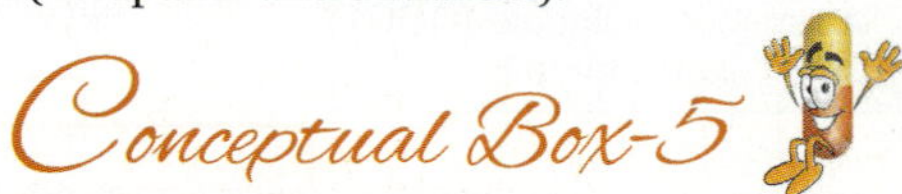

Classification of Calcium Channel Blockers

Nondihydropyridines:

CC block → ↑VD, ↑HR

Delay recovery of CC from block ↓ ⊝ Heart → ↓HR, AV ⊝

Net effect → ↑VD, Ⓝ HR, AV ⊝

Dihydropyridines:

CC block → ↑↑VD, ↑↑HR

Net effect → ↑↑VD, ↑↑HR

- Nondihydropyridines not only block calcium channels but also delay the recovery of channels from block (block calcium channels for a longer period), which causes inhibitory effect on blood vessels as well as heart. This maintains a normal heart rate along with vasodilation and block at AV node. Thus, nondihydropyridines are the antiarrhythmic calcium channel blockers.
- Dihydropyridines only block calcium channels without any effect on recovery and are more potent vasodilators, which results in reflex tachycardia. Hence, their uses are limited as vasodilators and is discussed in another section.

Nondihydropyridines

- The non-dihydropyridine class includes a phenylalkylamine i.e. **verapamil** (papaverine derivative) and a benzothiazepine i.e. **diltiazem**. Both the drugs have high plasma protein binding and first pass metabolism. Their effects are similar as described in the conceptual box, i.e. vasodilation (lesser than dihydropyridines), AV nodal block and a normal heart rate. Verapamil is more potent than diltiazem and hence is more preferred clinically and is associated more with side effects related to the class like hypotension and AV block. The L-isomer of verapamil blocks calcium channel, whereas the D-isomer can block sodium channel and accounts for local anesthetic activity.
- Since they block the conduction at AV node their primary use is in arrhythmias arising above the AV node i.e. SVT, PSVT, atrial fibrillation and flutter.
- Verapamil is the **drug of choice for treatment and prophylaxis of SVT and prophylaxis of PSVT**. It is second line drug for treatment of PSVT after vagal maneuvers and adenosine are ineffective. Diltiazem and verapamil are second line drugs for rate control in atrial fibrillation and flutter.
- Verapamil is also used for prophylaxis of migraine and HOCM.
- **Headache** is the **most common side effect** seen due to dilation of meningeal arteries. Verapamil is commonly associated with **constipation**. The class related side effects like hypotension, AV block, bradycardia and asystole are more common with verapamil than diltiazem. **Ankle edema** can be seen due to precapillary dilation and reflex post capillary contraction, which can be relieved by ACE inhibitors or ARBs by causing post capillary dilation. Decreased contraction of lower esophageal sphincter can cause GERD.
- Because of similar action on heart i.e. AV block and decreased ventricular contraction, **IV verapamil is contraindicated with an IV beta blocker**. As verapamil is a p-glycoprotein inhibitor it can decrease clearance of digitalis and hence is contraindicated for treatment of digitalis toxicity.

Class V: Miscellaneous Antiarrhythmic Drugs

Adenosine

- Adenosine is an endogenous nucleoside that is readily taken up by cells and immediately metabolized by adenosine deaminase. Hence, it has a very short half-life of around 1–5 seconds and a bolus of 6–12 mg by **rapid IV route** is required for clinical effect, as slow administration will result in complete uptake of drug by cells without any effect on heart.
- Stimulating Ach sensitive potassium channel (potassium channel opens), it shortens the action potential duration in the atrium, SA and AV node. Thus, it can **precipitate atrial fibrillation**.
- It also stimulates Gi subtype of GPCR that antagonizes the effects of catecholamines by decreasing intracellular cyclic AMP and calcium, which can increase refractoriness at AV node (block). Because it has a short half-life and blocks AV

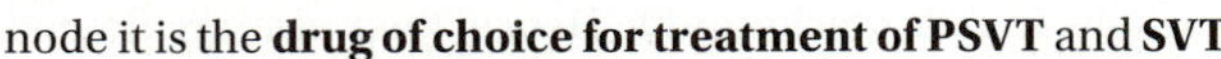

node it is the **drug of choice for treatment of PSVT** and **SVT**.

- However, the first thing to be done in case of SVT in an older child is to place face in **ice cold water** and in an infant an **ice bag** is placed on face. In adults **Valsalva maneuver** and **carotid sinus massage** can be done.
- Adenosine is also used for maintaining **controlled hypotension** in surgeries and for diagnosis of **coronary artery disease**.

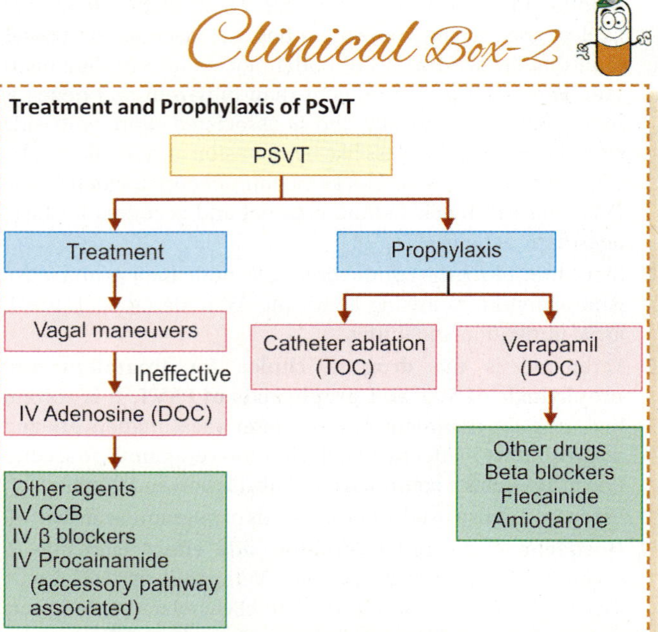

- The most common side effects are **flushing** and dyspnea. By stimulating adenosine receptors, it can cause **bronchoconstriction** and hence is contraindicated in patients of bronchial asthma and COPD. In such patients, IV verapamil is the drug of choice for PSVT.
- **Dipyridamole** is an adenosine reuptake inhibitor and hence to prevent toxicity dose of adenosine should be decreased by 50%. Methylxanthines are inhibitors of adenosine receptor and hence for patients on these drugs, IV verapamil is preferred.
- **Adenosine is contraindicated in patients with transplanted heart** as it is more sensitive to adenosine because of denervation supersensitivity.

Recent Advances

Regadenoson: It is an adenosine receptor agonist used as coronary vasodilator in angiography.

Digoxin

- The use of digoxin as an antiarrhythmic drug is because of its vagomimetic action, which decreases SA node automaticity, shortens atrial APD and blocks conduction at AV node. Hence, the use is limited as an adjunct for ventricular rate control in patients with atrial fibrillation and flutter. Since digoxin has a slow onset of action, it cannot be used in acute cases of arrhythmia.
- Digoxin is a proarrhythmic drug for which phenytoin (atrial tachyarrhythmia), lidocaine (ventricular tachyarrhythmia) and magnesium sulphate can be used for treatment.
- The other aspects of digitalis group of drugs is discussed elsewhere in this chapter.

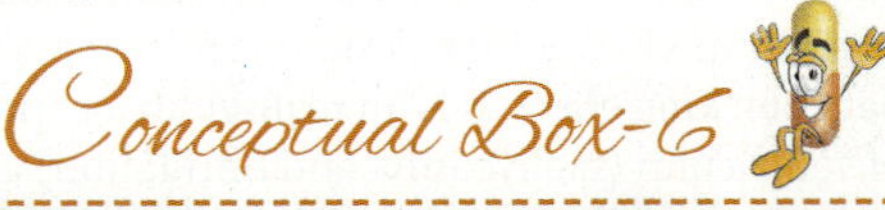

Effect of Antiarrhythmic Drugs on Refractoriness at Heart	
Accessory pathway	Class Ia sodium channel blocker
AV node	CCB (Verapamil > Diltiazem) β blockers Digitalis Adenosine
Both	Verapamil Class Ic sodium channel blocker

Magnesium Sulfate

- The antiarrhythmic effect of magnesium though not completely clear, is thought to be because of calcium channel block, that inhibits DAD (Delayed After Depolarization). There is no change in the duration of APD.

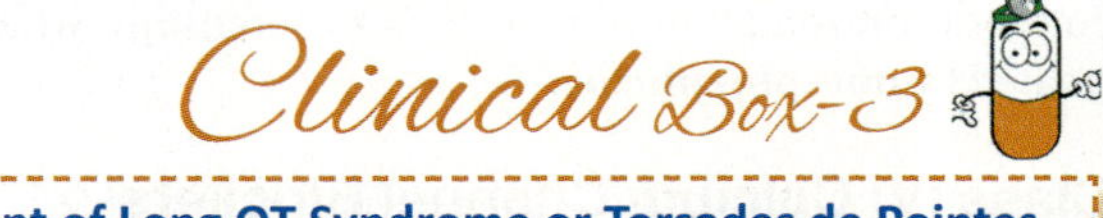

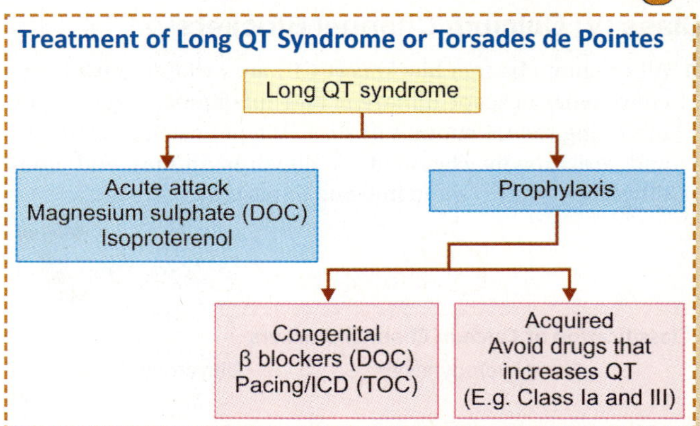

- IV magnesium sulphate is the **drug of choice for treatment of torsades de pointes** and it is also used for treatment of digitalis induced arrhythmia.

ACLS GUIDELINES 2017 ON CARDIAC ARREST AND ARRHYTHMIA

Cardiac Arrest Guidelines

- In case of cardiac arrest, start oxygen and attach monitor/defibrillator immediately. What is done next depends on the shockability of the rhythm.
- If rhythm is non-shockable and patient has asystole or PEA (Pulseless Electrical Activity), intravenous epinephrine is given every 3 to 5 minutes. If following this rhythm becomes shockable then cardioversion is done or else if rhythm is non-shockable then epinephrine is continued every 3 to 5 minutes.
- If rhythm is shockable i.e. patient has ventricular tachycardia or fibrillation, then cardioversion is done. If patient does not respond to cardioversion then epinephrine is given every

3 to 5 minutes and then if rhythm becomes shockable, then cardioversion is done. If patient still fails to respond then antiarrhythmic drug amiodarone is started.

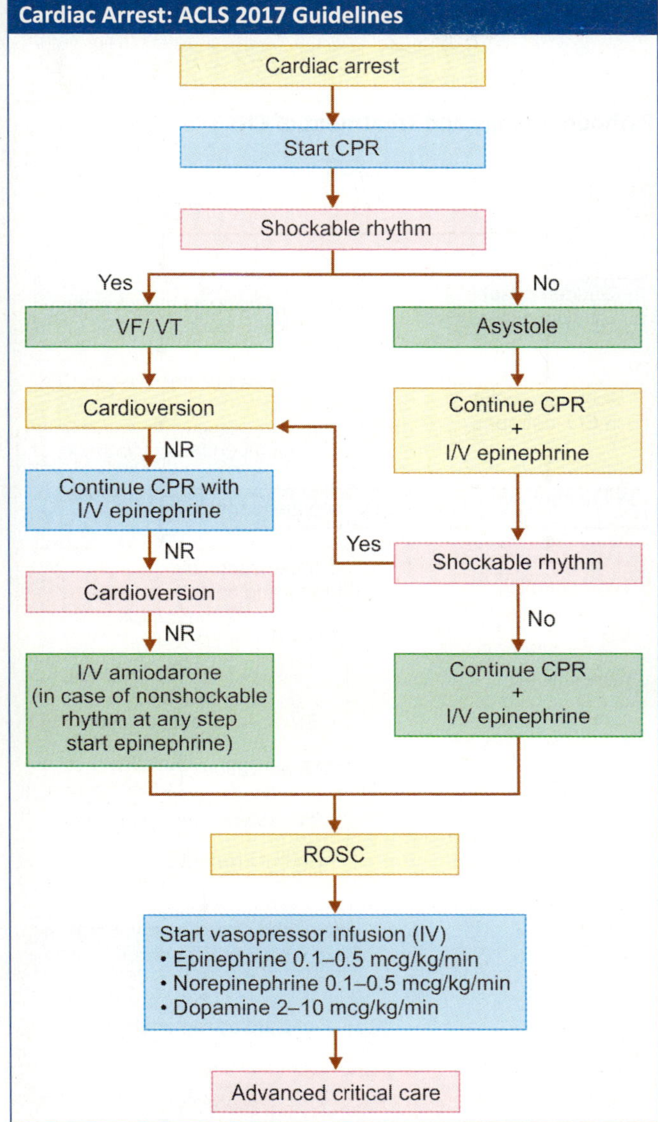

- After the patient responds to these therapies and there is return of spontaneous circulation (ROSC), postcardiac arrest management begins with optimal ventilation/oxygenation and administration of vasopressors (epinephrine/norepinephrine/dopamine) for hypotension. If the patient does not follow command after this, induced hypothermia can be tried. Finally, patient is offered advanced critical care.

Tachycardia Guidelines

- In case of tachycardia (HR > 150) the management depends if patient is symptomatic or asymptomatic.
- If patient is asymptomatic then management depends on the state of QRS complex. If there is wide QRS, then patient is started on antiarrhythmic drugs like procainamide, amiodarone or sotalol; if it is a case of regular monomorphic ventricular tachycardia then adenosine can be tried. If there is no QRS widening then vagal maneuvers can be tried and patient is started on AV nodal blocking agents like beta blockers or calcium channel blockers like verapamil; if it is regular ventricular tachycardia adenosine can be used.
- If patient is symptomatic with symptoms of hypotension, altered mental status, shock, ischemic pain or heart failure, then immediate cardioversion should be done. Adenosine can be used in case of narrow complex ventricular tachycardia.

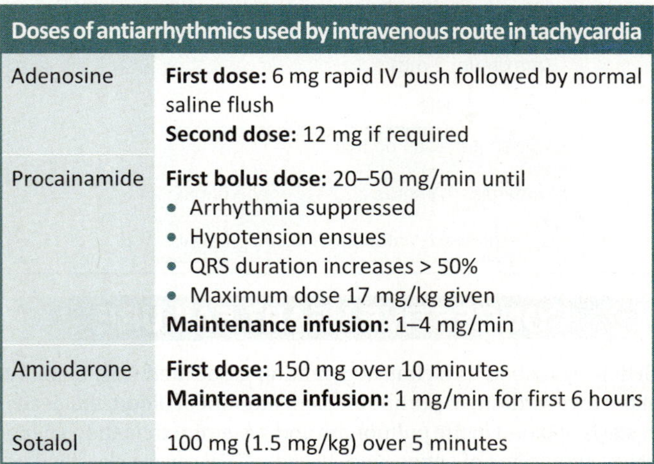

Doses of antiarrhythmics used by intravenous route in tachycardia	
Adenosine	**First dose:** 6 mg rapid IV push followed by normal saline flush **Second dose:** 12 mg if required
Procainamide	**First bolus dose:** 20–50 mg/min until • Arrhythmia suppressed • Hypotension ensues • QRS duration increases > 50% • Maximum dose 17 mg/kg given **Maintenance infusion:** 1–4 mg/min
Amiodarone	**First dose:** 150 mg over 10 minutes **Maintenance infusion:** 1 mg/min for first 6 hours
Sotalol	100 mg (1.5 mg/kg) over 5 minutes

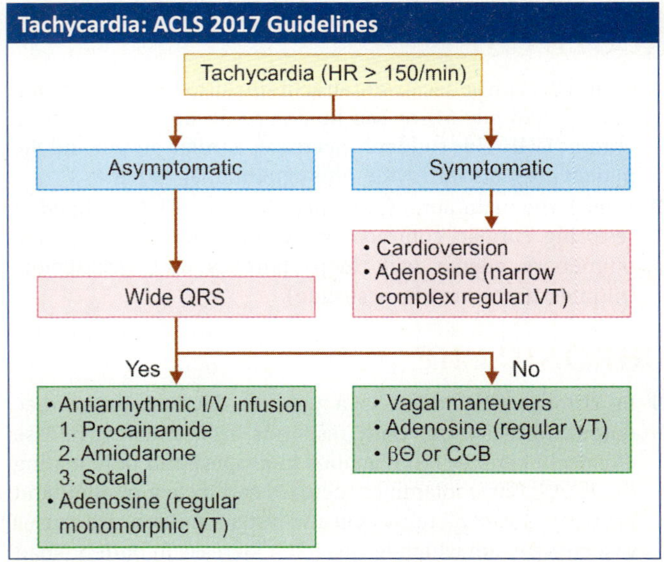

Bradycardia Guidelines

- In case of bradycardia (HR < 50) treatment depends if patient is symptomatic or asymptomatic.
- In case of an asymptomatic patient supportive care is given and patient is just monitored.
- In case patient is symptomatic with symptoms of hypotension, altered mental status, shock, ischemic pain or heart failure then, immediately atropine is started at a bolus dose of 0.5 mg and then repeated every 3 to 5 minutes. If patient does not respond to atropine then transcutaneous pacing can be done or dopamine or norepinephrine can be given at doses given in flowchart.

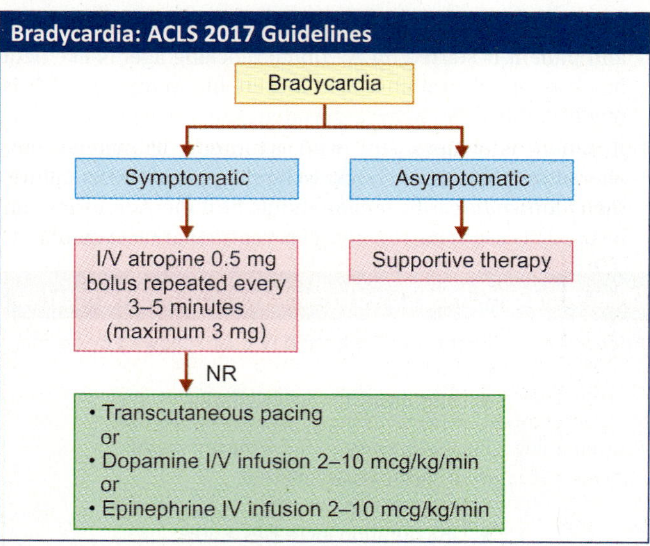

CONGESTIVE HEART FAILURE

CHF is described as a clinical condition associated with inability of the myocardium to pump sufficient amount of blood, that leads to stasis of blood in the pulmonary and systemic circulation giving rise to symptoms of congestion. Broadly CHF can be classified as acute and chronic.

ACUTE CHF

- Acute CHF can be because of an acute insult to the myocardium, most commonly MI or can be due to decompensation of a chronic CHF. This suddenly decreases cardiac output and the patient presents with symptoms of pulmonary edema.
- Hence, the main aim of treatment in acute CHF is aimed at restoring cardiac contractility by inotropes and resolving pulmonary edema with loop diuretics and vasodilators (nitrates, nitroprusside, nesiritide).

CHRONIC CHF

- In chronic CHF there is a gradual decrease in cardiac output, to which our body responds by stimulating release of catecholamines (endogenous inotropes) and potentiating the RAAS. Catecholamines increase cardiac contraction and heart rate. RAAS increases salt and water retention and causes vasoconstriction which results in an increase in both preload and afterload on the heart.
- If by above mentioned mechanisms cardiac output is maintained it is called as compensated chronic CHF. However, if the patient decompensates, symptoms of acute CHF appears and hence decompensated chronic CHF has been merged with acute CHF which makes a syndrome called as acute heart failure syndrome (AHFS). Thus, the term decompensated chronic CHF is obsolete and in current scenario chronic CHF means it is compensated one.
- In case of compensated chronic CHF or chronic CHF, catecholamines and RAAS, increase the stress significantly on myocardium and cause hypertrophy, thereby increasing its metabolic demands. This is called as cardiac remodeling, which is progressive with course of disease and is responsible for mortality. Hence, the main aim is to prevent mortality by inhibiting remodeling by drugs like beta blockers, ACEI, ARB, aldosterone antagonists, ivabradine and vasodilators.

Conceptual Box-7

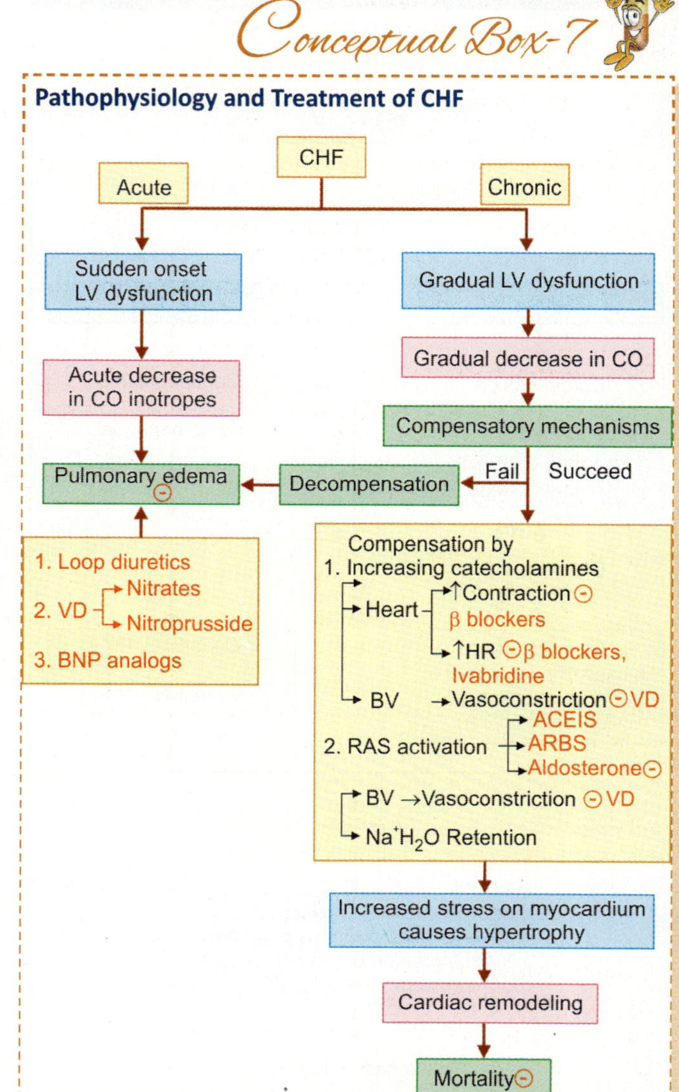

TREATMENT OF ACUTE CHF

Low Cardiac Output

Low cardiac output in acute CHF can be dealt with positive inotropic drugs like dopamine, dobutamine, milrinone and levosimendan.

Sympathomimetics

- Dobutamine is a nonselective β_1 and β_2 receptor agonist at normal doses and α_1 agonist at high doses. The net effect at clinically used doses is a strong positive inotropic and weak chronotropic effect with vasodilatation. It is used in acute CHF with decreased cardiac output to maintain the systolic function. It is the drug of choice for treatment of CHF associated with cardiogenic shock.

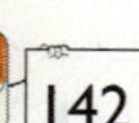

- Dopamine at low doses of <2 mcg/kg/min, has selective action on renal D_1 receptors causing vasodilatation and diuresis. Thus, it is used in CHF if GFR is not maintained even with diuretics. It is also used with dobutamine as, the latter can decrease renal perfusion.

PDE-3 Inhibitors

- PDE-3 inhibitors are called as inodilators due to their positive inotropic effect as well as vasodilatory effect. Inotropic effect increases cardiac output, whereas vasodilatation reduces both preload and afterload.
- Inamrinone, enoximone and **milrinone** are PDE-3 inhibitors, which increase cyclic AMP, responsible for positive inotropic effect and mixed vasodilatation i.e. of both arteries and veins. Inamrinone is not only longer acting than milrinone but also is associated with more **thrombocytopenia**.
- Hence, enoximone and milrinone are clinically more preferred for short-term management of advanced acute CHF. These are preferred to dobutamine, if the patient is on beta blockers. **Milrinone** and enoximone are also the inotrope of choice for treatment of **right sided heart failure**, as venodilation can reduce systemic congestion.
- Levosimendan apart from blocking PDE-3, also produces inotropic effect and vasodilatation by **sensitizing myocardium to calcium ions** and **opening potassium channels** respectively. Though not approved by FDA, it is approved by many countries for treatment of acute CHF not responding to other inotropes.

Recent Advances

Recent advances in heat failure treatment

Omecamtiv mecarbil: It is an inotrope with selective myosin activation, under trial for treatment of acute CHF.

Cinaciguat: It is a soluble guanylate cyclase stimulator that causes vasodilatation and is under trial for treatment of acute CHF.

Rolofylline: It is an adenosine receptor antagonist that increases renal blood flow and diuresis. In trials for treatment of acute CHF, no significant benefit was seen.

Istaroxime: It is an inhibitor of Na/K ATPase and stimulator of sarcoplasmic Ca-ATPase. In both mechanisms it increases cytosolic calcium and produces positive inotropic effect. It is under trial for treatment of acute CHF.

Serelaxin: It is a relaxin analogue that causes vasodilatation by increasing NO and endothelin receptor production. It is under trial for treatment of acute CHF.

Pulmonary Edema

Pulmonary edema can be resolved with diuretics, morphine, vasodilators and BNP analogues.

Diuretics

Loop diuretics are the first line drug for treatment of pulmonary edema, due to their high ceiling effect and ability to rapidly control volume overload. Thiazides are less effective but can be combined to loops in case of inadequate response. Potassium sparing diuretics are combined to combat hypokalemia and refractory edema.

Morphine

Morphine can be given in case of less severe decompensation. Apart from decreasing preload and afterload, it reduces associated anxiety and chest discomfort.

Vasodilators

Vasodilators can be used in combination with the first line drugs i.e. loop diuretics, when the patient continues to be symptomatic on the latter. Nitrates and sodium nitroprusside are the preferred vasodilators in pulmonary edema. They become more important, in case the heart failure is associated with hypertension.

Natriuretic Peptide Analogs

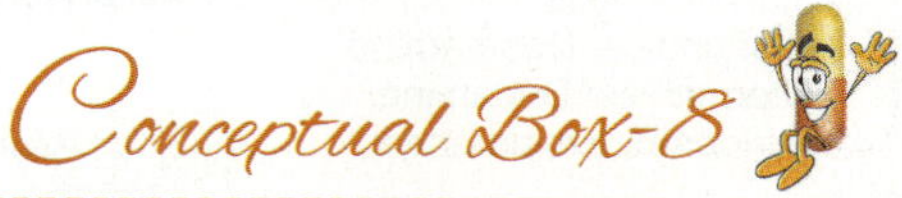

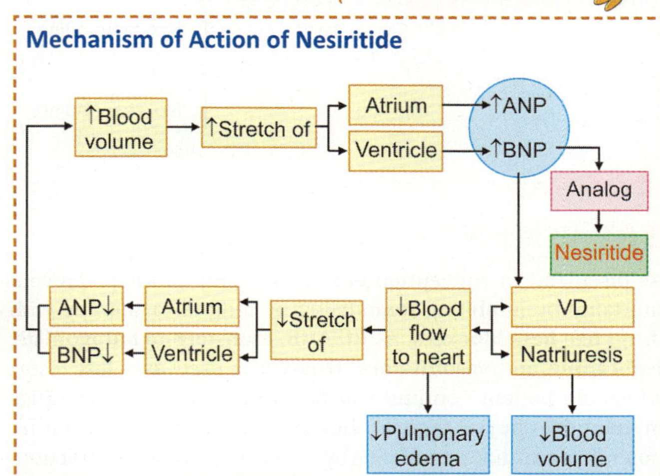

- ANP and BNP are endogenous peptides produced in response to increased stretch of ventricles due to increased blood volume. When released they cause **vasodilatation** along with **natriuresis** and diuresis, by increasing cyclic GMP in the inner medullary collecting ducts.
- Cyclic GMP inhibits the CNG (cyclic nucleotide gated) cationic channels and facilitates natriuresis. They also decrease synthesis of aldosterone and renin. The overall effect is a decrease in the amount of blood coming back to heart and hence relief in pulmonary edema. The most common side effect of these drugs is **hypotension**.
- Urodilatin is a renal natriuretic peptide that is an analog of ANP. It is synthesized in the distal renal tubule and then acts on the CNG in collecting duct like ANP. It induces more potent natriuresis and diuresis as compared to ANP.
- **Nesiritide** is a BNP analogue that has a short half-life (18 minutes), as it is rapidly metabolized by an enzyme **neutral endopeptidase** and eliminated also by NPR-C (natriuretic peptide receptor) and kidney. Since it is a peptide, it is given by **IV route** for treatment of pulmonary edema associated with acute CHF to patients who are still symptomatic with diuretics and nitrates.

- **Carperitide** is an ANP analog, approved only in Japan for treatment of acute CHF.
- **Ularitide** is an urodilatin analog in phase III trial for treatment of acute CHF.

Clinical Box-4

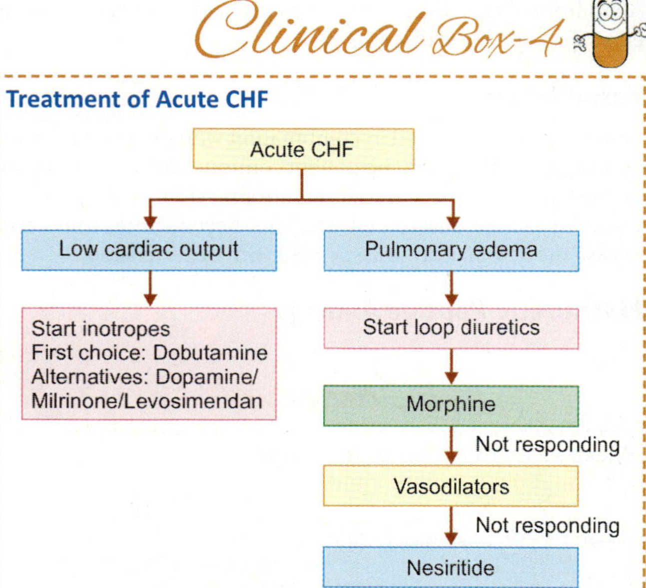

TREATMENT OF CHRONIC CHF

As discussed in conceptual box-7, the main aim is to prevent mortality by inhibiting remodeling by long-term therapy with drugs like **beta blockers, ACEI, ARB, aldosterone antagonists, ivabradine** and **vasodilators**. **Digoxin** is used as a last resort when the patient continues to be symptomatic on the drugs mentioned above. Digoxin however doesn't inhibit, rather potentiates cardiac remodeling by increasing cardiac contraction.

Drugs Inhibiting Cardiac Remodeling and Delaying Mortality

Mnemonics

SHIBA
- **S :** Spironolactone
- **H :** Hydralazine + IDN
- **I :** Ivabridine
- **B :** Beta blockers
- **A :** ACEI/ARB

ACEI/ARB

- ACEI/ARB are the first drug to be started in case of chronic compensated CHF. The preferred ARBs in CHF are **candesartan** and **valsartan**.
- Due to vasodilatation both preload and afterload is decreased on the heart. Moreover, by inhibiting RAAS and decreasing aldosterone, they can decrease blood volume by facilitating sodium and water loss, which further decreases preload. By these mechanisms they prevent cardiac remodeling and hence decrease hospitalization and mortality.
- Since they can cause hypotension that can worsen CHF, the starting dose is lesser, which is gradually up titrated every week to the maximum indicated dose in clinical trials.

Recent Advances

Sacubitril: It is a **neutral endopeptidase (neprilysin) inhibitor** that increases the endogenous BNP and hence causes vasodilatation along with natriuresis and diuresis. It is approved by FDA in 2015 along with **valsartan** for use in chronic CHF to decrease mortality. Valsartan + Sacubitril combination is more effective in reducing mortality as compared to ACEI or ARB. Thus, according to recent ACC/AHA guidelines if patient Is tolerating ACEI or ARB, these should be replaced with Valsartan + Sacubitril. The risk of postural hypotension is higher with this combination as compared to ACE inhibitors. Sacubitril should not be used along with ACEI or within last 36 hours of last dose of ACEI and in patients with history of angioedema.

Omapatrilat: It is a **vasopeptidase inhibitor**, which inhibits both ACE and neutral endopeptidase. Its development was stopped due to high risk of angioedema.

Beta Blockers

- Beta blockers are the second class of drugs to be started, before full target dose of ACEI/ARB is achieved. They block the action of excess catecholamines on heart and prevent mortality. A **maximum decrease in mortality i.e. 35% is seen with beta blockers**, followed by ACEI/ARB i.e. 23%.
- Three beta blockers with proven benefits are - **nebivolol, carvedilol, bisoprolol and metoprolol** (long acting formulation), however **carvedilol** has maximum effect on mortality.
- Beta blockers have negative inotropic effect and they can decompensate heart failure. Hence, the starting dose is lesser than 1/10th of normal dose (suboptimal dose), which is up titrated every 2 weeks to the maximum tolerable dose. Patients who are intolerant to beta blockers (10%), ivabradine can be given which is a drug with similar effect on heart.

Aldosterone Antagonist

- Aldosterone antagonists like spironolactone and eplerenone are the third line drugs and used when the patient is still progressive on ACEI/ARB and beta blockers.
- Aldosterone is upregulated in CHF and leads to sodium and water retention, thereby increasing preload. Hence, inhibition of aldosterone does give mortality benefits.
- Since these drugs can cause **hyperkalemia** serum potassium levels should be checked **after 1 and 4 weeks** of starting drug. According to recent ACC/AHA guidelines aldosterone antagonists can be used in patients only if GFR is >30 mL/min, serum creatinine is <2.5 mg/dL and **serum potassium is <5 mEq/L**. Aldosterone antagonists are more beneficial in patients with elevated BNP levels, ejection fraction ≥ 45% and heart failure admission within 1 year.

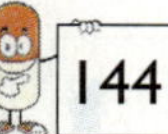

Ivabradine

- As discussed in conceptual box-1, I_f/I_h or funny current is responsible for the automaticity of SA node. Ivabradine inhibits I_f current and hence decreases automaticity of SA node and heart rate.
- By decreasing heart rate, it decreases the stress on myocardium and inhibits remodeling. Thus, it also has mortality benefit.
- It is a fourth line drug used after ACEI/ARB, beta blockers and aldosterone antagonist are ineffective. It is used in stable patients with a sinus rhythm and heart rate of 70 beats per minute or more.

Vasodilators

A combination of IDN and hydralazine decreases preload and afterload respectively, thereby decreasing mortality. This combination is the fifth line drug for disease progressive on the previous four classes of drugs.

Digitalis

- Digoxin in heart failure is used, when all the previous options are exhausted and the patient is still symptomatic, or CHF is associated with atrial fibrillation (for rate control).
- Digoxin is the only currently available cardiac glycoside derived from a plant called as digitalis lanata (white foxglove). Other drugs of this group like digitoxin and ouabain have been discontinued and hence not discussed here.
- Digoxin has a good oral absorption with a bioavailability of around 75%, has low plasma protein binding of around 25% and primarily excreted unchanged by **kidney**. The half-life is around **36–48 hours**. It is highly distributed in the skeletal muscles (high volume of distribution) and hence a loading dose is given according to the lean body mass.
- Though it can be given both by oral and intravenous route, oral route is more preferred due to its low therapeutic index and due to same reason, the serum digoxin level should be maintained below 1 ng/mL. Some patients with intestinal colonization with Eubacterium lentum can have inefficacy at normal doses due to metabolism by the same.
- The effect of digitalis on heart can be better understood by dividing it into cellular effect and organ effect as given below.
- **Cellular effect of digoxin**
  - In a myocardial cell, digitalis act by inhibiting phosphorylated Na/K ATPase pump, whose function is to reverse the effect of depolarization by pumping sodium out and potassium in. Thus, when this effect is inhibited, there is intracellular accumulation of sodium and extracellular potassium, and thus the side effect **hyperkalemia**.
  - Potassium which accumulates extracellularly, dephosphorylates Na/K ATPase pump and hence limits digitalis action. Thus, in case of **hypokalemia digitalis toxicity can be seen.**
  - Increased intracellular sodium blocks the Na/Ca exchanger pump, which leads to block of sodium movement in and calcium movement out. Thus, the calcium accumulated in cytoplasm is stored in the sarcoplasmic reticulum. Now when an action potential strikes the myocardial cell, a huge amount of calcium is released from the sarcoplasmic reticulum giving a strong positive **inotropic effect**.
  - The persistently high level of calcium in myocardial cells can generate small depolarization just after or in between repolarization and is known as **delayed after depolarization (DAD)**. Further it can take shape of a complete action potential, i.e. a cardiac contraction triggered by calcium alone (usually by Na in myocardial cells) and is known as an extra systole. If it's repetitive **bigeminy can be seen, which is the most common digitalis induced arrhythmia.**
  - Ventricular tachycardia can follow, which is self-sustained (by myocardial cell) and bidirectional and finally can precipitate fibrillation.

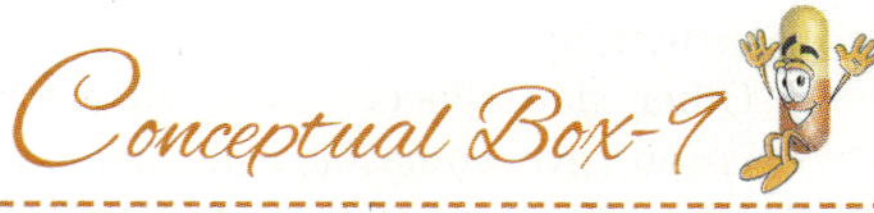

Cellular Effect of Digoxin

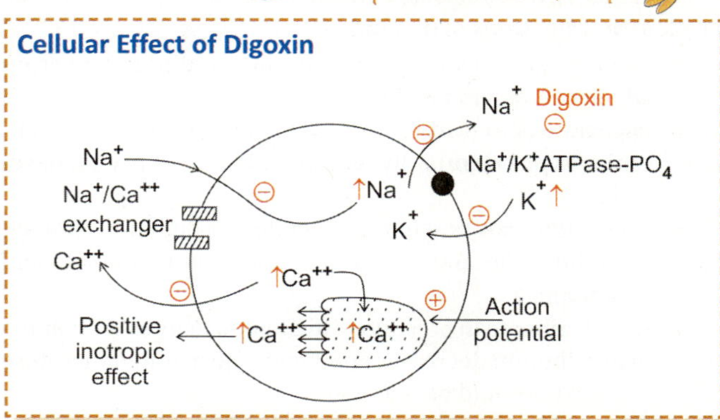

- **Organ effect of digoxin**
  - On the heart digitalis has a parasympathomimetic and sympatholytic effect at normal doses and sympathomimetic effect at toxic doses.
  - Thus, at normal doses it decreases automaticity at SA node **(bradycardia), increases refractoriness at AV node (AV block)**. In rare cases AV block can be associated with atrial tachycardia due to cellular effect of increase in calcium in **atrial cells. Such an arrhythmia called as atrial tachycardia with AV block is most specific arrhythmia associated with digitalis**, as is not seen with any other drug or disease.
  - Because of the effects mentioned above digitalis is used to convert atrial flutter into fibrillation as the latter can be easily controlled. Still there is no risk of ventricular arrhythmia due to AV block.
- **ECG changes with digoxin**

ECG changes	Cause
PR prolongation	Refractoriness at AV node
QT shortening	Shortening of action potential duration
T wave inversion ST segment depression	Accelerated repolarization of inner layers of myocardium

- **Uses of digoxin**
  - Digoxin though is a positive inotrope, it does not have any benefit in mortality and hence is used for treatment of CHF, if the first line drugs like ACEI/ARB, beta blockers

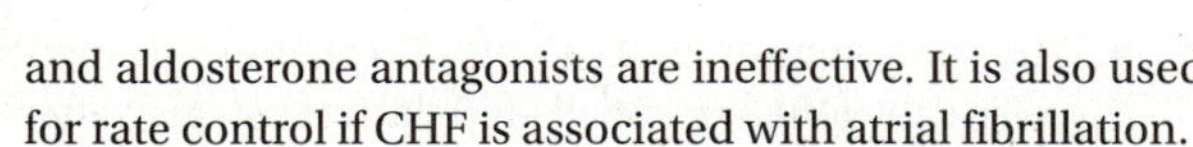

and aldosterone antagonists are ineffective. It is also used for rate control if CHF is associated with atrial fibrillation.
- It is the only inotrope used in chronic CHF, rest are used acute CHF.

- **Side effects of digoxin**
  - GIT upset in the form of **nausea**, vomiting and diarrhoea is the earliest and most common side effect.
  - Almost any **arrhythmia** can be seen with digitalis i.e. both tachyarrhythmia and bradyarrhythmia, but flutter and Mobitz II block are never seen. As discussed earlier ventricular bigeminy is the most common one, whereas atrial tachycardia with AV block is the most specific arrhythmia.
  - Other side effects associated are - xanthopsia (yellow vision), gynecomastia, hallucinations and **hyperkalemia**.
- **Contraindications of digoxin**
  - Digoxin is contraindicated in various conditions and drugs which can precipitate its toxicity.
  - Digoxintoxicity can be precipitated by **myocardial ischemia, hypokalemia, hypercalcemia** and **hypomagnesemia**.
  - Drugs that can precipitate digitalis toxicity are diuretics, quinidine, flecainide, propafenone, amiodarone and verapamil.
  - **Renal failure** can precipitate digitalis toxicity as the volume of distribution decreases and hence the maintenance dose of digoxin should be decreased.
  - Digoxin blocks conduction through AV node and hence can worsen WPW syndrome as it does not affect conduction through accessory pathway. Hence, it is contraindicated in **WPW syndrome** as well.
- **Treatment of digitalis toxicity**

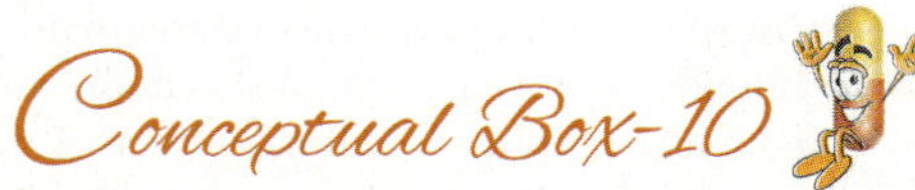

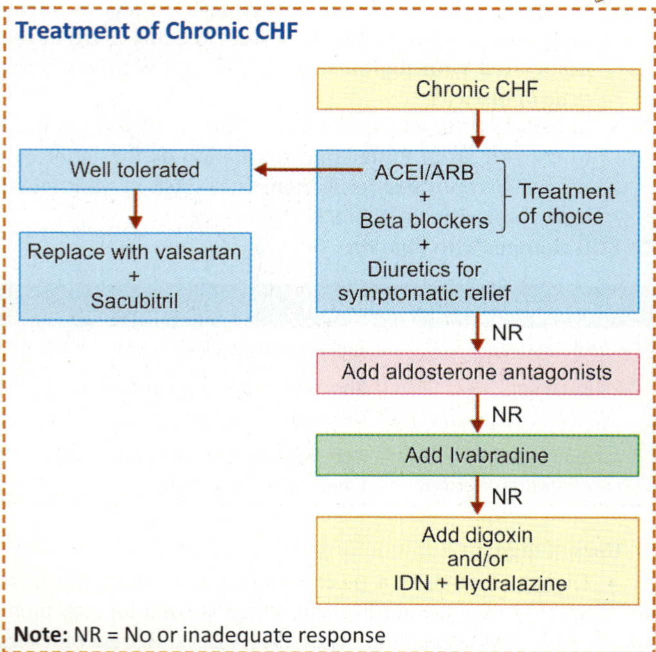

  - **Lidocaine** is the drug of choice for digitalis induced **ventricular tachyarrhythmias**, whereas **phenytoin** and **$MgSO_4$** are alternatives. Phenytoin is also effective for treatment of digitalis induced ventricular arrhythmias.
  - **Digiband**, an anti-digoxin antibody is the **most effective drug** and hence reserved for treatment of life-threatening arrhythmias induced by digoxin. The dose of digiband is calculated based on the total digoxin dose administered.
  - **Potassium** can be given for benign arrhythmias like atrial and AV junctional arrhythmias and ventricular ectopic rhythms, even if serum potassium levels are normal. Potassium dephosphorylates Na/K ATPase and limits digitalis action. Potassium is **contraindicated in case of AV block**, as it can be worsened.
  - **Atropine** is indicated in case of bradyarrhythmia and AV block, which are rarely seen.
  - Cardioversion can be problematic as it can itself induce arrhythmia in digitalis toxicity.

HYPERTENSION

- Hypertension is the most common CVS disorder, which on persistence can lead to damage of other organs and cause CHF, pulmonary edema, renal failure, retinopathy, MI and stroke.
- Thus, early diagnosis and treatment is of utmost importance to prevent or delay the mentioned disorders.
- ACEI/ARB, CCB and thiazides are considered as first line drugs for treatment of hypertension. Among these there is no single drug of choice according to current guidelines and a drug can be preferred based on age, race and associated comorbidities.
- The patient is started on a single drug and if the goal BP is not reached after one month, a second drug can be started and similarly a third drug. The adequate amount of BP decrease that can be achieved with a single drug is 10 mm Hg.
- If the patient is not responsive to 3 drugs with at least one of them being diuretic, it is termed as resistant hypertension for which spironolactone is the drug of choice.
- Other drugs like beta blockers, vasodilators, DRIs, alpha blockers and sympatholytics are second line drugs.

DIAGNOSIS OF HYPERTENSION

Classification	Criteria
Normal	BP <120/<80
Prehypertension	BP 120-129/<80
Hypertension (Stage I)	BP 130-139/80-89
Hypertension (Stage II)	BP ≥140/≥90
Hypertensive urgency	BP >220/125 without end organ damage
Hypertensive emergency	End organ damage (CHF, pulmonary edema, retinopathy, renal failure, MI, stroke, eclampsia, aortic dissection or unstable angina) irrespective of blood pressure
Malignant hypertension (Old term)	Hypertensive encephalopathy or nephropathy + retinopathy
Resistant hypertension	Persistently elevated BP >140/90 being on 3 drugs with at least 1 being diuretic

TREATMENT OF HYPERTENSION BASED ON DIFFERENT CRITERIA

Age

According to recent guidelines, **A**CEI/ARB designated as **A** and **B**eta blockers designated as B are more effective in young patients i.e. age <55 years. The reason being both these classes act on RAS and in young patients, hypertension is frequently associated with increased renin i.e. high renin hypertension. Out of both classes ACEI/ARB being first line drugs are drug of choice for hypertension in young patients.

CCB designated as **C** and **D**iuretics (thiazides) designated as **D**, are more effective in elderly i.e. age ≥55 years. The reason is low renin hypertension in elderly in which these drugs are more effective and CCB being the drug of choice.

Race

White people have predominantly high renin hypertension and hence again ACEI/ARB and beta blockers are more effective. Blacks have low renin hypertension and thus CCB and diuretics (thiazides) are preferred.

Comorbidities

Associated comorbidity with hypertension	Drugs preferred
DM CKD Scleroderma Nephrotic syndrome	ACEI/ARB
Angina Previous MI Hyperthyroidism Migraine Anxiety with somatic manifestations Essential tremor Atrial fibrillation and flutter Preoperative hypertension	Beta blockers
Osteoporosis	Thiazides
Raynaud's disease Cyclosporine induced hypertension	CCB
BPH Dyslipidemia	α_1 blockers

Contd...

Clinical Box-5

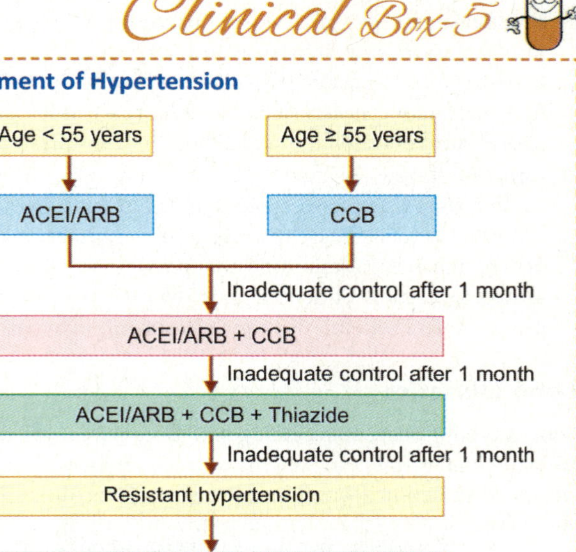

Antihypertensive Drugs Classification

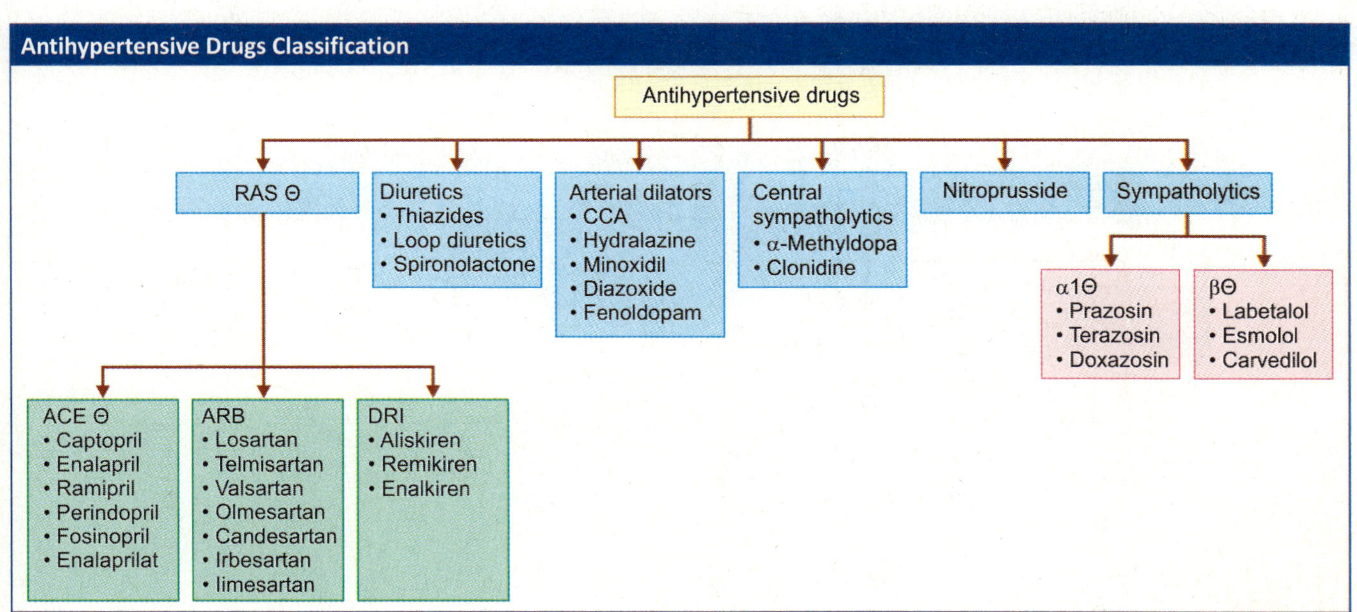

ANTIHYPERTENSIVE DRUGS

Diuretics

Thiazides

- Thiazides act by inhibiting Na/Cl cotransporter in DCT that facilitates diuresis and decreases blood pressure. But this mechanism is short lived as it is counteracted by potentiation of RAS.
- Thus, on long-term therapy **vasodilation is the main mechanism**, which is seen because of potassium channel opening and negative sodium balance. The latter mechanism is blunted in renal failure and hence diuretics become ineffective.
- **Thiazides** are one of the first line drugs for treatment of **mild to moderate hypertension** and drug of choice in hypertension associated with osteoporosis, as they can cause hypercalcemia. These are more effective in **older patients, obese, smokers** and other conditions with low plasma renin.
- **Chlorthalidone** being longest acting provides better 24 hour blood pressure control and is the thiazide of choice. Chlorthalidone decreases cardiovascular mortality in patients of hypertension. **Indapamide** has poor diuretic effect because of short duration of action, thus direct vasodilation is the primary effect with this drug and is used only in hypertension.

Loop Diuretics

Loop diuretics being short acting and more potent are reserved for acute management in patients with hypertensive emergency, kidney dysfunction (serum creatinine >2.5 mg/dL), CHF and edema seen due to fluid retention as with minoxidil.

Potassium Sparing Diuretics

- Potassium sparing diuretics are weak diuretics but combined with thiazides to prevent hypokalemia.
- **Spironolactone** is the drug of choice for **resistant hypertension** because the most common cause of resistant hypertension is elevated aldosterone levels.

RAS Inhibitors

- The renin-angiotensin system begins with production of angiotensinogen by liver, which is metabolized by renin from juxtaglomerular cells of kidney to angiotensin I (AT-I).
- AT-I is further metabolized by angiotensin converting enzyme (ACE) into angiotensin II (AT-II).
- AT-II has diverse target and causes **vasoconstriction** and constriction of glomerular efferent and afferent arterioles, and increases release of **aldosterone, vasopressin** and catecholamines (inhibits NE reuptake in synapse and stimulates catecholamine release in adrenals) and induces thirst and anorexia. In the nephron, AT-II stimulates Na/H exchanger in PCT and Na/K/2Cl transporter in thick ascending limb of loop.
- Angiotensin II is further metabolized into angiotensin III, which further forms angiotensin IV; both steps being catalyzed by amino peptidases. Angiotensin III has effects like angiotensin II, whereas angiotensin IV enhances cognition. Hence, angiotensin IV analogs are under development for treatment of Alzheimer's disease.
- RAS can be targeted at various levels by inhibiting renin (renin inhibitors), ACE (ACE inhibitors) and AT-1 receptors (angiotensin receptor blockers). The common effect seen will be a reduction in blood pressure, loss of solutes and water and retention of potassium i.e. hyperkalemia.

Conceptual Box-11

Renin-angiotensin System (RAS) System

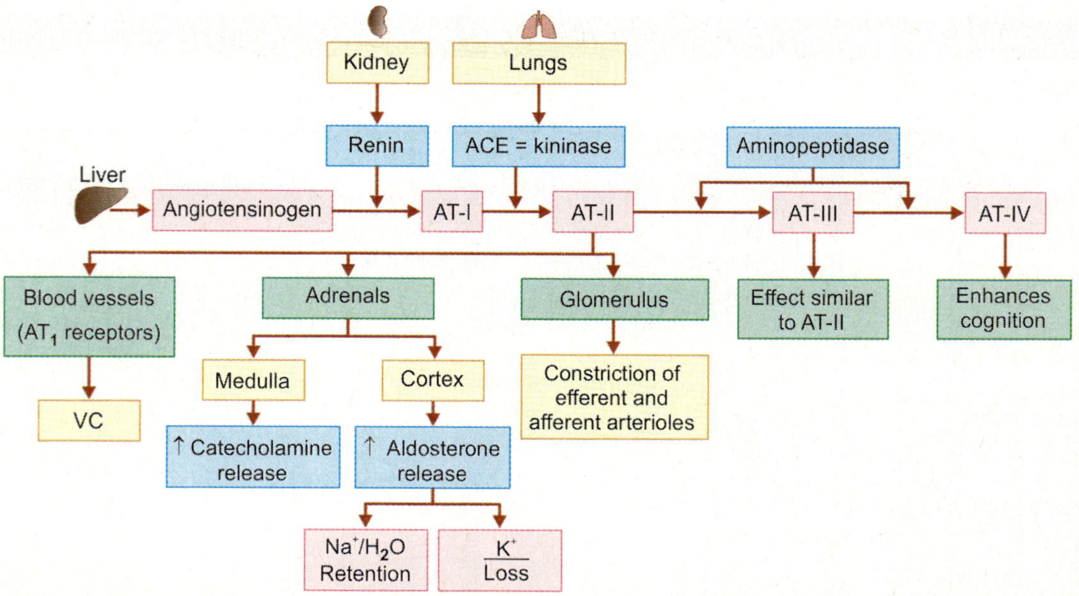

Kidney
Lungs
Renin
ACE = kininase
Aminopeptidase
Liver
Angiotensinogen
AT-I
AT-II
AT-III
AT-IV
Blood vessels (AT_1 receptors)
Adrenals
Glomerulus
Effect similar to AT-II
Enhances cognition
VC
Medulla
Cortex
Constriction of efferent and afferent arterioles
↑ Catecholamine release
↑ Aldosterone release
Na^+/H_2O Retention
K^+ Loss

Factors and Drugs Affecting Renin

Renin increased	Renin decreased
ATP	Loop diuretics
Adenosine	Beta blockers
ACEIs/ARBs/DRIs	Central sympatholytics (e.g. clonidine)
Prostaglandins	NSAIDS

ACE Inhibitors

ACE inhibitors (ACEI) produce vasodilation primarily be reducing production of vasopressor peptide AT-II from AT-I. Apart from that increase in bradykinin and prostaglandins (NSAIDs decrease antihypertensive effect of ACEIs) levels due to inhibition of its metabolism may contribute. Other effects are decrease in insulin resistance and incidence of DM, decrease in lipoprotein (a) and cholesterol.

- **All ACEIs are prodrugs except captopril and lisinopril**; the prodrugs being much less potent. The route of excretion is predominantly kidney for all ACEIs except fosinopril and spirapril, which are equally excreted by kidney and liver. Captopril was the first ACEI approved, which was followed by other drugs like enalapril, lisinopril (analog of enalaprilat), fosinopril, ramipril, trandolapril, quinapril and benazepril. All ACEI are given by oral route except enalaprilat, which is the active metabolite of enalapril given by intravenous route for treatment of hypertensive emergency. Food decreases absorption of captopril and hence should be given one hour before food intake. Captopril has maximum (75%), whereas lisinopril has minimum (25%) bioavailability.
- Many ACE inhibitors exhibit biphasic elimination i.e. one due to metabolism and second phase is because of high affinity binding for ACE. Such ACEI are enalapril, trandolapril, quinapril and perindopril. Ramipril has a triphasic elimination i.e. a third phase which is due to high tissue distribution. All these ACEIs are long acting because of slow dissociation from ACE. **Ramipril and perindopril are longest acting** whereas **captopril** is the **shortest acting** ACEI.
- Uses of ACEI are like angiotensin receptor blockers (ARBs), with the former given first preference. They are drugs of choice for treatment of heart failure and **hypertension associated with comorbidities like DM and chronic kidney disease (CKD)**. As discussed earlier in heart failure decrease in mortality is the primary gain. In case diabetes mellitus and chronic kidney disease they can afford nephroprotection and decrease proteinuria along with a decrease in progression of diabetic retinopathy. They are also beneficial in **scleroderma renal crisis** which is primarily caused by AT-II. ACE inhibitors should be started in acute phase of MI and continued in high risk patients i.e. large infarcts for mortality benefit. Long-term use of ACE inhibitors in patients with vascular disease or DM decreases the risk of MI and stroke. **Captopril** is used for **diagnosis of renovascular hypertension** prior to confirmation with renal angiography. An increase in renin with captopril is more in case of renovascular hypertension as compared to essential.
- **Dry cough** (females > males) is the most common side effect seen because of accumulation of bradykinin, substance P and prostaglandins in lungs, for which either dose is decreased, or drug changed to ARBs. NSAIDS and iron can reduce the cough. Bradykinin, substance P and prostaglandins being vasodilators can cause a rare side effect, angioedema which can be worsened by **thiazolidinediones** (inhibit substance P degradation). Other side effects encountered are hypotension, **hyperkalemia, dysgeusia** (maximum with **captopril**), neutropenia, glycosuria and rash with itch (maximum with captopril). Hypotension is more common in patients with elevated plasma renin as in case of heart failure and hence patients are started at low doses.

Mnemonics

Side effects of ACEIs – ACE INH
- **A** : Angioedema
- **C** : Cough
- **E** : Electrolyte imbalance (Hyperkalemia)
- **I** : Itch caused by rash
- **N** : Neutropenia
- **H** : Hypotension

ACE Inhibitor Induced Angioedema

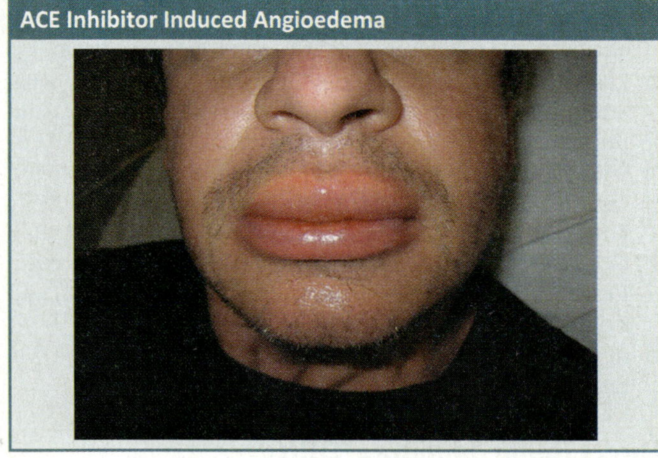

- ACEIs can dilate efferent arterioles and decrease the filtration pressure in glomerulus. Hence, they are contraindicated in a patient with **bilateral renal artery stenosis** or **single kidney with renal artery stenosis**, as renal failure can be precipitated. **Pregnancy** is an absolute contraindication as in first trimester cardiac and CNS defects can be seen. In second and third trimester renal defects can be seen due to interference with fetal RAS, which is required for renal development.
- **Drug interactions with ACEIs**

Drug	Interaction with ACEIs
Antacids	Decrease bioavailability
NSAIDS	Decrease antihypertensive effect
Thiazolidinediones	Increase angioedema
Allopurinol	Increased risk of hypersensitivity
Digoxin Lithium	Decreased clearance increases toxicity
Potassium sparing diuretics	Hyperkalemia

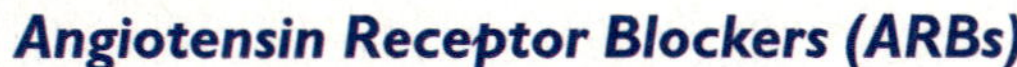

Angiotensin Receptor Blockers (ARBs)

Losartan was the first ARB developed and approved. ARBs are competitive inhibitors of AT1 receptors; candesartan and olmesartan being most potent, whereas losartan being least potent at AT1 receptor. Losartan was followed by other long acting ARBs like telmisartan, candesartan, irbesartan, ilmesartan and valsartan. Eprosartan is the shortest acting ARB, whereas telmisartan is longest acting. All ARBs have low oral bioavailability but high plasma protein binding. **Candesartan and olmesartan are prodrugs.** Food decreases absorption of valsartan and should be taken one hour before food intake.

- The uses of ARBs are like ACEIs like hypertension, hypertension with DM and CKD, MI and heart failure. Only difference is ACEIs are preferred first as compared to ARBs. Losartan is also used for treatment of portal hypertension and irbesartan can be used for maintaining sinus rhythm in atrial fibrillation.
- The class side effects like hyperkalemia are hypotension are commonly seen, whereas cough and angioedema are rarely associated with ARBs. Other side effects like alopecia, agranulocytosis, neutropenia and vasculitis (HSP) can also be seen. **Olmesartan** is associated with **sprue like syndrome** characterized by nausea, weight loss and abdominal pain.
- Like ACEIs these are contraindicated in bilateral renal artery stenosis, single kidney with renal artery stenosis and pregnancy.
- Some ARBs can stimulate PPAR-γ receptors and increase insulin sensitivity. This effect with ARBs is directly proportional to their lipid solubility, and based upon it, their order PPAR-γ agonist activity is **telmisartan > Irbesartan > Losartan. Losartan has antiaggregant (inhibits TX-A2) and uricosuric effect also.**
- ACE inhibitors also increases insulin sensitivity but via bradykinin pathway.

Direct Renin Inhibitors (DRIs)

The first generation DRIs like remikiren and enalikiren being less potent with poor bioavailability were not successful in trials. **The first and only DRI approved by FDA is aliskiren**. It has a low bioavailability of only 2.5%, but is long acting and highly potent. Absorption is reduced by fatty food and excretion is primarily by liver in unchanged form.

- Aliskiren is a second line drug for treatment of hypertension and used when the patient is intolerant to the first line drugs or it may be combined with other RAS inhibitors for added benefit. In trials it has been associated with a benefit in heart failure and hypertension associated with DM and CKD.
- Class side effects like hyperkalemia and hypotension are seen. Cough and angioedema though is rarely seen as compared to ACEIs. Other side effects associated are hyperuricemia, nephrolithiasis, diarrhoea and GERD.

Arterial Dilators

Vasodilators with selectivity for the resistance vessels are calcium channel blockers, hydralazine, minoxidil, diazoxide and fenoldopam.

Calcium Channel Blockers

- The non-DHPs have been discussed in detail in the topic of antiarrhythmics. DHP class has drugs like nifedipine, nimodipine, isaradipine, clevidipine, felodipine and nisoldipine.
- **Amlodipine** (t½ = 30–50 hours) is the **longest acting DHP** with maximum bioavailability, whereas **clevidipine** (t½ = 2 minutes) is the **shortest acting** as it is metabolized by plasma esterase.
- As discussed earlier, DHPs are more potent vasodilators but associated with reflex tachycardia, whereas non-DHPs are less potent vasodilators and maintain a normal heart rate. In classical angina DHPs and non-DHPs both can be used, but DHPs are always combined with beta blockers to counteract reflex tachycardia, which can increase oxygen demand. DHPs are also used for treatment of Prinzmetal angina.
- CCBs are first line drugs for treatment of hypertension. **Intravenous nicardipine**, which is the most potent and longest acting parenteral DHP, is the **drug of choice for hypertensive emergency**. Nifedipine by oral route can be used for treatment of hypertensive urgency. Intravenous clevidipine can be used for hypertensive emergency as well as perioperative hypertension.
- **Nimodipine** being a highly lipid soluble drug readily crosses blood brain barrier and is preferred for treatment of **cerebral vasospasm**.
- Nifedipine, amlodipine, felodipine and diltiazem are used for treatment of Raynaud's disease.
- Amlodipine is the only CCB safe in patients with severe heart failure.

Minoxidil

- Minoxidil is a **potassium channel opener** like hydralazine and diazoxide. Opening of potassium channel causes hyperpolarization of smooth muscles, which leads to potent vasodilatation.
- Associated side effects like fluid retention, reflex cardiac stimulation and hirsutism have discouraged the regular use of minoxidil.
- It is rather reserved for treatment of severe hypertension not responsive to other drugs. As it causes hirsutism, topic application is approved for treatment of androgenic alopecia.

Hydralazine

- Hydralazine primarily acts by inhibiting IP3 induced calcium release from sarcoplasmic reticulum. Other mechanisms are opening of potassium channel and an **increase in release of nitric oxide**.
- It is used along with IDN for treatment of CHF. For treatment of hypertensive emergency with pregnancy it is the most commonly used drug, however the drug of choice is labetalol.
- Apart from side effects related to vasodilatation like hypotension, headache, tachycardia etc. It can also cause **drug induced SLE**, which is more common in females and usually seen after at least 6 months of drug use. Peripheral neuropathy can be seen, which responds to pyridoxine.
- **Sweet's syndrome** or neutrophilic dermatosis is also seen with hydralazine; it has also been reported with OCP, minoxidil and cotrimoxazole.

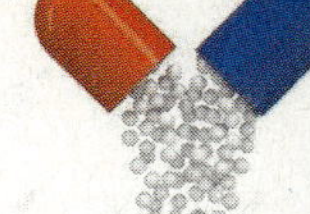

Diazoxide

- Diazoxide acts by opening potassium channel and was earlier used for treatment of hypertensive emergency. Its use in hypertension has been discontinued due to risk of severe hypotension.
- It inhibits insulin release and currently is the **drug of choice for insulinoma**.

Fenoldopam

- Fenoldopam activates D1 receptors and facilitates diuresis and decreases NE release by α_2 agonism.
- Due to collective effect it causes a significant decrease in blood pressure and can be used by IV route for treatment of hypertensive emergency.

Sodium Nitroprusside

- Nitroprusside is metabolized in RBC into nitric oxide, which causes dilation of both arteries and veins by cyclic GMP pathway as seen with nitrates.
- It is also metabolized into cyanide, which is further metabolized in liver to thiocyanate. Thiocyanate can cause neuropsychiatric side effects and hypothyroidism by inhibiting sodium iodide symporter in thyroid. It can also cause metabolic acidosis and methemoglobinemia.
- Nitroprusside is a **very short and fast acting** drug as the effect is seen within 30 seconds and terminates 3 minutes after infusion is stopped. It is **photosensitive** and hence should be covered with an opaque foil.
- Currently it is a second line drug for treatment of hypertensive emergency. It can be used for treatment of CHF (associated pulmonary edema), MI (decreases myocardial oxygen demand) and to induce controlled hypotension in anesthesia. In aortic dissection it is used along with beta blocker to prevent reflex tachycardia, which can worsen dissection.

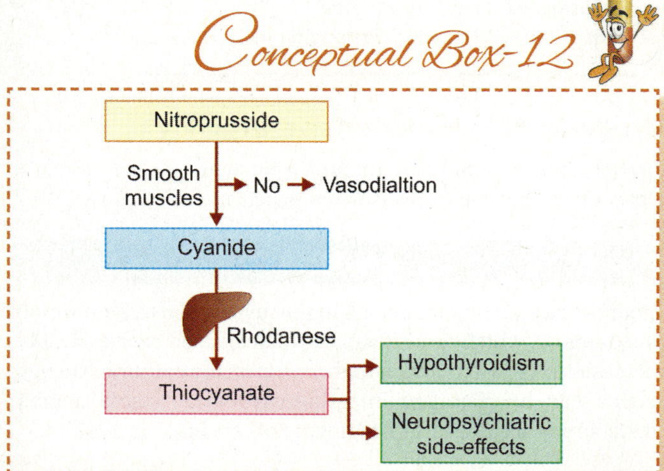

Sympatholytics

This class has drugs like α_1 blockers, β blockers, central sympatholytics (α methyldopa, clonidine, guanfacine and guanabenz), sympathetic neuronal blockers (guanethidine, guanadrel, reserpine and metyrosine) are mixed dilators.

α_1 Blockers

- The drugs in this class are prazosin, terazosin and doxazosin. For treatment of hypertension, these are second line drugs and used in combination with other drugs.
- These drugs have a positive effect on lipid profile (increase HDL/decrease LDL and triglycerides) and also dilate prostatic urethra. Hence are the drugs of choice for treatment of hypertension associated with BPH or dyslipidemia.
- These are also preferred for treatment of hypertension associated with nightmares caused by PTSD.
- The major side effect is **orthostatic hypotension** seen in 50% patients **only in the beginning** called as first dose effect and hence should be started at low doses given at bed time. Increased risk of CHF is also associated with this class.

β Blockers

- β blockers decrease blood pressure by decreasing cardiac output and inhibiting renin secretion in the JG cells.
- Currently β blockers are considered second line drugs as in trials they were associated with relatively more incidence of hypertension associated cardiovascular death (MI) and stroke. These are more effective in young and non-black patients.
- However, β blockers are still drug of choice if hypertension is associated with comorbidities like angina, chronic CHF, hyperthyroidism, migraine, essential tremor and anxiety with somatic manifestations.
- Intravenous beta blockers (labetalol > esmolol) are used for treatment of hypertensive emergency. Oral and IV labetalol are the drug of choice for treatment of hypertension and hypertensive emergency in pregnancy respectively.
- Carvedilol, bisoprolol and metoprolol are preferred for treatment of hypertension when associated with chronic CHF.
- In case of hypertension associated with bronchial asthma or COPD, the beta blocker of choice is bisoprolol.
- Though most of the antihypertensive drugs can cause **erectile dysfunction**, it is **maximum with beta blockers**. Other side effects associated are **nasal congestion**, AV block, Raynaud's phenomenon and CNS side effects like nightmares and depression.
- Sudden stoppage of beta blocker can cause **withdrawal hypertension** and hence dose should be gradually tapered down.
- Hypertension associated with cocaine use is a contraindication as block of beta2 receptors will cause unopposed vasoconstriction due to alpha adrenergic receptors. NSAIDs can decrease the antihypertensive effect due to inhibition of vasodilator prostacyclin synthesis and retention of sodium.

Central Sympatholytics

- This class decrease NE in the synapse and NE being a CNS stimulant, sedation is a common side effect seen. Apart from this, xerostomia, erectile dysfunction and postural hypotension may be seen.
- Methyldopa is a prodrug activated into α-methyl nor-epinephrine, which apart from displacing NE from vesicles

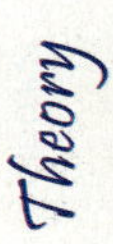

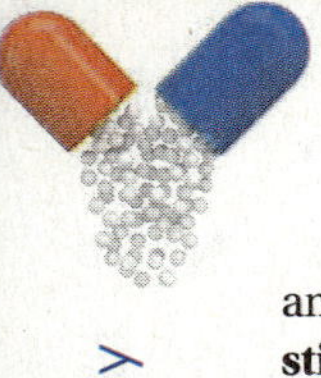

and depleting it, also **inhibits norepinephrine release by stimulating presynaptic α_2 receptors (primary mechanism in hypertension)**. Though it has a short half-life of 2 hours, it is long acting (24 hours) due to time required for transport into CNS, activation and depleting NE in vesicle. The use is limited to treatment of hypertension in pregnancy. The side effects associated are **coombs positive hemolytic anemia** due to anti-Rh antibodies, hepatitis and **decreased libido**. Decreased dopamine may cause parkinsonism and hyperprolactinemia. Mild **withdrawal hypertension** may be seen.

- Clonidine, guanfacine and guanabenz are α_2 agonists that act by inhibiting presynaptic NE release. Clonidine also acts by stimulating **imidazole I_1 receptors**. Oral clonidine is the drug of choice for treatment of **hypertensive urgency** and is also used for diagnosis of pheochromocytoma. Clonidine patches are used in incompliant patients. Immediate discontinuation of clonidine can cause **withdrawal hypertension**, which can be treated in non-life-threatening condition by restarting clonidine and in life-threatening condition by phentolamine, labetalol/carvedilol or nitroprusside. TCA can compromise the antihypertensive effect of clonidine.
- **Moxonidine** is an agonist at both alpha2 and imidazole receptors (I_1). It is used for treatment of resistant hypertension in elderly and for neuropathic pain and has been seen to reduce risk of atrial fibrillation as well. Another drug with similar properties is **rilmenidine**. Imidazole receptor I_1 stimulation releases norepinephrine into the alpha2 receptor and this produces central sympatholytic action.

Sympathetic Neuronal Blockers

- Reserpine is a natural alkaloid derived from a plant Rauwolfia serpentine. It blocks vesicular monoamine transporter (VMAT-2), required for vesicle movement and release of NE. The use is limited to treatment of hypertension along with diuretics in elderly patients. Side effects associated are sedation and depression.
- Metyrosine inhibits tyrosine hydroxylase, the rate limiting enzyme of NE synthesis. It can be used along with phenoxybenzamine for treatment and preoperative preparation of pheochromocytoma. Crystalluria is a specific side effect that is associated.
- Guanadrel and guanethidine act by depleting the vesicular NE like methyldopa. These drugs are rarely used for treatment of hypertension and are contraindicated in pheochromocytoma as they release NE. Postural hypotension is a persistent side effect seen due to sympathetic blockade even on **chronic administration**.

N_N Receptor Antagonists (Ganglionic Blockers)

- These are targeted at the ganglionic site which leads to inhibition of norepinephrine and acetylcholine release in the post ganglionic fibers. Hence, the effect that can be seen are vasodilation and mild reflex tachycardia associated with anticholinergic effects like dry mouth, constipation, urine retention etc.
- **Tetraethylammonium** (TEA), **trimethaphan, hexamethonium** and **mecamylamine** are the drugs in this class, also known as ganglionic blockers were the first class of drug to be used in hypertension. Though nowadays less preferred due to associated side effects.
- Mecamylamine an oral drug, is also used for treatment of Tourette's syndrome and as an adjunct to nicotine patch in smoking dependence.
- Trimethaphan is used by intravenous route for treatment of hypertensive emergency.
- These drugs can also be used in nicotine toxicity to block the NN receptors in ganglion.
- Tetraethylammonium is currently used as a research agent that selectively blocks potassium channel.

HYPERTENSIVE CRISIS

High blood pressure with end organ damage causing CHF, pulmonary edema, retinopathy, renal failure, MI, stroke, eclampsia, aortic dissection or unstable angina is known hypertensive emergency. Malignant is an old term which represents hypertensive encephalopathy or nephropathy along with retinopathy. Both are treated immediately by intravenous drugs. A blood pressure more than 220/125 mm Hg, without any end organ damage is known as hypertensive urgency, which is treated with oral drugs.

Drugs used in Hypertensive Emergency

DHPs (Nicardipine > Clevidipine) and beta blockers (Labetalol > Esmolol) are the most preferred drugs with the former being first choice. Hence, IV nicardipine is the drug of choice for hypertensive emergency. But in pregnancy intravenous labetalol is the drug of choice.

Mnemonics

HELEN Dance
- **H :** Hydralazine
- **E :** Esmolol
- **L :** Labetalol, Lasix
- **E :** Enalaprilat
- **N :** Nitroglycerine, Nitroprusside
- **Dance:** DHPs, D1 agonist (Fenodolpam)

Drugs used in Hypertensive Urgency

Oral clonidine is the drug of choice for hypertensive urgency. Other drugs that can be used are enalapril and nifedipine.

ANGINA

Angina is caused by a mismatch in the myocardial oxygen supply and demand, which can be because of decreased oxygen supply, increased oxygen demand or both. Based on the pathophysiology, angina can be classified into three types i.e. stable angina, unstable angina and variant (Prinzmetal) angina.

STABLE OR TYPICAL ANGINA

- Stable angina is caused by coronary atherosclerosis causing a progressive narrowing, which decreases coronary blood supply. In case of physical or emotional stress, there is an increase in heart rate and cardiac contraction that increases myocardial oxygen demand and precipitates angina. The

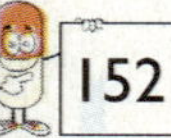

primary aim of treatment is to ameliorate an acute attack, prevent further attacks of angina and MI and decrease mortality (coronary death).

- For an acute attack sublingual nitroglycerine is the drug of choice. To prevent an acute attack in case of expected stress, sublingual NTG should be taken five minutes before. For long-term prevention, beta blockers, CCB, nitrates, ranolazine, ivabradine and nicorandil can be used. The only class of drug used for long-term prevention that also decreases mortality are beta blockers. Antiplatelet agents also decrease incidences of coronary events in patients of angina. Aspirin (81–325 mg) is preferred and in case of intolerance clopidogrel is used.
- Vasodilators like nitroglycerine, CCBs, dipyridamole and papaverine are used for assessment of coronary artery stenosis. Dipyridamole is an adenosine reuptake inhibitor that can cause coronary steal phenomenon. Papaverine is a short acting vasodilator that acts by inhibiting PDE.

UNSTABLE ANGINA

- Unstable angina is caused by atherosclerotic plaque rupture, that stimulates platelet aggregation and coagulation system that causes occlusion of coronary artery. In unstable angina, there is no ST elevation and along with MI without ST elevation, together it is known as acute coronary syndrome.
- Treatment of acute attack is with sublingual NTG. Then a patient is started on beta blockers and in case of ineffectiveness or intolerance, a CCB can be substituted or added.
- To decrease mortality on long-term basis patient is started on antiaggregant and high dose statins. Aspirin is immediately started at a loading dose of 162-325 mg and then continued at a dose of 81–162 mg. At the time of PCI (percutaneous intervention) a P2Y12 inhibitor (clopidogrel, prasugrel or ticagrelor) is added. Inhibitors of glycoprotein IIb/IIIa (abciximab, tirofiban and eptifibatide) are used as adjuncts to P2Y12 inhibitor during PCI in high risk patients i.e. with fluctuating ST segment.
- Anticoagulation with LMWH is preferred to prevent further ischemic attacks. Other alternatives are fondaparinux and direct thrombin inhibitor (bivalirudin).
- **Thrombolysis is absolutely contraindicated** in acute coronary syndrome (no ST segment elevation), as absolute coronary block is usually not seen and thus the risk of thrombolysis is more than benefit.

VARIANT (PRINZMETAL) ANGINA

Variant angina is caused by coronary vasospasm that acutely decreases coronary blood flow and precipitates angina. Sublingual nitroglycerine is the drug of choice for acute attack whereas both DHPs and nitrates can be used to for prophylaxis. These drugs give symptomatic relief by producing **endothelium independent coronary vasodilation**. Aspirin can worsen variant angina by decreasing prostaglandin synthesis and beta blockers by inhibiting beta-2 receptor mediated vasodilation.

DRUGS USED IN ANGINA

Nitrates

- A mitochondrial enzyme aldehyde dehydrogenase activates nitrates into nitric oxide (NO), which stimulates **guanylate cyclase** in smooth muscles to produce cyclic GMP. Cyclic GMP further activates protein kinase G, which dephosphorylates myosin light chain and results in vasodilatation. Cyclic GMP is metabolized by phosphodiesterase-5 (PDE-5). Hence, PDE-5 inhibitor like **sildenafil is contraindicated with nitrates** due to risk of severe hypotension.
- Dilatation of coronary arteries relieves angina pain and systemic veins decrease the preload on heart. A **decrease in cardiac preload** significantly **decreases the wall tension and oxygen demand of myocardium** is the most important mechanism for beneficial effect in classical angina as well as chronic CHF. Coronary vasodilation is the most important mechanism in variant angina.
- The other effects are relaxation of smooth muscles in GIT and inhibition of platelet aggregation. Antiaggregant effect contributes to its antianginal effect, whereas relaxation of GIT makes them useful to relieve **esophageal** and **biliary spasm**.
- The side effects are related to vasodilation and present as orthostatic hypotension and headache. These effects are seen in workers of industries with nitrate compounds particularly on resuming works after weekends on Monday and hence is called as **"Monday disease".**
- Downregulation of aldehyde dehydrogenase production can cause nitrate tolerance. To avoid it a nitrate free period of 8 hours is given at night.

Conceptual Box-13

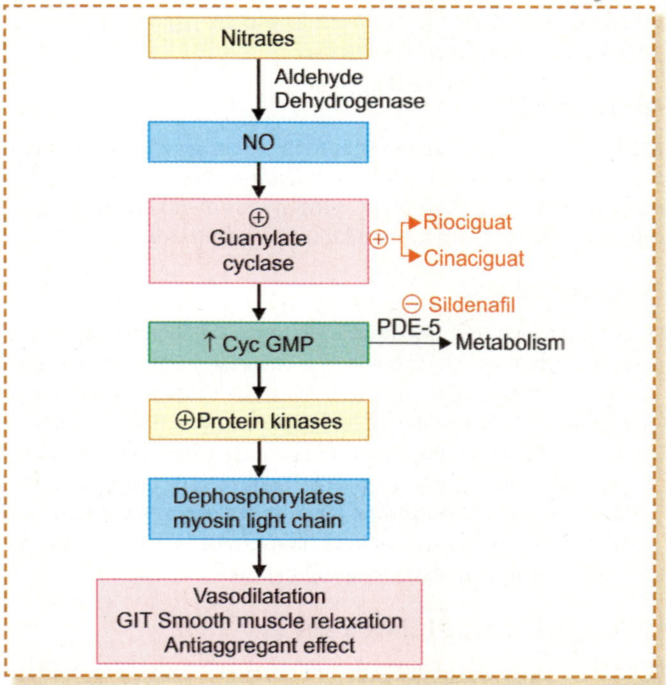

Nitroglycerine (NTG)

- Nitroglycerine undergoes significant first pass metabolism by nitrate reductase and hence is not effective by oral route.
- Sublingual nitroglycerine is the drug of choice for treatment of an **acute attack of stable and Prinzmetal (variant) angina,** for which a buccal spray can also be used. To prevent an acute attack in case of expected stress, sublingual NTG should be taken five minutes before.

- Sublingual NTG is also drug of choice for treatment of pain associated with MI.
- Buccal and transdermal route can be used for prophylaxis. Transdermal NTG is preferred for prophylaxis of nocturnal angina.
- Intravenous nitroglycerine is used for treatment of pulmonary edema associated with acute CHF and for hypertensive emergency.

Isosorbide Dinitrate (IDN)

- IDN also undergoes first pass metabolism but lesser than NTG. IDN is metabolized by denitration into IMN, the active form.
- It is administered by sublingual route for an acute attack and by oral route for long-term prophylaxis of angina.
- By oral route it is also used along with hydralazine for treatment of chronic CHF.

Isosorbide Mononitrate (IMN)

IMN has **no scope for first pass metabolism** and hence is the only nitrate with 100% oral bioavailability. IMN is used for long-term prophylaxis of angina.

Erythritol Tetranitrate and Pentaerythritol Tetranitrate

Pentaerythritol tetranitrate is the longest acting nitrate followed by erythritol tetranitrate. These are used by oral route for long-term prophylaxis of angina.

Molsidomine

Molsidomine is activated in liver to linsidomine which produces vasodilation by releasing NO, as it disintegrates. It is long acting and can be used for long-term prophylaxis of angina in place of nitrates. Its side effects are similar to that of nitrates.

Beta Blockers

- Beta blockers decrease heart rate, myocardial contraction and blood pressure, which leads to a decrease in oxygen demand by the myocardium. This decreases the number of ischemic episodes and hence is used for long-term prevention of angina.
- Apart from this **beta blockers are only class that decrease mortality on long-term use in angina** and progression to MI. Though care should be taken in a case of variant angina caused by vasospasm, as beta blockers can worsen it due to block of beta-2 mediated vasodilatation.

Calcium Channel Blockers

- In case of stable angina calcium channel blocker's beneficial effect is more due to a decrease in oxygen demand (due to decreased myocardial contraction, HR and BP) than increased coronary blood flow due to vasodilatation.
- They are indicated for long-term prevention, in case of beta blocker ineffectiveness, contraindication or intolerance.
- Diltiazem and verapamil can be used as monotherapy as they don't increase oxygen demand. DHPs can cause reflex tachycardia and worsen angina and hence are always used along with beta blockers. CCBs don't decrease mortality in angina.
- DHPs are also used for prophylaxis of variant or Prinzmetal angina.

Ranolazine

- **Ranolazine** acts by inhibiting the late **Na current** and **K channels** in the myocardial cells. A decrease in intracellular sodium secondarily stimulates the Na/Ca exchanger pumps, which based on the need of the hour pump sodium into the cell and calcium out of the cell. Thus, depletion of intracellular calcium decreases the contraction of myocardium and oxygen demand, but there is no effect on HR and BP.
- Ranolazine is indicated for long-term prevention of angina, when all other drugs i.e. beta blockers, CCBs and nitrates are ineffective.
- The other effects are **decrease incidence of atrial fibrillation** and **improved glucose profile (It decreases $HbA1_c$)**. It is under trial for treatment of atrial fibrillation along with dronedarone.
- It is contraindicated with other drugs increasing QT interval (it can prolong QT interval) and in **liver failure**.

Ivabradine

- **Ivabradine** inhibits the **funny channels (I_f current)** required for depolarization of cells in SA node that maintains its automaticity. Hence its inhibition decreases the heart rate and oxygen demand, thereby decreasing episodes of **angina**. It is also effective for treatment of **sinus tachycardia** and **chronic CHF**.
- It has a weak beta blocking effect and at high doses inhibits PFOX.
- It is used as a substitute for beta blockers, when the heart rate is more than 75 being on beta blockers.
- It should be avoided with verapamil and diltiazem.
- Side effects associated are bradycardia, luminous phenomena, QT prolongation and atrial fibrillation. Luminous phenomena or phosphenes are transient bright spots or haloes in the visual field.

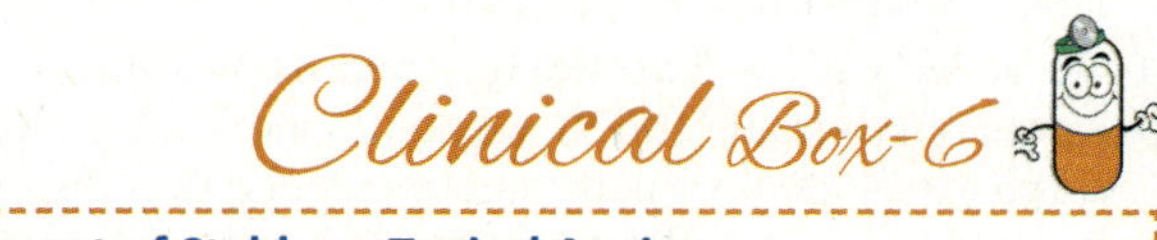

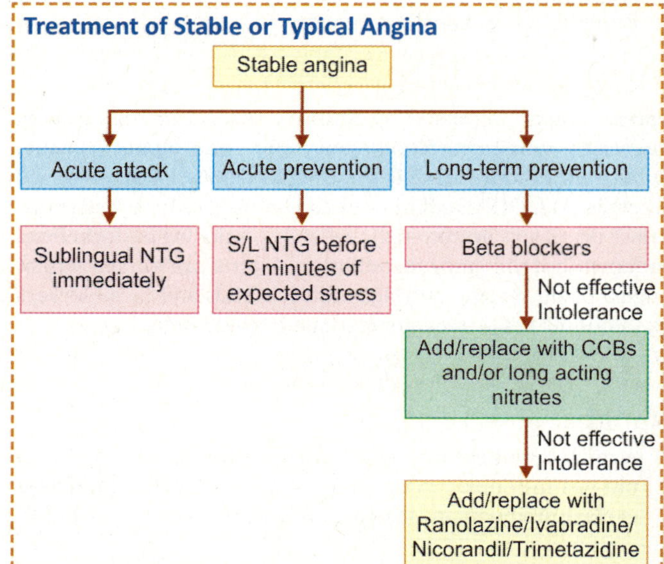

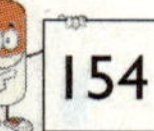

Recent Advances

Recent Advances in Treatment of Angina

Nicorandil: It **opens ATP sensitive potassium channel** in the blood vessels which leads to dilation of both arteries and veins. This follows a decrease in contraction of myocardium and oxygen demand. It has cardioprotective effect due to ischemic preconditioning. It can cause hypotension, headache and gastric ulcers. It is contraindicated with sildenafil.

Fasudil: It is a rho kinase inhibitor, that acts by inhibiting phosphorylation of smooth muscles and causes vasodilation. It is effective for treatment of angina, pulmonary hypertension and angina.

Metabolic agents: Trimetazidine and perhexiline are inhibitors of partial fatty acid oxidation (PFOX) that forces myocardium to use glucose as a source of energy. Glucose oxidation consumes less oxygen as compared to fatty acid oxidation and hence the oxygen demand by myocardium decreases. It increases risk of Parkinson's diseases.

MYOCARDIAL INFARCTION

Acute myocardial infarction is most commonly caused by plaque rupture that stimulates platelet aggregation and coagulation system leading to thrombosis. Occlusion can lead to STEMI or non-STEMI; the treatment for the later has been discussed in the section of angina. In case of STEMI, the aim is to ameliorate pain, facilitate perfusion into infarct area and prevent further attack of MI and death.

ANALGESIC THERAPY

Sublingual NTG is the drug of choice for ameliorating pain associated with MI. Apart from relieving pain it also decreases oxygen demand and increase oxygen supply to the myocardium. In case of ineffectiveness, morphine should be started, which also decreases associated pulmonary edema by decreasing preload and afterload. IV beta blockers can also relieve pain by decreasing oxygen demand of myocardium.

REPERFUSION THERAPY

- Reperfusion is the mainstay in STEMI to salvage the peri-infarct area of the myocardium and should be done **within 12 hours of symptom onset**.
- PCI is more preferred than fibrinolysis if the facility for PCI is available and has maximum benefit if done within **90 minutes** ("door to balloon time") of infarction.
- In case a patient is referred from a center without PCI availability, the time can be extended to 120 minutes.
- If fibrinolysis is done, then should be attempted within **30 minutes** ("door to needle time"). The thrombolytics used are tissue plasminogen activator or tPA (alteplase), genetically engineered tPA (reteplase and tenecteplase) and streptokinase. Alteplase is the most clot specific drug.

ANTICOAGULANT THERAPY

- Anticoagulant therapy maintains patency of the affected coronary artery and prevents rethrombosis.
- IN PCI stent placement is done with a LMWH or direct thrombin inhibitor bivalirudinto prevent thrombosis.
- After fibrinolytic infusion LMWH is given every 12 hours.
- Use of LMWH is associated with a significant decrease in reinfarction and mortality.

THERAPY AIMED AT MORTALITY BENEFIT

- **Antiaggregant therapy** decreases the chances of rethrombosis and prevents mortality. A patient of MI is immediately given aspirin at dose of 162–325 mg in chewable form and then given daily at dose of 75–162 mg. A patient with stent is started on dual antiaggregant combination i.e. aspirin and a P2Y12 inhibitor. Prasugrel and ticagrelor being longer acting and more potent are more preferred more than clopidogrel. However, P2Y12 inhibitor of choice during fibrinolysis is clopidogrel as there are no trials with the previous drugs. A glycoprotein IIb/IIIa inhibitor can be used along with LMWH or bivalirudin during PCI to prevent thrombosis.
- **Statins** decrease the risk of reinfarction and improves outcome after bypass surgery.
- **Beta blockers** show short-term mortality benefit and should be started with 24 hours of MI, unless they are contraindicated.
- **ACEI/ARB** show both long and short-term benefit and should be started early in patients with MI. They are more beneficial with EF<40%, large infarcts and associated CHF.
- **Aldosterone antagonist** are beneficial in case of associated CHF.

Clinical Box-7

Treatment of MI

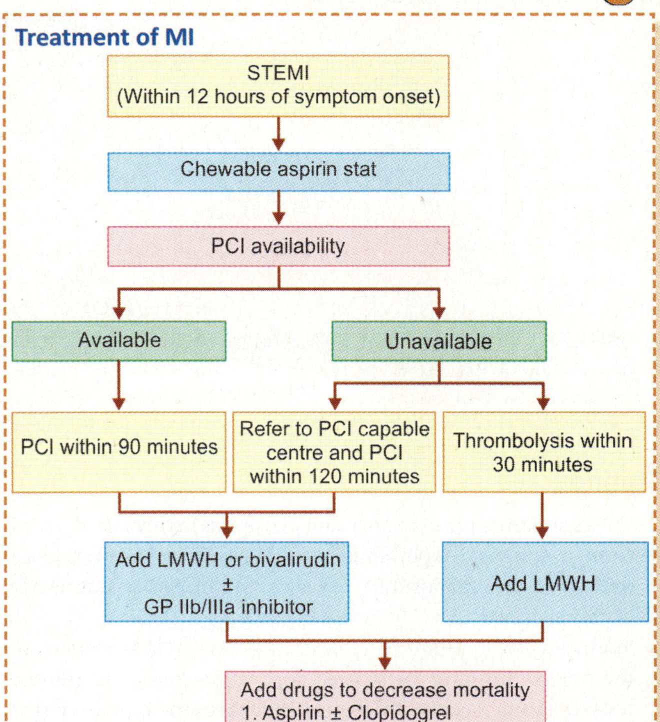

HYPOLIPIDEMICS

Lipids are an important source of energy, but on accumulation can cause atherosclerosis and result in ischemic heart and cerebrovascular disease and peripheral vascular disease. Hypolipidemic therapy in the former is an important part of treatment to decrease mortality.

- Triglycerides and cholesterol (by NPC1L1 protein) is absorbed from the intestine and then converted into chylomicrons and transported into systemic circulation.
- Endogenous triglycerides are synthesized in the liver and transported by MTP (Microsomal Triglyceride transfer Protein) to the site in rough endoplasmic reticulum where along with apo-B 100 proteins, VLDL is synthesized and secreted into systemic circulation.
- Chylomicrons and VLDL, while passing through the capillaries rich in lipoprotein lipase (LPL) in adipose tissue, cardiac and skeletal muscles and breast tissue in lactating mothers, triglycerides are hydrolyzed and taken up and utilized by these tissues.
- Thus, there is a decrease in VLDL, triglycerides and chylomicrons. The resultant LDL after this is metabolized by LPL and hepatic lipase (HL) into LDL, which is taken up by LDL receptors and metabolized.
- Another source of triglycerides in plasma is through lipolysis in adipocytes by hormone sensitive lipase.
- LDL is taken up and oxidized by macrophages that form foam cells, crucial for atherogenesis in arteries.
- HDL precursor is primarily synthesized in liver and intestine, which when released into systemic circulation acquires cholesterol and matures. Thus, HDL decreases plasma cholesterol and apart from that possesses antioxidant, antiaggregant, anti-inflammatory and anti-coagulant effect.
- These physiological pathways of lipid metabolism are targeted by hypolipidemic drugs and a decrease in LDL, triglycerides and increase in HDL are the important outcomes.

Conceptual Box-14

Lipid Metabolism and Drugs Acting on it

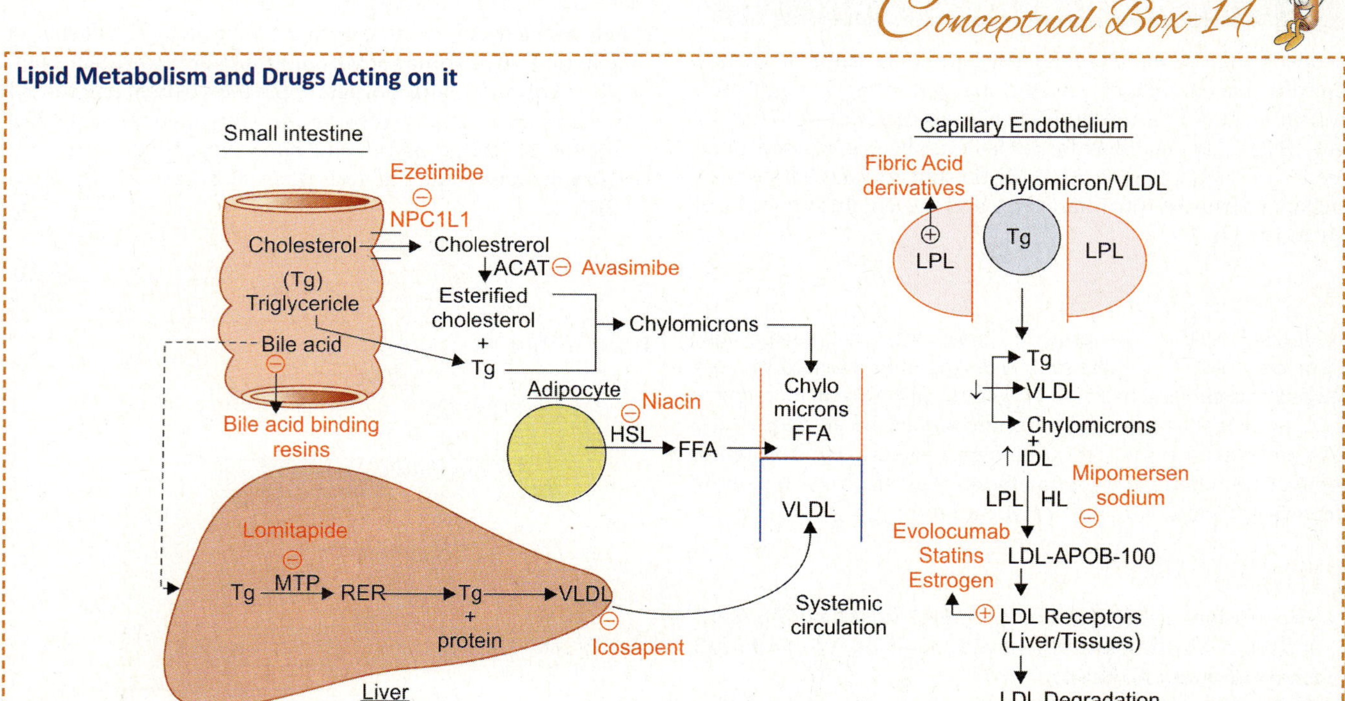

Statins

- The first statin approved for clinical use was **lovastatin** derived from a fungus (Aspergillus terreus), whose semisynthetic derivatives are pravastatin and simvastatin. Other statins are purely synthetic.
- Statins act by competitively inhibiting **HMG-CoA reductase**, the rate limiting enzyme for cholesterol synthesis. A decrease in plasma cholesterol, **increases the LDL receptor production** which lowers plasma LDL levels (except in familial homozygous hypercholesterolemia due to faulty LDL receptors). They also decrease triglyceride levels by inhibiting VLDL synthesis and another effect is an increase in HDL levels.
- The non-hypolipidemic activities of statins called as **pleiotropic effects** are **antiaggregant**, anticoagulant, anti-inflammatory (decreases CRP), vasodilatory (increases endothelial NO release) and atherosclerotic plaque stabilizing effect.
- Statins have a high first pass metabolism due to uptake by organic anionic transporter (OATP1B1). The metabolites of statins also inhibit HMG-CoA reductase except for fluvastatin and pravastatin. The only prodrug statins are **lovastatin** and

simvastatin, which are made **highly lipid soluble** to increase oral absorption. They have high plasma protein binding, with pravastatin being least. **Rosuvastatin** and **atorvastatin** are **longest acting** statins. **Pitavastatin and rosuvastatin (pitavastatin > rosuvastatin)** are most potent statins whereas simvastatin is the least potent one.

- Statins are the drug of choice for **dyslipidemia with raised LDL (type II hyperlipoproteinemia)** except in pregnancy and children, where the bile acid binding resins are preferred. They have a mortality benefit when used in patients/patients at risk of **CAD** and **stroke** and hence are preferred drugs. Since the activity of HMG-CoA reductase is maximum at night time, statins are **taken at bed time**. Only statins which **need not be taken at bed time** are **rosuvastatin** and **atorvastatin**, due to their long half-life.
- Side effects associated are hepatotoxicity and myopathy (maximum with simvastatin). Pretreatment measurement of ALT/AST and follow up testing every 3–6 months is recommended. Routine CK measurement is not recommended as myopathy can be delayed until years. **Pravastatin can decrease fibrinogen levels**. Statins also increase the risk of diabetes mellitus and hence patients on statin therapy should be evaluated for new onset diabetes mellitus; however, since the benefit of prevention of atherosclerotic cardiovascular disease outweighs the risk of diabetes mellitus, statins are routinely used.
- Increased risk of adverse reaction to statins is seen in patients with impaired hepatic and renal function, unexplained ALT elevations >3 times normal limit, age >75 years, history of hemorrhagic stroke and Asian population. The concomitant use of other drugs that affect statin metabolism can also precipitate statintoxicity and has been discussed below.
- Fibrates inhibit statin glucunoridation and increase the risk of myopathy. Maximum risk is seen with gemfibrozil (also inhibits OATP1B1) whereas it is least with fenofibrate. Niacin can also enhance the myopathy effect of statins by inhibiting cholesterol synthesis in skeletal muscles. As statins are metabolized by CYP_{450} enzymes, enzyme inhibitors also increase risk of myopathy. Bile acid binding resins can decrease absorption of pravastatin and fluvastatin.
- All statins are contraindicated in children less than 10 years of age except **pravastatin**, which is contraindicated in children only **less than 8 years of age**.

Important points regarding statins

Important points	Statins
Longest acting (No night time dosing required)	Rosuvastatin > Atorvastatin
Most potent	Pitavastatin > Rosuvastatin
Prodrugs and lipid soluble	Lovastatin and Simvastatin
Maximum myopathy	Simvastatin
Metabolites don't inhibit HMG-CoA reductase	Fluvastatin and Pravastatin

Bile Acid Binding Resins (Sequestrants)

- Bile acid binding resins inhibit the enterohepatic circulation of bile acids thereby decreasing the same in liver. This causes a compensatory increase in bile acid synthesis from cholesterol by upregulation of hepatic enzyme 7-α-hydroxylase. The resultant decrease in cholesterol increases LDL receptor synthesis and a decrease in LDL and increase in HDL. Though there is a compensatory increase in cholesterol synthesis by **potentiation of HMG-CoA reductase**.
- They also increase VLDL and triglycerides and **are contra-indicated in hypertriglyceridemia**. These are used in patients only if serum triglycerides level is lesser than 300 mg/dL.
- Cholestyramine, colestipol and colesevelam are the drugs in this class used as a second line defense in dyslipidemia if statins are ineffective. They are drug of choice for **dyslipidemia in pregnancy and children**. The dose is taken before food and should not be taken with drugs as the absorption can be decreased, except colesevelam. Colesevelam can be used for treatment of diabetes mellitus also.
- GIT side effects like bloating, dyspepsia and constipation are most common. Hyperchloremic alkalosis can also be seen as these drugs are given as chloride salts.

Dyslipidemia in Pregnancy

Bile acid binding resins are the hypolipidemic drugs of choice in pregnancy and lactation. Other drugs should be stopped at least one month before planned conception. Statins, niacin, lomitapide and ezetimibe are absolutely contraindicated during pregnancy and lactation. Other drugs like mipomersen and PCSK-9 inhibitors lack data on safety in pregnancy.

Niacin

- Niacin or nicotinic acid is a vitamin that shows hypolipidemic activity by stimulating a G_i subtype of GPCR in adipocytes. There is a decrease in cyclic AMP that decreases synthesis of hormone sensitive lipase in adipocytes. Decreased lipolysis results in decreased free fatty acid for triglyceride and VLDL synthesis in liver.
- The net effect is a decrease in VLDL, triglycerides and LDL with a maximum **increase in HDL** synthesis among all hypolipidemic drugs. It is the only hypolipidemic drug to **decrease the plasma lipoprotein-a levels**.
- Niacin is used for treatment of hypertriglyceridemia associated with low HDL levels. For treatment of dyslipidemia with high LDL, it can be combined with statins at 25% of maximal dose due to risk of myopathy.
- **Flushing** and dyspepsia are most common side effects. Niacin increases prostaglandins that can cause flushing and pruritus; the drug of choice for same is **aspirin**. It can **increase blood glucose (insulin resistance)** and uric acid levels and hence both are measured routinely. Hepatotoxicity can be seen, and ALT/AST should also be monitored. It can also cause gastric ulcers.

Fibric Acid Derivatives

- Fibric acid derivatives stimulate **PPAR**-α and **increase lipoprotein lipase (LPL) synthesis**. An increase in LPL in the capillary endothelial cell decreases plasma triglycerides, chylomicrons and VLDL. There is also an increase in both HDL and LDL (maximum with gemfibrozil). Fibrates have anticoagulant and fibrinolytic effect as well.

- Clofibrate, fenofibrate, bezafibrate, ciprofibrate and gemfibrozil are the drugs in this class, which are drug of choice for treatment of **hypertriglyceridemia (fasting triglyceride >500 mg/dL), chylomicronemia syndrome and type III hyperlipoproteinemia**. They are usually taken 30 minutes before food as **food increases their absorption**.
- **Fenofibrate** can also decrease serum uric acid levels and hence can be used for treatment of gout if associated with hypertriglyceridemia.
- Fibrates can themselves cause myopathy (except bezafibrate) and can increase statin induced myopathy as well and hence should not be combined. Fibrates competitively inhibit glucunoridation of statins and increase their plasma levels. The effect on glucunoridation is maximum with gemfibrozil and minimum with fenofibrate. Choledocholithiasis can be seen, which is maximum with clofibrate.
- Fibrates are excreted by kidney and hence are contraindicated in renal failure.

Ezetimibe

- **Ezetimibe** inhibits **cholesterol absorption** by inhibiting **NPC1L1 (Niemann Pick C1 Like 1) protein** in the intestine. This decreases cholesterol delivery to liver by chylomicrons and leads to an increase in LDL receptors and decrease in plasma LDL.
- It is used as an add-on therapy in patients with inadequate response to statins.
- Allergic reactions and GIT upset can be seen with ezetimibe.

Lomitapide

- Lomitapide inhibits microsomal triglyceride transfer protein, which is required for transport of triglycerides to endoplasmic reticulum for attachment of lipoprotein that synthesizes VLDL and chylomicrons. Thus, lomitapide inhibits VLDL and chylomicron synthesis in liver and intestine respectively.
- It is used for treatment of homozygous familial hypercholesterolemia as an add-on drug.

Icosapent

Icosapent selectively decreases triglycerides by inhibiting VLDL synthesis and secretion and increasing clearance of VLDL from plasma. Thus, it is used for treatment of severe hypertriglyceridemia.

Mipomersen Sodium

- Mipomersen sodium is an antisense oligonucleotide that binds to mRNA for ApoB-100 resulting in degradation of mRNA by RNase. This inhibits synthesis of ApoB-100 required for LDL synthesis.
- It is approved as an add-on drug for treatment of homozygous familial hypercholesterolemia. Side effects associated are injection site reactions and flu like symptoms.

Anti PCSK-9 Monoclonal Antibodies

- **Evolocumab** and **alirocumab** are currently approved anti PCSK-9 monoclonal antibodies in use. The development of a third drug in this class **bococizumab** was stopped due to lesser efficacy than the current approved ones.
- PCSK-9 (Proprotein Convertase Subtilisin Kexin-9) binds to LDL receptors and mediate their degradation. Hence, these drugs by inhibiting PCSK-9 inhibit LDL receptor degradation thereby increasing LDL receptors and decreasing plasma LDL.
- These are approved as an add-on therapy to statins in patients of familial hypercholesterolemia and atherosclerotic cardiovascular disease (ASCVD) and patients with LDL-C levels ≥190 mg/dL.
- Route of administration is by subcutaneous route every 2–4 weeks.
- Side effects associated are injection site reactions, nasopharyngitis and influenza.

Avasimibe

- **Avasimibe** is an **Acyl CoA Cholesterol Acyl Transferase (ACAT) inhibitor** currently under trial for treatment of dyslipidemia. ACAT1 present in macrophages causes cholesterol esterification and promotes development of foam cells and atherosclerosis.
- ACAT2 present in small intestine and liver is essential for cholesterol esterification for chylomicron and VLDL synthesis. Thus, ACAT is a novel target for treatment of dyslipidemia.

CETP Inhibitors

Cholesteryl Ester Transfer Protein transfers cholesterol from HDL to LDL and VLDL. Hence, its inhibition increases HDL. Trials of most drugs were discontinued either due to toxicity (Torcetrapib) or efficacy issues (Dalcetrapib, Evacetrapib and Anacetraparib).

Phytosterols and Fibers

- Phytosterols displace cholesterol form micelles and hence decrease intestinal absorption of cholesterol.
- Fibers trap cholesterol and bile acids in intestine and prevent their absorption.
- These drugs can be used along with statins in patients of atherosclerotic cardiovascular disease (ASCVD) in case the LDL-C lowering goals are not achieved with statins alone.

Effect of hypolipidemic drugs on lipid profile

Hypolipidemic drugs	Effects
Statins	↓LDL, Cholesterol, VLDL, Triglycerides ↑HDL
Bile acid binding resins	↓LDL, Cholesterol ↑VLDL, Triglycerides
Niacin (Nicotinic Acid)	↓LDL, VLDL, Triglycerides, Lipoprotein-a ↑HDL (Maximum among hypolipidemics)
Fibrates	↓VLDL, IDL, Triglycerides ↑HDL
Ezetimibe PCSK-9 Inhibitors	↓LDL
Lomitapide Icosapent	↓VLDL, Triglycerides

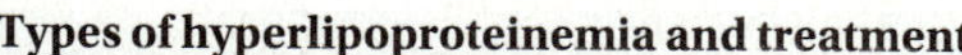

Types of hyperlipoproteinemia and treatment

Type of hyperlipoproteinemia	Lipoprotein increased	Treatment
Type I	Chylomicrons	No treatment required
Type IIa	LDL	Statins and Ezetimibe
Type IIb	LDL and VLDL	Fibrates, Statins and Nicotinic acid
Type III	VLDL	Fibrates
Type IV	Beta VLDL	Fibrates
Type V	Chylomicrons and VLDL	Fibrates, Niacin and Statins

ACC (AMERICAN COLLEGE OF CARDIOLOGY)/AHA (AMERICAN HEART ASSOCIATION) GUIDELINES

STATIN THERAPY

- According to ACC/AHA guidelines, there are four evidence- based statin benefit groups as given below:
  - Patients with clinical atherosclerotic cardiovascular disease (ASCVD). Clinical ASCVD includes acute coronary syndromes, history of myocardial infarction, stable or unstable angina, coronary or other artery revascularization, stroke, transient ischemic stroke (TIA) or peripheral arterial disease of atherosclerotic origin.
  - Patients aged ≥21 years with LDL-C ≥190 mg/dL; these patients are at high risk of ASCVD
  - Patients aged 40–75 years with diabetes mellitus and LDL-C 70–189 mg/dL
  - Patients aged 40–75 years with no diabetes mellitus and LDL-C 70–189 mg/dL
- Based on dose of statins administered, statin therapy is classified into three types i.e. high, moderate and low intensity statin therapy. The extent of reduction in risk of ASCVD is directly proportional to decreases in levels of LDL-C.

Statin therapy	Percentage reduction of LDL-C	Statins and doses	Indication
High Intensity	≥50%	Atorvastatin 40–80 mg Rosuvastatin 20–40 mg	• Patients age ≤75 years with clinical ASCVD • Patients age ≥21 years with LDL-C levels ≥190 mg/dL • Patients age 40–75 years with or without diabetes mellitus, LDL-C 70–189 and 10 years risk of ASCVD ≥7.5%
Moderate Intensity	30–49%	Atorvastatin 10–20 mg Rosuvastatin 5–10 mg Simvastatin 20–40 mg Pravastatin 40–80 mg Lovastatin 40 mg Pitavastatin 2–4 mg	• Patients age >75 years with clinical ASCVD • Patients age 40–75 years with or without diabetes mellitus, LDL-C 70–189 and 10 years risk of ASCVD <7.5%
Low intensity	<30%	Simvastatin 10 mg Pravastatin 10–20 mg Lovastatin 20 mg Pitavastatin 1 mg	Usually not preferred

NONSTATIN THERAPY

- Drugs other than statins like ezetimibe, PCSK-9 inhibitors and bile acid binding resins are used in case the desired LDL-C levels are not reached with statins alone. The guidelines can be broadly classified into two groups:
  - Patients with ASCVD or LDL-C levels ≥ 90 mg/dL
  - Patients without ASCVD or LDL-C levels <190 mg/dL
- Ezetimibe and bile acid binding resins can be used in both groups whereas PCSK-9 inhibitors are currently indicated only in the first group. PCSK-9 inhibitors are not indicated in patients of ASCVD with NYHA class II-III heart failure and in patients on dialysis.
- The flow chart describing the strategy of management in both groups is given below.

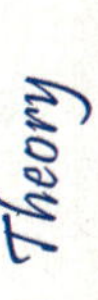

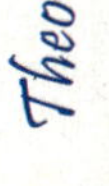

Patients with ASCVD or LDL-C Levels ≥190 mg/dL

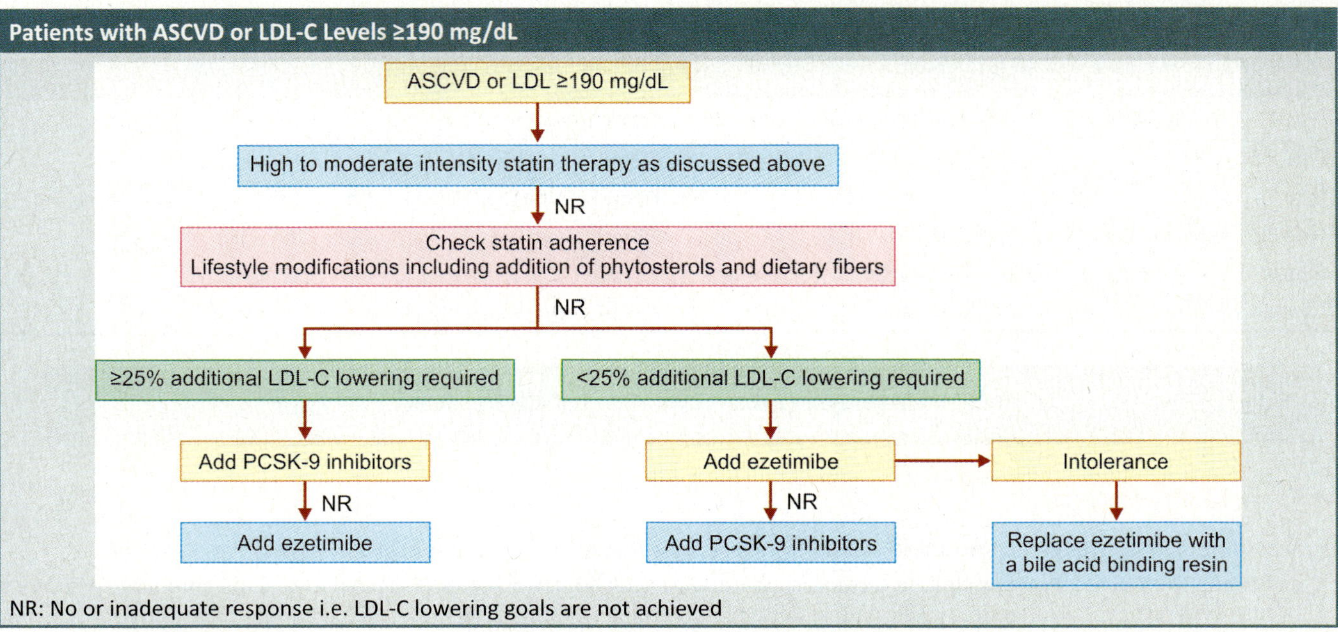

NR: No or inadequate response i.e. LDL-C lowering goals are not achieved

Patients without ASCVD or LDL-C Levels <190 mg/dL

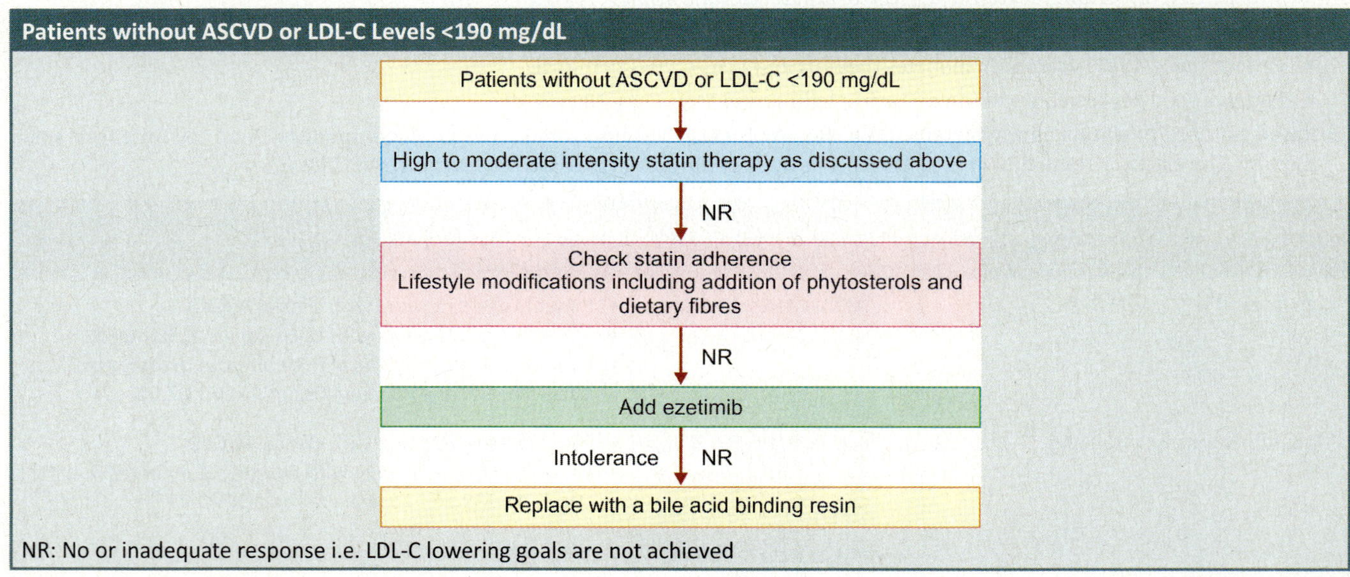

NR: No or inadequate response i.e. LDL-C lowering goals are not achieved

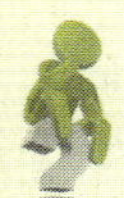

Image-based Questions

1. A patient was prescribed an antiarrhythmic drug which caused pigmentation as seen in the picture. Which of the following drugs might have done it?

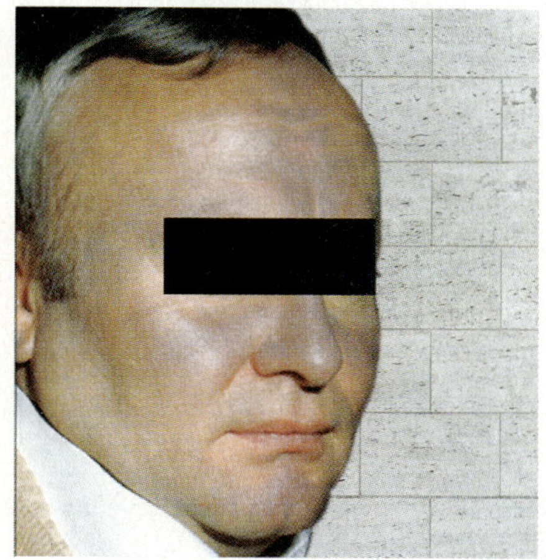

a. Lidocaine
b. Amiodarone
c. Procainamide
d. Bretylium

2. A patient of COPD presents to the emergency with recent onset of palpitation. The ECG revealed findings given below. Which of the following is drug of choice for chronic therapy?

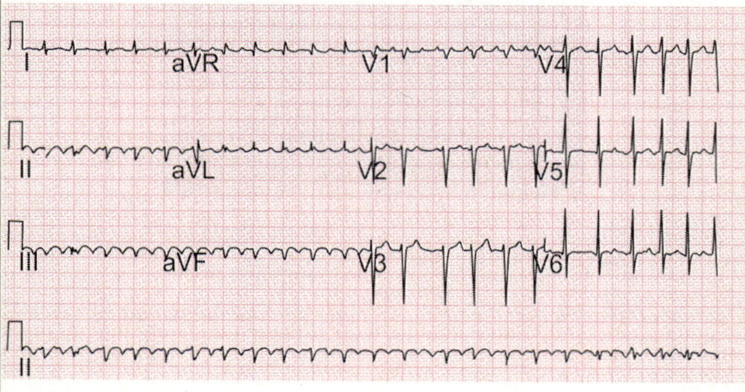

a. Amiodarone
b. Flecainide
c. Digoxin
d. Propranolol

3. A 25-year-old patient presents to the emergency with palpitation and shortness of breath. An ECG was advised, which gave the following finding. Which of the following is to be done immediately?

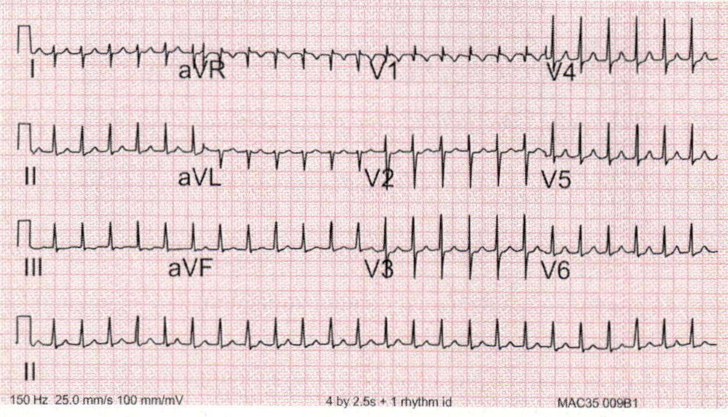

a. IV adenosine
b. IV Procainamide
c. Carotid sinus massage
d. IV Verapamil

4. The apparatus in the X-ray given below is the first line treatment option in all of the following except:

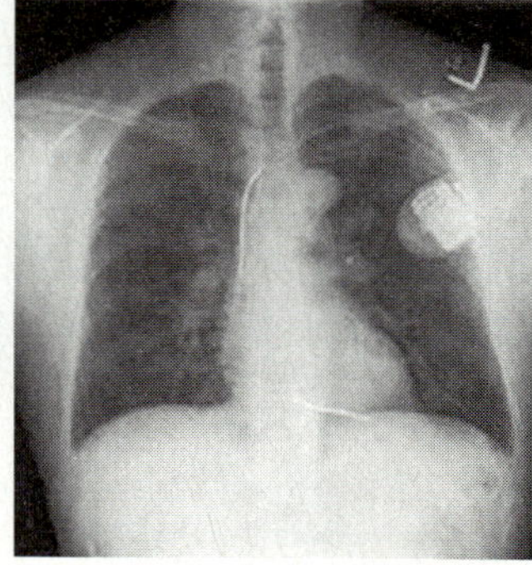

a. Congenital long QT syndrome
b. Ventricular fibrillation
c. Ventricular tachycardia
d. Atrial fibrillation

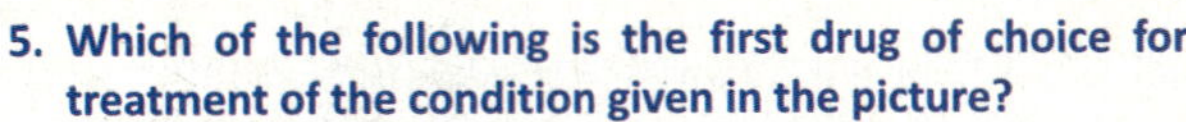

5. Which of the following is the first drug of choice for treatment of the condition given in the picture?

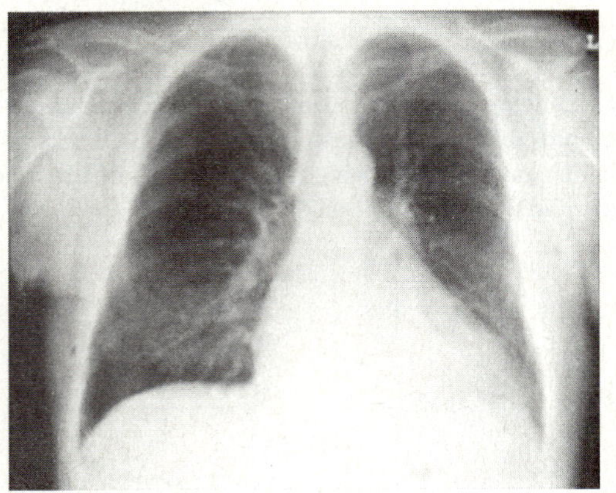

a. ACEI
b. Beta blockers
c. Spironolactone
d. Ivabradine

6. The plant in the picture is a source of:

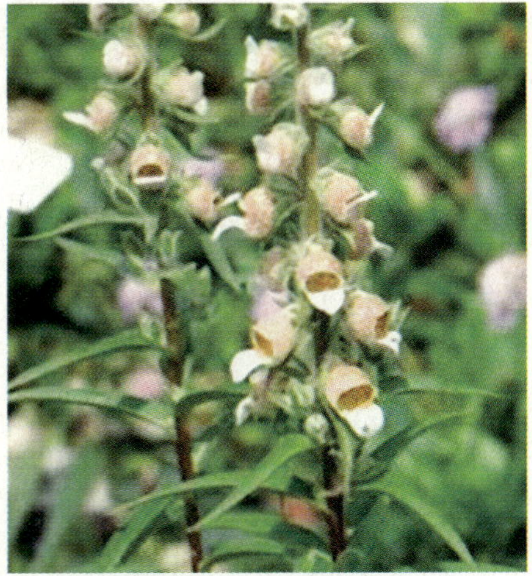

a. Digoxin
b. Atropine
c. Reserpine
d. Physostigmine

7. Which of the following drug is contraindicated in a patient with the given angiogram?

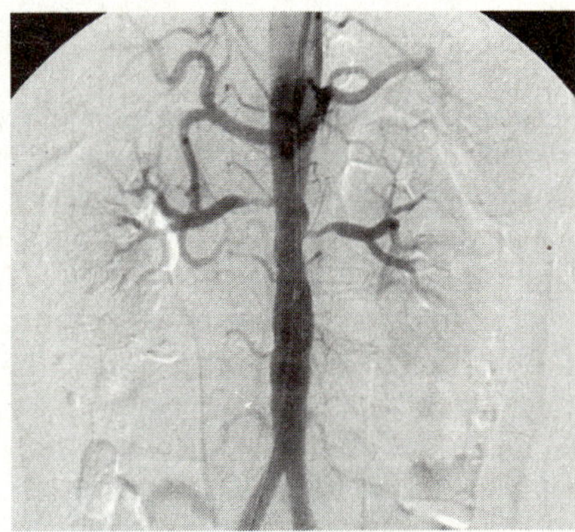

a. Chlorthalidone
b. Metoprolol
c. Captopril
d. Enalapril

8. Which of the following drug could have precipitated the condition in the angiography?

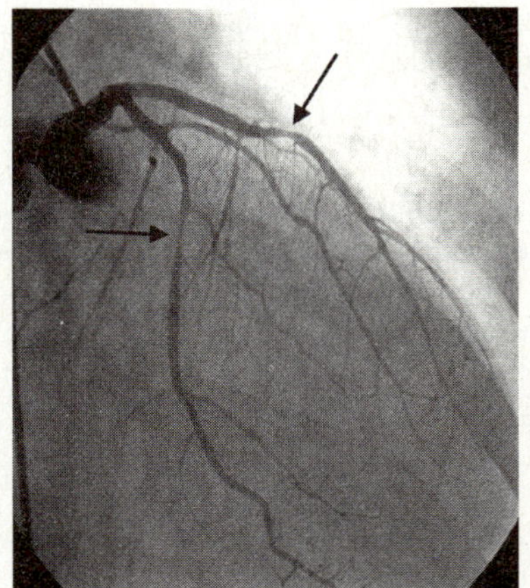

a. CCB
b. Beta blockers
c. ACEI
d. Nitroglycerine

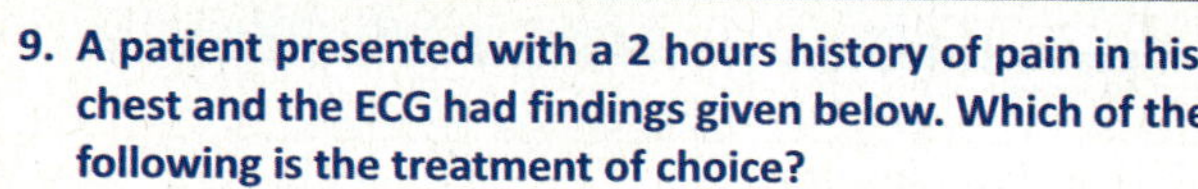

9. A patient presented with a 2 hours history of pain in his chest and the ECG had findings given below. Which of the following is the treatment of choice?

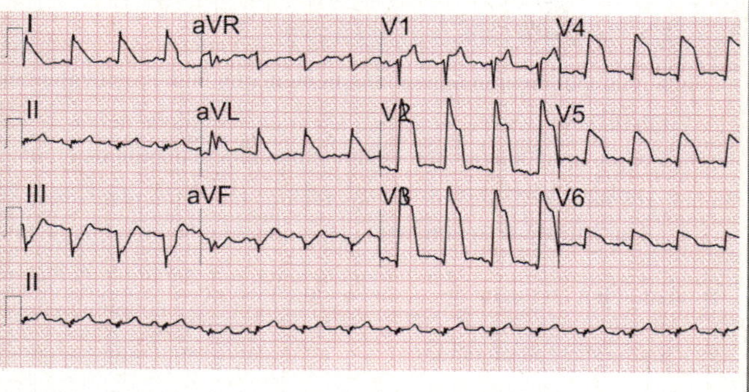

a. PCI
b. Thrombolysis
c. NTG
d. IV beta blocker

11. A patient 65-year-old presented with chest pain and the following ECG was recorded. Which of the following is not to be done?

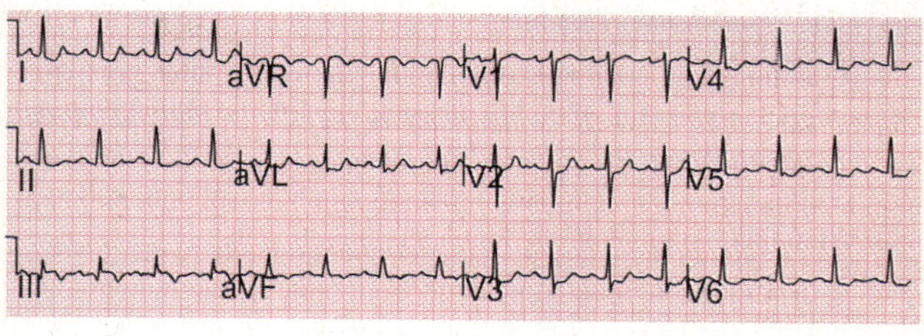

a. PCI
b. Thrombolysis
c. LMWH
d. Aspirin

10. Which of the following antiarrhythmic can cause the ocular changes in the picture?

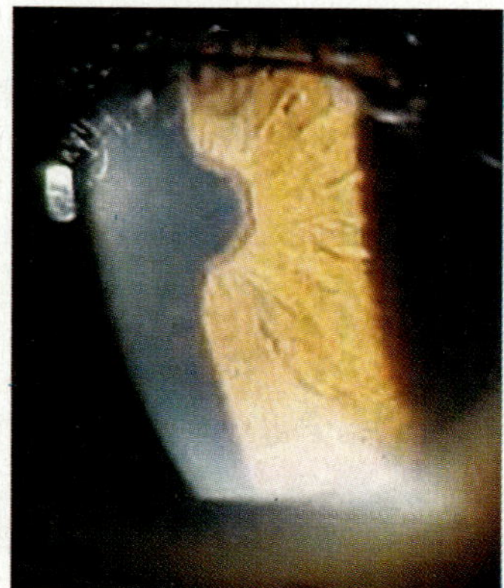

a. Procainamide
b. Verapamil
c. Amiodarone
d. Dronedarone

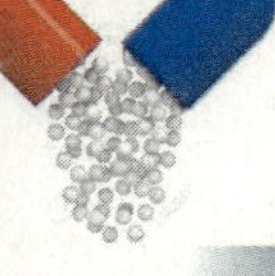

Answers with Explanations to Image-based Questions

1. Ans. (b) Amiodarone

(Ref: Braunwald's Cardiology 9th E/P723)

- Blue gray pigmentation, as seen in the picture is characteristic of amiodarone, which is also known as ceruloderma.

2. Ans. (a) Amiodarone

(Ref: CMDT 2015/P390)

- Sawtooth pattern in leads II, III and AVF and association of COPD confirms the diagnosis of atrial flutter. For chronic atrial flutter and to maintain sinus rhythm, amiodarone is the drug of choice.

3. Ans. (c) Carotid sinus massage

(Ref: CMDT 2015/P381)

- Narrow complex tachycardia with absent P waves at a young age is suggestive of PSVT. The first line of management is vagal maneuvers like carotid sinus massage. If the patient does not respond, then IV adenosine is given.

4. Ans. (d) Atrial fibrillation

(Ref: Goodman Gilman 12th E/P824)

- The patient has been implanted an ICD (Implanted cardiovert defibrillator) device, which is used for long-term management to prevent
- Congenital long QT syndrome
- Ventricular tachycardia associated with MI
- Ventricular fibrillation

5. Ans. (a) ACEI

(Ref: Goodman and Gilman 12th E/P 798)

- The given X-ray depicts, CHF with left ventricular hypertrophy.
- The first drug of choice to decrease mortality is ACEI/ ARB.

6. Ans. (a) Digoxin

(Ref: Goodman and Gilman 12th E/P 801)

- The plant in the picture is Digitalis lanata or white foxglove, which is the source for digoxin.

7. Ans. (c) Captopril

(Ref: Goodman Gilman 12th E/P778)

- The given angiogram depicts a case of bilateral renal artery stenosis.
- RAS inhibitors are absolutely contraindicated in a patient of bilateral renal artery stenosis, as they can precipitate renal failure.

8. Ans. (b) Beta blockers

(Ref: CMDT 2016/P363)

- This is a case of vasospastic angina precipitated by beta blockers.
- Beta blockers block beta-2 mediated vasodilation and cause unopposed alpha-1 receptor mediated vasoconstriction.
- Thus beta blockers are contraindicated in variant angina as it can be worsened.

9. Ans. (a) PCI

(Ref: Harrison 19th E/P1604)

- This is a case of STEMI and since the patient has presented before 12 hours, reperfusion should be performed at the earliest.
- PCI is more preferred as compared to thrombolysis for reperfusion.

10. Ans. (c) Amiodarone

(Ref: Goodman Gilman 12th E/P829)

- The streaks of deposits in cornea in a concentric circle is called as whorl like deposits, seen with amiodarone.
- It is seen in almost 100% patients with six months of drug exposure.

11. Ans. (b) Thrombolysis

(Ref: CMDT 2016/P364)

- ST segment depression in the precordial leads and minimal STE in avR. This is a case of NSTEMI.
- In case of NSTEMI thrombolysis is absolutely contraindicated.

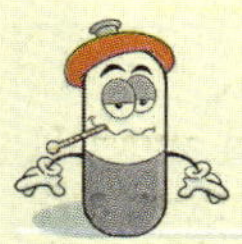

Annexures

Drugs of Choice

Angina	• Acute attack (All types of angina) – Sublingual Nitroglycerine • Long-term prophylaxis in stable angina – Beta blockers

Aortic dissection	Labetalol

Atrial Fibrillation and flutter	• Acute Attack – IV Ibutilide • Rhythm control – Amiodarone • Rate control – Beta blockers

Anticoagulation in Atrial fibrillation	Novel Oral anticoagulants • Dabigatran • Apixaban

Acute CHF	• First drug of choice – Furosemide • Inotrope of choice – Dobutamine

Chronic CHF	ACEIs/ARBs

• Hypertriglyceridemia • Chylomicronemia Syndrome • Type III hyperlipoproteinemia	• Fibrates

Hypercholesterolemia	• Statins • Pregnancy and Children – Bile Acid Sequestrants

Hypertension	• First line drugs ▪ ACE inhibitors or ARB ▪ CCB ▪ Thiazides • Resistant hypertension ▪ Aldosterone antagonists

Hypertension in age groups	• Elderly–CCB • Young–ACEIs/ARBs

Hypertension with comorbidities	
DM CKD Scleroderma Nephrotic syndrome	ACEI/ARB
Angina Previous MI Hyperthyroidism Migraine Anxiety with somatic manifestations Essential tremor Atrial fibrillation and flutter Preoperative hypertension	Beta blockers
Osteoporosis	Thiazides
Raynaud's disease Cyclosporine induced hypertension	CCB
BPH Dyslipidemia	α1 blockers
Hypertensive Emergency	I/V Nicardipine
Hypertensive Urgency	Clonidine

Hypertensive emergency with scleroderma	Captopril

PSVT **SVT**	• Treatment – I/V Adenosine • Prophylaxis – Verapamil or Beta blockers

Shock	• Anaphylactic – Epinephrine • Cardiogenic – Norepinephrine or Dopamine • Septic – Norepinephrine • Vasodilatory – Norepinephrine

SVT	• Treatment and prophylaxis – Verapamil > Beta blockers • Associated CHF – Digoxin

Torsades de pointes	Magnesium sulfate

Ventricular extrasystole (Symptomatic)	Beta Blockers
Ventricular Fibrillation	Amiodarone

Ventricular Tachycardia in MI and digitalis toxicity	Lidocaine
WPW Syndrome	IV procainamide

New Drugs

Drug	Mechanism of action	Use
Ivabradine	Inhibits current in SA node that decreases its automaticity and myocardial oxygen consumption	Decrease in oxygen demand is beneficial in • Angina • CHF
Cangrelor	P2Y12 platelet receptor inhibitor that blocks ADP-induced platelet activation and aggregation.	Antiaggregant
Vorapaxar	Protease-activated receptor-1 (PAR-1) antagonist, which inhibits thrombin-induced and thrombin receptor agonist peptide (TRAP)-induced platelet aggregation	Antiaggregant
Riociguat	Soluble guanylate cyclase stimulator, which increases cyc GMP and causes vasodilation	Pulmonary artery hypertension
Mipomersen sodium	Inhibits ApoB-100 protein and decreases LDL production	Homozygous familial hypercholesterolemia
Macitentan	Endothelin receptor antagonist	Pulmonary artery hypertension
Lomitapide	Microsomal triglyceride transport protein (MTP) inhibitor	Homozygous familial hypercholesterolemia
Icosapent	Decreases VLDL synthesis and secretion	Hypertriglyceridemia
Sacubitril	Inhibits Neutral endopeptidase	Chronic CHF along with ARBs
Omapatrilat	Vasopeptidase Inhibitor	Chronic CHF
Evolocumab	Anti PCSK-9 Ab	Hyperlipidemia

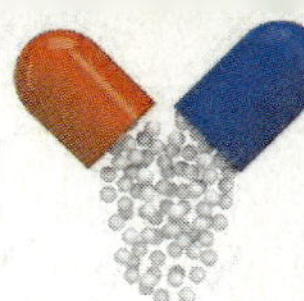

Multiple Choice Questions

ANTIARRHYTHMICS

1. The drug preferred in a patient with ischemic heart disease with VT ***(Recent Question 2019)***
a. Lignocaine b. Diltiazem
c. Propranolol d. Adenosine

2. QT prolongation is caused by: ***(Recent Question 2017)***
a. Quinidine b. Omeprazole
c. Lidocaine d. Penicillin

3. Which of the following is treatment of choice for the condition given in ECG (SVT) in a one year old child? ***(Recent Question Dec 2016)***

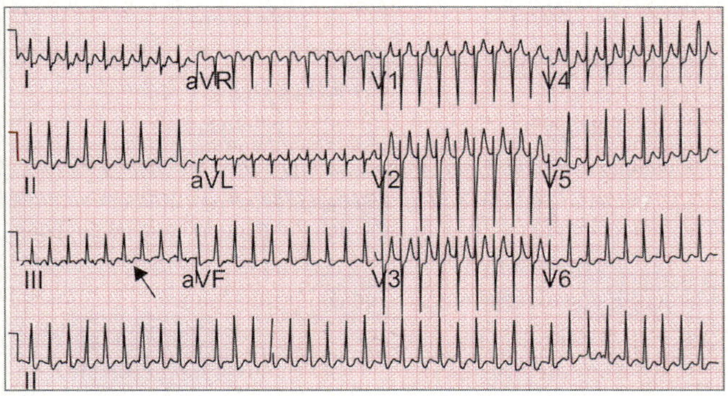

a. Fast adenosine
b. Slow adenosine
c. Synchronized cardioversion
d. Procainamide

4. Which of the following is used for treatment of 2 year old baby with supraventicular tachycardia? ***(Recent Question Dec 2016)***
a. Adenosine b. Verapamil
c. IV Nicardipine d. Synchronized DC

5. Quinidine toxicity cause ***(Recent Question Dec 2016)***
a. Torsades de pointes
b. Brugada syndrome
c. QT prolongation
d. Ventricular arrhythmias

6. Side effects of amiodarone are all except:- ***(Recent Question Dec 2016)***
a. Pulmonary fibrosis b. Hepatotoxicity
c. Hypothyroidism d. Nephrotoxicity

7. Which of the following ion causes delayed after depolarization? ***(Recent Question Dec 2016)***
a. Calcium b. Sodium
c. Potassium d. Magnesium

8. Digitalis causes all except ***(Recent Question Dec 2016)***
a. Heart block b. PSVT
c. Bradycardia d. Atrial flutter

9. All of the following drugs can cause whorl like corneal deposits except? ***(AIIMS May 2015)***
a. Aminodarone b. Chloroquine
c. Indomethacin d. Chlorpromazine

10. All are toxicities seen with amiodarone therapy except: ***(AIIMS May 2009)***
a. Pulmonary fibrosis b. Corneal microdeposits
c. Cirrhosis of liver d. Productive cough

11. Which of the following anti-arrhythmic agents does not belong to class Ic? ***(AIIMS Nov 2006)***
a. Tocainide b. Encainide
c. Flecainide d. Propafenone

12. Which of the following drugs is not used in the treatment of torsades de pointes? ***(Recent Question 2016)***
a. Isoproterenol b. Propanolol
c. Magnesium d. Amiodarone

13. Which of the following drugs is used for termination as well as prophylaxis of paroxysmal supraventricular tachycardia? ***(Recent Question 2016)***
a. Digoxin b. Verapamil
c. Propanolol d. Quinine

14. Patient on verapamil should not be given beta blocker as ***(Recent Question 2016)***
a. Conduction block b. Bronchospasm
c. Neurogenic shock d. Anaphylaxis

15. Digitalis produces which of the following changes in ECG? ***(Recent Question 2016)***
a. Tall T waves
b. ST segment elevation
c. Prolonged QT interval
d. Prolonged PR interval

16. All of the following are used in atrial arrhythmias except: ***(Recent Question 2016)***
a. Digoxin b. Verapamil
c. Quinidine d. Lignocaine

17. All the following statements regarding adenosine are true except: ***(Recent Question 2016)***
a. Dipyridamole potentiates its action
b. Used to produce controlled hypotension
c. Administered by slow IV injection
d. Administered by rapid IV injection

18. Adverse effects of quinidine are all except? ***(Recent Question 2016)***
a. SLE
b. Diarrhea
c. Bradycardia
d. Torsades de pointes

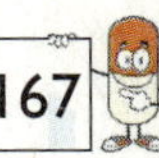

19. The antiarrythmic drug which causes myocardial depression is? ***(Recent Question 2016)***
a. Sotalol b. Quinine
c. Amiodarone d. None of these

20. Beta blockers are antiarrhythmic agents of type? ***(Recent Question 2016)***
a. I b. II
c. III d. IV

21. Amiodarone does not cause? ***(Recent Question 2016)***
a. Irreversible microdeposits on the cornea
b. Hypothyroidism
c. Photosensitization
d. Pulmonary fibrosis

22. Which drug can cause thyroid dysfunction? ***(Recent Question 2016)***
a. Amiodarone b. Ampicillin
c. Ibutillide d. Acyclovir

23. Drug of choice for supraventricular tachycardia is ***(Recent Question 2016)***
a. Verapamil b. Diltiazem
c. Digoxin d. Phenytoin

24. Which of the following drugs can cause torsades'de pointes? ***(Recent Question 2016)***
a. Quinidine b. Lignocaine
c. Esmolol d. Flecainide

25. Not an adverse effect of chronic amiodarone therapy ***(Recent Question 2016)***
a. Pulmonary fibrosis
b. Hypothyroideism
c. Hyperthyroidism
d. Systemic lupus erythematosus

26. Digoxin is not indicated in ***(Recent Question 2016)***
a. Atrial flutter b. Atrial fibrillation
c. High output failure d. PSVT

27. Racemic mixture of two enantiomers with different pharmacokinetic and pharmacodynamics properties is seen in ***(Recent Question 2016)***
a. Dilantin b. Digoxin
c. Verapamil d. Octerotide

28. The antiarrhythmic drug of choice in most of the cases of acute paroxysmal supraventricular tachycardia is ***(Recent Question 2016)***
a. Adenosine b. Amiodarone
c. Propranolol d. Quinidine

29. Which of the following has the maximum half-life? ***(Recent Question 2016)***
a. Adenosine b. Amiodarone
c. Esomolol d. Lidocaine

30. Which of the following antiarrhythmic drugs can decrease the slope of phase 0 and prolong the action potential duration? ***(Recent Question 2016)***
a. Lignocaine b. Propranolol
c. Quinidine d. Adenosine

31. The drug of choice for rapid correction of PSVT in known asthmatic is ***(Recent Question 2016)***
a. Adenosine b. Esmolol
c. Neostigmine d. Verapamil

32. Dofetilide is which class of antirrhythmic drug? ***(Recent Question 2016)***
a. Class 1 b. Class 2
c. Class 3 d. Class 4

33. Procainamide is a class___antiarrhythmic drug ***(Recent Question 2016)***
a. I b. II
c. III d. IV

34. Drug resembling thyroid hormone ***(Recent Question 2016)***
a. Amiodarone b. Captopril
c. Lithium d. Losartan

35. Drug used in teminating SVT ***(Recent Question 2016)***
a. Diltiazem b. Amlodipine
c. Vasopressin d. Verapamil

36. All of the following anti-arrhythmic drug are from class Ic EXCEPT: ***(Recent Question 2016)***
a. Encainide b. Hecainide
c. Tocainide d. Propafenone

37. Drug not causing edema ***(AIIMS Nov 2014)***
a. NSAID b. Digoxin
c. Estrogen d. Cyclosporine

38. Digoxintoxicity is enhanced by all of the following except: ***(AIIMS May 2010, AIIMS May 2009, Nov 2008; Recent Question 2008)***
a. Hyperkalemia b. Hypercalcemia
c. Hypomagnesemia d. Renal failure

39. Digoxin action is not affected in: ***(AIIMS May 2007)***
a. Hepatic disease b. Electrolyte disturbances
c. Renal failure d. MI

40. BNP is degraded by: ***(AIIMS May 2007)***
a. Neutral endopeptidase b. Elastase
c. Omapatrilat d. ACE

41. Which of the following conditions increases the risk of digoxintoxicity? ***(Recent Question 2016)***
a. Administration of quinidine
b. Hyperkalemia
c. Hypermagnesemia d. Hypocalcemia

42. Which of the following is not given in acute severe digitalis toxicity? ***(Recent Question 2016)***
a. Potassium b. Digibind
c. Lignocaine d. None of these

43. Which of the following is a monovalent cation that can reverse a digitalis induded arrhythmia? ***(Recent Question 2016)***
a. Digibind antibodies b. Lignocaine
c. Magnesium d. Potassium

44. Digitalis produces which of the following changes in ECG? ***(Recent Question 2016)***
a. Tall T waves b. ST segment elevation
c. Prolonged QT interval d. Prolonged PR interval

45. Mechanism of action of levosimendan is: ***(Recent Question 2016)***
a. Inoconstrictor b. Potassium channel opener
c. Sodium channel opener d. Beta blocker

46. Half-life of digoxin is: *(Recent Question 2016)*
a. 12 hours b. 24 hours
c. 36 hours d. 48 hours

47. Most effective method of treatment of digitalis toxicity is? *(Recent Question 2016)*
a. Hemodialysis b. Cardioversion
c. Digoxin antibody d. Atropine

48. Drug used in remodeling of heart in congestive cardiac failure are all except: *(Recent Question 2016)*
a. Beta blocker b. ACE inhibitor
c. Digoxin d. Aldosterone antagonist

49. Which among the following is the best inotrope drug for use in right heart failure? *(Recent Question 2016)*
a. Dobutamine b. Digoxin
c. Dopamine d. Milrinone

50. All of the following drugs are used for the treatment of congestive heart failure except: *(Recent Question 2016)*
a. Nitroglycerine b. Spironolactone
c. Nesiritide d. Trimetazidine

51. All of the following statements about nesiritide are true except: *(Recent Question 2016)*
a. It is a BNP analogue
b. It can be used in decompensated CHF
c. It can be administered orally
d. It causes loss of Na+ in the urine

52. The most important channel of elimination of digoxin is: *(Recent Question 2016)*
a. Glomerular filtration b. Tubular secretion
c. Hepatic metabolism d. Excretion in bile

53. Which of the following drugs can prolong survival in patients with CHF? *(Recent Question 2016)*
a. Furosemide b. Inamrinone
c. Losartan d. Digoxin

54. The diuretic of choice for rapid relief of congestive symptoms in a patient of CHF is: *(Recent Question 2016)*
a. Hydrochlorothiazide b. Furosemide
c. Metolazone d. Amiloride

55. All are useful for long-term treatment of congestive heart failure except: *(Recent Question 2016)*
a. Digoxin b. Ramipril
c. Dobutamine d. Spironolactone

56. The drug not useful in congestive heart failure is: *(Recent Question 2016)*
a. Adrenaline b. Digoxin
c. Hydrochlorothiazide d. Enalapril

57. Digibind is used to: *(Recent Question 2016)*
a. Potentiate the action of digoxin
b. Decrease the metabolism of digoxin
c. Treat digoxintoxicity
d. Rapidly digitalize the patient

58. Digitalis toxicity can cause: *(Recent Question 2016)*
a. Hyperkalemia
b. Nausea
c. Arrhythmias
d. All of the above

59. Drugs causing aferload reduction is: *(Recent Question 2016)*
a. Digoxin b. Captopril
c. Dobutamine d. Frusemide

60. Drug of choice in LVH: *(Recent Question 2016)*
a. ACE inhibitors
b. Beta blockers
c. Calcium channel blockers
d. Sodium channel blockers

61. Drug used in heart failure: *(Recent Question 2016)*
a. Celiprolol b. Carteolol
c. Carvediol d. All of the above

62. Mechanism of action of digoxin in CHF is: *(Recent Question 2016)*
a. Prolonged systole b. Shortened diastole
c. Increased HR d. Decreased HR

63. Digoxin increases refractoriness at: *(Recent Question 2016)*
a. SA node b. AV node
c. Ventricular cells d. Atrial cells

HYPERTENSION, ANGINA AND MI

64. For a patient of hypertension on metoprolol, verapamil was given; this will result in *(AIIMS Nov 2018)*
a. Atrial fibrillation
b. Bradycardia with AV block
c. Torsades de pointes
d. Tachycardia

65. Nitroprusside active metabolite act by *(AIIMS Nov 2018)*
a. Phosphokinase 1,2 b. Guanylyl cyclase
c. Phospholipase A d. Phospholipase B

66. Primary action of nitrates in a patient of angina is *(AIIMS Nov 2018)*
a. Coronary vasodilation b. Decreases preload
c. Decreases afterload d. Decreases heart rate

67. A patient having prinzmetal angina is started with isosorbide mononitrate. Patient got symptomatic relief from angina. what is the mechanism of action of nitrate? *(AIIMS Nov 2017)*
a. Endothelium independent coronary vasodilation
b. Reduced cardiac contractility
c. Increased left ventricular end diastolic volume
d. Decreased diastolic perfusion pressure

68. Which of the following drug is not used in pregnancy induced hypertension? *(Recent Question 2017)*
a. Atenolol b. Labetalol
c. Hydralazine d. Methyldopa

69. ARB inhibitor with additional PPAR-γ agonist activity is *(AIIMS May 2016)*
a. Losartan b. Candisartan
c. Telmesartan d. Eprosartan

70. Which of the following antihypertensive drug causes nasal congestion? *(Recent Question Dec 2016)*
a. Ace inhibitor b. Beta blockers
c. ARB d. CCB

71. Which of the following ARB is thromboxane A2 inhibitor with PPAR gamma stimulating property? *(Recent Question Dec 2016)*

a. Telmisartan b. Losartan
c. Candesartan d. Olmesartan

72. Not centrally acting antihypertensive are *(Recent Question Dec 2016)*

a. Methyl dope b. Clonidine
c. Minoxidil d. Guanabenz

73. Which of the following drug is contraindicated in a case of B/L renal artery stenosis *(Recent Question Dec 2016)*

a. Methyldopa b. Enalapril
c. Hydralazine d. Dopamine

74. Drug of choice for hypertension in eclampsia is:- *(Recent Question Dec 2016)*

a. MgSo4 b. Labetalol
c. Nifedipine d. Hydralazine

75. Which of the following is drug of choice for pregnancy-induced hypertension? *(AIIMS Nov 2015)*

a. Atenolol b. α-methyl dopa
c. Enalapril d. Nitroprusside

76. A 60-year-old man, chest pain since one day, with the following ECG. Which of the following drugs should not be used? *(AIIMS Nov 2015)*

a. Aspirin b. Thrombolytics
c. Morphine d. Statins

77. Which of the following antihypertensive is absolutely contraindicated in pregnancy? *(AIIMS May 2015)*

a. Enalapril b. Methyldopa
c. Nifedipine d. Labetalol

78. Diuretic which can be given in mild to moderate hypertension *(AIIMS May 2015)*

a. Loop diuretics b. Osmotic diuretics
c. Thiazide diuretics
d. Potassium sparing diuretics

79. All of the following drugs can worsen angina except: *(AIIMS May 2011)*

a. Dipyridamole b. Oxyphedrine
c. Thyroxine d. Sumatriptan

80. Which of the following statements regarding ACE inhibitors is true? *(AIIMS May 2008, 2011, Nov 2008)*

a. These inhibit the conversion of angiotensinogen to angiotensin-1
b. Omission of prior diuretic dose decreases the risk of postural hypotension
c. Lisinopril is shorter acting than enalapril
d. These are contraindicated in diabetic patients

81. Nitrates are used for all of the following conditions except? *(AIIMS Nov 2009)*

a. Congestive heart failure b. Cyanide poisoning
c. Esophageal spasm d. Renal colic

82. A man presents with chest pain. ECG shows ST segment depression in leads V1-V4. Which of the following should not be given? *(AIIMS May 2008)*

a. Beta blocker b. Thrombolytic
c. Morphine d. Aspirin

83. Hypertension is not seen with: *(AIIMS May 2007)*

a. Cyclosporine
b. NSAIDs
c. Erythropoietin
d. L-dopa

84. Renin is secreted from: *(AIIMS May 2007)*

a. Juxtaglomerular apparatus
b. PCT
c. DCT
d. Collecting ducts

85. Maximum incidence of impotence is seen with the following antihypertensive agent: *(AIIMS May 2007)*

a. CCBs b. Beta blockers
c. ARBs d. ACE inhibitors

86. The most significant adverse effect of ACE inhibition is: *(AIIMS May 2006)*

a. Hypotension b. Hypertension
c. Hypocalcemia d. Hypercalcemia

87. Preload of heart reduced by: *(Recent Question 2018)*

a. CCB b. Minoxidil
c. Hydralazine d. Nitroglycerine

88. Drug of choice for ventricular arrhythmias due to myocardial infarction (MI) is *(Recent Question 2016)*

a. Quinidine b. Amiodarone
c. Xylocaine d. Diphenylhydantoin

89. Ranolazine is a *(Recent Question 2016)*

a. Vasodilator b. Antianginal
c. Antihypertensive d. Antiarrhythmic

90. ACE inhibitors should not be used with *(Recent Question 2016)*

a. Amiloride b. Calcium channel blockers
c. Chlorthalidone d. Spironolactone

91. Antihypertensive drug contraindicated in pregnancy is *(Recent Question 2016)*

a. Enalapril
b. Cardio selective beta blockers
c. Methyl dopa
d. Hydralazine

92. Which of the following drug decreases plasma rennin activity? *(Recent Question 2016)*

a. Enalapril b. Nifedipine
c. Hydralazine d. Clonidine

93. ACE inhibitors cause *(Recent Question 2016)*

a. Hyperkalemia b. Hypokalemia
c. Hypocalcemia d. Hypernatremia

94. False about diazoxide is *(Recent Question 2016)*

a. It acts by causing prolonged opening of ATP depended K^+ channels in beta cells
b. It can cause severe hypoglycemia
c. It can be used to treat patients with insulinoma
d. It is used as an antihypertensive agent

95. Which of the following drugs is best for reducing proteinuria in a diabetic patient? *(Recent Question 2016)*

a. Metoprolol b. Perindopril
c. Chlorthiazide d. Clonidine

96. Alpha methyldopa is primarily used for: ***(Recent Question 2016)***

a. Pregnancy induced hypertension
b. endovascular hypertension
c. First line agent in hypertension
d. Refractory hypertension

97. Which of the following ACE inhibitor is not a prodrug? ***(Recent Question 2016)***

a. Fosinopril
b. Enalapril
c. Ramipril
d. Lisinopril

98. Nitroglycerine causes all except ***(Recent Question 2016)***

a. Hypotension and bradycardia
b. Methemoglobinemia
c. Hypotension and tachycardia
d. Vasodilation

99. Angiotensin II causes all except: ***(Recent Question 2016)***

a. Stimulates release of ADH
b. Increases thirst
c. Vasodilation
d. Stimulates aldosterone release

100. Calcium channel blocking agents of use in the treatment of hypertension include: ***(Recent Question 2016)***

a. Prazosin b. Lidoflazine
c. Captopril d. Nifedipine

101. All are true regarding losartan except

a. It is a competitive angiotensin receptor antagonist
b. It has a long acting metabolite ***(Recent Question 2016)***
c. Associated with negligible cough
d. Causes hyperuricemia

102. Coronary steal phenomenon is seen with: ***(Recent Question 2016)***

a. Dipyridamole b. Diltiazem
c. Propranolol d. Verapamil

103. Which of the following is not given alone in a patient of pheochromocytoma? ***(Recent Question 2016)***

a. Atenolol b. Prazosin
c. Nitroprusside d. Metyrosine

104. Not an adverse effect of ACE inhibitors: ***(Recent Question 2016)***

a. Cough b. Hypokalemia
c. Angioneurotic edema d. Skin rash

105. An elderly hypertensive has diabetes mellitus and bilateral renal artery stenosis. The best management is ***(Recent Question 2016)***

a. Enalapril b. Verapamil
c. Beta blockers d. Thiazides

106. Postural hypotension is the common side effect of ***(Recent Question 2016)***

a. ACE inhibitors b. Alpha receptor blockers
c. Arteriolar dilators d. Selective b1 blockers

107. Nitroglycerine exerts beneficial effects in classical angina pectoris primarily by ***(Recent Question 2016)***

a. Increase intotal coronary blood flow
b. Redistribution of coronary blood flow
c. Reduction of cardiac preload
d. Reduction of cardiac afterload

108. Nitroglycerine can be administered by all of the following routes except ***(Recent Question 2016)***

a. Oral b. Sublingual
c. Intramuscular d. Intravenous

109. The antihypertensive agent that should be avoided in young females and is used topically to treat alopecia is ***(Recent Question 2016)***

a. Hydralazine b. Prazosin
c. Minoxidil d. Indapamide

110. Which antihypertensive is a prodrug and is converted to its active form in brain? ***(Recent Question 2016)***

a. Clonidine b. Methyl dopa
c. Minoxidil d. Nitroprusside

111. Which of these anti-hypertensives do not have any central action? ***(Recent Question 2016)***

a. Propranolol b. Methyldopa
c. Clonidine d. Prazosin

112. When treating hypertension chronically, orthostatic hypotension is maximum with ***(Recent Question 2016)***

a. Clonidine b. Guanethidine
c. Prazosin d. Propranolol

113. Which of the following drugs is used in severe hypertension emergencies, is very short acting and must be given by i.v. infusion? ***(Recent Question 2016)***

a. Diazoxide b. Hydralazine
c. Labetolol d. Nitroprusside

114. Longest acting nitroglycerine preparation is ***(Recent Question 2016)***

a. Glyceryltrinitrate
b. Amyl nitrite
c. Pentaerythritol tetranitrate
d. Isosorbidedinitrate

115. A drug lacking vasodilatory properties that is effective in angina is ***(Recent Question 2016)***

a. Isosorbidedinitrate b. Metoprolol
c. Nifedipine d. Verapamil

116. Which of the following antihypertensive drug does not alter serum glucose and lipid levels? ***(Recent Question 2016)***

a. Propranolol b. Prazosin
c. Clonidine d. Thiazide diuretics

117. Drug not useful in hypertensive emergency is ***(Recent Question 2016)***

a. IV hydralazine b. Indapamide
c. Sublingual nifedipine d. Sodium nitroprusside

118. Nimodipine is used in ***(Recent Question 2016)***

a. Subarachnoid hemorrhage
b. Intracerebral hemorrhage
c. Extradural hemorrhage
d. Subdrual hemorrhage

119. Calcium channel blockers are used in all except ***(Recent Question 2016)***

a. Angina b. Arrhythmia
c. Congestive heart failure d. Hypertension

120. Sodium-nitroprusside act by activation of ***(Recent Question 2016)***

a. Guanylatecyclase b. K^+ channels
c. Ca^{++} channels d. Cyclic AMP

121. Drug not to be given in ischemic heart disease is *(Recent Question 2016)*
a. Atenolol b. ACE inhibitor
c. Isoproterenol d. Streptokinase

122. Cough is an adverse reaction seen with intake of *(Recent Question 2016)*
a. Thiazide b. Nifedipine
c. Enalapril d. Prazosin

123. An antihypertensive drug that causes positive coomb's test is *(Recent Question 2016)*
a. Methyl dopa b. Clonidine
c. Hydralazine d. Sodium-nitropruside

124. Potassium channel opener with anti-anginal activity is
a. Nicorandil b. Dipyridamole
c. Trimetazidine d. Oxyphedrine

125. Amy nitrite in used by which route? *(Recent Question 2016)*
a. Oral b. Inhalation
c. IV d. IM

126. ACE inhibitors are contraindicated in *(Recent Question 2016)*
a. Diabetes mellitus
b. Hypertension in old age groups
c. Scleroderma
d. Bilateral renal artery stenosis

127. All of the following are vasodilators except *(Recent Question 2016)*
a. Methyl dopa b. Nitroprusside
c. Hydralazine d. Diazoxide

128. Cough and angioedema in a patient receiving ACE inhibitors is due to *(Recent Question 2016)*
a. Bradykinin b. Renin
c. Angiotensin-II d. All

129. Enalapril increases the levels of *(Recent Question 2016)*
a. Bradykynin b. Interferon
c. PAF d. TNF

130. Treatment of choice in hypertension with diabetes mellitus is *(Recent Question 2016)*
a. B-Blockers b. Thiazides
c. ACE inhibitors d. Calcium channel blockers

131. Which of the following antihypertensives causes sedation *(Recent Question 2016)*
a. Clonidine b. Hydralazine
c. Losartan d. Amlodipine

132. Antidote for calcium channel blockers overdose *(Recent Question 2016)*
a. Atropine b. Calcium gluconate
c. Adrenaline d. Digoxin

133. Drug of choice for prinzmetal angina is *(Recent Question 2016)*
a. Nifedipine b. Propranolol
c. CCB d. GTN

134. In variant angina calcium channel blockers act by *(Recent Question 2016)*
a. Reducing coronary spasm
b. Increasing myocardial oxygen demand
c. Colonary vasoconstriction
d. All of the above

135. Most common side effect of ARB *(Recent Question 2016)*
a. Hypotension b. Hypokalemia
c. Edema d. Cough

136. Cerebro protective calcium-channel blocker *(Recent Question 2016)*
a. Nifedipine b. Amlodipine
c. Enalapril d. Nimodipine

137. Most commonly used drug in hypertensive emergencies *(Recent Question 2016)*
a. Clonidine b. Nifedipine
c. Sodium nitroprusside d. α-methyl dopa

138. Drug of choice for hypertension with angina pectoris *(Recent Question 2016)*
a. Atenolol b. ACE inhibitors
c. Verapamil d. Nitrates

139. ACE inhibitor not to be given along with *(Recent Question 2016)*
a. Amiloride b. Xipamide
c. Hydrochlorothiazide d. Chlorthalidone

140. Enalapril is a/an *(Recent Question 2016)*
a. Angiotensin receptor blocker
b. Angiotensin converting enzyme inhibitor
c. Renin inhibitor
d. Calcium channel blocker

141. Most common side effect of calcium channel blocker is *(Recent Question 2016)*
a. Headache b. Constipation
c. Diarrhea d. Muscle cramps

142. Adverse effect of angiotensin receptor blocker *(Recent Question 2016)*
a. Postural hypotension b. Urticaria
c. Bronchospasm d. Hypokalemia

143. Drug of choice for intermittent claudication
a. Atropine b. Paracetamol
c. Pentoxiphlline d. Phenytoin

144. SLE like reaction is caused by? *(Recent Question 2016)*
a. Hydralazine b. Rifampicin
c. Paracetamol d. Furozemide

145. Anti-hypertensive drug contraindicated in pregnancy is? *(Recent Question 2016)*
a. Enalapril
b. Cardio selective beta blockers
c. Methyldopa
d. Hydralazine

146. Adverse effects of losartan are all except: *(Recent Question 2016)*
a. Angioedema b. Cough
c. Hyperkalemia d. Headache

147. Which drug may aggravate renovascular hypertension? *(Recent Question 2016)*
a. ACE inhibitors b. Beta blockers
c. Calcium channel blockersd. Thiazide diuretics

148. Drug not given sublingually is: *(Recent Question 2016)*
a. Isosorbidedinitrate b. Buprenorphine
c. Ergotamine tartrate d. Isosorbide-5-mononitrate

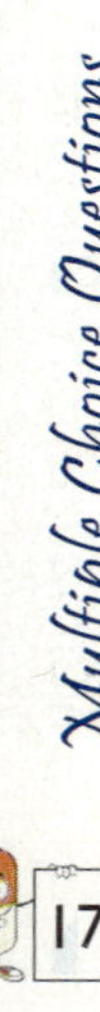

149. Drug not used in prinzmetal angina is? *(Recent Question 2016)*
a. Propranolol b. Verapamil
c. Nitrites d. Isosorbide dinitrate

150. The anti-hypertensive agent which decreases libido is? *(Recent Question 2016)*
a. Methyl dopa b. Captopril
c. Diazoxide d. Hydralazine

151. The antihypertensive which causes decreased libido and impotence is? *(Recent Question 2016)*
a. Atenolol b. Enalapril
c. Prazosin d. Diltiazem

152. Ivabradine is indicated in the management of: *(Recent Question 2016)*
a. Congestive heart failure b. Angina pectoris
c. Cardiomyopathy d. Irritable bowel syndrome

HYPOLIPIDEMICS

153. A patient of CAD with history of MI 2 months back, diabetes mellitus with LDL 126, HDL 32 and triglycerides 236. What should be given: *(AIIMS May 2017)*
a. Atorvastatin 80 mg
b. Rosuvastatin 10 mg
c. Fenofibrate
d. Fenofibrate and Rosuvastatin

154. Niacin is dangerous in diabetes mellitus because: *(Recent Question 2017)*
a. It causes insulin resistance
b. It causes sudden hypoglycemia
c. It decreases glucagon secretion
d. It decreases effect of other OHA

155. Dyslipedemic drug used in hyperurecemia and acute gout is *(Recent Question Dec 2016)*
a. Niacin b. Fenofibrate
c. Cholestyramine d. Statins

156. True about fibrates is all except: *(AIIMS Nov 2007)*
a. Drug of choice for type III hyperlipoproteinemia and hypertriglyceridemia
b. Activates PPAR to stimulate LPL
c. Absorbed good on empty stomach and absorption is delayed by fatty meals
d. Side effects are rash, urticarial, myalgia and impotence

157. All of the following are true regarding HMG-CoA reductase inhibitors except *(AIIMS May 2002)*
a. CNS accumulation of simvastatin and lovastatin is high and less for pravastatin and fluvastatin
b. Simvastatin is rapidly and pravastatin is least metabolized
c. Bioavailability is minimally modified when pravastatin is taken with food
d. Fibrinogen levels are increased by pravastatin

158. Hypolipidemic drugs act on all except *(Recent Question 2016)*
a. HMG Co A reductase
b. Lipoprotein lipase
c. Acyl CoA, cholesterol acyl transferase 1
d. Peripheral decarboxylase

159. Nicotinic acid *(Recent Question 2016)*
a. Increases HDL
b. Increased triglyceride synthesis
c. Type II hyperlipoproteinemia
d. Decreased hydrolysis of VLDL

160. Drug that decreasesLpA in blood *(Recent Question 2016)*
a. Statin b. Nicotinic acid
c. Ezetimibe d. CETP inhibitors

161. Mechanism of action of fibrates in treatment of hyperlipidemia is *(Recent Question 2016)*
a. Activator of lipoprotein lipase
b. PPAR alpha agonist
c. Decreased synthesis of VLDL
d. Inhibitor of CETP

162. Mechanism of action of cholestyramine is *(Recent Question 2016)*
a. Bind to bile acid
b. Decrease HMG-COA
c. Increase excretion of cholesterol
d. Decrease utilization of cholesterol

163. Drug that inhibits absorption of Cholesterol from intestine *(Recent Question 2016)*
a. Resins b. Ezetimibe
c. Niacin d. Orlistat

164. Which of the following is not a direct acting antiplatelet agent? *(Recent Question 2016)*
a. Aspirin b. Colpidogrel
c. Atorvastatin d. Alteplase

165. Competitive inhibition of rate limiting step in cholesterol synthesis is by *(Recent Question 2016)*
a. Bile acid sequestrants b. Fibric acid derivatives
c. Statins d. Nicotinic acid

166. Mechanism of action of lovastatin is by *(Recent Question 2016)*
a. Competitive inhibition of rate limiting step in cholesterol synthesis
b. Bile acid sequestration
c. Activate lipoprotein lipase
d. Inhibits lipolysis and triglyceride

167. Mechanism of action of statins is *(Recent Question 2016)*
a. Inhibition of HMG-CoA synthase
b. Stimulation of HMG-CoA reductase
c. Indirect increase of LDL receptors synthesis
d. Inhibition of intestinal cholesterol absorption

168. Mechanism of action of ezithimibe *(Recent Question 2016)*
a. Inhibit cholesterol absorption
b. Inhibit release of triglycerides in LDL
c. Inhibit HMG CoA reductase
d. Inhibit HMG CoA synthase

169. The vitamin which in large doses decreases the triglycerides and cholesterol levels *(Recent Question 2016)*
a. Vitamin B_{12} b. Nicotinic acid
c. Vitamin B_1 d. Retinol

170. Appropriate drug for a patient with high LDL level is ***(Recent Question 2016)***

a. Atorvastatin b. Rosuvastatin
c. Fenofibrate d. Nicotinic acid

171. Statins are used in ___type of dyslipidemia ***(Recent Question 2016)***

a. II b. III
c. IV d. I

172. Mechanism of action of clofibrate ***(Recent Question 2016)***

a. Inhibit HMGCoAreductase
b. Inhibit HMGCoA synthase
c. Inhibit absorption if cholesterol
d. Stimulates lipoprotein lipase

173. First dose syncope occurs with which of the following drug(s): ***(PGI May 2018)***

a. ACE inhibitor b. CCB
c. Alpha blockers d. Beta blockers
e. Thiazide diuretics

174. Drugs used in monomorphic ventricular tachycardia in hemodynamically stable patient: ***(PGI Nov 2017)***

a. Amiodarone b. Propranolol
c. Lignocaine d. Diltiazem
e. Procainamide

175. Among ACE inhibitors, which of the following is/are prodrug(s): ***(PGI May 2017)***

a. Perindopril b. Captopril
c. Lisinopril d. Ramipril
e. Enalapril

176. Drug(s) causing QT interval prolongation: ***(PGI May 2017)***

a. Amiodarone b. Cisapride
c. Calcium gluconate d. Magnesium therapy
e. Ketoconazole

177. Drug that can potentiate Torsades de pointes: ***(PGI Nov 2016)***

a. Amiodarone b. Sotalol
c. Chlorpromazine d. Cisapride
e. Aspirin

178. Drugs which can be used in gestational hypertension: ***(PGI Nov 2016)***

a. Metoprolol b. Labetalol
c. Methyldopa d. Sustained release nifedipine
e. Losartan

179. Peripheral neuropathy is/are caused by: ***(PGI Nov 2014)***

a. Vincristine b. Sulfonamide
c. Amiodarone d. Paclitaxel

180. Drug that increases QT interval: ***(PGI May 2012)***

a. Haloperidol b. Fexofenadine
c. Amiodarone d. Ebastine
e. Sotatol

181. MOA of Verapamil is: ***(PGI May 2012)***

a. Inhibition of Ca+2 channel
b. Inhibition of Na+ channel
c. Inhibition of K+ channel
d. Block membrane repolarisation
e. Membrane stabilisation

182. Which of the following is/are not calcium-channel blocking agent(s): ***(PGI May 2012)***

a. Verapamil b. Propranolol
c. Carvedilol d. Nicardipine
e. Nebivolol

183. Rebound hypertension is seen with: ***(PGI June 2009)***

a. Amlodipine b. Methyldopa
c. Clonidine d. Na nitroprusside
e. Atenolol

184. Beta Blockers used in CHF are: ***(PGI Nov 2008)***

a. Propranolol b. Bisoprolol
c. Carvedilol d. Nebivolol
e. Pindolol

185. Vasodilators are: ***(PGI Nov 2007)***

a. NO b. CO_2
c. Minoxidil d. ACE inhibitor

186. Digoxin is used in A/E: ***(PGI Nov 2007)***

a. Decompensated heart failure
b. HOCM
c. Supraventicular tachycardia
d. Myocarditis

187. ECG changes in digitalis toxicity are A/E: ***(PGI Nov 2007)***

a. T wave inversion
b. Diminished T wave amplitude
c. Conduction block
d. ST depression in proximal part

188. Side effects of directly acting vasodilators are: ***(PGI June 2007)***

a. Hypertrichosis b. Hypotension

189. Drugs used in CHF: ***(PGI June 2007)***

a. Nesiritide b. Digoxin
c. Spironolactone d. Losartan

190. Drugs of choice in lignocaine toxicity: ***(PGI June 2007)***

a. Bretylium b. Amiodarone
c. Isoprenaline d. Beta blocker

191. After inadvertent inj. of Bretylium, TOC is: ***(PGI June 2007)***

a. Bretylium b. Propranolol
c. Norepinephrine d. Lignocaine

192. Drugs which cause fetal renal anomalies: ***(PGI Nov 2006)***

a. Enalapril
b. Frusemide
c. Angiotensin receptor blocker
d. Amlodipine
e. Phenytoin

193. Mg++ administered in: ***(PGI June 2006)***

a. Eclampsia b. Cardiac arrhythmia
c. Seizure d. Tetani

194. Digoxintoxicity aggravated in: ***(PGI June 2006)***

a. Hypokalemia
b. Hyperkalemia
c. hypercalcemia
d. Hypermagnesemia

195. Action of Angiotensin II *(PGI June 2005)*
a. Systemic vasconstriction
b. Systemic vasodilatation
c. Renal vasodilatation
d. Re-absorbtion of Na in proximal renal tubule
e. Water reabsorbtion

196. A hypertensive patient with BP 160/90 mm of Hg presents with increased level of Lipoprotein a. Which Hypolipidemic drug will you prescribe? *(JIPMER May 2018)*
a. Fenofibrate b. Pitavastatin
c. Niacin d. Ezetimibe

197. A 60 years old hypertensive patient is on lithium for treatment of BPD. What is the antihypertensive of choice: *(JIPMER 2017)*
a. Ramipril
b. Amlodipine
c. Atenolol
d. Chlorthiazide

198. Which of the following statement is true regarding Sacubitril? *(JIPMER 2017)*
a. Used with ARB for treatment of CHF
b. BNP inhibitor
c. ACE inhibitor
d. Decreases BNP

199. Which of the following is a PCSK-9 inhibitor? *(JIPMER 2017)*
a. Evolocumab b. Bordalumab
c. Ramucirumab d. Bolosozumab

200. Which statin is given to an 8 years old child with heterozygous familial hypercholesterolemia? *(JIPMER, 2016/2014)*
a. Simvastain b. Pravastain
c. Atorvastain d. Lovastatin

201. A 50 years old man was recently diagnosed to be having coronary artery disease. There was no added risk factors except for a LDL value of 150-165mgs/dL. The single drug most appropriate for initial therapy is *(JIPMER 2016)*
a. Gemfibrozil
b. Nicotinic acid
c. Bile acid binding resins
d. Statins (Any)

202. A 49-year-old male is diagnosed with hypertension. He is a known asthmatic. His creatinine and potassium are both slightly elevated. Which of the following drugs would be appropriate in his case? *(JIPMER 2016)*
a. Amlodipine b. Spironolactone
c. Propranolol d. Hydrochlorthiazide

203. A 59 years old female patient taking medications for hypertension and congestive cardiac failure. She suddenly develops skin rashes along with swelling of tongue, lips as well as eyes, causing her breathing difficulty. Which one of the following medications is the reason for the untoward effects? *(JIPMER 2016)*
a. Propranolol b. Hydrochlorthiazide
c. Captopril d. Clonidine

204. A patient is brought to the emergency department with severe bradycardia, drowsiness, feeble pulse, and very low blood pressure. The patient was found to have consumed unknown quantity of his anti-hypertensive medication. Which of the following cannot be the medication? *(JIPMER 2016)*
a. Clonidine b. Hydralazine
c. Reserpine d. Digoxin

205. Which of the following drug has least value in heart failure? *(JIPMER 2014)*
a. Antiplatelet agents b. Beta blockers
c. Diuretics d. ACE inhibitors

206. Which is not a pleiotropic effect of statins? *(JIPMER 2014)*
a. Reduce LDL cholesterol
b. Improve endothelial stability
c. Anti inflammatory/anti oxidant
d. Reduce plaque rupture

207. Antiarrhythmic drug causing hypothyroidism is: *(JIPMER 2014)*
a. Lidocaine b. Propanolol
c. Amiodarone d. Procainamide

208. Which is not side effect of aminodarone? *(JIPMER 2012)*
a. Pulmonary fibrosis b Torsades de pointes
c. Atrial fibrillation d Bradycardia

209. Which of the following is a direct rennin inhibitor? *(JIPMER 2012)*
a. Aliskiren b. Losartan
c. Perindopril d. Vernakalant

210. Which of the following is a calcium sensitizing agent? *(JIPMER 2012)*
a. Levosimendan b. Cinacalcet
c. Alendronate d. Teriparatide

211. Drug contraindicated in severe hypertriglyceridemia is: *(JIPMER 2010)*
a. Fibrates b. Simvastatin
c. Niacin d. Cholestyramine

212. ACE inhibitors are contraindicated in all the following except: *(JIPMER 2008)*
a. Bilateral renal artery stenosis
b. Elderly hypertensive
c. Diabetic microalbuminuria
d. Severe renal failure

213. Calcium channel blocker which is usually used in subarachnoid hemorrhage is: *(JIPMER 2007)*
a. Nimodipine b. Diltiazem
c. Verapamil d. Flunarizine

214. Which is a characteristic adverse effect of chronic amiodarone therapy? *(JIPMER 2007)*
a. Corneal deposition
b. Cataract
c. Glaucoma
d. Retinal pigmentation

215. Drug used in the treatment of Congestive Heart Failure is *(NIMHANS 2013)*
a. ACE inhibitor b. Beta blocker
c. Art blocker d. All of the above

216. Verapamil belongs to which Class of Anti Arrhythmic Drugs? *(NIMHANS 2013)*

a. I
b. II
c. III
d. IV

217. All of the following are side effects of Hydralazine except *(NIMHANS 2007)*

a. Lupus syndrome
b. Rheumatoid arthritis
c. Postural hypotension
d. Teratogenicity

CHF

218. A 40-year-old man presents with NYHA 3 class, dyspnea, creatinine of 2.5 mg%, potassium level of 4.5 mEq/L. Drug contraindicated is: *(AIIMS May 2017)*

a. Carvedilol
b. Spironolactone
c. Enalapril
d. Digoxin

219. What is the mechanism of action of sacubitril? *(Recent Question 2017)*

a. ACE inhibitor
b. Neutral endopeptidase inhibitor
c. Endothelin antagonist
d. Angiotensin receptor blocker

Practice Questions & Answers from 220 to 264 are given at the end of the chapter.

Answers with Explanations to Multiple Choice Questions

1. Ans (a) Lignocaine

(Ref: Goodman Gilman 13th E/P555)

- Lidocaine is the drug of choice for treatment of ventricular tachycardia caused by myocardial infarction and digoxintoxicity.

2. Ans. (a) Quinidine

(Ref: Goodman Gilman 12th E/P821)

Drugs Causing QT Prolongation

- **Antiarrhythmics:** Class Ia (Quinidine) and Class III
- Cisapride
- **Antipsychotics:** Ziprasidone, Sertindol, Quitiapine, Haloperidol etc.
- **Antidepressants:** Tricyclic antidepressants like amitryptilline, SSRI like flluoxetine
- **Antibiotics:** Fluoroquinolones, Erythromycin
- **Antihistaminics:** Astemizole, Terfenadine
- **Antifungals:** Ketoconazole
- **Antimalarials:** Chloroquine, Quinine, Halofentrine
- **Antivirals:** Amantidine

3. Ans. (a) Fast adenosine

(Ref: Nelson 19th E/P1614)

- The ECG is characteristic of SVT.
- The first thing to be done in infant is place ice bag over the face and placing the face in ice water for older children. If it fails then pharmacotherapy is used.
- The drug of choice for SVT in children is adenosine by rapid IV administration.
- Verapamil is contraindicated in children less than 1 year.

4. Ans. (a) Adenosine

(Ref: Nelson 19th E/P1613)

5. Ans. (d) Ventricular arrhythmia

(Ref: Goodman Gilman 12th E/P844)

- Quinidine toxicity can present as ventricular tachycardia.
- QT prolongation and torsades with quinidine can be seen even at normal doses.

6. Ans. (b) Hepatotoxicity

(Ref: Goodman Gilman 12th E/P834)

7. Ans. (a) Calcium

(Ref: Goodman Gilman 12th E/P803-04)

Cellular effect of digoxin

- In a myocardial cell, digitalis act by inhibiting phosphorylated Na/K ATPase pump, whose function is to reverse the effect of depolarization by pumping sodium out and potassium in. Thus when this effect is inhibited, there is intracellular accumulation of sodium and extracellular potassium, and thus the side effect hyperkalemia. Potassium which accumulates extracellularly, dephosphorylates Na/K ATPase pump and hence limits digitalis action. Thus in case of hypokalemia digitalis toxicity can be seen.
- Intracellular sodium stimulates the Na/Ca exchanger pump, which extrudes sodium out and pumps calcium in, which is further stored in the sarcoplasmic reticulum. Now when an action potential strikes the myocardial cell, a huge amount of calcium is released from the sarcoplasmic reticulum giving a strong positive inotropic effect.
- The persistently high level of calcium in myocardial cells can generate small depolarization just after or in between repolarization and is known as delayed after depolarization (DAD). Further it can take shape of a complete action potential i.e. a cardiac contraction triggered by calcium alone (usually by Na in myocardial cells) and is known as an extra systole. If it's repetitive

bigeminy can be seen, which is the most common digitalis induced arrhythmia. Ventricular tachycardia can follow, which is self-sustained (by myocardial cell) and bidirectional and finally can precipitate fibrillation.

8. Ans. (d) Atrial flutter

(Ref: Goodman Gilman 12th E/P803-04)

9. Ans. (c) Indomethacin

(Ref: Copeland and Afshari's principles and practice of cornea)

- Whorl like corneal deposits can be seen with drugs like
  - **Chloroquine**
  - **Amiodarone**
  - **Chlorpromazine**
  - **Vandetanib**
  - **Indomethacin**
- Indomethacin being the least common cause in the options is the best answer.

10. Ans. (d) Productive cough

(Ref: Goodman Gilman 12th E/P837)

Side effects of Amiodarone

Mnemonics

Side effects of Amiodarone

Potassium : Pulmonary fibrosis
Channel : Corneal microdeposits
Blocker : Blue colored skin
Makes : Myocarditis
Liver : Liver toxicity
Nerve : Neuropathy
And : Alpha receptor block causes hypotension
Skin : Photosensitivity
Toxic : Thyroid (Hypothyroidism > Hyperthyroidism)

11. Ans. (a) Tocainide

(Ref: Goodman Gilman 12th E/P829)

Class I antiarrhythmics

Ia	Ib	Ic
Procainamide Quinidine Disopyramide	Lidocaine Mexiletine Phenytoin Tocainide	Flecainide Propafenone Moricizine

12. Ans. (d) Amiodarone

(Ref: CMDT 2015/P394)

Amiodarone being a class III drug itself causes torsades and hence should be avoided.

Treatment of Long QT Syndrome or Torsades de Pointes

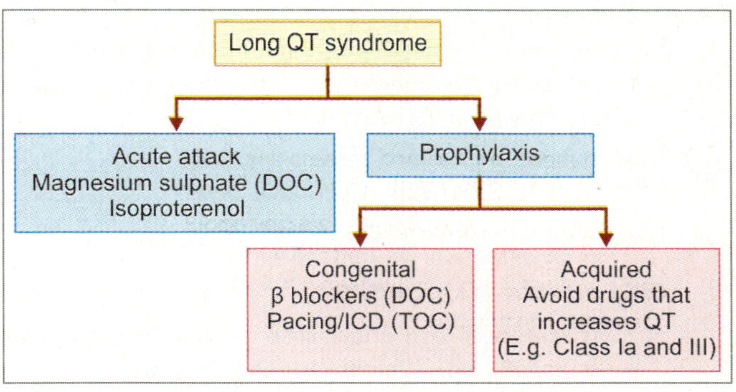

13. Ans. (b) Verapamil

(Ref: Goodman Gilman 12th E/P830)

- Verapamil is the drug of choice for prophylaxis of PSVT.
- Adenosine is the drug of choice for treatment of PSVT. As it causes bronchoconstriction, in patients of COPD and bronchial asthma, verapamil becomes the drug of choice for treatment of PSVT.

14. Ans. (a) Conduction block

(Ref: Goodman Gilman 12th E/P831)

- Both beta blockers and non-dihydropyridine CCBs i.e. diltiazem and verapamil block conduction at AV node and hence they have similar antiarrhythmic uses.
- However due to risk of severe conduction block IV verapamil should never be given with IV beta blocker.

15. Ans. (d) Prolonged PR interval

(Ref: Goodman Gilman 12th E/P838)

- The characteristic ECG change seen with digitalis is PR prolongation due to AV block.
- ST segment depression can be seen due to alteration in ventricular repolarization.

16. Ans. (d) Lignocaine

(Ref: Goodman Gilman 12th E/P830)

- Lignocaine is not effective in atrial arrhythmia, as it blocks sodium channel in a closed state.
- In atrium the action potential is short and the sodium channels are in closed state for a very short period of time.

17. Ans. (c) Administered by slow IV injection

(Ref: Goodman Gilman 12th E/P834)

- Adenosine is an endogenous nucleoside that is readily taken up by cells and immediately metabolized by adenosine deaminase. Hence it has a very short half-life of around 1-5 seconds and a bolus of 6-12 mg by **rapid IV route** is required for clinical effect, as slow administration will result in complete uptake of drug by cells without any effect on heart.

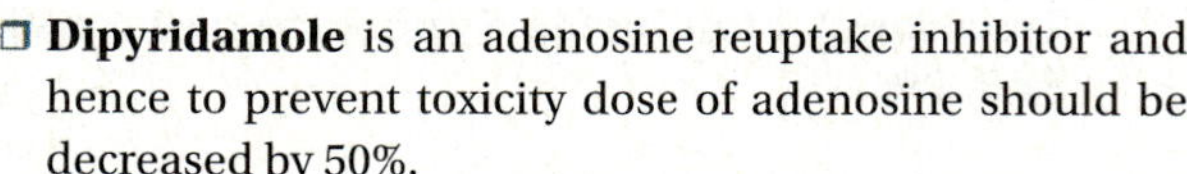

- **Dipyridamole** is an adenosine reuptake inhibitor and hence to prevent toxicity dose of adenosine should be decreased by 50%.
- Adenosine is used for maintaining **controlled hypotension** in surgeries and for diagnosis of **coronary artery disease**.

18. Ans. (c) Brdaycardia

(Ref: Goodman Gilman 12th E/P834)

Side effects of Quinidine

- Most common side effect seen is **diarrhea**, whereas most specific side effect is **cinnchonism**, which is dose dependent as it improves with decrease in dose.
- High doses of quinidine can precipitate **ventricular tachycardia**. Hypotension can be seen due to alpha receptor blockade.
- Unlike other drugs of this class, quinidine can causes **QT prolongation even at therapeutic and subtherapeutic doses**.

19. Ans. (c) Amiodarone

(Ref: Goodman Gilman 12th E/P837)

- Apart from blocking potassium channels, amiodarone also blocks sodium channels (in closed state), beta and alpha receptors and calcium channels.
- This is responsible of myocardial depression, which is usually seen with IV administration.

20. Ans. (b) II

(Ref: Goodman Gilman 12th E/P829)

Vaughan William's classification of antiarrhythmic drugs

Class I	Class II	Class III	Class IV
Sodium channel blockers	Beta blockers	Potassium channel blockers	Calcium channel blockers

21. Ans. (a) Irreversible microdeposits on cornea

(Ref: Goodman Gilman 12th E/P837)

- **Whorl like corneal microdeposits** (corneal verticillata) associated with amiodarone are usually **asymptomatic and reversible** on dose decrease or discontinuation of drug.
- The incidence is around 100% after six months of drug use.

22. Ans. (a) Amiodarone

(Ref: Goodman Gilman 12th E/P837)

- Amiodarone being an analog of thyroid hormone, has iodine which can cause thyroid related disorders.
- If it is given to patients living in euthyroid region, iodine inhibits release of thyroid hormones and causes hypothyroidism. However if it is given to patients living in endemic iodine deficiency region, the iodine is taken up by thyroid and accelerated production of thyroid hormones causes hyperthyroidism.
- Since most patients live in euthyroid region, **hypothyroidism is more common than hyperthyroidism**.

23. Ans. (a) Verapamil

(Ref: Goodman Gilman 12th E/P830)

- Verapamil is the drug of choice for treatment and prophylaxis of SVT and for prophylaxis of PSVT.
- IN case PSVT is associated with bronchial asthma or COPD verapamil is drug of choice for treatment of PSVT.

24. Ans. (a) Quinidine

(Ref: Goodman Gilman 12th E/P844)

Antiarrhythmics Causing Torsades

- Class Ia
- Class III

25. Ans. (d) Systemic lupus erythematosus

(Ref: Goodman Gilman 12th E/P834)

26. Ans. (c) High output failure

(Ref: Goodman Gilman 12th E/P838)

- The use of digoxin as an antiarrhythmic drug is because of its vagomimetic action, which decreases SA node automaticity, shortens atrial APD and blocks conduction at AV node.
- Hence the use is limited as an adjunct for ventricular rate control in patients with atrial fibrillation and flutter.
- Though not routinely indicated in PSVT, digoxin by blocking AV node can be helpful.
- Since it is a positive inotrope, it has no role in high output cardiac failure.

27. Ans. (c) Verapamil

(Ref: Goodman Gilman 12th E/P831)

- All calcium channel blockers are racemic mixture of enantiomers, except nifedipine and diltiazem.
- L-verapamil is more potent and undergoes more first pass metabolism than D-verapamil. Hence IV verapamil delivers a higher amount of L-verapamil, that significantly increases chances of toxicity.

28. Ans. (a) Adenosine

(Ref: Goodman Gilman 12th E/P834)

- Adenosine is the drug of choice for treatment of PSVT.
- As it causes bronchoconstriction, in patients of COPD and bronchial asthma, verapamil becomes the drug of choice for treatment of PSVT.

29. Ans. (b) Amiodarone

(Ref: Goodman Gilman 12th E/P837)

Pharmacokinetics of Amiodarone

- The average half-life of amiodarone is around 53 days and hence is the **longest acting antiarrhythmic**.
- It has high lipid solubility, which is responsible for its **high volume of distribution** (5000 liters) and hence a loading dose of 800-1600 mg/day is given for many weeks to achieve steady state concentration. For same reason its concentration is 20 times more in heart and 300 times more in fat as compared to plasma.

30. Ans. (c) Quinidine

(Ref: Goodman Gilman 12th E/P844)

- Quinidine being a class Ia drug blocks both sodium and potassium channel.
- Hence it can decrease slope of phase 0 as well as prolong the action potential duration.

31. Ans. (d) Verapamil

(Ref: Goodman Gilman 12th E/P831)

32. Ans. (c) Class 3

(Ref: Goodman Gilman 12th E/P829)

33. Ans. (a) I

(Ref: Goodman Gilman 12th E/P829)

34. Ans. (a) Amiodarone

(Ref: Goodman Gilman 12th E/P834)

- Amiodarone is an analog of thyroid hormone and it has iodine which can cause thyroid related disorders.
- If it is given to patients living in euthyroid region, iodine inhibits release of thyroid hormones and causes hypothyroidism. However if it is given to patients living in endemic iodine deficiency region, the iodine is taken up by thyroid and accelerated production of thyroid hormones causes hyperthyroidism.
- Since most patients live in euthyroid region, **hypothyroidism is more common than hyperthyroidism**.

35. Ans. (d) Verapamil

(Ref: Goodman Gilman 12th E/P831)

36. Ans. (c) Tocainide

(Ref: Goodman Gilman 12th E/P829)

37. Ans. (b) Digoxin

(Ref: Goodman and Gilman 12th E/P 803-04)

- Digoxin doesn't cause edema, rather is used for treatment of cardiogenic edema.
- Estrogen stimulates endothelial NO production, which causes vasodilation and edema.
- NSAID decrease Pg synthesis and hence inhibit Pg induced Cl loss and block of Vasopressin, which results in fluid retention and edema.
- Cyclosporine can cause nephrotoxicity, which leads to retention of solute and water followed by edema.

38. Ans. (a) Hyperkalemia

(Ref: Goodman and Gilman 12th E/P 803)

Digitalis toxicity can be precipitated by

- **Renal failure**
- **Myocardial ischemia**
- **Hypokalemia**
- **Hypercalcemia**
- **Hypomagnesemia**
- **Drugs**
  - **Diuretics**
  - **Quinidine**
  - **Verapamil**
  - **Flecainide**
  - **Propafenone**
  - **Amiodarone**

39. Ans. (a) Hepatic disease

(Ref: Goodman and Gilman 12th E/P 803)

40. Ans. (a) Neutral endopeptidase

(Ref: Goodman and Gilman 12th E/P 696)

- BNP is metabolized by neutral endopeptidase.
- Omapatrilat is a vasopeptidase inhibitor that inhibits both ACE and neutral endopeptidase.

41. Ans. (a) Administration of quinidine

(Ref: Goodman and Gilman 12th E/P 803)

42. Ans. (a) Potassium

(Ref: Goodman and Gilman 12th E/P 804)

Treatment of Digitalis Toxicity

- **Lidocaine** is the drug of choice for digitalis induced ventricular tachyarrhythmias. Other alternatives are phenytoin and MgSO4.
- **Digiband** is an anti-digoxin antibody reserved for treatment of life threatening arrhythmias induced by digoxin.
- **Potassium** can be given for benign arrhythmias like atrial, AV junctional and ventricular ectopic rhythms, even if serum potassium levels are normal. Potassium dephosphorylates Na/K ATPase and limits digitalis action. Potassium is **contraindicated in case of AV block**, as it can be worsened.
- Cardioversion can be problematic as it can itself induce arrhythmia in digitalis toxicity.

43. Ans. (d) Potassium

(Ref: Goodman and Gilman 12th E/P 804)

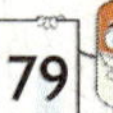

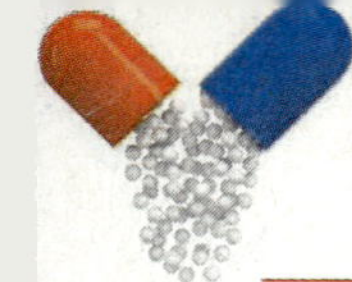

44. Ans. (d) Prolonged PR interval

(Ref: Goodman and Gilman 12th E/P 804)

ECG Changes with Digoxin

ECG changes	Cause
PR prolongation	Refractoriness at AV node
QT shortening	Shortening of action potential duration
T wave inversion ST segment depression	Accelerated repolarization of inner layers of myocardium

45. Ans. (b) Potassium channel opener

(Ref: Harrison 19th E/P1510)

- Levosimendan apart from blocking PDE-3, also produces inotropic effect and vasodilatation by **sensitizing myocardium to calcium ions** and **opening potassium channels** respectively.
- Though not approved by FDA, it is approved by many countries for treatment of acute CHF not responding to other inotropes.

46. Ans. (c) 36 hours

(Ref: Goodman and Gilman 12th E/P 803)

- Digoxin has a half-life of 36-48 hours. Though both are in options, 36 is a better answer as it is mostly lower in the limit for young patients with normal renal functions.

47. Ans. (c) Digoxin antibody

(Ref: Goodman and Gilman 12th E/P 804)

- **Digiband**, an anti-digoxin antibody is the **most effective drug** and hence reserved for treatment of life threatening arrhythmias induced by digoxin.
- **The dose of digiband is calculated based on the total digoxin dose administered.**

48. Ans. (c) Digoxin

(Ref: Goodman and Gilman 12th E/P 791)

Drugs inhibiting cardiac remodeling and delaying mortality in CHF

Mnemonics

SHIBA

S : Spironolactone
H : Hydralazine + IDN
I : Ivabridine
B : Beta blockers
A : ACEI/ARB

49. Ans. (d) Milrinone

(Ref: Goodman and Gilman 12th E/P 805)

- **In right sided heart failure milrinone has positive inotropic effect, as well as it decreases systemic congestion by venodilation.**
- **Hence it is the inotrope of choice.**

50. Ans. (d) Trimetazidine

(Ref: Goodman and Gilman 12th E/P 791)

51. Ans. (c) It can be administered orally

(Ref: Goodman and Gilman 12th E/P 696)

- **Nesiritide** is a BNP analogue that has a short half-life, as it is rapidly metabolized by an enzyme **neutral endopeptidase**. Since it is a peptide it is given by **IV route** for treatment of pulmonary edema associated with acute CHF to patients who are still symptomatic with diuretics and nitrates.
- It causes vasodilatation along with **natriuresis** and diuresis.

52. Ans. (a) Glomerular filtration

(Ref: Goodman and Gilman 12th E/P 803)

- The primary rout of excretion of digoxin is renal in unchanged form.
- Thus renal failure can precipitate digitalis toxicity.

53. Ans. (c) Losartan

(Ref: Goodman and Gilman 12th E/P 791)

54. Ans. (b) Furosemide

(Ref: Goodman and Gilman 12th E/P 790)

- **Loop diuretics are the first line dr**ug for treatment of pulmonary edema, due to their high ceiling effect and ability to rapidly control volume overload.
- Thiazides are less effective but can be combined to loops in case of inadequate response.
- Potassium sparing diuretics are combined to combat hypokalemia and refractory edema.

55. Ans. (c) Dobutamine

(Ref: Goodman and Gilman 12th E/P 791)

- **Dobutamine** is the inotrope of choice for acute CHF, but not used for long-term management.
- Drugs decreasing cardiac remodelling like ACEI/ARB, beta blockers, spironolactone, ivabridine and IDN + Hydralazine is used on long-term basis to decrease mortality.When these drugs are ineffective the patient is then maintained on digoxin.

56. Ans. (a) Adrenaline

(Ref: Goodman and Gilman 12th E/P 791)

57. Ans. (c) Treat digoxintoxicity

(Ref: Goodman and Gilman 12th E/P 804)

58. Ans. (d) All of the above

(Ref: Goodman and Gilman 12th E/P 804)

Side effects of Digitalis

- GIT upset (nausea, vomiting and diarrhea) - It is the earliest and most common side effect associated.
- Arrhythmias - Ventricular bigeminy is most common and atrial tachycardia with variable AV block is most specific arrhythmia.
- Xanthopsia (yellow vision)
- Gynecomastia
- Hallucinations
- Hyperkalemia.

59. Ans. (b) Captopril

(Ref: Goodman and Gilman 12th E/P 798)

- Captopril is an ACE inhibitor that is a mixed dilator and hence decreases both preload and after load.

60. Ans. (a) ACE inhibitors

(Ref: Goodman and Gilman 12th E/P 797)

- In case of LVH seen after CHF, the first class of drug started are ACEI or ARB to decrease mortality by inhibiting cardiac mortality.
- After ACEI/ARB, beta blockers are started.

61. Ans. (c) Carvedilol

(Ref: Goodman and Gilman 12th E/P 801)

Beta Blockers Used in CHF to Decrease Mortality

- Carvedilol - Maximum decrease in mortality
- Metoprolol (long acting formulation)
- Bisoprolol

62. Ans. (d) Decreased HR

(Ref: Goodman and Gilman 12th E/P 804)

- Digoxin is a positive inotropic drug and hence increases the force of contraction thereby shortening systole, which increases the duration of diastole and filling period.
- Because of vagomimetic and sympatholytic effect the HR decreases.

63. Ans. (b) AV node

(Ref: Goodman and Gilman 12th E/P 804)

64. Ans. (b) Bradycardia with AV block

(Ref: Goodman Gilman 13th E/P214)

- Beta blockers and calcium channel blockers like verapamil block both SA and AV node. Thus if both are combined, it will result in bradycardia and AV block.
- This is the reason why beta blockers should not be combined with verapamil.

65. Ans. (b) Guanylyl cyclase

(Ref: Goodman Gilman 13th E/P520)

- Sodium nitroprusside is metabolized into nitric oxide, which activates guanylyl cyclase and increases cyclic GMP.
- Cyclic GMP activates protein kinase G which dephosphorylates MLCP (Myosin Light Chain Phosphorylase) and relaxes the smooth muscles of blood vessels.
- Other drugs acting by similar mechanism are nitrates, hydralazine, riociguat and cinaciguat.
- Nitrates and hydralazine are also metabolized into nitric oxide and then they act by same mechanism.
- Riociguat and cinaciguat are direct stimulators of guanylyl cyclase.

66. Ans. (b) Decreases preload

(Ref: Goodman Gilman 13th E/P493)

- Dilatation of coronary arteries increases coronary blood flow and dilation of systemic veins decrease the preload on heart.
- A decrease in cardiac preload significantly decreases the wall tension and oxygen demand of myocardium is the most important mechanism for beneficial effect in classical angina as well as chronic CHF.
- Coronary vasodilation is the most important mechanism in variant angina.

67. Ans. (a) Endothelium independent coronary vasodilation

(Ref: Goodman Gilman 12th E/P749)

- In Prinz metal angina which is caused by contraction of coronary artery; endothelium independent coronary vasodilation is primary mechanism.
- In case of stable angina the primary mechanism is a decrease in preload, which decreases cardiac contraction and oxygen demand; hence in this case answer would have been b.

68. Ans. (a) Atenolol

(Ref: CMDT 2018/P826)

- Three drugs commonly used in pregnancy induced hypertension are
  - Methyldopa
  - Labetalol
  - Nifedipine
- Hydralazine is used for treatment of hypertensive emergency in pregnancy.
- Atenolol is avoided in pregnancy due to concerns about fetal growth retardation.

69. Ans. (c) Telmesartan

(Ref: Michael Schupp, Jürgen, JankeRonald, Clasen. Angiotensin Type 1

Receptor Blockers Induce Peroxisome Proliferator-Activated Receptor-Activity.
Circulation 2004;109: 2054-2057.)

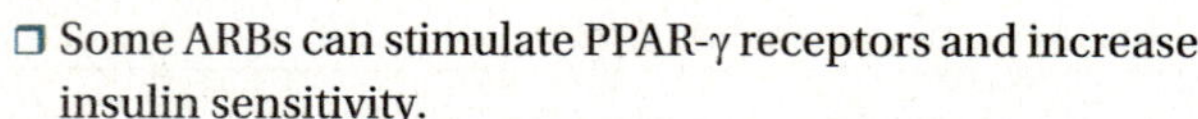

- Some ARBs can stimulate PPAR-γ receptors and increase insulin sensitivity.
- This effect with ARBs is directly proportional to their lipid solubility, and based upon it their order PPAR-γ agonist activity is telmisartan > Irbesartan > Losartan.
- ACE inhibitors also increase insulin sensitivity but via bradykinin pathway.

70. Ans. (b) Beta blockers

(Ref: CMDT 2017/P449)

Bradykinin increased by ACE inhibitors can cause nasal congestion and rhinitis.

71. Ans. (b) Losartan

(Ref: Goodman Gilman 12th E/P791)

72. Ans. (c) Minoxidil

(Ref: Goodman Gilman 12th E/P733)

73. Ans. (b) Enalapril

(Ref: Goodman Gilman 12th E/P736)

74. Ans. (b) Labetalol

(Ref: Goodman Gilman 12th E/P801)

- According to current OBG guidelines the drug of choice for hypertension in pregnancy is labetalol.

75. Ans. (b) α-methyl dopa

(Ref: Goodman Gilman 12th E/P773)

- According to older guidelines α-methyl dopa is the drug of choice for pregnancy induced hypertension.
- In newer OBG guidelines, oral labetalol is the drug of choice for pregnancy induced hypertension and IV labetalol is the drug of choice for hypertensive emergency in pregnancy.

76. Ans. (b) Thrombolytics

(Ref: CMDT 2016/P370)

- This is a case of acute myocardial infarction with ST elevation in the ECG.
- For such a case thrombolysis or PCI is indicated within 12 hours of symptom onset. In this case since it has been one day, thrombolysis is contraindicated.

77. Ans. (a) Enalapril

(Ref: Goodman and Gilman 12th E/P 736)

- RAS inhibitors like ACEIs, ARBs and DRIs are absolutely contraindicated in pregnancy.
- The teratogenic effects seen are

  1st trimester: CVS and CNS defects

  2nd and 3rd trimester: Renal defects

78. Ans. (c) Thiazide diuretics

(Ref: Goodman Gilman 12th E/P770)

- Thiazides are used for mild to moderate hypertension.
- Loops are indicated in hypertensive emergency with renal failure.
- Potassium sparing diuretics are used to prevent hypokalemia. Spironolactone is drug of choice in resistant hypertension.

79. Ans. (b) Oxyphedrine

(Ref: Goodman Gilman 12th E/P770)

- Oxyphedrine causes coronary vasodilation along with positive inotropic effect without an increase in oxygen demand or worsening of angina.
- Dipyridamole can cause coronary steal phenomenon and worsen angina.
- Thyroxine can increase the oxygen demand and sumatriptan can cause coronary vasoconstriction.

80. Ans. (b) Omission of prior diuretic dose decrease the risk of postural hypotension

(Ref: Goodman and Gilman 12th E/P 736)

- ACEIs can cause hypotension which can be augmented by diuretics and if not given the chances of hypotension are lesser.
- They inhibit conversion of AT-I to AT-II.
- Enalapril has a half-life of 1.3 hours, but its active metabolite enalaprilat has a half-life of 11 hours because of higher affinity for ACE that causes slow dissociation. Lisinopril is an analog of enalaprilat and hence has a longer half-life of 12 hours as compared to enalapril.
- ACEIs are the drug of choice for treatment of DM with hypertension, where they delay the progression of nephropathy as well as retinopathy.

81. Ans. (d) Renal colic

(Ref: Goodman Gilman 12th E/P753-54)

Uses of Nitrates

- Angina
- MI
- Esophageal and biliary spasm
- Cyanide toxicity (Nitrites preferred)
- CHF (IDN + Hydralazine)

82. Ans. (b) Thrombolytic

(Ref: CMDT 2016/P364)

- In case of NSTEMI and unstable angina thrombolysis is absolutely contraindicated.

83. Ans. (d) L-dopa

(Ref: Goodman Gilman 12th E/P616)

- Levodopa in periphery is metabolized to dopamine, which causes orthostatic hypotension.

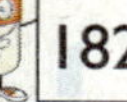

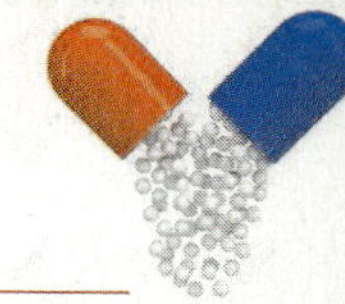

- NSAIDS can decrease prostaglandin synthesis and cause hypertension.
- Erythropoetin increases blood viscousity and cause hypertension.
- Cyclosporine also causes hypertension, though mechanism is not clear.

84. Ans. (a) Juxtaglomerulus apparatus

(Ref: Goodman and Gilman 12th E/P 722, 724)

85. Ans. (b) Beta blockers

(Ref: KDT 7th E/P563)

86. Ans. (a) Hypotension

(Ref: Goodman and Gilman 12th E/P 736)

Mnemonics

Side effects of ACEIs – ACE INH

- **A** : Angioedema
- **C** : Cough
- **E** : Electrolyte imbalance (Hyperkalemia)
- **I** : Itch caused by rash
- **N** : Neutropenia
- **H** : Hypotension

87. Ans. (d) Nitroglycerine

(Ref: Goodman Gilman 13th E/P491)

Arterial dilators: Decrease afterload	Vasodilators: Decrease preload	Mixed dilators: Decrease both preload and afterload
Calcium channel blockers Minoxidil Hydralazine Fenoldopam Diazoxide	Nitrates	Nitroprusside ACE Inhibitors ARBs DRIs Alpha blockers

88. Ans. (c) Xylocaine

(Ref: CMDT 2016 E/P375)

- Earlier lidocaine was prophylactically given to prevent ventricular arrhythmia in a patient of MI. But now prophylactic use has been discontinued due to no reduction in mortality.
- Currently to all patients of ventricular arrhythmia in MI, lidocaine is only given for treatment and is the drug of choice. Other alternatives are amiodarone and procainamide.

89. Ans. (b) Antianginal

Ref: (Goodman Gilman 12th E/P752)

90. Ans. (a) Amiloride, (d) Spironolactone

(Ref: Goodman Gilman 12th E/P736)

- **Potassium sparing diuretics are contraindicated with ACEIs due to risk of hyperkalemia. In the options both amiloride and spironolactone are potassium sparing diretics.**

91. Ans. (a) Enalapril

(Ref: Goodman Gilman 12th E/P736)

92. Ans. (d) Clonidine

(Ref: Goodman Gilman 12th E/P736)

Factors and drugs affecting renin

Renin increased	Renin decreased
ATP Adenosine NSAIDS ACEIs/ARBs/DRIs	Prostaglandins Loop diuretics Beta blockers Central sympatholytics (e.g. clonidine)

93. Ans. (a) Hyperkalemia

(Ref: Goodman Gilman 12th E/P736)

94. Ans. (b) It can cause severe hypoglycemia

(Ref: Goodman Gilman 12th E/P783,1248)

- Diazoxide is a potassium channel opener that inhibits insulin release and is drug of choice for treatment of insulinoma. Since it decreases insulin release it can cause hyperglycemia.
- By opening of potassium channels in blood vessels it can cause vasodilatation and was earlier used for treatment of hypertensive emergency.

95. Ans. (b) Perindopril

(Ref: Goodman Gilman 12th E/P735)

- ACEIs decrease proteinuria and the progression of nephropathy and retinopathy associated with DM.

96. Ans. (a) Pregnancy induced hypertension

(Ref: Goodman Gilman 12th E/P773)

97. Ans. (d) Lisinopril

(Ref: Goodman Gilman 12th E/P736)

- **All ACEIs are prodrugs except captopril and lisinopril.**

98. Ans. (c) Hypotension and tachycardia

(Ref: Goodman Gilman 12th E/P749)

- Hypotension and bradycardia can be seen with sublingual nitroglycerine due to activation of Bezold-Jarisch reflex.

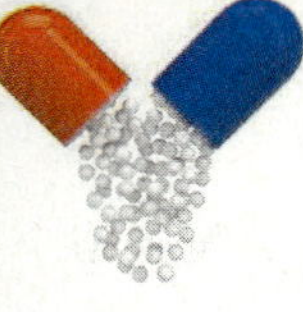

- Vasodilatation decreases preload on the heart. Methemoglobinemia can also be seen.
- Tachycardia due to vasodilatation can be seen only a high doses of nitrates.

99. Ans. (c) Vasodilation

(Ref: Goodman Gilman 12th E/P728)

Effects of Angiotensin II

- Vasoconstriction
- Constriction of afferent and efferent arterioles of glomerulus
- Increase in release of aldosterone, vasopressin and catecholamines
- Thirst
- Anorexia

100. Ans. (d) Nifedipine

(Ref: Goodman Gilman 12th E/P777)

101. Ans. (d) Causes hyperuricemia

(Ref: Goodman Gilman 12th E/P736)

- Losartan is a competitive inhibitor of angiotensin receptors AT1>AT2.
- It is metabolized into an active metabolite called as EXP 3174. Losartan has a half-life of 2.5 hours, whereas EXP 3174 has a half-life of 9 hours.
- Cough and angioedema are rarely seen with ARBs.
- Losartan has a uricosuric effect and causes hypouricemia.

102. Ans. (a) Dipyridamole

(Ref: KDT 7th E/P553)

- Dipyridamoledilates the blood vessels in non-ischemic area and diverts the blood from ischemic area known as coronary steal phenomenon.

103. Ans. (a) Atenolol

(Ref: Goodman Gilman 12th E/P772)

- Beta blockers are given only after alpha blockers in pheochromocytoma.
- If alone beta blocker is given then inhibition of beta-2 mediated vasodilatation can cause unopposed alpha-1 mediaded vasoconstriction and worsen pheochromocytoma.

104. Ans. (b) Hypokalemia

(Ref: Goodman Gilman 12th E/P736)

105. Ans. (b) Verapamil

(Ref: Goodman Gilman 12th E/P736)

- Enalapril cannot be used as ACEIs are contraindicated in bilateral renal artery stenosis.
- Beta blockers and thiazides are contraindicated in DM, as betablockers can cause hypoglycemic unawareness and thiazides cause hyperglycemia.
- Hence verapamil is the best drug in the options for the patients.

106. Ans. (b) Alpha receptor blocker

(Ref: Goodman Gilman 12th E/P772)

- Alpha blockers can cause postural hypotension in around 50% patients.
- ACE inhibitors can also cause postural hypotension but incidence is lesser than alpha blockers.
- Beta blockers don't cause postural hypotension.
- Arterial dilators don't cause postural hypotension as venodilation is essential for postural hypotension.

107. Ans. (a) Increase intotal coronary blood flow

(Ref: Goodman Gilman 12th E/P749)

- In classical angina the main mechanism of benefit is venodilatation, that decreases the preload and oxygen demand by the myocardium.
- In variant angina the main mechanism is coronary vasodilatation.

108. Ans. (c) Intramuscular

(Ref: Goodman Gilman 12th E/P753)

Routes of Administration for Nitroglycerine

- Sublingual
- Oral (Sustained release preparation)
- Transdermal
- Buccal spray
- Intravenous

109. Ans. (c) Minoxidil

(Ref: Goodman Gilman 12th E/P781)

- Minoxidil can cause hirsutism and hence is not used in females.
- Topical minoxidil is used for treatment of androgenic alopecia.

110. Ans. (b) Methyl dopa

(Ref: Goodman Gilman 12th E/P773)

- Methyl dopa is a prodrug converted into alpha methyl norepinephrine in CNS.

111. Ans. (d) Prazosin

(Ref: Goodman Gilman 12th E/P773)

- **Prazosin causes vasodilatation by blocking alpha 1 receptors in the peripheral blood vessels.**

112. Ans. (b) Guanethidine

(Ref: Goodman Gilman 12th E/P775)

- Guanethidine and guanadrel can cause postural hypotension due to sympathetic blockade even on chronic use.
- Alpha-1 blockers like prazosin and ACEIs cause postural hypotension only during initial doses.
- Beta blockers don't cause postural hypotension.

113. Ans. (d) Nitroprusside

(Ref: Goodman Gilman 12th E/P783)

- Nitroprusside is a very short and fast acting drug as the effect is seen within 30 seconds and terminates 3 minutes after infusion is stopped.

114. Ans. (c) Pentaerythritol tetranitrate

(Ref: KDT 7th E/P544)

115. Ans. (b) Metoprolol

(Ref: Goodman Gilman 12th E/P761)

- Beta blockers are not effective in angina because of vaso-dilatation, rather decrease oxygen demand on long-term use and decrease mortality.

116. Ans. (b) Prazosin

(Ref: Goodman Gilman 12th E/P773)

- Alpha-1 antagonist like prazosin have favourable effect on lipid profile i.e. increase HDL and decrease LDL. They don't have any effect on blood glucose level.

117. Ans. (b) Indipamide, (c) Sublingual nifedipine

(Ref: KDT 7th E/P573)

- Indipamide is used for treatment of mild to moderate hypertension but not hypertensive emergency.
- Sublingual nifedipine is used for treatment of hypertensive urgency but not emergency.

118. Ans. (a) Subarachnoid hemorrhage

(Ref: Goodman Gilman 12th E/P758)

119. Ans. (c) Congestive heart failure

(Ref: Goodman Gilman 12th E/P758-760)

- CCB are used for long-term prevention of angina. Verapamil and diltiazem can be used as monotherapyin stable angina, whereas DHPs are always used with beta blockers to prevent reflex tachycardia. DHPs are also used in variant angina and are drugs of choice.
- Vaerapamil>Diltiazem is used in PSVT and SVT.
- DHPs are commonly used first line drugs in hypertension.

120. Ans. (a) Guanylatecyclase

(Ref: Goodman Gilman 12th E/P782)

- Vasodilators stimulating guanylatecyclase by increasing NO are nitrates, nitroprusside and hydralazine.
- Direct stimulators of guanylatecyclase are recent drugs like riociguat and cinaciguat.

121. Ans. (c) Isoproterenol

(Ref: Goodman Gilman 12th E/P760)

- Beta blockers and ACEIs are used in MI to decrease mortality.
- Streptokinase is used for thrombolysis in STEMI.
- Isoproteronol in ischemic heart disease can increase oxygen demand by increasing force and rate of heart contraction. Hence it should be avoided.

122. Ans. (c) Enalapril

(Ref: Goodman Gilman 12th E/P736)

123. Ans. (a) Methyl dopa

(Ref: Goodman Gilman 12th E/P773)

124. Ans. (a) Nicorandil

(Ref: Harrison 19th E/P1590)

125. Ans. (b) Inhalation

(Ref: Katzung 11th E/P195)

- Amyl nitrite can be given by inhalational route for an acute attack of angina. Because of pungent odor it is not used nowadays.
- Sodium nitrite is used for treatment of cyanide toxicity.

126. Ans. (d) Bilateral renal artery stenosis

(Ref: Goodman Gilman 12th E/P736)

Absolute contraindications of ACEIs

- Bilateral renal artery stenosis
- Single kidney with renal artery stenosis
- Pregnancy
- Along with Potassium sparing diuretics

127. Ans. (a) Methyl dopa

(Ref: Goodman Gilman 12th E/P773)

128. Ans. (a) Bradykinin

(Ref: Goodman Gilman 12th E/P735)

- Cough and angioedema caused by ACEIs is primarily due to bradykinin. Other contributing factors are substance P and prostaglandins.

129. Ans. (a) Bradykinin

(Ref: Goodman Gilman 12th E/P735)

- Bradykinin is metabolized by kininase which is similar to ACE and hence ACEIs also inhibit kininase and metabolism of bradykinin.

130. Ans. (c) ACE inhibitors

(Ref: Goodman Gilman 12th E/P735)

- ACEIs are drug of choice for treatment of hypertension associated with DM and CKD.

131. Ans. (a) Clonidine

(Ref: Goodman Gilman 12th E/P774)

- Clonidine is a central sympatholytic that decreases NE release.
- NE being a CNS stimulant, its decrease can result in sedation.

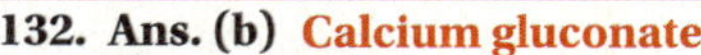

132. Ans. (b) Calcium gluconate

(Ref: Goodman Gilman 12th E/P759)

133. Ans. (d) GTN

(Ref: CMDT 2016/P363)

- **Drug of choice for an acute attack of Prinzmetal angina is nitroglycerine.**
- **Long acting nitrates and DHPs can be used for prophylaxis.**

134. Ans. (a) Reducing coronary spasm

(Ref: CMDT 2016/P363)

135. Ans. (a) Hypotension

(Ref: Goodman Gilman 12th E/P736)

- Hypotension with ARBs is much more common than cough and angioedema, which are rarely seen as compared to ACEIs.

136. Ans. (d) Nimodipine

(Ref: Goodman Gilman 12th E/P758)

137. Ans. (c) Sodium nitroprusside

(Ref: Goodman Gilman 12th E/P782)

- **In the given options only nitroprusside by IV route is used in hypertensive emergency.**
- **Clonidine and nifedipine are used in hypertensive urgency but not emergency.**
- α-methyl dopa is primarily used in pregnancy induced hypertension.

138. Ans. (a) Atenolol

(Ref: Goodman Gilman 12th E/P772)

Drug of Choice for Hypertension Associated with Comorbidities

Associated comorbidity with hypertension	Drugs preferred
DM CKD Scleroderma Nephrotic syndrome	ACEI/ARB
Angina Previous MI Hyperthyroidism Migraine Anxiety with somatic manifestations Essential tremor Atrial fibrillation and flutter Preoperative hypertension	Beta blockers
Osteoporosis	Thiazides
Raynaud's disease Cyclosporine induced hypertension	CCB
BPH Dyslipidemia	α_1 blockers

139. Ans. (a) Amiloride

(Ref: Goodman Gilman 12th E/P736)

140. Ans. (b) Angiotensin converting enzyme inhibitor

(Ref: Goodman Gilman 12th E/P736)

141. Ans. (a) Headache

(Ref: Goodman Gilman 12th E/P759)

142. Ans. (a) Postural hypotension

(Ref: Goodman Gilman 12th E/P739)

143. Ans. (c) Pentoxifylline

(Ref: Goodman Gilman 12th E/P764)

Drugs used in peripheral vascular disease

Drugs	Mechanism of action
Pentoxifylline	Rheological drug that acts by increasing deformability of RBCs
Cilostazole	PDE-3 inhibitor

144. Ans. (a) Hydralazine

(Ref: Goodman Gilman 12th E/P780)

145. Ans. (a) Enalapril

(Ref: Goodman Gilman 12th E/P736)

146. Ans. (d) Headache

(Ref: Goodman Gilman 12th E/P739)

147. Ans. (a) ACE inhibitors

(Ref: Goodman Gilman 12th E/P736)

- ACE inhibitors can worsen kidney function in renovascular hypertension by dilating the efferent arterioles, that can cause a decrease in filtration pressure in glomerulus.

148. Ans. (d) Isosorbide-5-mononitrate

(Ref: Goodman Gilman 12th E/P751)

- Isosorbide-5 mononitrate has lesser first pass metabolism and hence given by oral route.
- IDN and NTG can be given by sublingual route.

149. Ans. (a) Propranolol

(Ref: Goodman Gilman 12th E/P761)

150. Ans. (a) Methyl dopa

(Ref: Goodman Gilman 12th E/P774)

Antihypertensive Drugs Causing ED are

- Beta blockers (Maxiumum)

- Thiazides
- Methyl dopa

151. Ans. (a) Atenolol

(Ref: Goodman Gilman 12th E/P772)

152. Ans. (a) Congestive heart failure, (b) Angina pectoris

(Ref: CMDT 2016/P358)

- Ivabridine was first approved for treatment of angina.
- Recently in 2014 it has also been approved for CHF to decrease mortality.
- So when the MCQ was asked, angina was the answer but now both a and b are correct options.

153. Ans. (b) Atorvastatin 80 mg

(Ref: CMDT 2017/P1263-64)

- There is history of MI and hence in this case there is clinical atherosclerotic disease and hence high intensity statin therapy is indicated.
- Among given options atorvastatin 80 mg is high intensity statin therapy.
- **Note:** Moderate intensity statin can be used if patient is above 75 years of age.
- Hypertriglyceridemia above 150 association with CAD is not defined. Triglycerides above 500 is treated to prevent pancreatitis.

154. Ans. (a) It causes insulin resistance

(Ref: Goodman Gilman 12th E/P900)

- **Niacin causes insulin resistance and hence causes severe hyperglycemia in patients of diabetes mellitus.**
- **Hence it should be avoided in patients of diabetes mellitus.**

155. Ans. (b) Fenofibrate

(Ref: Goodman Gilman 12th E/P902)

156. Ans. (c) Absorbed good on empty stomach and absorption is delayed by fatty meals

(Ref: Goodman Gilman 12th E/P902)

- Fibrates are better absorbed with food and lesser on empty stomach.
- They activate PPAR alpha and increase LPL synthesis.
- Rash, urticarial, myalgia, impotence, alopecia, headache, anemia can be associated.

157. Ans. (d) Fibrinogen levels are decreased by pravastatin

(Ref: 9KDT 7th E/P637)

- Simvastatin and lovastatin are lipid soluble drugs and hence CNS accumulation is higher. The inverse is correct for pravastatin and fluvastatin.
- Fibrinogen levels are decreased by pravastatin and not increased.

158. Ans. (d) Peripheral decarboxylase

(Ref: Goodman Gilman 12th E/P893-903)

Hypolipidemics Mechanism of Action

Drugs	Mechanism of action
Statins	Inhibit HMG-CoA reductase
Bile acid binding resins	Deplete bile acid and result in decrease in cholesterol and triglycerides
Fibrates	Stimulate PPAR alpha and increase LPL synthesis
Niacin	Inhibits hormone sensitive lipase
Ezetimibe	Inhibits NPC1L1 protein in small intestine and inhibits cholesterol absorption
Lomitapide	Inhibits MTP
Icosapent	Inhibits VLDL synthesis/secretion by liver
Meopmersen sodium	Inhibits Apo-B100 synthesis
Evolocumab	Anti PCSK-9 antibody
Avasimibe	Acyl CoA Cholesterol Acyl Transferase (ACAT) inhibitor

159. Ans. (a) Increases HDL

(Ref: Goodman Gilman 12th E/P900)

160. Ans. (b) Nicotinic acid

(Ref: Goodman Gilman 12th E/P900)

161. Ans. (b) PPAR alpha agonist

(Ref: Goodman Gilman 12th E/P901)

162. Ans. (a) Bind to bile acid

(Ref: Goodman Gilman 12th E/P898)

163. Ans. (b) Ezetimibe

(Ref: Goodman Gilman 12th E/P903)

164. Ans. (c) Atorvastatin

(Ref: Goodman Gilman 12th E/P895)

- Atorvastatin is primarily hypolipidemic associated with pleiotropic effects, out of which one is antiaggregant effect.

165. Ans. (c) Statins

(Ref: Goodman Gilman 12th E/894)

166. Ans. (a) Competitive inhibition of rate limiting step in cholesterol synthesis

(Ref: Goodman Gilman 12th E/894)

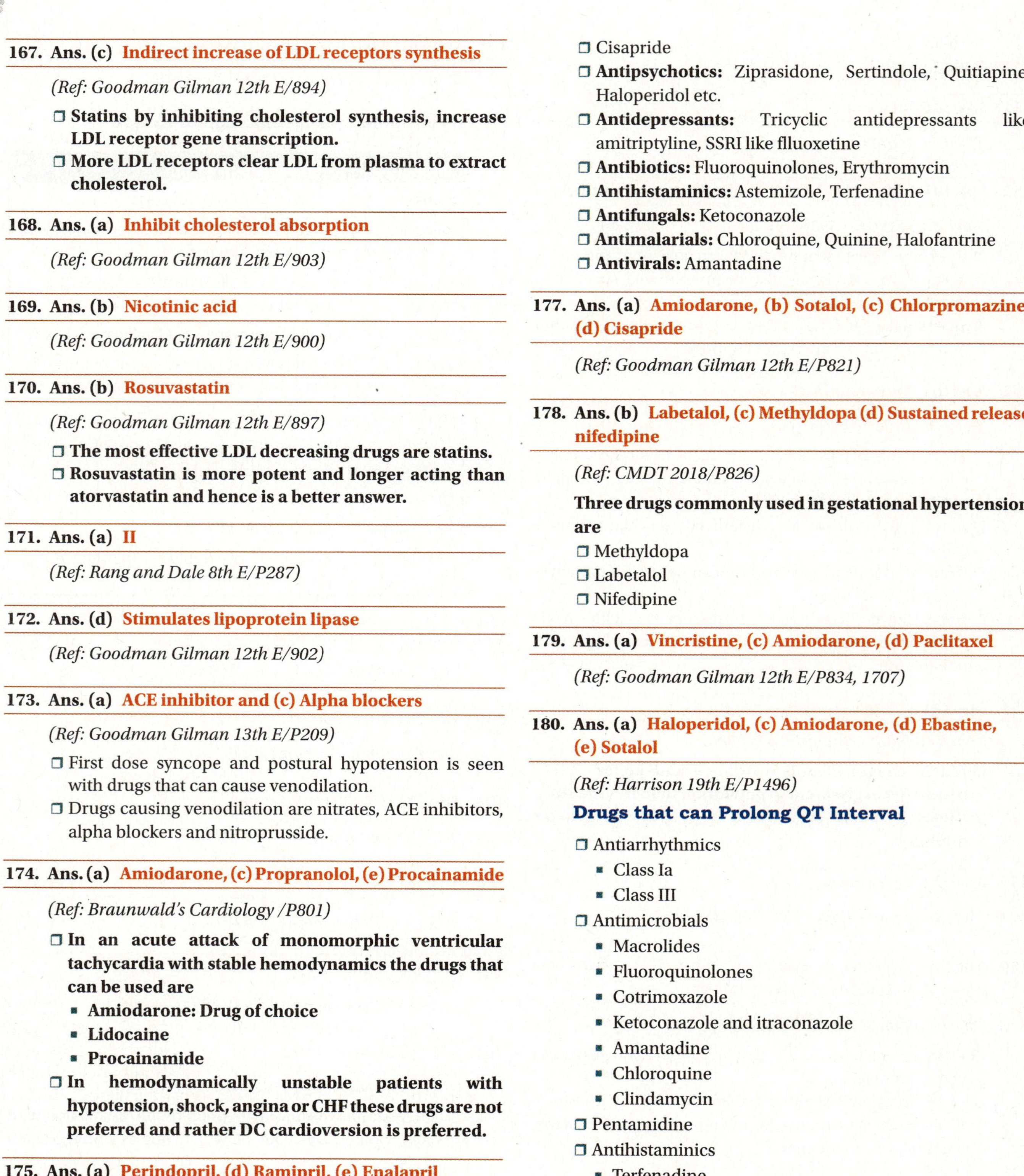

167. Ans. (c) Indirect increase of LDL receptors synthesis

(Ref: Goodman Gilman 12th E/894)

- **Statins by inhibiting cholesterol synthesis, increase LDL receptor gene transcription.**
- **More LDL receptors clear LDL from plasma to extract cholesterol.**

168. Ans. (a) Inhibit cholesterol absorption

(Ref: Goodman Gilman 12th E/903)

169. Ans. (b) Nicotinic acid

(Ref: Goodman Gilman 12th E/900)

170. Ans. (b) Rosuvastatin

(Ref: Goodman Gilman 12th E/897)

- **The most effective LDL decreasing drugs are statins.**
- **Rosuvastatin is more potent and longer acting than atorvastatin and hence is a better answer.**

171. Ans. (a) II

(Ref: Rang and Dale 8th E/P287)

172. Ans. (d) Stimulates lipoprotein lipase

(Ref: Goodman Gilman 12th E/902)

173. Ans. (a) ACE inhibitor and (c) Alpha blockers

(Ref: Goodman Gilman 13th E/P209)

- First dose syncope and postural hypotension is seen with drugs that can cause venodilation.
- Drugs causing venodilation are nitrates, ACE inhibitors, alpha blockers and nitroprusside.

174. Ans. (a) Amiodarone, (c) Propranolol, (e) Procainamide

(Ref: Braunwald's Cardiology /P801)

- **In an acute attack of monomorphic ventricular tachycardia with stable hemodynamics the drugs that can be used are**
  - **Amiodarone: Drug of choice**
  - **Lidocaine**
  - **Procainamide**
- **In hemodynamically unstable patients with hypotension, shock, angina or CHF these drugs are not preferred and rather DC cardioversion is preferred.**

175. Ans. (a) Perindopril, (d) Ramipril, (e) Enalapril

(Ref: Goodman Gilman 12th E/P731)

176. Ans. (a) Amiodarone, (b) Cisapride, (e) Ketoconazole

(Ref: Goodman Gilman 12th E/P821)

Drugs Causing QT Prolongation

- **Antiarrhythmics:** Class Ia and Class III (Amiodarone)
- Cisapride
- **Antipsychotics:** Ziprasidone, Sertindole, Quitiapine, Haloperidol etc.
- **Antidepressants:** Tricyclic antidepressants like amitriptyline, SSRI like flluoxetine
- **Antibiotics:** Fluoroquinolones, Erythromycin
- **Antihistaminics:** Astemizole, Terfenadine
- **Antifungals:** Ketoconazole
- **Antimalarials:** Chloroquine, Quinine, Halofantrine
- **Antivirals:** Amantadine

177. Ans. (a) Amiodarone, (b) Sotalol, (c) Chlorpromazine, (d) Cisapride

(Ref: Goodman Gilman 12th E/P821)

178. Ans. (b) Labetalol, (c) Methyldopa (d) Sustained release nifedipine

(Ref: CMDT 2018/P826)

Three drugs commonly used in gestational hypertension are

- Methyldopa
- Labetalol
- Nifedipine

179. Ans. (a) Vincristine, (c) Amiodarone, (d) Paclitaxel

(Ref: Goodman Gilman 12th E/P834, 1707)

180. Ans. (a) Haloperidol, (c) Amiodarone, (d) Ebastine, (e) Sotalol

(Ref: Harrison 19th E/P1496)

Drugs that can Prolong QT Interval

- Antiarrhythmics
  - Class Ia
  - Class III
- Antimicrobials
  - Macrolides
  - Fluoroquinolones
  - Cotrimoxazole
  - Ketoconazole and itraconazole
  - Amantadine
  - Chloroquine
  - Clindamycin
- Pentamidine
- Antihistaminics
  - Terfenadine
  - Astemisole
  - Diphenhydramine
  - Hydroxyzine
  - Ebastine
- Antipsychotics
  - Typical – Haloperidol, Phenothiazines
  - Atypical – Ziprasidone, sertindol and quitiapine

- TCA
- Cisapride
- Methadone
- Fluoxetine

181. Ans. (a) Inhibition of calcium channel

(Ref: Goodman Gilman 12th E/P831)

182. Ans. (b) Propranolo, (c) Carvedilol, (e) Nebivolol

(Ref: Goodman Gilman 12th E/P758)

183. Ans. (b) Methyl dopa, (c) Clonidine, (e) Atenolol

(Ref: KDT 7th E/P564,65,66)

Antihpertensives causing rebound hypertension

- Clonidine
- Beta blockers (On sudden withdrawal)
- Methyl dopa (Mild)

184. Ans. (b) Bisoprolol, (c) Carvedilol

(Ref: Goodman Gilman 12th E/P801)

Beta blockers with proven benefit in CHF are

- Metoprolol
- Carvedilol
- Bisoprolol

185. Ans. (a) NO, (b) CO_2, (c) Minoxidil, (d) ACE inhibitor

(Ref: Goodman Gilman 12th E/P735,747,781)

186. Ans. (b) HOCM, (d) Myocarditis

(Ref: Goodman Gilman 12th E/P803)

- Digoxin by increasing the force of contraction increases left outflow tract obstruction in HOCM and hence is contraindicated.
- It has no role in myocarditis.

187. Ans. None

(Ref: Goodman Gilman 12th E/P 804)

ECG Changes with Digoxin

ECG changes	Cause
PR prolongation	Refractoriness at AV node
QT shortening	Shortening of action potential duration
T wave inversion ST segment depression	Accelerated repolarization of inner layers of myocardium

188. Ans. (a) Hypertrichosis, (b) Hypotension

(Ref: Goodman Gilman 12th E/P 781)

189. Ans. (a) Nesiritide, (b) Digoxin, (c) Spironolactone, (d) Losartan

(Ref: Goodman Gilman 12th E/P 804)

190. Ans. (c) Isoprenaline

(Ref: Paul Barsh's Clinical Anesthesia/P545)

- The cardiosuppressive effects of lignocaine toxicity like bradycardia and hypotension can be reversed by catecholamines like isoprenaline.

191. Ans. (c) Norepinephrine

(Ref: Peter Bryson's comprehensive review of toxicology/P238)

- Hypotension due to NE depletion is the most common side effect of bretylium, which can be treated by norepinephrine.

192. Ans. (a) Enalapril, (c) Angiotensin receptor blockers

(Ref: Goodman Gilman 12th E/P736)

193. All

(Ref: Goodman Gilman 12th E/P 842, 1847)

194. Ans. (a) Hypokalemia, (c) Hypercalcemia

(Ref: Goodman Gilman 12th E/P 802-4)

Digitalis toxicity can be precipitated by

- **Myocardial ischemia**
- **Hypokalemia**
- **Hypercalcemia**
- **Hypomagnesemia**.

195. Ans. (b) Systemic vasodilation, (c) Renal vasodilation, (d) Reabsorption of Na in proximal tubules, (e) Water reabsorption.

196. Ans. (c) Niacin

(Ref: Goodman Gilman 13th E/P613)

- Niacin is the only hypolipidemic which can significantly decrease lipoprotein a levels. Hence is the answer in this question.

197. Ans. (b) Amlodipine

(Ref: Goodman Gilman 12th E/P446)

- **In old age hypertension (> 55 years age) the preferred first line drugs are calcium channel blockers and thiazides. Since thiazides can cause lithium toxicity by decreasing renal clearance, it is not advised in this situation. Hence the best drug in this case is calcium channel blocker amlodipine.**
- **Drugs that can precipitate lithium toxicity are**
  - **Diuretics:** Thiazides > Potassium sparing diuretics
  - **ACE Inhibitors:** Maximum with renally cleared drug like lisinopril
  - **NSAIDS:** Maximum with indomethacin

Note: Loop diuretics does not affect lithium clearance and osmotic diuretics increases lithium clearance.

198. Ans. (a) Used with ARB for treatment of CHF

(Ref: CMDT 2018/P414)

Sacubitril

- **It is a neutral endopeptidase (neprilysin) inhibitor that increases the endogenous BNP and hence causes vasodilatation along with natriuresis and diuresis.**
- **It is approved by FDA in 2015 along with valsartan for use in chronic CHF to decrease mortality.**

199. Ans. (a) Evolocumab

(Ref: CMDT 2018/P1276)

PCSK-9 Inhibitors

- Evolocumab
- Alirocumab
- Bococizumab

200. Ans. (b) Pravastatin

(Ref: Goodman Gilman 12th E/P894)

- All statins are contraindicated in children less than 8 years.
- Only pravastatin is contraindicated in children less than 10 years and hence can be used in a 8 year old child.

201. Ans. (d) Statins (Any)

(Ref: Goodman Gilman 12th E/P1246)

202. Ans. (d) Hydrochlorthiazide

(Ref: Goodman Gilman 12th E/P688)

- Propranolol cannot be used in this case as the patient has bronchial asthma and spironolactone cannot be used as there is hyperkalemia.
- Both amlodipine and hydrochlorthiazide can be used, but the latter is more preferred as it can cause hypokalemia and blunt the hyperkalemia.

203. Ans. (c) Captopril

(Ref: Goodman Gilman 12th E/P736)

204. Ans. (b) Hydralazine

(Ref: Goodman Gilman 12th E/P780)

- Hydralazine being an arterial dilator will cause reflex tachycardia and hence it is not a possibility here.
- Clonidine being a central sympatholytic can cause bradycardia and so is the case with reserpine which decreases NE synthesis.
- Digoxin can also cause given symptoms as it has parasympatholytic effect.

205. Ans. (a) Antiplatelet agents

(Ref: Goodman Gilman 12th E/P791)

Drugs Inhibiting Cardiac Remodelling and Delaying Mortality in Chronic CHF:

Mnemonics

SHIBA

- **S** : Spironolactone
- **H** : Hydralazine + IDN
- **I** : Ivabridine
- **B** : Beta blockers
- **A** : ACEI/ARB

206. Ans. (a) Reduce LDL cholesterol

(Ref: Goodman Gilman 12th E/P894)

The non hypolipidemic activities of statins called as **pleiotropic effects** are

- Antiaggregant
- Anticoagulant
- Anti-inflammatory (decreases CRP)
- Vasodilatory (increases endothelial NO release)
- Atherosclerotic plaque stabilizing effect.

207. Ans. (c) Amiodarone

(Ref: Goodman Gilman 12th E/P837)

208. Ans. (c) Atrial fibrillation

(Ref: Goodman Gilman 12th E/P837)

- Amiodarone increases cell refractoriness and hence is rather used for rhythm control in atrial fibrillation.
- It never causes atrial fibrillation.

209. Ans. (a) Aliskiren

(Ref: Goodman Gilman 12th E/P745)

210. Ans. (a) Levosimendan

(Ref: Harrison 19th E/P1510)

Mechanism of Action of Levosimendan

- PDE-3 Inhibition
- Opens potassium channel
- Sensitizes myocardial cells to calcium

211. Ans. (d) Cholestyramine

(Ref: Goodman Gilman 12th E/P899)

- Bile acid binding resins like cholestyramine can increase triglycerides and hence are contraindicated in patients of hypertriglyceridemia.

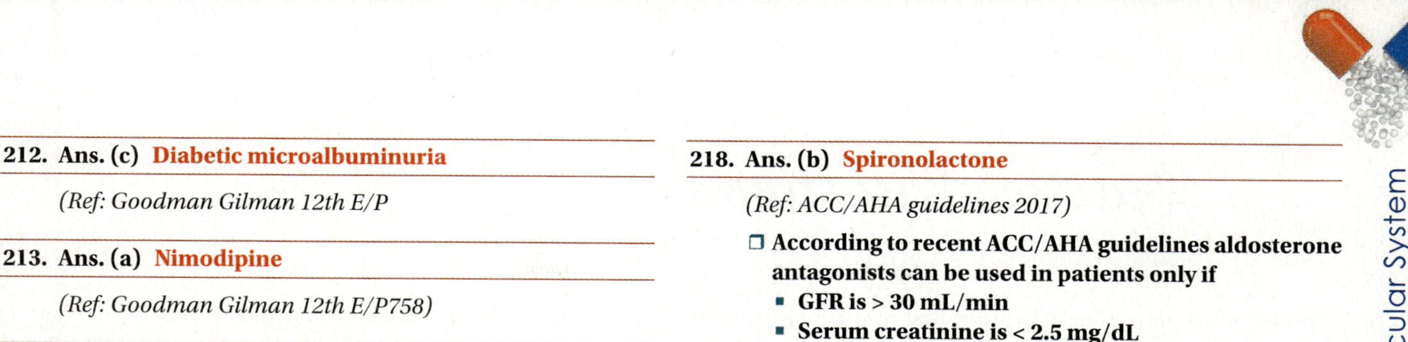

212. Ans. (c) Diabetic microalbuminuria

(Ref: Goodman Gilman 12th E/P

213. Ans. (a) Nimodipine

(Ref: Goodman Gilman 12th E/P758)

214. Ans. (a) Corneal deposits

(Ref: Goodman Gilman 12th E/P837)

215. Ans. (d) All of the above

(Ref: Goodman Gilman 12th E/P791)

216. Ans. (d) Class IV

(Ref: Goodman Gilman 12th E/P829)

217. Ans. (c) Postural hypotension

(Ref: Goodman Gilman 12th E/P780)

218. Ans. (b) Spironolactone

(Ref: ACC/AHA guidelines 2017)

- **According to recent ACC/AHA guidelines aldosterone antagonists can be used in patients only if**
  - **GFR is > 30 mL/min**
  - **Serum creatinine is < 2.5 mg/dL**
  - **Serum potassium is < 5 mEq/L**
- **Since in this case serum creatinine is 2.5, spironolactone can not be used.**

219. Ans. (b) Neutral endopeptidase inhibitor

(Ref: CMDT 2018/P414)

Scubitril is a neutral endopeptidase or neprylisin inhibitor approved for treatment of chronic CHF in combination with angiotensin receptor blocker like valsartan.

Practice Questions

220. Lidocaine dose should be decreased in a patient with all except

a. Shock
b. Liver failure
c. Concomitant beta-blocker use
d. MI

Ans. (d) MI

(Ref: Goodman Gilman 12th E/P842)

Lidocaine dose should be decreased with

- Heart failure: As volume of distribution decreases.
- Liver failure
- Concomitant cispride or beta-blocker therapy
- Prolonged infusions

Lidocaine dose should be increased in

- MI: As lidocaine binds to beta-1 acidic glycoprotein, which is increased in MI. The free drug decreases and hence for the same clinical effect dose needs to be increased.

221. A maximum decrease in V_{max} is caused by:

a. Procainamide
b. Amiodarone
c. Lidocaine
d. Flecainide

Ans. (d) Flecainide

(Ref: Goodman Gilman 12th E/P829)

- Since the recovery from block is delayed maximum i.e. >10 sec by Class Ia antiarrhythmic, they have maximum delaying effect on V_{max} or the rate of rise of action potential.

222. Which of the following is the most preferred drug for treatment of atrial fibrillation associated with WPW syndrome?

a. Ibutilide
b. Amiodarone
c. Lidocaine
d. Procainamide

Ans. (d) Procainamide

(Ref: Goodman Gilman 12th E/P824)

- The drug preferred for atrial fibrillation with functional re-entry is ibutilide, but if its associated with anatomical re-entry as in case of WPW syndrome, then procainamide is preferred which blocks conduction in the accessory pathway.

223. Which of the following drug increases PR interval?

a. Lidocaine
b. Procainamide
c. Flecainide
d. Quinidine

Ans. (c) Flecainide

(Ref: Goodman Gilman 12th E/P828)

- Among sodium channel blockers, only class Ic blocks conduction at AV node and hence prolongs PR interval.
- Class Ia increases conduction at AV node due to parasympatholytic effect and hence shortens PR interval.
- Class Ib has no effect on conduction at AV node and PR interval.

224. Which of the following is the most preferred class for treatment of idiopathic ventricular tachycardia?

a. Class I
b. Class II
c. Class III
d. Class IV

Ans. (b) Class II

(Ref: Harrison 19th E/P1496)

- Class II or beta blockers are the first line drugs for idiopathic VT.
- Class IV or CCB are the second line drugs.

225. A patient of atrial fibrillation was to be given a drug to control ventricular rate. Which of the following is the most preferred drug?

a. Beta blocker
b. Amiodarone
c. Adenosine
d. MgSO4

Ans. (a) Beta blocker

(Ref: Harrison 19th E/P1496)

226. Pulmonary fibrosis associated with amiodarone is due to depletion of

a. Macrophages
b. Type I pneumocytes
c. Type II pneumocytes
d. Lymphocytes

Ans. (c) Type II pneumocytes

(Ref: Goodman Gilman 12th E/P837)

227. Corneal vertcillata is associated with

a. Chloroquine
b. Ethambutol
c. Amiodarone
d. Vigabatrin

Ans. (c) Amiodarone

(Ref: Goodman Gilman 12th E/P829)

228. Which of the following is the drug of choice for digitalis induced atrial arrhythmia?

a. Lidocaine
b. Verapamil
c. Amiodarone
d. Phenytoin

Ans. (d) Phenytoin

(Ref: Braunwald's cardiology 9th E/P728)

229. Dronedarone is better than amiodarone in that

a. It has more efficacy
b. It has more potency
c. It has less toxicity
d. It is cheaper

Ans. (c) It has less toxicity

(Ref: Goodman Gilma 12th E/P839)

- Dronedarone does not have iodine and hence is devoid of iodine related toxicities seen with amiodarone.
- However it is less efficacious than amiodarone.

230. Which of the following is more potent?

a. L-Verapamil b. D-Verapamil
c. L-Diltiazem d. D-Diltiazem

Ans. (a) L-Verapamil

(Ref: Goodman Gilman 12th E/P831)

- All CCB are racemic mixtures of L and D isomers except diltiazem and nifedipine.
- Verapamil is more potent than diltiazem and L isomer of verapamil is more potent than D isomer.
- However L-isomer undergoes more significant first pass metabolism than D isomer.

231. All of the following drugs can increase digitalis toxicity except

a. Quinidine b. Verapamil
c. Chlorthiazide d. Enalapril

Ans. (d) Enalapril

(Ref: Goodman and Gilman 12th E/P 803)

- Drugs increasing digitalis toxicity are:
  - **Diuretics**
  - **Quinidine**
  - **Verapamil**
  - **Flecainide**
  - **Propafenone**
  - **Amiodarone**
- As potassium limits the action of digitalis, hyperkalemia as associated with ACEI can prevent digitalis toxicity.

232. The dose of digibind in digoxintoxicity is calculated based on digoxin's

a. Loading dose b. Maintenance dose
c. Total dose d. Last dose

Ans. (c) Total dose

(Ref: Goodman and Gilman 12th E/P 804)

- Digibind, an anti-digoxin antibody is the most effective drug and hence reserved for treatment of life threatening arrhythmias induced by digoxin.
- The dose of digibind is calculated based on the total digoxin dose administered.

233. All of the following are used in digitalis induced arrhythmia except

a. Dialysis b. Digibind
c. $MgSO_4$ d. Phenytoin

Ans. (a) Dialysis

(Ref: Goodman and Gilman 12th E/P 804)

- Dialysis is not effective for treatment of digoxin induced arrhythmia, as it has a high volume of distribution.

234. Loading dose of digoxin is calculated based on:

a. Total body mass b. Lean body mass
c. Adipose tissue mass d. None

Ans. (b) Lean body mass

(Ref: Goodman and Gilman 12th E/P 803)

- Digoxin is highly distributed in the skeletal muscles (high volume of distribution), and hence a loading dose is given according to the lean body mass.

235. TDM is done to maintain the plasma digoxin level below

a. 3 ng/mL b. 2 ng/mL
c. 1 ng/mL d. 0.5 ng/mL

Ans. (c) 1 ng/mL

(Ref: Goodman and Gilman 12th E/P 803)

- Digoxin has a low therapeutic index. Hence TDM is done to keep the plasma concentration below 1 ng/mL to prevent toxicity.

236. Nesiritide is eliminated by following mechanisms except

a. Liver b. Kidney
c. Neutral endopeptidase d. NPR-C

Ans. (a) Liver

(Ref: Goodman and Gilman 12th E/P 696)

Three mechanisms of nesiritide elimination are:

- Neutral endopeptidase
- NPR-C
- Kidney

237. Ularitide is an analog of:

a. ANP b. BNP
c. Urodilantin d. Uricase

Ans. (c) Urodilantin

(Ref: Goodman and Gilman 12th E/P 696)

238. Carperitide is an analog of:

a. ANP b. BNP
c. Urodilantin d. Caspase

Ans. (a) ANP

(Ref: Goodman and Gilman 12th E/P 696)

239. Omapatrilat is an inhibitor of:

a. ACE
b. Neutral endopeptidase
c. Vasopeptidase
d. All of the above

Ans. (d) All of the above

(Ref: Goodman and Gilman 12th E/P 932)

- Omapatrilat is a vasopeptidase inhibitor, which inhibits ACE as well as neutral endopeptidase.

240. The dose of beta blocker is uptitrated in CHF every:

a. 1 week b. 2 weeks
c. 3 weeks d. 4 weeks

Ans. (b) 2 weeks

(Ref: Goodman and Gilman 12th E/P 800)

241. **All of the following are indicated for treatment of CHF except:**
a. Propranolol b. Carvedilol
c. Metoprolol d. Bisoprolol

Ans. (a) Propranolol

(Ref: Goodman and Gilman 12th E/P 800)

242. **The class of drug with maximum mortality benefit in CHF is:**
a. ACEI b. Beta blocker
c. Spironolactone d. Digoxin

Ans. (b) Beta blocker

(Ref: Goodman and Gilman 12th E/P 800)

243. **The first ARB to be used clinically was:**
a. Valsartan b. Losartan
c. Telmisartan d. Candesartan

Ans. (b) Losartan

(Ref: Goodman and Gilman 12th E/P 736)

244. **Which of the following is not a prodrug:**
a. Enalapril b. Candesartan
c. Olmesartan d. Lisinopril

Ans. (d) Lisinopril

(Ref: Goodman and Gilman 12th E/P 738)

- All ACEIs are prodrugs except captopril and lisinopril.
- Only candesartan and olmesartan are ARBs which are prodrugs.

245. **Which of the following ARB is not taken with food?**
a. Valsartan b. Telmisartan
c. Candesartan d. Olmesartan

Ans. (a) Valsartan

(Ref: Goodman and Gilman 12th E/P 738)

246. **ARB with antiaggregant effect is:**
a. Telmisartan b. Losartan
c. Valsartan d. Candesartan

Ans. (b) Losartan

(Ref: Goodman and Gilman 12th E/P 738)

247. **ACEI used for diagnosis of renovascular hypertension before renal angiography is:**
a. Captopril b. Lisinopril
c. Fosinopril d. Ramipril

Ans. (a) Captopril

(Ref: KDT 7th E/P505)

248. **Which of the following is shortest acting ACEI?**
a. Enalapril b. Captopril
c. Lisinopril d. Fosinopril

Ans. (b) Captopril

(Ref: Goodman and Gilman 12th E/P 732)

249. **Angioedema caused by ACEI can be worsened by:**
a. Diuretics b. Lithium
c. Glitazones d. Digoxin

Ans. (c) Glitazones

(Ref: Braunwald's cardiology/P967)

250. **ACEI with triphasic elimination is:**
a. Enalapril b. Captopril
c. Lisinopril d. Ramipril

Ans. (d) Ramipril

(Ref: Goodman and Gilman 12th E/P 733)

251. **Which of the following beta blockers can be used, when beta blockade is contraindicated?**
a. Labetalol b. Carvedilol
c. Esmolol d. Propranolol

Ans. (c) Esmolol

(Ref: Harrison 19th E/P1589)

- Esmolol is shortest acting beta blocker which is given by continuous IV infusion.
- Because of its rapid offset of action it is preferred in case beta blockade is contraindicated as the side effects of cardiosuppression will be short lived.

252. **Antiaggregant of choice in myocardial infarction:**
a. Clopidogrel b. Aspirin
c. Prasugrel d. Ticagrelor

Ans. (b) Aspirin

(Ref: Harrison 19th E/P1606)

- Antiaggregant of choice in MI is aspirin.
- Two drug therapy i.e. aspirin plus a P2Y12 inhibitor is preferred in patients with stent placement.

253. **All of the following drugs decrease mortality in a patient of MI except:**
a. CCB b. ACEI
c. Beta blockers d. Aspirin

Ans. (a) CCB

(Ref: Harrison 19th E/P1607)

Drugs decreasing mortality in MI
- Aspirin
- ACEI/ARB
- Beta blockers
- Aldosterone antagonist

254. **Which of the following drug decreases mortality in a patient of angina?**
a. ACEI
b. Nitrates
c. Beta blockers
d. Ranolazine

Ans. (c) Beta blockers

(Ref: Harrison 19th E/P1588)

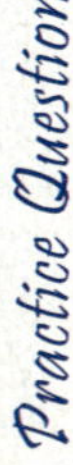

255. Which of the following is the drug of choice to decrease pain of angina?

a. NTG b. Morphine
c. Pethidine d. Beta blockers

Ans. (a) NTG

(Ref: CMDT 2016/P373)

Drugs used to decrease pain of MI
- S/L NTG – First drug of choice
- IV opioids (Morphine > Pethidine)
- IV Beta blockers

256. Which of the following is the drug of choice for an acute attack of angina?

a. NTG b. IDN
c. IMN d. CCB

Ans. (a) NTG

(Ref: CMDT 2016/P357)

257. Which of the following cannot be used as monotherapy in angina?

a. Verapamil b. Nifedipine
c. Ranolazine d. Metoprolol

Ans. (b) Nifedipine

(Ref: CMDT 2016/P357)

- DHPs cannot be used as monotherapy in angina due to reflex tachycardia that can increase oxygen demand of myocardium and worsen angina.
- They are always used with beta blockers.

258. A maximum decrease in LDL is caused by:

a. Simvastatin b. Rosuvastatin
c. Pitavastatin d. Fluvastatin

Ans. (b) Rosuvastatin

(Ref: CMDT 2016/P1246)

259. Which of the following is preferred for treatment of niacin induced flushing?

a. Indomethacin b. Aspirin
c. Cortisol d. Dexamethasone

Ans. (b) Aspirin

(Ref: Goodman Gilman 12th E/P900)

- Flushing caused by niacin is due to prostaglandins, which can be prevented by NSAIDs. The preferred NSAID is aspirin.

260. Which of the following fibrates increases the risk of statin induced myopathy?

a. Clofibrate b. Fenofibrate
c. Bizafibrate d. Gemfibrozil

Ans. (d) Gemfibrozil

(Ref: Goodman Gilman 12th E/P903)

- Among fibrates the risk of myopathy with statins is increased maximum by gemfibrozil as it not only inhibits glucunoridation of statins but also hepatic uptake by inhibiting OATP1B1.
- Fibrate with least effect on glucunoridation and statin induced myopathy is fenofibrate.

261. Which of the following fibrate does not cause myopathy?

a. Gemfibrozil b. Clofibrate
c. Bizafibrate d. Fenofibrate

Ans. (c) Bizafibrate

(Ref: Goodman Gilman 12th E/P900)

262. A patient on statins should be routinely screened for

a. Myopathy b. Hepatotoxicity
c. Nephrotoxicity d. Agranulocytosis

Ans. (b) Hepatotoxicity

(Ref: Goodman Gilman 12th E/P896)

- A patient on statins should be routinely monitored ALT/AST because of hepatotoxicity.
- CK monitoring for myopathy is not done as myopathy can be delayed for years.

263. Statins are derived from:

a. Bacteria b. Fungus
c. Plant d. Animal

Ans. (b) Fungus

(Ref: Goodman Gilman 12th E/P893)

- The first statin lovastatin was derived from fungus, Aspergillus terrus.

264. Intestinal cholesterol absorption is inhibited by:

a. Cholestyramine b. Bizafibrate
c. Lomitapide d. Ezitimibe

Ans. (d) Ezitimibe

(Ref: Goodman Gilman 12th E/P903)

NOTES

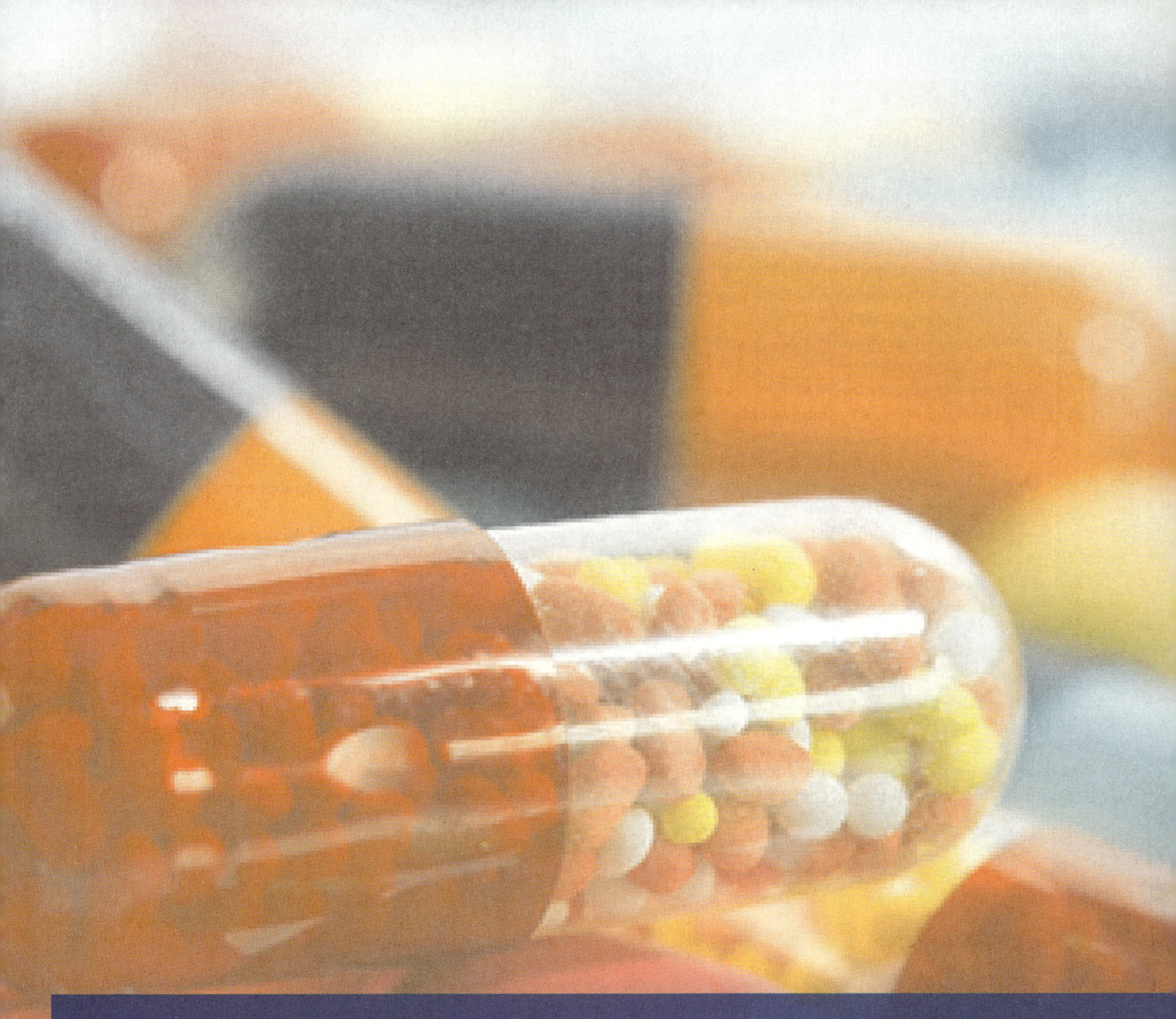

Kidney

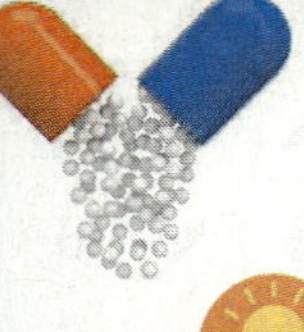

One Liners

- Loop diuretics act on **thick ascending limb** by inhibiting **Na/K/2Cl** cotransporter.
- **Bumetanide** is most potent whereas **torsemide** is longest acting loop diuretic.
- **Ototoxicity** with loop diuretics is usually reversible and maximum with **ethacrynic acid**.
- Hyperglycemia, hyperuricemia and hypokalemia are more common with **thiazides** as compared to loop diuretics.
- Carbonic anhydrase (CA) inhibitors and K sparing diuretics cause metabolic acidosis, whereas loop diuretics and thiazides cause metabolic alkalosis.
- Nonsteroidal anti-inflammatory drugs **(NSAIDs)** can decrease diuretic effect of both thiazides and loop diuretics by inhibiting prostaglandin synthesis.
- Hypokalemia is caused by all diuretics except K sparing diuretics.
- All loop diuretics except **bumetanide** and thiazides except **indapamide** have weak CA inhibiting effect.
- Carbonic anhydrase inhibitors, loop diuretics (except **ethacrynic acid** and **bumetanide**) and thiazides are sulphonamide derivatives.
- **Glomerular filtration rate (GFR) is decreased** by CA inhibitors > thiazides, **increased** by loop diuretics and not changed by potassium sparing diuretics.
- Carbonic anhydrase **inhibitors** increase free water clearance but **thiazides** and **loop diuretics** decrease free water clearance.
- **Spironolactone** is the diuretic of choice in liver cirrhosis, whereas amiloride is contraindicated due to folic acid deficiency caused by both.
- **Octreotide** is the drug of choice for bleeding esophageal varices; terlipressin is more preferred than vasopressin.

DIURETICS

Diuretics are drugs that primarily cause loss of water from the body, though solute loss (Na/Cl) is also associated. Natriuretics (ANP/BNP/Urodilatin analogs) cause sodium loss and aquaretics (osmotic diuretics) cause water loss without solutes. Diuretics act along the length of nephron at various sites and encompass drugs like carbonic anhydrase inhibitors, loop diuretics, thiazides, osmotic diuretics and potassium sparing diuretics. The primary usefulness of diuretics is by decreasing extracellular fluid volume due to decrease in Na and Cl.

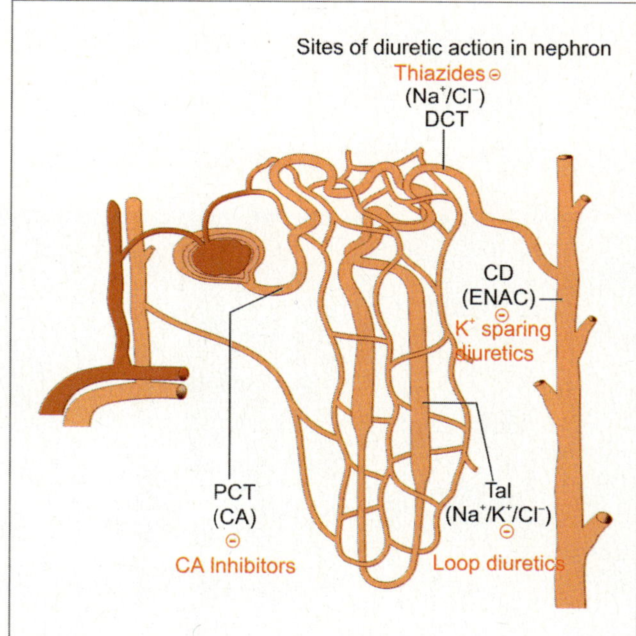

Site of diuretic action in nephron

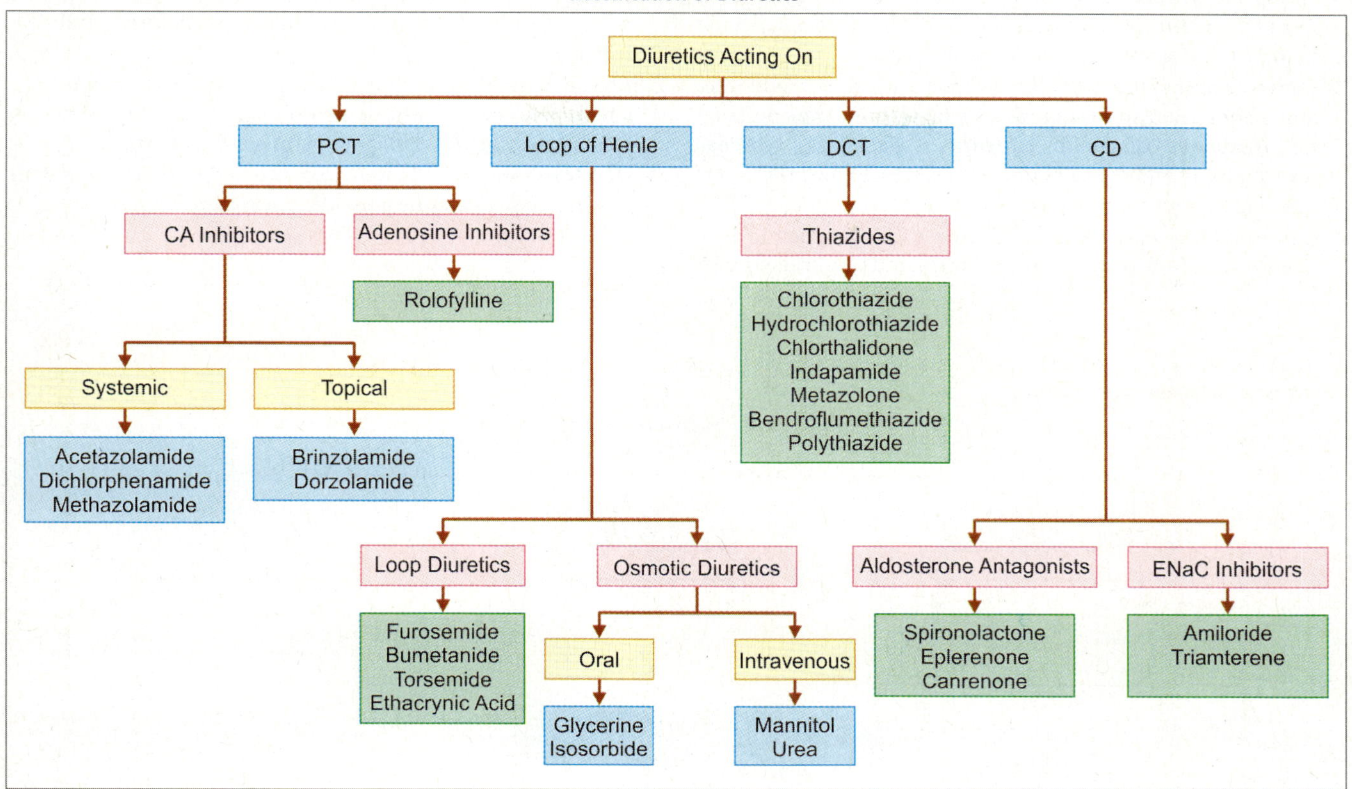

DIURETICS ACTING ON PCT

- In the proximal convoluted tubule (PCT) maximum filtered sodium is absorbed along with water, glucose and amino acids.
- The luminal membrane and cytoplasm of PCT epithelial cell contains an enzyme called as carbonic anhydrase.
- In the lumen the filtered H_2CO_3 splits into H_2O and CO_2 due to carbonic anhydrase.
- CO_2 diffuses into epithelial cell, where it combines with H_2O to make H_2CO_3 with the help of carbonic anhydrase.
- H_2CO_3 breaks into H^+ and HCO_3^-. HCO_3^- is transported along with Na by the Na/HCO_3^- symporter into interstitium. H^+ is exchanged with the luminal Na^+ by the Na^+/H^+ antiporter.

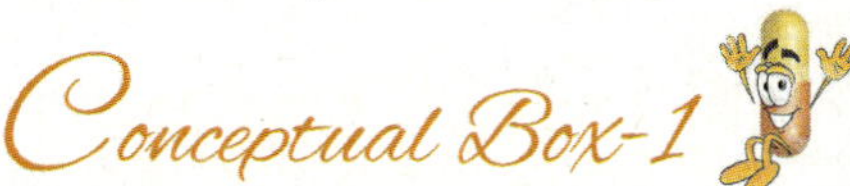

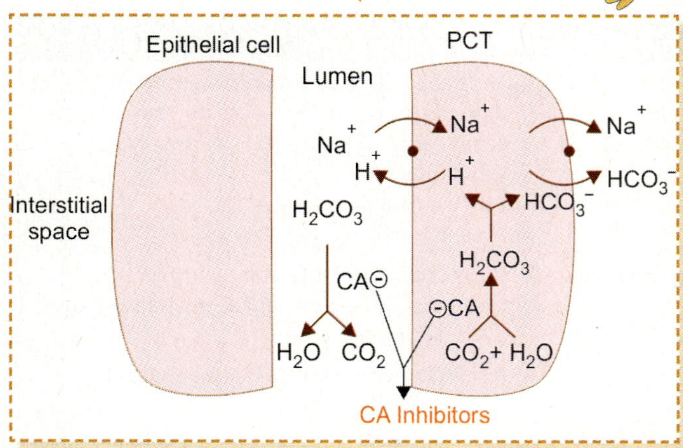

Carbonic Anhydrase Inhibitors

- Carbonic anhydrase inhibitors are **noncompetitive reversible inhibitors**. By inhibiting luminal carbonic anhydrase, there is an increase in urine H_2CO_3.
- Inhibition of cytoplasmic carbonic anhydrase inhibits H_2CO_3 production and hence H^+ ions are not synthesized.
- This causes a block of **Na^+/H^+ antiporter** and hence Na^+ is not absorbed. The maximum load of sodium lost is reabsorbed in the loop, which limits the Na loss (5%) and diuretic effect.
- Delivery of excess Na^+ to loop, stimulates macula densa to release renin from JG cells that cause afferent arteriole constriction and **decreases GFR**.
- The lost sodium in the collecting duct stimulates ENaC (Epithelial Na Channels) and causes absorption of some amount of sodium and loss of potassium and protons.
- Carbonic anhydrase inhibitors also inhibit NH_4^+ and H^+ secretion in collecting duct.
- Carbonic anhydrase inhibitor class contains drugs like **acetazolamide, dichlorphenamide, methazolamide** for systemic use and **brinzolamide** and **dorzolamide** for topical (ocular) use. Acetazolamide is most potent, whereas methazolamide is the longest acting drug. Acetazolamide and methazolamide have 100% bioavailability.

Uses

- Acetazolamide is used for treatment of **metabolic alkalosis** as it causes metabolic acidosis. A decrease in CSF PH stimulates medullary ventilation centre and hence it can be used in **mountain sickness** and **sleep apnea**.

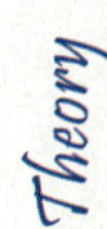

- Acetazolamide causes alkalization of urine and hence used in **cystinuria** to prevent cysteine stone formation. Cysteine being an acid is more soluble in alkaline urine.
- Carbonic anhydrase inhibitors decrease aqueous production and hence used in **glaucoma**. Acetazolamide can be used for treatment of acute congestive glaucoma, whereas brinzolamide and dorzolamide are used by topical routes for treatment of open angle glaucoma.
- Carbonic anhydrase inhibitors decrease CSF production also. Acetazolamide is drug of choice for treatment of **raised CSF pressure headache** and used in dural ectasia, idiopathic intracranial hypertension, **and mountain sickness** and CSF leakage.
- Acetazolamide by inhibiting CA in neurons, increase CO_2, which releases inhibitory neurotransmitters and hence is used in **catamenial epilepsy** and **absence seizure**.
- **Dichlorphenamide** is the drug of choice for treatment of **familial hyperkalemic periodic paralysis**.

Clinical Box-1

Treatment of High Altitude illness

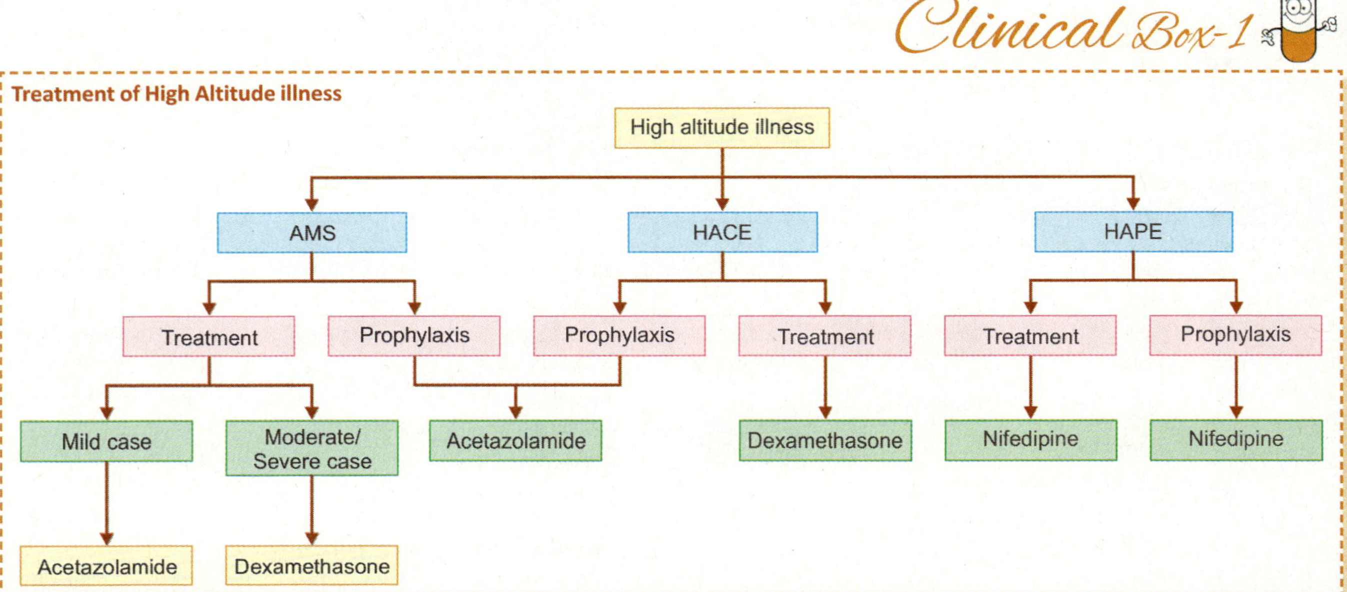

Abbreviations: AMS: Acute Mountain Sickness, HACE: High Altitude Cerebral Edema, HAPE: High Altitude Pulmonary Edema

Side Effects

- Loss of H_2CO_3 and retention of H^+ and NH_4^+ causes metabolic acidosis. NH_4^+ retention can cause encephalopathy and hence CA inhibitors are contraindicated in patients of **liver cirrhosis**. CA inhibitors are contraindicated in **metabolic** and **respiratory acidosis (COPD)**.
- Increased H_2CO_3 and decreased H^+ and NH_4^+ in urine makes it alkaline. In alkaline urine calcium salts are insoluble and can lead to **renal stones**.
- All carbonic anhydrase inhibitors are sulphonamide derivatives and hence retain their side effects like hypersensitivity, **bone marrow suppression** and crystalluria.
- Other associated side effects are hypokalemia, hypophosphatemia, paraesthesia and somnolence.

Correlation of Effects with Side effects and uses

Effects of CA inhibitors	Side effects	Uses
• Loss of H_2CO_3 from body • H^+ and NH_4^+ retention in body	• Metabolic acidosis • Hyperammonemia: Can cause hepatic encephalopathy and hence contraindicated in patients of cirrhosis	• Metabolic alkalosis: Primarily caused by diuretics and correction of respiratory acidosis • Sleep apnea: Decrease CSF pH stimulates ventilation. • Familial periodic paralysis • Mountain sickness
• Increased H_2CO_3 in urine • Decreased H^+ and NH_4^+ in urine • Increased PO_4 IN urine	Nephrolithiasis: Alkaline urine precipitates calcium salts	• Prevention of cysteine stone formation in cystinuria: Cysteine is soluble in alkaline urine
Increased K excretion	Hypokalemia	• Familial hyperkalemic periodic paralysis

Contd...

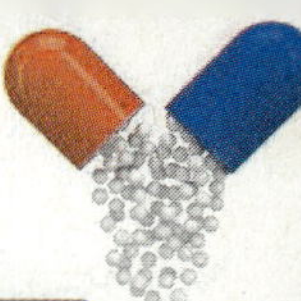

Effects of CA inhibitors	Side effects	Uses
Decreased aqueous humor production		• Open angle glaucoma: Brinzolamide and dorzolamide are used topically. • Closed angle glaucoma: Acetazolamide is drug of choice for an acute attack
Decreased CSF production		• Acetazolamide is drug of choice for treatment of raised CSF pressure headache. • Dural ectasia • Idiopathic intracranial hypertension • CSF leakage
Increased CO_2 in neurons releases inhibitory neurotransmitters	Paraesthesia Somnolence	Catamenial epilepsy: The use is limited due to development of tolerance

Adenosine Antagonist

- Adenosine by acting on A1 receptors in kidney, increases Na^+ absorption in the PCT by stimulating the action of Na^+/H^+ exchanger and increases K^+ excretion in the collecting duct.
- Hence adenosine antagonists are being developed as diuretics that can not only cause Na^+ and water loss but also prevent hypokalemia by inhibiting K^+ excretion.
- The later effect is significant as all other diuretics acting before collecting duct cause hypokalemia.
- **Rolofylline**, an adenosine antagonist was withdrawn from trial due to neurotoxicity, whereas other new agents are currently under trial as diuretics.

DRUGS ACTING ON LOOP OF HENLE

- The PCT extends to form loop of Henle, which comprises of a descending thin limb (DTL), ascending thin limb (ATL) and a thick ascending limb (TAL).
- The DTL absorbs only water and hence tubular fluid Na^+/Cl^- concentration increases. This facilitates concentration dependent absorption of Na^+/Cl^- in ATL, which is impermeable to water.
- In the TAL $Na^+/K^+/2Cl^-$ symporter absorbs all the solutes with maximum contribution in loop for Na^+ absorption (25%).
- Na^+/Cl^- are accommodated in epithelial cell and transported to interstitium.
- Potassium being an intracellular ion is already high inside cell and hence is repelled back into lumen. This loss of positive ion creates a gradient for absorption of other positively charged ions like calcium and magnesium.

Conceptual Box-2

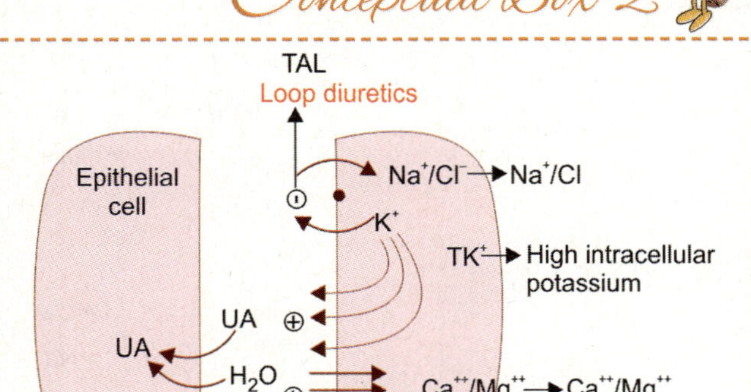

Loop Diuretics

- **Furosemide, bumetanide, ethacrynic acid** and **torsemide** are the commonly used drugs in this class. All of them are sulphonamide derivatives (except **ethacrynic acid**) and hence retain the side effect of hypersensitivity. **Bumetanide** is the **most potent** whereas **torsemide** is the **longest acting** loop diuretic. Ethacrynic acid has 100% bioavailability. The route of administration is both oral and parenteral. Organic mercurial compounds like **mersalyl** are also inhibitors of **Na+/K+/2Cl-** symporter, but not used currently due to toxicity.
- Loop diuretics inhibit **Na+/K+/2Cl- pump** in the TAL and hence cause a maximum loss of Na (25%) among diuretics and are also known as high ceiling diuretics. They induce prostaglandin synthesis, which causes vasodilation and inhibits solute absorption in TAL. **NSAIDs can decrease diuretic effect** by inhibiting prostaglandin synthesis. In part weak carbonic anhydrase inhibiting effect (except **bumetanide**) also contributes.
- This significant loss of solute and water decreases osmotic pressure in plasma and there is compensatory reabsorption of uric acid **(hyperuricemia)**, which has osmotic power.
- Apart from this inhibition of potassium absorption inhibits the gradient for absorption of calcium and magnesium resulting in **hypomagnesemia** and **hypocalcemia**.
- The filtered load of sodium stimulates ENaC in collecting duct that causes loss of potassium and protons and leads to **hypokalemia** and **metabolic alkalosis**.

Uses

- Loop diuretics are first drug of choice for treatment of **pulmonary edema** associated with acute CHF. In pulmonary edema the effect is seen first because of decrease in preload on heart due to **venodilation** by prostaglandins followed by diuresis. Torsemide is more effective than furosemide in treatment of pulmonary edema seen with CHF.
- They are used in hypertensive emergency and hypertension associated with renal failure (oliguria).
- Other uses are for treatment of hyperkalemia, anion toxicity (bromide, fluoride and iodide), hypercalcemia, **cerebral edema, edema associated with liver cirrhosis** and CKD and life threatening hyponatremia (with hypertonic saline).

Side Effects

- **Ototoxicity** is maximum with **ethacrynic acid** and is usually reversible on drug discontinuation. It is precipitated at high doses, rapid IV administration and use with ototoxic drugs like aminoglycosides, cisplatin and vancomycin.
- Other side effects like hyperlipidemia, hyperglycemia, hyperuricemia along with **hypokalemia, alkalosis,** hypomagnesemia and hypocalcemia can be seen. Compensatory reabsorption of calcium from intestine can compensate for its loss and hence **hypocalcemia is not a common side effect.**

Correlation of the Effects with Side effects and uses

Effects	Side effects/drug interaction	Uses
Maximum loss of solute and water	• Dehydration • Electrolyte depletion	High ceiling diuretics • Pulmonary edema • Cerebral edema • Hypertensive emergency with renal failure • Edema in CKD and liver cirrhosis
Compensatory reabsorption of uric acid	Hyperuricemia	
Loss of calcium and magnesium	• Hypocalcaemia • Hypomagnesemia	Hypercalcemia
Induce prostaglandin synthesis	NSAIDs decrease prostaglandin synthesis and diuretic effect	First effect in pulmonary edema due to vasodilation
Loss of potassium	Hypokalaemia	Hyperkalaemia

Osmotic Diuretics

The effect of osmotic diuretics can be divided into their effects on cells in body and on nephrons. This class contains oral drugs like glycerin, isosorbide and intravenous drugs like mannitol and urea.

Cellular Effect

Osmotic diuretics are distributed into extracellular space, where they absorb water from the cells.

Renal Effects

- In the kidney the major site of action of loop diuretics is loop followed by PCT. Presence of osmotic diuretics in the PCT lumen prevents absorption of water.
- The cellular effect increases plasma volume and renal blood flow that removes Na^+/Cl^- and urea from medulla, thereby decreasing medullary osmolarity.
- Thus, water is not absorbed from descending thin limb to medulla. This dilutes the tubular fluid decreasing solute concentration and hence Na^+/Cl^- are not absorbed in thick ascending limb.
- They inhibit absorption of magnesium also in thick ascending limb.

Uses

- The cellular effect described above makes them effective in treatment of **cerebral edema (diuretic of choice), acute congestive glaucoma (DOC), raised ICT, impending acute renal failure** and dialysis disequilibrium syndrome.
- Apart from this they can also be used in bronchial hyper reactivity test (inhalational route), in drug toxicity to increase excretion and urologic irrigation in transurethral prostatectomy to prevent hemolysis.
- The renal effect makes them effective as a diuretic in case other diuretics are ineffective due to compensatory Na/Cl reabsorption (diuretic braking) on long term use.

Side Effects

- Cellular effects can increase plasma volume and cause **hyponatremia** and **pulmonary edema**. Hyponatremia causes the common side effects like nausea, vomiting and headache.
- Renal effects can cause excessive water loss that leads to **hypernatremia**, hyperkalemia and dehydration. Inhibition of magnesium absorption causes hypomagnesemia.
- Urea is not used routinely due to side effects like pain and thrombosis; it is contraindicated in liver failure. Mannitol and urea are contraindicated in active **cranial hemorrhage**. Glycerin causes hyperglycemia, as it is metabolized into glucose.

DRUGS ACTING ON DISTAL CONVOLUTED TUBULE

- Distal convoluted tubule **(DCT)** is subjected only to 10% of filtered Na as 90% is absorbed in the prior segments. Both Na and Cl are absorbed in the DCT by Na/Cl cotransporter.
- Calcium is also absorbed in DCT by calcium channels, which are then pumped into interstitium by Na/Ca exchanger.

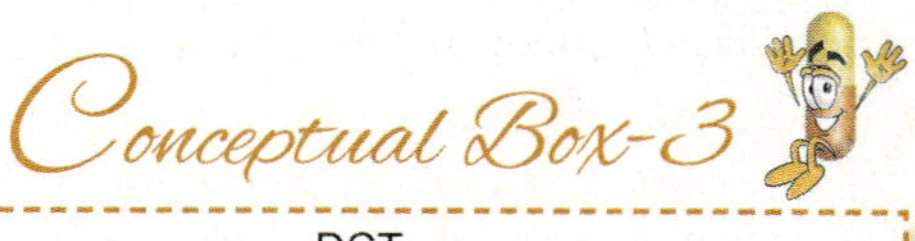

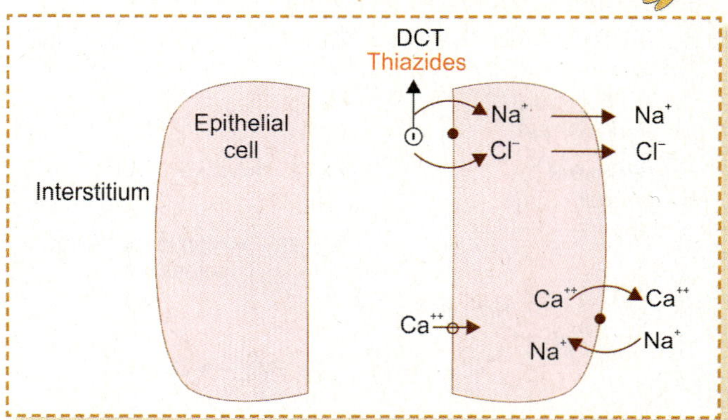

Thiazides and Thiazide like Diuretics

- This class contains sulphonamide derivative drugs like chlorothiazide, hydrochlorothiazide, indapamide, metolazone, chlorthalidone, polythiazide and bendroflumethiazide. Chlorthalidone is the longest acting, whereas chlorothiazide is the shortest acting drug in this class. The route of administration is only oral, except chlorothiazide which can be given be parenteral route also. Thiazides with 100% bioavailability are polythiazide and bendroflumethiazide.
- Thiazides are secreted in proximal convoluted tubule (PCT) by pumps and then they act in the DCT by inhibiting **Na^+/Cl^- cotransporter** and as the maximum possible loss of solutes and water is limited, i.e. only 10%, these are moderately effective diuretics.
- In part diuretic effect is also seen because of weak carbonic anhydrase inhibiting effect (except **indapamide**) and prostaglandin synthesis **(NSAIDs decrease effect)**.
- Inhibition of **Na^+/Cl^-** cotransporter decreases intracellular sodium in DCT epithelium. This stimulates Na^+/Ca^{++} exchanger to pump Na+ in and Ca++ out of epithelial cell into interstitium, which stimulates Ca absorption from the lumen. Calcium absorption is also stimulated in the PCT, due to volume depletion.
- Since thiazides are moderately effective diuretics, effect is not seen if GFR is below **30 mL/min**, except **indapamide** and **metolazone**.

Uses

- **Hypertension:** Apart from diuresis on long term therapy **vasodilation is the main mechanism** for antihypertensive effect, which is seen because of potassium channel opening and negative sodium balance. The latter mechanism is blunted in renal failure and hence diuretics become ineffective. **Thiazides** are one of the first line of drugs for treatment of **mild to moderate hypertension** and drug of choice in hypertension associated with osteoporosis, as they can cause hypercalcemia. **Chlorthalidone** being longest acting provides better 24 hour BP control and is the thiazide of choice. **Indapamide** has poor diuretic effect because of short duration of action, thus **direct vasodilation** is the primary effect with this drug and is used only in hypertension.
- **Edema:** Thiazides can be used for treatment of edema associated with various systemic disorders like CHF (primarily), liver cirrhosis, nephrotic syndrome etc. Metolazone is primarily used in edema.
- **Nephrogenic diabetic insipidus:** Thiazides are used in lithium induced diabetic insipidus. Volume depletion causes secondary water reabsorption in the PCT and decreases free water clearance.
- **Calcium stones:** As thiazides increase Calcium absorption, they are effective in treatment of nephrolithiasis associated with hypercalciuria.

Side Effects

- **Erectile dysfunction:** Volume depletion can cause ED, which is **maximum among the antihypertensives followed by beta blockers**.
- **Hypercalcemia:** The cause has been described above.
- **Hyperuricemia:** Uric acid (UA) is excreted by pumps into the lumen, which is also utilized by thiazides. Hence they competitively inhibit UA excretion.
- **Hyperglycemia:** Thiazides **decrease insulin release** due to hypokalemia and patients on long term therapy are at risk of diabetes mellitus.
- **Hypokalemia and metabolic alkalosis:** Increased Na load to collecting ducts (CD), stimulates loss of K and H. Hypokalemia increases the risk of torsades, if thiazides are used with drugs increasing QT interval like class Ia and Class III antiarrhythmics.
- Other side effects associated are hyponatremia, hypomagnesemia, hyperlipidemia and hypersensitivity (sulphonamide derivatives).
- Hyperglycemia, hyperuricemia and hypokalemia is seen more frequently with thiazides as compared to loop diuretics.

DRUGS ACTING ON COLLECTING DUCT

- Collecting ducts are made up of two types of cells, i.e. principal and type A intercalated cells.
- Principal cells have ENaC (Epithelial Na Channels) and ROMK (K channels) and intercalated cells have H^+ ATPase pump.
- Aldosterone forms a complex with aldosterone receptor in the cytoplasm which then translocates into nucleus and increases transcription factor for ENaC synthesis.
- Only 2% of filtered Na^+ reaches collecting duct, where it is absorbed by ENaC.
- Influx of Na depolarizes luminal membrane and activates ROMK and H ATPase pumps that secretes K^+ and H^+ respectively into the lumen.

Conceptual Box-4

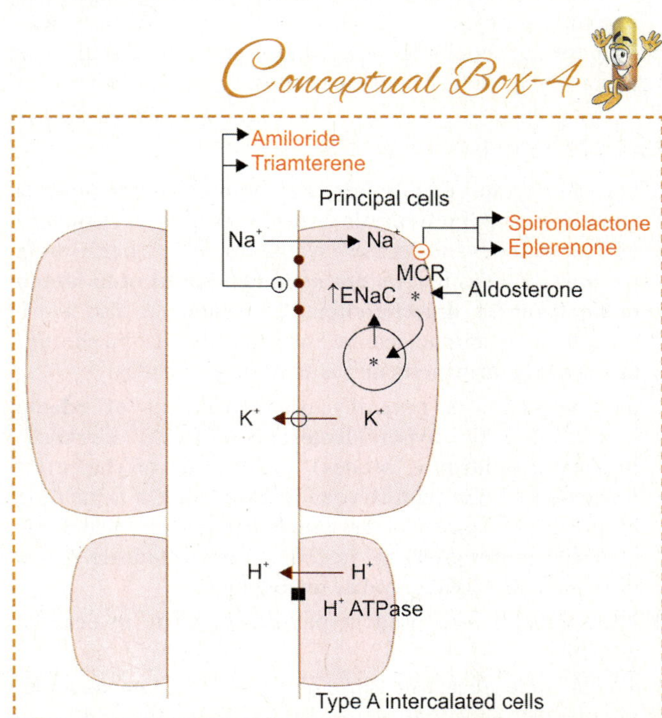

Potassium Sparing Diuretics

- Inhibitors of ENaC and aldosterone antagonists are the drugs in this class, which inhibit potassium loss and hence are known as potassium sparing diuretics.
- The end effect of this class is loss of very minimal Na (2%) and retention of K^+ and H^+. Thus, the diuretic effect is very less and these drugs are commonly used as add on diuretics to loop diuretics and thiazides.
- Hyperkalemia is caused by K^+ retention and hence these are combined with other diuretics also to prevent hypokalemia.
- For the same reason they are contraindicated in renal failure and along with drugs causing **hyperkalemia** like **RAS inhibitors**, digoxin and other drugs that inhibit ENaC (pentamidine and trimethoprim).
- **Metabolic acidosis** is also a common side effect of this class due to H^+ retention.

ENaC Inhibitors

- **Amiloride** and **triamterene** are ENaC inhibitors available. Amiloride is excreted unchanged by kidney, whereas triamterene is highly metabolized by liver (short acting) into active metabolite and excreted by kidney.
- **Amiloride** inhibits lithium absorption by ENaC in CD and hence is the drug of choice for **lithium induced diabetes insipidus**.
- **Liddle syndrome** is associated with raised ENaC overexpression and hence can be treated with amiloride.
- In **cystic fibrosis** inhalational amiloride is used to increase Na^+ and water in secretions and improve mucociliary clearance.
- Most common side effects of this class drugs is GIT upset, i.e. nausea and vomiting. Triamterene can cause folic acid deficiency, hyperglycemia, photosensitivity, interstitial nephritis and nephrolithiasis; hence is not used commonly. Triamterene should not be used in liver cirrhosis as there is already folic acid deficiency in cirrhosis.

Aldosterone Antagonists

- **Spironolactone, eplerenone, canrenone** and its prodrug **canreonate** inhibit mineralocorticoid receptor in cytoplasm of principal cells and decrease synthesis of ENaC; hence these are only diuretics that **do not need to be present in lumen of nephron for diuretic effect. Canrenone** is also active metabolite of spironolactone. Spironolactone is the shortest acting drug and canreonate has 100% bioavailability.
- Spironolactone is primarily used treatment of **edema** associated with **hyperaldosteronism (CHF, cirrhosis, nephrotic syndrome, ascites)** and is drug of choice for **refractory edema (aldosterone level is high)**. It is the drug of choice for treatment of **resistant hypertension** and diuretic of choice in **liver cirrhosis**. In CHF, spironolactone decreases mortality by inhibiting cardiac remodeling.
- Eplerenone is also used in patients of acute myocardial infarction.
- Specific side effects of spironolactone like **gynecomastia**, impotence, menstrual abnormalities, hirsutism and voice change are seen due to inhibition of androgen and progesterone. Because of same effect it is used for treatment of hirsutism and acne seen in polycystic ovary syndrome (PCOS).
- Eplerenone is more specific for mineralocorticoid receptors and is devoid of these side effects.

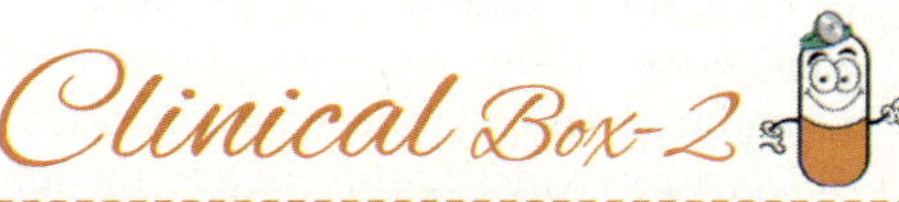

Drug of choice for various types of edema	
Pulmonary edema with CHF	Furosemide
Edema caused by liver cirrhosis	Spironolactone
Resistant edema	Spironolactone
Cerebral edema	Mannitol

VASOPRESSIN AGONISTS AND ANTAGONISTS

- Vasopressin is synthesized in the hypothalamus and released by pituitary in response to plasma hyperosmolarity and hypovolemia.
- Once released it acts on V1 receptors in blood vessels and GIT and V2 receptors renal collecting duct and vascular endothelium.
- V1 receptors are G_q subtype of GPCR, which when stimulated increase Ca^{++} in the smooth muscles of blood vessels causing vasoconstriction and GIT increasing contraction.
- V2 receptors are G_s subtype of GPCR which increase cyclic AMP that results in movement of aquaporin 2 to the luminal side of principal cells in collecting duct. Aquaporins 2 mediate absorption of water and urea in medullary CD. The latter contributes to medullary hyperosmolarity.
- V2 receptors in thick ascending limb and collecting duct also increase effect of $Na^+/K^+/2Cl^-$ and ENaC channels respectively which leads to Na+ absorption.
- V2 receptors in vascular endothelium stimulate release of factor VIII and von Willebrand factor.
- Most of the solutes are reabsorbed in the nephron till collecting duct and the tubular fluid has water in excess of solutes. The medullary hyperosmolarity due to counter current mechanism and urea, extracts water from dilute tubular fluid.

VASOPRESSIN AGONISTS

Vasopressin acts non selectively on both V1 and V2 receptors whereas desmopressin is highly selective for V2 receptors and terlipressin for V1 receptors. They are readily metabolized in plasma by peptidases and thus have a short half-life. Their primary site of action in kidney is **medullary CD**.

Vasopressin

- **Vasopressin** being a vasopressor can be used for treatment of **bleeding esophageal varices**, however the recent drug **terlipressin is more preferred** due to better side effect profile.

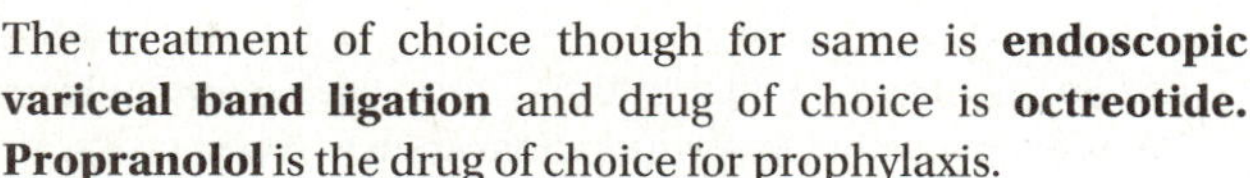

The treatment of choice though for same is **endoscopic variceal band ligation** and drug of choice is **octreotide. Propranolol** is the drug of choice for prophylaxis.

- Other uses of vasopressors are to decrease bleeding in various surgeries, hemorrhagic cystitis with cyclophosphamide and ifosfamide, bleeding gastric ulcer and in NE resistant vasodilatory shock.
- Vasopressin increases GIT contraction and hence used in postoperative ileus and abdominal distention.
- Vasopressin though can be used in central diabetes insipidus, but is less preferred than desmopressin due to side effects.
- Vasoconstriction causes facial pallor whereas GIT stimulation causes nausea and cramps.

Desmopressin

- Desmopressin is the drug of choice for treatment of **central (neurogenic) diabetes insipidus** and nocturnal enuresis in children. Oral route is preferred for nocturnal enuresis as intranasal desmopressin was associated with hyponatremic seizures.
- Imipramine though can be used in nocturnal enuresis is less preferred and the treatment of choice is bed alarm therapy.
- Desmopressin is used for treatment of **von Willebrand's disease type I** and **hemophilia A** (mild to moderate).
- Other uses are bleeding disorders seen in uremia, liver cirrhosis and HIT (Heparin Induced thrombocytopenia).
- Water intoxication, facial flushing and headache can be seen with desmopressin.

VASOPRESSIN ANTAGONISTS

- Vasopressin antagonists can be nonselective like **conivaptan** and selective V2 antagonists like **tolvaptan** and **mozavaptan**. Conivaptan can be used by intravenous route for short term management in admitted patients, whereas tolvaptan and mozavaptan by oral route for long term management. Demeclocycline, fludrocortisone and lithium can also be used.
- Tolvaptan is the most potent drug and is drug of choice for treatment of **euvolemic hyponatremia (SIADH)** and used in hypervolemic hyponatremia caused by CHF.
- The initial **treatment of choice** though for SIADH is **free water restriction** and **3% normal saline is used** in patients with neurological symptoms of hyponatremia.
- **Tolvaptan** has been recently approved to slow kidney function decline in adults at risk of rapidly progressing **autosomal dominant polycystic kidney disease**. V2 inhibition decreases cyclic AMP which results in decreased water secretion and proliferation of cells, resulting in decreased growth of cysts. Other possible use under investigation is congenital X-linked nephrogenic diabetes insipidus.
- Rapid correction of hyponatremia by these drugs can cause osmotic demyelination. Other side effects seen are headache, hyperglycemia, **hypokalemia and hepatotoxicity (only with tolvaptan)**. Due to hepatotoxicity tolvaptan is contraindicated in liver cirrhosis and should not be used for more than 1 month in a patient.

Clinical Box-3

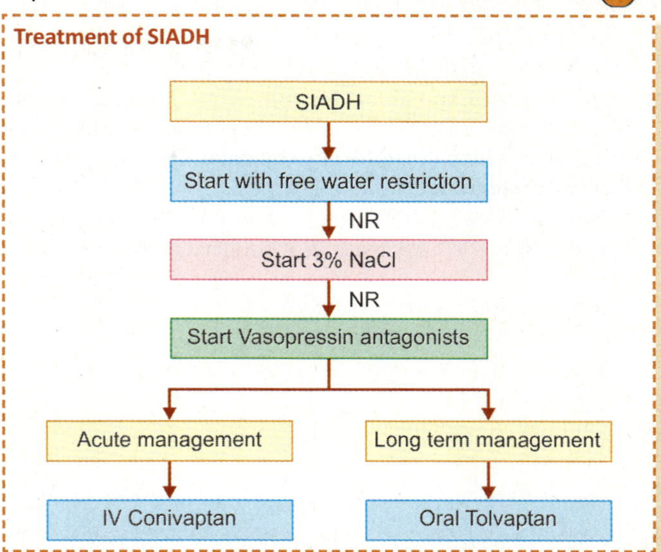

Drugs Causing SIADH

Mnemonics

CHIVAS

- **C :** Chlorpropamide, Clonidine
- **H :** Haloperidol
- **I :** Ifosfamide and cyclophosphamide
- **V :** Vincristine
- **A :** ACEI (Enalapril)
- **S :** SSRI and TCA

Recent Advances

Relcovaptan: Selective V1 receptor antagonist for dysmenorrhea, Raynaud's disease and tocolysis.

Nelivaptan: Selective V1b (V3) receptor antagonist under trial as anxiolytic.

Satavaptan and Lixivaptan: Selective V2 antagonist awaiting approval by FDA for hyponatremia.

Free Water Clearance

- Free water clearance is the amount of solute free water generated by the kidney.
- This solute free water is generated in the thick ascending limb and distal convoluted tubule, which are permeable to solutes but impermeable to water. Thus, this solute free water generated in the lumen is called as **positive free water clearance**.
- Solutes absorbed in thick ascending limb gives rise to medullary hyperosmolarity which absorbs the free water in collecting duct in response to vasopressin. Thus, here solute

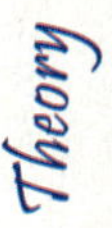

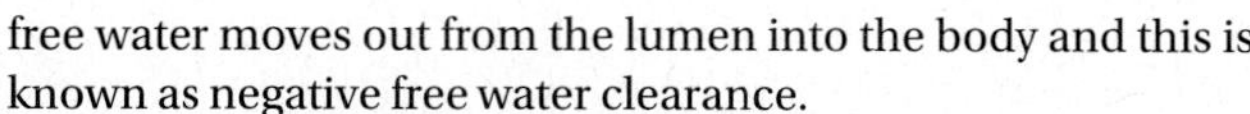

free water moves out from the lumen into the body and this is known as negative free water clearance.

- **Carbonic anhydrase inhibitors** deliver more Na+ and water to thick ascending limb and distal convoluted tubule, where only Na+ is absorbed and water remains in lumen. Thus there is an **increase in positive free water clearance**.
- **Loop diuretics** and **thiazides** inhibit Na^+ absorption and hence there is more Na than before in lumen as compared to water. Hence **loop diuretics** and **thiazides decrease positive free water clearance.**
- **Loops** decrease Na^+/Cl^- absorption in thick ascending limb and thus there is a decrease in medullary hyperosmolarity. This decreases absorption of solute free water from the lumen of collecting duct into the body. Hence loop diuretics **decrease negative free water clearance** as well.

Effect of diuretics on free water clearance	
Carbonic anhydrase inhibitors	Increase positive free water clearance
Thiazides	Decrease positive free water clearance
Loop diuretics	Decrease positive free water clearance Decrease negative free water clearance

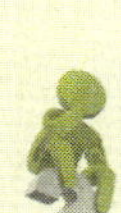

Image-based Questions

1. **Which of the following diuretic prevents formation of renal stone given in the picture?**

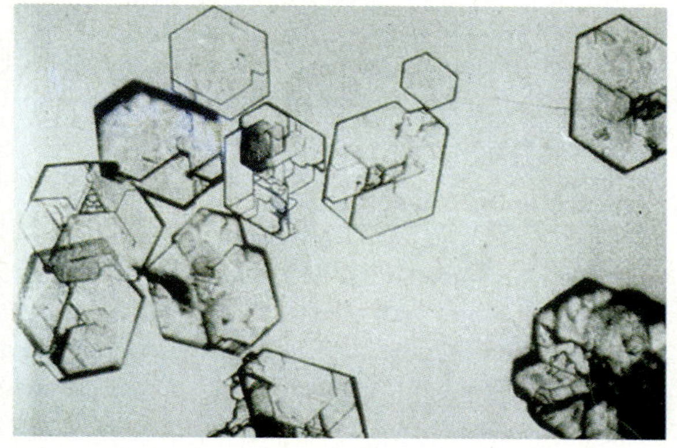

a. Furosemide b. Chlorthalidone
c. Acetazolamide d. Mannitol

2. **Which of the following diuretic is preferred in the condition presented in the X-ray?**

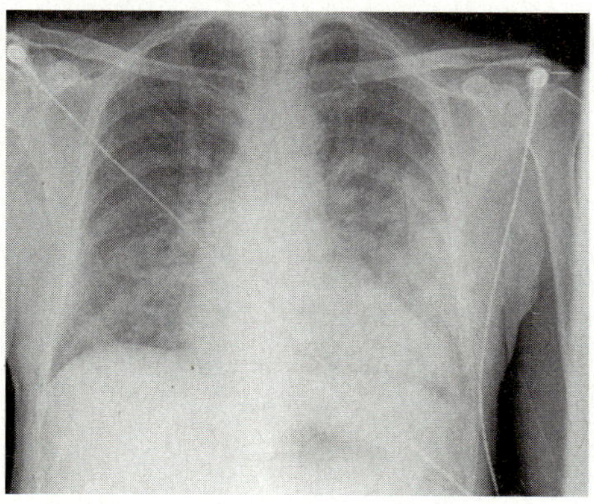

a. Acetazolamide b. Furosemide
c. Chlorthalidone d. Mannitol

3. **Which of the following diuretic is preferred in the condition given in the NCCT given below?**

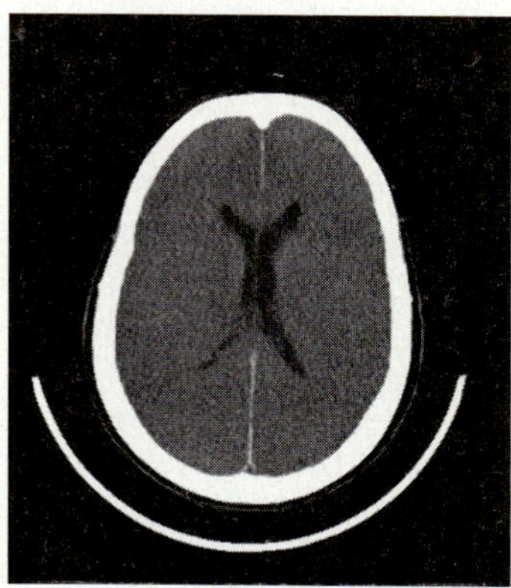

a. Furosemide b. Spironolactone
c. Thiazides d. Mannitol

4. **Which of the following drug is used for treatment of the stones given in the picture?**

a. Acetazolamide b. Furosemide
c. Chlorothiazide d. Spironolactone

5. **Which of the following is preferred in the condition given in the picture?**

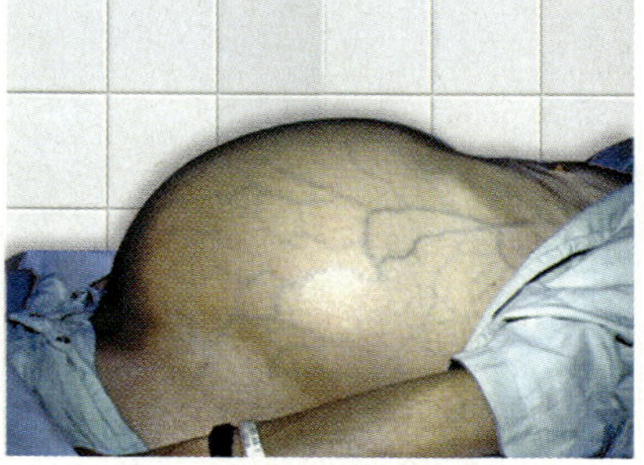

a. Amiloride b. Spironolactone
c. Furosemide d. Thiazides

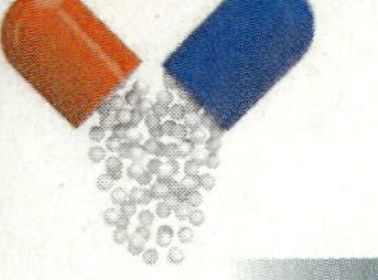

Answers with Explanations to Image-based Questions

1. Ans. (c) Acetazolamide

(Ref: Goodman Gilman 12th E/P 680)

- The hexagonal stones in the picture are cysteine stones associated with cystinuria.
- Acetazolamide alkalinizes urine and increases solubility of cysteine and decreases chances of stone formation.

2. Ans. (b) Furosemide

(Ref: Goodman Gilman 12th E/P686)

- The presence of Kerley lines and peribronchial cuffing is suggestive of pulmonary edema in the patient.
- The diuretic of choice in pulmonary edema is furosemide.

3. Ans. (d) Mannitol

(Ref: Goodman Gilman 12th E/P682)

- The loss of grey and white matter differentiation is suggestive of cerebral edema.
- The diuretic of choice in cerebral edema is mannitol.

4. Ans. (c) Chlorothiazide

(Ref: Goodman Gilman 12th E/P690)

- Envelope shaped stones in the picture are calcium oxalate stones.
- These calcium stone formations can be treated by thiazides as they can increase calcium absorption and decrease it in urine.

5. Ans. (b) Spironolactone

(Ref: Goodman Gilman 12th E/P695)

- Massive ascites with dilated and prominent superficial veins of the abdomen are suggestive of cirrhotic ascites.
- In cirrhotic ascites there is upregulation of aldosterone synthesis and hence it best responds to aldosterone antagonists like spironolactone.

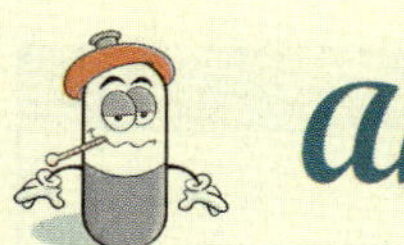

Annexures

Drug of Choice

Cystinuria	• Cystine binding agent – Tiopronin Plus • Urine alkalinizer – Potassium citrate as sodium salt

Edema	
Pulmonary edema with CHF	Furosemide
Edema caused by liver cirrhosis	Spironolactone
Resistant edema	Resistant edema
Cerebral edema	Mannitol

Lupus nephritis Rapidly progressive glomerulonephritis (RPGN)	• Cyclophosphamide Plus • Glucocorticoids

Nephrotic syndrome	• Nephrotic syndrome (NS): Steroids • Steroid resistant NS: Cyclosporine • Steroid dependent NS: Cyclophosphamide • NS with frequent relapses: Cyclophosphamide

Urine incontinence	• Overflow incontinence: Cholinergics (Bethanechol) • Urge incontinence: Anticholinergics (Darifenacin) • Stress incontinence: SNRI (Duloxetine) • Urinary tract infection (UTI) Cystitis: Cotrimoxazole • Pyelonephritis: Ciprofloxacin

Drug-Induced Ion Abnormalities

Ion abnormality	Causative drugs
Hypokalemia	• Beta 2 agonists • Alpha blockers • Insulin • Theophylline/Caffeine • B12/Folic acid • Amphotericin B

Contd...

Ion abnormality	Causative drugs
	• Diuretics except K sparing ones ■ CA inhibitors ■ Loops ■ Thiazides ■ Osmotic diuretics • Penicillin • Fludrocortisone
Hyperkalemia	• Beta blockers (Nonselective) • Digoxin • Sch • Renin-angiotensin-aldosterone system (RAAS) inhibitors ■ ACEI ■ ARB ■ Renin inhibitors ■ Aldosterone antagonists • Amiloride/Triamterene • Trimethoprim • Pentamidine • Nonsteroidal anti-inflammatory drugs (NSAIDs) • Cyclosporine/Tacrolimus • Heparin
Hypomagnesemia	• PPI • Ethanol • Diuretics ■ Loops ■ Thiazides ■ Osmotic • Pentamidine • Foscarnet • Cyclosporine • Aminoglycosides • Amphotericin B • Cetuximab
Hypermagnesemia	• Cathartics • Urologic irrigants • Antacids • Enemas • Laxatives • Lithium • Theophylline
Hyponatremia	• Chlorpropamide • Vincristine • Cyclophosphamide • Nicotine • Clofibrate • SSRI

Contd...

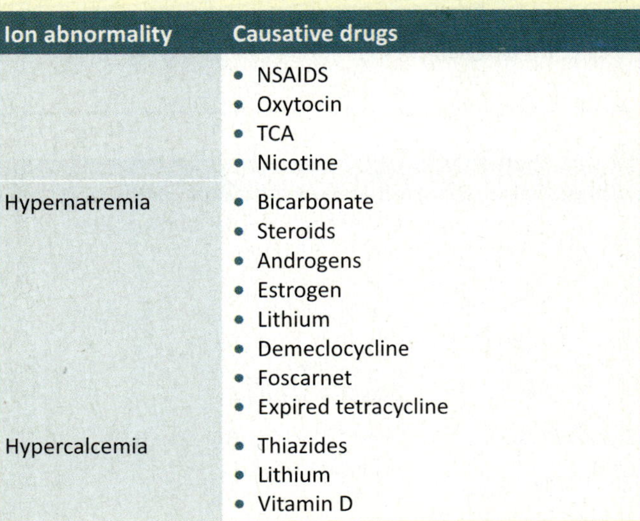

Ion abnormality	Causative drugs
	• NSAIDS • Oxytocin • TCA • Nicotine
Hypernatremia	• Bicarbonate • Steroids • Androgens • Estrogen • Lithium • Demeclocycline • Foscarnet • Expired tetracycline
Hypercalcemia	• Thiazides • Lithium • Vitamin D

Contd...

Ion abnormality	Causative drugs
	• Vitamin A intoxication • Aluminium intoxication • Theophylline • Estrogen • Tamoxifen
Hypocalcemia	• Bisphosphonates • Cisplatin • Foscarnet • Calcitonin • Loops • Glucocorticoids • Antiepileptics • PPI • PTU • Colchicine toxicity

Multiple Choice Questions

1. **Which of the following drug is used to prevent acute mountain sickness** ***(AIIMS Nov 2018)***
   a. Acetazolamide b. Dexamethasone
   c. Diltiazem d. Digoxin
2. **Mannitol is used for treatment of** ***(Recent Question 2019)***
   a. Acute congestive glaucoma
   b. CHF
   c. Pulmonary edema
   d. Hepatic encephalopathy
3. **A patient of hypercalcemia with serum calcium level, 16 mg/dL. What is the immediate management?** ***(AIIMS Nov 2016)***
   a. Subcutaneous calcitonin
   b. IV fluids and diuretics
   c. Phosphate injection
   d. Corticosteroid injection
4. **The site of action of the loop diuretic furosemide is** ***(AIIMS May 2014)***
   a. Thick ascending limb of loop of Henle
   b. Descending limb of loop of Henle
   c. Proximal tubule
   d. Distal tubule
5. **Vasopressin antagonists act on:** ***(AIIMS May 2013)***
   a. Cortical collecting tubule
   b. Medullary collecting duct
   c. DCT
   d. PCT
6. **Thiazides can cause:** ***(AIIMS Nov 2009)***
   a. Hyperkalemic paralysis b. Hypouricemia
   c. Hypolipidemia d. Impotence
7. **Hypomagnesemia due to increased excretion by the kidney is caused by all except:** ***(AIIMS May 2010)***
   a. Furosemide b. Digitalis
   c. Aminoglycoside d. Cisplatin
8. **Free water clearance is decreased by:** ***(AIIMS May 2008)***
   a. Vincristine b. Vinblastine
   c. Chlorpropamide d. Furosemide
9. **Hypercalcemia is caused by all except:** ***(AIIMS Nov 2007)***
   a. Loop diuretics b. Lithium
   c. Vitamin D intoxication d. Thiazides
10. **Thiazides diuretics causes all except:** ***(AIIMS Nov 2007)***
    a. Hyperglycemia
    b. Increased calcium excretion
    c. Useful in congestive heart failure
    d. Decreased uric acid excretion
11. **Regarding furosemide true statement is:** ***(AIIMS Nov 2007)***
    a. Acute pulmonary edema is an indication
    b. Acts on PCT
    c. Mild diuresis
    d. Given only by parental route
12. **Tolvaptan is used for treatment of** ***(Recent Question 2019)***
    a. Central DI b. SIADH
    c. Shock d. Von Willebrand's disease
13. **Vasopressin acts through which receptors in collecting duct** ***(Recent Question 2019)***
    a. V1 b. V2
    c. ENaC d. SGLT
14. **Side effect of carbonic anhydrase inhibitors is:** ***(Recent Question 2018)***
    a. Bone marrow suppression
    b. Weight gain
    c. Hyperkalemia
    d. Insomnia
15. **Mannitol is not useful for** ***(Recent Question 2016)***
    a. Glaucoma b. Raised ICT
    c. Impending renal failure d. Pulmonary edema
16. **Following are the side effects of thiazides except** ***(Recent Question 2016)***
    a. Hypokalemia b. Hypocalcemia
    c. Hepatic coma d. Impotence
17. **Mechanism of action thiazide is** ***(Recent Question 2016)***
    a. Na + Cl^- symport inhibitor
    b. Na + K^+ symport inhibitor
    c. Carbonic anhydrase inhibitor
    d. Osmotic diuresis
18. **Spironolactone is effective in** ***(Recent Question 2016)***
    a. Cardiac edema b. Ascitic edema
    c. Nutritional edema d. All of the above
19. **Complication of long-term thiazide administration** ***(Recent Question 2016)***
    a. Metabolic alkalosis b. Metabolic acidosis
    c. Hypermagnesemia d. Hypocalcemia
20. **Vasopressin cannot correct** ***(Recent Question 2016)***
    a. Nephrogenic DI b. Neurogenic DI
    c. GI bleeding d. Nocturnal enuresis
21. **Lithium induced diabetes insipidus respond to** ***(Recent Question 2016)***
    a. Diclofenac b. Vasopressin
    c. Amiloride d. Indapamide
22. **Most common complication of loop diuretics** ***(Recent Question 2016)***
    a. Hypocalcemia b. Hypokalemia
    c. Hyperkalemia d. Hypercalcemia
23. **Drug causing metabolic acidosis** ***(Recent Question 2016)***
    a. Acetazolamide
    b. Thiazide
    c. Torsemide
    d. Spironolactone

24. Treatment of hypercalcemia are all except ***(Recent Question 2016)***

a. Thiazides b. Loop diuretics
c. Calcitonin d. All of the above

25. Hypercalciuria with renal stones are treated by ***(Recent Question 2016)***

a. Thiazides b. Loop diuretics
c. Calcitonin d. All of the above

26. Drug of choice for neurogenic diabetes insipidus is ***(Recent Question 2016)***

a. Lypressin b. Terlipressin
c. Desmopressin d. Pralipressin

27. True regarding acetazolamide is ***(Recent Question 2016)***

a. Irreversible inhibitor of carbonic anhydrase
b. Structural resemblance to sulfonamides
c. It decrease Na, K and glucose excretion
d. It causes metabolic alkalosis

28. Thiazide diuretic used when GFR<30 mL/min? ***(Recent Question 2016)***

a. Metolazone b. Benzthiazide
c. Chlorothiazide d. Hydrochlorothiazide

29. All the following adverse effects can be caused by loop diuretics except ***(Recent Question 2016)***

a. Hypercalcemia b. Hyperglycemia
c. Hypomagnesemia d. Hyperuricemia

30. Treatment of choice for SIADH is ***(Recent Question 2016)***

a. Lithium carbonate b. Demeclocycline
c. Vasopressin d. Hypertonic saline

31. Drug of choice in lithium induced polyuria is? ***(Recent Question 2016)***

a. Amiloride b. Demeclocycline
c. Thiazide diuretics d. Indomethacin

32. Brinzolamide is ***(Recent Question 2016)***

a. Competitive and reversible carbonic anhydrase inhibitor
b. Noncompetitive and reversible carbonic anhydrase inhibitor
c. Competitive and irreversible carbonic anhydrase inhibitor
d. Non-competitive and irreversible carbonic anhydrase inhibitor

33. Drug causing gynecomastia is ***(Recent Question 2016)***

a. Spironolactone b. Rifampicin
c. Penicillin d. Bumetanide

34. Which of the following drugs increases the concentration of sodium and chloride ions in the urine with normal bicarbonate excretion? ***(Recent Question 2016)***

a. Ethacrynic acid b. Furosemide
c. Acetazolamide d. Bumetanide

35. Thiazides diuretics causes all except ***(Recent Question 2016)***

a. Hyperglycemia
b. Increased calcium excretion
c. Useful in congestive heart failure
d. Decreased uric acid excretion

36. Aldosterone antagonists are not useful in the treatment of ***(Recent Question 2016)***

a. Hypertension b. Congestive heart failure
c. Gynecomastia d. Hirsutism

37. Amiloride can cause hyperkalemia due to its action on ***(Recent Question 2016)***

a. Electrogenic K^+ channels
b. Electrogenic Na^+ channels
c. Non electrogenic Na^+ -Cl^- symporter
d. $H^+ - K^+ -$ ATPase

38. Selective V2 receptor agonist useful for the treatment of central diabetes insipidus is ***(Recent Question 2016)***

a. Arginine vasopressin b. Desmopressin
c. Lypressin d. Terlipressin

39. Desmopressin can be used for all of the following conditions except ***(Recent Question 2016)***

a. Neurogenic diabetes insipidus
b. Nephrogenic diabetes insipidus
c. Bed wetting in children
d. Bleeding due to hemophilia

40. Not associated with thiazide diuretics ***(Recent Question 2016)***

a. Hypercalciuria b. Hyponatremia
c. Hypokalemia d. Hyperuricemia

41. Furosemide should not be administered with NSAIDs because latter ***(Recent Question 2016)***

a. Prevent platelet aggregation
b. Inhibit prostacyclin synthesis
c. Decrease sodium reabsorption
d. Increases the secretion of furosemide in urine

42. All of the following diuretics inhibit Na^+ -K^+- $2Cl^-$ symporter, except ***(Recent Question 2016)***

a. Furosemide b. Thiazide
c. Ethacrynic acid d. Mersalyl

43. In cirrhotic ascites, which diuretic is preferred? ***(Recent Question 2016)***

a. Furosemide b. Acetazolamide
c. Spironolactone d. Any of the above

44. Potassium sparing diuretics acts on ***(Recent Question 2016)***

a. Na^+ K^+ pump b. Aldosterone receptor
c. Carbonic anhydrase d. Na+ Cl- symporter

45. Drug causing deafness is ***(Recent Question 2016)***

a. Thiazide b. Spironolactone
c. Ethacrynic acid d. Triamterene

46. Which of the following is aldosterone antagonist? ***(Recent Question 2016)***

a. Eplerenone b. Deoxycorticosterone
c. Fenoldopam d. Furosemide

47. Canrenone is a metabolite of ***(Recent Question 2016)***

a. Ampicillin b. Spironolactone
c. Furosemide d. Acetazolamide

48. Acetazolamide can be used in all except ***(Recent Question 2016)***

a. Epilepsy b. Acute mountain sickness
c. Cirrhosis d. Glaucoma

49. Furosemide causes all except *(Recent Question 2016)*
a. Hyperglycemia b. Hypomagnesemia
c. Hypokalemia d. Acidosis

50. Thiazide diuretics do not produce *(Recent Question 2016)*
a. Hypoglycemia b. Hyponatremia
c. Hypokalemia d. Hyperuricemia

51. Furosemide is used in Rx of all except *(Recent Question 2016)*
a. Cerebral edema
b. Generalised edema
c. Pulmonary edema
d. Pulmonary hypertension

52. Diuretics are the first choice as antihypertensive therapy in all except *(Recent Question 2016)*
a. Asthma
b. Elderly systolic hypertension
c. Low renin hypertension
d. Pregnancy-induced hypertension

53. True about Acetazolamide is? *(Recent Question 2016)*
a. Decreased GFR
b. Action similar to sulphonamide
c. It decreases Na, K, Glucose excretion
d. It causes metabolic alkalosis

54. Spironolactone is the first drug to be given for? *(Recent Question 2016)*
a. Cirrhotic edema b. Cardiac edema
c. Idiopathic edema d. Nutritional edema

55. Main side effects of acetazolamide is? *(Recent Question 2016)*
a. Hyperglycemia
b. Increased intracranial pressure
c. Metabolic alkalosis
d. Metabolic acidosis

56. Which of the following diuretics is/are carbonic anhydrase inhibitors: *(PGI 2018)*
a. Acetazolamide b. Topiramate
c. Thiazide d. Spironolactone
e. Bumetanide

57. Carbonic anhydrase inhibitor(s) is/are: *(PGI Nov. 2016)*
a. Acetazolamide b. Amiloride
c. Nitrofurantoin d. Topiramate

58. True about osmotic diuretics: *(PGI Nov. 2016)*
a. Osmotic diuretics have their major effect in the distal convoluted tubule
b. Contraindicated in congestive heart failure
c. Causes hyperkalemia
d. Increases renal blood flow

59. Desmopressin is/are used in: *(PGI June 2015)*
a. Diabetes insipidus b. Esophageal varices
c. Haemophilia A d. Von Willebrand disease

60. All are true about hydrochlorothiazide except: *(PGI Nov 2014)*
a. Cause hyperglycemia
b. Inhibit Na-Cl symport
c. Increases calcium excretion in urine
d. Cause hyperuricaemia
e. Used in treatment of renal stone

61. Mineralocorticoid receptors antagonist(s) is/are: *(PGI May 2014/Nov 2010)*
a. Spironolactone b. Triamterene
c. Eplerenone d. Amiloride
e. Acetazolamide

62. Hypokalemia occurs in use of: *(PGI Nov 2013)*
a. Thiazide b. ACE inhibitor
c. Amphotericin B d. Heparin
e. Insulin

63. Which of the following drugs is/are contraindicated/ warning in sulphonamide allergy: *(PGI May 2013)*
a. Brinzolamide b. Levobunolol
c. Bumetanide d. Nitrate
e. Acetazolamide

64. Loop diuretics act by *(PGI Dec 2008)*
a. Inhibition of Na^+–Cl^- Symport
b. Inhibition of Na^+–K^+–2 Cl^- cotransport
c. Inhibition of Na^+–K^+ ATPase
d. Inhibition of H^+–K^+ ATPase
e. Inhibition of renal epithelial Na+ channel

65. Carbonic anhydrase inhibitor not given in: *(PGI Nov 2006)*
a. Sulfonamide hypersensitivity
b. Glaucoma
c. Contraindicated in high altitude sickness
d. Contraindicated in metabolic acidosis
e. COPD

66. Which of the following drug need not be present in tubular lumen for diuretic action *(JIPMER 2018)*
a. Chlorothiazide b. Acetazolamide
c. Mannitol d. Eplerenone

67. Which of the following drug is contraindicated in cirrhosis? *(JIPMER 2017)*
a. Spironolactone b. Furosemide
c. Acetazolamide d. Eplerenone

68. Which of the following is false regarding diabetes insipidus (DI)? *(JIPMER 2017)*
a. Thiazides useful in both pituitary and nephrogenic cause
b. Desmopressin is not effective in nephrogenic type
c. Terlipressin is more effective than desmopressin in DI
d. Amiloride is the drug of choice for lithium induced DI

69. Only thiazide used in renal failure when GFR is less than 30-40 mL/min: *(JIPMER 2014)*
a. Chlorothiazide b. Chlorthalidone
c. Metolazone d. Methyclothiazide

70. Which should not be given in Liver failure? *(JIPMER 2012)*
a. Acetazolamide b. Frusemide
c. Eplerenone d. Spironolactone

71. Which of the following is not seen with thiazide diuretics? *(JIPMER 2010)*
a. Hypokalemia b. Hypercalcemia
c. Hyperuricemia d. Metabolic acidosis

72. Maximum bicarbonate loss occurs with: *(JIPMER 2010)*
a. Acetazolamide b. Furosemide
c. Thiazide d. Spironolactone

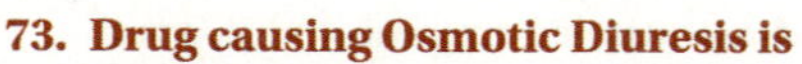

73. **Drug causing Osmotic Diuresis is** *(NIMHANS 2013)*
a. Mannitol b. Isosorbide
c. Glycerol d. All of the above

74. **Use of diuretics in pulmonary edema leads to all except** *(NIMHANS 2010)*
a. Na abnormal blockage
b. Increased renal blood flow
c. Increased venous capacitance
d. Increased sensitivity of adrenergic alpha receptors

75. **Treatment indicated for refractory SIADH includes** *(NIMHANS 2007)*
a. Demeclocycline b. Carbamazepine
c. Phenytoin d. Desmopressin

76. **The Loop diuretic acts at** *(NIMHANS 2007)*
a. PCT b. DCT
c. Ascending loop d. Descending loop

Practice Questions & Answers from 77 to 86 are given at the end of the chapter.

Answers with Explanations to Multiple Choice Questions

1. Ans. (a) Acetazolamide

(Ref: Goodman Gilman 13th E/P451)

2. Ans. (a) Acute congestive glaucoma

(Ref: Goodman Gilman 13th E/P452)

- IV mannitol is preferred for treatment of acute congestive glaucoma. It removes water from tissues and hence is effective in acute congestive glaucoma and cerebral edema.
- The water removed from tissues comes to plasma and an increased plasma volume can increase load on heart and cause pulmonary edema. Hence it is never used in CHF or pulmonary edema.

3. Ans. (b) IV fluids and diuretics

(Ref: Harrison 19th E/P2481)

In case of severe hypercalcemia i.e. > 13 mg/dL, primary aim is to restore normal hydration. The patients are started on IV fluids along with diuretics and calcitonin.

4. Ans. (a) Thick ascending limb of loop of Henle

(Ref: Goodman Gilman 12th E/P682)

Diuretics	Site of action
CA inhibitors	PCT
Loop diuretics	Thick ascending limb
Thiazides	DCT
Potassium sparing diuretics	Medullary CD
Vasopressin antagonist	Medullary CD

5. Ans. (b) Medullary collecting duct

(Ref: Goodman Gilman 12th E/P673)

6. Ans. (d) Impotence

(Ref: Goodman Gilman 12th E/P689)

- Among the antihypertensives maximum impotence is seen with thiazides followed by beta blockers.
- Thiazides cause impotence due to volume depletion.

7. Ans. (b) Digitalis

(Ref: Harrison 19th E/P2462)

Drugs Causing Hypomagnesemia

- PPI
- Ethanol
- Diuretics
  - Loops
  - Thiazides
  - Osmotic
- Pentamidine
- Foscarnet
- Cyclosporine
- Aminoglycosides
- Amphotericin B
- Cetuximab
- Cisplatin

8. Ans. (d) Furosemide

(Ref: KDT 7th E/P577)

9. Ans. (a) Loop diuretics

(Ref: Goodman Gilman 12th E/P686)

- Loop diuretics cause hypocalcemia.

Causes of Drug Induced Hypercalcemia

- Thiazides
- Lithium
- Vitamin D
- Vitamin A intoxication
- Aluminium intoxication
- Theophylline
- Estrogen
- Tamoxifen

10. Ans (b) Increased calcium excretion

(Ref: Goodman Gilman 12th E/P689)

- Thiazides decrease calcium excretion and hence cause hypercalcemia.
- Hyperglycemia and hyperuricemia are more commonly seen with thiazides as compared to loop diuretics.

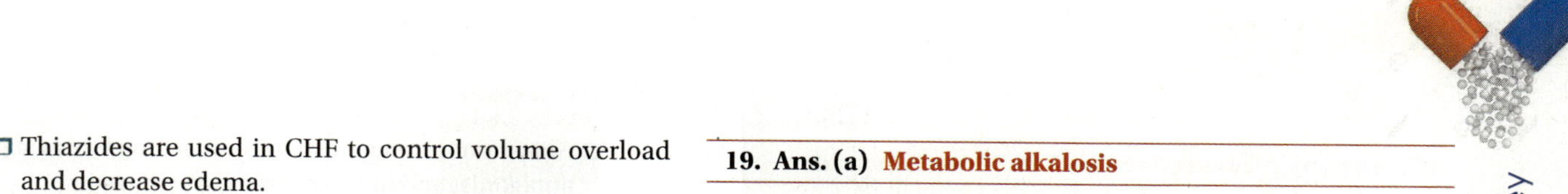

- Thiazides are used in CHF to control volume overload and decrease edema.

11. Ans. (a) Acute pulmonary edema is an indication

(Ref: Goodman Gilman 12th E/P686)

- Furosemide is the drug of choice for treatment of acute pulmonary edema.
- The site of action is thick ascending limb in the loop of Henle.
- Maximum solute and water loss gives powerful diuretic effect and hence this class is known as high ceiling diuretic.
- Furosemide is given by both oral and parenteral route.

12. Ans. (b) SIADH

(Ref: Goodman Gilman 13th E/P466)

- V2 receptor antagonist like conivaptan, tolvaptan and mozavaptan are used for treatment of SIADH.
- Demeclocycline is also an inhibitor of V2 receptor and used for treatment of SIADH.

13. Ans. (b) V2

(Ref: Goodman Gilman 13th E/P461)

- Vasopressin acts on V2 receptors in medullary collecting duct.
- V2 receptors are Gs subtype of GPCR and hence increase cyclic GMP, which activates aquaporins.

14. Ans. (a) Bone marrow suppression

(Ref: Goodman Gilman 13th E/P451)

15. Ans. (d) Pulmonary edema

(Ref: Goodman Gilman 12th E/P682)

- Mannitol is contraindicated in pulmonary edema as it can worsen it by increasing the plasma volume.
- In cerebral edema it is effective by extracting water from the neurons into the extracellular space.

16. Ans. (b) Hypocalcemia

(Ref: Goodman Gilman 12th E/P689)

- Thiazides cause hypercalcemia and not hypocalcemia.
- Thiazides are the antihypertensives associated with maximum impotence.

17. Ans. (a) Na+Cl- symport inhibitor

(Ref: Goodman Gilman 12th E/P687)

18. Ans. (d) All of the above

(Ref: Goodman Gilman 12th E/P695)

Spironolactone is primarily used for treatment of edema associated with hyperaldosteronism in conditions like

- CHF
- Ascites
- Nephrotic syndrome
- Liver cirrhosis

19. Ans. (a) Metabolic alkalosis

(Ref: Goodman Gilman 12th E/P689)

- CA inhibitors and potassium sparing diuretics cause metabolic acidosis.
- Thiazides and loop diuretics cause metabolic alkalosis.

20. Ans. (a) Nephrogenic DI

(Ref: Goodman Gilman 12th E/P712)

- Vasopressin is used in central DI, which is due to decreased ADH.
- In nephrogenic DI, as the site of action V2 receptors are blocked.

21. Ans. (c) Amiloride

(Ref: Goodman Gilman 12th E/P692)

- Amiloride is the drug of choice for treatment of lithium induced DI.
- Thiazides can also be used for same.

22. Ans. (a) Hypokalemia

(Ref: Goodman Gilman 12th E/P686)

- Na loss by loop diuretics stimulate ENaC in CD, that leads to absorption of Na and loss of K, thus making hypokalemia a common side effect.
- Hypocalcemia though can be seen is not as common, because GIT compensates by increasing Ca absorption.

23. Ans. (a) Acetazolamide

(Ref: Goodman Gilman 12th E/P680)

24. Ans. (a) Thiazides

(Ref: Goodman Gilman 12th E/P689)

- Thiazides cause hypercalcemia and hence cannot be used or treatment of same.
- Loop diuretics cause hypocalcemia and can be used for treatment of hypercalcemia.
- Calcitonin prevents bone resorption and decrease serum calcium level and hence applied for treatment of hypercalcemia.

25. Ans. (a) Thiazides

(Ref: Goodman Gilman 12th E/P670)

- Thiazides decrease calcium excretion and hence used for treatment of renal stones associated with hypercalciuria.

26. Ans. (c) Desmopressin

(Ref: Goodman Gilman 12th E/P712)

Desmopressin is the Drug of Choice for

- Central or neurogenic DI
- Von Willebrand's disease type I
- Hemophilia A
- Nocturnal enuresis

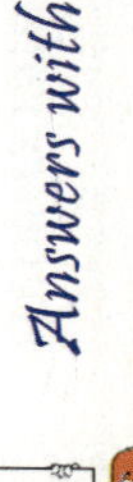

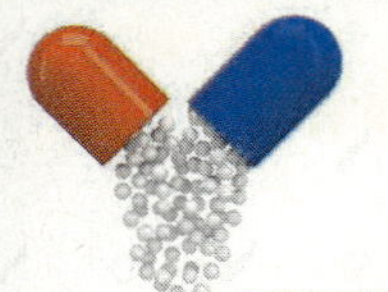

27. Ans. (b) Structural resemblance to sulfonamides

(Ref: Goodman Gilman 12th E/P678)

Sulfonamide Derivative Diuretics

- **CA inhibitors**
- Loop diuretics (except ethacrynic acid)
- Thiazides

28. Ans. (a) Metolazone

(Ref: Goodman Gilman 12th E/P689)

- Thiazides being moderate diuretics are ineffective if GFR is below 30 mL/min, with the exception of indapamide and metolazone.
- Both can be used along with loop diuretics in renal failure when loop diuretics alone are ineffective.

29. Ans. (a) Hypercalcemia

(Ref: Goodman Gilman 12th E/P686)

Side effects of Loop Diuretics

Hyperlipidemia	Hypokalemia
Hyperglycemia	Hypomagnesemia
Hyperuricemia	Hypocalcemia

30. Ans. (d) Hypertonic saline

(Ref: Harrison 19th E/P2282)

- 3% hypertonic saline is the treatment of choice for SIADH.
- Drug of choice are vaptans currently, but demeclocycline can also be used.

31. Ans. (a) Amiloride

(Ref: Goodman Gilman 12th E/P692)

32. Ans. (b) Noncompetetitive reversible inhibitors

(Ref: Goodman Gilman 12th E/P678)

33. Ans. (a) Spironolactone

(Ref: Goodman Gilman 12th E/P694)

- Spironolactone can inhibit androgen receptors and cause gynecomastia and impotence.

34. Ans. (d) Bumetanide

(Ref: Goodman Gilman 12th E/P692)

- All loop diuretics except bumetanide and thiazides except indapamide have weak CA inhibiting action.

35. Ans. (b) Increased calcium excretion

(Ref: Goodman Gilman 12th E/P689)

36. Ans. (c) Gynecomastia

(Ref: Goodman Gilman 12th E/P695)

- Aldosterone antagonist, spironolactone is also androgen antagonist and hence causes gynecomastia.
- Thus, it cannot be used in gynecomastia.

37. Ans. (b) Electrogenic Na^+ channels

(Ref: Goodman Gilman 12th E/P690)

- Amiloride inhibit ENaC, which are electrogenic as Na influx depolarizes the luminal membrane, which leads to activation of K and H ATPase pumps in CD.

38. Ans. (b) Desmopressin

(Ref: Goodman Gilman 12th E/P712)

39. Ans. (b) Nephrogenic diabetes insipidus

(Ref: Goodman Gilman 12th E/P712)

40. Ans. (a) Hypercalciuria

(Ref: Goodman Gilman 12th E/P689)

41. Ans. (b) Inhibit prostacyclin synthesis

(Ref: Goodman Gilman 12th E/P685)

- Furosemide inhibits prostaglandin synthesis which is responsible for vasodilatation and partly for solute loss.
- Hence NSAIDs by inhibiting prostaglandin synthesis blunt both these effects.

42. Ans. (b) Thiazide

(Ref: Goodman Gilman 12th E/P683)

- Na^+ -K^+- $2Cl^-$ symporter is inhibited by loop diuretics like furosemide, bumetanide, torsemide and ethacrynic acid.
- Organic mercurial compounds like mersalyl are also inhibitors of Na^+ -K^+- $2Cl^-$ symporter, but not used currently due to toxicity.

43. Ans. (c) Spironolactone

(Ref: Goodman Gilman 12th E/P694)

- In case of cirrhotic ascites, aldosterone level is high and hence spironolactone is preferred.

44. Ans. (b) Aldosterone receptor

(Ref: Goodman Gilman 12th E/P692)

Potassium Sparing Diuretics Act On

- Aldosterone receptor
- ENaC

45. Ans. (c) Ethacrynic acid

(Ref: Goodman Gilman 12th E/P686)

- Loop diuretics can cause ototoxicity when used by rapid IV route and is mostly reversible.
- Maximum ototoxicity is associated with ethacrynic acid.

46. Ans. (a) Eplerenone

(Ref: Goodman Gilman 12th E/P690)

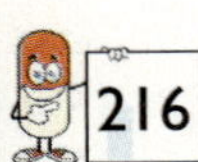

Aldosterone Antagonists

- Eplerenone
- Spironolactone

47. Ans. (b) Spironolactone

(Ref: KDT 7th E/P588)

- Spironolactone is metabolized into its active components like canrenone.
- Canrenone is also used as a drug along with its prodrug canrenoate.

48. Ans. (c) Cirrhosis

(Ref: Goodman Gilman 12th E/P680)

- Acetazolamide is contraindicated in liver cirrhosis, as it causes retention of ammonia and can increase chances of encephalopathy.

49. Ans. (d) Acidosis

(Ref: Goodman Gilman 12th E/P685)

50. Ans. (a) Hypoglycemia

(Ref: Goodman Gilman 12th E/P689)

- Thiazides cause hyperglycemia due to inhibition of insulin release.

51. Ans. (d) Pulmonary hypertension

(Ref: Goodman Gilman 12th E/P686)

Uses of Furosemide

- Pulmonary edema
- Cerebral edema
- Edema associated with CKD and liver cirrhosis
- Hypertensive emergency
- Hypertension with renal failure
- Hypercalcemia
- Hyponatremia (Along with hypertonic saline)
- Hyperkalemia

52. Ans. (d) Pregnancy induced hypertension

(Ref: Goodman Gilman 12th E/P690)

- Labetalol is the current drug of choice in pregnancy induced hypertension.
- In low renin hypertension ACEI/ARB and beta blockers are not effective and hence CCB and thiazide diuretics are first line. In elderly hypertensives renin level is low and hence again same drugs are preferred.

53. Ans. (a) Decrease GFR

(Ref: Goodman Gilman 12th E/P680)

54. Ans. (a) Cirrhotic edema

(Ref: KDT 7th E/P588)

55. Ans. (d) Metabolic acidosis

(Ref: Goodman Gilman 12th E/P680)

56. Ans. (a) Acetazolamide, (b) Topiramate and (c) Thiazide

(Ref: Goodman Gilman 13th E/P

Drugs inhibiting carbonic anhydrase

- Acetazolamide/Brinzolamide/Dorzolamide
- Topiramate/Zonisamide
- Thiazides except indapamide
- Loop diuretics except bumetanide

57. Ans. (a) Acetazolamide, (d) Topiramate

(Ref: Goodman Gilman 12th edition, Page 677)

58. Ans. (b) Contraindicated in congestive heart failure, (c) Causes hyperkalemia, (d) Increases renal blood flow

(Ref: Goodman Gilman 12th edition, Page 681)

Osmotic diuretics have major action on the loop of Henle followed by proximal convoluted tubules

59. Ans. (a) Diabetes insipidus, (c) Hemophilia A, (d) von Willebrand's disease

(Ref: Goodman Gilman 12th E/P712)

60. Ans. (c) Increase calcium excretion in urine

(Ref: Goodman Gilman 12th E/P689)

- Thiazides cause decrease calcium absorption and hence used for treatment of calcium renal stones associated with hypercalciuria.
- They act in DCT by inhibiting Na/Cl cotransporter.
- Hyperglycemia is caused by a decrease in insulin release.
- Hyperuricemia is caused by competitive inhibition of UA excretion in PCT.

61. Ans. (a) Spironolactone, (c) Eplerenone

(Ref: Goodman Gilman 12th E/P692)

- Spironolactone and eplerenone are mineralocorticoid receptor antagonist.
- Amiloride and triamterene are ENaC inhibitors.

62. Ans. (a) Thiazide, (c) Amphotericin B, (e) Insulin

(Ref: Goodman Gilman 12th E/P687)

Drugs Causing Hypokalemia

- Beta 2 agonists
- Alpha blockers
- Insulin
- Theophylline/Caffeine
- B_{12}/Folic acid
- Amphotericin B
- Diuretics except K sparing ones
  - CA inhibitors

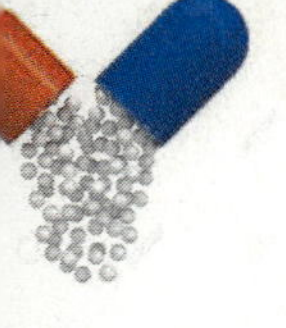

- Loops
- Thiazides
- Osmotic diuretics

❒ Penicillin

❒ Fludrocortisone

63. Ans. (a) Brinzolamide, (c) Bumtenide, (e) Acetazolamide

(Ref: Goodman Gilman 12th E/P680)

Diuretics not used in Sulfonamide Allergy, as they are Sulfonamide Derivatives are

❒ CA Inhibitors

❒ Loop diuretics except ethacrynic acid

❒ Thiazides

64. Ans. (b) Inhibition of Na^+-K^+-2 Cl^- cotransport

(Ref: Goodman Gilman 12th E/P684)

65. Ans. (a) Sulfonamide hypersensitivity, (d) Containdicated in metabolic acidosis, (e) COPD

(Ref: Goodman Gilman 12th E/P680)

66. Ans. (d) Eplerenone

(Ref: Goodman Gilman 13th E/P456)

67. Ans. (c) Acetazolamide

(Ref: Goodman Gilman 12th edition, Page 680)

Carbonic anhydrase inhibitors can cause hyperammonemia and hence can cause hepatic encephalopathy. Thus these drugs are contraindicated in cirrhosis.

68. Ans. (c) Terlipressin is more effective than desmopressin in DI

(Ref: Katzung 12th edition, Page 303)

❒ Thiazides are effective both in central and nephrogenic diabetes insipidus. Being diuretic still they are effective in diabetes insipidus because by increasing water loss, thiazides cause compensatory reabsorption of solute and water in the proximal convoluted tubule (PCT).

❒ Desmopressin is not effective in nephrogenic diabetes insipidus as for it to be effective the V2 receptors must be free and functional.

❒ Terlipressin is a vasopressin analog which is more selective for V1 receptors and hence causes vasoconstriction. Thus, it is used for treatment of acute variceal bleeding and not diabetes insipidus.

❒ Amiloride prevents absorption of lithium in the collecting duct and hence is the drug of choice for treatment of lithium induced diabetes insipidus.

69. Ans. (a) Metolazone

(Ref: Goodman Gilman 12th E/P689)

70. Ans. (a) Acetazolamide

(Ref: Goodman Gilman 12th E/P680)

71. Ans. (d) Metabolic acidosis

(Ref: Goodman Gilman 12th E/P689)

72. Ans. (a) Acetazolamide

(Ref: Goodman Gilman 12th E/P680)

73. Ans. (d) All of the above

(Ref: Goodman Gilman 12th E/P681)

74. Ans. (a) Na abnormal blockage

(Ref: Goodman Gilman 12th E/P696)

75. Ans. (a) Demeclocycline

(Ref: Goodman Gilman 12th E/P711)

76. Ans. (c) Ascending loop

(Ref: Goodman Gilman 12th E/P682)

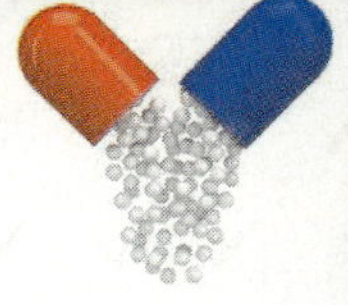

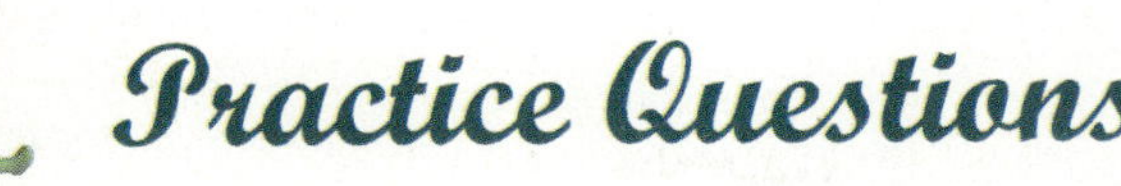

Practice Questions

77. Thiazides induced hyperglycemia is because of

a. Hyperglycemia
b. Hypokalemia
c. Hyperuricemia
d. Alkalosis

Ans. (b) Hypokalemia

(Ref: Goodman Gilman 12th E/P689)

- Hypokalemia caused by thiazides decreases insulin release by beta islet cells due to a secondary decrease in intracellular calcium.

78. The diuretic used in dural ectasia is

a. Furosemide
b. Chlorthalidone
c. Acetazolamide
d. Mannitol

Ans. (c) Acetazolamide

(Ref: Goodman Gilman 12th E/P680)

79. GFR is not altered by

a. Furosemide
b. Thiazides
c. Spironolactone
d. Acetazolamide

Ans. (c) Spironolactone

(Ref: Goodman Gilman 12th E/P96)

80. Rolofylline has diuretic action by acting on

a. PCT
b. DCT
c. Cortical CD
d. TAL

Ans. (a) PCT

(Ref: Katzung 8th E/P258)

- Rolofylline is an adenosine receptors antagonist, which acts by decreasing effect of Na/H exchanger in the PCT.

81. Which of the following is not a sulfonamide derivative?

a. Acetazolamide
b. Dorzolamide
c. Ethacrynic acid
d. Brinzolamide

Ans. (c) Ethacrynic acid

(Ref: Goodman Gilman 12th E/P689)

- All CA inhibitors are sulfonamide derivatives except ethacrynic acid and bumetanide.
- Loop diuretics and thiazides are also sulfonamide derivatives.

82. Which of the following diuretic is contraindicated in active cranial hemorrhage?

a. Mannitol
b. Furosemide
c. Thiazides
d. Spironolactone

Ans. (a) Mannitol

(Ref: Goodman Gilman 12th E/P682)

83. Osmotic diuretics can cause all except

a. Hypernatremia
b. Hyponatremia
c. Both
d. None

Ans. (c) Both

(Ref: Goodman Gilman 12th E/P682)

- Osmotic diuretics can withdraw water from cells and increase plasma volume causing hyponatremia.
- Excessive use of osmotic diuresis can decrease plasma volume causing hypernatremia.
- So both can be seen.

84. Thiazide that does not inhibit CA is

a. Indapamide
b. Metolazone
c. Chlorthalidone
d. Chlorothiazide

Ans. (a) Indapamide

(Ref: Goodman Gilman 12th E/P584)

- All thiazides are CA inhibitors except Indapamide.

85. Antihypertensive associated with maximum incidence of erectile dysfunction is

a. Beta blockers
b. Thiazides
c. ACEIs
d. CCBs

Ans. (b) Thiazides

(Ref: Goodman Gilman 12th E/P689)

- Thiazides cause maximum erectile dysfunction followed by beta blockers.

86. Which of the following diuretic is contraindicated in cirrhosis?

a. Spironolactone
b. Amiloride
c. Thiazide
d. Furosemide

Ans. (b) Amiloride

(Ref: Goodman Gilman 12th E/P682)

- In cirrhosis folic acid deficiency can be seen. Hence amiloride as contraindicated as it can also cause folic acid deficiency.

NOTES

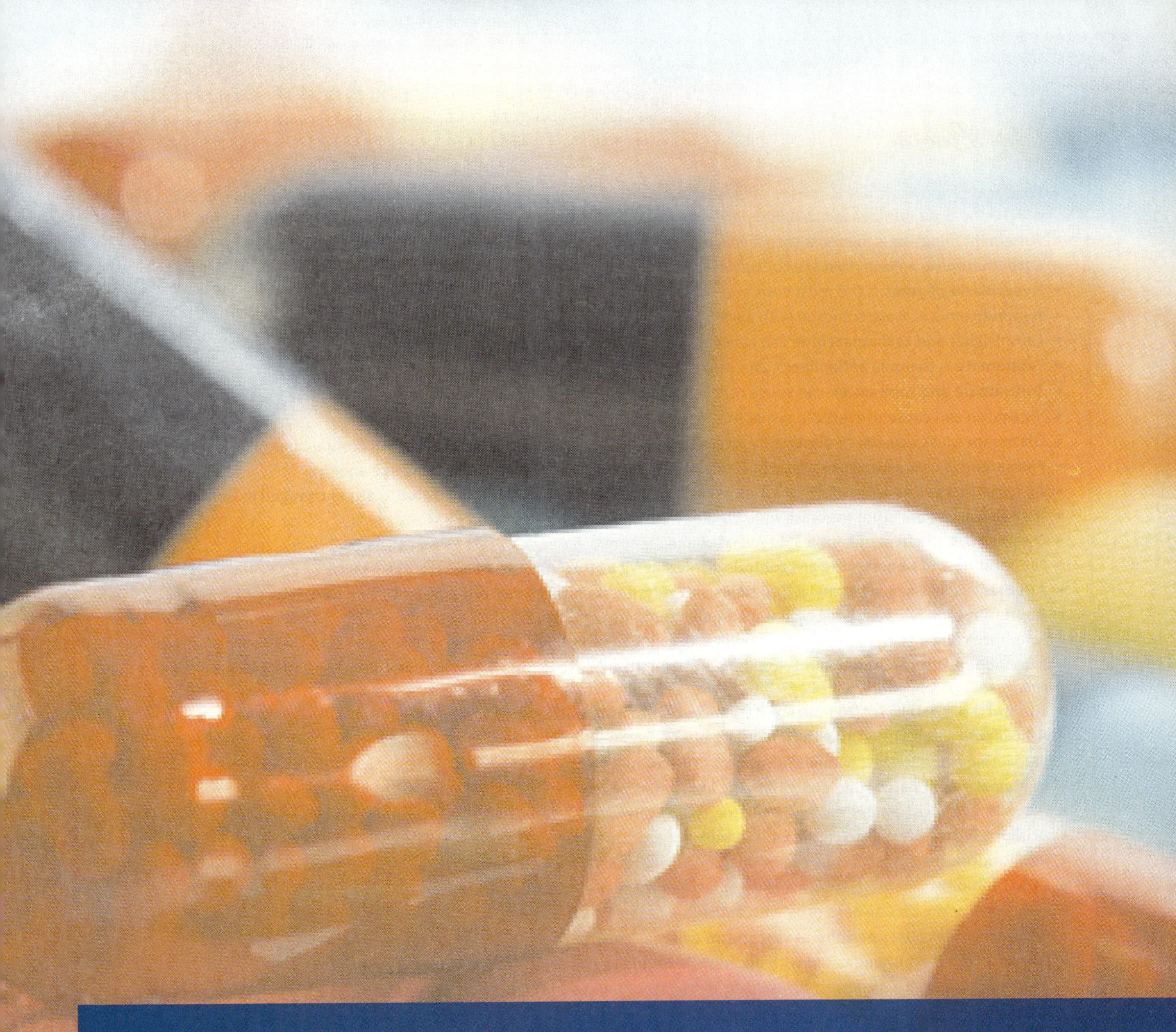

Central Nervous System

One Liners

- Folic acid prophylactically is started at least **one month** before planned pregnancy at a dose of **400 μg/day**; in case of history of NTD the dose is increased to **4,000** μg/day.
- **Fulminant hepatitis** is the most severe side effect whereas nausea and vomiting are the most common side effect of valproate.
- **Carbamazepine > Phenytoin** are contraindicated in myoclonic seizures.
- **Hyperplasia of gums** is the most common side effect of phenytoin.
- **Hyponatremia** is more common with oxcarbazepine than carbamazepine and more common in elderly.
- **Lamotrigine and carbamazepine** can cause Steven Johnson syndrome.
- **Topiramate** is the only antiepileptic and molindone is the only antipsychotic to cause weight loss.
- **Zonisamide and topiramate** can cause renal stones by inhibiting carbonic anhydrase.
- Vigabatrin can cause irreversible visual field defects.
- **Diazepam** causes **coronary dilation** by increasing adenosine and **midazolam** decreases cerebral blood flow.
- **Flumazenil** is benzodiazepine antagonist whereas β-**carboline** is benzodiazepine inverse agonist.
- All barbiturates are completely metabolized except **phenobarbital**, which is excreted 1/4th unchanged in urine.
- **Ramelteon** is a melatonin agonist with **2% bioavailability** and 2 hours of half-life.
- **Dysphoria** is an effect of **kappa** subtype of opioid receptor.
- **Meperidine** and **pentazocine** are **contraindicated in MI** as they can cause tachycardia.
- **Alfentanil** is 20 times, **fentanyl** is 100 times and **sufentanil** is 1000 times more potent than morphine.
- **Buprenorphine** is a partial agonist at μ and antagonist at k receptor.
- Tolerance can be seen to all effects of opioids except **constipation**, **convulsion** and **miosis**.
- **Methadone, buprenorphine and clonidine** are used to decrease withdrawal symptoms whereas **naltrexone** is used to prevent relapse in opioid deaddiction.
- **Lithium** has a half-life of **24 hours** and it should be **discontinued 24 hours before surgery**.
- **Amoxapine** is the only TCA with D_2 blocking effect.
- **Fluoxetine** is the longest acting SSRI whereas **fluvoxamine** is the shortest acting SSRI.
- **Venlafaxine** and **paroxetine** are commonly associated with withdrawal symptoms on discontinuation.
- **Paroxetine** is most potent enzyme inhibitor, is only teratogenic SSRI and causes maximum erectile dysfunction.
- **Aripiprazole** is only antipsychotic with D_2 partial agonistic effect.
- **Penfluridol** is the longest acting oral antipsychotic whereas **haloperidol decanoate** is the longest acting injectable antipsychotic.
- **COMT inhibitors** increase bioavailability of levodopa and are drug of choice for on-off phenomena.
- Only anti-Parkinson's disease drug with antioxidant effect is **selegiline**.
- **Bromocriptine** causes **peripheral vasospasm** whereas cabergoline and pergolide cause cardiac valve fibrosis.
- **Ondansetron** is contraindicated with **apomorphine** due to risk of severe hypotension.
- **Anticholinergics** are preferred for mild to moderate whereas **memantine** is preferred for moderate to severe Alzheimer's disease.
- Only drugs approved by FDA for ALS are **riluzole** and **edaravone**.
- Maximum decrease in EDSS is caused by **mitoxantrone** followed by **natalizumab**.
- **Natalizumab** can cause progressive multifocal **leukoencephalopathy**.

ANTIEPILEPTICS

Abnormal excessive firing of a group of neurons in central nervous system (CNS) leads to an event called as **seizure**. If these seizures are repetitive due to a chronic underlying pathology, then it is called as **epilepsy**. Epilepsy can be broadly classified into **generalized** and **partial epilepsy**, both having distinct pathophysiology as well as management strategy. The aim in treatment of epilepsy is to prevent attacks of seizure and for that antiepileptics are continued for at least **2 years** of complete seizure free period. However, in case of **JME** and **post infarction seizures**, there is a high risk of relapse after stopping drug and hence **lifelong treatment** is required.

GENERALIZED EPILEPSY

- Spontaneous firing of **T type calcium channels** in thalamus generates an action potential that depolarizes the cortical neurons. The activated cortical neurons when depolarized start firing and generate an action potential that is propagated to the spinal cord by **sodium channels**
- This leads to generalized contraction of muscles in the body and leads to an epilepsy called as **GTCS or grand mal epilepsy**
- Similar mechanisms lead to other generalized epilepsies like **myoclonic, tonic, atonic and absence seizures**

- Thus, the cause for most of generalized epilepsy is Ca^{++} followed by Na^{+}, except **absence seizure** in which cortex is not involved and only Ca^{++} channels are responsible
- Hence, the **first line drugs for all generalized seizures are Ca^{++} channel blockers and Na^{+} channel blockers**, whereas for **absence seizure only Ca^{++} channel blockers** are effective.

PARTIAL SEIZURE

- The cause of a partial seizure lies in the cortex itself and it is a **space occupying lesion (SOL)** like NCC, tumor or gliosis caused by an infarct or trauma
- This SOL depolarizes the nearby neurons in the cortex, which generate an action potential and propagate by **Na^{+} channel** opening. This action potential moves to a segment in spinal cord and depolarizes a group of muscle represented by the SOL in cortex. This is called as partial seizure
- Since the primary cause of partial epilepsy is **Na^{+} channels, the blockers of the same are first line drugs**.

CLASSIFICATION OF ANTIEPILEPTICS

Apart from **blocking Na^{+} and Ca^{++} channels**, the primary cause for epilepsy, the other ways to block the action potential propagating down is by **opening K^{+} channels, increasing effect of inhibitory neurotransmitter GABA and decreasing effect of excitatory neurotransmitter glutamate**. Thus, this gives us **five classes** of antiepileptics currently available.

Conceptual Box-1

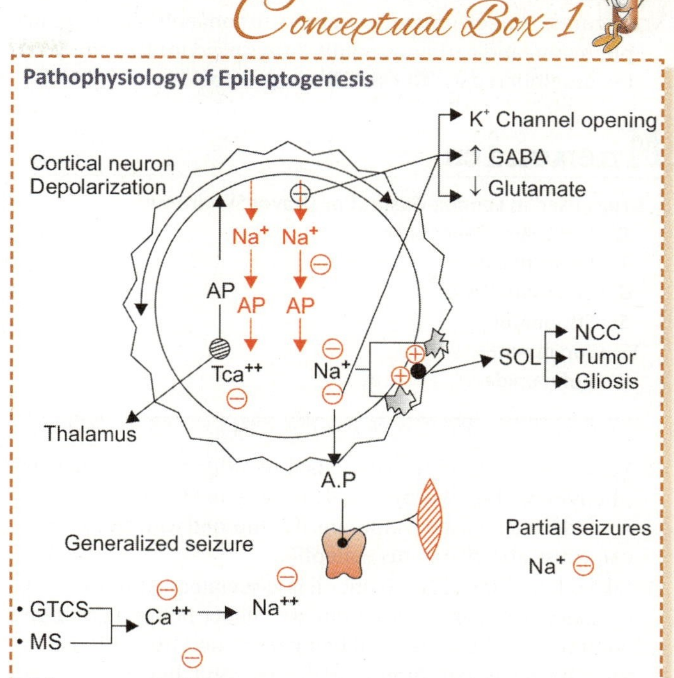

Classification of Antiepileptic Drugs

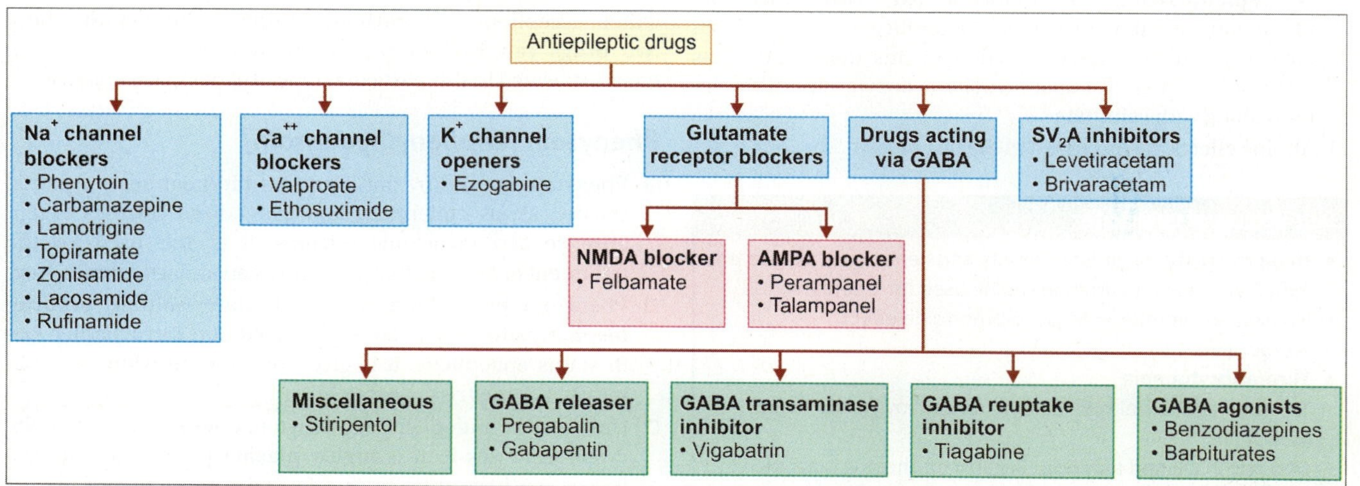

Calcium Channel Blockers

Valproate

- Valproate is the widest spectrum antiepileptic, as apart from blocking Ca^{++} channels it also blocks **Na^{+} channels** and **increases GABA** by stimulating synthesis and inhibiting metabolism. It is an **inhibitor of histone deacetylase** as well, which might contribute to its antiepileptic effect.
- It is the drug of choice for the treatment of **generalized seizures like GTCS, myoclonic (JME), tonic, atonic, clonic and absence seizures**. Though, it is contraindicated for absence seizure in children less than 2 years due to hepatotoxicity. It is also drug of choice for the treatment of **rheumatic chorea, Lennox-Gastaut syndrome** and **rapid cyclers in bipolar disorder**. For Lennox-Gastaut syndrome **ketogenic diet** is also prescribed. For prophylaxis of migraine and partial seizure it can be used as a second line drug.

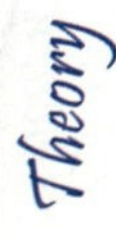

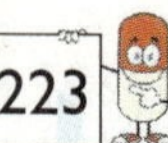

- Lennox-Gastaut syndrome is a childhood multi-seizure syndrome characterized by **cluster** of different types of seizures. The seizures are refractory to conventional drugs like phenytoin and carbamazepine. Drugs used for treatment can be remembered as **"CLUSTER"** as given below.

Mnemonics

Drugs used in Lennox-Gastaut or Dravet Syndrome

- **C** : Clobazam, Cannabidiol
- **L** : Lamotrigine
- **U** : Valproate (DOC)
- **S** : Stiripentol
- **TE** : TopiramatE
- **R** : Rufinamide

- Valproate can inhibit metabolism of other antiepileptics like phenytoin, phenobarbital and lamotrigine; hence their doses should be decreased. Valproate, if combined with clonazepam can cause absence status epilepticus.
- Like other older antiepileptics it is associated with wide range of toxicity. The most common side effect being nausea and vomiting and the most fatal being fulminant hepatitis. Neural tube defect is commonly associated and hence folic acid prophylactically is started at least **1 month** before planned pregnancy at a dose of **400 µg/day**; in case of history of neural tube defect (NTD) the dose is increased to **4,000** µg/day.
- Valproate is metabolized by CYP_{450} enzymes into a minor metabolite **2-propyl-4-pentenoic acid (4-ene-VPA) which is hepatotoxic**.Enzyme inducers like **carbamazepine**, phenytoin and phenobarbital can induce the microsomal enzymes and increase production of this metabolite. This increases the risk of hepatotoxicity if enzyme inducers are used along with valproate.
- All side effects are discussed in the box below.

Side effects of valproate

- **Hepatotoxicity:** Most fatal toxicity and hence contraindicated in below 2 years. L carnitine can be used for treatment.
- **Nausea and vomiting:** Most common side effect
- **Tremor (Fine)**
- **Thrombocytopenia**
- **Teratogenic:** Neural tube defect and cardiovascular defect associated
- **Obesity, PCOS and alopecia:** Because of these it is avoided in migraine prophylaxis in females
- **Pancreatitis**
- **Hyperammonemia.**

- Valproate is contraindicated in children less than 2 years and in pregnancy. However, if a female being pregnant is already on an antiepileptic drug, the **drug is never changed** because switching of drug can precipitate seizure. In case of valproate the drug is **continued along with therapeutic drug monitoring (TDM)** to lessen the teratogenic effect.

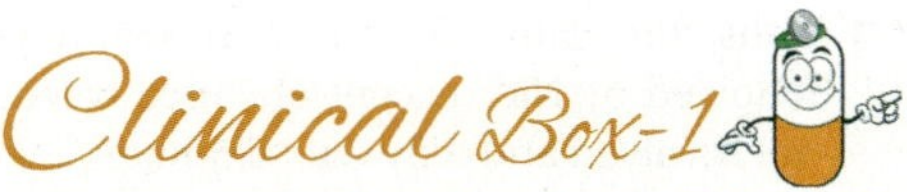

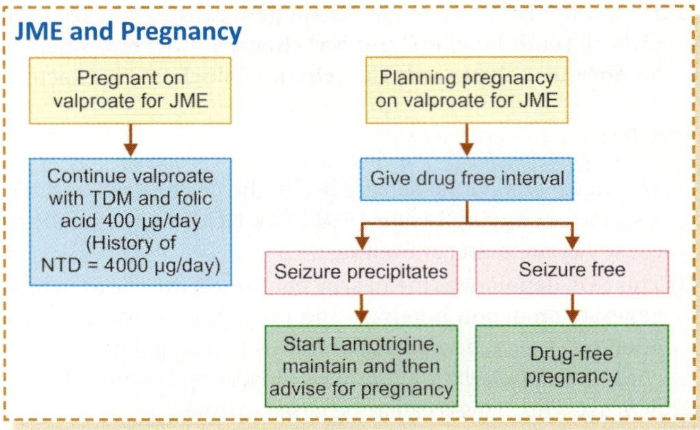

Ethosuximide

- Ethosuximide is only a Ca^{++} channel blocker without any other effect. Hence, it is used **only or treatment of absence seizure** and is drug of choice in children less than 2 years.
- Most common side effect is nausea and vomiting; other associated are neurotoxicity, bone marrow suppression or pancytopenia, rash, systemic lupus erythematosus (SLE) and parkinsonism.

Sodium Channel Blockers

As discussed earlier Na^{+} channel blocker is effective in partial seizures and all generalized seizures except absence seizure. Other exceptions are **carbamazepine** > **Phenytoin**; these two drugs can **worsen myoclonic seizures** and hence are contraindicated in this particular type of generalized epilepsy.

Phenytoin (Diphenylhydantoin)

- Phenytoin is used by oral route for the treatment of partial seizure, status epilepticus and generalized seizures except absence and myoclonic seizures. It is also used for the treatment of neuropathic pain and as an antiarrhythmic drug.
- Phenytoin being lipid soluble, a **water-soluble prodrug fosphenytoin** has been synthesized for **intravenous use** in status epilepticus. It is given by **slow infusion**, as rapid infusion carries risk of asystole.
- Unlike other antiepileptics phenytoin **does not depress CNS**, rather activates it. It is **highly plasma protein bound** and hence can have drug interaction with other highly plasma protein bound drugs like **valproate**. It is metabolized in liver by CYP2C9.
- Phenytoin follows zero order kinetics and hence with a slight change of dose the chances of acute toxicity are high. Phenytoin is one of the most commonly used antiepileptic drug and hence its side effects can be frequently seen.
- **Hyperplasia of gums is the most common side effect associated**. **Hirsutism** and **acne are** common in young females. CNS side effects like ataxia and diplopia are

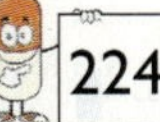

incompatible with normal life and hence in this case TDM is done to adjust dose. The therapeutic range of phenytoin is **10–20 µg/mL**. However, if nystagmus is seen it is compatible with normal life and dose is not altered. **Rash** can also be seen with phenytoin, which on rechallenge appears on the **first day** itself due to immunological memory. Lymphadenopathy is associated with a reduced IgA and it resembles Hodgkin's lymphoma.

- Phenytoin causes abnormal metabolism of vitamin D and causes hypocalcemia. Being enzyme inducer, it induces metabolism of vitamin K and decreased vitamin K decreases bone matrix synthesis. Together this results in severe softening of bone or **osteomalacia**.
- Phenytoin inhibits folic acid absorption by inhibition enzyme deconjugase in intestine and hence cause **megaloblastic anemia**. Intestinal deconjugase is also inhibited by primidone and barbiturates.
- Teratogenic effect that can be seen is called as **fetal hydantoin syndrome** which encompasses **facial cleft**, **microcephaly**, **IUGR**, **hypertelorism** and **triphalangeal thumb**. Fetal hydantoin syndrome can be seen with carbamazepine as well. Phenytoin decreases vitamin K and associated coagulating factors and hence can cause **hemorrhagic disease of newborns**. Hence, **vitamin K, 10 mg/day** is given prophylactically to all pregnant females on enzyme inducing antiepileptics like phenytoin and carbamazepine in the last month of pregnancy.

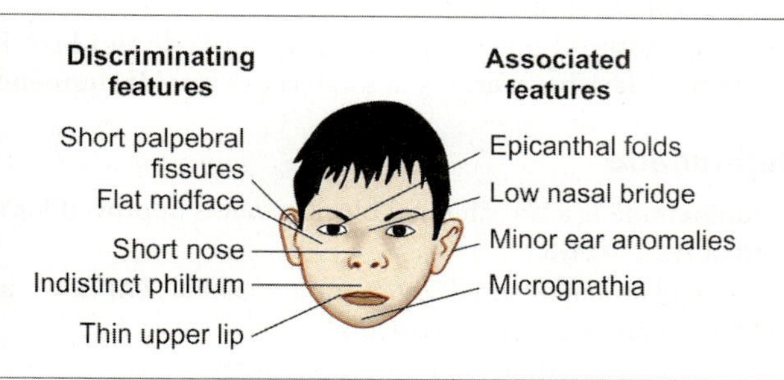

Fetal Hydantoin Syndrome

Side effects of phenytoin

H : **H**irsutism, **H**yperplasia of gums, **H**yperglycemia
Y : L**Y**mphadenopathy with reduced IgA
D : **D**iplopia, Vitamin D metabolism abnormality (Hypocalcemia)
A : **A**taxia, **A**trophy of cerebellum (Acute toxic dose)
N : **N**ystagmus
T : **T**eratogenic (Fetal hydantoin syndrome)
O : **O**steomalacia
I : **I**nduces metabolism of vitamin K = Decreased vitamin K = Decreased coagulation factors and bone matrix synthesis = Hemorrhagic disease of newborn
N : **N**eutropenia and anemia (megaloblastic)

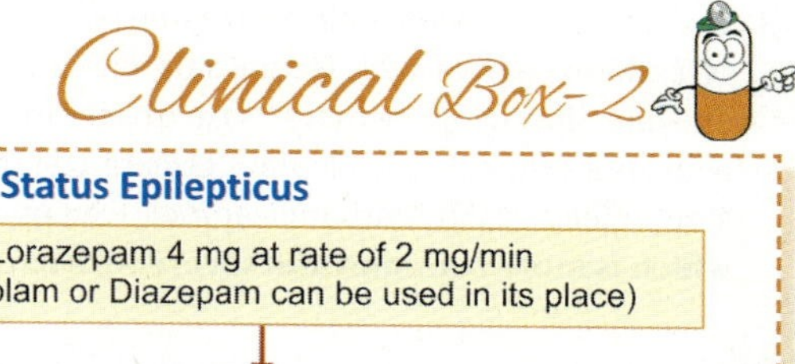

Treatment of Status Epilepticus

Lorazepam 4 mg at rate of 2 mg/min
(Midazolam or Diazepam can be used in its place)

↓

Phenytoin or Valproate or Levetiracetam 20 mg/kg

↓ NR

Phenobarbital 10–20 mg/kg

↓ NR

Propofol 1–2 mg/kg bolus followed by 2–15 mg/kg/hr
Or
Pentobarbital 15 mg/kg bolus followed by 0.5 mg/kg/hr

Carbamazepine

Carbamazepine is the drug of choice for the treatment of **partial seizures** and can be used in generalized seizures except myoclonic and absence seizures. It is also drug of choice for **trigeminal and glossopharyngeal neuralgia** and used as a second-line drug in **BPD**.

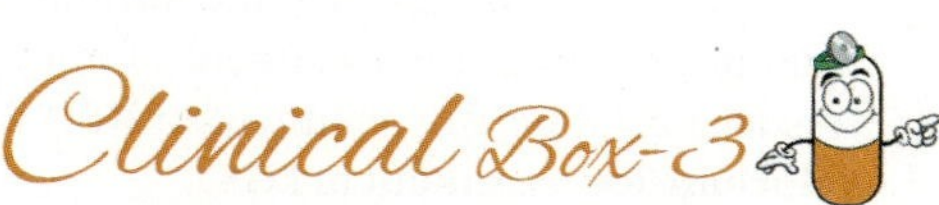

Drugs used in Trigeminal Neuralgia

- Carbamazepine (DOC) > Oxcarbazepine (Not FDA approved)
- Phenytoin
- Topiramate
- Lamotrigine
- Baclofen
- Gabapentin

- Carbamazepine follows first order kinetics and hence acute toxicity is rarely seen. Central nervous system (CNS) side effects like ataxia and diplopia if seen, **TDM is done to adjust dose**.
- **Agranulocytosis** is the gravest side effect seen and hence is contraindicated with clozapine, as it can also cause agranulocytosis.
- Hypersensitivity reaction like SJS, lymphadenopathy and splenomegaly can be seen. Unlike phenytoin which cause megaloblastic anemia, carbamazepine causes **aplastic anemia**. The risk of Steven Johnson's syndrome with carbamazepine and phenytoin is higher in Asians carrying ***HLA B1502*** gene and Caucasians carrying ***HLA A3101*** gene.
- **Dilutional hyponatremia** due to syndrome of inappropriate antidiuretic hormone secretion (SIADH) is a **delayed side effect** seen particularly in **elderly patients**.

- Oxcarbazepine and eslicarbazepine are recent congeners of carbamazepine with better side effect profile and lesser enzyme inducing activity. Oxcarbazepine is a prodrug activated into eslicarbazepine. Oxcarbazepine causes lesser side effects than carbamazepine, except **hyponatremia, which is more common and severe with oxcarbazepine**.

Mnemonics

Carbamazepine Side Effects

H : Hyponatremia, Hepatotoxic
E : Eosinophilia
A : Agranulocytosis, Ataxia, Aplastic anemia
D : Diplopia
S : SJS, Splenomegaly

Lamotrigine

- Lamotrigine is also a wide spectrum antiepileptic as apart from **blocking Na$^+$ channels**, it also **inhibits Ca^{++} channels** and **decreases release of glutamate**.
- Lamotrigine is approved by FDA and is a first-line drug for treatment of partial seizure and all types of generalized epilepsy except absence seizure, where it is used off label. Since it is the **least teratogenic antiepileptic drug**, it is the drug of choice for the treatment of **epilepsy in pregnancy**. It is also used for the treatment of **BPD** and **preferred after valproate for treatment of LGS**.
- Side effects associated are **SJS**, nausea and vomiting and CNS side effects like diplopia and ataxia. To prevent the fatal side effect, i.e. SJS, lamotrigine should be **started at low doses**. Since it is started at low doses it cannot be used in emergency conditions.
- Valproate inhibits metabolism of lamotrigine and hence the dose of lamotrigine should be decreased if both drugs are combined.

Topiramate

- Topiramate is also a wide spectrum antiepileptic as apart from blocking **Na$^+$ channels**, it also **opens K$^+$ channels**, **stimulates GABA$_A$ receptors** and **inhibits glutamate receptors (AMPA, Kainate)**.
- Topiramate is used for the treatment of all types of partial and generalized epilepsy except absence seizure. It is also used for treatment of **BPD**, **prophylaxis of migraine** and treatment of **LGS**. As it inhibits carbonic anhydrase it can be used for the treatment of **pseudotumor cerebri (idiopathic intracranial hypertension)**.
- Side effects associated are **weight loss**, taste change, speech or language problem and memory loss. Carbonic anhydrase inhibition can cause nephrolithiasis, metabolic acidosis and hypohidrosis. Bilateral acute secondary **angle closure glaucoma** can be seen with topiramate and hence an **ophthalmological examination** should be done prior starting this drug.

Recent Advances

Topiramate + Phentermine: This combination has been approved recently for the treatment of obesity.

Zonisamide

- Zonisamide is not only a **Na$^+$ channel blocker**, but also a **Ca^{++} channel blocker**. It is a **free radical scavenger** and thus prevention of free radical damage to neurons, might contribute to its antiepileptic effect.
- It is approved as an add on drug only for the treatment of **partial seizures**.
- Like topiramate it also inhibits **carbonic anhydrase** and can cause **renal stones, metabolic acidosis** and hypohidrosis. Thus, serum bicarbonate levels should be monitored to prevent acidosis.

Lacosamide

- Lacosamide is a derivative of amino acid L-serine approved for the treatment of **partial seizures** in adults. Route of administration is both oral and intravenous.
- Lacosamide is the only Na$^+$ channel blocker which acts by enhancing **slow inactivation of sodium channels**; all other Na$^+$ channel blockers act by enhancing fast inactivation. It also binds to collapsing response mediator protein-2, though its significance is not known yet.
- It can cause PR interval prolongation in ECG and FDA has issued a black box warning as it can cause **suicidal tendency**.

Rufinamide

- Rufinamide is a Na$^+$ channel blocker that is approved for the treatment of **LGS**.
- Metabolism sponsored by nonmicrosomal enzymes and hence there is no drug interaction.
- It can cause QT shortening and leukopenia.

Potassium Channel Opener

- The only approved drug in this class is called as **ezogabine**, that has been approved in 2012 as an add on drug for the treatment of partial seizures.
- It is associated with side effects like **blue skin/lip and nail pigmentation**, QT prolongation, retinal abnormalities and tremor.
- Because of the ocular side effect, ophthalmological examination should be done every 6 months.

Glutamate Receptor Blockers

NMDA Inhibitor

- Felbamate apart from antagonizing NMDA is also though to act via GABA.
- Tonicclonic It can be used for the treatment of partial and generalized tonic-clonic seizures and LGS but is not preferred due to side effects like aplastic anemia and hepatotoxicity.
- It can also cause weight loss and insomnia.

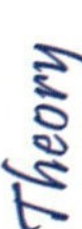

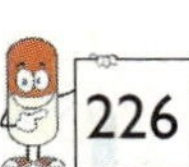

AMPA Inhibitors

- AMPA inhibitor class was approved by FDA in 2012 as an add on class for the treatment of **partial seizures**. The drugs approved in this class are **perampanel** and **telampanel**.
- These drugs are more effective inhibitors of seizure propagation than generation. Both drugs are metabolized by microsomal enzymes and hence drug interaction can take place.
- Side effects associated are somnolence, weight gain and mood abnormality.

Drugs Acting on GABA

Pregabalin and Gabapentin

- Both drugs act by binding to the $\alpha_2\delta1$ subunit of presynaptic calcium channels and preventing its endocytosis. Persistence of calcium channels increase **exocytosis of GABA into the synapse**.
- The drugs are approved for the treatment of **partial seizure** and are first-line drugs for **peripheral neuropathy**.
- Gabapentin is also approved for **prophylaxis of migraine**, treatment of **BPD, phobia** and **GAD**.
- Side effects associated with gabapentin are **weight gain** and edema. Both these drugs are not metabolized and **excreted unchanged in urine**.
- Since these are not metabolized, they **do not have any interaction with other antiepileptic drugs**.

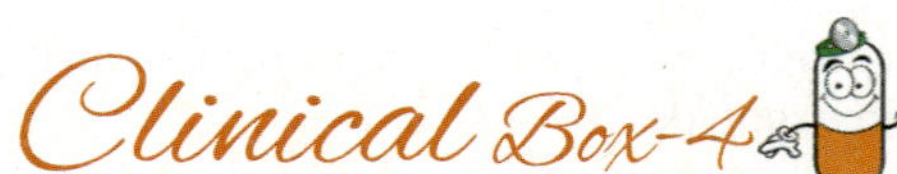

First-Line Drugs for the Treatment of Peripheral Neuropathy

- Pregabalin and Gabapentin
- TCA (Nortriptyline)
- SNRI (Duloxetine)

Tiagabine

- Tiagabine inhibits reuptake of GABA by inhibiting transporter GAT-1 and hence increases GABA in the synapse
- It is approved as an add-on drug or **partial seizure** treatment
- It causes seizure in a nonepileptic patient and psychosis.

Vigabatrin

- Vigabatrin is a GABA analog that causes **irreversible inhibition of GABA transaminase** the enzyme that metabolizes GABA.
- It is used in **refractory partial seizures** and is drug of choice for treatment of **infantile spasm associated with tuberous sclerosis**, because in this case ACTH is not effective.
- Hence, otherwise ACTH is the drug of choice for treatment of infantile spasm, because vigabatrin is associated with **irreversible visual field defects.**
- Since vigabatrin is excreted unchanged by kidney, dose modification is essential in renal failure.

Ganaxolone

Ganaxolone is a $GABA_A$ agonist that can be used for treatment of partial seizure and infantile spasm. It is under trial for migraine prophylaxis.

Stiripentol

- Stiripentol acts by increasing GABA (inhibits reuptake and metabolism of GABA) and by $GABA_A$ receptor agonism like barbiturates.
- It is an orphan drug to be used in patients of Dravet syndrome as an add-on to drugs like valproate and clobazam. Valproate is the drug of choice in Dravet syndrome.
- Being **enzyme inhibitor,** it can interact with other drugs metabolized by microsomal enzymes.
- Side effects associated are anorexia, insomnia and weight loss.

$GABA_A$ Agonists

- $GABA_A$ agonists like benzodiazepine and barbiturates are discussed in detail in the topic of sedative and hypnotics.
- **Lorazepam** is the first drug of choice for treatment of **status epilepticus and alcohol withdrawal seizures.**
- **Rectal diazepam** is the drug of choice both for **treatment** and **prophylaxis of febrile seizures.**
- **Phenobarbital** is the drug of choice for **seizures in neonates.**
- **Clobazam** can be used for **LGS** and **clonazepam** is indicated in **myoclonic, absence seizures and infantile spasm** and **clorazepate** for **partial seizures.**
- Clonazepam can be used by intranasal route also for acute repetitive seizures (ARS) or **crescendo seizures.**

Table 1: Therapeutic Range of Commonly used Antiepileptic Drugs

Antiepileptic drug	Normal therapeutic range in µg/mL
Clonazepam	0.01–0.07
Lamotrigine	2–7
Carbamazepine	4–12
Primidone	5–12
Phenytoin	10–20
Phenobarbital	15–40
Levetiracetam	15–45
Valproate	50–100
Ethosuximide	50–100

Miscellaneous Drugs

Levetiracetam

- Levetiracetam is an inhibitor of synaptic vesicular protein SV_2A subtype and it also blocks N type calcium channels.
- It is approved for treatment of **partial seizure, GTCS** and **myoclonic seizures (JME)**. It can also be used for treatment of status epilepticus and levodopa induced dyskinesia.
- Side effects associated are anemia, leucopenia and mood changes. Since it is less teratogenic, it **can be used in pregnancy** as well.

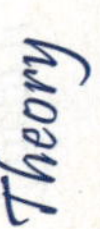

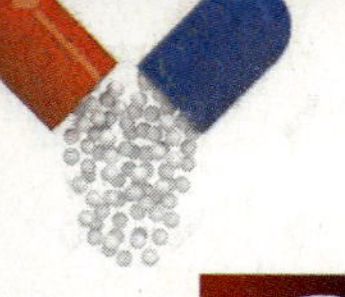

Recent Advances

Brivaracetam is an SV2A inhibitor recently approved for treatment of partial seizure. It also blocks sodium channels.

ACTH and Corticosteroids

These are the drug of choice for treatment of **infantile spasm**.

Recent Advances

Cannabidiol: It is a cannabinoid recently approved for treatment of **LGS or Dravet syndrome** in children more than 2 years of age. Its mechanism of action is not known. Liver function test is done prior to drug therapy as it is hepatotoxic.

SEDATIVE HYPNOTICS

A sedative drug has calming effect on the patient that **decreases anxiety** and a hypnotic drug is one that **facilitates sleep**. The first sedative hypnotic to be used was **bromide**. That followed discovery and use of various other drugs like $GABA_A$ agonists, melatonin agonists, chloral hydrate, meprobamate, etc.

$GABA_A$ RECEPTOR MODULATORS

- GABA receptors are of three subtypes, i.e. **A, B and C**. The A subtype is a chloride ion channel, that cause hyperpolarization of neurons and relaxation and hence the sedative and hypnotic effect. The B subtype is a G_i subtype of GPCR that decreases cyclic AMP and opens K^+ channels in the spinal cord neurons and facilitates **muscle relaxation**. The C subtype is also chloride ion channel receptor located in the retina, pituitary, spinal cord and superior colliculus.
- The $GABA_A$ receptor is a pentameric structure made up of three protein subunits, i.e. α, β and γ. α **subunit** is most important and is common site for action of all drugs, as this subunit closes the lumen.
- GABA binds to its site located in between α and β subunits and forces α subunit to withdraw the part closing the lumen, thereby opening the chloride ion channel. The $GABA_A$ agonists like **muscimol** and **gaboxadol** and antagonists like **bicuculline**, **gabazine** and **picrotoxin** are used as experimental drugs. **Alcohol** is also an agonist at $GABA_A$ receptors.
- α subunit is further sub classified into α_1 and α_2 subtypes; α_1 is primarily responsible for **sedation and hypnosis** and α_2 for other effects like muscle relaxation and antiepileptic effect.
- **Barbiturates** bind to subunits and modulate GABA effect by **increasing the duration of chloride channel opening**. In presence of barbiturate GABA can open chloride ion channels for more duration.
- **Benzodiazepines** bind to a site in between α and γ subunit and modulate GABA effect by **increasing the frequency of chloride channel opening**. In presence of benzodiazepines GABA opens chloride ion channels for more number of times.
- Thus, benzodiazepines and barbiturates facilitate opening of chloride ion channel opening by GABA and hence are known as **GABA facilitating agents**. However, at high doses barbiturates have **GABA mimetic effect** as well.

GABA	Alpha and beta
Benzodiazepine	Alpha and gamma
Barbiturates	Beta
Z compounds	$Alpha_1$

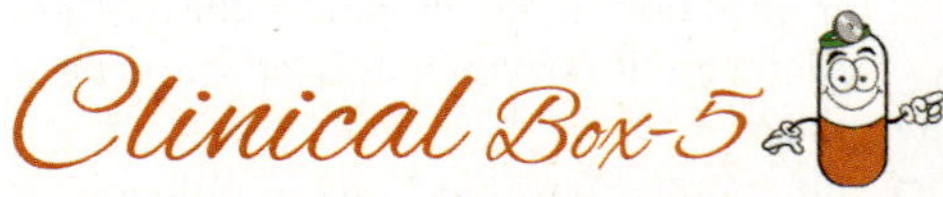

$GABA_A$ Receptor

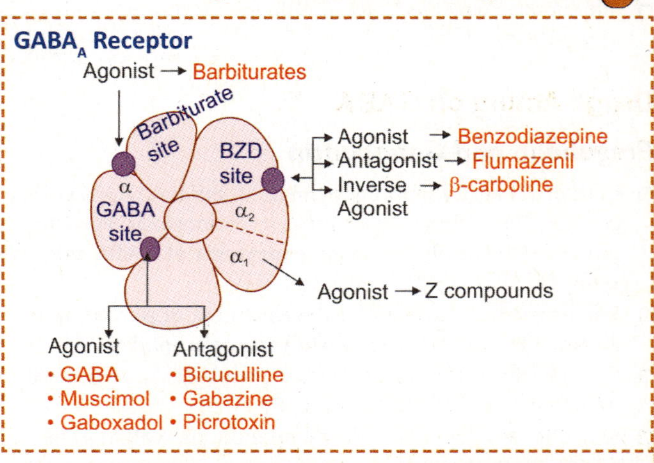

Benzodiazepines

Classification

Benzodiazepine can be classified based on their metabolism into three subtypes.

Table 2: Classification of Benzodiazepine

Class I	Class II	Class III
Metabolized by • Phase I - CYP3A4 • Phase II – Glucunronidation	Metabolized by • Phase I – CYP3A4 • Phase II – Fast glucuronidation	Metabolized by • Only Phase II – Direct glucuronidation
Long-acting	**Ultrashort-acting**	**Short-acting**
• **Minimum dependence and withdrawal symptoms** as it is inversely proportional to duration of action • **Maximum duration of sedation and amnesia**	Maximum dependence and withdrawal symptoms	**Safest in liver failure** because of direct glucuronidation
Metabolites after phase I are active compounds	Metabolites after phase I are active compounds	Metabolites after phase II are inactive compounds
Diazepam Clonazepam Clorazepate Flurazepam Quazepam	**Midazolam (overall shortest acting)** **Triazolam (Best in insomnia)**	Lorazepam Temazepam Oxazepam Estazolam

Effects and Uses of Benzodiazepines

- **Hypnosis:** The short and shortest acting drugs available by oral route like **quazepam, triazolam, temazepam, flurazepam and estazolam** are used for treatment of insomnia. **Triazolam is the best benzodiazepine for insomnia** because of its fast onset, adequate effect without any residual effect, though in some patients it can cause early morning insomnia. Benzodiazepines **increase duration of NREM stage 2 sleep** and decrease duration of all other NREM stages and REM, though the number of REM cycles is increased.
- **Sedation:** Oral Diazepam, lorazepam, oxazepam, alprazolam and clorazepate are used for treatment of **anxiety disorders**.
- **Muscle relaxation: Diazepam** is used as a muscle relaxant in muscle spastic disorder like multiple sclerosis.
- **Antiepileptic effect:** The antiepileptic uses of benzodiazepines have been discussed in previous topic.
- **Anterograde amnesia:** Intravenous or intramuscular **diazepam, lorazepam and midazolam** are used as preanesthetic medications.
- **Anticraving effect:** Long-acting benzodiazepines like **diazepam, clorazepate and chlordiazepoxide** are used in alcohol dependence. Intravenous benzodiazepines like **lorazepam and diazepam** are preferred for treatment of acute alcohol withdrawal syndrome.
- **Acute mania:** Clonazepam is used as an adjunct to atypical antipsychotics and lithium for treatment of acute mania.
- **Analgesic effect: Intrathecal midazolam** can be used for postoperative pain relief.
- **Miscellaneous effects: Diazepam** causes **coronary dilation** by increasing adenosine and **midazolam** decreases cerebral blood flow.
- **Flunitrazepam** is a tasteless benzodiazepine abused for **date rape**. It is abused by drug abusers as well and is known as **"roofie"**.

Side Effects of Benzodiazepines

- CNS depression presents as confusion, anterograde amnesia, ataxia and over sedation.
- Flurazepam is associated with night mares and triazolam can cause abnormal behavioral symptoms.
- A paradoxical side effect of benzodiazepines is **seizure worsening** seen in some patients.

Table 3: Benzodiazepine Withdrawal Symptoms

• Nightmares • Insomnia • Dysphoria • Sweating • Tremor • Anorexia • Dizziness

Flumazenil

- **Flumazenil** is a benzodiazepine antagonist used for treatment of **benzodiazepine and Z compounds toxicity only**. It also antagonizes the effect of **benzodiazepine inverse agonist called as beta carboline**.
- 0.2 mg is administered by slow intravenous route over 30–60 seconds and gradually increased up to a total **maximal dose of 5 mg**. The duration of action lasts for **30–60 minutes, i.e. average of 45 minutes**.
- Flumazenil though is of no use in alcohol or barbiturate poisoning because their site of action is different.

Z Compounds

- Z compounds are selective agonist at α_1 **subunit** of the $GABA_A$ receptors and hence associated **only with sedative and hypnotic effect**. These drugs are associated with **lesser dependence and CNS depression** as compared to benzodiazepines. REM is less affected with these drugs and hence are better than benzodiazepines in insomnia.
- **Zaleplon** is the shortest acting and hence drug of choice for **sleep induction in insomnia and jet lag.**
- Zolpidem is intermediate acting and used for short-term treatment of insomnia.
- **Eszopiclone** is longest acting and hence is drug of choice for **sleep maintenance in insomnia and is also preferred for long-term treatment of insomnia**.
- Toxicity of these compounds can be treated by flumazenil.

Barbiturates

Barbiturates are derived from barbituric acid, which is made up of **urea** and **malonic acid**.

Mechanism of Action

- Apart from modulating $GABA_A$ receptors as described earlier, barbiturates also **inhibit glutamate receptors of AMPA subtype** and at high doses have **GABA mimetic action,** i.e. act on GABA site and open chloride ion channels.
- Because of this multiplicity of site of action barbiturates are **highly unsafe at high doses** and hence not preferred as sedative hypnotics nowadays.

Classification of Barbiturates

Barbiturates are classified based on duration of action into ultra-short, short and long-acting.

Table 4: Classification of Barbiturates

Ultrashort-acting	Short-acting barbiturates	Long-acting barbiturates
• Thiopental • Methohexital	• Butobarbital • Secobarbital • Pentobarbital	• Phenobarbital • Mephobarbital

Uses of Barbiturates

- Short-acting barbiturates like secobarbital, butobarbital and pentobarbital are used for preoperative sedation and insomnia.
- Thiopental and methohexital are ultrashort-acting due to their high lipid solubility that causes **redistribution**. These are used as intravenous anesthetic agents.
- Phenobarbital and mephobarbital are used for seizure disorders and day time sedation. Phenobarbital is the drug of

choice for treatment of **seizures in neonates** and is also used for treatment of status epilepticus.

- Phenobarbital being an enzyme inducer is also used for treatment of **Crigler-Najjar syndrome type II.**

Side Effects of Barbiturates

- All the barbiturates are completely metabolized in liver by CYP_{450} enzymes followed by glucuronidation and then excretion by kidney and hence elderly are more prone to toxicity due to impaired liver function. **Phenobarbital** is not completely metabolized, and **1/4th part is excreted unchanged in urine**.
- CNS side effects and **paradoxical seizures** can be seen with barbiturates just like benzodiazepines, except it can additionally cause euphoria.
- Barbiturates block autonomic ganglion and hence can cause vasodilatation and **hypotension** in case of toxicity.
- Being enzyme inducers barbiturates can increase activity of ALA synthase and precipitate **acute intermittent porphyria**.
- Barbiturates can also cause hyperalgesia.

Barbiturate Toxicity

- The patient can develop shock with oliguria and hence hypovolemia should be corrected.
- Phenobarbital toxicity can be treated by **urine alkalization**.
- **Picrotoxin** can be given until the **pupillary reflex normalizes**.

MELATONIN AGONISTS

Melatonin is synthesized in the pineal gland in response to darkness. Melatonin then acts on MT_1 and MT_2 receptors in the hypothalamus and induces sleep and maintains circadian rhythm.

Conceptual Box-2

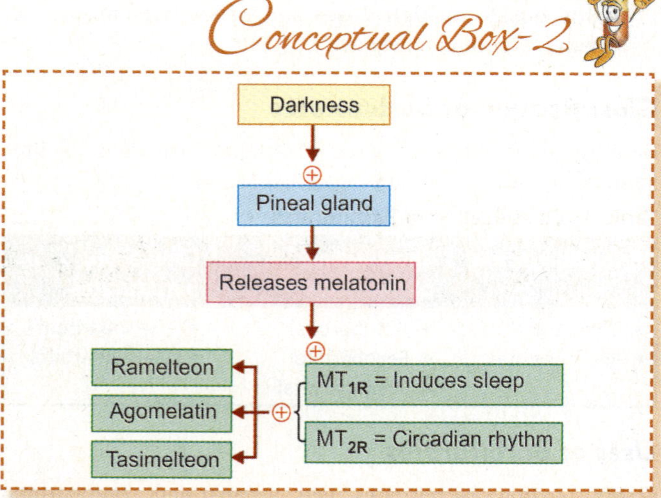

Ramelteon

- **Ramelteon** is a melatonin agonist approved for sleep induction in insomnia and jet lag taken at a dose of 8 mg half an hour before sleep.
- Good oral absorption is followed by a high first pass metabolism and hence the **bioavailability is just 2%**, but enough to induce sleep. It has a half-life of 2 hours and plasma protein binding of 80%.
- The best part is **tolerance and withdrawal symptoms are not seen** as with benzodiazepines or Z compounds, but are less efficacious.

Recent Advances

Agomelatine: It is a recent melatonin agonist approved for treatment of major depressive disorder.
Tasimelton: It is a recent melatonin agonist approved for treatment of sleep-awake disorder in blinds.

CHLORAL HYDRATE

Chloral hydrate is metabolized into trichloroethanol, which has modulatory effect on $GABA_A$ receptors. It can be used for treatment of paradoxical seizures associated with benzodiazepines. It was a drug of abuse to make people unconscious by adding to alcohol to make **Mickey Finn cocktail** and is also known as **knock out drops**.

MEPROBAMATE

Meprobamate is a drug with properties like benzodiazepines. It is used as an anxiolytic. **Carisoprodol is a prodrug of meprobamate** used as a muscle relaxant. These drugs are associated with abuse potential and meprobamate can cause gastric bezoars.

SUVOREXANT

- **Suvorexant** is an inhibitor of **orexin 1 and 2 receptors**; since orexins produce wakefulness by acting on these receptors, inhibition produces sedation.
- It can worsen depression and cause suicidal tendency.

OPIOIDS

RECEPTORS

The opioid receptors are primarily of 3 subtypes, i.e. μ, k and δ. The effects produced by each of these receptors are given.

Table 5: Effects Produced by Opioid Receptors

μ	k	δ
M : Miosis U : Urine retention S : Sedation C : Constipation A : Analgesia R : Respiratory depression I : Increased muscle rigidity N : No bile flow (Oddi contraction) E : Euphoria	C: Constipation A: Analgesia P: psychotomimetic effect = **Dysphoria**	Analgesia Increases release of • Prolactin • Somatostatin • Cortisol • Testosterone • GH

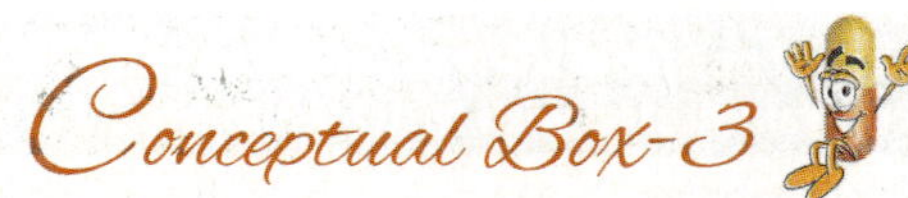

Analgesic Effect of Opioids

Opioids produce analgesic effect by acting on μ receptors, which inhibit presynaptic calcium channels and inhibit nociceptive NT release. In post synaptic membrane opioids open K^+ channels and hyperpolarize it thereby blunting action potential.

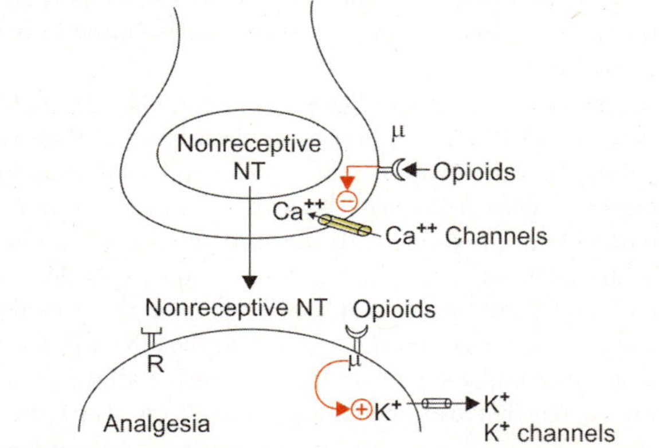

ENDOGENOUS OPIOIDS

These receptors given above are acted upon by endogenous opioids like **endorphins, enkephalins and dynorphins**, which are most potent at δ, μ and k receptors respectively.

EXOGENOUS OPIOIDS

Exogenous opioids can be classified based on source and opioid receptor interaction.

Classification Based on Source

Based on source opioids can be sub classified as natural, semisynthetic and purely synthetic opioids.

Table 6: Classification of Exogenous Opioids

Natural	Semisynthetic	Synthetic
• Morphine • Codeine • Thebaine • Papaverine • Noscapine	• Heroin (Diacetyl morphine) • Apomorphine • Etorphine • Oxycodone • Hydrocodone • Buprenorphine	• Fentanyl • Alfentanil • Sufentanil • Methadone

- The natural opioids also known as opiates are derived from poppy plant *Papaver somniferum*. The maximum content in the plant is that of **morphine** followed by others like noscapine, codeine, thebaine and papaverine.
- **Papaverine lacks opioid activity** and is used as smooth muscle relaxant in GIT, urethral and biliary colic.
- **Apomorphine** is a morphine derivative without any opioid effect, rather it is agonist at D_1 and D_2 receptors and is used in Parkinsonism.
- **Heroin** is a more potent opioid than morphine and is primarily a substance of abuse.
- **Codeine** and noscapine are used as antitussives. Codeine is also used as an analgesic alone or along with NSAIDs. It is a prodrug metabolized partially (10%) by CYP2D6 to morphine which produces analgesic effect, whereas rest 90% is inactivated by glucuronidation and CYP3A4 and is not responsible for analgesic effect. Codeine is the opioid with least plasma protein binding of less than 10% followed by morphine with 33%.
- **Oxycodone** and **hydrocodone** are used as analgesics and combined with NSAIDs for treatment of mild to moderate pain.

Classification Based on Opioid Receptor Interaction

Based on interaction of opioids with it receptors, they can be classified as full agonists, mixed agonist antagonists and pure antagonists.

Full Agonists

The full agonist class contains opioids like morphine, pethidine, methadone, codeine, tramadol, loperamide, etc.

Morphine

- Morphine is used by **both oral and parenteral route** as an **analgesic in labor, terminally ill cancer patients** and **myocardial infarction**. In **pulmonary edema** it is effective by decreasing both preload and afterload. As an antitussive it is used for **severe persistent cough associated with bronchial cancer**.
- Morphine is **metabolized in liver** to an active metabolite excreted by kidney. Hence, the dose should be decreased both in renal and liver failure. It has a half-life of 2 hours, but the effect can be seen up to **24 hours** due to a long-acting active metabolite.
- It is contraindicated in patients with **head injury** as it can raise the intra cranial tension and interfere with assessment of patient outcome by causing miosis. It is also to be **avoided in bronchospastic disorders** as it can release histamine and cause bronchoconstriction. It can cause contraction of sphincter of Oddi and hence contraindicated in **biliary colic**.
- There are some common effects of opioids apart from the receptor effect described earlier.

Effects of morphine and related opioids

- **Nausea and vomiting:** Due to stimulation of CTZ area and vestibular component as well.
- **Muscle rigidity:** Muscle tone is increased at high doses.
- **Temperature:** μ receptor causes hyperthermia, whereas k receptor causes hypothermia.
- **ICT:** Opioids cause hypoventilation that increases CO_2 in plasma which causes vasodilation and increases cerebral blood flow.
- **CVS:** Opioids cause bradycardia except pethidine and pentazocine which cause tachycardia.
- **GIT:** Constipation and contraction of sphincter of Oddi.
- **Blood Pressure:** Hypotension due to histamine release and depression of vasomotor centre, except pentazocine which increases blood pressure.
- **Bronchoconstriction:** Due to histamine release and hence opioids are avoided in bronchial asthma and COPD.

Contd...

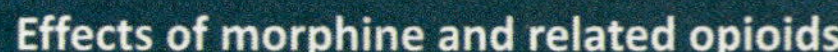

Effects of morphine and related opioids

- **Pruritus:** Due to histamine release.
- **Immunomodulatory action**
- **Respiratory depression:** Neonates are more prone to respiratory depression due to immature blood brain barrier.
- **Bladder:** Inhibits voiding reflex and increases tone of external sphincter
- **Sphincter of Oddi contraction**: Opioids are contraindicated in biliary colic.

Meperidine (Pethidine)

- **Meperidine** is drug of choice for treatment of **postanesthetic chills** and infusion related chills associated with drugs like amphotericin-B and monoclonal antibodies. It is used only for **acute analgesia in obstetrics (labor pain)**, postsurgical patients, migraine, etc. with a maximum duration of use being **48 hours** due to risk of toxicity. In postanesthetic chills it is effective by acting on α_2 receptors.
- Meperidine is 10 times less potent than morphine, but onset of analgesia is faster. Side effects like constipation and urine retention are less common with meperidine as compared to morphine. Unlike other opioids meperidine causes **mydriasis and tachycardia** due to anticholinergic effect.
- Meperidine is metabolized in liver by hydrolysis and N-demethylation into meperidinic acid and normeperidine. Normeperidine further undergoes hydrolysis into normeperidinic acid. Out of these metabolites only **normeperidine** is active and long-acting, which can cause **neurotoxicity in the form of seizures**, tremors, hallucinations and mydriasis on accumulation.
- MAO inhibitors interfere with meperidine metabolism by inhibiting hydrolysis and hence increase amount of **normeperidine** and its toxicity and hence **MAO inhibitors are contraindicated**. Meperidine inhibits serotonin reuptake and MAO inhibits serotonin metabolism and hence **serotonin syndrome** is another complication that can be seen.

Conceptual Box-4

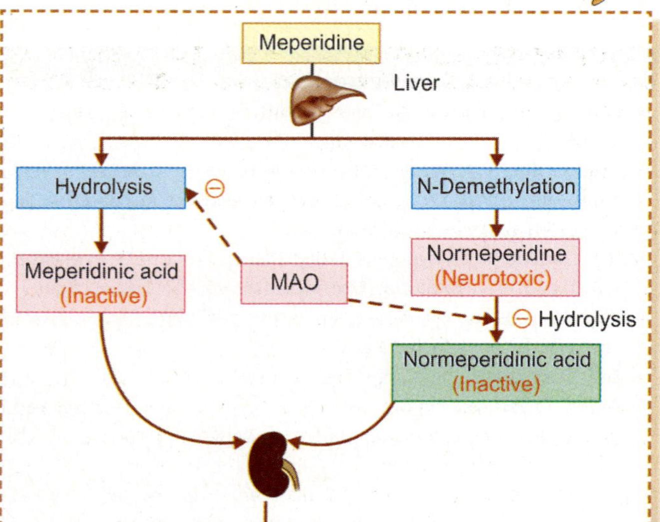

Opioid or opioid derivatives that Inhibit 5HT reuptake and contraindicated with MAO inhibitors

- Meperidine
- Tramadol
- Dextromethorphan
- Tapentadol

- Since meperidine is metabolized by liver and excreted by kidney, the duration of action and toxicity increases in both renal and liver failure. Hence, it is **contraindicated in liver and renal failure**.
- **Loperamide** and **diphenoxylate** are meperidine derivatives with weak opioid effect and used for treatment of **diarrhea**. Loperamide is the drug of choice for treatment of **diarrhea associated with IBS** and **anticancer drug irinotecan**. Loperamide is combined with **simethicone** for treatment of diarrhea and flatulence simultaneously. Loperamide does not cross blood brain barrier and hence has no abuse potential. Diphenoxylate crosses blood brain barrier, has abuse potential and hence formulated with atropine to prevent abuse; patient will not abuse due to anticholinergic side effects of atropine.

Methadone

- Methadone is a racemic mixture of enantiomers with the R isomer producing primary effect. It is used for treatment of **chronic pain** and to **decrease withdrawal symptoms in opioid addicts**.
- Methadone is sequestrated into tissues and slowly eliminated and hence does not cause acute withdrawal on discontinuation, as it is slowly eliminated.
- Methadone can be given by oral, IM, SC and IV routes. It is **rapidly absorbed by oral route within 30 minutes**. The time for onset of analgesia seen after these routes is given in Table.

Table 7: Time for Onset of Analgesia

Route of methadone	Time for onset of analgesia
Parenteral	10–20 minutes
Oral	30–60 minutes

- Side effects are like other opioids, with the exception of **QT prolongation** and anticholinergic effects seen with methadone.

Levorphanol

- Levorphanol is an opioid used primarily as an analgesic. Apart from opioid receptors agonism, it also inhibits reuptake of norepinephrine and serotonin and inhibits NMDA receptors.
- Its D-isomer **dextromethorphan** has no effect on opioid receptors, rather is an NMDA antagonist and used as **antitussive**. Dextromethorphan is a poor antitussive as compared to opioids.

Tramadol

- Tramadol is used for the treatment of **mild to moderate pain** as it is a weak opioid agonist.

- It has been derived from codeine and apart from opioid action, it also **inhibits reuptake of 5HT and NE** that contributes to analgesic effect.
- **Tapentadol** is similar in all ways to tramadol.

Fentanyl

- **Fentanyl is 100** times more potent than morphine. It is used along with droperidol in neuroleptic analgesia and anesthesia. Fentanyl together with pentazocine is used for sequential analgesic anesthesia.
- Fentanyl and sufentanil are the fastest acting opioids used in anesthesia. These opioids are highly lipid soluble opioids and hence effect is seen faster.

Table 8: Uses of Fentanyl by Different Routes

• Epidural • Spinal • Intravenous	• Analgesics in anesthesia
• Transdermal patch	• Chronic pain
• Buccal tablets • Buccal films • Lozenges	• Acute pain

- It causes maximum muscle rigidity and is associated with "wooden chest syndrome". Seizures can also be seen with fentanyl.

Alfentanil

- **Alfentanil is 20 times** more potent than morphine.
- It is combined with propofol intotal intravenous anesthesia (TIVA) for day care surgery.

Sufentanil

- **Sufentanil** is **1,000 times** more potent than morphine. It is the opioid with maximum potency and plasma protein binding.
- It is the drug of choice to prevent stress response to laryngoscopy and intubation.

Remifentanil

- Remifentanil has **fastest onset of effect and recovery** and hence is the opioid of choice in day care surgery.
- As it is metabolized by plasma esterase it is the **shortest acting** opioid and hence given by continuous intravenous infusion.
- It is not used in spinal analgesia as its formulation contains an inhibitory neurotransmitter glycine.

Mixed Agonist Antagonists

- This class contains drugs like dezocine, nalbuphine and butorphanol which are agonist at k receptor and antagonist at μ receptor, whereas **pentazocine is also an agonist at kappa receptor but partial agonist/antagonist at μ receptor**. Buprenorphine is a partial agonist at μ receptor and antagonist at k receptor.

Mnemonics

Mixed Agonist Antagonists

Do : Dezocine
Not : Nalbuphine
Mix : Agonist antagonists
Pani with : Pentazocine
Bodka : Butorphanol, Buprenorphine

- The logic behind synthesizing such a class of drug was that analgesic effect can be achieved by stimulating any of the opioid receptors, but μ antagonism along with it will minus the related side effects like respiratory depression. Hence these are **more benign analgesics with lesser side effects**.
- **Pentazocine** is used as an analgesic, preanesthetic medication and along with fentanyl in sequential opioid anesthesia. Unlike other opioids it causes an **increase in BP and tachycardia**.
- **Nalbuphine** is used only as an analgesic and can be used in MI as it is cardio stable.
- **Butorphanol** can be used for treatment of postoperative pain and migraine. In migraine it can be given by **intranasal route** for prompt relief.
- **Buprenorphine** is used as an **analgesic** by intramuscular route and in **opioid dependence to decrease withdrawal symptoms** by sublingual route. It is used only for treatment of mild to moderate pain due to **ceiling effect,** i.e. analgesic effect does not increase with increasing dose. For opioid dependence it is combined with **naloxone** to prevent abuse. Buprenorphine is around **50 times more potent than morphine**. It slowly dissociates from μ receptor and hence has prolonged effect; because of slow dissociation **naloxone is ineffective in antagonizing its effect**. For same reason it is gradually cleared off the body and hence withdrawal symptoms are mild after discontinuation.

Pure Opioid Antagonists

Naloxone, nalmefene and naltrexone are centrally acting antagonists at **all opioid receptors** with nalmefene being more selective for mu receptors. Methyl naltrexone and alvimopan are quaternary compounds which do not cross blood brain barrier and hence **antagonise only mu receptors** in the periphery.

- **Naloxone** is the shortest acting and **nalmefene** is intermediate acting antagonist used by **intravenous route** for treatment of opioid poisoning or toxicity. **Naloxone** being shortest acting is the **drug of choice**; it reverses all effects completely **except sedation**. Naloxone is also used for treatment of respiratory depression in neonates due to opioids; but is **contraindicated if the mother was dependent on opioids** as it can precipitate withdrawal symptoms in neonates. Naloxone by inhibiting opioid action cause tachypnea (overshoot phenomenon) and by releasing catecholamines causes hypertension, arrhythmia and pulmonary edema.

- **Naltrexone** is **more potent and longer acting** than naloxone and nalmefene; it is used by **oral route** for **relapse** prevention in **opioid and alcohol dependence**. It is also used for treatment of **obesity** in combination with **bupropion**. It is used along with morphine to prevent abuse. High doses can cause **hepatic necrosis** and hence is contraindicated in patients with liver dysfunction.
- **Naloxegol**, **methylnaltrexone** being peripherally acting mu antagonists, are used for treatment of opioid associated **constipation**. Alvimopan is approved for treatment of **postoperative ileus**.

Recent Advances

Naldemedine is a recently approved opioid antagonist for the treatment of opioid associated constipation.

OPIOID ADDICTION

Tolerance

- Abusers consume opioids or euphoric effect, but due to tolerance gradually a higher dose of opioid is required to produce same euphoric effect.
- Thus, by the time addicts decide to leave opioid they are on a high dose.
- Tolerance can be seen to all effects of opioids except **constipation**, **convulsion** and **miosis**.

Withdrawal Symptoms

- Abrupt discontinuation of opioids leads to withdrawal symptoms. The severity of withdrawal symptoms is directly proportional to dose and potency of opioid.
- As discussed intolerance addicts are on a high dose. The opioid of abuse like heroin is a very potent opioid. Hence, these patients end up developing severe withdrawal symptoms.

Mnemonics

P Withdrawal Symptoms

W-M : Mydriasis
I : Increased yawning, piloerection
T : Temperature increased
H : Hyperventilation
D : Diarrhea
R : Rhinorrhea
A : Anxiety
W-M : Myalgia
L : Lacrimation

OPIOID DEADDICTION

Maintenance Phase

- The first aim in opioid de addiction is to **decrease the severity of withdrawal symptoms** and hence the patient is started on opioids associated with lesser withdrawal symptoms like **methadone** and **buprenorphine**.
- **Clonidine** can also be used for maintenance phase as monotherapy or with methadone or naltrexone. Clonidine with naltrexone combination is used for rapid opioid detoxification. An addition of anesthetic agent to both drugs makes an ultra-rapid detoxification regimen.
- When tapered down the lesser severity withdrawal symptom can be managed symptomatically.

Recent Advances

Lofexidine: It is a central alpha-2 agonist approved to decrease withdrawal symptoms in opioid dependence.

Relapse Prevention Phase

- The patient though is de addicted, if left in this situation will always find his old friends and one episode of opioid consumption will push him back to the circle of tolerance, dependence and withdrawal symptoms, i.e. patient will relapse.
- One cannot stop him from taking opioid, but it can be ensured that opioid does not act on opioid receptor; this can be done by blocking opioid receptors with an oral, potent and long-acting opioid antagonist like **naltrexone**.

AFFECT DISORDER

- Mania and depression are two extreme poles of same disorder and hence according to recent hypothesis it is related to a common factor known as **brain-derived neurotropic factor (BDNF)**.
- An increase in BDN causes **mania**, whereas a decrease causes **depression**.
- In some patients the level of BDNF keeps on fluctuating and patient keeps swinging from mania to depression. Such a disorder is known as **bipolar disorder (BPD)**. If the patient swings from one pole to another more than 4 times in a year, i.e. has **mania and depression** episodes **more than 4 times in a year**, then the patient is known as **rapid cycler**.

Conceptual Box-5

Affect Disorder and BDNF

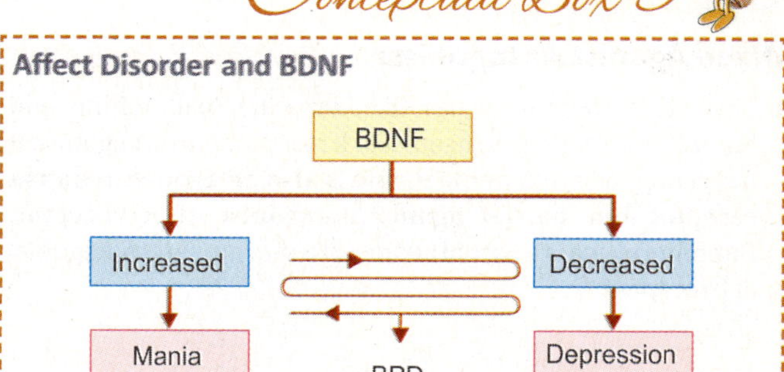

BDNF SYNTHESIS

- The most accepted hypothesis of BDNF synthesis are the IP3 and GSK-3 pathway. When PIP-2 is activated, IP-3 increases there by increasing BDNF production. BDNF increases **neuroplasticity** and **neuroprotection** of the CNS neurons.
- When GSK-3 is activated it breaks down intracellular β-catenin, which is responsible for BDNF synthesis by increasing transcription factors in nucleus. Hence, GSK-3 activation decreases BDNF production.
- The aim of CNS is to selectively activate these pathways to maintain BDNF levels at centre so that mood is stable.

Conceptual Box-6

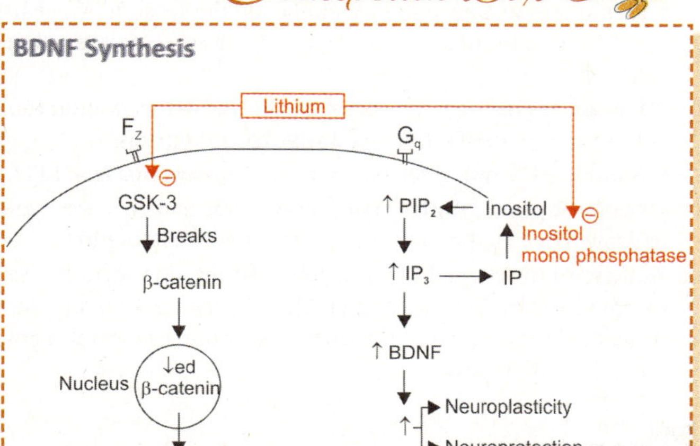

MANIA AND BPD

Lithium

Lithium has a good oral absorption and has a poor plasma protein binding. The primary rout of elimination is by **kidney** and it has a **half-life of 24 hours**. Thus, steady state concentration is achieved after **5 days** (5 $T_{1/2}$). Hence, TDM is done after 5 days of starting drug.

Mechanism of Action

- Lithium acts by inhibiting both pathways of BDNF synthesis depending on the levels of BDNF in CNS. It can both increase and decrease BDNF and control both mania and depression and hence is known as a mood stabilizer.
- Lithium inhibits **inositol monophosphatase** and hence decreases inositol for IP-3 synthesis. A decrease in IP-3 decreases BDNF followed by a decrease in neuroplasticity and neuroprotection. This is when mania is controlled, but for all this to happen at least 2 weeks are required. Hence, lithium is **not much effective in acute mania**, but once its effects are seen it is best drug to prevent further attack.
- Lithium by inhibiting GSK-3 increases β-catenin levels and increases BDNF synthesis. Hence, lithium is also effective in unipolar depression and bipolar disorder.

Uses of Lithium

- Lithium is drug of choice for **prophylaxis of mania** and **treatment of BPD,** and along with that it also **decreases suicidal tendency**. It is also drug of choice for treatment of **hypnic headache**.
- It is also used for treatment of **resistant depression** and **leukopenia**.
- In acute mania though it is started, so that its effect can be seen as soon as possible, it is not much effective. Hence, the **drug of choice for treatment of acute mania are atypical antipsychotics (Aripiprazole is DOC)**, which are the fastest acting anti-mania drugs. Benzodiazepines can be added for symptomatic relief of symptoms like insomnia and anxiety. Once lithium's effect has completely kicked in, typical antipsychotics are stopped generally after **2-4 months**.
- **Atypical antipsychotics** by parenteral route **(aripiprazole > risperidone > olanzapine)** are more preferred than **parenteral haloperidol** in acute mania.
- The other drugs that can be given in acute mania are antiepileptics like **carbamazepine** and **valproate**. **Lamotrigine is not used** in acute mania because of risk of SJS if used at high doses.

Clinical Box-6

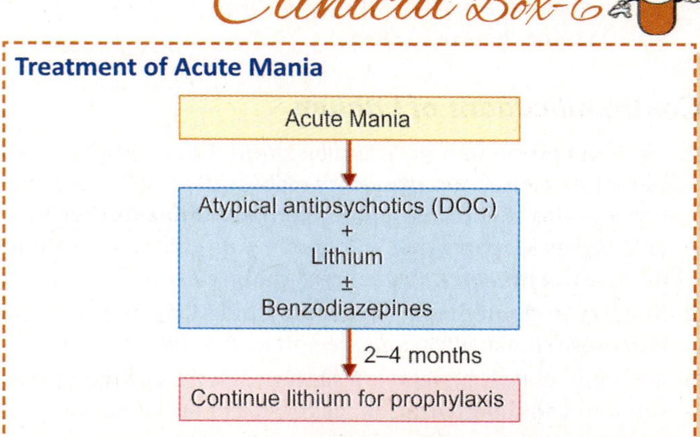

Side Effects of Lithium

- As lithium inhibits a GPCR pathway in its mechanism of action, it nonselectively inhibits other GPCRs like TSH_R and V_{2R} and hence causes **hypothyroidism** and **diabetes insipidus (thirst)** respectively.
- **High frequency fine tremors of 6–10 Hz** are most common side effect seen with lithium at normal doses. It can also cause **leucocytosis**, seizure, weight gain, alopecia, **hypercalcemia** (increases PTH) and ECG changes (T wave flattening and U waves).

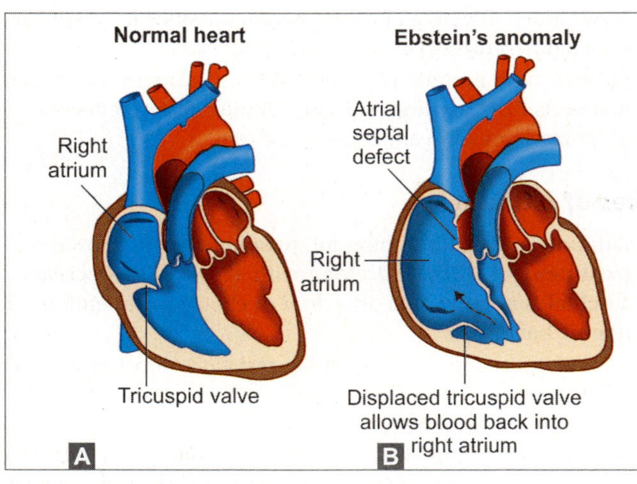

(A) Normal heart; (B) Ebstein's anomaly

- Lithium use in pregnancy can cause **cardiac malformations (Ebstein's anomaly)**, floppy infant syndrome and fetal goiter. Thus, in first trimester of pregnancy the drug of choice for mania are **atypical antipsychotics**, however in second and third trimester since benefit of lithium is more than risk it is preferred for maintenance therapy. Another important aspect to consider during lithium therapy is that, the baby can have toxicity to lithium even at normal lithium plasma concentration in the mother.
- Lithium can worsen psoriasis in some patients. Long-term therapy can cause EPS like cog wheel rigidity.
- Lithium can block transmission at neuromuscular junction and increase effect of NDMR. Hence, it should be stopped at least **24 hours before surgery**.

Contraindications of Lithium

- Lithium and sodium have similar properties and hence loss of sodium causes compensatory reabsorption of lithium and toxicity. This effect is most prominent with **thiazide diuretics** followed by K^+ sparing ones. Loops have no effect and osmotic diuretics on the contrary increase lithium clearance.
- **NSAIDS (Indomethacin maximum)** and **ACE inhibitors** can also cause similar effect and precipitate toxicity.
- For same reason patients on lithium should take **adequate salt** and **avoid dehydration**, as these can also contribute to lithium retention and toxicity.
- Lithium excretion is increased by sodium bicarbonate, theophylline and osmotic diuretics (mannitol). Valproate decreases plasma lithium levels.

Lithium Toxicity and Therapeutic Drug Monitoring

- Acute lithium toxicity presents with earliest symptoms like nausea and vomiting, **ataxia**, **dysarthria** and **coarse tremors** which can progress to **cardiac arrhythmias**, hypotension and coma. To prevent acute toxicity TDM is done.
- TDM is done for lithium as it is a drug with low therapeutic index. The plasma concentration is measured first **after 5 days** of starting therapy and **sample is drawn 12 hours after the last dose**.

Table 9: Therapeutic Drug Monitoring (TDM) for Lithium

Plasma concentration of lithium (mEq/L)	Relevance
1–1.5	Acute attack of mania
0.6–1.0	Prophylaxis of mania, BPD
>2	Indicator of toxicity
>3	Permanent neurological damage Absolute indication for dialysis
>4	Death

Drugs Used in BPD

- **Valproate** is the drug of choice for **rapid cyclers**, i.e. patients with more than 4 episodes of mania and depression in a year. It is also used for treatment of acute mania and is faster acting than lithium.
- **Carbamazepine** is used for treatment of acute mania and BPD in case patient is not responsive to other drugs.
- **Lamotrigine** is only effective for the depressive phase of BPD.
- **Oxcarbazepine, topiramate and gabapentin** are not approved by FDA but used off label for treatment of BPD.
- **Antipsychotics** are fastest acting anti mania drugs and hence preferred in acute mania. They are also used in bipolar disorder; atypical antipsychotics are more preferred than typical antipsychotics.

Mnemonics

Drugs used in BPD

V : Valproate
O : Oxcarbazepine (Non-FDA), Carbamazepine
L : Lamotrigine, Lithium
T : Topiramate (Non-FDA)
A : Antipsychotics (Atypical>Typical)
GE : Gabapentin

DEPRESSION

Depression is characterized by depressed mood for at **least 2 weeks** along with associated symptoms of insomnia, decreased libido and energy etc. The hypothesis of depression upon which most of the current drugs are based is the monoamine hypothesis. The latest hypothesis is that of BDNF discussed earlier.

Monoamine Hypothesis

- In patients of depression there is a decreased amount of monoamines, i.e. **5HT, NE and dopamine in the limbic system**. These monoamines either undergo metabolism by MAO A and B or undergo reuptake into the presynaptic neuron.
- Hence, the aim of treatment was to increase the monoamines by inhibiting either metabolism or reuptake by giving **MAO inhibitors or TCA** respectively. These are **first generation** drugs with a lot of side effects and hence the search for better drugs was on.

- TCA nonselectively inhibit reuptake of all monoamines and hence selective reuptake inhibitors were synthesized like SSRI and SNRI which belong to second generation drugs with lesser side effects.
- An increase in monoamines in the synapse, increases BDNF production and there is increase in neuroplasticity and neuroprotection. This takes around **2 weeks** and hence there is a **lag period** in the antidepressant effect seen.

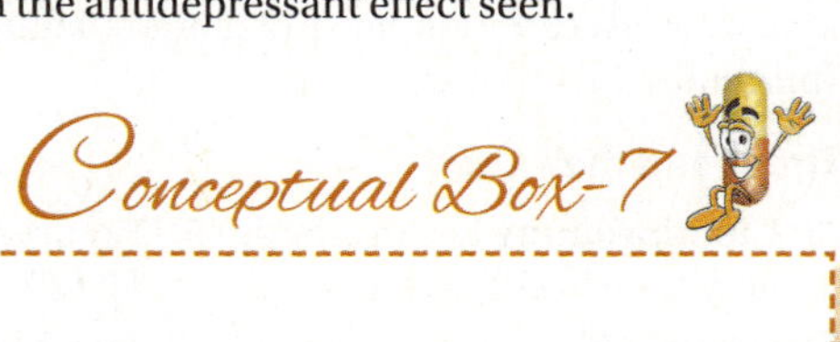

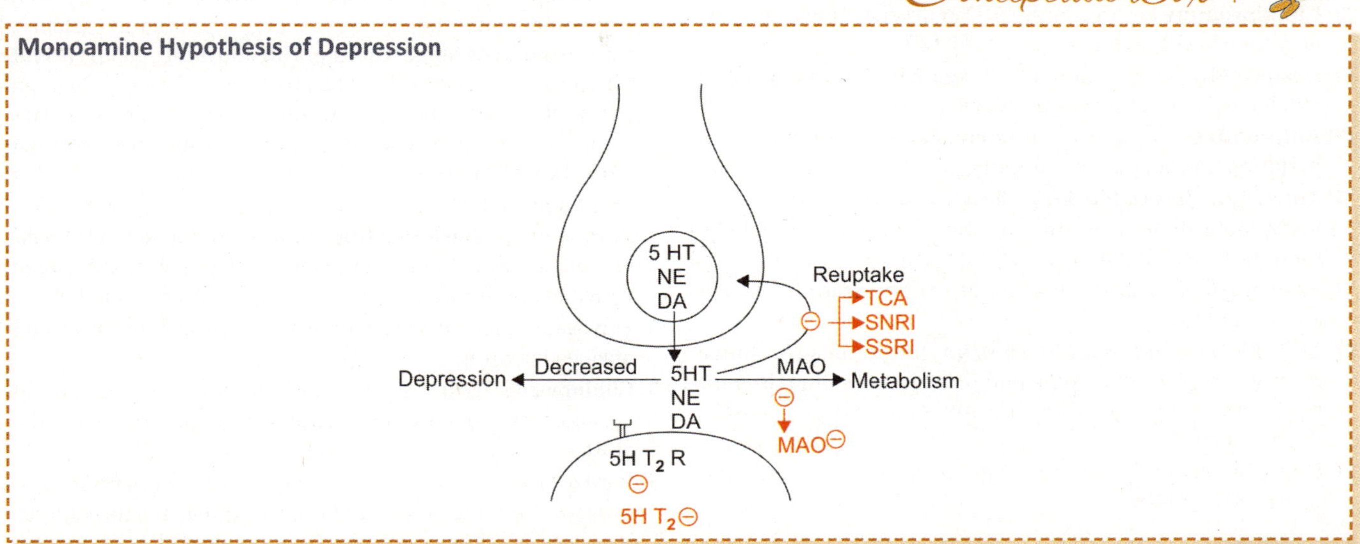

Classification of Antidepressant Drugs

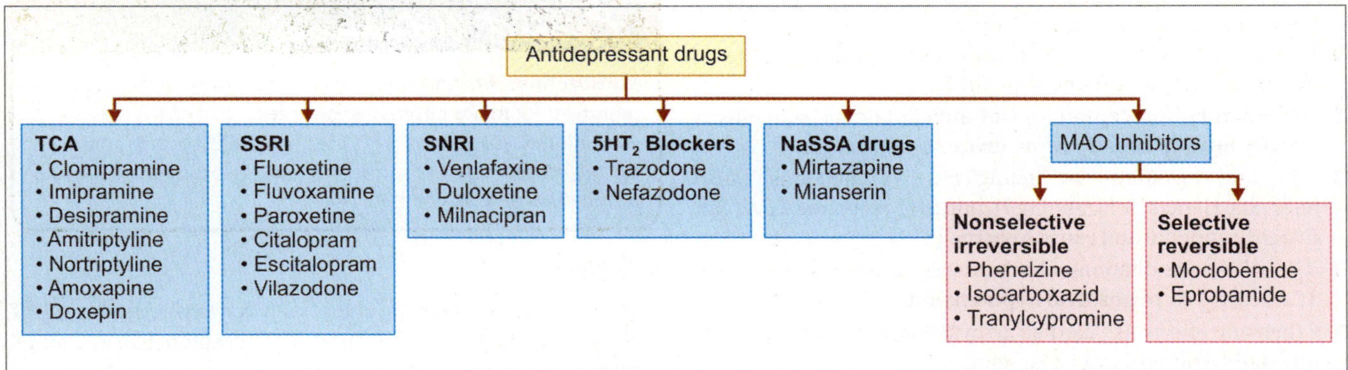

MAO Inhibitors

- **Monoamine oxidase (MAO)** is a mitochondrial enzyme of two subtypes, i.e. A and B. MAO A is present throughout the body and metabolizes all monoamines, whereas MAO B present in brain metabolizes dopamine.
- Nonselective MAO inhibitors are irreversible inhibitors of both MAO A and B. The drugs in this class are **phenelzine, isocarboxazid** and **tranylcypromine**. Selective and reversible MAO A inhibitors are **moclobemide** and **eprobemide**.
- MAO inhibitors are more effective than TCA in atypical depression. These drugs are not preferred nowadays due to wide range of side effects and drug interactions. MAO inhibitors can inhibit metabolism of tyramine in tyramine containing food and drinks like cheese and red wine and precipitate hypertensive crisis, i.e. **cheese reaction**. The MAO inhibitors are also **hepatotoxic**.
- MAO inhibitors can inhibit metabolism of **meperidine** and cause **seizures** due to accumulation of neurotoxic metabolite normeperidine. They inhibit 5HT metabolism and any class of drug that can increase 5HT in the synapse is contraindicated due to risk of **serotonin syndrome**. The drugs that can increase 5HT are **SSRI, SNRI, TCA, opioids (meperidine, tramadol and tapentadol), amphetamine, dextromethorphan, methylphenidate, etc**. Benzodiazepines are used for mild serotonin syndrome, whereas cyproheptadine or chlorpromazine is used for treatment of moderate to severe serotonin syndrome.

Tricyclic Antidepressants (TCA)

Tricyclic antidepressants (TCAs) are reuptake inhibitor of 5HT and NE and currently second line drugs in depression due to toxicity. Most common cause of therapy failure is inadequate trial (minimum for 6 weeks).

Drugs and their Uses

- **Clomipramine** has maximum 5HT reuptake inhibiting effect and is the best TCA for treatment of OCD.
- **Desipramine** has maximum NE reuptake inhibiting effect and is used in **cocaine dependence.**
- **Imipramine** can be used in **nocturnal enuresis** but is not preferred nowadays due to toxicity.
- **Amoxapine has D_2 blocking effect** as well and hence is used in psychotic depression and can cause **EPS**. An antipsychotic loxapine has been synthesized from amoxapine.
- **Amitriptyline** causes maximum antimuscarinic action among all TCAs.
- **TCAs like nortriptyline and amitriptyline** are **drug of choice for post herpetic neuralgia** and used as a first line drug for peripheral neuropathy. Nortriptyline is also used in smoking dependence.
- **Doxepin** was initially synthesized as an antihistaminic but now used as a TCA.

Side Effects

TCAs being nonselective inhibit group of **other receptors in the body like H_1, M, α_1 and 5HT**. These receptors are also inhibited by **typical and atypical antipsychotics**.

- Inhibition of H_1 and M receptors cause **sedation**. TCAs can also be used for treatment of insomnia.
- Inhibition of M receptors causes anticholinergic side effects like **dry mouth, constipation, urine retention,** etc.
- 5HT and histamine by acting on hypothalamus cause anorexia. Hence, by inhibiting H_1 and 5HT receptors TCAs can increase appetite and cause **obesity**.
- α_1 block causes dilation of both arteries and veins and hence TCAs carry risk of **postural hypotension**.
- Other side effects like cardiac arrhythmia, lowering of seizure threshold, **tremor** etc. can be seen.

Drug Interaction

- TCAs can also cause serotonin syndrome like SSRIs.
- They can also decrease antihypertensive effect of clonidine.

TCA Toxicity and Treatment

- TCA and antipsychotics toxicity present with anticholinergic symptoms along with cardio toxicity (QRS widening, arrhythmia and hypotension), convulsions and coma.
- Treatment is aimed at reversing the cardiac effects and acidosis by **sodium bicarbonate**.

Selective Serotonin Reuptake Inhibitors (SSRI)

SSRIs are the most effective and least toxic antidepressants and hence are the drug of choice currently. The first SSRI developed was **zimelidine**. The antidepressant effects of SSRIs are seen only after 4–6 weeks of drug therapy and this period is called as lag period.

Drugs and their Uses

- SSRIs are the drug of choice for treatment of **depression, premenstrual syndrome and neurotic disorders like OCD, phobia, PTSD, anorexia nervosa, bulimia and GAD**. The dose is higher, and duration of treatment is longer for OCD than depression with SSRIs.
- Fluoxetine ($T_{1/2}$ = 50 hours) is a **prodrug** metabolized into active metabolite nor fluoxetine ($T_{1/2}$ = 200 hours). Hence, **fluoxetine is the longest acting SSRI** and is the preferred SSRI for all conditions mentioned above. Being longest acting, on abrupt discontinuation its concentration gradually decreases in plasma and hence **withdrawal symptoms are not seen with fluoxetine**. Once in a week formulation are available only for fluoxetine.
- **Paroxetine is shortest acting** followed by due to a short half-life and it has no active metabolites. Hence, it is associated with maximum withdrawal symptoms on discontinuation.
- Fluvoxamine is approved only for treatment of OCD and anxiety disorders.
- **Citalopram** is used specifically in premenstrual syndrome and agitation. Its S **enantiomer escitalopram is the most specific SSRI**.
- **Paroxetine** is the most potent enzyme inhibitor and associated with teratogenic effect, i.e. cardiac malformations. It causes maximum erectile dysfunction and is associated with anticholinergic effects as well.

> **Recent Advances**
>
> **Vortioxetine:** Vortioxetine is an SNRI and $5HT_{1/3}$ agonist approved for major depressive disorder.
> **Vilazodone:** Vilazodone is an SSRI and $5HT_1$ agonist approved for major depressive disorder. It is not associated with sexual dysfunction and weight gain.

Side Effects

Side effects with SSRIs are primarily seen due to an increase in 5HT in the body, which acts on various 5HT receptors like 2, 3 and 4 subtypes.

- **$5HT_2$ in brain:** Increased stimulation of postsynaptic $5HT_2$ receptors in brain causes **anxiety and insomnia**. These effects persist for initial 2 weeks and then disappear due to receptor down regulation, i.e. $5HT_2$ receptors move into the neurons. So, after 2 weeks anxiolytic effect is seen. To negate anxiety in initial days, SSRIs are always started with a benzodiazepine.
- **$5HT_2$ in spinal cord:** Increased stimulation of $5HT_2$ receptors in spinal cord causes **erectile dysfunction and delayed ejaculation**. Hence, SSRIs are used off label for **treatment of premature ejaculation**. These effects are maximum with **paroxetine** and are **most common long-term side effects**.
- **$5HT_3$ in CTZ area:** Increased stimulation of $5HT_3$ in CTZ area causes **nausea and vomiting** which is by far the **most common acute side effect of SSRIs followed by anxiety**.
- **$5HT_4$ in GIT:** Increased stimulation of $5HT_4$ in GIT increases acetylcholine release, which increases contraction and causes **loose stools**.

- Citalopram can cause **QT prolongation**. Akathisia and bleeding (increase in platelet serotonin) can also be seen; **sertraline** and **citalopram** have least effect on bleeding.
- Most SSRIs are enzyme inhibitors and thus can increase effect of drugs like benzodiazepines and warfarin. The safest drugs with lesser enzyme inhibition are sertraline and citalopram.
- All SSRIs can cause serotonin syndrome characterized by autonomic instability, delirium, myoclonus, hyperthermia and coma.
- SSRIs as well as SNRIs, TCAs and MAO inhibitors can increase suicidal tendency.
- Withdrawal of SSRIs can cause nausea, insomnia, fatigue, paresthesia and **flu like symptoms**, which is maximum with **paroxetine** due to its short half-life and no active metabolite.

Drug interactions

- SSRIs are metabolized by CYP2D6 and are enzyme inhibitors of CYP2D6. Because of this they can inhibit metabolism of other drugs metabolized by CYP2D6.
- MAO inhibitors if given with SSRI can cause **serotonin syndrome**. Hence, a wash off period of **2 weeks** at least is required before shifting from MAO inhibitors to SSRIs or vice versa. Only exception is fluoxetine for which **5 weeks wash off period** is required before starting MAO inhibitors, due to longer duration of action of fluoxetine.

Serotonin Norepinephrine Reuptake Inhibitor (SNRI)

SNRIs act just like TCAs with the only difference that they don't act on other receptors in the body and hence are devoid of TCA associated side effects. However, they retain the side effects of SSRIs caused by elevated 5HT levels. These drugs are second line for treatment of anxiety and depression. SNRI and TCA are more preferred than SSRI for treatment of melancholic depression.

- These drugs are used as second line drugs in depression currently after SSRIs.
- **Venlafaxine** is used for PTSD and panic disorder. It is associated with **perinatal complications** and hence should not be used in pregnancy. **Diastolic hypertension** can be seen with venlafaxine and hence should be preferred in patients with hypotension and depression. Desvenlafaxine is a D isomer of venlafaxine and is longer acting than venlafaxine.
- **Duloxetine** is used for fibromyalgia, stress incontinence, autism, hot flashes, bulimia, premenstrual syndrome and peripheral neuropathy. It is the longest acting SNRI.
- **Milnacipran** is approved only for treatment of fibromyalgia.
- Side effects seen with these drugs are similar to the side effects of SSRIs**. Duloxetine** and **milnacipran** do block muscarinic receptors and cause mydriasis and hence are contraindicated in uncontrolled angle closure glaucoma**.**
- The wash off period with MAO inhibitors is of only one week.
- Withdrawal symptoms like SSRI are seen with **venlafaxine** due to it short half-life.

Selective NE Reuptake Inhibitor

Atomoxetine is the drug of choice for treatment of **ADHD associated with Tourette's syndrome** and **ADHD associated with family history of drug abuse.**

5HT2 Antagonists

In depression a decreased synaptic 5HT, causes up regulation of the postsynaptic $5HT_2$ receptors. Hence, inhibition of these receptors also has antidepressant effect.

- Trazodone and nefazodone are older drugs in this class. **Nefazodone** has been banned due to **hepatotoxicity**. Trazodone causes sedation and is used along with SSRIs and SNRIs for treatment of associated **insomnia**. It can also cause **priapism** and has been used in erectile dysfunction.
- Mirtazapine and mianserin are the newer drugs in this class which **increase NE by α_2 block** and **serotonin by $5HT1_A$** block and hence are known as NaSSA (Noradrenergic and Specific Serotonergic Antidepressant). These drugs also block **H1 (sedation)**, 5HT2 and **5HT3 receptors (antiemetic effect)**. **Mirtazapine is the drug of choice for treatment of depression associated with insomnia and is given at bed time.** It has lesser sexual side effects as compared to SSRIs. Mirtazapine can cause obesity, sedation and agranulocytosis (rare).

Bupropion

- **Bupropion** not only **inhibits reuptake**, but also **induces release of NE and dopamine** from presynaptic neuron. It structurally resembles amphetamine.
- It is used for treatment of **atypical depression**, **smoking dependence**, ADHD, peripheral neuropathy and obesity.
- It can cause **seizures**, specifically at high doses. It is the **most anxiogenic antidepressant** and hence not used for treatment of anxiety.

ANTIPSYCHOTICS

TYPICAL ANTIPSYCHOTICS

Dopamine Hypothesis

- The first hypothesis of psychosis was established after an increased amount of dopamine was found in the limbic system of psychotic patients. This dopamine acts on D_2 receptors which are G_i subtype to GPCRs and inhibit the action potential transmission.
- A block in the limbic system blocks the thought process and affect in the patient. Based on this hypothesis the first class of drugs was synthesized to be D_2 antagonists and hence are known as **typical antipsychotics**.

Conceptual Box-8

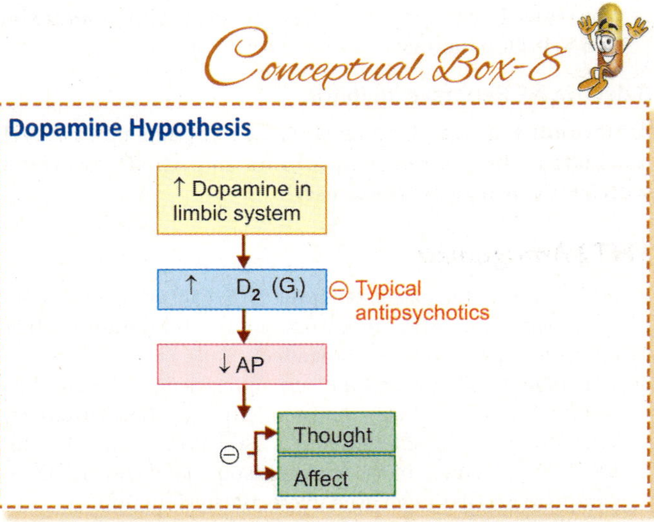

Classification

Typical antipsychotics can be classified based on their potency at D_2 receptors **as low and high potency drugs** as given in the conceptual box below:

Conceptual Box-9

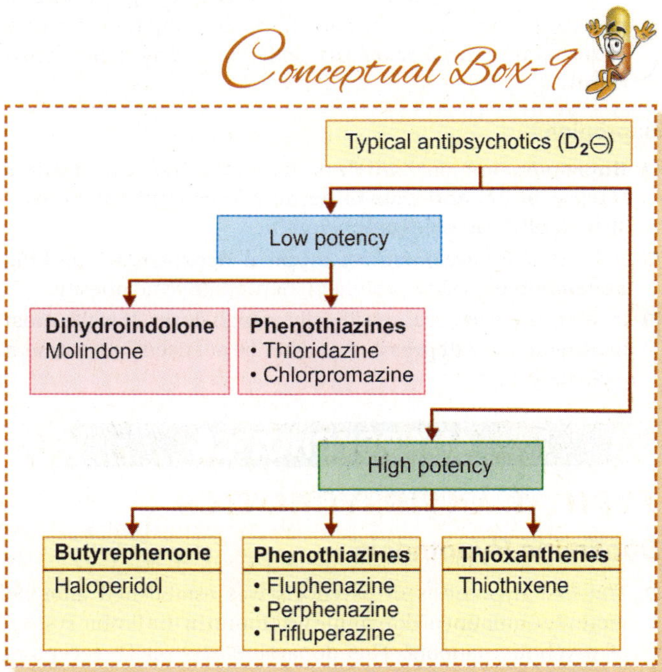

Correlation of Potency with Side Effects

Side effects of typical antipsychotics are seen because of inhibition of D_2 receptors and a group of other receptors like M, H_1, α_1 and 5HT. The more potent drugs at D_2 receptors will be less potent at other receptors and vice versa. D_2 block side effects like EPS will be seen more with potent drugs, whereas other receptor side effects will be more with less potent drugs.

ATYPICAL ANTIPSYCHOTICS

Serotonin Hypothesis

- A group of researchers were studying patients on LSD, which is a hallucinogen. Accidentally they found increased amount of 5HT in the urine of those patients.
- Then the hypothesis began; LSD is a hallucinogen (symptom of psychosis) and it increases 5HT, then is it a possibility that 5HT is increased in psychosis. Thus, a new class of drug was synthesized **that inhibits 5HT2$_A$ receptors** and since it deviates from first hypothesis it is known as **atypical antipsychotic**.
- But when the drugs were analyzed it was found that atypical antipsychotics have **some amount of D_2 block** as well, though it is very less as compared to typical antipsychotic.
- **Aripiprazole** and **brexpiprazole** are **partial agonist at D_2 receptor**, whereas **aripiprazole, brexpiprazole, ziprasidone and clozapine** are **partial agonists at 5HT1$_A$ receptor**. Thus, **aripiprazole** and brexpiprazole are the only atypical antipsychotic that are **partial agonist at both D_2 and 5HT1$_A$ receptor**.
- Cariprazine is a partial agonist whereas amisulpride is an antagonist at D_2 and D_3 receptor.
- **Quetiapine is an antagonist at α_2 receptor as well.**

Conceptual Box-10

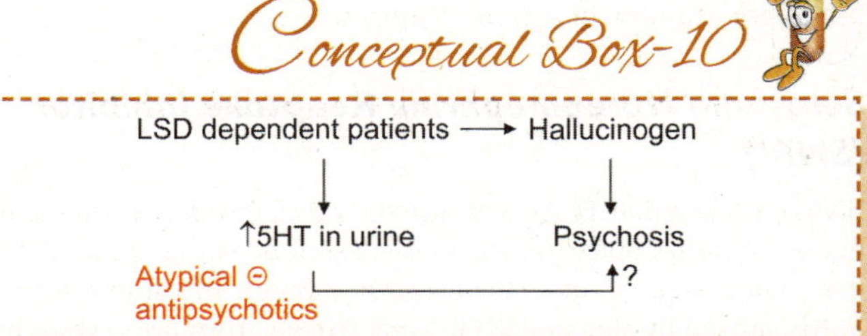

Recent Advances

- Glutamate being an excitatory neurotransmitter has been implicated in psychosis. Hence, glutamate antagonist are currently under development.
- Glycine is required along with glutamate to bind to NMDA receptors and hence a decrease in glycine can also have antipsychotic effect. Thus, glycine transporter 1 receptor inhibitors like **bitopertin** and sarcosine are under trial as antipsychotics.

USES OF TYPICAL AND ATYPICAL ANTIPSYCHOTICS

- **Schizophrenia: Atypical antipsychotics** are the current drugs of choice for treatment of schizophrenia. The drugs with lesser metabolic side effects like **aripiprazole and ziprasidone** are preferred for initial treatment. Typical antipsychotics are used if these atypical drugs are not effective. **Clozapine** is a reserve drug and is the drug of choice for **refractory schizophrenia**. It is the only drug that has been effective in **suicidal tendency**. **Typical antipsychotics** are more effective against **positive** symptoms, whereas **atypical antipsychotics** are effective against **both negative and positive symptoms** of psychosis. Asenapine though is more effective in treatment of negative symptoms. Lurasidone is an atypical antipsychotic used in acute decompensation of schizophrenia.

Recent Advances

Pimavanserin: It is a recently approved atypical antipsychotic for the treatment of hallucination and delusion associated with Parkinson's disease. It is an inverse agonist at $5HT_{2A}$ receptors.

Conceptual Box-11

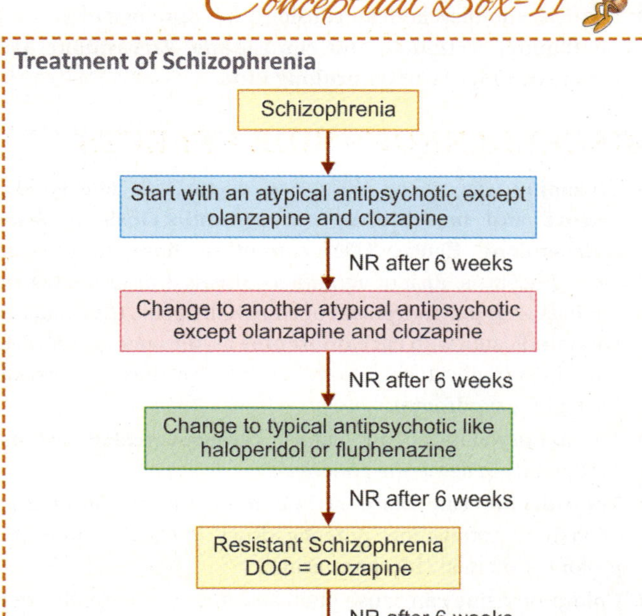

- **Depression:** Atypical antipsychotics like aripiprazole, olanzapine and risperidone are used as add on drugs to antidepressants for treatment of **resistant depression**. The only atypical antipsychotic effective as monotherapy in depression is **quetiapine**, because its metabolite norquetiapine inhibits NE reuptake.
- **Mania and BPD**: The uses of antipsychotics in mania and BPD have been discussed in the previous section.
- **Huntington's chorea:** Tetrabenazine being the drug of choice, atypical and typical antipsychotic are second- and third-line drugs respectively.
- **Tics associated with Tourette's syndrome:** Clonidine or guanfacine being the drug of choice, atypical and typical antipsychotic are second- and third-line drugs respectively.
- **Autism associated irritability:** Risperidone and aripiprazole are approved for this indication.
- **Antiemetic:** All typical antipsychotics **except thioridazine** are used as antiemetics. The antiemetic effect is because of D_2 receptor block in the CTZ area. **Promethazine is a phenothiazine used only as an antiemetic**.
- **Antipruritic:** Low potency phenothiazines can be used as antipruritic drugs due to potent H_1 inhibition.
- **Insomnia: Quetiapine** is not approved by FDA, but used off label for treatment of insomnia.
- **Hiccups: Chlorpromazine is the drug of choice for hiccups.**

SIDE EFFECTS OF TYPICAL AND ATYPICAL ANTIPSYCHOTICS

D_2 Block Side Effects

- Side effects due to D_2 receptor block are known as **extrapyramidal side effects (EPS)**. Overall typical antipsychotics cause more EPS than atypical antipsychotics.
- Among typical antipsychotics the highly potent drugs like **thioxethene, haloperidol, fluphenazine, trifluoperazine and perphenazine cause maximum EPS,** while low potency drugs like **thioridazine and chlorpromazine cause minimum EPS**.
- Among atypical antipsychotics **aripiprazole < ziprasidone have lowest risk**, whereas **risperidone has highest risk of EPS**. Aripiprazole has lowest risk due to partial agonism at D_2 receptors and because of this it can cause nausea and vomiting.
- The cause for most of EPS is D_2 block except akathisia and tardive dyskinesia. The cause of akathisia is not known, and **tardive dyskinesia is D_2 receptor upregulation and supersensitivity** due to prolonged block for many years. The risk factors for tardive dyskinesia are old age, years of drug use, diabetes and smoking.

EPS	Presentation	Treatment
Acute dystonia **Earliest EPS**	Head, neck, tongue, extraocular (oculogyric crisis), laryngeal muscle spasm Seen in younger patients	**Anticholinergics (M1 antagonists)** – For long-term management after acute crisis. Trihexyphenidyl Benztropine Biperiden Antihistaminics with maximum anticholinergic effect – For acute crisis Promethazine Diphenhydramine **Amantadine** can be used in parkinsonism
Parkinsonism	Symptoms of Parkinson's disease and perioral tremor (rabbit syndrome) Seen in elderly	

Contd...

EPS	Presentation	Treatment
Akathisia: **Most common EPS**	Desire to move around (Restlessness) Aggravated by smoking	β blockers – Drug of choice Benzodiazepines
Tardive dyskinesia	Stereotype repetitive choreiform movements of facial muscles Seen in elderly	Change to atypical antipsychotics VMAT-2 Inhibitors Deutetrabenazine Valbenazine
Neuroleptic malignant syndrome	Severest form of EPS presents with Muscle rigidity Raised plasma CPK Hypotension Hyperthermia	Dantrolene is the drug of choice D_2 agonist like bromocriptine is the most specific drug

Other Receptor Block Side Effects

Other receptors in the body like **H_1, M, α_1 and 5HT** can be blocked by typical and atypical antipsychotics. These other receptor side effects are **maximum with less potent typical antipsychotics like thioridazine and chlorpromazine**. Among atypical antipsychotics these side effects are **least with aripiprazole, asenapine and ziprasidone and maximum with clozapine and olanzapine.**

- Inhibition of H_1 and M receptors cause **sedation**.
- Inhibition of M receptors cause **anticholinergic side effects** like dry mouth, constipation (clozapine), urine retention etc.
- 5HT and histamine by acting on hypothalamus cause anorexia. Hence, by inhibiting H_1 and 5HT receptors antipsychotics can increase appetite and cause **obesity**. **The only antipsychotic that causes weight loss is molindone. Among atypical antipsychotics obesity is maximum with clozapine > olanzapine and minimum with aripiprazole < ziprasidone.**
- α_1 block causes dilation of both arteries and veins and hence antipsychotics carry risk of **postural hypotension**.

Insulin Resistance, DM and Hyperlipidemia

- Antipsychotics cause insulin resistance and this facilitates lipolysis and results in hypertriglyceridemia.
- These side effects are again **maximum with less potent typical antipsychotics like thioridazine and chlorpromazine.** Among atypical antipsychotics these side effects are **least with aripiprazole, asenapine, cariprazine and ziprasidone and maximum with clozapine and olanzapine**.

Hyperprolactinemia

- **Hyperprolactinemia** is directly proportional to the potency of typical antipsychotics and hence is maximum with **haloperidol**.
- Among atypical ones it is maximum with **risperidone and paliperidone** as these are most potent blockers of D_2 receptors.
- Aripiprazole, brexpiprazole and cariprazine due to D_2 agonism cause **hypoprolactinemia**.

QT Prolongation

- Most typical antipsychotics cause QT prolongation and the **risk is much higher with typical antipsychotics** as compared to atypical ones.
- Atypical antipsychotics causing QT prolongation are **quetiapine, sertindole and ziprasidone. Ziprasidone has the maximum risk of QT prolongation.**

MISCELLANEOUS SIDE EFFECTS

- **Clozapine** can cause dose dependent side effects like **seizure and myocarditis**, but **agranulocytosis is dose independent**. Hence, **TDM cannot be done** to prevent agranulocytosis. Risk of agranulocytosis is 3 times higher in patients with polymorphism of HLADQB1 gene. Clozapine is contraindicated with **carbamazepine** as, the later also carries risk of agranulocytosis. Clozapine can also cause sialorrhea (wet pillow syndrome).
- All antipsychotics can cause **cerebrovascular events** particularly in dementia patients.
- **Thioridazine** can cause **retinal deposits and browning of vision**. Among low potency drugs it causes more QT prolongation than chlorpromazine.
- Chlorpromazine can cause photosensitivity, retinopathy and lens pigmentation (melanin deposits).
- In **pregnancy** the safest antipsychotic overall is **haloperidol** and the **most unsafe with maximum placental passage is olanzapine**.

ROUTES OF ADMINISTRATION

- Almost all antipsychotics can be given by oral route for maintenance therapy. **Penfluridol** is the longest acting oral antipsychotic given once in a week.
- Intravenous haloperidol can be used for acute management of a psychotic episode.
- IM formulations can be used for acute management and IM depot formulations which are long-acting are preferred incompliant patients for long-term management. Haloperidol decanoate is the longest acting injectable antipsychotic given once in a month.
- **Loxapine** can be given by **intranasal route** for management of agitation.
- **Asenapine** has a high first pass metabolism of 98% and hence is available only as **oral disintegrating tablets (ODT)**.

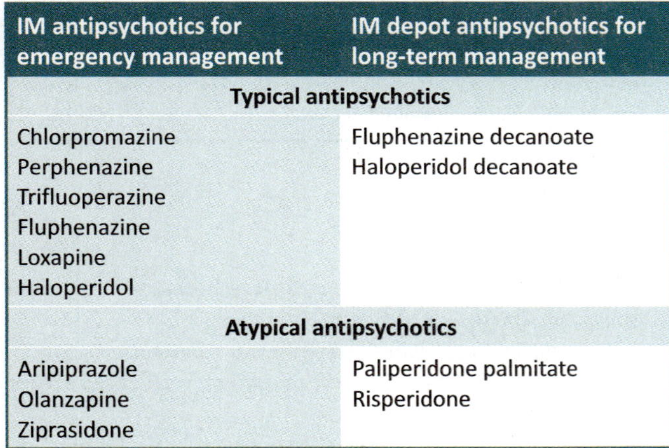

IM antipsychotics for emergency management	IM depot antipsychotics for long-term management
Typical antipsychotics	
Chlorpromazine Perphenazine Trifluoperazine Fluphenazine Loxapine Haloperidol	Fluphenazine decanoate Haloperidol decanoate
Atypical antipsychotics	
Aripiprazole Olanzapine Ziprasidone	Paliperidone palmitate Risperidone

NEURODEGENERATIVE DISORDERS

PARKINSON'S DISEASE

- Parkinson's disease is caused by progressive depletion of dopaminergic neurons in corpus striatum.
- Dopamine acts on D_2 (G_i) receptors in the corpus striatum and inhibits the action potential flow from cortex to spinal cord motor neurons. This has a physiological inhibitory effect on the movements.
- In the absence of dopamine this inhibition is absent, and the movements are increased and leads to movement disorder called as Parkinson's disease.

Conceptual Box-12

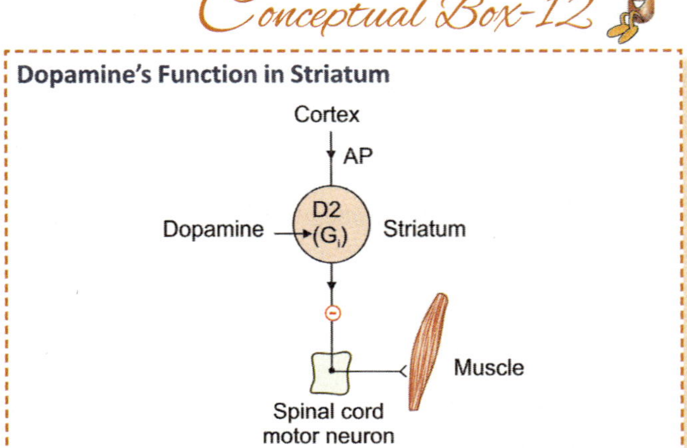

Thus, for treatment of PD either the level of dopamine can be restored or D_2 receptor can be stimulated (D_2 agonists). Dopamine level is restored by either giving a prodrug of dopamine, i.e. levodopa or by inhibiting metabolism of dopamine by MAO and COMT inhibitors.

Conceptual Box-13

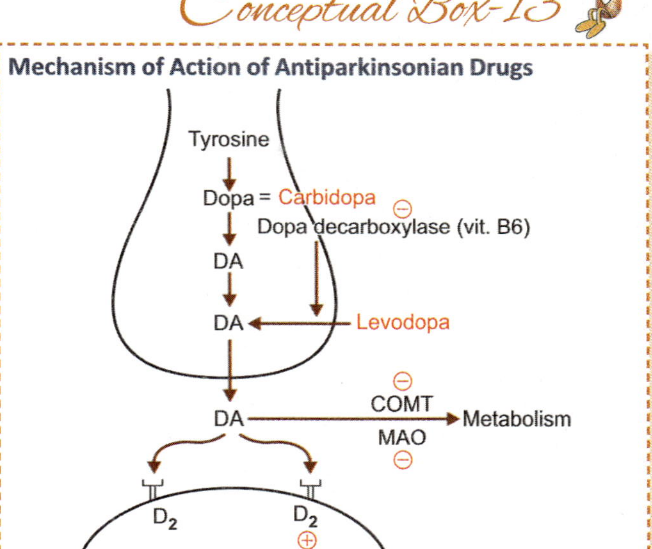

Levodopa

- **Levodopa is a prodrug of dopamine** that is metabolized by dopa decarboxylase (DD) into dopamine, which has beneficial effect in PD. But since dopa decarboxylase is present throughout the body major chunk is metabolized outside the CNS, which not only decreases central effect but also increases dopamine related peripheral side effects.
- **Carbidopa** and **benserazide** are inhibitors of dopa decarboxylase and since these are lipid insoluble, they do not cross the blood brain barrier. Levodopa is always combined with carbidopa or benserazide, so that maximum levodopa moves to CNS, where it is activated to dopamine. The carbidopa and levodopa dose ratio is 1:10 or 1:4. Carbidopa by preventing metabolism of levodopa in periphery also prevents peripheral side effects like nausea, arrhythmia and postural hypotension, however it does not prevent central side effect like psychosis.
- Vitamin B6 is a cofactor for DD and can increase peripheral metabolism of levodopa. Hence, **vitamin B6 is contraindicated with levodopa**.
- Levodopa is the drug of choice for treatment of Parkinson's disease (PD). The patient is started on normal formulation and in case of motor fluctuations can be shifted to sustained release, extended release or intestinal gel formulation.
- Side effects are related to elevated dopamine levels which cause side effects by acting on dopamine receptors. Clozapine and quetiapine are best for treatment of levodopa induced psychosis. Nausea, vomiting and hypotension are most common side effects.

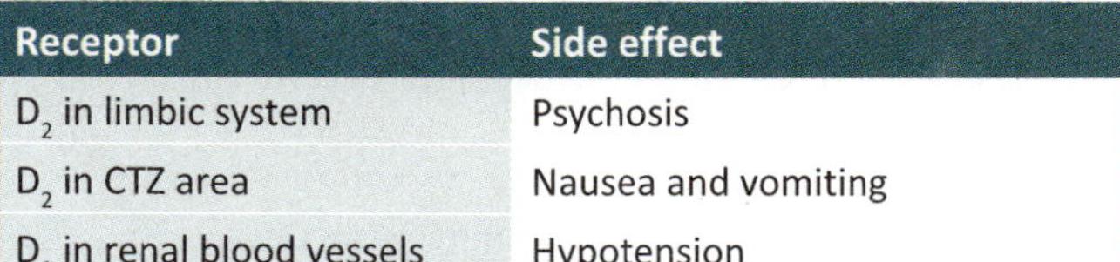

Receptor	Side effect
D_2 in limbic system	Psychosis
D_2 in CTZ area	Nausea and vomiting
D_1 in renal blood vessels	Hypotension

- Levodopa induced **dyskinesia** produces most troublesome side effects seen with high doses. This limits the use of levodopa beyond a particular dose. Levetiracetam and amantadine can be used for treatment of dyskinesia.
- **On-off phenomena** is another drawback that develops because of progressive nature of disease. Let us suppose a patient is diagnosed with PD and he has only 60% dopamine in striatum. For treatment 40% of dopamine is given in the form of levodopa. After 6 months the dopamine of patient further decreases to 50%, but exogenous dose is still 40%. Thus, because of 10% dopamine deficit the patient will have intermittent symptomatic (off) periods in between asymptomatic (on) periods. This is called as on-off phenomena.
- Levodopa can also worsen **melanoma** and **peptic ulcer disease**.
- Levodopa is contraindicated in closed angle glaucoma but can be used in well controlled open angle glaucoma. As it causes psychosis it is **contraindicated in psychosis** as well.

COMT Inhibitors

- In the presence of carbidopa, levodopa is primarily metabolized in the periphery by COMT. Hence, inhibition of COMT not only **increases the half-life of levodopa** but also **bioavailability by inhibiting metabolism in liver**.
- These drugs can cause **diarrhea. Tolcapone** is longer acting inhibitor of both peripheral and central COMT but is less preferred due to **hepatotoxicity**.
- Entacapone is a specific peripheral COMT inhibitor that is **drug of choice for on-off phenomena or wearing-off symptoms** associated with levodopa. It is also available in a fixed dose combination with levodopa and carbidopa.
- Side effects related to increase in dopamine are like levodopa as discussed earlier.

MAO-B Inhibitors

- MAO-B present only in CNS is responsible for dopamine metabolism in the striatum. Thus, this class has only central effect.
- **Selegiline** and **rasagiline** are used for treatment of **young onset PD** and for **on-off phenomena** associated with levodopa.
- MAO-B inhibitors also have **antioxidant effect,** and this gives some prevention of neurodegeneration in PD by **antiapoptotic** effect on dopaminergic neurons.
- Selegiline is metabolized into amphetamine, which can cause CNS stimulation and lead to agitation and insomnia. By D_2 stimulation it can also cause dyskinesia and psychosis.
- MAO-B inhibitors are contraindicated with **meperidine** due to risk of toxicity.

Recent Advances

Safinamide: It is a MAO-B inhibitor recently approved for the treatment of on-off phenomena seen with levodopa therapy.

D_2 Agonists

Ergot Agonists

- **Bromocriptine, cabergoline and pergolide** are rarely used nowadays due to side effects.
- Bromocriptine can cause **peripheral vasoconstriction** of end arteries and pergolide and cabergoline can cause **cardiac valve fibrosis**.
- By D_2 receptor agonism these drugs can cause dyskinesia and psychosis.

Nonergot Agonists

- **Pramipexole, ropinirole and rotigotine** are non-ergot agonists which are **longer acting** than levodopa. **Rotigotine** is the only anti PD drug given by topical route, i.e. **transcranial patch** and is an agonist at both D_2 and D_1.
- These drugs being longer acting than dopamine, are associated with **lesser chances of on-off phenomena and dyskinesia**. Thus, they are used either as **monotherapy to begin treatment of PD or used along with levodopa**.
- These are also used for treatment of **on-off phenomena** and are drug of choice for **restless leg syndrome** as well.
- Apart from the dopamine related side effects discussed earlier, these drugs can also cause fatigue, **somnolence, peripheral edema and impulse control disorders (gambling and sexual activities).**

Apomorphine

- Apomorphine is an opioid derivative with D_2 agonistic activity.
- It is used by subcutaneous route as a **last resort (rescue therapy)** for treatment of **on-off phenomena**, when COMT and MAO inhibitors and synthetic alkaloids are ineffective.
- Significant nausea can be seen due with apomorphine and hence patient is prophylactically given trimethobenzamide. **Ondansetron is contraindicated with apomorphine** due to risk of severe hypotension.

Amantadine

- **Amantadine** acts in PD by its anticholinergic effect, increasing dopamine release and by inhibiting NMDA receptors.
- It has limited effect and is used only for mild PD and for dyskinesia associated with levodopa.
- Side effects associated are **ankle edema** and **livedo reticularis.**

Anticholinergics

- Anticholinergics like **benztropine, biperiden and trihexyphenidyl** and antihistaminics with maximum anticholinergic effect like promethazine and diphenhydramine are also effective in PD.

- Anticholinergics by inhibiting muscarinic receptors in striatum increase dopamine release.
- These are rarely used for PD purpose but are drug of choice for **treatment of drug induced parkinsonism e.g. with typical antipsychotics**.

ALZHEIMER'S DISEASE

- Alzheimer's disease is characterized by progressive depletion of cholinergic neurons of the cortex. Decreased acetylcholine in cortex decreases cognition.
- Cholinergic drugs like **donepezil, rivastigmine and galantamine** are the preferred drugs for mild to moderate Alzheimer's disease. Donepezil is also approved for severe disease and is the drug of choice for Alzheimer's disease. Tacrine is not preferred now days due to hepatotoxicity. These drugs can be used for treatment of vascular and Lewy body dementia as well.
- NMDA antagonist **memantine** is preferred for treatment of moderate to severe Alzheimer's disease.
- Associated abnormal behaviors and psychosis is treated with atypical antipsychotics.
- Depression if associated can be treated with SSRIs.
- Drugs that are used as memory enhancers but not approved by FDA are **nootropic drug piracetam**, cerebrolysin, piribedil, pyritinol and citicoline.

Recent Advances

Alzheimer's Disease

Tarenflurbil: It is a gamma secretase modulator under trial as a disease modifying agent for Alzheimer's disease.

Etazolate/Bryostatin: These are alpha secretase modulator under trial as a disease modifying agent for Alzheimer's disease.

Aducanumab: It is an anti-beta amyloid monoclonal antibody under trial for treatment of Alzheimer's disease.

HUNTINGTON'S DISEASE

- Huntington's disease is a genetic disorder characterized by jerky movements known as chorea.
- **Tetrabenazine is the drug of choice** for treatment of Huntington's chorea. Patient not responding to tetrabenazine can be given atypical antipsychotics (aripiprazole) or typical antipsychotic (haloperidol).
- Psychosis and depression if associated requires atypical antipsychotics and SSRIs.

AMYOTROPHIC LATERAL SCLEROSIS (ALS)

- ALS is a motor neuron disease characterized by progressive depletion of upper and lower motor neurons. The patient presents with motor weakness, muscle atrophy, dysarthria and muscle spasticity.
- **Riluzole** is the only drug approved by FDA for ALS and is the drug of choice. It acts by inhibiting glutamate release as well as by antagonizing NMDA and kainite receptors and by blocking sodium channels. It inhibits neurodegeneration by inhibiting glutamate induced oxidative damage and prolongs survival. Side effects associated are nausea, diarrhea and hepatotoxicity (LFT monitoring required).
- Apart from riluzole **non-invasive ventilation** for 4 hours a day can also prevent neurodegeneration.
- **Baclofen is the drug of choice for spasticity** associated with ALS. Other drugs that can be used are clonazepam, dantrolene and tizanidine.
- **Anticholinergics** are used for drooling and **dextromethorphan + quinidine** combination for pseudobulbar symptoms.

Recent Advances

Edaravone: It is a free radical scavenger approved as an orphan drug for treatment of **ALS** by intravenous route recently. It can also be used in **acute stroke**. Side effects associated are hypersensitivity (due to sodium bisulfite in solution), gait disturbance, contusion and headache.

MULTIPLE SCLEROSIS

- Multiple sclerosis is an autoimmune demyelinating disorder of the CNS.
- The myelin basic protein (MBP) present in the oligodendrocytes behave as foreign protein and are presented by MHC to the local immune cells. The local immune cells produce inflammatory mediators that stimulate CD-8 cell proliferation in lymph node and spleen.
- These CD-8 cells are released into the plasma and they adhere to the blood brain barrier with the help of their $\alpha_4\beta_1$ integrin and then transmigrate into CNS. In the CNS they damage the MBP and cause an inflammatory reaction leading to demyelination.
- Demyelination is a problem because in myelinated segments the conduction o action potential is faster, i.e. 70 meters/sec, whereas in unmyelinated segment it reduces to 1 meter/sec.

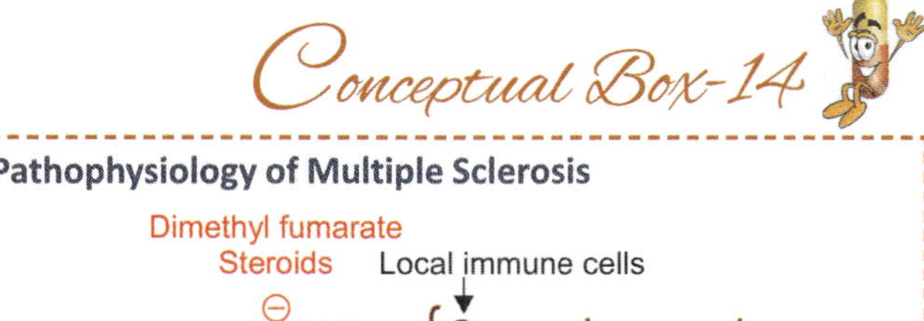

Conceptual Box-14

Pathophysiology of Multiple Sclerosis

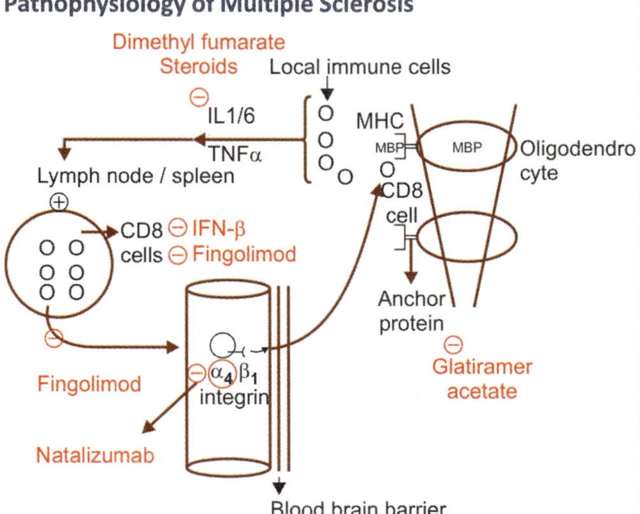

Types of Multiple Sclerosis

- **RRMS:** Relapsing remitting multiple sclerosis presents with various attacks of MS between which patient remains normal. The aim of therapy is to decrease the frequency and severity of attacks.

Conceptual Box-15

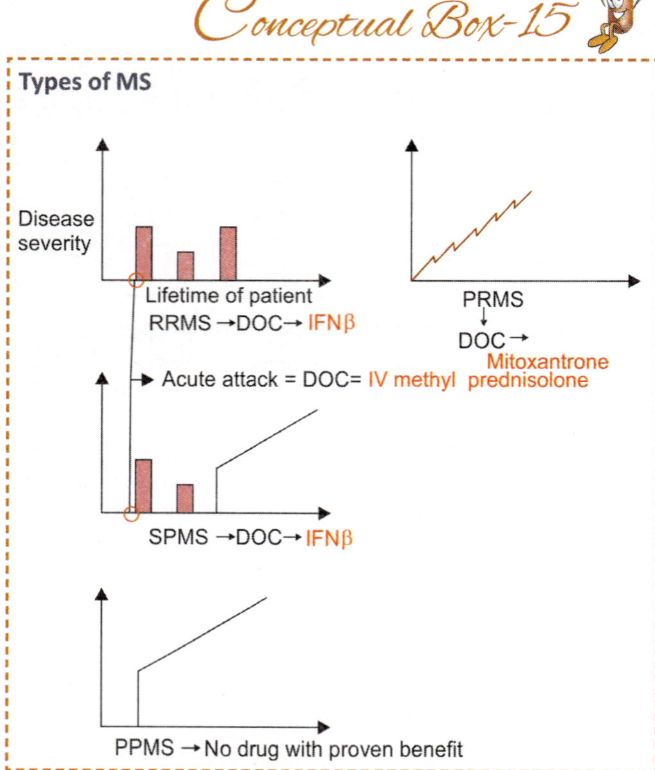

- **SPMS and PPMS:** Secondarily progressive multiple sclerosis is the one in which the patient begins as RRMS but become progressive with time. Primarily progressive multiple sclerosis is the one in which the disease is progressive from the beginning. The main aim of treatment here is to decrease the progression of disease. Progression of disease is measured clinically by expanded disability severity scale (EDSS). Hence, in other words the aim is to decrease the EDSS score.

Steroids

- Steroids act by inhibiting the inflammatory mediators, which ultimately decreases CD-8 cell proliferation.
- **Intravenous methylprednisolone is the drug of choice for treatment of an acute attack of multiple sclerosis.**

Interferon β

- Interferon β inhibits CD-8 cell proliferation and also has inhibitory effect on the inflammatory mediators.
- **Interferon β1a and 1b are the drug of choice for treatment of RRMS and relapses in SPMS**.s
- They can cause hepatotoxicity, flu like symptoms and injection site reactions.

Fingolimod

- Fingolimod inhibits the release of CD-8 cells by the central lymphoid organs like lymph node and spleen.
- It is an oral drug effective in RRMS and associated with cardiac side effects.

Natalizumab

- **Natalizumab** inhibits the α_4 **subunit of** $\alpha_4\beta_1$ **integrins** and hence inhibits transmigration of CD-8 cells through the blood brain barrier.
- Its use has been associated with **progressive multifocal leukoencephalopathy**. Hence, it is reserved for patients with JC antibody negative patients not responding to other drugs.
- It is given once in a month by injectable route.

Glatiramer Acetate

- Glatiramer acetate is a polypeptide made up of four amino acids Glutamate, Lysine, Alanine and Tyrosine. It competitively displaces the anchor protein of MHC receptor and changes MHC structure. Hence, MHC cannot present the abnormal MBP to local immune cells.
- It can be used in RRMS for patients not responding or intolerable to interferon beta.

Dimethyl Fumarate

- Dimethyl fumarate produces anti-inflammatory effect by inhibiting the inflammatory mediators.
- It is used by oral route for treatment of RRMS.
- Its use has also been associated with progressive multifocal leukoencephalopathy.

Teriflunomide

- Teriflunomide is a metabolite of immunomodulator leflunomide. It acts by inhibiting dihydroorotate dehydrogenase which leads to inhibition of de novo pyrimidine synthesis. This has a depleting effect on lymphocytes as they lack salvage pathway.
- It is also given by oral route for RRMS.

Mitoxantrone

- Mitoxantrone is an anticancer drug approved for treatment of RRMS, SPMS and PRMS. It is the **only drug approved for PRMS**.
- **A maximum decrease in EDSS is seen with mitoxantrone followed by natalizumab**.

Alemtuzumab

- Alemtuzumab is a anti CD-52 monoclonal antibody recently approved for treatment of RRMS.

- Alemtuzumab and fingolimod have been associated with **disseminated varicella zoster infection.**

Miscellaneous Drugs

- Methotrexate, cyclophosphamide, azathioprine and IVIG though not approved by FDA are used off label for treatment of multiple sclerosis.
- Modafinil is the drug of choice for treatment of fatigue associated with multiple sclerosis.
- Dalfampridine is used for improving timed gait in multiple sclerosis.

Recent Advances

Recent Advances in Multiple Sclerosis

- **Daclizumab** is an anti-IL-2 receptor or CD-25 monoclonal antibody approved recently for the treatment of relapsing remitting multiple sclerosis (RRMS).
- Ocrelizumab is an anti-CD-20 monoclonal antibody recently approved for the treatment of both RRMS and PPMS.

ALCOHOLS

ETHANOL

- Ethanol has a good oral absorption but undergoes first pass metabolism in stomach and liver by alcohol dehydrogenase. 90% of alcohol is metabolized by alcohol dehydrogenase into acetaldehyde, which is further metabolized into acetic acid by aldehyde dehydrogenase. 10% of alcohol is metabolized by CYP2E1. Acute ethanol consumption causes competitive inhibition of CYP2E1, whereas chronic ethanol consumption causes induction of CYP2E1.
- Ethanol consumption can cause various side effects as mentioned in the mnemonic box below. However, consumption of ethanol below 30 gm/day increases HDL and decreases cholesterol and hence decreases risk of atherosclerotic cardiovascular disease like coronary artery disease and stroke.

Mnemonics

Side Effects of Ethanol

A : Arrhythmia
L : Liver toxicity (Hepatitis and cirrhosis)
C : Cancer (Esophageal, liver and breast), Cardiomyopathy
O : Osteoporosis
H : Hypertension
O : Esophageal reflux
L : Leukopenia and anemia
P : Pancreatitis (Diabetes), Psychosis (Wernicke-Korsakoff)
E : Erectile dysfunction

Conceptual Box-16

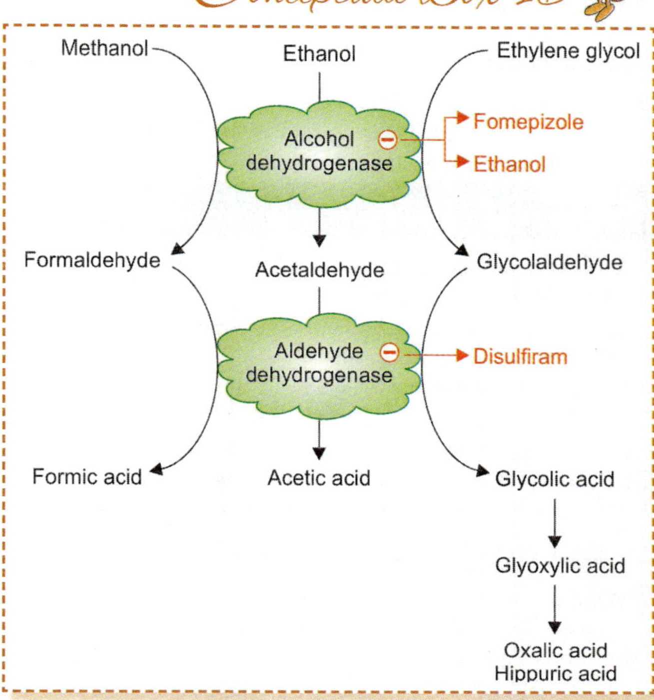

Uses

- Ethanol is clinically used for treatment of chronic intractable pain associated with trigeminal neuralgia and cancer.
- Ethanol is used for treatment of **methanol** and **ethylene glycol poisoning**. Ethanol competitively inhibits metabolism of methanol by inhibiting **alcohol dehydrogenase**. The drug of choice though for poisoning of both is **fomepizole**.

Alcohol Dependence

The FDA approved drugs for alcohol dependence are **disulfiram, naltrexone and acamprosate**.

Disulfiram

- Disulfiram is an aversive agent which acts by inhibiting **aldehyde dehydrogenase** the enzyme for alcohol metabolism. This leads to accumulation of acetaldehyde, toxic metabolite of alcohol which causes **vomiting, flushing, hypotension, chest pain and other uncomfortable symptoms.**
- Disulfiram does not decrease craving. It is less preferred than naltrexone and acamprosate. It is given to patient with **abstinence from alcohol for at least 12 hours.**
- Such a disulfiram like reaction can also be seen with other drugs like **metronidazole, chlorpropamide and cephalosporins.**

Naltrexone

- Naltrexone is an opioid antagonist used to **decrease craving in alcoholics.**
- It can be given by oral route 50 mg daily or once monthly depot injection or as subcutaneous implant for 6 months.

- Side effects seen are nausea, dysphoria and hepatotoxicity (cirrhosis). Hence, it is contraindicated in patients of depression and hepatic dysfunction.

Acamprosate

- Acamprosate is a GABA analog which inhibits NMDA receptors and is used to decrease craving in alcoholics.
- It can cause diarrhea as a side effect.

Recent Advances

Ondansetron: Ondansetron is under trial for alcohol dependence to decrease craving.

Nalmefene: Nalmefene is under trial for alcohol dependence to decrease craving.

Topiramate: Topiramate is under trial for codependence on alcohol and smoking.

Gabapentin, **Varenicline** and **Baclofen**: These are drugs under trial to decrease craving in alcohol dependence.

Alcohol Withdrawal and Toxicity

- Alcohol withdrawal causes symptoms like seizures, tremors, anxiety, delirium tremens etc. **Benzodiazepines** are the drug of choice for treatment of alcohol withdrawal. For withdrawal seizures intravenous lorazepam or diazepam is used, whereas for others long-acting oral drug like chlordiazepoxide is preferred for detoxification. After detoxification drugs for treatment of alcohol dependence can be started.
- Alcohol toxicity can present with agitation, **hypoglycemia**, arrhythmia and respiratory depression. Treatment begins with **glucose** and **thiamine** along with basic life support.

Alcohol and Pregnancy

Alcohol use in pregnancy is associated with fetal alcohol syndrome, which contains three features as given below:

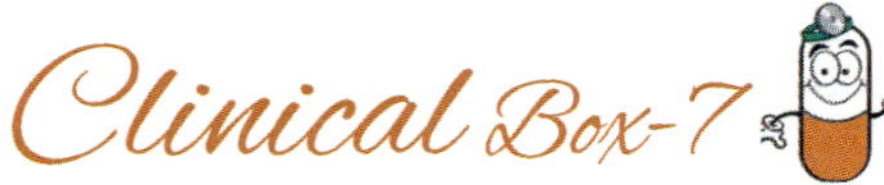

Fetal Alcohol Syndrome

- **Dysmorphic facial features (All 3 are required)**
  - Small palpebral fissures
  - Thin vermilion border
  - Smooth philtrum
- **Prenatal and/or postnatal growth impairment**
- **Central nervous system abnormalities (1 required)**
  - Structural: head size <10th percentile, significant brain abnormality on imaging
  - Neurological
  - Functional: global cognitive or intellectual deficits functional deficits in at least three domains

METHANOL

- Methanol is the simplest alcohol used as a solvent and antifreeze. It is metabolized in the human body into formaldehyde and formic acid which are toxic compounds.
- Accidental consumption of methanol can cause ocular toxicity (optic nerve atrophy and blindness), metabolic acidosis, pancreatic necrosis, respiratory depression and coma.
- Fomepizole (DOC) and ethanol being competitive inhibitors of alcohol dehydrogenase can block synthesis of the toxic compounds and hence are used for methanol poisoning. Bicarbonate can also be used for treatment of metabolic acidosis and dialysis to remove methanol, formaldehyde and formic acid.

ETHYLENE GLYCOL

- Ethylene glycol is also used as a solvent and antifreeze. It is metabolized in the human body into toxic compounds like glycolaldehyde, glycolic acid, glyoxylic acid, oxalic acid and hippuric acid.
- Accidental consumption can cause renal failure due to renal tubule block by oxalate crystals and associated metabolic acidosis.
- Treatment is exactly same as methanol poisoning.

SMOKING DEPENDENCE

Smoking is a very common preventable cause of mortality worldwide. Nicotine stimulates **$\alpha_4\beta_2$ subtype of nicotinic receptor on dopaminergic neurons** in ventral tegmental area. This releases dopamine into the nucleus accumbens and prefrontal cortex giving reward. Nicotine withdrawal can cause anxiety, depression, weight gain and irritability.

First-line Drugs

- **Nicotine replacement**, **bupropion** and **varenicline** are first-line drugs for smoking dependence.
- Nicotine replacement therapy (gums, patch, inhaler or lozenge) is commonly used and inhaler being the most effective one.
- **Bupropion** is an antidepressant approved for treatment of smoking dependence.
- **Varenicline**, a **nicotinic receptor agonist** is more effective than bupropion. Varenicline is also associated with suicidal and cardiovascular risk. The primary effect of varenicline in smoking dependence is seen via **$\alpha_4\beta_2$ subtype of nicotinic receptor**.

Second-line Drugs

- **Clonidine** and **nortriptyline** are second-line drugs for smoking dependence.
- **Cytisine** is a plant derivative which is partial agonist at $\alpha_4\beta_2$ subtype of nicotinic receptor. Varenicline has been synthesized from cytisine.
- **Rimonabant** a **cannabinoid receptor inverse agonist/antagonist** has been banned due to depression and suicide risk.

Treatment of smoking dependence

- **First-line drugs**
  - Nicotine replacement
  - Bupropion
  - Varenicline
- **Second-line drugs**
  - Nortriptyline
  - Clonidine
  - Cytisine

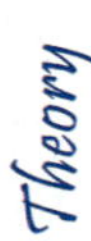

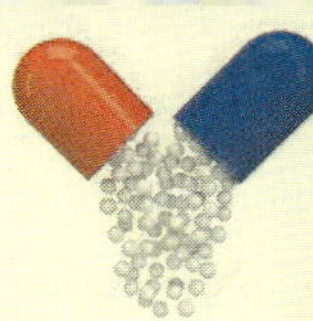

Image-based Questions

1. **A patient with symptoms of epilepsy was advised for EEG. He returned to the OPD with the following finding in the picture. What is the most appropriate treatment?**

   a. No treatment required
   b. Vigabatrin
   c. Valproate
   d. Carbamazepine

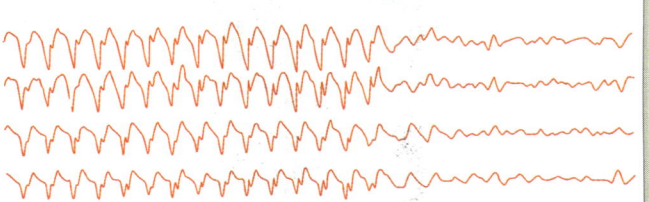

2. **An epileptic patient on regular medications presents with c/o easy fatigability, dizziness and palpitations. The peripheral smear blood picture is given below. The most probable associated drug is**

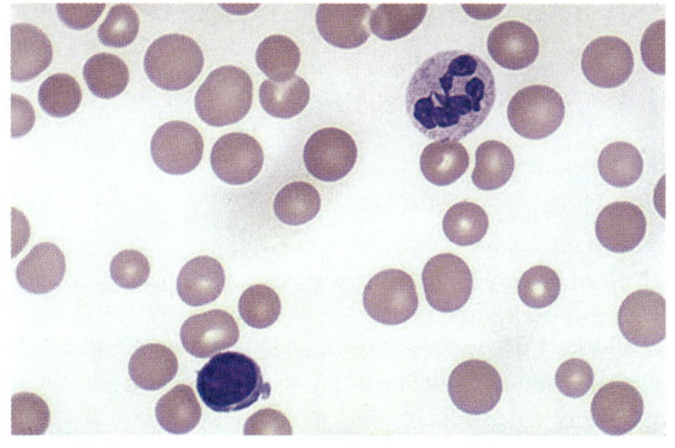

   a. Valproate
   b. Lamotrigine
   c. Carbamazepine
   d. Phenytoin

3. **Which of the following antiepileptics might have caused the side effect given in the picture?**

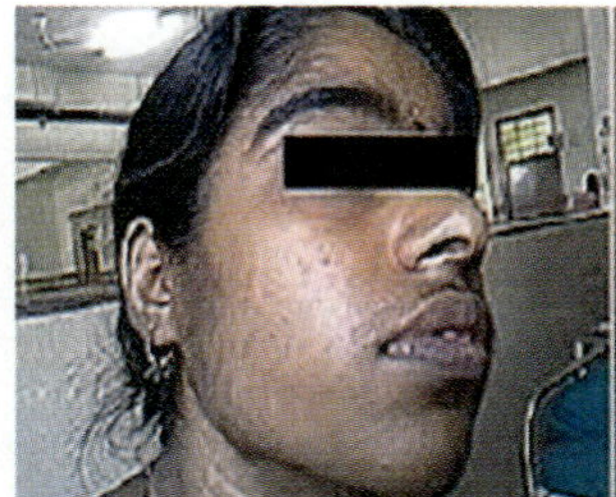
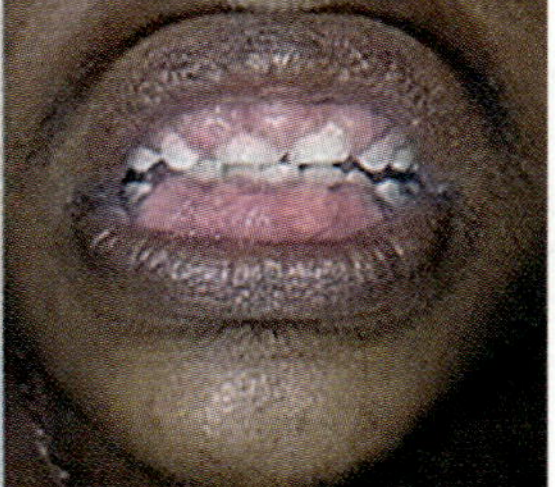

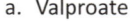

   a. Valproate
   b. Lamotrigine
   c. Carbamazepine
   d. Phenytoin

4. **A patient started on carbamazepine started for partial seizure treatment develops the side effect given in the picture? What is the next best step?**

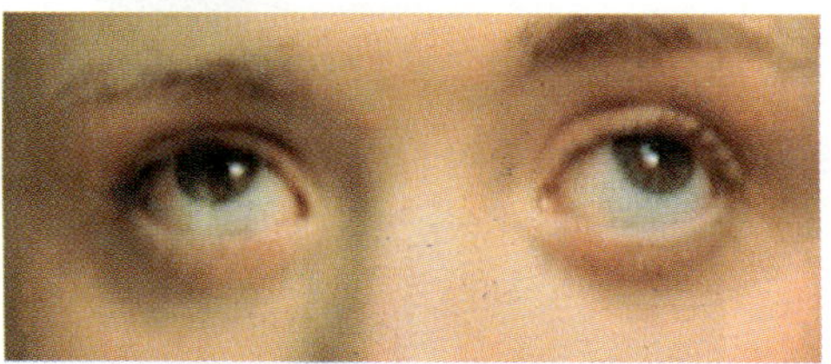

   a. Decrease dose of carbamazepine
   b. Change to phenytoin
   c. First do TDM
   d. Nothing is to be done

5. **Which of the following antiepileptics might have caused the skin reaction given in the picture?**

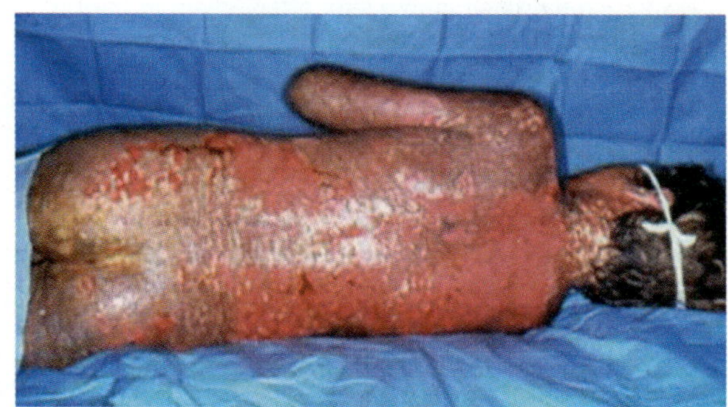

   a. Valproate
   b. Topiramate
   c. Lamotrigine
   d. Zonisamide

6. **Which of the following barbiturate is useful in the procedure given in the picture?**

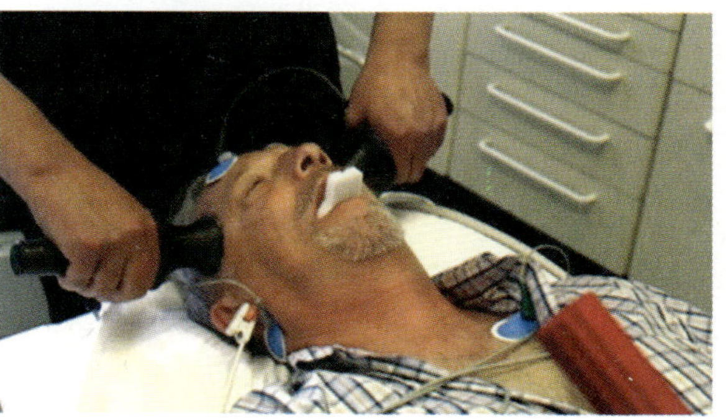

   a. Phenobarbital
   b. Secobarbital
   c. Thiopental
   d. Methohexital

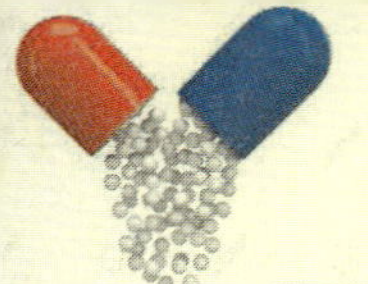

7. The plant given in the picture is a source for:

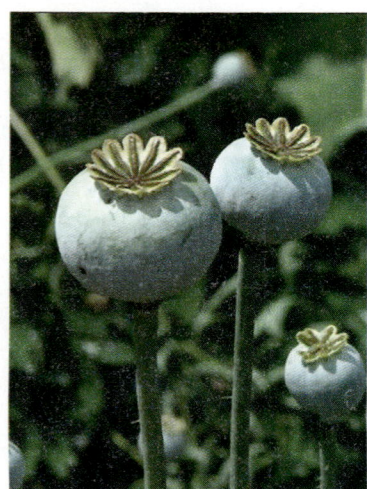

a. Buprenorphine
b. Methadone
c. Fentanyl
d. Pentazocine

8. A female was started on a drug after which she immediately developed a side effect given in the picture. Which of the following drug would have caused it?

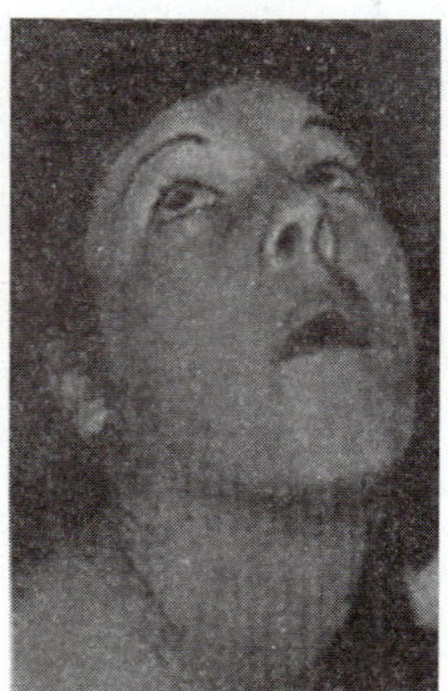

a. Clozapine
b. Chlorpromazine
c. Thioridazine
d. Haloperidol

9. Which of the following drug used early can delay the onset of gait given in the picture?

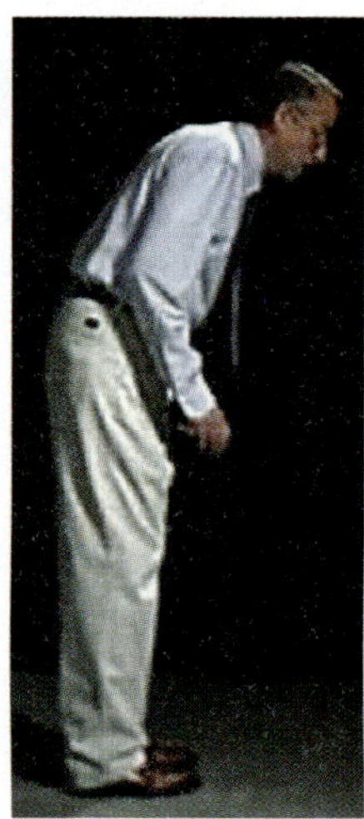

a. Levodopa
b. Pramipexole
c. Amantadine
d. Selegiline

10. A patient having score of 13 in the test given in the picture. Which of the following drug is used for treatment?

MINI MENTAL STATE EXAMINATION (MMSE)

Name:
DOB:
Hospital Number:

One point for each answer — DATE:

a. Riluzole
b. Interferon beta
c. Donepezil
d. Tetrabenazine

11. Which of the following drug has maximum effect on the scale given in the picture?

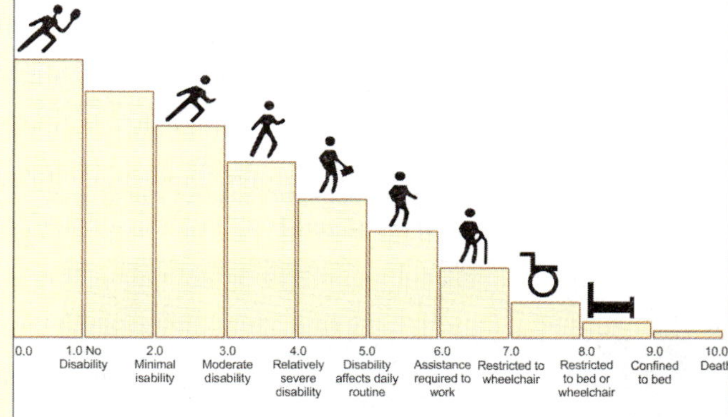

a. Natalizumab
b. Mitoxantrone
c. IFN beta
d. Methyl prednisolone

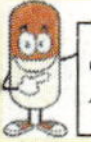

Answers with Explanations to Image-based Questions

1. Ans. (c) Valproate

(Ref: Goodman Gilman 12th E/P597)

- The EEG with 3 Hz spike is confirmatory of absence seizure.
- Valproate is the drug of choice for absence seizure and hence is the best answer.

2. Ans. (d) Phenytoin

(Ref: Goodman Gilman 12th E/P591)

- The presence of large RBCs and hypersegmented neutrophils in the picture are confirmatory of megaloblastic anemia.
- Among the options megaloblastic anemia is specifically seen with phenytoin.

3. Ans. (d) Phenytoin

(Ref: Goodman Gilman 12thE/P592)

- The female in the picture has hirsutism and hyperplasia of gums, which are characteristic of phenytoin.

4. Ans. (d) Nothing is to be done

(Ref: Goodman Gilman 12th E/P595)

- If a patient develops ataxia and diplopia, then TDM is done and dose is adjusted to bring plasma concentration under therapeutic range.
- If nystagmus develops and epilepsy is controlled then nothing is to be done.

5. Ans. (c) Lamotrigine

(Ref: Goodman Gilman 12th E/P600)

- Lamotrigine and carbamazepine can cause Steven Jhonson syndrome.
- To prevent it lamotrigine is started at low doses and then dose is gradually increased.

6. Ans. (d) Methohexital

(Ref: Goodman Gilman12th E/P473)

- The procedure given in the picture is ECT.
- Methohexital is a barbiturate anesthetic agent that paradoxically causes seizures.
- Hence, it is the anesthetic agent of choice in ECT.

7. Ans. (a) Buprenorphine

(Ref: Goodman Gilman 12th E/P499)

- The plant given in the picture is Papaver Somniferum.
- It is a source for thebaine and thebaine is the source for buprenorphine.

8. Ans. (d) Haloperidol

(Ref: Goodman Gilman 12th E/P437)

- The female is having acute dystonia in the picture.
- All the drugs in the options can cause acute dystonia but the risk is higher with potent typical antipsychotic like haloperidol.

9. Ans. (d) Selegiline

(Ref: Goodman Gilman 12th E/P618)

- The stooping gait given in the picture is characteristic of Parkinson's disease.
- Selegiline is the only drug that has inhibitory effect on neurodegeneration.

10. Ans. (c) Donepezil

(Ref: Goodman Gilman 12th E/P621)

- MMSE test is done for diagnosis of Alzheimer's disease.
- Thus, the best answer is donepezil.

11. Ans. (b) Mitoxantrone

(Ref: Goodman Gilman 12th E/P1026)

- The disability scale given in the picture is known as EDSS.
- Drug with maximum effect on EDSS is mitoxantrone followed by natalizumab.

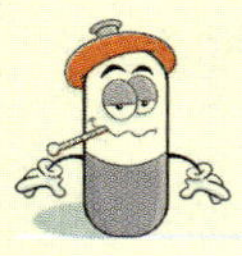

Annexures

Drugs of Choice

Condition	Drug of Choice
ADHD	Methylphenidate
ADHD with Tourette syndrome ADHD with family history of drug abuse	Atomoxetine
Amyotrophic Lateral Sclerosis	Riluzole
Alzheimer's disease	Donepezil
Bell's Palsy	Prednisolone
Bipolar Disorder Prophylaxis of mania	Lithium
Depression	SSRI
Epilepsy	
Generalized • GTCS • Absence seizure • Myoclonic Seizure	Valproate
Partial	Carbamazepine
Lennox Gastaut Syndrome	Valproate
Infantile Spasm	ACTH
Infantile spasm with tuberous sclerosis	Vigabatrin
Rolandic Epilepsy (Benign epilepsy of childhood)	Carbamazepine
Seizures in Pregnancy	$MgSO_4$
Seizures in Neonates	Phenobarbital
Dravet Syndrome (Severe myoclonic epilepsy of childhood)	Valproate
West Syndrome (Infantile spasm + MR)	ACTH
Status Epilepticus	Lorazepam
Essential Tremor	Propranolol
Guillain Barre syndrome	IVIG
Headache (Other Than Migraine) • Cluster headache – Triptans • Raised CSF Pressure – Acetazolamide • Paroxysmal Hemicrania – Indomethacin • Primary Cough Headache – Indomethacin • Hypnic Headache – Lithium	
Huntington's chorea	Tetrabenazine
Insomnia	Z Compounds • Sleep induction – Zaleplon (Shortest acting) • Sleep Maintenance – Eszopiclone (Longest acting)
Jet Lag	Short-acting Z Compounds (Zaleplon)
Mania	• Acute attack of Mania – Atypical Antipsychotics • Prophylaxis of mania – Lithium
Migraine	• Acute attack – Triptans • Prophylaxis – Propranolol
Multiple Sclerosis	• Acute attack – I/V Methyl Prednisolone • RRMS – IFN β • SPMS – IFN β • PRMS – Mitoxantrone
Myasthenia Gravis	• Treatment – Pyridostigmine • Diagnosis – Edrophonium
Narcoanalysis	Thiopental sodium
Narcolepsy	Modafinil
Neuralgia • Glossopharyngeal Neuralgia • Trigeminal Neuralgia	Carbamazepine
Parkinson's Disease	Levodopa
Young onset PD	Selegiline
Motor fluctuation of levodopa	Pramipexole
On-off phenomena associated with levodopa	Entacapone
Neuroprotection in PD	MAO inhibitors (Rasagiline and Selegiline)
Peripheral Neuropathy	• TCA (Nortriptyline and Desipramine) or • SNRI (Duloxetine) or • GABA releasing drugs (Gabapentin and Pregabalin)

Rapid Cyclers	Valproate

Restless leg syndrome	Dopamine Agonists • Pramipexole or • Ropinirole

Schizophrenia	Atypical antipsychotics (Aripiprazole)

Suicidal Tendency Resistant Schizophrenia	Clozapine

Tourette syndrome	α_2 agonists • Clonidine or • Guanfacine

New Drugs

Drug	Mechanism of Action	Use
Cannabidiol	Unknown	LGS or Dravet syndrome
Stiripentol	GABA Modulator	LGS or Dravet syndrome
Patisiran	Double stranded SiRNA which degrades mutant and wild type transthyretin (TTR) mRNA and decreases deposition of transthyretin in tissues	Hereditary transthyretin mediated amyloidosis associated polyneuropathy
Inotersen	Antisense oligonueotide that degrades wild and mutant type TTR mRNA and decreases TTR protein deposits in tissues	Hereditary transthyretin mediated amyloidosis associated polyneuropathy
Amifampridine	Potassium channel blocker	Lambert Eaton Myasthenic Syndrome

Multiple Choice Questions

ANTIEPILEPTICS

1. **If carbamazepine is added to valproate, which of the following side effect increases? *(AIIMS Nov 2018)***
   a. Thrombocytopenia
   b. Hepatotoxicity
   c. Hyperammonemia
   d. Pancreatitis

2. **A 16-year-old girl was on antiepileptic for treatment of seizure episodes while asleep. She had no seizure for 6 months and NCCT and EEG was normal. What is further management? *(AIIMS Nov 2018)***
   a. Stop treatment
   b. Continue for 2 years
   c. Lifelong treatment
   d. Stop treatment and follow up with 6 monthly EEG

3. **1. 30 year old epileptic was on levetrecetam 1gm BD was experiencing anger and aggression as adverse effect and it was affecting his quality of life and has come to you. He had a two year seizure free period. What is to be done?**
   a. Taper levetrecetam and stop it after 6 months
   b. Stop immediately *(AIIMS May 2017)*
   c. Wait till the 5 year clearance period of seizure
   d. Change the anti-epileptic

4. **Idiosyncratic reactions associated with carbamazepine are all except: *(AIIMS May 2017)***
   a. Steven Jhonson syndrome
   b. Rash
   c. Agranulocytosis
   d. Blurred vision

5. **Drug of choice for severe rheumatic chorea is: *(Recent Question 2017)***
   a. Valproate   b. Haloperidol
   c. Immunoglobulin   d. Diazepam

6. **Which of the following pair does not match? *(AIIMS Nov 2016)***

	Epilepsy	1st line	2nd line
a.	Absence	Lamotrigine Carbamazepine	Ethosuximide Valproate
b.	Myoclonic	Valproate Lamotrigine	Clonazepam
c.	GTCS	Valproate Lamotrigine	Carbamazepine Topiramate
d.	Partial	Lamotrigine Carbamazepine	Valproate

7. **A female patient suffered from exanthematous rashes 4 weeks after being started on phenytoin and valproate for epilepsy. After how many days of rechallenge rash will reappear again if drug is started after rash subsides?**
   a. 1 day   b. 1 week *(AIIMS Nov 2016)*
   c. 2 weeks   d. 4 weeks

8. **The adverse drug reaction of phenytoin in the picture is *(Recent Question Dec 2016)***

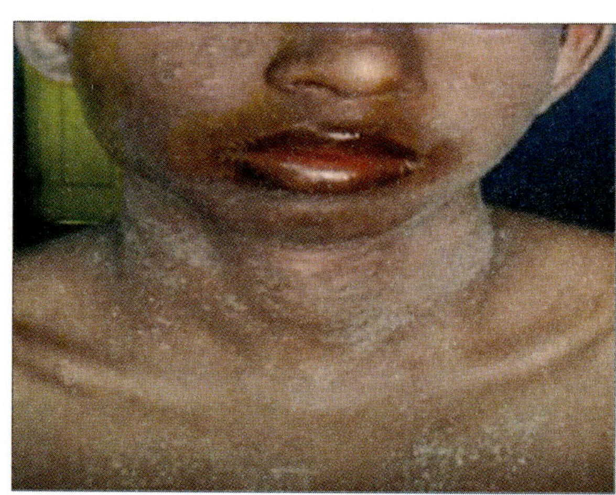

   a. TEN
   b. Acute exanthematous pustulosis
   c. SJS
   d. Hyperpigmentation

9. **Recent treatment combination along with phentermine approved for weight reduction in obesity? *(Recent Question Dec 2016)***
   a. Lamotrigine   b. Topiramate
   c. Valproate   d. Gabapentin

10. **Which of the following antiepileptic drug use requires ophthalmological consultation? *(Recent Question Dec 2016)***
    a. Carbamazepine   b. Topiramate
    c. Valproate   d. Lamotrigine

11. **Drug for migraine which is antiepileptic *(Recent Question Dec 2016)***
    a. Topiramate   b. Lamotrigine
    c. Carbamazepine   d. Vigabatrin

12. **Most common antiepileptic causing toxic epiderm necrosis *(Recent Question Dec 2016)***
    a. Carbamazepine
    b. Valproate
    c. Phenytoin
    d. Gabapentin

13. **Which of the following is a gender specific side effect caused by valproate? *(AIIMS Nov 2015)***
    a. PCOS   b. Tremor
    c. Alopecia   d. Weight gain

14. **Which drug can cause progressive visual field constriction? *(AIIMS Nov 2015)***
    a. Phenobarbitone   b. Vigabatrin
    c. Ethosuximide   d. Valproate

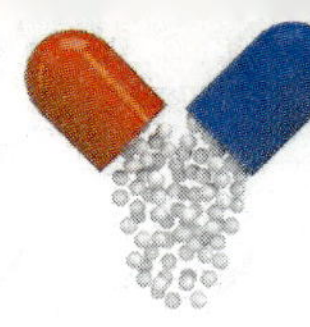

15. When to start folic acid in a patient on antiepileptics? *(AIIMS Nov 2015)*
- a. Any woman who can potentially be pregnant
- b. 3 months before planning pregnancy
- c. At confirmation of pregnancy
- d. After pregnancy

16. A female with history of previous pregnancy associated with neural tube defect. What should be the prophylactic dose of folic acid given in microgram? *(AIIMS May 2015)*
- a. 4
- b. 40
- c. 400
- d. 4,000

17. Prolonged use of which of the following anticonvulsants can produce weight loss? *(Recent Question 2016)*
- a. Gabapentin
- b. Oxcarbazepine
- c. Topiramate
- d. Valproic acid

18. Carbamazepine in elderly causes: *(Recent Question 2016)*
- a. Hypernatremia
- b. Hyponatremia
- c. Hyperkalemia
- d. Hypokalemia

19. Which statement is true about carbamazepine? *(Recent Question 2016)*
- a. Used in trigeminal neuralgia
- b. Carbamazepine is an enzyme inhibitor
- c. Can cause megaloblastic anemia
- d. It is the drug of choice for status epilepticus

20. Which among the following is the mechanism of action of Carbamazepine? *(Recent Question 2016)*
- a. Prolongation of inactivated state of Na^+ channels
- b. Facilitates GABA
- c. Inhibition of Ca^{2+} channels
- d. NMDA receptor blockade

21. Cleft lip is caused by which of the following drug? *(Recent Question 2016)*
- a. Levetiracetum
- b. Phenytoin
- c. Sodium Valproate
- d. Phenobarbitone

22. Which antiepileptic drug is least secreted in breast milk – *(Recent Question 2016)*
- a. Ethosuximide
- b. Clonazepam
- c. Gabapentin
- d. Carbamazepine

23. Patient of juvenile myoclonic epilepsy on valproate comes to you at 5 months of pregnancy with level II scan normal what will you advise- *(Recent Question 2016)*
- a. Change the drug
- b. Continue the drug in same dose
- c. Decrease the dose of drug
- d. Increase the dose of drug

24. Felbamate is used in *(Recent Question 2016)*
- a. Epilepsy
- b. Anxiety
- c. Social phobia
- d. Depression

25. Antiepileptic drug not associated with enzyme induction or inhibition property is *(Recent Question 2016)*
- a. Phenytoin
- b. Valproate
- c. Carbamazepine
- d. Ethosuximide

26. Most serious side effect of valproate is *(Recent Question 2016)*
- a. Fulminant hepatitis
- b. Spina bifida
- c. Weight gain
- d. Thrombocytopenia

27. Oxcarbazepine true is all except *(Recent Question 2016)*
- a. Metabolises itself
- b. Less chances of hyponatremia than carbamazepine
- c. It is less enzyme inducer than carbamazepine
- d. Less chances of hepatotoxicity than carbamazepine

28. Which of the following is not an antiepileptic agent? *(Recent Question 2016)*
- a. Phenytoin
- b. Flunarizine
- c. Topiramate
- d. Carbamazepine

29. Fetal hydantoin syndrome is seen if following drug is used in pregnancy? *(Recent Question 2016)*
- a. Phenytoin
- b. Alcohol
- c. Ethosuximide
- d. Phenobarbitone

30. Ethosuximide can be used for the treatment of *(Recent Question 2016)*
- a. Generalized tonic clonic seizures
- b. Absence seizures
- c. Complex seizures
- d. Myoclonic seizures

31. All of the following are adverse effects of sodium valproate except *(Recent Question 2016)*
- a. Weight gain
- b. Alopecia
- c. Liver damage
- d. Osteomalacia

32. Which antiepileptic drug does not act via inhibition of sodium channels? *(Recent Question 2016)*
- a. Vigabatrin
- b. Carbamazepine
- c. Lamotrigine
- d. Phenytoin

33. The drug used in absence seizures and having a narrow spectrum of antiepileptic activity is *(Recent Question 2016)*
- a. Lamotrigine
- b. Ethosuximide
- c. Sodium valproate
- d. Primidone

34. Status epilepticus is managed best with the use of which of the following drugs? *(Recent Question 2016)*
- a. Intravenous diazepam
- b. Intravenous phenytoin sodium
- c. Intramuscular phenobarbitone
- d. Rectal diazepam

35. Antiepileptic drug implicated in causing toxic epidermal necrolysis is *(Recent Question 2016)*
- a. Felbamate
- b. Gabapentin
- c. Lamotrigine
- d. vigabatrin

36. Carbamazepine in elderly causes *(Recent Question 2016)*
- a. Hypernatremia
- b. Hyponatremia
- c. Hyperkalemia
- d. Hypokalemia

37. Drug of choice for rapid cyclers in manic-depressive psychosis is *(Recent Question 2016)*
- a. Carbamazepine
- b. Valproate
- c. Phenytoin
- d. Lithium

38. Osteomalacia is adverse effect of: *(Recent Question 2016)*

a. Primidone b. Phenytoin
c. Carbamazepine d. Valproic acid

39. Which drug is contraindicated in pregnancy? *(Recent Question 2016)*

a. Phenytoin b. Insulin
c. Heparin d. All

40. Folate deficiency occurs due to *(Recent Question 2016)*

a. Phenytoin b. Phenobarbitone
c. Primidone d. All

41. Not true about fosphenytoin is *(Recent Question 2016)*

a. Used for GTCS b. Prodrug of phenytoin
c. Lipid soluble d. Highly protein bound

42. Dilantin causes *(Recent Question 2016)*

a. Folic acid deficiency
b. Thiamine deficiency
c. Nicotinamide deficiency
d. Riboflavin deficiency

43. Valproic acid *(Recent Question 2016)*

a. It is an enzyme inducer
b. It causes obesity
c. It causes hirsutism
d. It causes neural tube defects

44. Drug of choice for absence seizure is *(Recent Question 2016)*

a. Ethosuximide b. Valproic acid
c. Carbamazepine d. Phenytoin

45. Regarding phenytoin all the following are correct except *(Recent Question 2016)*

a. It acts on voltage sensitive neuronal Na^+ channels
b. Used by slow IV injection in status epilepticus
c. Kinetics change from 1st order to zero order over therapeutic range
d. It inhabits microsomal enzymes

46. Clonazepam is used in all except *(Recent Question 2016)*

a. Absence seizure b. Infantile spasms
c. Myoclonic seizure d. Eclampsia

47. Drug of choice for myoclonic seizures *(Recent Question 2016)*

a. Vigabatrin b. Phenytoin
c. Valproate d. Carbamazepine

48. Fosphenytoin is given *(Recent Question 2016)*

a. Oral b. IM
c. IV d. SC

49. DOC for prophylaxis of febrile seizures *(Recent Question 2016)*

a. Rectal diazepam b. Valproate
c. Phenytoin d. Carbamazepine

50. Felbamate was discontinued due to *(Recent Question 2016)*

a. Aplastic anemia
b. Renal impairment
c. Gastrointestinal disorder
d. Seizures

51. Topiramate-major side effect is *(Recent Question 2016)*

a. Renal stone b. Agranulocytosis
c. Nephrotoxicity d. Retinal detachment

52. DOC for seizures in tuberous sclerosis *(Recent Question 2016)*

a. Vigabatrin b. Topiramate
c. Lamotrigine d. Levitiracetam

53. The drug of choice for a patient presenting with H/O lennox gastaut syndrome *(Recent Question 2016)*

a. Vigabatrin b. Topiramate
c. Lamotrigine d. Levetiracetam

54. Drug indicated in absence seizures *(Recent Question 2016)*

a. Valproate b. Vigabatrin
c. Topiramate d. Lamotrigine

SEDATIVE HYPNOTICS

55. Which of the following benzodiazepine can be used as a muscle relaxant? *(Recent Question Dec 2016)*

a. Diazepam b. Nitrazepam
c. Clonazepam d. Flurazepam

56. Barbiturates have *(Recent Question Dec 2016)*

a. GABA mimetic b. GABA facilitatory
c. Both d. None

57. Which of the following is not used as a sedative, but causes sedation as a side effect: *(AIIMS Nov 2007)*

a. Digitalis, anti-arrhythmics
b. Antihistaminics, antidepressants
c. Macrolides
d. Benzodiazepines

58. Inverse agonist is: *(Recent Question 2016)*

a. Buspirone b. β carboline
c. Flumazenil d. Zolpidem

59. Which of the following is a non-benzodiazepine hypnotic acting on benzodiazepine receptor that has no muscle relaxant property? *(Recent Question 2016)*

a. Zaleplon b. Beta-carboline
c. Bicuculline d. Ramelteon

60. Antagonist of benzodiazepine is? *(Recent Question 2016)*

a. Naltrexone b. Flumazenil
c. Naloxone d. N-Acetyl cysteine

61. IV diazepam has which of the following effect which is not seen by other routes *(Recent Question 2016)*

a. Analgesia b. Sedation
c. Hypotension d. Coronary dilatation

62. All of the following drugs require dose reduction in cirrhosis except *(Recent Question 2016)*

a. Lorazepam b. Diazepam
c. Metronidazole d. Rifampicin

63. Agents not acting via GABA-A receptors *(Recent Question 2016)*

a. Zopiclone b. Benzodiazepines
c. Thiopentone d. Prometazine

64. Increased tendency to fall asleep at night without causing central nervous system depression is a property exhibited by *(Recent Question 2016)*

a. Pyridoxine
b. Diphenhydramine
c. Melatonin
d. Ethanol

65. Drug contraindicated in acute intermittent porphyria *(Recent Question 2016)*

a. Thiopentone b. Ketamine
c. Propofol d. Etomidate

66. Action of flumazenil on benzodiazepine receptor is *(Recent Question 2016)*

a. Agonist b. Partial agonist
c. Inverse agonist d. Antagonist

67. Drug used in postoperative pain relief *(Recent Question 2016)*

a. Naloxone b. Alprazolam
c. Naltrexone d. Midazolam

68. Drug not affecting GABAA receptor is? *(Recent Question 2016)*

a. Muscimol b. Alcohol
c. Picrotoxin d. Buspirone

69. Bioavailability of ramelteon is *(Recent Question 2016)*

a. 2% b. 7%
c. 10% d. 30%

70. Which amongst the following is an on-benzodiazepine hypnotic *(Recent Question 2016)*

a. Clobazam b. Alprazolam
c. Chlordiazepoxide d. Meprobamate

71. Which of the following drug is not metabolized by liver *(Recent Question 2016)*

a. Fluntirazepam b. Diazepam
c. Oxazepam d. Nitrazepam

OPIOIDS

72. Morphine should not be given in a patient with: *(AIIMS Nov 2018)*

a. Ischemic pain b. Cancer pain
c. Biliary colic d. Postoperative pain

73. A patient presented with right lower quadrant pain. He was already treated for right renal stone disease. Which of the following opioid is partial agonist at mu and full agonist at kappa? *(AIIMS Nov 2017)*

a. Pentazocin b. Buprenorphine
c. Tramadol d. Fentanyl

74. A patient in labor ward was given opioid analgesic. Which drug should be kept ready for emergency? *(AIIMS Nov 2017)*

a. Naloxone b. Lignocaine
c. Diphenhydramine d. Fentanyl

75. Which of the following is a full opioid agonist? *(Recent Question Dec 2016)*

a. Methadone b. Buprenorphine
c. Flumazenil d. Naloxone

76. Which of the following is seen due to opioid withdrawal? *(Recent Question Dec 2016)*

a. Pupil dilation b. Constipation
c. Sedation d. Respiratory depression

77. Drug used for labour pain *(Recent Question Dec 2016)*

a. Meperidine b. Pentazocine
c. Methadone d. Buprenorphine

78. True statement regarding methadone are all except: *(AIIMS May 2014)*

a. It is a long-acting μ-receptor agonist
b. It is rapidly absorbed from the gastrointestinal tract and is detected in plasma 30 minutes after oral administration
c. The primary use of methadone is relief of chronic pain
d. The onset of analgesia is 30–60 minutes after parenteral administration and 1–2 hours after oral administration

79. Opioid receptor which is responsible for dysphoria: *(AIIMS May 2013)*

a. Mu b. Kappa
c. Delta d. Sigma

80. Which is the mechanism of action of Buprenorphine? *(Recent Question 2016)*

a. Partial agonist at mu and antagonist at kappa
b. Partial agonist at kappa and antagonist at mu and delta
c. Partial agonist at mu and kappa and antagonist at delta
d. Partial agonist at mu kappa and delta

81. Drugs for paralytic ileus forbowel resection surgery are all except *(Recent Question 2016)*

a. Alvimopan b. Dihydroergotamine
c. Naloxone d. Methylnaltrexone

82. Buprenorphine partial agonist at which opioid receptor? *(Recent Question 2016)*

a. Mu b. Kappa
c. Delta d. Lambda

83. Which among the following drug is contraindicated in renal failure? *(Recent Question 2016)*

a. Pethidine b. Morphine
c. Fentanyl d. Atracurium

84. Buprenorphine is *(Recent Question 2016)*

a. Partial agonist at μ receptor
b. Partial agonist kreceptor
c. Full agonist at μ receptor
d. Full agonist at κ receptor

85. Tolerance develops to all of the following actions of opioids except *(Recent Question 2016)*

a. Miosis b. Analgesia
c. Euphoria d. Nausea and vomiting

86. A new-born developed respiratory depression in a postoperative ward. It can result from the use of *(Recent Question 2016)*

a. Opioid b. Propofol
c. Furosemide d. Heparin

87. Which of the following is least narcotic opioid? *(Recent Question 2016)*

a. Morphine b. Codeine
c. Heroin d. Papaverine

88. Buprenorphine is *(Recent Question 2016)*
a. Pure agonist b. Pure antagonist
c. Partial agonist d. None

89. The following symptoms may be seen in opium withdrawal *(Recent Question 2016)*
a. Tremors
b. Lacrimation
c. Constipation
d. Dry nose and mouth constipation

90. Naltrexone is used in opioid dependence
a. To treat withdrawal symptoms *(Recent Question 2016)*
b. To prevent relapse
c. To treat overdose
d. For opioid rotation therapy

91. Morphine can be used in all except *(Recent Question 2016)*
a. Head injury b. Asthma
c. Hypothyroidism d. Diabetes

92. Naloxone is contraindicated in neonatal resuscitation if the mother is on *(Recent Question 2016)*
a. Cocaine b. Amphetamine
c. Methadone d. Phencyclidine

93. Which of the following opioids has maximum plasma protein binding capacity? *(Recent Question 2016)*
a. Morphine b. Sufentanil
c. Fentanyl d. Pethidine

94. Long-term use of pethidine is avoided because a metabolite of pethidine is associated with *(Recent Question 2016)*
a. Constipation b. Dependence
c. Seizures d. Respiratory depression

95. Drug of choice for controlling severe pain in cancer patients is *(Recent Question 2016)*
a. Morphine b. Diclofenac
c. Ibuprofen d. Codeine

96. In acute morphine poisoning, the drug of choice is *(Recent Question 2016)*
a. Atropine b. Methadone
c. Naloxone d. Alcohol

97. Naltrexone is used for poisoning of *(Recent Question 2016)*
a. Heroin b. Atropine
c. Cannabis d. Diazepam

98. Tolerance occurs to all actions of morphine except *(Recent Question 2016)*
a. Miotic action b. Analgesic action
c. Euphoric action d. All of the above

99. Actions of opiates include all except *(Recent Question 2016)*
a. Constipation b. Vomiting
c. Analgesia d. Mydriasis

100. Endogenous opioid peptide includes *(Recent Question 2016)*
a. Encephalin b. Endorphins
c. Dynorphins d. All of the above

101. Tramadol is: *(Recent Question 2016)*
a. Antiflatulent b. Antireflux drug
c. Beta-blocker d. Opioid analgesic

102. The effect of morphine which has least tolerance is *(Recent Question 2016)*
a. Analgesia b. Respiratory depression
c. Constipation d. Bradycardia

103. Opioid with monoamine action is *(Recent Question 2016)*
a. Tramadol b. Pentazocine
c. Pethidine d. Meperidine

104. Morphine causes all except *(Recent Question 2016)*
a. Increased prolactin secretion
b. Diarrhea
c. Analgesia
d. Sedation

105. Morphine is contraindicated in all except *(Recent Question 2016)*
a. Hepatic insufficiency b. Bronchial asthma
c. Head injury d. Preanesthetic medication

106. Drugs with agonist action to any opioid receptors are all except *(Recent Question 2016)*
a. Pentazocine b. Buprenorphine
c. Levallorphan d. Naloxone

107. The pain in a terminal cancer patient is best relieved by *(Recent Question 2016)*
a. Diclofenac sodium b. Pethidine
c. Morphine d. Diazepam

108. Opioid withdrawal is characterized by all except *(Recent Question 2016)*
a. Miosis b. Salivation
c. Diarrhea d. Lacrimation

109. Piloerection is seen with withdrawal of *(Recent Question 2016)*
a. Opioids b. LSD
c. Alcohol d. Phenytoin

ANTIDEPRESSANTS

110. Discontinuation of which of the following drug results in anxiety and insomnia? *(AIIMS May 2018)*
a. Venlafaxine b. Imipramine
c. Valproate d. Olanzapine

111. Which of the following is not an adverse effect of escitalopram? *(AIIMS May 2018)*
a. Sialorrhea b. Vivid dreams
c. Nausea d. Anorgasmia

112. Which of the following mood stabilizer has antisuicidal effect? *(AIIMS May 2017)*
a. Lithium b. Valproate
c. Carbamazepine d. Lamotrigine

113. Which of the following drug increases serotonin and nor epinephrine and is also an alpha 2 antagonist? *(Recent Question Dec 2016)*
a. Venlafaxine b. Mirtazapine
c. Duloxetine d. Fluoxetine

114. **Fluoxetine is given for a patient and after 5 days there is no improvement in symptoms. What is the next step?** *(Recent Question Dec 2016)*
a. Double the doses
b. Add lithium
c. Wait as it takes 2-6 weeks to respond
d. Change to TCA

115. **SSRIs are indicated in?** *(Recent Question Dec 2016)*
a. Impotence b. Retrograde ejaculation
c. Premature ejaculation d. Oligospermia

116. **First line treatment in tachycardia due to amitriptyline:** *(Recent Question Dec 2016)*
a. $CaCl_2$ b. Insulin + glucagon
c. IV $NaHCO_3$ d. Amiodarone

117. **A girl with history of getting medications prescribed by psychiatrist for depression presents with altered sensorium. ECG shows QRS widening and rt axis deviation >120° in terminal part. What is the management?** *(AIIMS Nov 2015)*
a. Haemodialysis b. IV Flumazenil
c. Charcoal d. IV sodium bicarbonate

118. **Best agent for premenstrual syndrome management:** *(AIIMS Nov 2012)*
a. Progesterone b. Anxiolytics
c. SSRI d. Vitamin E

119. **Dextromethorphan should not be given with which drug?** *(Recent Question 2016)*
a. SSRIs b. MAO inhibitors
c. Atropine d. Paracetamol

120. **Which is the antidepressant with no anticholinergic effects?** *(Recent Question 2016)*
a. Imipramine b. Mianserine
c. Fluvoxamine d. Amitriptyline

121. **Which of the following SSRI is a prodrug?** *(Recent Question 2016)*
a. Fluoxetine b. Paroxetine
c. Citalopram d. Fluvoxamine

122. **Which of the following agent is not a serotonin and dopaminergic blocker?** *(Recent Question 2016)*
a. Doxepin b. Amisulpride
c. Sertindole d. Zotepine

123. **Antidepressant drug that can be used in nocturnal enuresis is?** *(Recent Question 2016)*
a. Imipramine b. Fluvoxamine
c. Phenelzine d. Bupropion

124. **What is the drug of choice for obsessive compulsive disorder?** *(Recent Question 2016)*
a. Imipramine b. Fluoxetine
c. Benzodiazepines d. Alprazolam

125. **Which of the following is not a serotonin-norepinephrine reuptake inhibitor?** *(Recent Question 2016)*
a. Venlafaxine b. Duloxetine
c. Milnacipran d. Tianeptine

126. **Not a side effect of paroxetine** *(Recent Question 2016)*
a. Premature ejaculation b. Erectile dysfunction
c. Decreased libido d. Diarrhea

127. **Increased suicidal tendency is associated with alteration in the brain levels of** *(Recent Question 2016)*
a. Noradrenaline b. Serotonin
c. Dopamine d. GABA

128. **Antidepressant drug that can be safely used in children is** *(Recent Question 2016)*
a. Imipramine b. Fluoxetine
c. Dothiepin d. Rispiridone

129. **Which of the following is not a SSRI?** *(Recent Question 2016)*
a. Escitalopram b. Sertraline
c. Paroxetine d. Amitriptyline

130. **Drug with both antidepressant and antipsychotic properties is** *(Recent Question 2016)*
a. Buspirone b. Amoxapine
c. Trazodone d. Mianserine

131. **Atomoxetine inhibits the reuptake of** *(Recent Question 2016)*
a. Serotonin b. Dopamine
c. Norepinephrine d. Epinephrine

132. **Serotonin syndrome is caused by** *(Recent Question 2016)*
a. Linezolid b. Selegiline
c. Meperidine d. All of the above

133. **Atomoxetine is used for treatment of:** *(Recent Question 2016)*
a. ADHD b. Seasonal affective disorder
c. Depression d. OCD

MANIA AND BPD

134. **Lithium use in pregnancy leads to which effect on baby?** *(AIIMS Nov 2018)*
a. CVS defect b. Urogenital defect
c. Neural tube defect d. Facial defects

135. **A pregnant female with manic episode for 2 weeks; previously 3 episodes of mania in 5 years and 1 episode of depression. What should be given for treatment?** *(AIIMS Nov 2015)*
a. Lithium b. Clonazepam
c. Haloperidol d. Promethazine

136. **Toxic dose of lithium** *(AIIMS Nov 2014)*
a. 8 mEq/L b. 6 mEq/L
c. 4 mEq/L d. 2 mEq/L

137. **Lithium potentiates the action of non-depolarizing muscle relaxants. How many days before administration of the muscle relaxant should lithium be stopped?**
a. 1 day b. 2 days *(AIIMS May 2014)*
c. 3 days d. 4 days

138. **Earliest sign of lithium toxicity is:** *(Recent Question 2016)*
a. Renal shutdown b. Thyroid insufficiency
c. Cardiac arrhythmias d. Ataxia and dysarthria

139. **Most common renal sequel of lithium toxicity is** *(Recent Question 2016)*
a. Nephrogenic DI b. Renal tubular acidosis
c. Glycosuria d. MPGN

140. Lithium use in pregnancy may result in fetal ***(Recent Question 2016)***
a. Cardiac malformation b. Cranial abnormality
c. Cleft lip and cleft palate

141. Half-life of lithium is ***(Recent Question 2016)***
a. 8 hours b. 16 hours
c. 24 hours d. 36 hours

142. Coarse tremors, dysarthria and ataxia are side effects of ***(Recent Question 2016)***
a. Lithium b. Haloperidol
c. Imipramine d. None

143. Lithium causes all except ***(Recent Question 2016)***
a. Exaggeration of psoriasis b. Nephropathy
c. Ebstein's anomaly d. Hyperthyroidism

144. Frequency of lithium induced tremors ***(Recent Question 2016)***
a. 8–10 Hz b. 6–7 Hz
c. 1–2 Hz d. 4–8 Hz

145. Lithium cause which cardiac side effects ***(Recent Question 2016)***
a. Bradycardia b. Cardiac myopathy
c. T wave inversion d. Cardiac arrhythmia

146. Drug not used in chronic bipolar disorder ***(Recent Question 2016)***
a. Lithium b. Haloperidol
c. Valproate d. Topiramate

147. Toxic levels of serum lithium more than ***(Recent Question 2016)***
a. 2 mEq b. 4 mEq
c. 6 mEq d. 8 mEq

ANTIPSYCHOTICS

148. A patient was treated with haloperidol, later he develops symptoms of Parkinsonism. what is the best treatment: ***(Recent Question 2018)***
a. Cholinesterase inhibitors
b. Histamine inhibitors
c. M1 antagonist
d. Alpha 1 adrenergic

149. Maximum increase in prolactin level is caused by: ***(Recent Question 2017)***
a. Risperidone b. Clozapine
c. Olanzapine d. Aripiprazole

150. Which of the following is true regarding typical antipsychotics? ***(Recent Question Dec 2016)***
a. Increases seizure threshold
b. Antiemetic property
c. Pruritic effect
d. Diarrhea

151. A patient of Psychosis started on haloperidol, immediately develops rigidity and tremors but was able to speak normally. Which of the following drug should be administered immediately? ***(AIIMS May 2015)***
a. Diazepam b. Lorazepam
c. Promethazine d. Haloperidol

152. A 24 year old male with 10 years history of abnormal excessive blinking and grunting. He says about no control over his symptoms which have risen in frequency of late. This has started affecting his social life making him depressed. Which of the following medications would you prescribe him? ***(AIIMS May 2015)***
a. Methylphenidate b. Risperidone
c. Carbamazepine d. Imipramine

153. Which one of the following causes least sedation ***(Recent Question 2016)***
a. Olanzapine b. Quetiapine
c. Aripiprazole d. Risperidone

154. A patient, Hari has been diagnosed to have schizophrenia, which of the following acts as a limiting factor in the use of clozapine as an anti psychotic drug in this patient? ***(Recent Question 2016)***
a. Its potential to cause agranulocytosis
b. Its inability to benefit negative symptoms of schizophrenia
c. High incidence of extrapyramidal side effects
d. Productionof hyperprolactinemia

155. A patient an antipsychotic drugs develops temperature of 104°C, BP about 150/100 and abnormal behavior. What is the likely diagnosis? ***(Recent Question 2016)***
a. Aggravation of psychosis
b. Dystonia
c. Neuroleptic malignant syndrome
d. Akathisia

156. A phenothiazine which is used as an antiemetic is: ***(Recent Question 2016)***
a. Chlorpromazine b. Promethazine
c. Trifluoperazine d. Fluphenazine

157. Which of the following has the highest potential to cause metabolic syndrome? ***(Recent Question 2016)***
a. Clozapine b. Risperidone
c. Quetiapine d. Aripiprazole

158. Weight gain is seen with all of the following antipsychiatric medications except ***(Recent Question 2016)***
a. Quitiapine b. Resperidone
c. Clozapine d. Molindone

159. Most common receptor for typical antipsychotics is ***(Recent Question 2016)***
a. D1 b. D2
c. D3 d. D4

160. Drug causing agranulocytosis ***(Recent Question 2016)***
a. Pimozide b. Clozapine
c. Risperidone d. Olanzapine

161. Following is false about aripiprazole except ***(Recent Question 2016)***
a. Only antipsychotic with D1 agonistic activity
b. It has 5HT1A antagonistic action
c. It has maximum sedating potential
d. It is the drug of choice in treatment of acute mania

162. Which of the following has highest potential to cause metabolic syndrome? ***(Recent Question 2016)***
a. Clozapine b. Risperidone
c. Quetiapine d. Aripiprazole

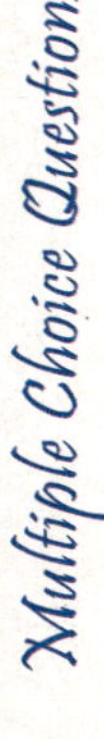

163. **Which of the following adverse effect can occur even after the offending drug has been withdrawn a long time back?** *(Recent Question 2016)*
   a. Paradoxical tachycardia
   b. Tardive dyskinesia
   c. Malignant hyperthermia
   d. Gynaecomastia

164. **Drug of choice in intractable hiccups is** *(Recent Question 2016)*
   a. Metoclopramide b. Haloperidol
   c. Thioridazine d. Chlorpromazine

165. **Akathisia is treated by all except** *(Recent Question 2016)*
   a. Trihexyphenidyl b. Diazepam
   c. Haloperidol d. Promethazine

166. **Which of the following drug causes sedation but no extra pyramidal side effect** *(Recent Question 2016)*
   a. Clozapine b. Pimozide
   c. Fluphenazine d. Haloperidol

167. **Schizophrenia can be treated with A/E** *(Recent Question 2016)*
   a. Pemoline b. Olanzapine
   c. Sulpiride d. Chlorpromazine

168. **Antipsychotic drug with least extra pyramidal side effects is** *(Recent Question 2016)*
   a. Triflupromazine b. Thioridazine
   c. Pimozide d. Trifluperazine

169. **Antipsychotic drug is** *(Recent Question 2016)*
   a. Doxepin b. Fluoxetine
   c. Clozapine d. All

170. **Which antipsychotic has partial agonist action of both D2 and 5HT1A?** *(Recent Question 2016)*
   a. Risperidone b. Olanzapine
   c. Clozapine d. Aripiprazole

171. **Clozapine** *(Recent Question 2016)*
   a. Has D2 agonist activity
   b. Cause agranulocytosis
   c. Cause hyperprolactinemia
   d. Anti-seizure property

172. **Haloperidol acts on which receptor** *(Recent Question 2016)*
   a. Adrenaline b. Glutamate
   c. Dopamine d. Nonadrenergic receptors

173. **A patient on antipsychotic treatment has an inability to sit at a place. He has to keep on moving to relieve his discomfort** *(Recent Question 2016)*
   a. Akathisia
   b. Tardive dyskinesia
   c. Malignant hypertharmia
   d. Neuroleptic malignant syndrome

NEURODEGENERATIVE DISORDERS

174. **Recent drug approved for amyotrophic lateral sclerosis?** *(AIIMS May 2018)*
   a. Doxycycline b. Ceftriaxone
   c. Edaravone d. Piracetam

175. **The use of levodopa is contraindicated in** *(Recent Question 2018)*
   a. Alzheimer's disease b. Psychosis
   c. Glaucoma d. ALS

176. **Drug used for Alzheimer's disease acting on NMDA receptor is** *(Recent Question Dec 2016)*
   a. Donepezil b. Memantine
   c. Tacrine d. Galantamine

177. **Which of the following statement regarding selegeline is FALSE?** *(Recent Question Dec 2016)*
   a. May be used in on-off phenomenon
   b. Does not cause cheese reaction
   c. It is used in parkinsonism
   e. It is a MAO-A inhibitor

178. **Tolcapone is** *(Recent Question Dec 2016)*
   a. Hepatotoxic b. Nephrotoxic
   c. Ototoxic d. Neurotoxic

179. **Peripheral vasospasm is observed with which of the following anti-Parkinsonian drugs?** *(AIIMS May 2014)*
   a. Ropinirole b. Levodopa
   c. Bromocriptine d. Entacapone

180. **Which of the following is a pro drug is** *(Recent Question 2016)*
   a. Levodopa b. Poiglitazone
   c. Dexamethasone d. Captopril

181. **Which drug is used in amytrophic lateral sclerosis?** *(Recent Question 2016)*
   a. Riluzole b. Glatirame
   c. Tacrine d. Olanzapine

182. **Rotigotine is** *(Recent Question 2016)*
   a. Dopamine agonist b. Dopamine antagonist
   c. GABA agonist d. GABA antagonist

183. **Patient on treatment on carbidopa + levodopa for 10 years now has weaning off effect. What should be added to restore action** *(Recent Question 2016)*
   a. Tolcapone b. Amantadine
   c. Rasagiline d. Benzhexol

184. **Natalizumab is used in treatment of** *(Recent Question 2016)*
   a. Muliple sclerosis b. Breast carcinoma
   c. Psoriasis d. B cell lymphoma

185. **Drug of choice for relapsing remitting multiple sclerosis is** *(Recent Question 2016)*
   a. α IFN b. β IFN
   c. γ IFN d. Natalizumab

186. **Which of the following drug is used as transcrranial patch for parkinson's disease?** *(Recent Question 2016)*
   a. Levodopa b. Rotigotine
   c. Selegiline d. Carbidopa

187. **Which of the following agents enhances the bioavailability of levodopa in patients with parkinson's disease** *(Recent Question 2016)*
   a. Amantadine b. Ropinirole
   c. Entacapone d. Selegiline

188. False statement about selegiline is
a. It is a MAO-A inhibitor *(Recent Question 2016)*
b. Does not cause cheese reaction
c. May be used in "on-off" phenomenon
d. It is used in parkinsonism

189. Anti-Parkinsonism drug that is a selective COMT inhibitor *(Recent Question 2016)*
a. Entacapone b. Ropinirole
c. Pergolide d. Pramipexole

190. All are dopaminergic angonists used for parkinsonism except *(Recent Question 2016)*
a. Bromocriptine b. Ropinirole
c. Pramipexole d. Selegiline

191. Antiparkinson's drug with anti-apoptotic activity *(Recent Question 2016)*
a. Levodopa b. Selegiline
c. Entacapone d. Ropinirole

192. All are side effects of ropinirole except *(Recent Question 2016)*
a. Sedation b. Nausea
c. Retroperitoneal fibrosis d. Hallucination

193. Antiparkinson drug known to cause cardiac valvular fibrosis is *(Recent Question 2016)*
a. Bromocriptine b. Ropinirole
c. Pramiprexole d. Pergolide and cabergoline

194. Galantamine is used in *(Recent Question 2016)*
a. Alzheimer's disease
b. Parkinson's disease
c. Emesis
d. Chorea

195. Drug of choice for restless leg syndrome *(Recent Question 2016)*
a. Diazepam b. Risperidose
c. Valproate d. Ropinirole

196. All are ergot derivatives used in parkinsonism except *(Recent Question 2016)*
a. Bromocriptine b. Pergolide
c. Trihexyphenidyl d. Cabergoline

197. Which is hepatotoxic *(Recent Question 2016)*
a. Entacapone b. Ropinirole
c. Tolcapone d. Trihexyphenidyl

DEPENDENCE

198. Drug used for smoking and tobacco chewing is *(Recent Question 2019)*
a. Varenicline b. Acamprosate
c. Bupropion d. Naltrexone

199. Which of the following drug is used for treatment of acute alcohol withdrawal? *(Recent Question Dec 2016)*
a. Chlorodiazepoxide b. Diazepam
c. Clorazepate d. Alprazolam

200. Which of the following drug is not used in nicotine withdrawal? *(Recent Question 2016)*
a. Buspirone b. Bupropione
c. Vernaceline d. Nicotine

201. What is not used in detoxification of chronic alcohol dependence? *(AIIMS Nov 2015)*
a. Acamprosate b. Flumazenil
c. Naltrexone d. Disulfiram

202. Drug not given in alcohol dependency syndrome *(AIIMS Nov 2014)*
a. Disulfiram b. Acamprosate
c. Naltrexone d. Phenytoin

203. Drugs used in alcohol withdrawal during maintenance phase are all except: *(Recent Question 2016)*
a. Naltrexone b. Naloxone
c. Acamprosate d. Disulfiram

204. CB 1 antagonist used in smoking cessation is *(Recent Question 2016)*
a. Naloxona b. Rimonabant
c. Vareniloline d. Bupripion

205. Drugs used in alcohol dependence to prevent relapse are all except *(Recent Question 2016)*
a. Nalmefene b. Topiramate
c. Ondansetron d. Fluoxetine

206. Varenicline acts by *(Recent Question 2016)*
a. Partial nicotine receptor agonist
b. Nicotine receptor antagonist
c. Both agonist and antagonist at nicotine receptor
d. None of the above

207. Which of the following is not a feature of fetal alcohol syndrome? *(Recent Question 2016)*
a. Microcephaly b. Low intelligence
c. Large proportionate body
d. Septal defects of heart

208. Anti-craving agents for alcohol dependence are all except *(Recent Question 2016)*
a. Lorazepam b. Acamprosate
c. Topiramate d. Naltrexone

209. In alcohol withdrawal, drug of choice is *(Recent Question 2016)*
a. TFP b. Chlormethazole
c. Chlordiazepoxide d. Buspirone

210. Which of the following is used to maintain abstinence in alcohol dependence? *(Recent Question 2016)*
a. Naltrexone b. Clonidine
c. Disulfiriam d. Naloxone

211. The combination of alcohol and disulfiram results in nausea and hypotension as a result of accumulation of *(Recent Question 2016)*
a. Acetaldehyde b. Acetate
c. Methanol d. NADH

212. Disulfiram like reaction is not seen with *(Recent Question 2016)*
a. Amoxicillin b. Metronidazole
c. Cefoperazone d. Disulfiram

213. Antabuse *(Recent Question 2016)*
a. Inhibitis glucuronide conjugation
b. Inhibits oxidation of alcohol
c. Inhibits excretion of alcohol through kidney
d. None of the above

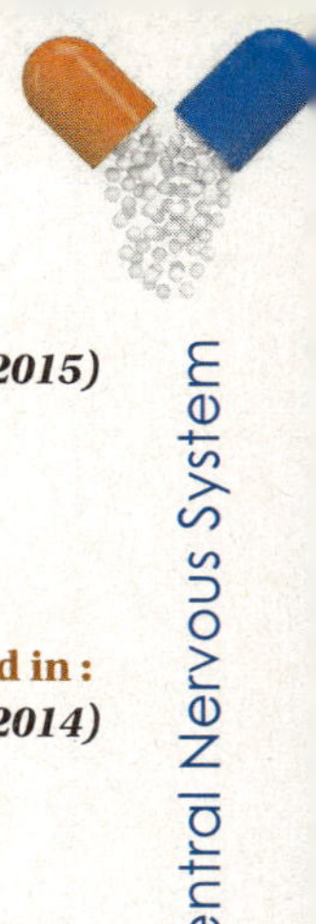

214. Nicotine replacement therapy is available in all forms except ***(Recent Question 2016)***

a. Chewing gum b. Lozenges
c. Patch d. Tablets

215. Which of the following is/are adverse effect(s) of tricyclic antidepressants (TCA): ***(PGI May 2018)***

a. Tremor
b. Hypertension
c. Weight loss
d. Diarrhea
e. Urinary retention

216. Which of the following antiseizure drug(s) is/are sodium channel blocker: ***(PGI May 2018)***

a. Ethosuximide b. Felbamate
c. Phenytoin d. Levetiracetam
e. Ezogabine

217. Nor epinephrine reuptake inhibitor: ***(PGI Nov 2017)***

a. Fluoxetine b. Duloxetine
c. Paroxetine d. Atomoxetine
e. Milnacipran

218. Drugs given in mania: ***(PGI Nov 2017)***

a. Mood stabilizers
b. Anti-psychotics
c. Anti-depressants
d. Antiepileptics
e. Sedative hypnotics

219. Clozapine S/E: ***(PGI Nov 2017)***

a. Seizures b. Sedation
c. Dry mouth d. Hypothermia
e. Constipation

220. Which of the following is true statement(s) about codeine:

a. Used as anti-tussive agent ***(PGI May 2017)***
b. Analgesic potency is equivalent to morphine
c. Causes respiratory depression
d. Partly metabolized to morphine
e. Completely metabolized to morphine

221. Adverse effects of mirtazapine is/are: ***(PGI NOV 2016)***

a. Insomnia b. Sedation
c. Sexual dysfunction d. Vomiting
e. Weight gain

222. Mechanism of action of gabapentin is/are:

a. Enhances GABA release ***(PGI June 2015)***
b. Agonist at GABAA receptor
c. Act on NMDA receptor
d. Prolongation of Na^+ Channel Inactivation
e. Inhibition of voltage-gated Ca^{2+} channels

223. Levetiracetam is commonly used for: ***(PGI June 2015)***

a. Juvenile myoclonic epilepsy
b. Absence seizure
c. Generalized Tonic clonic seizure
d. Complex partial seizure
e. Act through GABA

224. Which of the followings are feature of benzodiazepine withdrawal except: ***(PGI June 2015)***

a. Anxiety b. Hypersomnia
d. Bad dreams e. Tremor

225. In comparison to haloperidol, clozapine causes:

a. Weight gain ***(PGI June 2015)***
b. Agranulocytosis
c. Sedation
d. Severe extrapyramidal symptoms
e. Less eliptogenic potential

226. Fomepizole can be used in : Fomepizole can be used in :

a. Methanol poisoning ***(PGI May 2014)***
b. Organophosphorus poisoning
c. Ethylene glycol poisoning
d. Barbiturate poisoning

227. Unwanted interactions of MAO inhibitors occur with: ***(PGI May 2014)***

a. Levodopa b. Hydrochlorothiazide
c. Reserpine d. Pethidine

228. Weight gain is not seen with: ***(PGI May 2014)***

a. Clozapine b. Risperidone
c. Olanzapine d. SSRI
e. Zotepine

229. True about morphine: ***(PGI May 2014)***

a. Act as antagonist μ receptor with no agonist action
b. Activation in liver
c. Half life 4 hr
d. Cause miosis
e. Clearance time is around 20 hr

230. Which of the following is/are true about phenytoin

a. Inactivation by Liver enzyme ***(PGI May 2014)***
b. Causes Vit B12 deficiency
c. Causes thiamine deficiency
d. Gum hypertrophy is the most side effect
e. Inhibitor of CYP3A4/5

231. Which of the following is not atypical antipsychotic: ***(PGI Nov 2013)***

a. Aripiprazole b. Amoxapine
c. Clozapine d. Zotepine
e. Asenapine

232. Morphine exert action through which receptors: ***(PGI Nov 2012)***

a. μ receptor b. δ receptor
c. κ receptor d. α receptor
e. β receptor

233. Which of the following drug-receptor pair(s) correctly matched: ***(PGI May 2012)***

a. Buspirone : 5HT-1 agonist
b. Granisetron: 5HT-2 antagonist
c. Cisapride: 5 HT-3 agonist
d. Methysergide: 5 HT-4 antagonist
e. Imipramine:TNF-α inhibitor

234. Phenytoin causes: ***(PGI May 2012)***

a. Red cell aplasia b. Megaloblastic anemia
c. Aplastic anemia d. Hemolytic anemia
e. Thrombocytopenia

235. Amitriptyline overdose cause all except: ***(PGI Nov 2011)***

a. Conduction defect b. Diarrhea
c. Metabolic acidosis d. Orthostatic hypotensiion
e. Urinary retention

236. Which of following are not selective serotonin reuptake inhibitors (SSRI): *(PGI Nov 2011)*
a. Venlafaxine
b. Mirtazapine
c. Duloxetine
d. Paroxetine
e. Escitalopram

237. True about buprenorphine: *(PGI Nov 2010)*
a. Naloxone cannot reverse its effects
b. Agonist at δ receptor
c. Long-acting
d. More potent than morphine
e. Partial μ receptor agonist

238. Which is opioid: *(PGI Nov 2010)*
a. Pethidine
b. Diacetylmorphine
c. Naloxone
d. Pentazocine
e. Morphine

239. True statement about pethidine w.r.t morphine: *(PGI Nov 2010)*
a. Cause more bradycardia
b. Constipation less marked
c. Cough more suppressed
d. More potent
e. Rapid onset

240. True statements about Antiparkinsonism drugs: *(PGI Nov 2009)*
a. Off & on phenomenon is seen with levodopa because up & down regulation of dopamineric receptor
b. Tolcapone cause greenish discolouration of urine
c. Apomorphine is used in treatment
d. Quinagolide is an ergot derivative
e. Ropinirole is used in restless leg syndrome

241. SNRI is/are: *(PGI Nov 2009)*
a. Escitaleprom
b. Venlafaxine
c. Mirtazepine
d. Duloxetine
e. Paroxetine

242. True about anticonvulsants: *(PGI Nov 2009)*
a. Carbamazepine safe in pregnancy
b. Lamotrigine is safe
c. Monotherapy is recommended
d. Newer drugs are safe

243. Anticonvulsant drugs, which are also used to cure psychiatric disorders are: *(PGI Dec 2008)*
a. Phenytoin
b. Na valproate
c. Lamotrigine
d. Topiramate
e. Levetiracetam

244. Antiparkinsonism drugs are : *(PGI Dec 2008)*
a. Rotigotine
b. Rivastigmine
c. Quinagolide
d. Ropinirole
e. Amantadine

245. Phenytointoxicity includes: *(PGI June 2007)*
a. Gum hypertrophy
b. Acne rosacea
c. Exacerbation of acne vulgaris
d. Loss of hair

246. Risperidone is asso. with ↑ risk of: *(PGI Dec 2006)*
a. Cerbrovascular accidents
b. ↑ EPS
c. Agranulocytosis
d. Diabetes insipidus
e. Gout

247. True about Zolpidem *(PGI Dec 2005)*
a. Act on Benzodiazipine receptor 1 and 2
b. Action not reversed by flumazenil
c. Sedation is less than diazepam
d. Only sedation and hypnosis
e. Duration of action less than diazepam

248. A Pt. is on antipsychotics develops temperature of 104°C and BP 150/100 and abnormal behavior. What is the diagnosis *(PGI Dec 2005)*
a. Aggravation of psychosis
b. Parkinsonism
c. Dystonia
d. Neuroleptic malignant syndrome
e. Akathesia

249. In OCD Rx of choice is/are *(PGI Dec 2005)*
a. Fluoxetine
b. Imipramine
c. Diazepam

250. Therapeutic level of phenytoin *(PGI Dec 2005)*
a. 0.9 μg/mL
b. 10–19 μg/mL
c. 20–29 μg/mL
d. 30–39 μg/mL
e. >40 μ g/mL

251. In a child of infantile spasm with visual defect, which drug is not used even though it is highly effective? *(JIPMER Nov 2018)*
a. Lamotrigine
b. Topiramate
c. ACTH
d. Vigabatrin

252. A 20 years old primigravidae, 33 weeks pregnant lady had 2 episodes of seizures. The drug of choice is *(JIPMER Nov 2018)*
a. Furosemide
b. Mannitol
c. Carbamazepine
d. Nifedipine

253. Inverse agonist of benzodiazepine is: *(JIPMER 2017)*
a. Flumazenil
b. Beta carboline
c. Bicuculine
d. Phenobarbital

254. Which of the following is a new drug for treatment of tardive dyskinesia: *(JIPMER 2017)*
a. Valbenazine
b. Deutetrabenazine
c. Tetrabenazine
d. Ropinirole

255. Which of the following is a new drug approved for treatment of ALS? *(JIPMER 2017)*
a. Edaravone
b. Baclofen
c. Riluzole
d. Rivociclib

256. Which of the following is a mu receptor antagonist? *(JIPMER 2017)*
a. Alvimopan
b. Naloxone
c. Tramadol
d. Buprenorphine

257. New Drug used to treat on off phenomena in Parkinson's disease is: *(JIPMER 2017)*
a. Safinamide
b. Telotristat
c. Niraparib
d. Amantidine

258. A known patient of seizure disorder was started on carbamazepine, following which he developed Steven Johnson's syndrome. The associated gene is: *(JIPMER 2017)*
a. HLA B51
b. HLA B1502
c. HLA B1507
d. HLA B27

259. Incorrect therapeutic range of antiepileptic drug: *(JIPMER 2017)*
a. Phenytoin 10–20 mcg/mL
b. Phenobarbitone 5–10 mcg/mL
c. Carbamazepine 4–12 mcg/mL
d. Levetiracetam 15–45 mcg/mL

260. Levodopa and carbidopa combination does not prevent which side effect: *(JIPMER 2017)*
a. Psychosis b. Severe vomiting
c. Arrhythmia d. Postural hypotension

261. A 34-year-old male presents to the outpatient department with a complaint of pain in the right sided jaw pain. Each episode of pain is lasting for around 30 seconds. The present complaint was present for the past one month but the increased in the number of episodes per day brought her to the clinic. Those episodes are increasing especially when she walks out in the cold. The mechanism of action of drug of choice in this patient is?
a. Prevention of Na^+ influx *(JIPMER 2016)*
b. Increase the time of Cl^- channel opening
c. Increase the frequency of Cl^- channel opening
d. Decrease in the Ca^{+2} influx

262. Pregnant woman is on valproate for juvenile myoclonic epilepsy. Alternative monotherapy of choice: *(JIPMER 2014)*
a. Carbamazepine b. Phenytoin
c. Leviteracitam d. Lacasomide

263. Administration of disulfiram in an alcoholic can cause all these side effects except: *(JIPMER 2014)*
a. Flushing b. Headache
c. Hypertension d. Nausea

264. Ethanol is used in Ethylene glycol poisoning. What is the mechanism of action? *(JIPMER 2013)*
a. Competitive inhibiton of Alchohol dehydrogenase
b. Competitive inhibition of Aldehyde dehydrogenase
c. Competitive inhibition NADPH oxidase
d. Non-competitive inhibition of Aldehyde dehydrogenase

265. Highly plasma protein bound opioid among the following is: *(JIPMER 2012)*
a. Pethidine b. Fentanyl
c. Sufentanyl d. Meperidine

266. Anticraving drug used in alcohol dependence: *(JIPMER 2012)*
a. Naltrexone b. Methadone
c. Vareniciline d. Rimonabant

267. Antiepileptic drug of choice in child treated with ketogenic diet? *(JIPMER 2012)*
a. Carbamazipine b. Phentoin
c. Valproate d. Lamotrigine

268. Phenobarbitone in mother causes all in baby except: *(JIPMER 2012)*
a. Hypoglycemia b. Ataxia
c. Neonatal drowsiness d. Vitamin K deficiency

269. Seizures are caused by all except: *(JIPMER 2012)*
a. Cyclosporine b. Olanzapine
c. Tramodol d. Propofol

270. Which drug can be administered through all routes? *(JIPMER 2012)*
a. Fentanyl b. Paracetamol
c. Penicillin G d. Azithromycin

271. Which antipsychotic has maximum hypotensive side effect: *(JIPMER 2011)*
a. Flufenazine b. Trifluoperazine
c. Thioridazine d. Haloperidol

272. Vasopressin inhibited by: *(JIPMER 2011)*
a. Alcohol b. Carbamazepine
c. Clofibrate d. Chlorpropamide

273. Which of the following is least protein bound? *(JIPMER 2011)*
a. Morphine b. Sufentanyl
c. Meperidine d. Fentanyl

274. Which of the following is not true regarding morphine?
a. Causes cerebral vasodilation *(JIPMER 2010)*
b. Inhibits urinary voiding reflex
c. Causes direct stimulation of chemoreceptor trigger muscle tone in high doses
d. Reduces muscle tone in high doses

275. Which is not true regarding disulfiram? *(JIPMER 2010)*
a. It irreversibly inhibits aldehyde dehydrogenase
b. It has several active metabolites
c. It can be given to a patient who has abstained from alcohol for atleast 6 hours
d. Sensitization to alcohol can last as long as 14 days after last intake of disulfiram

276. True statement regarding bromocriptine is: *(JIPMER 2009)*
a. It acts as agonist to dopamine receptors
b. It can be used in active peptic ulceration
c. It does not cause postural hypotension
d. It has possible neuroprotective effect

277. Which of the following is contraindicated in early pregnancy? *(JIPMER 2009)*
a. Heparin b. Phenytoin
c. Chloroquine d. Penicillin

278. All the following are anticonvulsants except: *(JIPMER 2009)*
a. Lamotrigine b. Methylphenidate
c. Vigabatrin d. Topiramate

279. Side effect of valvular heart disease is seen with: *(JIPMER 2009)*
a. Pergolide b. Methylphenidate
c. Amphetamine d. Pramipexole

280. Selective decrease in IgA is seen with administration of: *(JIPMER 2009)*
a. Phenytoin b. Diazepam
c. Clonazepam d. Phenobarbitone

281. Which of the following drugs is found to be effective in both epilepsy and migraine? *(JIPMER 2008)*
a. Valproate b. Lamotrigine
c. Vigabatrin d. Flunarizine

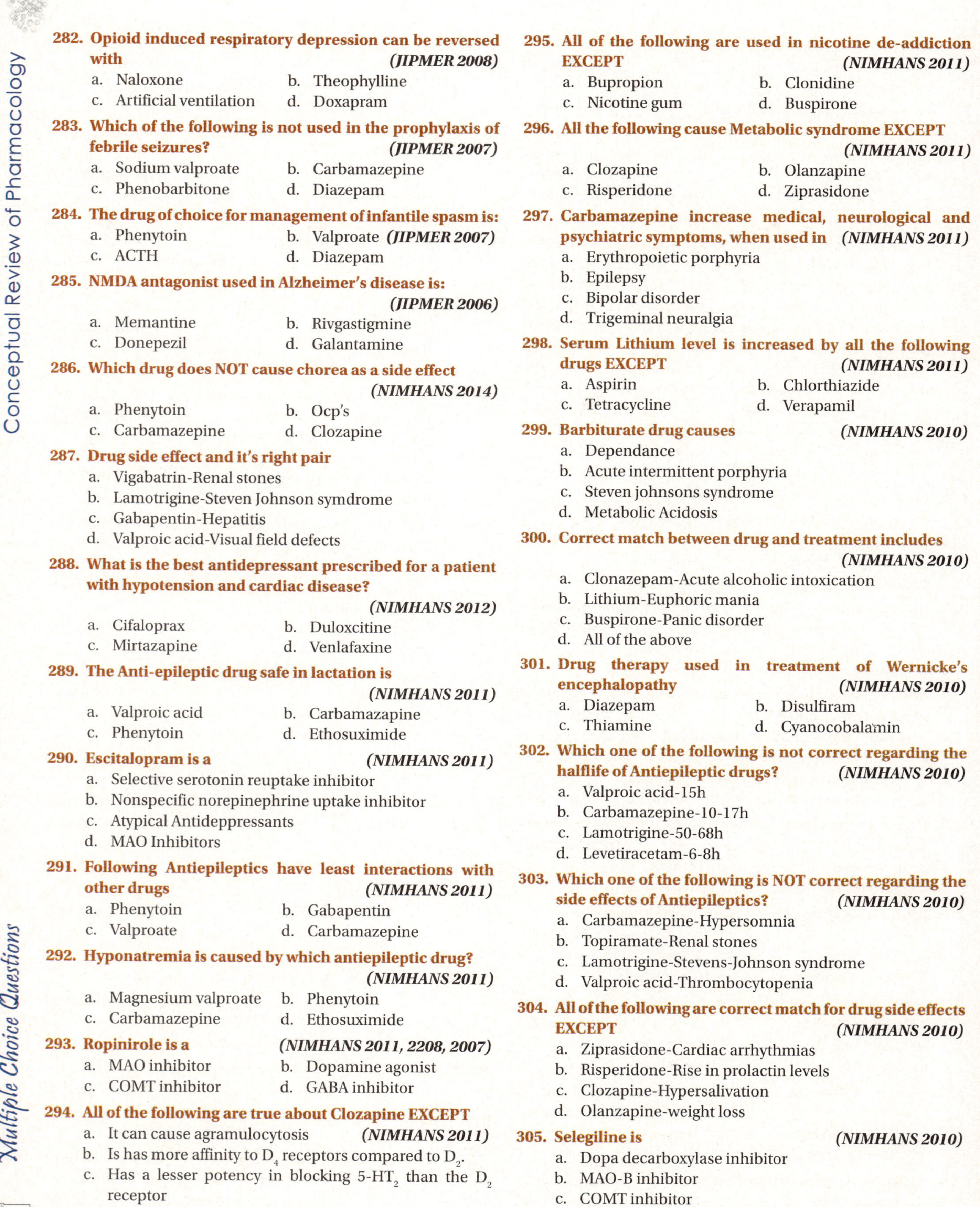

282. Opioid induced respiratory depression can be reversed with *(JIPMER 2008)*
a. Naloxone b. Theophylline
c. Artificial ventilation d. Doxapram

283. Which of the following is not used in the prophylaxis of febrile seizures? *(JIPMER 2007)*
a. Sodium valproate b. Carbamazepine
c. Phenobarbitone d. Diazepam

284. The drug of choice for management of infantile spasm is: *(JIPMER 2007)*
a. Phenytoin b. Valproate
c. ACTH d. Diazepam

285. NMDA antagonist used in Alzheimer's disease is: *(JIPMER 2006)*
a. Memantine b. Rivgastigmine
c. Donepezil d. Galantamine

286. Which drug does NOT cause chorea as a side effect *(NIMHANS 2014)*
a. Phenytoin b. Ocp's
c. Carbamazepine d. Clozapine

287. Drug side effect and it's right pair
a. Vigabatrin-Renal stones
b. Lamotrigine-Steven Johnson symdrome
c. Gabapentin-Hepatitis
d. Valproic acid-Visual field defects

288. What is the best antidepressant prescribed for a patient with hypotension and cardiac disease? *(NIMHANS 2012)*
a. Cifaloprax b. Duloxcitine
c. Mirtazapine d. Venlafaxine

289. The Anti-epileptic drug safe in lactation is *(NIMHANS 2011)*
a. Valproic acid b. Carbamazapine
c. Phenytoin d. Ethosuximide

290. Escitalopram is a *(NIMHANS 2011)*
a. Selective serotonin reuptake inhibitor
b. Nonspecific norepinephrine uptake inhibitor
c. Atypical Antideppressants
d. MAO Inhibitors

291. Following Antiepileptics have least interactions with other drugs *(NIMHANS 2011)*
a. Phenytoin b. Gabapentin
c. Valproate d. Carbamazepine

292. Hyponatremia is caused by which antiepileptic drug? *(NIMHANS 2011)*
a. Magnesium valproate b. Phenytoin
c. Carbamazepine d. Ethosuximide

293. Ropinirole is a *(NIMHANS 2011, 2208, 2007)*
a. MAO inhibitor b. Dopamine agonist
c. COMT inhibitor d. GABA inhibitor

294. All of the following are true about Clozapine EXCEPT *(NIMHANS 2011)*
a. It can cause agramulocytosis
b. Is has more affinity to D_4 receptors compared to D_2.
c. Has a lesser potency in blocking 5-HT_2 than the D_2 receptor
d. An atypical antipsychotic agent

295. All of the following are used in nicotine de-addiction EXCEPT *(NIMHANS 2011)*
a. Bupropion b. Clonidine
c. Nicotine gum d. Buspirone

296. All the following cause Metabolic syndrome EXCEPT *(NIMHANS 2011)*
a. Clozapine b. Olanzapine
c. Risperidone d. Ziprasidone

297. Carbamazepine increase medical, neurological and psychiatric symptoms, when used in *(NIMHANS 2011)*
a. Erythropoietic porphyria
b. Epilepsy
c. Bipolar disorder
d. Trigeminal neuralgia

298. Serum Lithium level is increased by all the following drugs EXCEPT *(NIMHANS 2011)*
a. Aspirin b. Chlorthiazide
c. Tetracycline d. Verapamil

299. Barbiturate drug causes *(NIMHANS 2010)*
a. Dependance
b. Acute intermittent porphyria
c. Steven johnsons syndrome
d. Metabolic Acidosis

300. Correct match between drug and treatment includes *(NIMHANS 2010)*
a. Clonazepam-Acute alcoholic intoxication
b. Lithium-Euphoric mania
c. Buspirone-Panic disorder
d. All of the above

301. Drug therapy used in treatment of Wernicke's encephalopathy *(NIMHANS 2010)*
a. Diazepam b. Disulfiram
c. Thiamine d. Cyanocobalamin

302. Which one of the following is not correct regarding the halflife of Antiepileptic drugs? *(NIMHANS 2010)*
a. Valproic acid-15h
b. Carbamazepine-10-17h
c. Lamotrigine-50-68h
d. Levetiracetam-6-8h

303. Which one of the following is NOT correct regarding the side effects of Antiepileptics? *(NIMHANS 2010)*
a. Carbamazepine-Hypersomnia
b. Topiramate-Renal stones
c. Lamotrigine-Stevens-Johnson syndrome
d. Valproic acid-Thrombocytopenia

304. All of the following are correct match for drug side effects EXCEPT *(NIMHANS 2010)*
a. Ziprasidone-Cardiac arrhythmias
b. Risperidone-Rise in prolactin levels
c. Clozapine-Hypersalivation
d. Olanzapine-weight loss

305. Selegiline is *(NIMHANS 2010)*
a. Dopa decarboxylase inhibitor
b. MAO-B inhibitor
c. COMT inhibitor
d. MAO-A inhibitor

306. Steven Johnson's syndrome is caused by (NIMHANS 2010, 2008)

a. Sodium-valporate b. Lamotrigine
c. Phenobarbitone d. Gabapentine

307. Weight gain is not a side effect by using the following drug? (NIMHANS 2007)

a. Sodium valproate b. Olanzapine
c. Topiramate d. Lithium carbonate

308. Find out the incorrect match (NIMHANS 2007)

a. Fatty liver-Tetracycline
b. Hepatitis-Halothane
c. Granuloma-Chlorpromazine
d. Cholestasis-Erythromycin

309. Which one of the following is a Benzodizapine Antagonist? (NIMHANS 2007)

a. Flumazenil b. Methadone
c. Atropine d. Naloxone

Answers with Explanations to Multiple Choice Questions

1. Ans. (b) Hepatotoxicity

(Ref: Goodman Gilman 13th E/P319, https://www.ncbi.nlm.nih.gov/pubmed/2119269/)

- Valproate is metabolized by CYP_{450} enzymes into a minor metabolite 2-propyl-4-pentenoic acid (4-ene-VPA) which is hepatotoxic.
- Enzyme inducers like carbamazepine, phenytoin and phenobarbital can induce the microsomal enzymes and increase production of this metabolite. This increases the risk of hepatotoxicity if carbamazepine is used along with valproate.

2. Ans. (c) Lifelong treatment

(Ref: Adam's Neurology)

- This is a classic case of juvenile myoclonic epilepsy. JME has an onset typically around 15 years of age. Parents often notice myoclonic jerks of arm and trunk seen during NREM stage I and II of sleep. These jerks can also be precipitated by fatigue and alcohol consumption.
- Valproate is the drug of choice and treatment is continued life long, as discontinuation can cause relapse.
- The treatment duration for various types of epilepsy is given below.

Juvenile myoclonic epilepsy Post infarction seizures	Lifelong treatment
Other epilepsies	Drug can be discontinued after 2 years of seizure free period

3. Ans. (a) Taper levetiracetam and stop it after 6 months

(Ref: CMDT 2018/P995)

- The patient had been antiepileptic for 2 years and there is a possibility if he is tapered off he might not develop seizure.
- Hence option a is best answer.

4. Ans. (d) Blurred vision

(Ref: Goodman Gilman 12th E/P595)

- There is genetic predisposition to carbamazepine induced hypersesitivity related to HLA-B 1502 gene and hence its screening can be done.
- Hypersensitivity associated with carbamazepine presents as SJS, TEN, rash, lymphadenopathy, eosinophilia and splenomegaly.
- Other idiosyncratic reactions associated are agranulocytosis, hepatic failure, serum sickness and pancreatitis.
- Blurred vision though can be seen is not a idiosyncratic reaction.

5. Ans. (c) Immunoglobulin

(Ref: Harrison 19th E/P2153)

- The drugs of choice for rheumatic chorea are valproate and carbamazepine.
- Haloperidol can be used but is less preferred as compared to mentioned drugs above.
- Steroids faster acting and more effective than other drugs and preferred in severe chorea refractory to valproate/carbamazepine and haloperidol.
- **In case no drug is effective** IVIG can be used for treatment of severe and refractory chorea **as a last resort.**

6. Ans. (a)

(Ref: Harrison 19th E/P2552)

- As lamotrigine and valproate are first line drugs in absence seizure, option a is incorrect.
- All other options are correct as valproate and lamotrigine are first line drugs in myoclonic and GTCS, whereas lamotrigine and carbamazepine are first line drugs in partial seizure.

7. Ans. (a) 1 day

(Ref: Meyler's Drug side effect/P229)

- Due to immunological memory rash on rechallenge will be immediate in 1-2 doses.

8. Ans. (b) Acute erythematous pustulosis

(Ref: Goodman Gilman 12th E/P606)

- Acute generalized exanthematous pustulosis is a rare side effects seen with antiepileptics like carbamazepine, phenobarbital and rarely with phenytoin.
- There is a sudden onset of fever with sterile pustules on an exanthematous skin all ver the body.

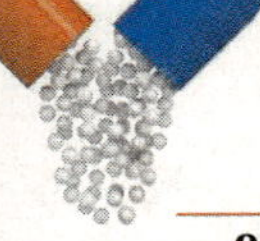

9. Ans. (b) Topiramate

(Ref: Harrison 19th E/P2396)

- Phenteramine is an anorexic agent and topiramate causes weight loss.
- Hence the combination has been recently approved for treatment of obesity.

10. Ans. (d) Lamotrigine

(Ref: Harrison 19th E/P2555)

- Topiramate can cause glaucoma and hence opthalmological consultation is necessary.

11. Ans. (a) Topiramate

(Ref: Harrison 19th E/P2594)

12. Ans. (a) Carbamazepine

(Ref: Harrison 19th E/P2555)

13. Ans. (a) PCOS

(Ref: Goodman Gilman 12th E/P597)

- Valproate causes weight gain and hence PCOS can be seen in young females.
- Hepatotoxicity is more common in children age less than 2 years and hence is contraindicated.

14. Ans. (b) Vigabatrin

(Ref: Goodman Gilman 12th E/P603)

15. Ans. (b) 3 months before pregnancy

(Ref: William's Obstetrics 24th E/P1189)

> "Women with epilepsy should undergo education and counseling before pregnancy. Folic acid supplementation with 0.4 mg per day is begun at least 1 month before conception."

- Folic acid prophylactically is started at least **one month** before planned pregnancy at a dose of **400 μg/day**.
- Sine one month is not in the option three is a better option.
- In case of history of NTD the dose is increased to **4000 μg/day**.

16. Ans. (d) 4,000

(Ref: Goodman Gilman 12th E/P1095)

Prophylactic doses of Folic Acid

Condition	Dose of folic acid
Pregnancy	400 μg/day
Pregnancy with H/O NTD	4000 μg/day
Homocystinemia	1000 μg/day

17. Ans. (c) Topiramate

(Ref: Harrison 19thE/P 2396, Goodman Gilman 12th E/P 601)

> Phentermine/Topiramate combination was approved by FDA in 2012 for treatment of obesity.

18. Ans. (b) Hyponatremia

(Ref: Harrison 19th E/P 2553, Goodman Gilman 12th E/P 595)

19. Ans. (a) Used in trigeminal neuralgia

(Ref: Harrison 19th E/P 2553, Goodman Gilman 12th E/P 595)

20. Ans. (a) Prolongation of inactive state of Na^+ channel

(Ref: Goodman Gilman 12th E/P 594,Harrison 19th E/P 2553)

21. Ans. (b) Phenytoin

(Ref: Harrison 19th E/P 2554, Goodman Gilman 12th E/P 606)

22. Ans. (b) Clonazepam

(Ref: Goodman Gilman 12th E/P598)

- Highly plasma protein bound drugs like phenytoin, valproate and benzodiazepines are less secreted in breast milk.
- Clonazepam has 85% and carbamazepine has 75% plasma protein binding and hence clonazepam is a better answer.
- Gabapentin and ethosuximide have negligible plasma protein binding.

23. Ans. (b) Continue drug in same dose

(Ref: Goodman Gilman 12th E/P606)

- For a pregnant female on antiepileptic drug the dose or drug is not changed as, it carries a risk of an acute attack of seizure.
- Hence the drug is continued along with TDM to decrease teratogenic effect.

24. Ans. (a) Epilepsy

(Ref: Goodman Gilman 12th E/P601)

- Felbamate is an NMDA antagonist used for treatment of partial and secondary generalized seizures.

25. Ans. (d) Ethosuximide

(Ref: Goodman Gilman 12th E/P596)

26. Ans. (a) Fulminant hepatitis

(Ref: Goodman Gilman 12th E/P597)

- Most common side effect is nausea and vomiting with valproate whereas fulminant hepatitis is the most grave side effect.

27. Ans. (b) Less chances of hyponatremia than carbamazepine

(Ref: KDT 7th E/P416)

- Oxcarbazepine and eslicarbazepine are recent congeners of carbamazepine with better side effect profile and lesser enzyme inducing activity.
- Oxcarbazepine causes lesser side effects than carbamazepine, except **hyponatremia, which is more common and severe with oxcarbazepine**.

28. Ans. (b) Flunarizine

(Ref: Goodman Gilman 12th E/P595-600)

29. Ans. (a) Phenytoin

(Ref: Goodman Gilman 12th E/P595-600)

- Fetal hydantoin syndrome can be seen with both phenytoin and carbamazepine.

30. Ans. (b) Absence seizures

(Ref: Goodman Gilman 12th E/P596)

31. Ans. (d) Osteomalacia

(Ref: Goodman Gilman 12th E/P597)

- Osteomalacia is a side effect of phenytoin and not valproate.

32. Ans. (a) Vigabatrin

(Ref: Goodman Gilman 12th E/P603)

- Vigabatrin is an irreversible inhibitor of GABA transaminase.

33. Ans. (b) Ethosuximide

(Ref: Goodman Gilman 12th E/P596)

- Ethosuximide is a calcium channel blocker approved only for treatment of absence seizure.

34. Ans. (a) Intravenous diazepam

(Ref: Goodman Gilman 12th E/P605)

- Intravenous benzodiazepines (lorazepam>diazepam) are the first drug of choice for treatment of status epilepticus.

35. Ans. (c) Lamotrigine

(Ref: Goodman Gilman 12th E/P600)

36. Ans. (b) Hyponatremia

(Ref: Goodman Gilman 12th E/P595)

- **Dilutional hyponatremia** due to SIADH is seen particularly in **elderly patients on carbamazpine**.
- Oxcarbazepine and eslicarbazepine are recent congeners of carbamazepine with better side effect profile and lesser enzyme inducing activity. Oxcarbazepine causes lesser side effects than carbamazepine, except **hyponatremia, which is more common and severe with oxcarbazepine**.

37. Ans. (b) Valproate

(Ref: Goodman Gilman 12th E/P598)

38. Ans. (b) Phenytoin

(Ref: Goodman Gilman 12th E/P593)

- Phenytoin causes abnormal metabolism of vitamin D and hence is associated with hypocalcemia.
- It induces metabolism of vitamin K, and hence decrease in vitamin K decreases bone matrix synthesis.
- A decrease in mineral and matrix causes severe depletion of bone known as osteomalacia.

39. Ans. (a) Phenytoin

(Ref: Goodman Gilman 12th E/P593)

- Phenytoin is contraindicated in pregnancy as it can cause fetal hydantoin syndrome.
- Fetal hydantoin syndrome encompasses facial cleft, microcephaly, IUGR, hypertelorism and triphalangeal thumb. Fetal hydantoin syndrome can be seen with carbamazepine as well.

40. Ans. (d) All

(Ref: Goodman Gilman 12th E/P606)

- Folic acid supplementation for all females with epilepsy is mandatory and started at least one month before pregnancy.
- Enzyme inducing antiepileptics like phenytoin and carbamazepine can cause vitamin K deficiency and hence same is given 10 mg/day in the last month of pregnancy.

41. Ans. (c) Lipid soluble

(Ref: Goodman Gilman 12th E/P591)

- **Fosphenytoin** is water soluble form of phenytoin synthesized, so that it can be given by intravenous route.
- **It is used for tratement of status epilepticus.**

42. Ans. (a) Folic acid deficiency

(Ref: Goodman Gilman 12th E/P591)

43. Ans. (d) It causes neural tube defects

(Ref: Goodman Gilman 12th E/P597)

44. Ans. (b) Valproic acid

(Ref: Goodman Gilman 12th E/P597)

Absence Seizure Treatment

- Valproic acid: DOC in children > 2 years
- Ethosuximide : DOC in children < 2 years

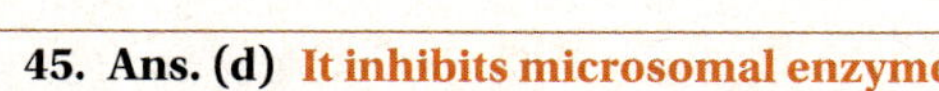

45. Ans. (d) It inhibits microsomal enzyme

(Ref: Goodman Gilman 12th E/P591)

- Phenytoin is an enzyme inducer.
- It is a sodium channel blocker used by oral route for treatment of partial and generalized seizure except absence seizure.
- Intravenous prodrug phenytoin is used in treatment of status epilepticus. It is given by slow intravenous infusion, as rapid infusion can cause asystole.

46. Ans. (d) Eclampsia

(Ref: Goodman Gilman 12th E/P598)

47. Ans. (c) Valproate

(Ref: Goodman Gilman 12th E/P597)

Valproate is Drug of Choice for

- GTCS
- Tonic seizures
- Atonic seizures
- Myoclonic seizures
- Absence seizures

48. Ans. (c) IV

(Ref: Goodman Gilman 12th E/P591)

49. Ans. (a) Rectal diazepam

(Ref: Goodman Gilman 12th E/P605)

- Rectal diazepam is the drug of choice for both treatment and prophylaxis of febrile seizures.

50. Ans. (a) Aplastic anemia

(Ref: Goodman Gilman 12th E/P602)

- Felbamate was discontinued due to high risk of aplastic anemia and hepatotoxicity.

51. Ans. (a) Renal stone

(Ref: Goodman Gilman 12th E/P601)

- Topiramate and zonisamide can cause renal stones due to inhibition of carbonic anhydrase.

52. Ans. (a) Vigabatrin

(Ref: Goodman Gilman 12th E/P603)

- Infantile spasm associated with tuberous sclerosis responds poorly to ACTH or corticosteroids.
- Hence vigabatrin is preferred for seizures associated with tuberous sclerosis.

53. Ans. (c) Lamotrigine

(Ref: Harrison 19th E/P2556)

- Valproate is the drug with widest spectrum and is drug of choice for mixed seizure syndrome like LGS.
- Another drug with wider spectrum lamotrigine is also preferred in LGS but second to valproate.
- Hence here lamotrigine is the better answer.

54. Ans. (a) Valproate

(Ref: Goodman Gilman 12th E/P597)

55. Ans. (a) Diazepam

(Ref: Goodman Gilman 12th E/P465)

56. Ans. (c) Both

(Ref: Goodman Gilman 12th E/P470)

57. Ans. (b) Antihistaminics, antidepressants

(Ref: Goodman Gilman 12th E/P457)

- Antihistaminics, antidepressants and antipsychotics can cause sedation due to antihistaminic and antimuscarinic effect on CNS.

58. Ans. (b) β carboline

(Ref: Goodman Gilman 12th E/P 468)

Benzodiazepine inverse agonist	β carboline
Benzodiazepine antagonist	Flumazenil

59. Ans. (a) Zaleplon

(Ref: Goodman Gilman 12th E/P 467)

60. Ans. (b) Flumazenil

(Ref: Goodman Gilman 12th E/P 468)

Benzodiazepine inverse agonist	β carboline
Benzodiazepine antagonist	Flumazenil

61. Ans. (d) Coronary dilation

(Ref: Goodman Gilman 12th E/P462)

- Diazepam causes coronary dilation by increasing adenosine and midazolam decreases cerebral blood flow.

62. Ans. (a) Lorazepam

(Ref: Goodman Gilman 12th E/P463)

- Benzodiazepines metabolized by direct gluconoridation (short acting class) are safest in patients of liver failure. The list of benzodiazepines safe in liver failure is given below.

• Lorazepam	• Temazepam
• Oxazepam	• Estazolam

63. Ans. (d) Promethazine

(Ref: Goodman Gilman 12th E/P457)

- Promethazine is an antihistaminic; other drugs in the options are $GABA_A$ agonists.

64. Ans. (c) Melatonin

(Ref: Goodman Gilman 12th E/P469)

- Darkness stimulates melatonin synthesis and induces sleep and maintains circadian rhythm.

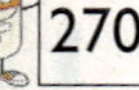

65. Ans. (a) Thiopentone

(Ref: Goodman Gilman 12th E/P472)

- Barbiturates like thiopentone are contraindicated in acute intermittent porphyria as they can induce ALA synthase and induce porphyrin synthesis.

66. Ans. (d) Antagonist

(Ref: Goodman Gilman 12th E/P468)

67. Ans. (d) Midazolam

(Ref: Goodman Gilman 12th E/P466)

- **Intrathecal midazolam** can be used for postoperative pain relief.

68. Ans. (d) Buspirone

(Ref: Goodman Gilman 12th E/P457)

- GABA binds to its site located in between α and β subunits and forces α subunit to withdraw the part closing the lumen, thereby opening the chloride ion channel.
- The $GABA_A$ agonists like muscimol and gaboxadol and antagonists like bicuculline, gabazine and picrotoxin are used as experimental drugs.
- Alcohol is also an agonist at $GABA_A$ receptors.

69. Ans. (a) 2%

(Ref: Goodman Gilman 12th E/P469)

Pharmacokinetics of Ramelteon

- Bioavailability = 2%
- Half-life = 2 hours
- Plasma protein binding = 80%

70. Ans. (d) Meprobamate

(Ref: Goodman Gilman 12th E/P475)

71. Ans. (c) Oxazepam

(Ref: Goodman Gilman 12th E/P463)

72. Ans. (c) Biliary colic

(Ref: Goodman Gilman 13th E/P368)

- Morphine can cause contraction of sphincter of Oddi and biliary spasm; hence it can worsen pain of biliary colic and is not used for same.
- In other conditions mentioned i.e. ischemic pain (myocardial infarction), cancer pain and postoperative pain, morphine is commonly used.
- Other conditions where morphine should not be used are
  - Bronchial asthma or severe hypotension: Morphine releases histamine which can cause bronchoconstriction and vasodilation.
  - Head injury: Morphine can increase intracranial pressure.

73. Ans. (a) Pentazocin

(Ref: Goodman Gilman 12th E/P508)

Pentazocin effect on opioid receptors

- Mui: Antagonist or Partial agonist
- Kappa: Full agonist

74. Ans. (a) Naloxone

(Ref: Goodman Gilman 12th E/P512)

- Naloxone which is an opioid antagonist is the drug of choice for treatment of opioid toxicity.
- Hence it should be kept ready to deal with possible toxicity.

75. Ans. (a) Methadone

(Ref: Goodman Gilman 12th E/P498)

76. Ans. (a) Pupil dilation

(Ref: Goodman Gilman 12th E/P510)

77. Ans. (a) Meperidine

(Ref: Goodman Gilman 12th E/P501)

Opioids Used in Labour Pain are

- Morphine
- Meperidine

78. Ans. (d) The onset of analgesia is 30-60 minutes after parenteral administration and 1-2 hours after oral administration

(Ref: Goodman Gilman 12th E/P506)

- Methadone can be given by oral, IM, SC and IV routes. It is rapidly absorbed by oral route within 30 minutes. The time for onset of analgesia seen after these routes is given below.

Route of methadone	Time for onset of analgesia
Parenteral	10-20 minutes
Oral	30-60 minutes

79. Ans. (b) Kappa

(Ref: Katzung 12th E/P544)

80. Ans. (a) Partial agonist at mu and antagonist at kappa

(Ref: Goodman Gilman 12th E/P 508)

81. Ans. (c) Naloxone

(Ref: Goodman Gilman 12th E/P512)

- Ergotamine is a nonselective 5HT agonist and has prokinetic effect due to stimulation of 5HT4 receptors.
- Alvimopan and methylnaltrexone are opioid antagonists used for treatment of opioid induced constipation and post operative ileus.
- Naloxone is a short acting, intravenous drug used for opioid toxicity.

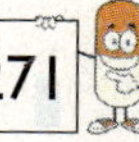

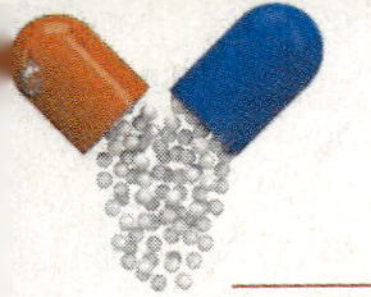

82. Ans. (a) Mu

(Ref: Goodman Gilman 12th E/P510)

83. Ans. (a) Pethidine

(Ref: Goodman Gilman 12th E/P502)

- Pethidine is contraindicated in renal failure because it can cause accumulation of norpethidine which is neurotoxic.

84. Ans. (a) Partial agonist at μ receptor

(Ref: Goodman Gilman 12th E/P510)

85. Ans. (a) Miosis

(Ref: Goodman Gilman 12th E/P488)

- Tolerance is not developed to actions of opioids like miosis, constipation and convulsion.

86. Ans. (a) Opioid

(Ref: Goodman Gilman 12th E/P510)

- Neonates are more prone to respiratory depression caused by opioids due to immature blood brain barrier.

87. Ans. (d) Papaverine

(Ref: Goodman Gilman 12th E/P496)

- **Papaverine** is a natural opioid that doesn't have opioid effect, rather causes relaxation of smooth muscles.

88. Ans. (c) Partial agonist

(Ref: Goodman Gilman 12th E/P510)

89. Ans. (b) Lacrimation

(Ref: Goodman Gilman 12th E/P510)

Mnemonics

P Withdrawal Symptoms

- **W-M** : Mydriasis
- **I** : Increased yawning, piloerection
- **T** : Temperature increased
- **H** : Hyperventilation
- **D** : Diarrhea
- **R** : Rhinorrhea
- **A** : Anxiety
- **W-M** : Myalgia
- **L** : Lacrimation

90. Ans. (b) To prevent relapse

(Ref: Goodman Gilman 12th E/P512)

91. Ans. (a) Head injury

(Ref: Goodman Gilman 12th E/P501)

- It is contraindicated in patients with **head injury** as it can raise the intracranial tension and interfere with assessment of patient outcome by causing miosis.

92. Ans. (c) Methadone

(Ref: Goodman Gilman 12th E/P511)

- If the mother is on methadone the baby is also dependent on methadone.
- Hence if naloxone is used in the baby, it can precipitate severe withdrawal symptoms.

93. Ans. (b) Sufentanil

(Ref: Goodman Gilman 12th E/P505)

94. Ans. (c) Seizures

(Ref: Goodman Gilman 12th E/P504)

95. Ans. (a) Morphine

(Ref: Goodman Gilman 12th E/P515)

96. Ans. (c) Naloxone

(Ref: Goodman Gilman 12th E/P512)

97. Ans. (a) Heroin

(Ref: Goodman Gilman 12th E/P512)

98. Ans. (a) Miotic action

(Ref: Goodman Gilman 12th E/P488)

- Tolerance occurs to all effects of opioids except miosis, constipation and convulsion.

99. Ans. (d) Mydriasis

(Ref: Katzung 12th E/P551)

100. Ans. (d) All of the above

(Ref: Goodman Gilman 12th E/P482)

101. Ans. (d) Opioid analgesic

(Ref: Goodman Gilman 12th E/P508)

102. Ans. (c) Constipation

(Ref: Katzung 12th E/P551)

103. Ans. (a) Tramadol

(Ref: Goodman Gilman 12th E/P504)

- Meperidine inhibits 5HT reuptake, whereas tramadol inhibits reuptake of both 5HT and NE.
- Thus both have monoamine action, but here pethidine would be a better answer.

104. Ans. (b) Diarrhea

(Ref: Katzung 12th E/P552)

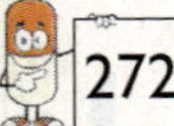

105. Ans. (d) Preanaesthetic medication

(Ref: Goodman Gilman 12th E/P501)

106. Ans. (d) Naloxone

(Ref: Goodman Gilman 12th E/P510)

107. Ans. (c) Morphine

(Ref: Goodman Gilman 12th E/P515)

108. Ans. (a) Miosis

(Ref: Goodman Gilman 12th E/P504)

109. Ans. (a) Opioids

(Ref: Goodman Gilman 12th E/P504)

110. Ans. (a) Venlafaxine

(Ref: Goodman Gilman 13th E/P273)

- Withdrawal symptoms like anxiety, insomnia, headache, nausea and dizziness are seen with paroxetine and venlafaxine due to their short half-lives.

111. Ans. (a) Sialorrhea

(Ref: Goodman Gilman 13th E/P273)

112. Ans. (a) Lithium

(Ref: Amercian Psychiatric textbook of Mood disorder/P492)

- Apart from its effect on mania and BPD, lithium is also associated with decreased suicidal events in patients with BPD and resistant depression.
- Antiepileptics are yet to be proved that they have antisuicidal effects.

113. Ans. (b) Mirtazapine

(Ref: Goodman Gilman 12th E/P407)

Mirtazapine and mianserin increase NE by α_2 block and serotonin by $5HT1_A$ block and hence are known as NaSSA (Noradrenergic and Specific Serotonergic Antidepressant)

114. Ans. (c) Wait as it takes 2-6 weeks to respond

(Ref: Goodman Gilman 12th E/P405)

115. Ans. (c) Premature ejaculaton

(Ref: Goodman Gilman 12th E/P405)

SSRIs can cause delayed ejaculation and hence are used off label for treatment of premature ejaculation.

116. Ans. (c) IV $NaHCO_3$

(Ref: Goodman Gilman 12th E/P411)

- TCA and antipsychotics toxicity presents with anticholinergic symptoms along with quinidine like effects (QRS widening, arrhythmia and hypotension), seizures.
- Treatment is aimed at reversing the cardiac effects and acidosis by sodium bicarbonate.

117. Ans. (d) IV sodium bicarbonate

(Ref: CMDT 2016/P1583)

- This is a case of TCA toxicity as evident from the ECG changes and history of antidepressant intake.
- The drug of choice in TCA toxicity is sodium bicarbonate.

118. Ans. (c) SSRI

(Ref: Goodman Gilman 12th E/P405)

119. Ans. (b) MAO inhibitors

(Ref: Goodman Gilman 12th E/P 504)

120. Ans. (c) Fluvoxamine

(Ref: Goodman Gilman 12th E/P 411)

121. Ans. (a) Fluoxetine

(Ref: Goodman Gilman 12th E/P 405)

- Fluoxetine is a prodrug that is activated to norfluoxetine.

122. Ans. (a) Doxepin

(Ref: Goodman Gilman 12th E/P 400)

- Doxepin is a TCA that inhibits NE and 5HT reuptake.
- Other drugs in the options are atypical antipsychotics and hence block D_2 and $5HT2_A$ receptors.

123. Ans. (a) Imipramine

(Ref: Goodman Gilman 12th E/P 533)

124. Ans. (b) Fluoxetine

(Ref: Goodman Gilman 12th E/P 405)

125. Ans. (d) Tianeptin

(Ref: Goodman Gilman 12th E/P 405)

- **Tianeptin is a selective serotonin reuptake enhancer also used as an antidepressant.**

126. Ans. (a) Premature ejaculation

(Ref: Goodman Gilman 12th E/P 410)

- SSRI cause delayed ejaculation and anorgasmia.

127. Ans. (b) Serotonin

(Ref: Goodman Gilman 12th E/P 418)

128. Ans. (a) Imipramine

(Ref: Goodman Gilman 12th E/P 405)

- Fluoxetine in children and adolescents is associated with increased suicidal risk, though fluvoxamine is approved in children.
- Risperidone is an atypical antipsychotic with metabolic side effects.

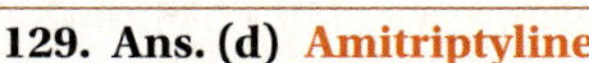

129. Ans. (d) Amitriptyline

(Ref: Goodman Gilman 12th E/P 403)

130. Ans. (b) Amoxapine

(Ref: Goodman Gilman 12th E/P 408)

- Amoxapine is a TCA with D_2 antagonistic action and hence has both antidepressant and antipsychotic properties.

131. Ans. (c) Norepinephrine

(Ref: Goodman Gilman 12th E/P 405)

- Atomoxetine is a selective NE reuptake inhibitor used for treatment of ADHD.

132. Ans. (d) All of the above

(Ref: Goodman Gilman 12th E/P412)

133. Ans. (a) ADHD

(Ref: Goodman Gilman 12th E/P 404)

Drug of choice for ADHD	Methylphenidate
Drug of choice for ADHD with tics	Atomoxetine (NE reuptake inhibitor)

134. Ans. (a) CVS defect

(Ref: Goodman Gilman 13th E/P298)

- Lithium use in pregnancy in the first trimester can lead to CVS defect i.e. Ebstein's anomaly.
- Hence the drug of choice in first trimester is atypical antipsychotics like aripiprazole; ECT is also an option.
- In second and third trimester lithium is preferred. Lithium use in pregnancy can cause hypotonia (floppy infant) and goiter in the neonate.
- Another important aspect to consider during lithium therapy is that, the baby can have toxicity to lithium even at normal lithium plasma concentration in the mother.

135. Ans. (c) Haloperidol

(Ref: CMDT 2016/P1067)

- This is a case of acute mania, for which atypical antipsychotics are drug of choice.
- Typical antipsychotics like **haloperidol** can also be used.

136. Ans. (d) 2 mEq/L

(Ref: Goodman and Gilman 12th E/P 447)

Plasma concentration of lithium (mEq/L)	Relevance
1–1.5	Acute attack of mania
0.6–1	Prophylaxis of mania, BPD
>2	Indicator of toxicity
>3	Permanent neurological damage Absolute indication for dialysis
>4	Death

137. Ans. (a) 1 day

(Ref: Nicholas Principle of Ambulatory Medicine 7th E/P1633, Greenstein Concise Clinical Pharmacology/p148)

- Lithium is discontinued one day before surgery as it can cause neuromuscular blockade and increase effect of NDMRs

138. Ans. (d) Ataxia and dysarthria

(Ref: Goodman Gilman 12th E/P 450)

139. Ans. (a) Nephrogenic DI

(Ref: Goodman Gilman 12th E/P 449)

140. Ans. (a) Cardiac malformation

(Ref: Goodman Gilman 12th E/P 449)

141. Ans. (c) 24 hours

(Ref: Goodman Gilman 12th E/P446)

- Lithium is completely absorbed within 8 hours.
- Peak plasma concentration is seen after 2–4 hours.
- Half-life is 24 hours.
- Steady state concentration is achieved after 5 days.

142. Ans. (a) Lithium

(Ref: Goodman Gilman 12th E/P450)

143. Ans. (d) Hyperthyroidism

(Ref: Goodman Gilman 12th E/P450)

144. Ans. (a) 8–10 Hz

(Ref: Michael's Clinical Neurology/P123)

145. Ans. (d) Cardiac arrhythmia

(Ref: Goodman Gilman 12th E/P450)

146. Ans. (d) Topiramate

(Ref: Goodman Gilman 12th E/P448)

- Though topiramate is used in bipolar disorder, it is not approved by FDA and hence is a better answer.
- All other drugs in the options are FDA approved drugs for BPD.

147. Ans. (a) 2 mEq

(Ref: Goodman Gilman 12th E/P450)

148. Ans. (c) M1 antagonist

(Ref: Goodman Gilman 13th E/P291)

149. Ans. (a) Risperidone

(Ref: Goodman Gilman 12th E/P439)

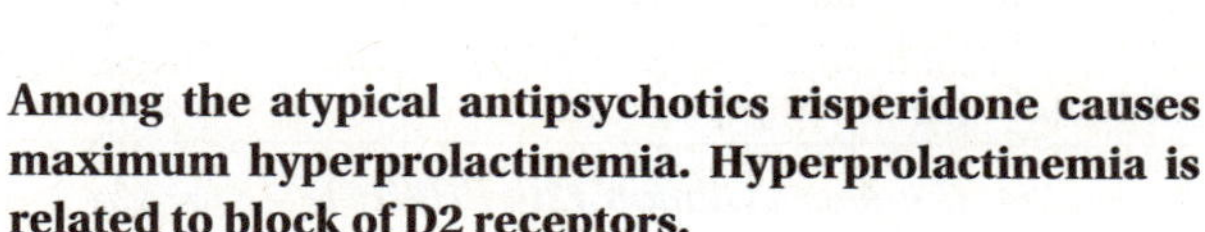

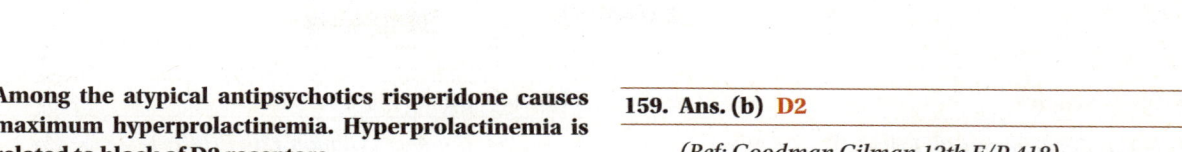

Among the atypical antipsychotics risperidone causes maximum hyperprolactinemia. Hyperprolactinemia is related to block of D2 receptors.

150. Ans. (b) Antiemetic property

(Ref: Goodman Gilman 12th E/P438)

151. Ans. (c) Promethazine

(Ref: Goodman Gilman 12th E/P437)

- The symptoms of rigidity and tremors after starting typical antipsychotic haloperidol are indicating towards EPS, parkinsonism.
- For this anticholinergics or antihistaminics with anticholinergic effect are preferred.
- Hence promethazine is the answer here.

152. Ans. (b) Risperidone

(Ref: Goodman Gilman 12th E/P436)

- The presence of motor and vocal tics in the patient is confirmatory of Tourette's syndrome.
- Alpha-2 agonist are first line and atypical antipsychotics are second line drugs.
- Hence risperidone is the answer in the given options.

153. Ans. (c) Aripiprazole

(Ref: Goodman Gilman 12th E/P 427,439)

Minimum sedation, obesity, hyperlipidemia and hyperglycemia	Maximum sedation, obesity, hyperlipidemia and hyperglycemia
Aripiprazole Asenapine Ziprasidone	Clozapine Olanzapine.

154. Ans. (a) Its potential to cause agranulocytosis

(Ref: Goodman Gilman 12th E/P 427)

- Clozapine can cause agranulocytosis and hence is contraindicated with carbamazepine.
- Atypical antipsychotics are more effective against the negative symptoms.
- Extrapyramidal side effects are not seen with clozapine and aripiprazole among atypical antipsychotics.

155. Ans. (c) Neuroleptic malignant syndrome

(Ref: Goodman Gilman 12th E/P 439)

156. Ans. (b) Promethazine

(Ref: Goodman Gilman 12th E/P 924)

157. Ans. (a) Clozapine

(Ref: Goodman Gilman 12th E/P 427)

158. Ans. (d) Molindone

(Ref: Goodman Gilman 12th E/P 440)

- All antipsychotics can cause weight gain except molindone which causes weight loss.

159. Ans. (b) D2

(Ref: Goodman Gilman 12th E/P 418)

160. Ans. (b) Clozapine

(Ref: Goodman Gilman 12th E/P 442)

161. Ans. (d) It is the drug of choice in treatment of acute mania

(Ref: Goodman Gilman 12th E/P 420)

- Aripiprazole is the only antipsychotic with D2 partial agonistic action.
- It has 5HT1A antagonistic action.
- It has minimal sedating potential.
- Atypical antipsychotics are the drug of choice for treatment of acute mania, with aripiprazole being the most preferred agent due to lesser side effects.

162. Ans. (a) Clozapine

(Ref: Goodman Gilman 12th E/P 440)

163. Ans. (b) Tardive dyskinesia

(Ref: Goodman Gilman 12th E/P 438)

164. Ans. (d) Chlorpromazine

(Ref: Goodman Gilman 12th E/P 436)

165. Ans. (c) Haloperidol

(Ref: Goodman Gilman 12th E/P 437)

- For akathasia the drugs of choice are either benzodiazepines or beta blockers.
- Anticholinergics or antihistaminics with anticholinergic effect though can be used are less effective.
- Haloperidol causes akathasia and not used for it.

166. Ans. (a) Clozapine

(Ref: Goodman Gilman 12th E/P 443)

- Risk of EPS is lesser with atypical antipsychotics like clozapine.

167. Ans. (a) Pemoline

(Ref: Goodman Gilman 12th E/P 427)

- Pemoline is a stimulant drug related to methylphenidate.
- It was approved for treatment of ADHD and narcolepsy.
- It has been banned due to risk of hepatotoxicity.

168. Ans. (b) Thioridazine

(Ref: Goodman Gilman 12th E/P 438)

- Among typical antipsychotics risk of EPS is minimal with less potent drugs like thioridazine and chlorpromazine and maximum with high potency drugs like haloperidol and thioxethene.

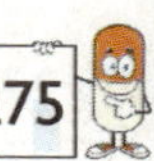

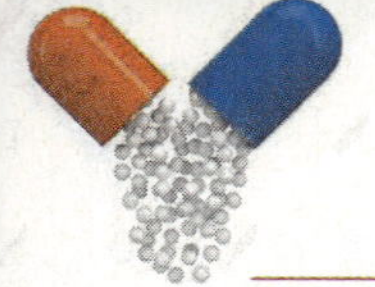

169. Ans. (c) Clozapine

(Ref: Goodman Gilman 12th E/P 427)

170. Ans. (d) Aripiprazole

(Ref: Goodman Gilman 12th E/P 442)

- Aripiprazole is a partial agonist at D_2 receptor, whereas aripiprazole, ziprasidone and clozapine are partial agonists at $5HT1_A$ receptor.
- Thus aripiprazole is the only atypical antipsychotic that is partial agonist at both D_2 and $5HT1_A$ receptor.

171. Ans. (b) Causes agranulocytosis

(Ref: Goodman Gilman 12th E/P 442)

172. Ans. (c) Dopamine

(Ref: Goodman Gilman 12th E/P 418)

173. Ans. (a) Akathasia

(Ref: Goodman Gilman 12th E/P 438)

- The desire to move around or restlessness called as akathasia is seen with antipsychotics.
- Benzodiazepines and beta blockers are used for treatment.

174. Ans. (c) Edaravone

(Ref: Goodman Gilman 13th E/P335)

175. Ans. (b) Psychosis

(Ref: Katzung 13th E/P477)

- Levodopa is metabolized into dopamine, which by acting on D2 receptors can cause psychosis and hence is contraindicated in psychosis.
- It can cause mydriasis and hence is contraindicated in angle closure glaucoma, however in open angle glaucoma it can be used.
- Hence the best answer in the given option is psychosis.

176. Ans. (b) Memantine

(Ref: Goodman Gilman 12th E/P622)

177. Ans. (e) It is a MAO-A inhibitor

(Ref: Goodman Gilman 12th E/P618)

- Selegeline is a selective MAO-B inhibitor used in Parkinson;s disease.
- It is used in on-off phenomenon and young onset PD.

178. Ans. (a) Hepatotoxic

(Ref: Goodman Gilman 12th E/P617)

179. Ans. (c) Bromocriptine

(Ref: Goodman Gilman 12th E/P617)

180. Ans. (a) Levodopa

(Ref: Goodman Gilman 12th E/P615)

- Levodopa is a prodrug of dopamine.

181. Ans. (a) Riluzole

(Ref: Goodman Gilman 12th E/P625)

182. Ans. (a) Dopamine agonist

(Ref: Goodman Gilman 12th E/P617)

183. Ans. (a) Tolcapone

(Ref: Goodman Gilman 12th E/P617)

- Though tolcapone and selegeline both are effective in weaning off period, the drug of choice is COMT inhibitor entecapone.
- Hence another drug of this class tolcapone is the best answer here.

184. Ans. (a) Multiple sclerosis

(Ref: Goodman Gilman 12th E/P1027)

185. Ans. (b) β IFN

(Ref: Goodman Gilman 12th E/P1025)

186. Ans. (b) Rotigotine

(Ref: Goodman Gilman 12th E/P617)

187. Ans. (c) Entecapone

(Ref: Goodman Gilman 12th E/P615)

- Selegeline inhibits MAO-B, which is present in the brain and thus it has nothing to do with bioavailability.
- Entecapone inhibits COMT, which is present in the both brain and periphery. By binhibiting COMT in liver and intestine entecapone can increase bioavailability of levodopa.

188. Ans. (a) It is a MAO-A inhibitor

(Ref: Goodman Gilman 12th E/P618)

- Selegeline and rasageline are MAO-B inhibitors.

189. Ans. (a) Entacapone

(Ref: Goodman Gilman 12th E/P617)

190. Ans. (d) Selegeline

(Ref: Goodman Gilman 12th E/P618)

191. Ans. (b) Selegeline

(Ref: Goodman Gilman 12th E/P618)

192. Ans. (c) Retroperitoneal fibrosis

(Ref: Goodman Gilman 12th E/P616)

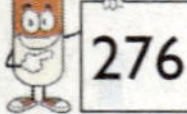

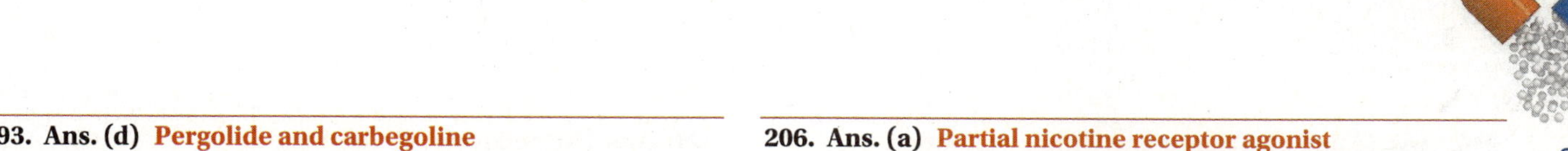

193. Ans. (d) Pergolide and carbegoline

(Ref: Goodman Gilman 12th E/P617)

194. Ans. (a) Alzheimer's disease

(Ref: Goodman Gilman 12th E/P621)

195. Ans. (d) Ropinirole

(Ref: Goodman Gilman 12th E/P617)

196. Ans. (c) Trihexphenydil

(Ref: Goodman Gilman 12th E/P617)

197. Ans. (c) Tolcapone

(Ref: Goodman Gilman 12th E/P617)

198. Ans. (a) Varenicline

(Ref: Goodman Gilman 13th E/P188)

199. Ans. (b) Diazepam

(Ref: Goodman Gilman 12th E/P643)

- For treatment of acute alcohol withdrawal IV benzodiazepines like lorazepam and diazepam are used.
- Clorazepate, diazepam, chlordiazepoxide by oral route are used for treatment of alcohol dependence.

200. Ans. (a) Buspirone

- Bupropion is an anxiolytic and not used in smoking dependence.

201. Ans. (b) Flumazenil

(Ref: Goodman Gilman 12th E/P643)

- Flumazenil is used for benzodiazepine toxicity.
- Acamprosate, naltrexone and disulfiram are FDA approved drugs for chronic alcohol dependence.

202. Ans. (d) Phenytoin

(Ref: Goodman and Gilman 12th E/P 643-44)

203. Ans. (b) Naloxone

(Ref: Goodman Gilman 12th E/P 643)

204. Ans. (b) Rimonabant

(Ref: Goodman Gilman 12th E/P 643)

- Rimonabant is acannabinoid receptor inverse agonist used in smoking dependence.
- This drug has been banned due to risk of depression and suicidal tendancy.

205. Ans. (d) Fluoxetine

(Ref: Goodman Gilman 12th E/P 642-44)

- Nalmefene, Topiramate and Ondansetron are currently under trial for alcohol dependence.

206. Ans. (a) Partial nicotine receptor agonist

(Ref: Goodman Gilman 12th E/P 643)

207. Ans. (c) Large proportionate body

(Ref: Goodman Gilman 12th E/P641)

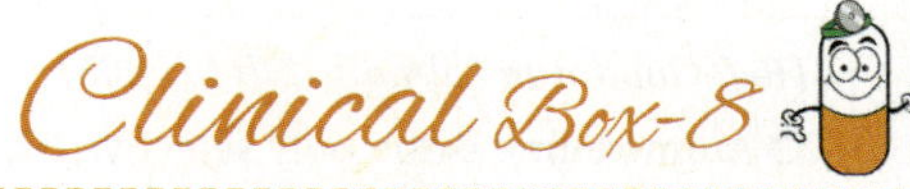

Fetal Alcohol Syndrome

- **Dysmorphic facial features (All 3 are required)**
  - Small palpebral fissures
  - Thin vermilion border
  - Smooth philtrum
- **Prenatal and/or postnatal growth impairment**
- **Central nervous system abnormalities (1 required)**
  - Structural: head size < 10th percentile, significant brain abnormality on imaging
  - Neurological
  - Functional: global cognitive or intellectual deficits functional deficits in at least three domains

208. Ans. (a) Lorazepam

(Ref: Goodman Gilman 12th E/P643)

209. Ans. (c) Chlordiazepoxide

(Ref: Harrison 19th E/P2727)

- Benzodiazepines are the drug of choice for alcohol withdrawal and toxicity.

210. Ans. (a) Naltrexone

(Ref: Goodman Gilman 12th E/P643)

- Out of the given options both naltrexone and disulfiram can be used in alcohol dependence.
- But naltrexone is a better answer as disulfiram is clinically less preferred.

211. Ans. (a) Acetyldehyde

(Ref: Goodman Gilman 12th E/P643)

212. Ans. (a) Amoxicillin

(Ref: Goodman Gilman 12th E/P643)

213. Ans. (b) Inhibits oxidation of alcohol

(Ref: Goodman Gilman 12th E/P643)

- Antabuse is disulfiram which inhibits oxidation of alcohol by inhibiting the enzyme alcohol dehydrogenase.

214. Ans. (d) Tablets

(Ref: Goodman Gilman 12th E/P658)

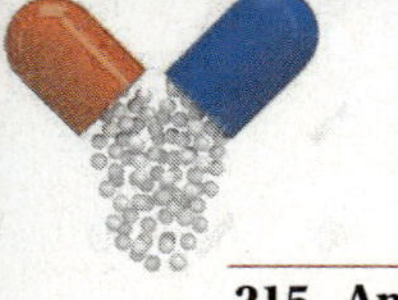

215. Ans. (a and e) Tremor and Urinary retention

(Ref: Goodman Gilman 13th E/P273)

216. Ans. (c) Phenytoin

(Ref: Goodman Gilman 13th E/P311)

217. Ans. (d) Atomoxetine

(Ref: Goodman Gilman 12th E/P405)

- Atomoxetine is the only selective NE inhibitor available and is used for treatment of ADHD.
- Fluoxetine and paroxetine are selective serotonin reuptake inhibitors.
- Duloxetine and milnacipran are serotonin norepinephrine reuptake inhibitors.

218. Ans. (a) Mood stabilizers, (b) Antipsychotics, (d) Antiepileptics, (e) Sedative hypnotics

(Ref: Goodman Gilman 12th E/P448)

Drugs used in Mania

- Mood stabilizers: Lithium is the best drug available for mania and is the drug of choice for prevention of mania and bipolar disorder.
- Antipsychotics: These are the fastest acting antimania drugs and are drug of choice for treatment of an acute attack of mania.
- Antiepileptics: Valproate, carbamazepine, topiramate and gabapentin are the antiepileptics that are used in mania and bipolar disorder.
- Sedative hypnotics: Benzodiazepines are used in an acute attack of mania.

Note: Antidepressants increase brain derived neurotropic factors (BDNF) and hence can precipitate mania. Thus antidepressants are contraindicated in mania.

219. Ans. (a) Seizures, (b) Sedation, (c) Dry mouth, (d) Hypothermia, (e) Constipation

(Ref: Goodman Gilman 12th E/P436-42)

- Clozapine blocks H1 receptors which can cause sedation.
- It also blocks muscarinic receptors which results in constipation and dry mouth.
- Seizures, hypothermia, agranulocytosis and myocarditis can also be seen with clozapine.

220. Ans. (a) Used as anti-tussive agent, (c) Causes respiratory depression, (d) Partly metabolized to morphine

(Ref: Goodman Gilman 12th E/P501)

- Codeine is primarily used as an antitussive agent.
- It is a natural opioid derived from poppy plant.
- Codeine is metabolized by liver into inactive metabolites and excreted by kidney, however 10% codeine is metabolized to morphine.
- It causes lesser analgesia and respiratory depression than morphine.

221. Ans. (b) Sedation (d) Vomiting

(Ref: Goodman Gilman 12th E/P411)

222. Ans. (a) Enhances GABA release

(Ref: Goodman Gilman 12th E/P599)

- Pregablin and gabapentin act by binding to the $\alpha_2\delta1$ subunit of presynaptic calcium channels and preventing its endocytosis. Persistence of calcium channels increase **exocytosis of GABA into the synapse**.
- Gabapentine does not inhibit the channel per se.

223. Ans. (a) Juvenile myoclonic epilepsy, (c) Generalized Tonic clonic seizure, (d) Complex partial seizure

(Ref: Goodman Gilman 12th E/P584)

224. Ans. (b) Hypersomnia

(Ref: Goodman Gilman 12th E/P465)

Benzodiazepine Withdrawal Symptoms

• Nightmares	• Insomnia
• Dysphoria	• Sweating
• Tremor	• Anorexia
• Dizziness	

225. Ans. (a) Weight gain, (b) Agranulocytosis, (c) Sedation

(Ref: Goodman Gilman 12th E/P 442)

- Clozapine and olanzapine cause maximum weight gain and sedation.
- Clozapine also causes agranulocytosis and seizures
- EPS is less common with atypical than typical antipsychotics.

226. Ans. (a) Methanol poisoning, (c) Ethylene glycol poisoning

(Ref: Goodman Gilman 12th E/P640)

227. Ans. (a) Levodopa, (c) Reserpine, (d) Pethidine

(Ref: Goodman Gilman 12th E/P412)

228. Ans. (d) SSRI

(Ref: Goodman Gilman 12th E/P 440)

- TCAs cause weight gain but SSRI and SNRI don't cause weight gain.
- All other drugs in the options are antipsychotics which can cause weight gain.

229. Ans. (b) Activation in liver, (d) Cause miosis, (e) Clearance time is around 20 hr

(Ref: Goodman Gilman 12th E/P504)

- Morphine is a μ receptor agonist.
- It has a half-life of 2 hours and clearance time is around 24 hours.
- It is activated in liver to morphine-6-glucunoride which is a long-acting active metabolite.

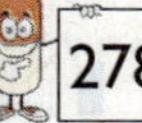

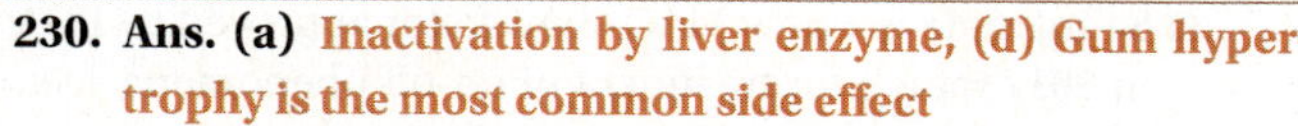

230. Ans. (a) Inactivation by liver enzyme, (d) Gum hypertrophy is the most common side effect

(Ref: Goodman Gilman 12th E/P591)

231. Ans. (b) Amoxapine

(Ref: Goodman Gilman 12th E/P 427)

- Amoxapine is a TCA that has got D_2 blocking effect.
- Loxapine is a typical antipsychotic synthesized from amoxapine.

232. Ans. (a) μ receptor, (b) δ receptor, (c) k receptor

(Ref: Goodman Gilman 12th E/P486)

233. Ans. (a) Buspirone : 5HT-1 agonist

234. Ans. (a) Red cell aplasia, (b) Megaloblastic anaemia, (c) Aplastic anaemia, (d) Hemolytic anaemia, (e) Thrombocytopenia

(Ref: Goodman Gilman 12th E/P593)

- Megaloblastic anemia is quite common with phenytoin.
- Other side effects mentioned are seen due to hypersensitivity and are very rare but seen with phenytoin.

235. Ans. (b) Diarrhea

(Ref: Goodman Gilman 12th E/P411)

- Amitriptyline is a TCA, which causes constipation, urine retention etc. due to anticholinergic side effects.
- Quinidine like cardiac effects like arrhythmia, QRS widening and hypotension is seen.

236. Ans. (a) Velnafexine, (b) Mirtazapine, (c) Duloxetine

(Ref: Goodman Gilman 12th E/P409)

237. Ans. (a) Naloxone cannot reverse its effects, (c) Long-acting, (d) More potent than morphine, (e) Partial μ receptor agonist

(Ref: Goodman Gilman 12th E/P510)

- Buprenorphine is a partial agonist at μ receptor, and is around 50 times more potent than morphine.
- It slowly dissociates from μ receptor and hence has prolonged effect; because of slow dissociation naloxone is ineffective in antagonizing its effect.

238. Ans. (a) Pethidine, (b) Diacetylmorphine, (d) Pentazocine, (e) Morphine

(Ref: Goodman Gilman 12th E/P498)

239. Ans. (b) Constipation less marked, (e) Rapid onset

(Ref: Goodman Gilman 12th E/P502)

240. Ans. (a) Off & on phenomenon is seen with levodopa because up & down regulation of dopaminergic receptor, (b) Tolcapone cause greenish discolouration of urine, (c) Apomorphine is used in treatment, (e) Ropinirole is used in restless leg syndrome

(Ref: Goodman Gilman 12th E/P615-620)

241. Ans. (b) Velnafexine, (d) Duloxetine

(Ref: Goodman Gilman 12th E/P409)

242. Ans. (b) Lamotrigine is safe, (c) Monotherapy is recommended, (d) Newer drugs are safe

(Ref: Goodman Gilman 12th E/P605-606)

- During pregnancy monotherapy is recommended as, the risk of teratogenicity is higher with polytherapy.
- The newer drugs like lamotrigine, topiramate and levetiracetam are less teratogenic than the older ones.
- Overall lamotrigine is least teratogenic and safest in pregnancy and hence is the drug of choice for epilepsy in pregnancy.

243. Ans. (b) Na valproate, (c) Lamotrigine, (d) Topiramate

(Ref: Goodman Gilman 12th E/P597-600)

244. Ans. (a) Rotigotine, (d) Ropinirole, (e) Amantadine

(Ref: Goodman Gilman 12th E/P615)

245. Ans. (a) Gum hypertrophy, (c) Exacerbation of acne Vulgaris

(Ref: Goodman Gilman 12th E/P592)

246. Ans. (a) Cerebrovascular events, (b) ↑ EPS

(Ref: Goodman Gilman 12th E/P 442)

247. Ans. (c) Sedation is less than diazepam, (d) Only sedation and hypnosis, (e) Duration of action less than diazepam

(Ref: Goodman Gilman 12th E/P467)

- Z compounds are selective agonist at $\boxtimes_1$ subunit of the $GABA_A$ receptors and hence associated **only with sedative and hypnotic effect**.
- These drugs are associated with **lesser dependence and CNS depression** as compared to benzodiazepines.

248. Ans. (d) Neuroleptic malignant syndrome

(Ref: Goodman Gilman 12th E/P 437)

249. Ans. (a) Fluoxetine

(Ref: Goodman Gilman 12th E/P 405)

250. Ans. (b) 10–19 μg/mL

(Ref: Goodman Gilman 12th E/P593)

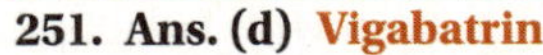

251. Ans. (d) Vigabatrin

(Ref: Goodman Gilman 13th E/P320)

- ACTH is the drug of choice for treatment of infantile spasm but is not effective in case it is caused by tuberous sclerosis.
- Vigabatrin is as effective as ACTH for treatment of infantile spasm, limitation though is irreversible visual field defects that can be seen.
- Hence it is reserved for cases not responding to ACTH, as in case of infantile spasm caused by tuberous sclerosis.

252. Ans. (c) Carbamazepine

(Ref: Goodman Gilman 13th E/P313)

- Carbamazepine though teratogenic (neural tube defect and fetal hydantoin syndrome) is safe in third trimester. Since it is the only antiepileptic in options, it is the best answer here.
- Other options i.e. diuretics and nifedipine have no role in epilepsy.

253. Ans. (b) Beta carboline

(Reg: Goodman Gilman 12th E/P468)

- Inverse agonist of benzodiazepine is beta carboline.
- Antagonist of benzodiazepine is flumazenil.

254. Ans. (a) Valbenazine

(Ref: CMDT 2018/P1082)

- Valbenazine is a VMAT 2 (Vesicular Monoamine Transporter 2) inhibitor, which acts by inhibiting release of catecholamines into the synapse.
- It has been approved in 2017 for treatment of tardive dyskinesia in adults.

255. Ans. (a) Edaravone

(Ref: https://www.centerwatch.com/drug-information/fda-approved-drugs/drug/100204/radicava-edaravone)

- Edaravone is a free radical scavenger approved in 2017 for treatment of amyotrophic lateral sclerosis (ALS).
- It prevents neurodegeneration and hence improves outcome.
- Route of administration is by intravenous infusion of 60 mg administered over a 60-minute for 14 days followed by a 14 days drug free period. Thereafter it is given for 10 days in a 14 days cycle followed by a 14 days drug free period.
- Side effects like contusion, headache and gait disturbances were seen in clinical trials.

256. Ans. (a) Alvimopan

(Ref: CMDT 2018/P648)

257. Ans. (a) Safinamide

(Ref: https://www.centerwatch.com/drug-information/fda-approved-drugs/drug/100191/xadago-safinamide)

- Safinamide is a new MAO-B inhibitor approved by FDA in 2017 march for treatment of on-off phenomena seen with levodopa.
- It is started at dose of 50 mg once daily by oral route and after two weeks the dose can be increased to maximal dose of 100 mg once daily.

258. Ans. (b) HLA B1502

(Ref: Adam's Neurology 10th E/P348, CMDT 2018/P997)

The risk of Steven Johnson's syndrome with carbamazepine and phenytoin is higher in

- Asians carrying HLA B1502 gene
- Caucasians carrying HLA A3101 gene

259. Ans. (b) Phenobarbitone 5-10 mcg/mL

(Ref: Adam's Neurology 10th E/P345)

Therapeutic Range of Commonly used Antiepileptic Drugs

Antiepileptic drug	Normal therapeutic range in mcg/mL
Clonazepam	0.01 – 0.07
Lamotrigine	2 – 7
Carbamazepine	4 – 12
Primidone	5 – 12
Phenytoin	10 – 20
Phenobarbital	15 – 40
Levetiracetam	15 – 45
Valproate	50 – 100
Ethosuximide	50 – 100

260. Ans. (a) Psychosis

(Ref: Goodman Gilman 12th E/P615)

- Levodopa is metabolized to dopamine by an enzyme dopa decarboxylase and hence if given alone most of the levodopa will be metabolized in the periphery.
- Hence a lipid insoluble (does not cross blood brain barrier) inhibitor of dopa decarboxylase i.e. carbidopa is combined with levodopa to inhibit this peripheral metabolism.
- By inhibiting activation of levodopa in the periphery it also prevents peripheral side effects like
  - Nausea and vomiting: Caused by action of dopamine on D2 receptors in CTZ area
  - Arrhythmia: By action of dopamine on beta-1 receptors
  - Postural hypotension: By action of dopamine on D1 receptors in renal blood vessels
- In presence of carbidopa, levodopa is metabolized into dopamine in CNS beyond the blood brain barrier which gives therapeutic effect by action of dopamine on D2 receptors in corpus striatum. Dopamine also acts on D2 receptors of limbic system which gives psychosis as a side effect.

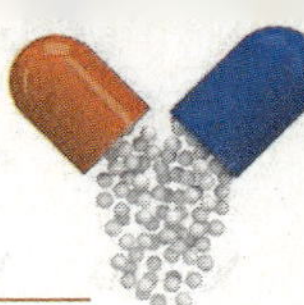

261. Ans. (a) Prevention of Na^+ influx

(Ref: Goodman Gilman 12th E/P595)

- The clinical picture given in the question is that of trigeminal neuralgia, for which carbamazepine is the drug of choice.
- As carbamazepine is a sodium channel blocker, option a is correct answer.

262. Ans. (c) Levetiracetam

(Ref: Harrison 19th E/P2553)

- Alternative monotherapy of JME in pregnancy are lamotrigine and levetiracetam.

263. Ans. (c) Hypotension

(Ref: Goodman Gilman 12th E/P643)

- Disulfiram is an aversive agent which acts by inhibiting aldehyde dehydrogenase the enzyme for alcohol metabolism.
- This leads to accumulation of acetyldehyde, toxic metabolite of alcohol which causes vomiting, flushing, hypotension, chest pain and other uncomfortable symptoms.

264. Ans. (a) Competitive inhibition of Alcohol dehydrogenase

(Ref: Goodman Gilman 12th E/P640)

265. Ans. (c) Sufentanyl

(Ref: Goodman Gilman 12th E/P504)

266. Ans. (a) Naltrexone

(Ref: Goodman Gilman 12th E/P643)

267. Ans. (c) Valproate

(Ref: Goodman Gilman 12th E/P597)

- Ketogenic diet is prescribed in children with Lennox Gastaut Syndrome.
- In LGS, the drug of choice is valproate.

268. Ans. (a) Hypoglycemia

(Ref: Goodman Gilman 12th E/P474)

269. Ans. (b) Olanzapine

(Ref: Harrison 19th E/P2547)

Drugs causing seizure	
• Beta lactam antibiotics	• Quinolones
• Cylosporine	• Meperidine
• Clozapine	• Fentanyl
• Tramadol	• Bupropion
• Tacrolimus	• Cocaine
• Acyclovir	• Methylphenidate
• Isoniazid	• Amphetamine

270. Ans. (a) Fentanyl

(Ref: Goodman Gilman 12th E/P505)

Uses of fentanyl by different routes	
Epidural Spinal Intravenous	Analgesics in anesthesia
Transdermal patch	Chronic pain
Buccal tablets Buccal films Lozenges	Acute pain

271. Ans. (c) Thioridazine

(Ref: Goodman Gilman 12th E/P

272. Ans. (a) Alcohol

273. Ans. (a) Morphine

(Ref: Goodman Gilman 12th E/P501)

- Codeine is the opioid with least plasma protein binding of less than 10% followed by morphine with 33%.

274. Ans. (d) Reduces muscle tone in high doses

(Ref: Goodman Gilman 12th E/P495)

Effects of morphine and related opioids

- **Nausea and vomiting:** Due to stimulation of CTZ area and vestibular component as well.
- **Muscle rigidity:** Muscle tone is increased at high doses.
- **Temperature:** μ receptor causes hyperthermia, whereas k receptor causes hypothermia.
- **ICT:** Opioids cause hypoventilation that increases CO_2 in plasma which causes vasodilation and increases cerebral blood flow.
- **CVS:** Opioids cause bradycardia except pethidine and pentazocine which cause tachycardia.
- **GIT:** Constipation and contraction of sphincter of Oddi.
- **Blood Pressure:** Hypotension due to histamine release and depression of vasomotor center, except pentazocine which increases blood pressure.
- **Bronchoconstriction:** Due to histamine release and hence opioids are avoided in bronchial asthma and COPD.
- **Pruritus:** Due to histamine release.
- Immunomodulatory action
- **Respiratory depression:** Neonates are more prone to respiratory depression due to immature blood brain barrier.
- **Bladder:** Inhibits voiding reflex and increases tone of external sphincter

275. Ans. (c) It can be given to a patient who has abstained from alcohol for atleast 6 hours

(Ref: Goodman Gilman 12th E/P644)

Abstinence should be at least 12 hours to start disulfiram.

276. Ans. (a) It acts as agonist to dopamine receptors

(Ref: Goodman Gilman 12th E/P617)

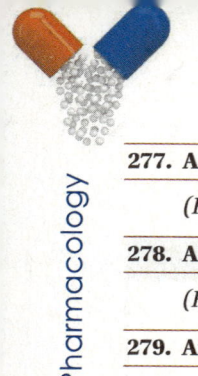

277. Ans. (b) Phenytoin

(Ref: Goodman Gilman 12th E/P606)

278. Ans. (b) Methylphenidate

(Ref: Goodman Gilman 12th E/P592)

279. Ans. (a) Pergolide

(Ref: Goodman Gilman 12th E/P617)

280. Ans. (a) Phenytoin

(Ref: Goodman Gilman 12th E/P593)

281. Ans. (a) Valproate

(Ref: Goodman Gilman 12th E/P597)

282. Ans. (a) Naloxone

(Ref: Goodman Gilman 12th E/P511)

283. Ans. (b) Carbamazepine

(Ref: Goodman Gilman 12th E/P595)

284. Ans. (c) ACTH

(Ref: Goodman Gilman 12th E/P605)

285. Ans. (a) Memantine

(Ref: Goodman Gilman 12th E/P622)

286. Ans. (d) Clozapine

(Ref: Goodman Gilman 12th E/P442)

287. Ans. (b) Lamotrigine-Steven Johnson syndrome

(Ref: Goodman Gilman 12th E/P600)

288. Ans. (d) Venlafaxine

(Ref: Goodman Gilman 12th E/P411)

289. Ans. (a) Valproic acid

(Ref: Goodman Gilman 12th E/P597)

290. Ans. (a) Selective serotonin reuptake inhibitor

(Ref: Goodman Gilman 12th E/P400)

291. Ans. (b) Gabapentine

(Ref: Goodman Gilman 12th E/P599)

292. Ans. (c) Carbamazepine

(Ref: Goodman Gilman 12th E/P595)

293. Ans. (b) Dopamine agonist

(Ref: Goodman Gilman 12th E/P617)

294. Ans. (c) Has a lesser potency in blocking 5-HT_2 than the D_2 receptor

(Ref: Goodman Gilman 12th E/P429)

Atypical antipsychotics are more potent 5-HT_2 inhibitors as compared to D_2.

295. Ans. (d) Buspirone

(Ref: Goodman Gilman 12th E/P658)

296. Ans. (d) Ziprasidone

(Ref: Goodman Gilman 12th E/P442)

- Among atypical antipsychotics obesity is maximum with clozapine > olanzapine and minimum with aripiprazole < ziprasidone.

297. Ans. (a) Erythropoietic porphyria

(Ref: Goodman Gilman 12th E/P595)

Carbamazepine being an enzyme inducer can increase porphyrin synthesis and precipitate acute attack of porphyria.

298. Ans. (d) Verapamil

(Ref: Goodman Gilman 12th E/P448)

299. Ans. (b) Acute intermittent porphyria

(Ref: Goodman Gilman 12th E/P473)

300. Ans. (b) Lithium-Euphoric mania

(Ref: goodman Gilman 12th E/P448)

301. Ans. (c) Thiamine

(Ref: Goodman Gilman 12th E/P640)

302. Ans. (c) Lamotrigine-50–68 h

(Ref: Goodman Gilman 12th E/P600)

Lamotrigine has a half life of 24-30 hours.

303. Ans. (a) Carbamazepine- Hypersomnia

(Ref: Harrison 19th E/P2555)

304. Ans. (d) Olanzapine – Weight loss

(Ref: Goodman Gilman 12th E/P442)

305. Ans. (b) MAO-B Inhibitor

(Ref: Goodman Gilman 12th E/P618)

306. Ans. (b) Lamotrigine

(Ref: Goodman Gilman 12th E/P600)

307. Ans. (c) Topiramate

(Ref: Goodman Gilman 12th E/P601)

308. Ans. (c) Granuloma – Chlorpromazine

(Ref: Goodman Gilman 12th E/P442)

309. Ans. (a) Flumazenil

(Ref: Goodman Gilman 12th E/P468)

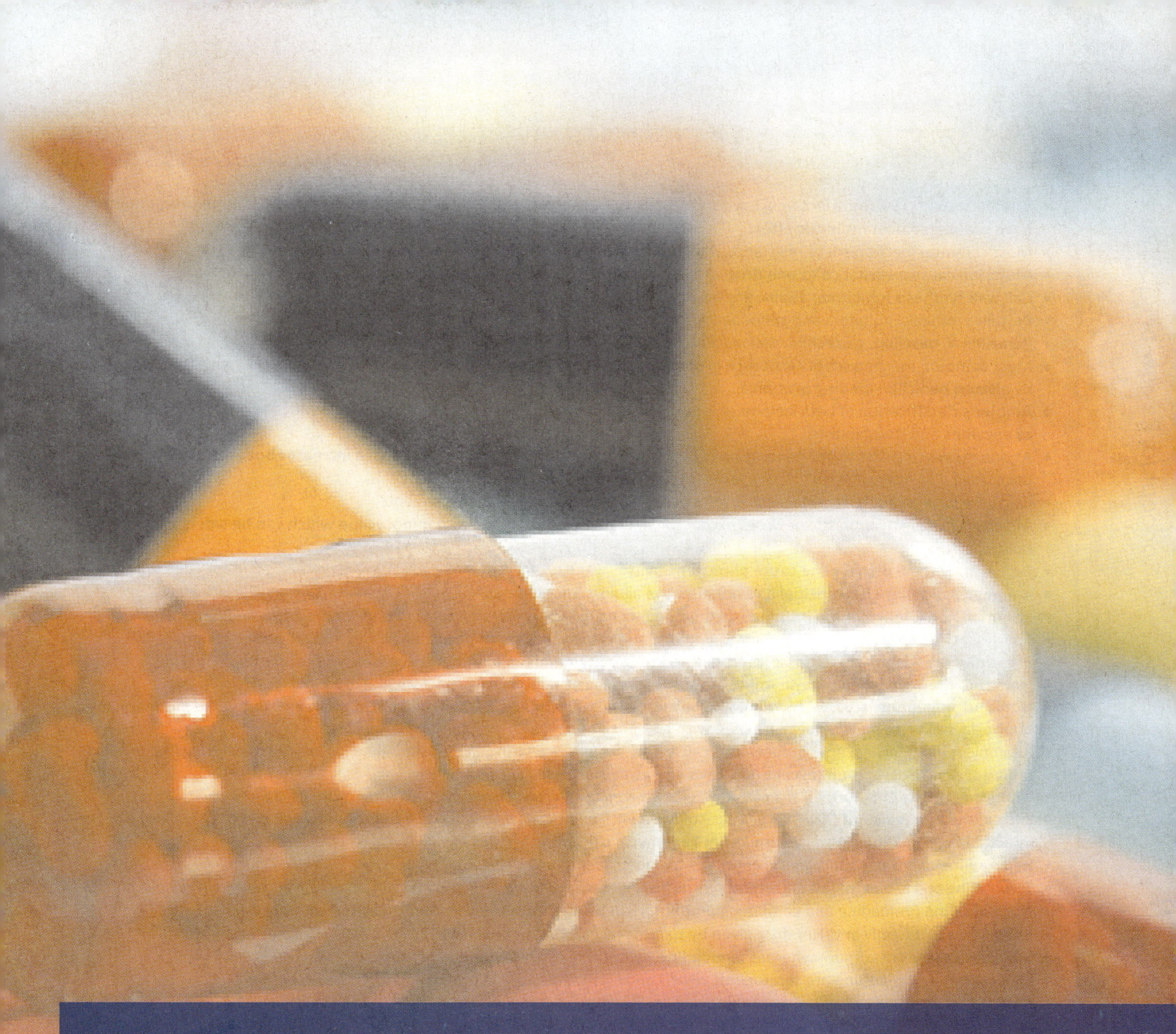

Antimicrobial Drugs

One Liners

- Antibiotics with **TDK (beta lactams) have short PAE**, whereas those **with CDK (aminoglycosides) and CTDK (fluoroquinolones) have prolonged postantibiotic effect**.
- Most common mechanism of resistance transfer in bacteria is through **plasmids by conjugation.**
- **Mutation** causes resistance to **one drug** whereas **plasmid** can cause **multidrug resistance**.
- Cell wall synthesis inhibitors, antibiotics acting on cell membrane, cotrimoxazole and DNA gyrase inhibitors are **bactericidal**.
- Protein synthesis inhibitors and sulfonamides are **bacteriostatic**.
- **Penicillin V, oxacillin, cloxacillin, dicloxacillin, ampicillin and amoxicillin** are oral penicillins.
- Most common mechanism of resistance in staphylococcus is by **penicillinase production**, whereas resistance to methicillin is by **altered penicillin binding protein**.
- **Ambler's classification** of beta lactamase is based on **structure of enzyme**, whereas **Bush's classification** is based on **substrate of enzymes** and its inhibitors.
- As one moves from **1st to 3rd generation** of cephalosporins **effect against gram-negative increases but against gram-positive decreases.**
- **Cefoperazone and cefpiramide** are the safest cephalosporins in **renal failure** patients.
- All tetracyclines are nephrotoxic drugs except for **tigecycline, doxycycline and minocycline which can be safely used in renal failure**.
- **Demeclocycline > doxycycline** cause photosensitivity.
- Aminoglycosides are **bactericidal** and not effective against **anaerobes**.
- **Enzymatic drug inactivation** is the most common mechanism of drug resistance, except for **amikacin** and **netilmicin**.
- **Sparfloxacin** is the longest acting fluoroquinolone and causes **maximum photosensitivity and QT prolongation.**
- **Pyrazinamide > isoniazid > rifampicin** cause hepatotoxicity, whereas **ethambutol** causes nephrotoxicity.
- **Isoniazid, rifampicin and pyrazinamide** are **static** whereas **ethambutol** is a **bactericidal** drug.
- **Isoniazid maximum crosses blood brain barrier** and is associated with **neuropsychiatric symptoms like memory loss, euphoria, hallucinations** etc. can be seen with **psychosis.**
- Rifampicin being an enzyme inducer can cause OCP failure, warfarin failure and failure of antiretroviral drugs of **protease inhibitor and NNRTI group (except efavirenz and etravirine)**.
- **Multidrug resistant (MDR) TB** is a case of TB that is resistant to both **isoniazid and rifampicin.**
- **Extremely drug resistant (XDR) TB** is a case of **MDR** with additional resistance to a **fluoroquinolone** and to at least one of the **injectable second line drugs like amikacin, kanamycin or capreomycin.**
- **Bedaquiline** and **delamanid** are recent drugs for treatment of MDR TB.
- **Terbinafine** and **azoles inhibit ergosterol synthesis** whereas amphotericin B and nystatin act on the ergosterol in cell membrane.
- **Normal saline** preloading and combining **amphotericin B** with **liposome** give **nephroprotective effect.**
- **Enfuvirtide** is the only anti-HIV drug given by **parenteral (subcutaneous)** route.
- **Stavudine** causes maximum whereas **lamivudine** causes minimum peripheral neuropathy.
- **Efavirenz** and **primaquine** are **teratogenic** NNRTI and contraindicated in pregnancy.
- **Ritonavir** is most potent, whereas **saquinavir** is least potent enzyme inhibitor.
- **Primaquine** is used for **radical cure** and **terminal prophylaxis** in vivax and ovale.
- **Artemisinin group** drugs are **fastest acting schizontocidal drugs**.
- Order of hemolysis in G6PD deficiency with antimalarials is **primaquine > chloroquine > quinine.**
- **Miltefosine** is the only **oral drug** for kala-azar, but compliance is poor due to **vomiting and diarrhea.**
- **Ivermectin** and **piperazine** cause **flaccid paralysis** in helminths.
- **Praziquantel, metrifonate and pyrantel pamoate** cause **spastic paralysis** in helminths.
- **Nitrofurantoin** and **methenamine** are urinary tract antiseptics used in UTI.
- **Phenazopyridine** is a urinary tract analgesic used to treat dysuria and burning associated with UTI.
- **Abacavir** and **NNRTI** are not effective against **HIV-2**.

GENERAL ASPECTS OF ANTIMICROBIAL DRUGS

Theory

ANTIMICROBIAL DRUG EFFECT

The effect of antimicrobial drugs depends on three aspects as given below:

Minimum Inhibitory Concentration (MIC)

MIC is the lowest possible concentration of a drug that inhibits visible growth after 24 hours of incubation. Thus, a drug with lesser MIC is more potent and vice versa.

Optimal Dose

Optimal dose is the dose of antimicrobial drug that inhibits growth of 90% of organisms (IC-90) at the site of infection.

Concentration-Time Curve (CTC)

CTC is a graph drawn in between the time of drug therapy in X-axis to the plasma concentration on Y-axis.

Time Dependent Killing (TDK) with Short Postantibiotic Effect (PAE)

- Antimicrobial effect is directly proportional to the **time** for which the drug concentration is above the MIC. Hence, these antimicrobials are said to have **TDK**.
- Since the effect is seen above MIC and vanishes as plasma concentration drops below MIC, clearly these drugs do not have effect after they are cleared from plasma, i.e. they have **short PAE**.
- The efficacy of these drugs depends on the **time period** the plasma concentration of drug is above MIC. Thus, to maintain a continuously higher PC than MIC for a longer time, these drugs require to be given at **multiple doses or continuous infusion**.
- Drugs with TDK and short PAE are **beta-lactams, vancomycin and flucytosine.**

Time Dependent Killing (TDK) with Prolonged Postantibiotic Effect (PAE)

- Most of the protein synthesis inhibitors belong to this class, which have a bacteriostatic effect. At high doses these drugs have bactericidal effect which continues till the time the high plasma concentration is maintained above MIC. Hence, these can also be said to be having **TDK**.
- But unlike the previous class, in this case the bacteriostatic effect persists even after the plasma concentration falls below MIC and hence are said to have prolonged **PAE**.
- The efficacy of these drugs depends on **AUC** above MIC. Thus, to get a bigger AUC, **maximum permissible amount (dose)** of drug should be used.
- Drugs having **TDK and prolonged PAE** are erythromycin, clarithromycin, clindamycin, tetracyclines, tigecycline, streptogramins, **linezolid** and triazoles.

Concentration Dependent Killing (CDK) with Prolonged Postantibiotic Effect (PAE)

- Antimicrobial effect is directly proportional to the magnitude of **plasma concentration** achieved even once above the MIC. Hence, these antimicrobials are said to have **CDK**.
- Since the effect is seen even after the plasma concentration falls below MIC, these drugs have effect even after they are cleared from plasma, i.e. they have **prolonged postantibiotic effect (PAE)**. The logic is simple, e.g. antitubercular drug rifampicin's entry into mycobacterium is concentration dependent and hence once the drug enters into the bacteria it produces effect even if drug is not in plasma.
- The efficacy of these drugs depends on both the **maximum plasma concentration (C_{max}) and AUC** above MIC. Thus, to get a maximum plasma concentration hike than the MIC, these drugs need to be given as **single dose**. The secondary benefit of single dosing is lesser toxicity as well.
- Drugs with CDK and prolonged postantibiotic effect are **aminoglycosides, fluoroquinolones, daptomycin, azithromycin, telithromycin, metronidazole, amphotericin B, echinocandins and rifampicin**.

TDK with short PAE	TDK with prolonged PAE	CDK with prolonged PAE
Beta-lactams	Erythromycin	**Aminoglycosides**
Vancomycin	Clarithromycin	Fluoroquinolones
Flucytosine	**Lincosamide (Clindamycin)**	Daptomycin
	Tetracyclines	Telithromycin
	Tigecycline	Azithromycin
	Streptogramins	Metronidazole
	(Oxazolidinidiones)	Amphotericin B
	linezolid	Echinocandins
	Triazoles	Rifampicin

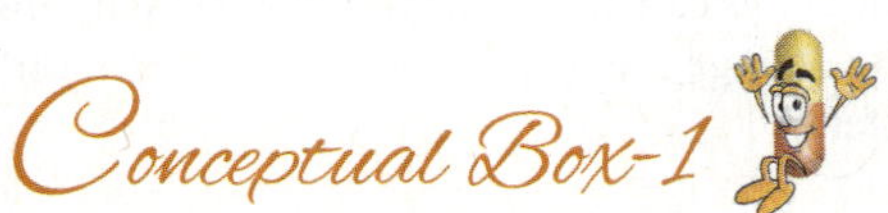

Concentration Time Curve

Important parameter:
TDK - Time over MIC

Concentration
MIC
T > MIC
Time (T)

Time dependent killing

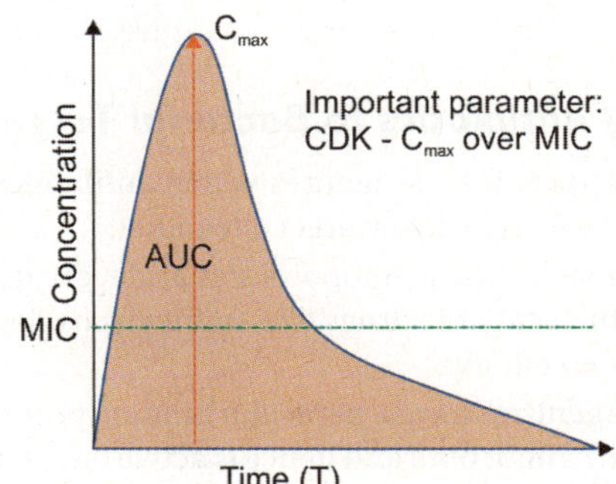

Concentration dependent killing

ANTIMICROBIAL DRUG SYNERGISM AND ANTAGONISM

Synergism

- **Sequential enzyme block:** Drugs blocking enzymes sequentially like DHPS with **sulfamethoxazole** and DHFR with **trimethoprim** gives a synergistic effect in the form of bactericidal effect. On the contrary given as monotherapy, these drugs are bacteriostatic.
- **Facilitation of drug uptake by microbes:** Cell wall synthesis inhibitors like **penicillins** and **vancomycin** increase uptake and effect of **aminoglycosides**. Thus, for treatment of **pseudomonas, enterococcus and gram-positive cocci endocarditis (*Staphylococcus* and *Streptococcus*) penicillins are combined with aminoglycoside, and for enterococcus vancomycin is combined with aminoglycosides**. Similarly, **amphotericin B** forms pores in fungus and increases entry of **flucytosine** and hence both are combined for induction therapy in cryptococcal meningitis.
- **Block of drug inactivating enzymes:** Combination of a **beta lactamase inhibitor with beta lactams like penicillins and cephalosporins** increases the spectrum. Combination of **cilastatin with imipenem** inhibits metabolism of imipenem and increases its effect. **Ritonavir combined with other protease inhibitors** increases the duration of action.

Antagonism

- Bacteriostatic drugs like **tetracyclines** and **macrolides** can inhibit the effect of cell wall synthesis inhibitors like **penicillins** which are more effective against rapidly dividing bacteria.
- Antibiotics like **ampicillin, cefoxitin and imipenem** can **induce beta lactamase production** and increase degradation of other beta lactam drugs.
- **Penicillins can inactivate aminoglycosides in solutions** and hence decrease its effect.

ANTIMICROBIAL DRUG RESISTANCE

Resistance to antimicrobial drugs can be either intrinsic or acquired.

Intrinsic Mechanisms

Intrinsic mechanism is natural ability of the bacteria to avoid a class of drugs due to specific functional or structural abilities as described below. These microbes were never susceptible to these antibiotics.

Poor Affinity of Antibiotics to Bacterial Targets

- Some bacterial targets have structures which antibiotics can do bind to or some even lack the target altogether.
- Burkholderia cepacia has a lipopolysaccharide on its cell membrane to which cationic drugs like aminoglycosides and polymyxins have no affinity.
- Gram-positive organisms have a penicillin binding protein, to which aztreonam cannot bind and hence is active only against gram-negatives.
- Similarly, enterococci have penicillin binding proteins, to which cephalosporins cannot bind.
- **Mycoplasma** does not have a cell wall and hence antibiotics inhibiting cell wall synthesis like beta lactams are not effective.

Poor Entry of Antibiotics Through Cell Wall

- Vancomycin has a huge size and hence it cannot enter through the small porins present on the cell wall of gram-negatives.
- Aminoglycosides require oxygen for entry into bacteria, as oxygen generates a transmembrane potential that attracts aminoglycosides through the cell wall. Hence, aminoglycosides are not effective against anaerobes.

Drug Efflux of Antibiotics

Efflux pumps which are chromosomally coded in Burkholderia cepacia can pump out antibiotics like tetracyclines, chloramphenicol and ciprofloxacin.

Production of Drug Inactivating Enzymes

These enzymes are intrinsically present in the bacteria and not formed after exposure.

- *Klebsiella* produces beta lactamase that destroys ampicillin and *S. maltophilia* produces beta lactamase that destroys imipenem.

Acquired Mechanisms

Acquired resistance is a typical example of fight back by the microorganisms to survive in the presence of antibiotics. Bacteria gradually develop different mechanism that makes them resistant to antibiotics to which they were earlier susceptible. The genetic elements in the bacteria are responsible for generation or transfer of resistance which will be discussed under **"genetic basis of resistance"**. These genetic changes bring about some biomechanical changes which will be discussed under **"biomechanical basis of resistance"**.

Genetic Basis of Resistance

Acquired resistance by genes can be of two types based upon the mechanism of genetic change, i.e. chromosome mediated and horizontal gene transfer.

Chromosome Mediated

Chromosome mediated resistance can be because of spontaneous mutation, hypermutation and adaptive mutation.

- **Spontaneous mutation** is a result of faulty DNA replication or repair of DNA damage seen during bacteria replication. This can bring about changes in the bacteria as described below:
  - **Change of a target for the antibiotics that gene codes:** *RpoB* gene mutation changes structure of RNA polymerase targeted by rifampicin.
  - **Decreased or absence of gene for porin production in gram-negatives:** Decreased activity or absence of *oprD* gene in pseudomonas decreases porins and entry of antibiotics.

- **Activation of efflux pumps:** *E. coli* mar gene mutation increases AcrAB pumps which cause efflux of beta lactams, fluoroquinolones and tetracyclines.
- **Upregulation of beta lactamase production due to mutation:** Resistance to cephalosporins in gram, negative organisms.

❐ **Hypermutation** is defined as an elevated mutation rate in bacteria that changes genes causing drug resistance e.g. multi-drug resistance TB of Beijing genotype.

❐ **Adaptive mutation** unlike spontaneous mutation is seen in nonreplicating bacteria. For example, exposure of quinolones causes mutation in *E. coli*.

Horizontal Gene Transfer

A gene containing drug resistance can be transferred either between bacteria or within a bacterium between chromosomes and plasmid.

❐ Transfer of resistance between bacteria, i.e. from one bacterium to another can happen by three mechanisms conjugation, transduction and transformation.

- **Conjugation:** In conjugation there is a cell to cell transfer of genes present in plasmid through a sex pilus. This is the most common mechanism of drug resistance transfer.
- **Transduction:** In transduction, the gene containing resistance is transferred by a bacteriophage from one bacterium to another.
- **Transformation:** In transformation a naked DNA part containing resistance genes, released due to lysis of a bacteria is taken up and integrated to its DNA by another bacterium.

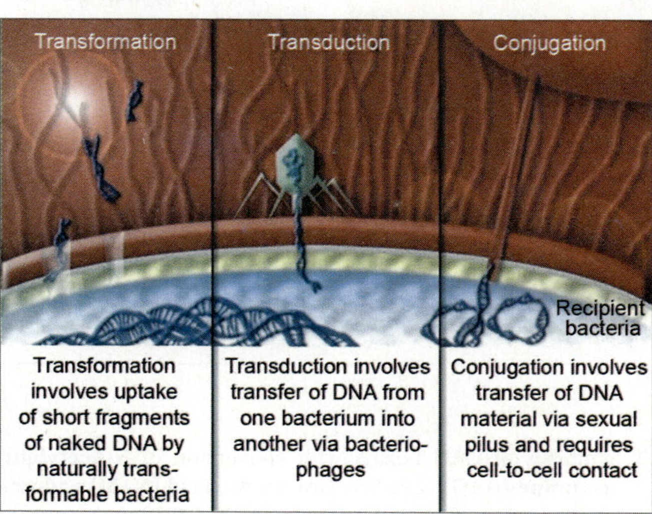

Transformation
Transduction
Conjugation
Recipient bacteria
Transformation involves uptake of short fragments of naked DNA by naturally trans-formable bacteria
Transduction involves transfer of DNA from one bacterium into another via bacterio-phages
Conjugation involves transfer of DNA material via sexual pilus and requires cell-to-cell contact

❐ Transfer of resistance within a bacterium between its chromosomes and plasmids with the help of transposons and integrons.

- **Integrons** are elements present in bacterial DNA or plasmid, which with the help of integrase can integrate gene cassettes containing drug resistance into DNA or plasmid.
- **Transposons** are part of chromosome in DNA or plasmid which can contain integrons. These transposons can breakdown from DNA or plasmid and get themselves incorporated into another plasmid. Hence, they will carry with them the integrons and transfer resistance from a chromosome of DNA to plasmid or vice versa and from one plasmid to anther plasmid as well.

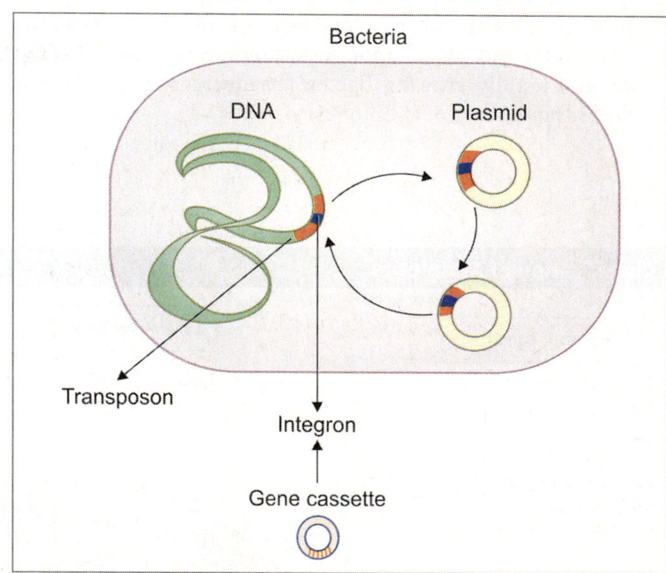

Biomechanical Basis of Resistance

The genetic mechanisms can bring about biomechanical changes in the bacteria that can cause resistance. The various mechanisms are discussed below:

Drug Inactivating Enzymes

Drug inactivating enzymes are produced against **beta lactams, chloramphenicol, aminoglycosides and tetracyclines**.

Alteration of Drug Target

Resistance can be seen in **methicillin, erythromycin, fluoroquinolones, rifampicin** can be seen due to alteration of their targets, i.e. **penicillin binding protein, 50S subunit, DNA gyrase and RNA polymerase respectively**.

Drug Efflux

Drug efflux is an important mechanism of resistance to **antimalarials, tetracyclines, erythromycin and fluoroquinolones** because these drugs must be present in the cytoplasm of bacteria to exert their effects.

Biofilm Mediated Drug Resistance

A biofilm is a population of bacteria enclosed in an exopolysaccharide matrix, growing on a surface of a medical device like catheter. Quorum sensing is a bacterium to bacterium signaling to coordinate among themselves for contribution in biofilm synthesis. This biofilm contributes to resistance to antibiotics by various mechanisms as given below:

❐ **Mechanical barrier:** The exopolysaccharide matrix serves as a mechanical barrier to diffusion of antibiotics through the biofilm.

❐ **Efflux pumps:** Biofilms develop efflux pumps that can actively pump the drug out of the biofilm.

- **Enzymatic inactivation:** Biofilms can produce drug inactivating enzymes like pseudomonas biofilms producing beta lactamase.
- **Decreased growth rate:** Decreased oxygen and nutrients passage through the biofilms slows down the metabolism of bacteria and growth rate. As antibiotics are most effective against rapidly growing bacteria, a decreased growth rate decreases efficacy of antibiotics.
- **Persisters:** Some bacteria undergo phenotypic modification into dormant, spore like structure and survive antibiotic insult. These are called as persisters which are activated later.

ANTIBIOTICS

Antibiotics can be broadly classified into **cell wall synthesis inhibitors, antibiotics acting on cell membrane, protein synthesis inhibitors, DNA gyrase inhibitors and antifolate antibiotics.**

Classification of Antibiotics

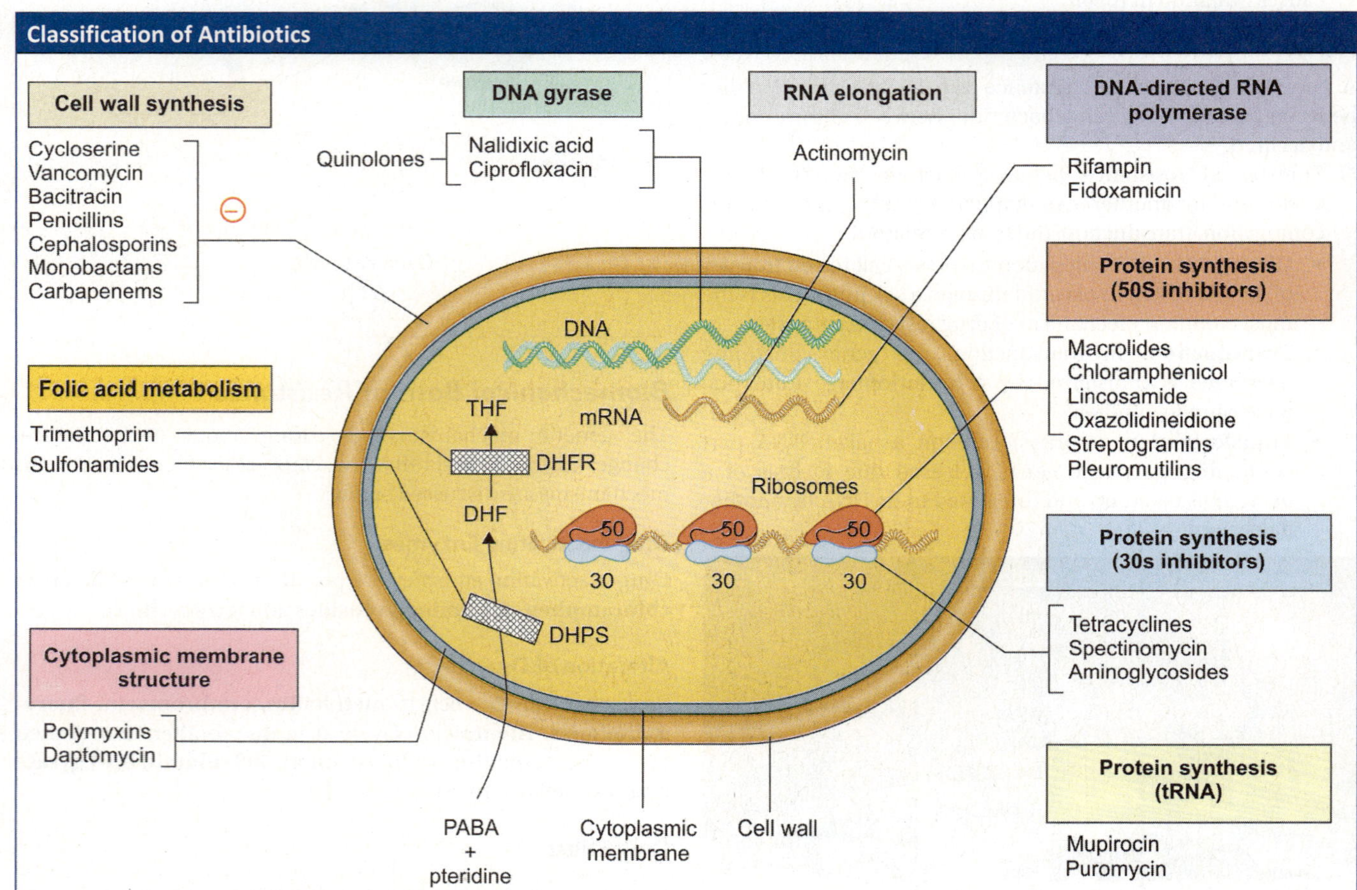

CELL WALL SYNTHESIS INHIBITORS

Gram-positive bacteria are made up of cell membrane and cell wall, whereas a gram-negative is made up of a cell membrane, cell wall and a capsule (contains pores). If cell wall synthesis is inhibited, the cell membrane of bacteria is exposed to hypertonic environment in our body, hence solute and water enter through the permeable cell membrane and bacteria undergo lysis. Thus, cell wall synthesis inhibitors are **bactericidal drugs**. Bactericidal drugs are preferred in infections seen in **neutropenic patients**.

Cell Wall Synthesis

- Cell wall, also known as **peptidoglycan** is made up of peptides, i.e. amino acids and glycosaminoglycans (GAG).
- Synthesis of GAG begins with conversion of **N-Acetylglucosamine (NAG)** to **N-Acetylmuramic acid (NAM)** with the incorporation of **phosphoenolpyruvate (PEP)** with the help of enzyme **enol pyruvate transferase (EPT)**.
- After this the peptides **d-alanine and glycine** are attached to NAM followed by attachment of NAM. This complete structure is one unit of cell wall.
- This unit moves out of the cell membrane with the help of a lipid carrier. Once the units come out a peptide bond forms in between one unit's glycine and another unit's d-alanine with the help of enzyme **transpeptidase**; the process being known as **cross linking**.

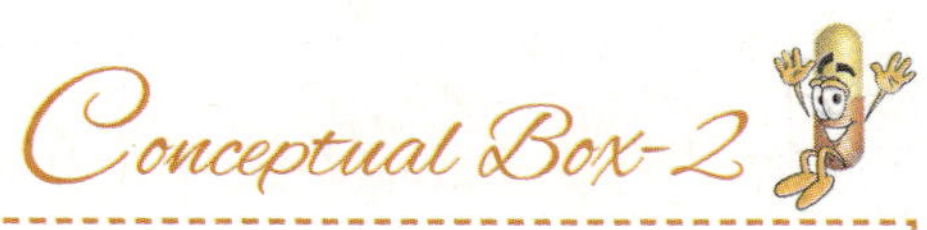

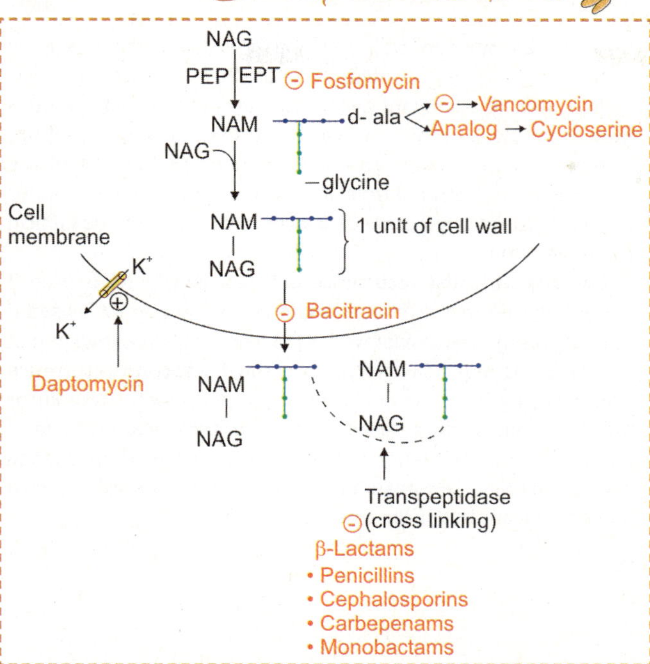

Fosfomycin

- **Fosfomycin** is an analog of PEP and hence competitively **inhibits EPT** and synthesis of NAM. It enters into the bacteria by glucose-6-phosphate transporters present in bacteria.
- These glucose-6-phosphate transporters are present in the gram-negative organisms like ***E. coli, Klebsiella* and *Serratia***; hence **fosfomycin is more effective against gram-negative as compared to gram-positive**.
- Fosfomycin is excreted unchanged in urine and hence approved for treatment of **urinary tract infection (UTI) in females** at a single dose of 3 g. It is free of grave side effects and is safe in pregnancy and can be used for **UTI in pregnant females**.
- **Fosmidomycin** is also a PEP analog with similar characteristics.

Glycopeptides

- This class contains the most commonly used drug **vancomycin** and others like **teicoplanin, dalbavancin, telavancin and oritavancin**.
- Glycopeptides inhibit **d-alanine** because of which peptide bond cannot be formed with glycine and crosslinking is inhibited.
- They have a large molecular size and hence have **poor oral absorption** and **poor penetration through capsule of gram-negatives**. Thus, these are used only for **gram-positive organisms.**

Vancomycin

- **Intravenous vancomycin** is the drug of choice for the treatment of **systemic MRSA infection (sepsis and endocarditis), *Enterococcus faecium* and ampicillin resistant *Enterococcus faecalis***. Vancomycin is synergistic with aminoglycosides and hence gentamicin or streptomycin is added to vancomycin for the treatment of *Enterococcus*.
- **Oral vancomycin** is the current drug of choice for the treatment of **pseudomembranous enterocolitis;** metronidazole is used in case oral vancomycin is not available. In case of vancomycin resistant cases **fidaxomicin** and **rifaximin** can be used.
- **Vancomycin** can cause **nephrotoxicity** and **ototoxicity**. It stimulates histamine release, which causes vasodilation, flushing and a red discoloration of patient known as **red man syndrome**.

Vancomycin Associated Red Man Syndrome

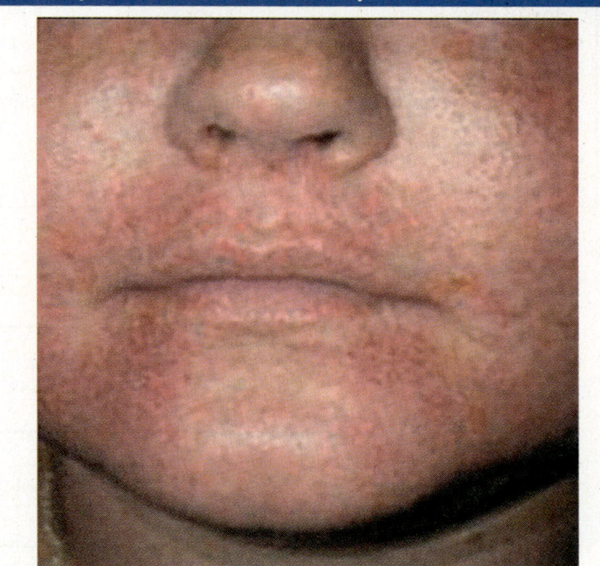

- Resistance to vancomycin is caused by change of **d-alanine to d-lactate** by van A transposon present in **plasmids**. This leads to vancomycin resistance in *Staphylococcus aureus* (VRSA) and *Enterococcus* (VRE). Vancomycin intermediate *Staphylococcus aureus* (VISA) are seen due to increased thickness of murein layer.

Other Glycopeptides

- Other drugs in this class like teicoplanin, dalbavancin, telavancin and oritavancin are used by intravenous route for treatment of skin and soft tissue infection caused by **MRSA**.
- Apart from inhibiting d-alanine, telavancin and oritavancin bind to the cell membrane and disrupt it and hence are more bactericidal than vancomycin.
- Delavancin and oritavancin are very long-acting and can be used once weekly by intravenous route.

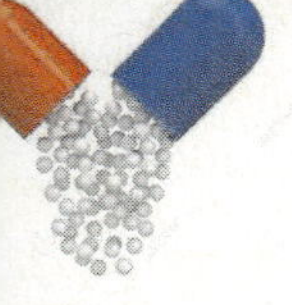

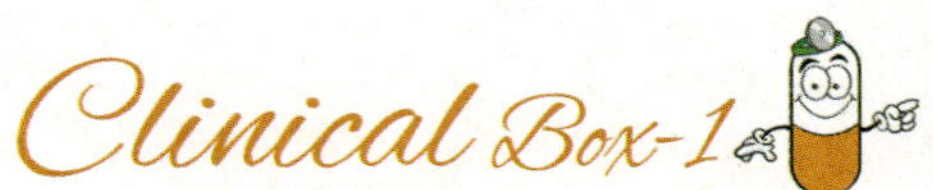

Pseudomembranous Enterocolitis (Updated Guidelines)

- Pseudomembranous enterocolitis is caused by gram-positive bacteria clostridium difficile. The precipitating factor is suppression of normal microbiota of colon by prolonged use of antibiotics like cephalosporins, ampicillin, fluoroquinolones and clindamycin. The most common cause currently are 3rd generation cephalosporins like ceftriaxone.
- The only FDA approved drugs for treatment are oral **vancomycin** and oral **fidaxomicin**. Other drugs that can be used off-label are metronidazole, rifaximin, nitazoxanide, bacitracin, tigecycline and fusidic acid.

Doses of drugs used

- **Vancomycin R1 (Regimen 1):** Oral vancomycin 125 mg QID for 10 days
- **Vancomycin R2 (Regimen 2):** Oral vancomycin 125 mg QID for 10–14 days → BD for 7 days → OD for 7 days → Every 2–3 days once for 2–8 weeks. This is a prolonged tapered and pulsed regimen.
- **Fidaxomicin:** 200 mg BD for 10 days
- **Rifaximin:** 400 mg TDS for 20 days

- In an **initial episode** oral vancomycin is the current drug of choice for treatment of mild/moderate/severe cases. In severe complicated or fulminant cases oral vancomycin + intravenous metronidazole is used. If the patient dose not respond to drugs in fulminant cases, then colectomy is done to save life of the patients. Oral metronidazole as single agent is used in mild/moderate cases only if other drugs like vancomycin or fidaxomicin is not available.
- In patients with **first recurrence** oral vancomycin R1 is used if patient was on metronidazole and oral vancomycin R2 is used if patient was on oral vancomycin R1. The other alternative in first recurrence is oral fidaxomicin. In case of a **second recurrence** oral vancomycin R2 or oral vancomycin R1 + oral rifaximin or oral fidaxomicin can be used. In case of **third recurrence** fecal microbiota transplantation is done. To prevent recurrence along with antibiotics, bezlotoxumab (anticlostridium difficile toxin B monoclonal antibody) can be used.

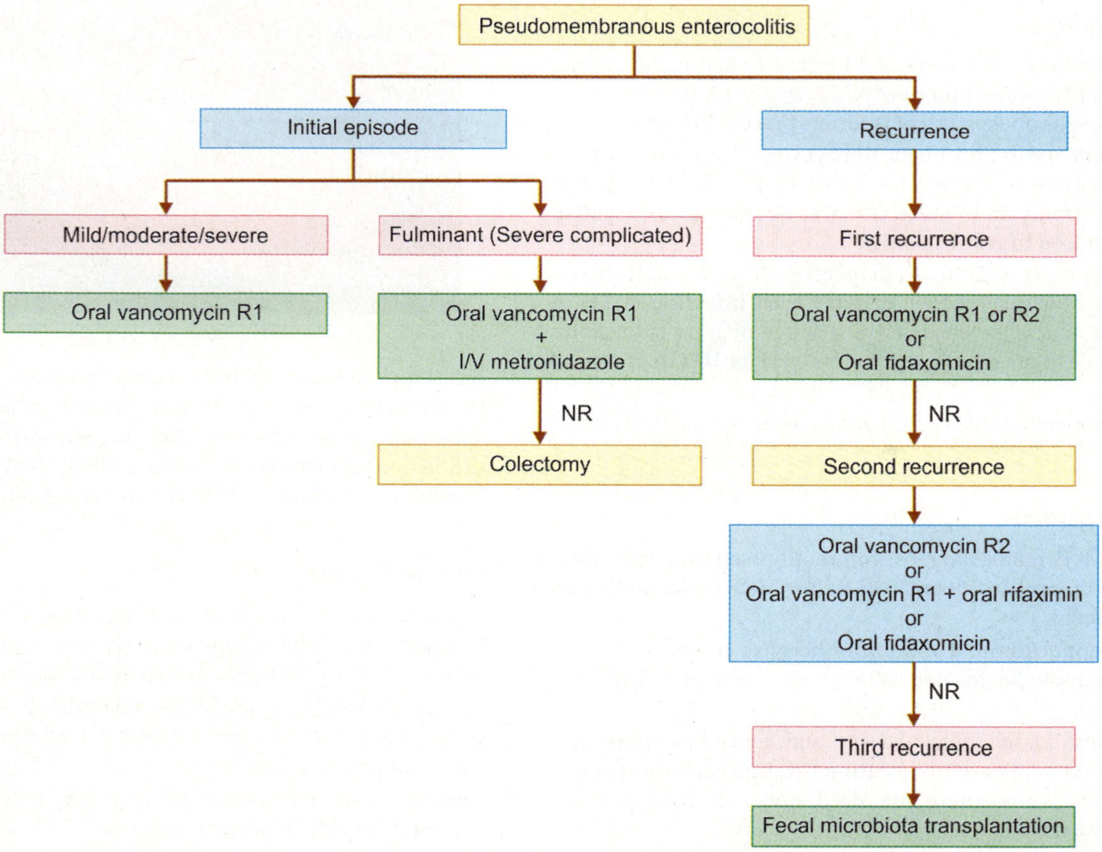

Pseudomembranous enterocolitis

- Initial episode
  - Mild/moderate/severe → Oral vancomycin R1
  - Fulminant (Severe complicated) → Oral vancomycin R1 + I/V metronidazole → NR → Colectomy
- Recurrence
  - First recurrence → Oral vancomycin R1 or R2 or Oral fidaxomicin → NR → Second recurrence → Oral vancomycin R2 or Oral vancomycin R1 + oral rifaximin or Oral fidaxomicin → NR → Third recurrence → Fecal microbiota transplantation

Recent Advances

- **Bezlotoxumab** is anti C. difficile toxin B monoclonal antibody recently approved for prophylaxis of pseudomembranous enterocolitis in patients on antibiotics.
- **Actoxumab** is an anti C. difficile toxin A monoclonal antibody under trial for prophylaxis of pseudomembranous enterocolitis in patients on antibiotics.

Antibiotic Associated Pseudomembranous Enterocolitis

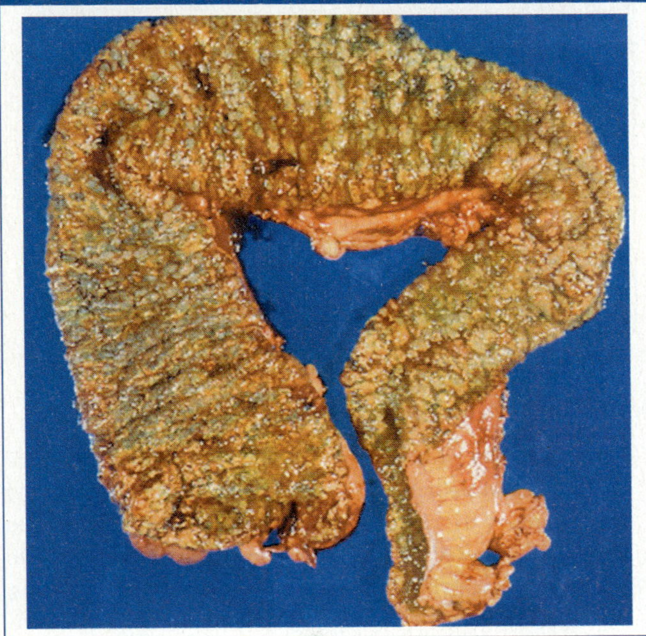

Cycloserine

- **Cycloserine** is an analog of d-alanine and irreversibly inhibits enzymes alanine racemase and ligase, which convert l-alanine to d-alanine and join d-alanine to d-alanine respectively.
- Cycloserine is used for treatment of MDR tuberculosis.
- Side effects associated are **neuropsychiatric** ones like seizures, peripheral neuropathy and psychosis.

Bacitracin

- Bacitracin inhibits transport of the cell wall units by inhibiting action of a lipid carrier called as **bactoprenol**.
- Systemic route is abandoned because of side effects like **nephrotoxicity and bone marrow suppression**. It is used as a topical antibiotic.
- Since it has poor oral absorption, it can be used by oral route for treatment of **pseudomembranous enterocolitis and VRE**.

BETA LACTAM ANTIBIOTICS

The beta lactam class contains four groups of antibiotics, i.e. **penicillins, cephalosporins, carbapenems and monobactams.**

Penicillins

Penicillins can be subclassified based on spectrum into narrow spectrum, penicillinase resistant and wide-spectrum penicillins. **Lipid soluble penicillins** like penicillin G and PRPs can penetrate through the cell wall of **gram-positives**, however they cannot enter into the gram-negatives through porins. Wide-spectrum penicillins are **water soluble** and hence can enter through cell wall of **gram-positives** as well through porins of gram-negatives.

Narrow Spectrum Penicillins

Penicillin G and penicillin V are lipid soluble, narrow spectrum penicillins with activity only against gram-positive organisms, anaerobes and only some gram-negative cocci like meningococci. They are not active against gram-negative organisms because of the capsule. The capsule has pores which allow only water soluble drugs of small size to enter.

Penicillin G

- **Penicillin G (aqueous)** has **poor oral absorption** as it is rapidly broken down by gastric acid, hence it is given by parenteral route. **Intravenous route is more preferred** than intramuscular route due to injection site reactions seen with intramuscular injections. Penicillin G is measured in international units, with each mg of penicillin G having 1600 international units.
- After parenteral administration it is rapidly eliminated due to tubular secretion by pumps and thus penicillin G per se is **very short acting (T1/2 of 30 minutes)**.
- To increase its duration of action either an inhibitor of pumps, i.e. **probenecid** is combined or salts like **benzathine or procaine** are combined which make penicillin G more water soluble and is slowly released from the intramuscular site of injection. Procaine being a local anesthetic, injections of procaine penicillin G are painless. These penicillins are not given by intravenous route due to risk of toxicity.
- **Benzathine penicillin G is the longest acting penicillin** with duration of action around 28 days, hence is more preferred. It is the drug of choice for prophylaxis of **rheumatic fever** given once in a month.
- In **syphilis benzathine penicillin G** is drug of choice for all stages except **CNS stage**, where **aqueous penicillin G** is more preferred. In pregnancy as there are no alternatives, in case of penicillin allergy the female is **desensitized to penicillin** and then administered. In patients of **secondary syphilis**, penicillin associated release of spirochetal antigen can cause hypersensitivity reaction known as **Jarisch-Herxheimer reaction**, characterized by fever, arthralgia, myalgia and **worsening of cutaneous lesions**.

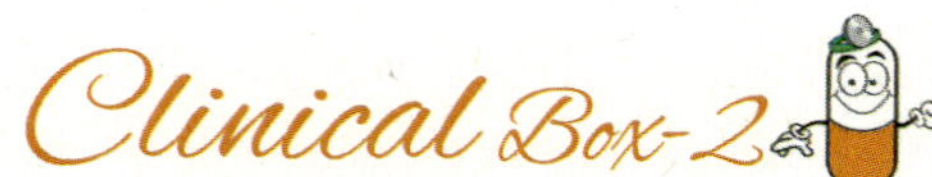

Treatment of Syphilis

Primary Secondary Early latent	Intramuscular benzathine penicillin G 2.4 million unit single dose
Tertiary without CNS involvement **Cardiovascular involvement** Late latent	**Intramuscular benzathine penicillin G 2.4-million-unit three doses (one dose/week)**
Neurosyphilis	Intravenous aqueous penicillin G 18-24-million-unit as continuous infusion or every 4 hours for 10–14 days

- In gram-negative bacilli, **pasteurella multocida** wound infection caused by dog or cat bite **penicillin G** is drug of choice but for meningitis **ceftriaxone** is preferred.
- Other conditions for which penicillin G is still the drug of choice is given below in the mnemonic box.

Mnemonics

Penicillin G is drug of choice for following infections:

B : Bacillus (Anthrax)
L : Leptospira (Rat bite fever)
A : Actinomyces
S : Streptococcus
T : Treponema pallidum (Syphilis)
Penicillin : Pertunae (Yaws), Pasteurella multocida
G : Gas gangrene

Clinical Box-3

Treatment of *Staphylococcus Aureus*

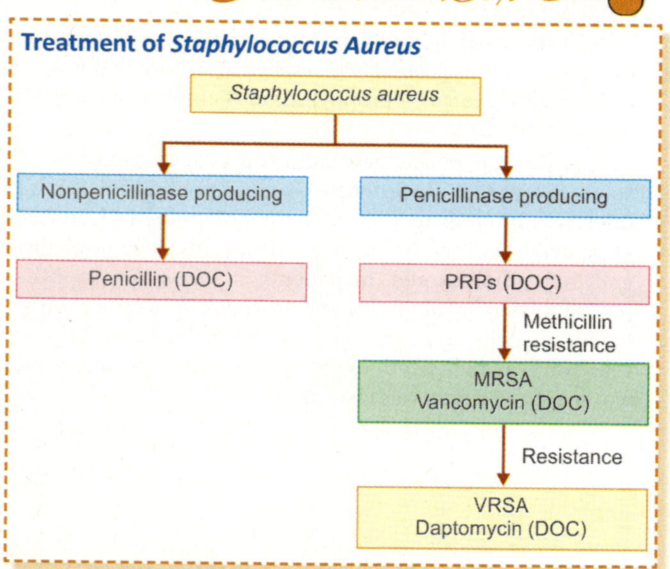

Penicillin V

- **Penicillin V** is an **acid stable** penicillin synthesized from penicillin G. It is given by oral route four times a day (QID dosing).
- The uses are like penicillin G and is the oral penicillin of choice for infections mentioned above.

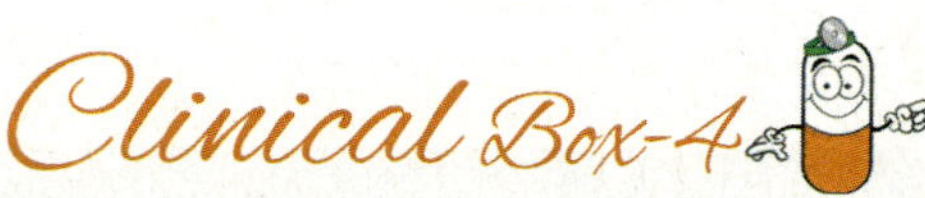

Alternative Antibiotics for MRSA and VRSA

MRSA and VRSA	MRSA
Linezolid Tedizolid Streptogramins Tigecycline 5th generation cephalosporins Other glycopeptides (dalbavancin, telavancin, oritavancin)	Clindamycin Minocycline Doxycycline Cotrimoxazole

Penicillinase Resistant Penicillins (PRP)

- Penicillinase is a beta lactamase that breaks down the beta lactam ring of penicillins. The structure of beta lactam ring was changed by changing structure of side chain R and hence this altered beta lactam ring became resistant to penicillinase, specifically produced by *Staphylococcus*. Thus, these penicillinase resistant penicillins are also called as **anti-staphylococcal penicillins**.
- The side chain R is broken down by an enzyme called as amidase to change the structure of penicillins.
- **Oxacillin, cloxacillin and dicloxacillin** are structurally similar, **acid stable penicillins** and hence are given by oral route. **Nafcillin and methicillin** are acid labile and hence given by parenteral route.
- **Dicloxacillin** is most active PRP against *Staphylococcus*, whereas **nafcillin** is most active PRP against organisms other than *Staphylococcus*.
- **Oxacillin can cause liver toxicity** which is reversible on drug stoppage.
- Cloxacillin is drug of choice for treatment of **mastitis**.
- **Nafcillin can cause agranulocytosis (neutropenia)** and interstitial nephritis.
- **Methicillin** use has been banned due to risk of **severe interstitial nephritis**. Methicillin currently is used as a marker and *Staphylococcus* resistant to methicillin are marked as **methicillin resistant *Staphylococcus aureus* (MRSA)**. In MRSA there is an altered penicillin binding protein or transpeptidase and hence none of the beta lactam drugs are effective.

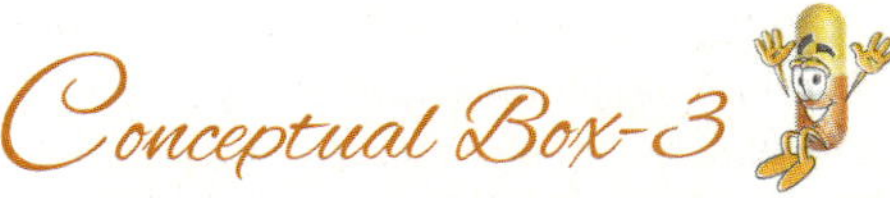

Structure of Penicillin

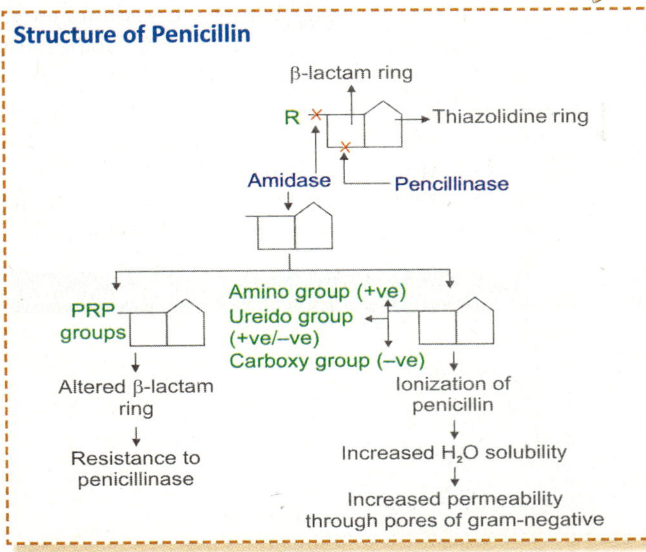

Clinical Box-5

Treatment of *Enterococcus*

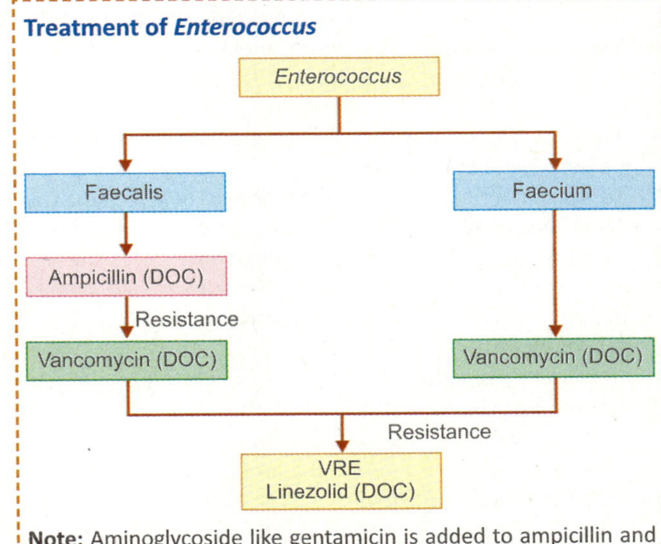

Note: Aminoglycoside like gentamicin is added to ampicillin and vancomycin and to get treatment of choice.

Wide-spectrum Penicillins

These are water soluble penicillins which can enter the pores in capsules and hence are effective against **gram-negative organisms** as well.

Aminopenicillins

- Substituting the side chain R by a positively charged amino group makes these penicillins ionized or water soluble that can easily pass through the pores in capsules of gram-negative organisms. However, these are still broken down by beta lactamases.
- **Amoxicillin and ampicillin** have **good oral absorption** and in other oral penicillins like, **dicloxacillin, penicillin V, cloxacillin and oxacillin** food interferes with absorption and hence should be given 1–2 hours before or after food. The only oral penicillin which is not affected by and can be given with food is **amoxicillin**.
- These are active against both gram-positive and negative organisms. Ampicillin is the drug of choice for ***Listeria, Enterococcus faecalis, H.ifluenzae pneumonia and otitis,* and infective endocarditis (enterococcal and streptococcal)**. *Enterococcus faecium*, however is universally resistant to ampicillin and hence **vancomycin** is preferred. Aminoglycosides have synergistic action with penicillins, as inhibition of cell wall synthesis increases entry of aminoglycosides into gram-negatives. For adequate coverage, **gentamicin** is added to **ampicillin and vancomycin** for *Enterococcus*.
- Ampicillin is active against *Shigella* but not amoxicillin.
- Amoxicillin is the drug of choice for the treatment of mild diverticulitis (for moderate ceftriaxone and in severe meropenem is drug of choice), asymptomatic bacteriuria, Ludwig's and Vincent angina, rhinosinusitis and cellulitis.

Carboxy and Ureido Penicillins

- **Carbenicillin and ticarcillin** are synthesized by addition of carboxy group in place of side chain R that gives a negative charge and makes penicillin water soluble.
- **Piperacillin, azlocillin and mezlocillin** are synthesized by addition of ureido group in place of side chain R that gives both negative and positive charge to penicillin and makes penicillin even more water soluble than carboxy penicillins. Being more water soluble these can enter more easily into gram-negatives and are more potent than carboxy penicillins.
- All of these are active against ***pseudomonas* and *enterobacter*** and hence these are also known as antipseudomonal penicillins. Piperacillin and mezlocillin are effective against ***Klebsiella* and *Enterococcus*** as well.

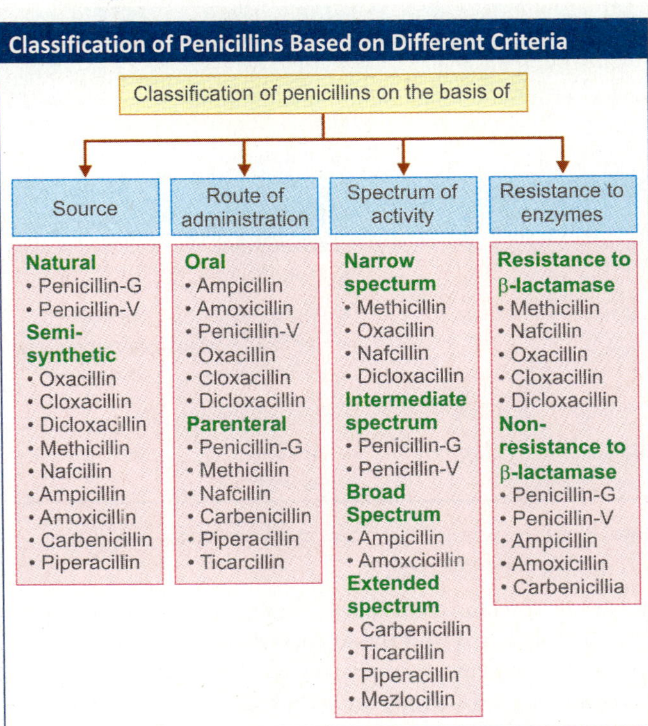

Side Effects of Penicillins

- **Hypersensitivity** is the most common side effect associated with penicillins; the most common one is **rash** whereas the least common but most severe is **anaphylaxis**. Penicillin break down products bind with proteins and form haptens which are antigenic. Stimulation of IgE production leads to hypersensitivity.
- Ampicillin if given in **EBV** infection can cause macular rash and hence should be avoided.
- Cross reactivity is seen with penicillins to all beta lactam drugs except **monobactams**. Monobactam cross reactivity is seen only with one cephalosporin, i.e. ceftazidime.
- Oral penicillins can cause GIT side effects like nausea, vomiting and **pseudomembranous enterocolitis (maximum with ampicillin)**.
- Intravenous penicillins can cause seizures and thrombophlebitis and intrathecal administration can cause arachnoiditis and encephalopathy.

Resistance to Penicillins

Resistance to penicillins can be seen by four mechanisms described below. The most common mechanism of resistance to penicillins is by **beta lactamase production**.

Beta-lactamase Production

Beta-lactamase can be classified by **Ambler's molecular classification and Bush's functional classification.**

- Ambler's molecular classification is based on **structure, i.e. protein sequence of enzymes**; class A, C and D use serine for beta lactam hydrolysis, whereas class B are metalloenzymes which use zinc ion for beta lactam hydrolysis.
- Bush's functional classification is based on the **substrates of enzymes and the inhibitors of enzymes.**

Ambler's classification	Bush's classification	Substrates	Inhibition by beta lactamase
Class A	Class 2	ESBL • Penicillins • Cephalosporins • (Except 5th generation) • Monobactams	Yes
Class B	Class 3	• Penicillins • Cephalosporins • Carbapenems	Variable carbapenems - No
Class C	Class 1	• Cephalosporins	No
Class D	Class 4	• Cloxacillin • Carbenicillin	No

Note: Recently some ESBL contains **carbepenemase**, which is difficult to treat.

- ESBL production is detected by the ability of the microorganisms to hydrolyze **3rd generation cephalosporins**. Since ESBL is not effective against carbapenems and 4th and 5th generation cephalosporins, **carbapenems are the drug of choice for ESBL** producing organisms and **4th and 5th generation** can also be used for the same. The plasmids for ESBL also have mutations that confer resistance to other antibiotics like **aminoglycosides, cotrimoxazole and fluoroquinolones. Piperacillin—tazobactam** and **cefoperazone sulbactam** can be used for mild infections caused by ESBL organisms.
- Most common cause of resistance to penicillins is because of **penicillinase** production.
- Beta-lactamase inhibitors have been developed to counteract this mechanism of resistance. **Sulbactam** has also got antimicrobial effect and is used for the treatment of ***Acinetobacter***.

Beta lactamase inhibitor	Beta lactam drug combined with
Clavulanic acid	Amoxicillin Ticarcillin
Sulbactam	Ampicillin
Tazobactam	Piperacillin
Avibactam	Ceftazidime
Vaborbactam	Meropenem

Recent Advances

- **New Delhi metallo beta-lactamase-1 (NDM-1) gene** codes for a beta-lactamase that can degrade all the beta-lactam drugs, i.e. penicillins, cephalosporins, monobactams and carbapenems. Apart from this, organisms with NDM-1 gene have also genes for drug efflux and enzymes that can metabolize other drugs like fluoroquinolones, macrolides and chloramphenicol.
- The drugs effective against NDM-1 gene containing bacteria are **tigecycline** and **colistin**.
- This gene was initially found in *Klebsiella*, which is present in plasmid. Now this is being seen in other bacteria like *Enterobacter*, *Salmonella* and *Providencia*.

Alteration of Penicillin Binding Protein (PBP)

- An alteration in the PBP is responsible for resistance particularly in gram-positive organism *Staphylococcus*.
- A **high molecular weight PBP** results in resistance of ***Staphylococcus aureus* to methicillin (MRSA)** and it is **plasmid mediated**. Thus, resistance to penicillins in *Staphylococcus* is due to penicillinase and to PRPs like methicillin is due to altered PBP mediated by ***meca gene***.

Decreased Porin Production

- Porins are the gateway for entry of beta lactams into the gram-negative organisms.
- ***Pseudomonas*** can selectively decrease porin production and deny entry to the penicillins.

Drug Efflux

- Microorganisms can develop drug efflux active pumps, which can pump drug out against concentration gradient.
- This mechanism is present in gram-negative organisms like ***Pseudomonas*, *E. coli* and *Gonococcus***.

Cephalosporins

The most accepted classification of cephalosporins is based on generations ranging from first to fifth. With each generation the spectrum and resistance to beta-lactamse kept on increasing.

First Generation Cephalosporins

- The first-generation drugs have primary activity against **gram-positive organisms** and some activity against gram-negatives (Proteus, *E. coli* and *Klebsiella*) and **anaerobes (except *Bacteroides*)**.
- Cefazolin by intravenous route is the drug of choice for **surgical prophylaxis**. It is the preferred agent among first generation because it is longest acting. Prophylactic antibiotic is given **60 minutes** before incision and continued for at least **24 hours** after surgery.
- Oral drugs like cefadroxil and cephalexin are well concentrated in urine and are active against *E. coli*, *Klebsiella* and Proteus. Hence, these are used for the treatment of UTI.

Mnemonics

First Generation Cephalosporins	Route
Dr : CefaDroxil **Reddy's** : CephRADine **X in** : CephaleXin	Oral
Zoo : CefaZolin	IV/IM

Second Generation

- The second generation are primarily active against **gram-negative** organisms (*H. influenza*, Moraxella, *E. coli*, *Klebsiella*, *Proteus* etc.) and anaerobes including *Bacteroides*. These are less effective against gram-positive as compared to first generation.
- **Cefotetan is the most active second-generation drug against anaerobes like *Bacteroides*** and hence used for prophylaxis of anaerobic infections in colorectal surgery.
- **Cefoxitin** is second most active agent against anaerobes and is used for the treatment if pelvic inflammatory disease and lung abscess.
- **Cefuroxime** has good activity against *H. influenza*, *Moraxella* and *Pneumococcus*; hence it is used for the treatment of community acquired pneumonia, otitis and sinusitis. It is the only second-generation drug **not active against *Bacteroides***. It can be used for surgical prophylaxis as well.

Mnemonics

Second Generation Cephalosporins	Route
Fa : CeFaclor **Lo** : Loracarbef	Oral
Ma : CefoMandole **Ur** : CefUroxime **Ta** : CefoteTan **Xi** : CefoXitin	IV/IM
Pr : CefProzil	Oral
Fa Lo (Follow) Ma Ur (mayur = peacock) Ta Xi (taxi) Pr (per = on).	

Note: Cefuroxime can be given by oral route as well.

Third Generation Cephalosporins

- The third generation drugs are more active against **gram-negative** organisms as compared to gram-positive.
- **Ceftriaxone** is the **longest acting** third-generation drug, requires less frequent dosing and hence more preferred. **Cefotaxime** is the **shortest acting** third-generation drug.
- Ceftriaxone is the most commonly used drug given by parenteral route and is drug of choice for the treatment of **Gonorrhea, *E. coli, Klebsiella, Providencia,*** Proteus, ***Shigella, Salmonella* (typhoid) and *H. influenzae* meningitis.** It is also drug of choice for empirical treatment of **acute bacterial meningitis** and for treatment of **osteomyelitis. Cefotaxime** can be used for treatment of meningitis as well.
- Ceftriaxone is not effective against listeria and hence ampicillin is drug of choice in listeria meningitis. In case of penicillin resistant pneumococcal meningitis, efficacy of ceftriaxone decreases and hence vancomycin is combined to ceftriaxone.

Recent Advances

Gonorrhea: Current TOC is ceftriaxone high doses + azithromycin/Doxycycline.

Due to increasing resistance to ceftriaxone, it is advised to combine azithromycin or doxycycline to high doses of ceftriaxone for gonorrhea treatment even if chlamydia infection is not coexistent.

- **Cefixime** is the **oral drug of choice for typhoid** and is preferred in ambulatory patients. It is also used for the treatment of otitis and UTI.

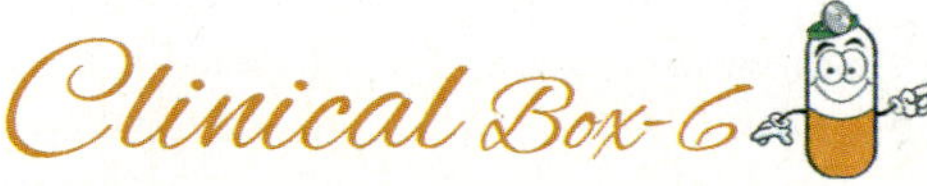

Drugs Used in Typhoid

- **Ceftriaxone: Drug of choice**
- **Cefixime: Oral drug of choice**
- **Ciprofloxacin: Drug of choice for carriers**
- Cefepime
- Cefpodoxime
- Azithromycin
- **Cotrimoxazole/Amoxicillin/Ampicillin/Chloramphenicol:** Widespread resistance

- The only two drugs from this class effective against *Pseudomonas* are **ceftazidime and cefoperazone**. **Ceftazidime** is the drug of choice for treatment of ***Pseudomonas*, febrile neutropenia and melioidosis**. An aminoglycoside like **gentamicin** is combined to ceftazidime for treatment of *Pseudomonas*. **Ceftolozane** is an analog of ceftazidime and hence is also used against *Pseudomonas*.
- Ceftolozane is combined with tazobactam and ceftazidime is combined with avibactam to counteract gram-negatives producing beta-lactamase. Both these combinations are used for treatment of complicated abdominal infections and UTI. Ceftazidime/Avibactam is the only cephalosporin

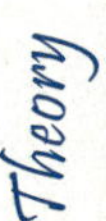

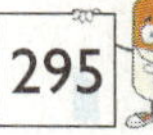

combination active against carbapenemase (KPC) producing gram-negatives.

Mnemonics

Third Generation Drugs	Route
Delhi : Cef**D**inir, Cef**D**itoren, Cefpo**D**oxime	Oral
P : Cefo**P**erazone **M** : **M**oxalactam **T** : Cef**T**riaxone, Cef**T**izoxime, Cefo**T**axime, Cef**T**azidime	IV/IM
EXam : Cefi**X**ime	Oral

Clinical Box-7

Treatment of H. influenza Infection

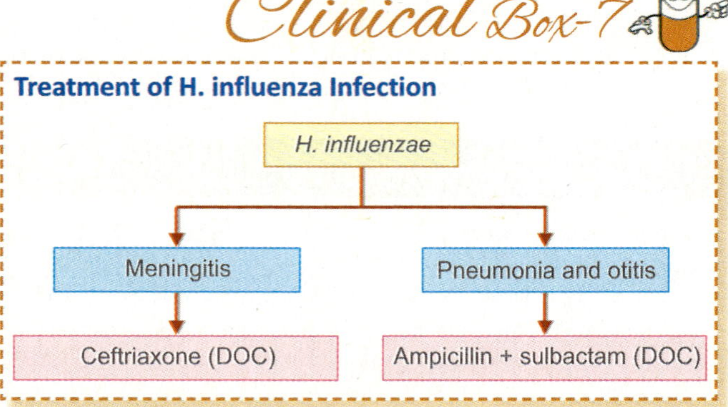

Fourth and Fifth Generation Cephalosporins

- The fourth-generation drugs are more active than third-generation drugs with added activity against gram-negatives like ***Enterobacter*, *Pseudomonas*** and gram-positives like *Staphylococcus* and *Streptococcus*.
- The fifth-generation drugs are as effective as third-generation drugs against gram-negatives. The striking feature is their activity against gram-positive organisms like **MRSA** and hence used for skin and soft tissue infections and community acquired pneumonia caused by MRSA.

Fourth generation cephalosporins	Route	Fifth generation cephalosporins	Route
Cefepime	IV/IM	Ceftobiprole	IV
Cefpirome	IV/IM	Ceftaroline	IV

Side Effects of Cephalosporins

- Hypersensitivity reaction like penicillins can be seen with cephalosporins as well. Cross-sensitivity to penicillins is seen usually with the first-generation drugs. Parenteral cephalosporins can cause pain on injection and thrombophlebitis.
- Nephrotoxicity can be seen with cephalosporins like **cephaloridine > cephalothin, which cause renal tubular necrosis.**
- Most cephalosporins are excreted by kidney except **ceftriaxone (50%)**, **cefpiramide (100%)** and **cefoperazone (100%)** which are excreted by liver. Thus, these are **safe in renal failure**. Because of significant biliary excretion these drugs can cause **diarrhea**. As ceftriaxone is highly concentrated in bile and has high affinity for calcium, it precipitates as calcium salts mimicking gall stones; this phenomenon being known as biliary **pseudolithiasis**.
- Some cephalosporins like **cefamandole, cefotetan, moxalactam and cefoperazone** have an extra group called as methylthiotetrazole (MTT) group which is responsible for **disulfiram like reaction, hypoprothrombinemia** and **bleeding**. Vitamin K given prophylactically twice weekly can prevent bleeding.
- **Ceftriaxone** and **cefamandole** are associated with thrombocytopenia. Cefixime can cause encephalopathy and nonconvulsive status epilepticus.
- **Ceftriaxone** has high albumin binding and hence can displace bilirubin and cause **kernicterus in new borns**. Thus, cefotaxime is preferred third generation drug in newborns.

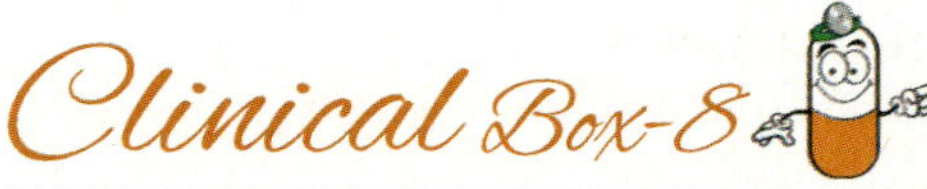

Empirical Treatment of Meningitis

Age	Drugs used
0–3 months	Ampicillin + cefotaxime
3 months – 55 years	Vancomycin + cefotaxime/ceftriaxone/cefepime
>55 years	**Vancomycin + cefotaxime/ceftriaxone/cefepime + ampicillin**

Carbapenems

- **Carbapenems** are the widest spectrum drugs active against gram-positive, gram-negative as well as anaerobic microorganisms. Route of administration is parenteral.
- Carbapenems are the drugs of choice for the treatment of **ESBL producing organisms, *Enterobacter* and *Serratia***. In case of carbapenem resistant *Enterobacter* colistin, tigecycline and fosfomycin can be used. These are reserved for the treatment of ceftriaxone resistant gram-negative oprganisms and ceftazidime resistant *Pseudomonas*.
- **Imipenem** was the first drug in this class but was disappointing due to its short duration of action because it is rapidly broken down by **renal dehydropeptidase**. Hence, **cilastatin**, an inhibitor of this enzyme is always combined with imipenem.
- The other carbapenems like ertapenem, meropenem and doripenem that were developed after imipenem are not substrates for dehydropeptidase.
- **Ertapenem** is the longest acting carbapenem but is **less effective than others against *Acinetobacter* and *Pseudomonas*.** It is used for the treatment of abdominal infections and pelvic inflammatory disease.
- Doripenem and meropenem are more active against gram-negatives but less effective against gram-positives as compared to imipenem. Doripenem is most active against pseudomonas.
- Side effects like **nausea/vomiting (most common)**, hypersensitivity reactions and phlebitis can be seen with all carbapenems. **Imipenem can cause seizures**.

Recent Advances

Meropenem has been recently approved along with a beta- lactamase inhibitor **vaborbactam** for the treatment of complicated urinary tract infections (UTI).

Monobactams

- Aztreonam is a narrow spectrum drug that is active against only **gram-negative** organisms, as it cannot bind to the transpeptidase of gram-positive organisms. Its spectrum against gram-negatives is simiar to third generation cephalosporins and covers *Enterobacter* and *Pseudomonas* as well.
- As it has **no cross reactivity with other beta lactams except ceftazidime**, it is used for the treatment of gram-negatives in penicillin allergic patients.
- **Hepatotoxicity** can be seen in pediatric patients.

ANTIBIOTICS ACTING ON CELL MEMBRANE

Polymyxins

- **Polymyxins** are amphipathic drugs that bind to lipids and disrupt the cell membrane. It also binds to endotoxin of gram-negative organism and neutralizes it. These are narrow spectrum drugs with activity only against **gram-negative organisms**.
- **Polymyxin B and E (colistin)** are used as topical antibiotics for gram-negative infections ***(Pseudomonas)*** of skin and mucous membranes.
- **Colistin** can be given by intravenous route for treatment of **multidrug resistant gram-negative organisms *like Pseudomonas, Klebsiella, Acinetobacter*** etc.
- Polymyxins are not effective against **Burkholderia cepacia** due to decreased binding to the lipopolysaccharide in cell membrane.
- Polymyxins can cause nephrotoxicity, neuromuscular block and paraesthesia. Hence, these are avoided with **aminoglycosides** which can also cause nephrotoxicity and neuromuscular block.

Daptomycin

- Daptomycin is a **lipopeptide** that binds to and depolarizes the bacterial cell membrane that causes K^+ efflux and **bactericidal** effect on microorganisms. Resistance is seen in cases of enterococcal endocarditis due to alteration of cell membrane charge. Beta lactams can counter this mechanism of resistance if given along with daptomycin.
- Daptomycin is the current drug of choice for treatment of **vancomycin resistant *Staphylococcus aureus* (VRSA)**. Though it is **not used for the treatment of pneumonia as it is inactivated by pulmonary surfactant. It can be used for treatment of VRE** but is not FDA approved for same.
- It has **poor oral absorption** and hence given by intravenous route.
- It can cause **myopathy,** neuropathy and allergic pneumonitis. Since it is **excreted by kidney**, dose is decreased in renal failure.

PROTEIN SYNTHESIS INHIBITORS

Proteins are an integral component of all bacteria required for replication and hence inhibition has a bacteriostatic effect.

Protein Synthesis

- Protein synthesis in bacteria takes place the 30S and 50S subunits of ribosomes.
- There are three sites named **A (acceptor), P (peptidyl)** and **E (ejection)** present on the ribosome. The A site accepts a new t-RNA that contains a new amino acid. The P site contains the growing peptide chain on an old t-RNA and the E site is for ejection of an unwanted t-RNA.
- Once new t-RNA binds at A site after the codon and anticodon interaction, the peptides at P site break from old t-RNA and jump to A site, a process called as transpeptidation.
- After this the unwanted old t-RNA jumps to E site from where it is ejected, and P site becomes free.
- Once P site is free the t-RNA at A site jumps to P site, a process called as translocation.

Conceptual Box-4

Protein Synthesis in Bacteria

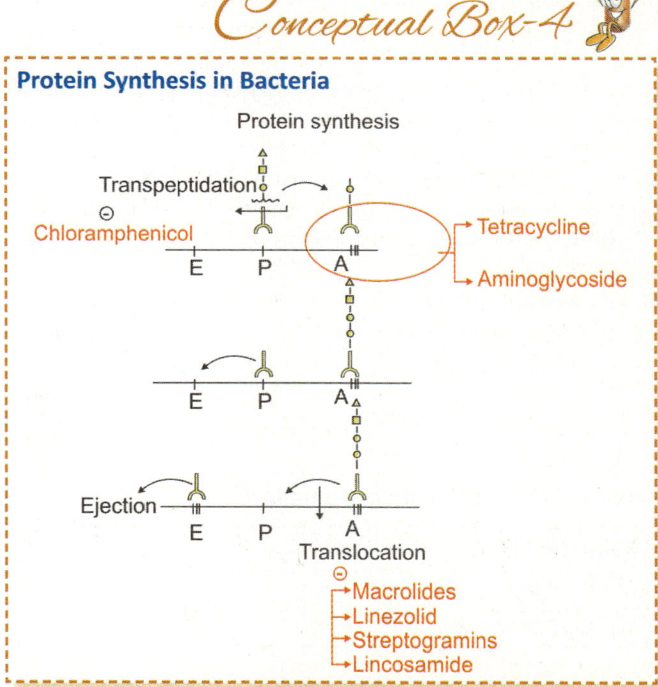

Classification of Protein Synthesis Inhibitors Based on Spectrum

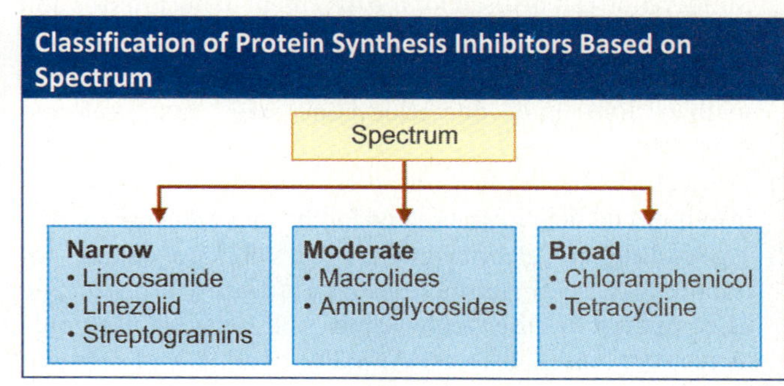

Tetracyclines

- Tetracyclines and glycylcydines (tigecycline) are analogs of t-RNA and hence cause competitive reversible inhibition at the A site of **30 S** subunit.
- These are active against both **gram-positive as well as negative organisms with some exceptions; tetracyclines and tigecycline are not effective against some gram-negatives like *Pseudomonas, Providencia, Morganella* and Proteus.**
- **Tetracyclines** have a variable oral absorption, the amount being maximum for minocycline (100%) followed by doxycycline. Tigecycline has poor oral absorption and hence is used only by intravenous route, whereas tetracyclines can be used by both oral and intravenous route. Intramuscular route is not preferred due to injection site reactions like pain and inflammation.

Uses

- Due to growing resistance to tetracycline the more preferred drug in this class nowadays is **doxycycline**. Tetracycline can be used in inflammatory acne.
- Doxycycline is the drug of choice for the treatment of **mycoplasma hominis, rickettsia, borrelia, brucella, chlamydia and cholera and for prophylaxis of plague**. It is also effective for the treatment of lymphogranuloma venereum, syphilis, Lyme disease and anthrax.
- It is also drug of choice for **pleurodesis and pericardiocentesis** in recurrent pneumothorax and cardiac tamponade; doxycycline when injected into pleural and pericardial cavity causes inflammation, fibrosis and obliteration of space.
- Doxycycline is also drug of choice for **prophylaxis of chloroquine resistant malaria** in patients traveling for less than 6 weeks.
- Tetracycline by topical route is used in prevention of ophthalmia neonatorum.

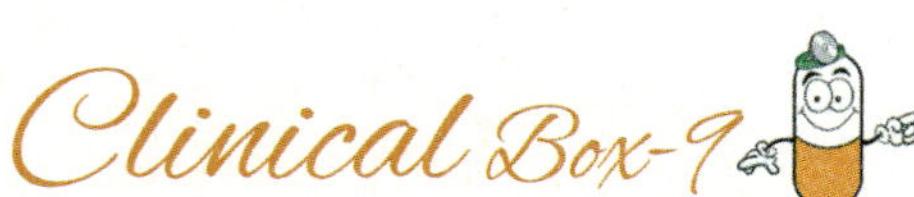

Prevention of Ophthalmia Neonatorum

Silver nitrate solution	1%
Erythromycin	0.5%
Tetracycline	1%

- Minocycline can be used for the treatment of nocardiosis and leprosy.
- The other drugs in this class oxytetracycline, chlortetracycline, methacycline and demeclocycline are less preferred nowadays.
- **Demeclocycline** is the most potent inhibitor of V_2 receptors in kidney and hence can be used for the treatment of **SIADH**.
- **Tigecycline**, a glycylcydine is a synthetic analog of minocycline. There is an increased risk of death with tigecycline as compared to other tetracyclines and hence is used only in resistant cases. It is used for the treatment of resistant gram-positive organisms like **MRSA and VRSA** infections and carbapenem resistant gram-negative organisms like *Acinetobacter, Klebsiella, E. coli* and *Enterobacter*. It can also be used for the treatment of anaerobes unlike tetracyclines. It is poorly concentrated in urine and serum and hence should be avoided for the treatment of urinary tract infection, bacteremia and meningitis.

Mnemonics

Doxycycline is DOC for

- **My :** Mycoplasma hominis (urogenital)
- **Pink :** Plague prophylaxis
- **R :** Rickettsia
- **B :** Borrelia, Brucella
- **C :** Chlamydia, Cholera

Recent Advances

Eravacycline: It is a parenteral tetracycline approved for treatment of complicated abdominal infections.

Omadacycline: It is a parenteral tetracycline approved for treatment of community acquired pneumonia and acute bacterial skin infection. It has a wide spectrum covering gram-positive and negative as well as atypical organisms. It is effective even in case of tetracycline resistance due to drug efflux or ribosomal protective protein.

Sarecycline: It is an oral tetracycline approved for the treatment of inflammatory non-nodular acne in age group >9 years.

Side Effects and Contraindication

- **Nausea and vomiting are the most common side effect** responsible for incompliance. They can also cause esophageal ulcers and hence patient is advised to take drug with a full glass of water and not to lie down for 30 minutes.
- All tetracyclines are nephrotoxic drugs except for **tigecycline, doxycycline and minocycline which can be safely used in renal failure.**

Mnemonics

Tetracyclines Safe in Renal Failure

- **T :** Tigecycline
- **D :** Doxycycline
- **M :** Minocycline

- Tetracyclines can bind to ions like calcium present in milk and magnesium and aluminum present in antacids; hence these are given on **empty stomach**. Further in systemic circulation they bind to calcium in bone and teeth and hence cause bone growth abnormality and are **contraindicated in pregnancy and children.**
- Tetracycline can absorb UV light and hence can cause discoloration of teeth and skin pigmentation or photosensitivity **(maximum with demeclocycline > doxycycline)**.
- **Demeclocycline** can inhibit V_2 receptors and hence cause **diabetes insipidus**.

- **Hepatotoxicity** is more commonly seen in pregnant females.
- **Minocycline specifically produces vestibular toxicity** and brown discoloration of skin.
- Other side effects seen are Fanconi syndrome (outdated tetracycline), pseudotumor cerebri, thrombophlebitis and leukocytosis.

Mnemonics

Side Effects of Tetracycline

F : Fanconi syndrome
L : Liver toxicity
O : Os growth abnormality
P : Photosensitivity, Pseudotumor cerebri
D : Diabetes insipidus
P : Pseudotumor cerebri
T : Teeth discoloration
Vaccine : Vestibulotixicity

Teeth Discoloration with Tetracycline

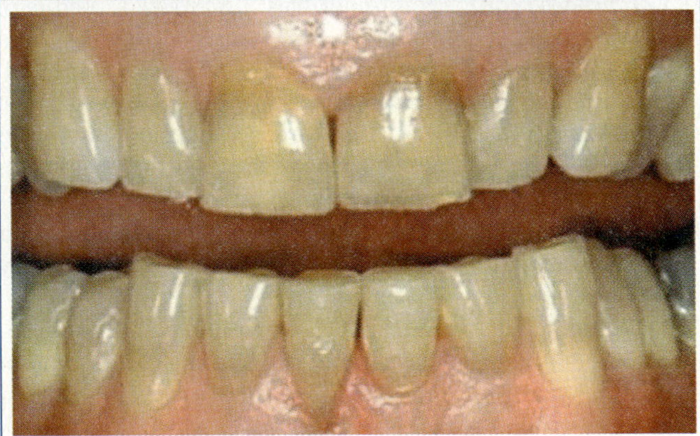

Mechanism of Resistance

- Resistance can be seen due to drug efflux, enzymatic inactivation and production of protective protein for 30S ribosome.
- Tigecycline is resistant to drug efflux.

Aminoglycosides

- Aminoglycosides are limited spectrum drugs with activity only against gram-negative organisms.
- After entering through the porins of capsule, the entry of aminoglycosides through the cell membrane requires an action potential generation with the help of **ATP and oxygen**. Hence, aminoglycosides are **not effective against anaerobes**.
- Once in the cytoplasm of gram-negatives, aminoglycosides cause misreading of m-RNA, which leads to a faulty protein synthesis which is toxic to the bacteria and causes **bactericidal effect**.
- Aminoglycosides are ionized or water soluble and hence have **poor oral absorption**. Hence, these are given by intravenous or intramuscular route. Once a day dosing is more effective as they follow concentration dependent killing and have a prolonged postantibiotic effect. Once a day doing is less toxic as well.
- Cell wall synthesis inhibitors like penicillin and vancomycin increase entry of aminoglycosides into bacteria and hence are frequently combined. However, in a solution **penicillins can inactivate aminoglycosides** and hence should not be mixed together.

Uses of Aminoglycosides

- **Gentamicin** > **streptomycin** is **the drug of choice for treatment of plague and tularaemia**. Gentamicin is also added on drug in ***Pseudomonas* and *Enterococcus***. Gentamicin and streptomycin are used for the treatment of **endocarditis *(Enterococcus, Staphylococcus, Streptococcus)*** with a cell wall synthesis inhibitor like **penicillin or vancomycin**.
- **Gentamicin** can be used for resistant gram-negatives like *Enterobacter, Klebsiella, Serratia, E. coli, Acinetobacter* etc. Gentamicin is also used as a topical antibitotic for bacterial skin infection, ocular infection (intraocular route) and meningitis (intrathecal route).
- **Tobramycin** is used by inhalational route for the treatment of ***Pseudomonas*** associated with cystic fibrosis and as eye drops for ocular infection. It has a spectrum similar to gentamicin except it is more effective against *Pseudomonas* and not effective against *Enterococcus faecium*.
- Netilmycin and amikacin have spectrum similar to gentamicin and used in case of resistance to gentamicin by enzymatic degradation.
- **Neomicin** is used by oral route for **gut sterilization** in patients of hepatic encephalopathy; the current drug of choice for same is **rifaximin**. It is also used for bladder irrigation and skin infections. Paromomycin is used by intravenous route for leishmaniasis and oral route for intestinal amebiasis.
- Streptomycin, amikacin, capreomycin and kanamycin are used as second line TB drugs.
- **Spectinomycin** is a structurally related drug to aminoglycosides, which act on 30S subunit and inhibits translocation. It is the **drug of choice for the treatment of resistant gonorrhea**.

Mnemonics

Antipseudomonal Drugs

C : Carbepenems
Colistin
Ciprofloxacin
Cephalosporins
1. 3rd gen: Ceftazidime, Cefoperazone
2. 4th gen: Cefepime, Cefpirome
3. 5th gen: Ceftobiprole, Ceftaroline

A : Aminoglycosides
P : Penicillins
1. Piperacillin
2. Azlocillin
3. Mezlocillin
4. Carbenicillin
5. Ticarcillin

Side Effects of Aminoglycosides

- **Nephrotoxicity:** Aminoglycosides get concentrated in and damage the proximal tubular cells of nephron and since these cells can regenerate, nephrotoxicity is **reversible**. Both nephrotoxicity and ototoxicity are seen usually after 5 days of starting the drug and more common in elderly and patients of renal failure. The most common finding is a raised serum creatinine level. To prevent nephrotoxicity aminoglycosides should be given as once a day dosing, as multiple dosing or continuous infusion is associated with more nephrotoxicity. **Neomycin** is the most nephrotoxic whereas **streptomycin** is the least nephrotoxic aminoglycoside.
- **Ototoxicity: Direct outer hair cell damage** causes irreversible high frequency hearing loss which is bilateral. Auditory toxicity is maximum with kanamycin, amikacin and neomycin whereas vestibular toxicity is maximum with streptomycin and gentamicin. Netilmicin is least ototoxic aminoglycoside. Thus, aminoglycosides should not be used with other ototoxic drugs like loop diuretics and cisplatin.

Mnemonics

Auditory Toxicity
K : Kanamycin
A : Amikacin
N : Neomycin

- **Neuromuscular toxicity:** Neuromuscular toxicity is caused by inhibition of N_M receptors and decrease in acetylcholine release. Neomycin causes maximum neuromuscular toxicity whereas it is least with tobramycin. Because of this side effect aminoglycosides can increase **effect of muscle relaxants** and worsen myasthenia gravis. The drug of choice for treatment of neuromuscular toxicity causing respiratory failure is **intravenous calcium**, however neostigmine can also be used.
- Accidental intraocular administration of gentamicin can cause **maculopathy** and blindness.

Resistance to Aminoglycosides

- **Enzymatic drug inactivation** is the most common mechanism of drug resistance, except for **amikacin** and **netilmicin**. However, *Enterococcus* produces enzyme that can inactivate all aminoglycosides except streptomycin. Hence, in case of gentamicin resistant enterococcus, streptomycin is used.
- Altered 30S ribosomal structure is specific for **streptomycin**.

Recent Advances

Plazomicin: It is an aminoglycoside recently approved for treatment of complicated UTI including pyelonephritis caused by gram-negative organisms in patients more than 18 years of age. It is resistant to enzymatic degradation and hence can be used in cases resistant to other aminoglycosides.

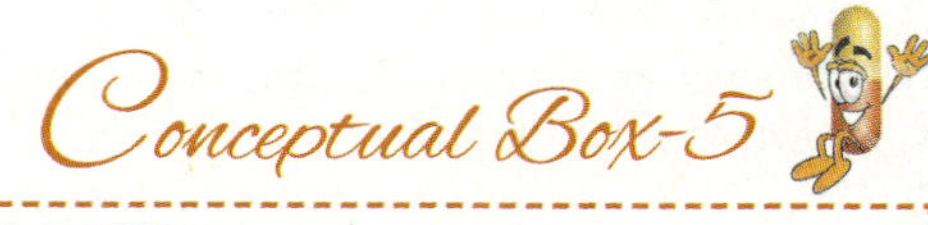

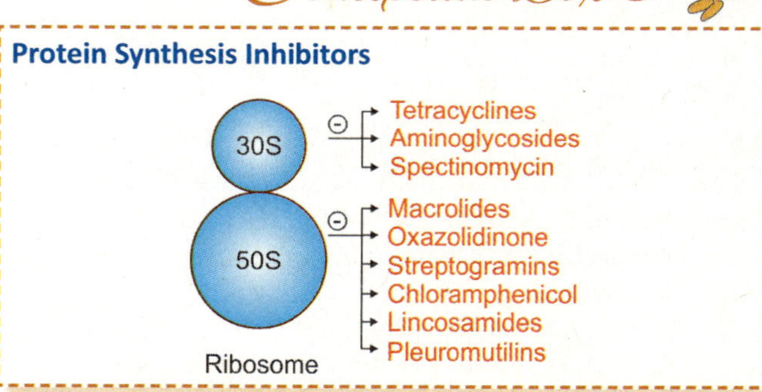

Macrolides

- Macrolides inhibit translocation of the t-RNA by acting on 50S subunit of ribosome. They are primarily bacteriostatic drugs but can be bactericidal at high doses.
- They are active against some gram-positives *(Streptococcus, Corynebacterium)*, gram-negatives (*Bordetella pertussis, Campylobacter, Bartonella* and *Mycobacterium*) and atypical organisms (Chlamydia, *Mycoplasma*, *Legionella*). Azithromycin and clarithromycin are more active against Mycobacterium as comparted to erythromycin. Spiramycin is specifically used intoxoplasmosis and is drug of choice in pregnancy.
- Resistance to macrolides can be seen by either **mutation of ribosome**, **drug efflux** and **enzymatic break down by esterases.**
- The binding site for macrolides, lincosamides and streptogramin B is same in 50S subunit of ribosome. Acquisition of erythromycin ribosome methylase (ERM) gene by bacteria can lead to methylase production, which methylates binding site in 50S ribosome and decreases binding of not only macrolides, but also lincosamides and $streptogramin_B$ (quinupristin). Hence, this mechanism is also known as **MLS_B type of resistance**.
- Macrolides decrease inflammatory mediators and have anti-inflammatory and immunomodulatory effect as well. Thus, low dose macrolide therapy is under trial for the treatment of chronic airway inflammatory disorders.
- Certain important aspects of pharmacokinetics and dosing of macrolides and ketolides is given below in the table.

Pharmacokinetics	Erythromycin	Azithromycin	Clarithromycin	Telithromycin
Oral bioavailability	↑ (Minimum)	↑	↑	↑ (Maximum)
Route	Oral/IV	Oral/IV	Oral	Oral
$T_{1/2}$	1.5 hours **(Shortest acting)**	68 hours **(Longest acting)**	6 hours	10 hours
Dosing	QID	OD	BD	OD

Erythromycin

- **Erythromycin** is the drug of choice for the treatment of **diphtheria and pertussis**. It is also drug of choice for prophylaxis of **rheumatic fever in penicillin allergic patients**. As it can stimulate **motilin receptors**, it is also used for the treatment of **gastroparesis and paralytic ileus**.
- Side effects associated are **cholestatic jaundice (estolate formulation), hypertrophic pyloric stenosis**, QT prolongation and diarrhea due to stimulation of motilin receptors.
- QT prolongation can be seen with all macrolides with order of **erythromycin > clarithromycin > azithromycin**.
- Erythromycin is an enzyme inhibitor and hence can cause drug interactions. It is a short-acting drug (T½ of 1.5 hours) and is broken down by gastric acid. Hence, it is given by intravenous route or oral route as enteric coated capsules four times a day (QID dosing).

Azithromycin

- Azithromycin is the drug of choice for treatment of **mycoplasma pneumoniae and genitalium, campylobacter, legionella and chancroid**. Overall it is the drug of choice for treatment of **atypical pneumonia** and commonly used for community acquired pneumonia.
- Azithromycin is also drug of choice for the treatment of **cholera and chlamydia in pregnancy,** as doxycycline is teratogenic.
- It can be substituted for clarithromycin in **MAC infection**.
- Azithromycin at a dose of 1 g (single dose) is combined along with ceftriaxone 250 mg is the current treatment of choice for gonorrhea due to growing resistance to monotherapy with ceftriaxone (drug of choice). In case of gonococcal and nongonococcal (mycoplasma and chlamydia) infection the same combination is preferred; alternatively, **2 grams of azithromycin** can also be used.
- Azithromycin is extensively distributed, sequestered in tissues and slowly released. Hence, it is the most active and **longest acting** macrolide. This is the reason why a single dose azithromycin of 1 or 2 grams is effective and it is used as OD dosing.

Clarithromycin

- Clarithromycin is used in the regimens for treatment of tuberculosis, nontuberculous mycobacteria (MAC and *M. kansasii*) and leprosy. It is also used in the regimen of *H. pylori*.
- It is longer acting than erythromycin and hence used as BD dosing by oral route.

Telithromycin

- Telithromycin is a ketolide with spectrum like macrolides but has **higher affinity for 50S subunit**. It is resistant to drug efflux and methylase mediated resistance as well. Hence, it is **effective in macrolide resistant cases** and used in community acquired pneumonia.
- It is less preferred due to hepatotoxicity, visual problems and neuromuscular blockade. Because of neuromuscular blockade it can **worsen myasthenia gravis** and hence contraindicated in such patients.
- It is long acting and hence used as OD dosing by oral route.

Recent Advances

Solithromycin is a new ketolide under trial for treatment if community acquired pneumonia.

Oxazolidinones

Oxazolidinediones bind to **50S subunit** and inhibit translocation. Resistance is seen due to **mutation of the binding site** on ribosome. It is a bacteriostatic drug but is bactericidal against *Streptococcus*.

Linezolid

- Spectrum is limited to gram-positive organisms**. Linezolid** is used for the treatment of **MRSA, VRSA and is drug of choice for VRE infections**. It is also used as a second line **TB** drug and for the treatment of nocardiosis.
- Its use is associated with bone marrow suppression that can cause thrombocytopenia, anemia and leucopenia. **Thrombocytopenia is most common side effect** and hence regular **platelet count monitoring** is advised. Mitochondrial toxicity can present as optic neuritis, peripheral neuropathy and lactic acidosis. This is the reason, it should be used only in resistant cases and it should not be given for long duration.
- It has nonspecific MAO inhibiting effect and hence can cause serotonin syndrome if used with drugs like SSRI, TCA, SNRI and MAO inhibitors.
- It is metabolized by nonenzymatic oxidation and has no effect on CYP-450 enzymes. It is a **good oral absorption (100% bioavailability)** and can be given by both oral and parenteral route by BD dosing.

Tedizolid

- **Tedizolid** is the latest drug in this class for the treatment of MRSA and VRSA infections. It causes lesser bone marrow suppression.
- It is longer acting than linezolid and hence given by OD dosing by oral or intravenous route.

Recent Advances

Sutezolid is another drug of this class currently under trial for the treatment of tuberculosis.

Streptogramins

- Streptogramins contains drugs like **quinupristin (streptogramin B)** and **dalfopristin (streptogramin A)**. Quinupristin binds to erythromycin binding site whereas dalfopristin binds nearby and facilitates quinupristin binding. Because of same site of binding for macrolides and quinupristin, there can be cross resistance due to altered binding site by methylase production in the MLS_B type of resistance.
- Quinupristin and dalfopristin are always given together at a ratio of 30:70 because of synergistic and bactericidal action.

- They are effective against **gram-positive cocci** *(Staphylococcus, Streptoccus, Enterococcus faecium)* and **atypical organisms** (mycoplasma, chlamydia, legionella) but not effective against gram-negatives.
- Streptogramins are used by parenteral route for treatment of **MRSA, VRSA and VRE (Only E. faecium) infections.**
- Most common side effects are injection site reactions like pain and phlebitis. These are enzyme inhibitors as well and hence can cause drug interactions.
- Route of elimination is primarily hepatic and hence **dose adjustment is required in liver diseases.**

Lincosamides

- **Clindamycin** also inhibits translocation by binding to P site of 50S subunit. It can be given by oral, parenteral and topical route. Spectrum covers gram-positive aerobes *(Staphylococcus, Streptococcus, Nocardia)* and anaerobes *(Actinomyces, Clostridium)*, gram-negative anaerobes *(Bacteroides, Prevotella)*. Clindamycin is not effective against gram-negative aerobes due to poor penetration through cell wall. It is also active against toxoplasma, plasmodium and pneumocyctis.
- Clindamycin is drug of choice for treatment of **supradiaphragmatic anaerobic infections** like anaerobic infection of the lung, pleural cavity and oral cavity (periodontal abscess). It can be used for treatment of infradiaphragmatic anaerobic infection (DOC is metronidazole) of abdomen and pelvis (PID and septic abortion).

Clinical Box-10

Treatment of Anaerobic Infections

Anaerobes
- Supradiaphragmatic (Prevotella) → Clindamycin
- Infradiaphragmatic (Bacteroides) → Metronidazole

- Clindamycin inhibits toxin synthesis in staphylococcus and streptococcus and hence is the **drug of choice for treatment of toxic shock syndrome (TSS)**; for complete antimicrobial coverage **vancomycin** is also added. For same reason it is also preferred in gas gangrene treatment as it can inhibit toxin synthesis by *C. perfringens*. It can also be used by topical route for treatment of bacterial vaginosis and acne. Clindamycin is used for treatment of osteomyelitis due to **excellent bone penetration** and good effect against staphylococcus.
- Side effects associated are **pseudomembranous enterocolitis**, neuromuscular blockade, Steven Johnson syndrome and thrombophlebitis. Because of neuromuscular block, they can potentiate effect of muscle relaxants.
- Resistance can be seen due to enzymatic inactivation, methylase production and ribosomal mutation like macrolides.

Fidaxomicin

- Fidaxomicin is a macrolide which inhibits RNA synthesis by blocking RNA polymerase. It is a bactericidal drug and active against clostridia species including Clostridium difficile.
- It has poor oral absorption and is FDA approved by oral route for treatment of **pseudomembranous enterocolitis**.

Chloramphenicol

- Chloramphenicol inhibits the **transpeptidation** reaction by acting on 50S subunit of ribosome.
- It is a **wide spectrum** drug with activity against both gram-positive and negative organisms, but use is limited by grave side effects like **bone marrow suppression and grey baby syndrome.**
- It is used as a reserved drug for treatment of **resistant meningitis** (***H. influenza, Meningococcus* and *Pneumococcus*) and severe rickettsial disease.** It can be used in **typhoid** but is less preferred due to availability of better drugs.
- Resistance can be seen due to decreased entry of drug and enzymatic inactivation.

Rifaximin

- Rifaximin is a rifamycin which acts by inhibiting RNA polymerase like rifampicin. It is a wide spectrum drug active against both gram-positive and negative organisms.
- It has a poor oral absorption and hence used for infections of the gut by oral route. It is used for gut sterilization in hepatic encephalopathy and for treatment of traveler's diarrhea, diarrhea of IBS and vancomycin resistant pseudomembranous enterocolitis.

Topical Antibiotics

Pleuromutilins

- Pleuromutilins also bind to the P site and inhibits translocation.
- **Retapamulin** is used as a topical antibiotic for skin infections.

Mupirocin

- Mupirocin acts by inhibiting **t-RNA synthase** and is active against gram-positives and some gram-negatives.
- Mupirocin is a topical antibiotic of choice for **staphylococcal nasal carriage** and impetigo infected with staphylococcus and streptococcus. It is the **topical drug of choice for MRSA.**

Fusidic Acid

- Fusidic acid inhibits protein synthesis by inhibition of the polypeptide elongation.
- It is used for treatment of bacterial skin infection caused by staphylococcus and streptococcus. It is also effective in MRSA.

DNA GYRASE INHIBITORS

- These drugs act by inhibiting **DNA gyrase** or topoisomerase II and topoisomerase IV. DNA gyrase is present in the **gram-negative** bacteria responsible for nicking of the torsional stress area in DNA. Persistence of this torsional stress leads to break down of DNA and hence these drugs give **cidal effect**.

- Resistance is seen due to mutation of topoisomerase II or IV, drug efflux and production of topoisomerase protective proteins. Resistance to any fluoroquinolone gives cross resistance to other drugs in this class.

Quinolones

Quinolones like **nalidixic acid** is active against gram-negatives, maximum concentrated in the urine and is used for treatment of **UTI** only.

Fluoroquinolones

- The fluoroquinolones are fluorinated quinolones with good activity against gram-negatives and moderate activity against gram-positives.
- Some important pharmacokinetic parameters of fluoroquinolones are given in the table below:

Pharmacokinetics	Maximum	Minimum
Bioavailability	Levofloxacin	Norfloxacin
Plasma protein binding	Gemifloxacin	Norfloxacin
T½	Sparfloxacin > Moxifloxacin	Ciprofloxacin < Norfloxacin

- Most of the fluoroquinolones are excreted by kidney except **pefloxacin** and **moxifloxacin** and hence these are **contraindicated in liver failure and are safe in renal failure**. Since they are not excreted by kidney, their concentration is urine is low and are not effective for treatment of UTI.
- Fluoroquinolones can be given by oral, intravenous and topical route. Moxifloxacin, gemifloxacin, prulifloxacin and levofloxacin being long-acting are given once a day, whereas others are given twice a day.

Oral	Oral/IV	Topical (eye drops)
Gemifloxacin Norfloxacin Prulifloxacin	Ciprofloxacin Ofloxacin Pefloxacin Levofloxacin Moxifloxacin	Gatifloxacin Levofloxacin Moxifloxacin

Uses of Fluoroquinolones

- Fluoroquinolones are well concentrated in urine, prostate, bone, soft tissue and lungs. Hence, these are commonly used for treatment of UTI, prostatitis, osteomyelitis, diabetic foot infection and pneumonia.
- **Ciprofloxacin** is the most active fluoroquinolone and is drug of choice for **anthrax, traveler's diarrhea, pyelonephritis, prophylaxis of contacts and mass chemoprophylaxis in meningococcal meningitis and carriers of typhoid**. In case of **acute diarrhea** ciprofloxacin is drug of choice and **used only if patient is febrile**; otherwise rehydration is sufficient in form of **ORS or IV fluids**. Ciprofloxacin however is not effective against Burkholderia cepacia.

Mnemonics

Uses of Ciprofloxacin

C : Contacts of meningococcal meningitis, Carriers of typhoid
A : Anthrax
P : Pyelonephritis
T : Traveler's diarrhea
A : Acute diarrhea
IN : INeffective in Burkholderia cepacia

- Ciprofloxacin is most active against pseudomonas, whereas moxifloxacin is most active against anaerobes (used in abdominal anaerobic infections). Levofloxacin and ciprofloxacin are the only fluoroquinolones used in pseudomonas, anthrax and plague.
- **Norfloxacin** is the least active fluoroquinolone and is used for treatment of **UTI, traveler's diarrhea and prostatitis.** Because of its low tissue distribution, it is not effective in systemic infections.
- **Levofloxacin, gemifloxacin, gatifloxacin and moxifloxacin** are active against gram-positive organism like *pneumococcus*, gram-negative organism like *klebsiella* and atypical organisms like chlamydia, mycoplasma and *legionella*. This interesting spectrum covers almost all respiratory pathogens and hence these drugs are **first line drugs for empirical treatment of pneumonia** and are also known as **respiratory quinolones**.
- Moxifloxacin, ofloxacin and ciprofloxacin are used as second line drugs for treatment of tuberculosis. Ofloxacin is used for treatment of resistant leprosy, however the most effective fluoroquinolone for leprosy is moxifloxacin.
- **Pefloxacin** is the most lipid soluble fluoroquinolone and hence **crosses blood brain barrier maximum** and is preferred for treatment of meningitis.
- Fluoroquinolones can be used as second line drugs for sexually transmitted diseases as mentioned below:

Gonorrhea	Gemifloxacin + azithromycin (Gemifloxacin can be used in place of ceftriaxone)
Chlamydia	Levofloxacin Ofloxacin
Chancroid	Ciprofloxacin

- Gatifloxacin, levofloxacin and moxifloxacin eye drops are used for the treatment of bacterial conjunctivitis.

Recent Advances

- **Delafloxacin** is a new systemic fluoroquinolone recently approved for treatment of acute bacterial skin and skin structure infections (ABSSSI) caused by both gram-positive and negative organisms.
- **Ozenoxacin** is a topical fluoroquinolone approved recently for treatment of impetigo caused by *Staphylococcus aureus* and *Streptococcus pyogenes*.

Side Effects of Fluoroquinolones

- Fluoroquinolones can noncompetitively inhibit GABA and hence cause **neurotoxicity** which manifests as peripheral neuropathy, hallucinations, delirium and seizures. NSAIDs are also noncompetitive inhibitors of GABA and hence worsen neurotoxicity. Theophylline by antagonizing adenosine receptors in brain can worsen neurotoxicity like seizure.
- **Nausea and vomiting** is the most common side effect. **Pseudomembranous enterocolitis** can be seen and is maximum with **ciprofloxacin**.
- **Cartilage defect** in joints can cause arthropathy; hence is **contraindicated in children and pregnancy. Tendinitis** is a side effect that is common in elderly and is aggravated by steroids.
- **QT prolongation** is maximum with **sparfloxacin > moxifloxacin** followed by other drugs like lomefloxacin, levofloxacin, gemifloxacin and gatifloxacin. The risk of QT Prolongation is least with **ciprofloxacin.**
- **Photosensitivity** is also maximum with sparfloxacin followed by lomefloxacin and pefloxacin. Most side effects of fluoroquinolones can be remembered as the "PQRST" waves of ECG.

Mnemonics

Side Effects of Fluoroquinolones

P : Photosensitivity, Pseudomembranous enterocolitis
Q : QT prolongation
R : Rash
S : Seizure
T : Tendinitis

- Many fluoroquinolones have been banned due to grave side effects mentioned below:

Fluoroquinolones Banned	Cause
Gatifloxacin	Both hypo and hyperglycemia
Sparfloxacin and lomefloxacin	QT prolongation and photosensitivity
Trovafloxacin	Hepatotoxicity
Grepafloxacin	Cardiotoxicity
Clinafloxacin	Photosensitivity
Temafloxacin	Autoimmune hemolytic anemia

ANTIFOLATE ANTIBIOTICS

Folic Acid Synthesis and Activation

- Folic acid synthesis begins with joining of PABA and pteridine to form dihydropteroic acid (DHPA) with the help of enzyme dihydropteroate synthase (DHPS). After this glutamate is incorporated to synthesize dihydrofolic acid (DHFA). DHFA is activated into tetrahydrofolate (THF) by dihydrofolic acid reductase (DHFR).
- **Sulfonamides** are PABA analogs which cause **competitive reversible inhibition of dihydropteroate synthase (DHPS).** Resistance to sulfonamides can be seen due to increased production or changed structure of PABA.
- DHPS is also inhibited by PAS and dapsone. DHFR is inhibited by pyrimethamine, proguanil, methotrexate and trimethoprim.

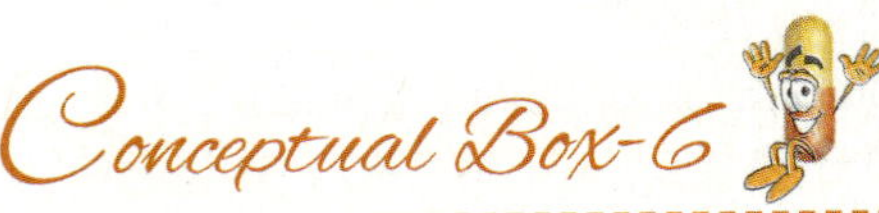

Antifolate Drugs

Mnemonic: First do schooling in delhi public school (DPS) and then appear for PMT to be a doctor

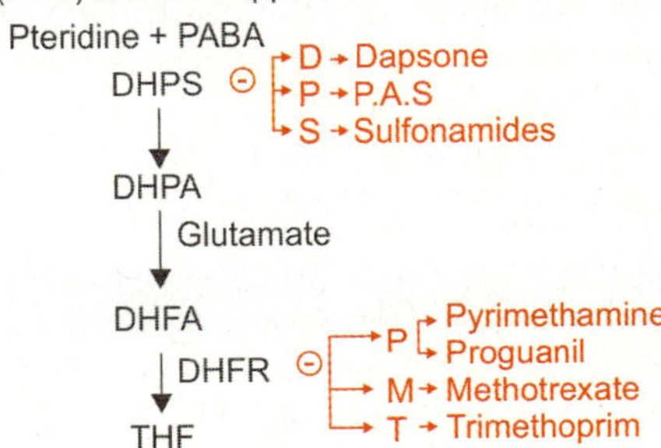

Note: DHPS= Dihydropteroate synthase
DHPA = Dihydropteroic acid
DHFA = Dihydrofolic acid
DHFR = Dihydrofolic acid reductase
THF = Tetrahydrofolate

- Inhibition of one enzyme causes bacteriostatic effect, whereas sequential inhibition of both enzymes causes bactericidal effect. Thus, sulfonamides are bacteriostatic, but if combined with DHFR inhibitors like pyrimethamine or trimethoprim, it becomes bactericidal.
- DHFR inhibitors can cause folic acid deficiency in human body and cause side effects like megaloblastic anemia and teratogenicity like neural tube defects. Hence, all these DHFR inhibitors are contraindicated in pregnancy and folic acid deficiency states like cirrhosis of liver.

Sulfonamides

Sulfonamides have good activity against gram-positives and negatives **(except pseudomonas and enterococcus)** but not active against anaerobes. They are not active against rickettsia, rather growth of rickettsia increases in presence of sulfonamides.

Uses

- **Sulfamethoxazole** is combined with trimethoprim to gain bactericidal effect. The combination is known as cotrimoxazole and is discussed ahead.
- **Sulfadoxine** is the longest acting sulfonamide. **Sulfadoxine along with pyrimethamine** and **artesunate**, together known as artesunate combination therapy (ACT) is used for treatment of **chloroquine resistant malaria**.
- **Sulfadiazine along with pyrimethamine** is the treatment of choice for treatment of **toxoplasmosis**. Since antifolate drugs

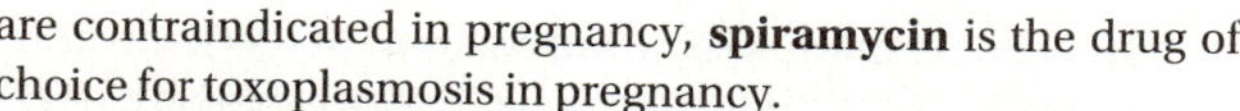

are contraindicated in pregnancy, **spiramycin** is the drug of choice for toxoplasmosis in pregnancy.

- **Sulfisoxazole** has the most rapid oral absorption and is most water soluble sulphonamide. Hence, it causes least crystalluria and nephrotoxicity. It is used for treatment of lower urinary tract infection and otitis media.
- **Sulfasalazine** has poor oral absorption and is used for treatment of **ulcerative colitis**. Its active component for anti-inflammatory activity is **5-ASA**.
- **Silver sulfadiazine, sulfacetamide and mafenide** are used as topical antibiotics. **Sulfadiazine** > **mafenide** is the topical drug of choice to prevent infection in burn patients and as it has antifungal effect, is used in **fungal keratomycosis**. Sulfacetamide solution is used by ocular route for treatment of bacterial conjunctivitis and trachoma. Mafenide is most toxic of the three and hence not preferred. Side effects associated with mafenide are allergy, pain on application and **metabolic acidosis** (inhibits carbonic anhydrase).

Side Effects of Sulfonamides

- Sulfonamides and drugs with sulfonamide group like diuretics (carbonic anhydrase inhibitors, loop diuretics except ethacrynic acid, thiazides), sulfonylureas and diazoxide can cause hypersensitivity characterized by rash, Steven Johnson syndrome and bone marrow suppression.
- Crystalluria seen with these drugs can be prevented by bicarbonate, which alkalinizes urine and increases solubility of sulfonamides.
- Other side effects are given in the mnemonic box below:

Mnemonics

Side Effects of Sulfonamides

B : Bone marrow suppression
I : Insoluble in urine (Crystalluria)
K : Kernicterus in newborns
A : AIP, Agranulocytosis
S : SJS, Rash
H : Hemoglobin (Met), Hemolysis in G6PD deficiency

Trimethoprim

As described in the conceptual box above, trimethoprim is a bacteriostatic drug which acts by inhibiting DHFR. It has a spectrum like sulfonamides but is significantly more potent and hence requires lesser dose than sulfonamides. As a single drug its use is limited to treatment of **UTI**, however along with sulfamethoxazole it is used for a wide range of infections. Side effects seen with trimethoprim are **megaloblastic anemia** (inhibits DHFR) and **hyperkalemia** (inhibits ENaC in collecting duct). It is contraindicated in pregnancy as it can cause neural tube defect.

Cotrimoxazole

- Cotrimoxazole is combination of **trimethoprim and sulfamethoxazole** in a ratio of **1:5**, however in plasma the ratio becomes 1:20 due to high distribution of trimethoprim. Since trimethoprim is 20 times more potent than sulfamethoxazole this ratio of 1:20 is desirable in plasma.
- Due to sequential blockade of DHPS and DHFR, cotrimoxazole produces a bactericidal effect. The spectrum is like sulfonamides and cotrimoxazole is considered drug of choice in many conditions.
- **Cotrimoxazole** is the drug of choice for treatment of **prostatitis, pneumocystis, nocardiosis, burkholderia cepacia, isosporiasis, cyclosporiasis, sarcocystosis and cystitis**. It is also effective in **carriers of typhoid** and treatment of **prostatitis, MRSA**. It can be given by oral and intravenous route (serious infections).

Mnemonics

Cotrimoxazole is DOC for

P : Pneumocystis, Prostatitis
I : Isosporiasis
C : Cyclosporiasis, Cystitis
NI : Nocardlosis
C : Cepacia burkholderia
S : Sarcocystosis

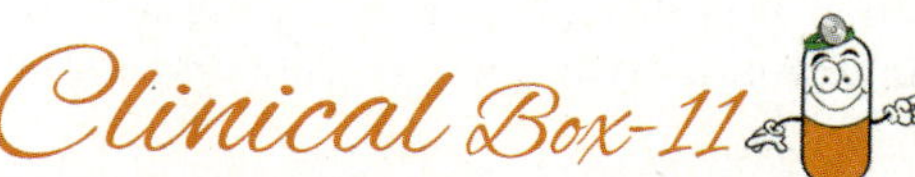

Drugs used in Prophylaxis of Pneumocystis in HIV (In Descending Order of Preference)

- **Cotrimoxazole**
- Dapsone
- Atovaquone
- Pentamidine

URINARY ANTISEPTIC AGENTS

Urinary antiseptic agents are antibiotics which have excellent concentration in urine but poor concentration in tissues. Hence, these are primarily used for treatment of lower UTI and should never be used in prostatitis or pyelonephritis.

Methenamine

- Methenamine is metabolized into **formaldehyde** and **ammonia** in acidic urine and hence it is formulated with mandelic acid (Methenamine Mandelate) or hippuric acid (Methanamine hippurate). A urine pH of less than 5 is crucial for this metabolism. Hence, to make the urine further acidic, ascorbic acid or ammonium chloride can also be given to the patient.
- The active component of methenamine is formaldehyde, which has bactericidal effect on gram-negative organisms. It can be used for **prophylaxis of UTI** and not for the treatment of an acute attack of UTI.
- Proteus makes the urine pH basic and hence methenamine is not effective in UTI caused by proteus.

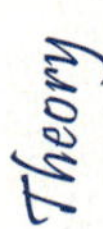

- It is usually free from side effects except GIT upset. It is contraindicated in patients of cirrhosis (ammonia produced in metabolism), renal failure (mandelic and hippuric acid retention and toxicity) and along with sulfonamides (sulfonamides bind to and inactivate formaldehyde).

Nitrofurantoin

- Nitrofurantoin is metabolized by the bacterial reductase into reactive metabolites that interfere with synthesis of neucleic acids and protein. It is bactericidal against most gram-positive and negative organisms (except pseudomonas and proteus).
- It can be used for treatment of uncomplicated lower UTI and asymptomatic bacteriuria.
- Most common side effect is GIT upset (nausea, vomiting, diarrhea) followed by others like hemolysis in G6PD deficiency, neuropathy, pneumonitis and pulmonary fibrosis. It is absolutely contraindicated in renal failure, pregnancy and neonates.

Miscellaneous Drugs

There are other antibiotics like fosfomycin and nalidixic acid which are well concentrated in urine and used only for UTI. Both these drugs have been discussed in detail in cell wall synthesis inhibitors and DNA gyrase inhibitors sections respectively.

ANTIMYCOBACTERIAL DRUGS

The pathogenic mycobacterium that need to be target are *mycobacterium tuberculosis, mycobacterium leprae* and *mycobacterium avium* complex.

MYCOBACTERIUM TUBERCULOSIS

Mycobacterium is an acid fast bacillus, with a thick cell wall made up of **mycolic acid** linked to **arabinogalactan and peptidoglycan.** This thick layer makes it difficult for antibiotics to enter. Mycobacterium can be slow and rapid replicators; the specific first line drugs like isoniazid rifampicin, pyrazinamide and ethambutol are effective against both slow and rapid replicators, whereas the second line drugs are more effective in rapid replicators.

First Line Drugs

Isoniazid

Isoniazid is metabolized by liver and excreted by kidney.

Mechanism of Action and Resistance

- Isoniazid (INH) passively diffuses in the *mycobacterium*. INH is a prodrug activated by **mycobacterial catalase peroxidase (Kat G)** and the activated INH inhibits two enzymes, i.e. **acyl protein carrier reductase (Inh A) and acyl protein carrier kinase (Kas A),** required for mycolic acid synthesis.
- Thus, by **inhibiting mycolic acid synthesis** INH produces **bactericidal** effect.
- Resistance can be seen due to mutation of Kat G gene and Kas A gene or overexpression of Inh A gene.
- **Kat G gene mutation** is the **most common** mechanism and is responsible for the most severe **form of resistance**. It might be associated with **ethambutol resistance**.
- **Inh A gene over expression** increases production of acyl protein carrier reductase (Inh A), which is a target for a second line drug ethionamide. Hence, this mechanism leads to **cross resistance to ethionamide**.
- Inh A gene over expression and Kas A gene mutation leads to low level of resistance.

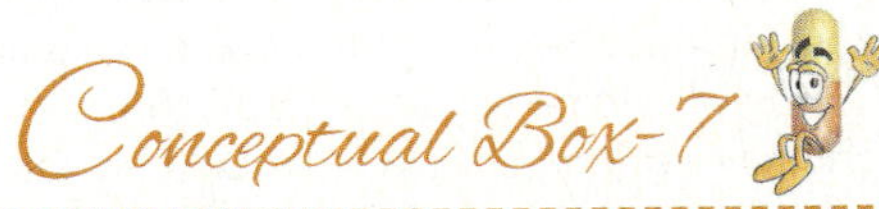

Mechanism of Action and Resistance to Isoniazid

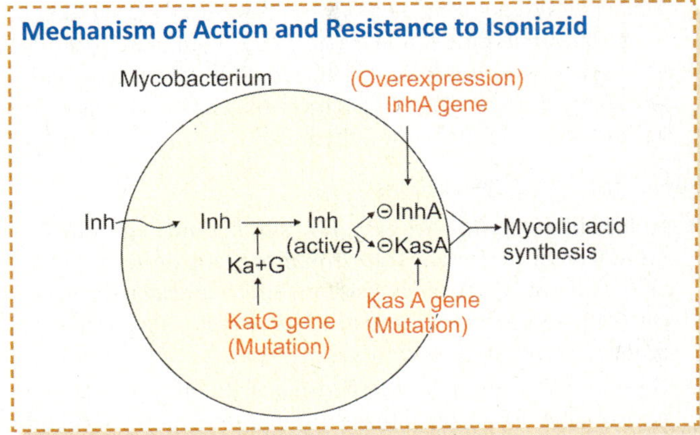

Uses of INH

- INH is a first line drug for TB and is **drug of choice for treatment of LTBI (latent tubercular infection) and prophylaxis of TB**.
- It is a **bactericidal drug against both intra and extracellular fast growing** mycobacterium however has static effect on slow growers.
- Among the first line drugs it is the drug that **makes the patient non infective earliest**.
- It is not effective against *mycobacterium avium* complex.

Side Effects of INH

- **Isoniazid maximum crosses blood brain barrier** and is associated with **neuropsychiatric symptoms like memory loss, euphoria, hallucinations** etc. can be seen with **psychosis.** Isoniazid **inhibits pyridoxine phosphokinase** required to convert pyridoxine to pyridoxal 5 phosphate; isoniazid also **directly inhibits pyridoxal 5 phosphate**. Since pyridoxal 5 phosphate is required for GABA synthesis, isoniazid thus inhibits synthesis of inhibitory neurotransmitter GABA.
- In slow acetylators **peripheral neuropathy** is more common, whereas in fast acetylators **hepatotoxicity** is more common. **Rifampicin** can **increase hepatotoxicity** of isoniazid by enzyme induction and increase in production of hepatotoxic metabolite **acetyl hydrazine**.
- Isoniazid can inhibit delta-amino levulinate synthase, which leads to decrease in haem synthesis and **sideroblastic anemia. Pyridoxine** being a cofactor for the enzyme can be used for treatment.

- **Pyridoxine replacement** can improve symptoms of peripheral neuropathy, neuropsychiatric side effects and anemia as well. The dose of pyridoxine is 10–20 mg daily in adults and 5 mg day in infants.
- Arthritis involving the upper limb known as **shoulder hand syndrome** can be seen.
- Patients with isoniazid toxicity present with drug refractory seizures, metabolic acidosis and coma. Intravenous pyridoxine is the drug of choice for treatment; dose of pyridoxine is 1 g for each gm of isoniazid and the maximum dose is 5 g. Antiepileptics like benzodiazepines and barbiturates are effective for seizure but conventional drugs like phenytoin are not effective.

Mnemonics

Side Effects of INH

- **C** : Change in memory
- **H** : Hepatotoxic, Hallucinations
- **A** : Anemia, Arthritis
- **N** : Neuropathy
- **G** : Gynaecomastia
- **E** : Euphoria, Epilepsy

Rifampicin

- Rifampicin is rifamycin derived from **Streptomyces mediterranei**.
- It is metabolized and **primarily excreted by liver**; only 30% is excreted by kidney and hence is the **safest first line drug in renal failure**.
- The semisynthetic derivatives of rifamycin are rifapentine and rifabutin which can be used in place of rifampicin.
- Rifabutin (45 hours) has the longest half-life followed by rifapentine (13 hours) and rifampicin (2-5 hours). However, **rifapentine is the longest acting** rifamycin owing to its high lipid solubility and tissue distribution and hence can be used **once weekly** for prophylaxis of LTBI.
- The order of effectiveness against intracellular mycobacterium is rifapentine > rifabutin > rifampicin and on extracellular is just opposite. The order of enzyme induction is rifampicin > rifapentine > rifabutin.
- Food decreases rifampicin absorption, increases rifapentine absorption (fatty food) and has no effect on absorption of rifabutin. Hence, rifabutin and rifapentine are taken with food and rifampicin is taken on empty stomach.
- Rifabutin is more effective than rifampicin against microorganisms like MAC. It can cause **anterior uveitis (iridocyclitis), polymyalgia** and yellow skin discolouration known as **pseudojaundice**.
- Rifaximin is the drug of choice for gut sterilization in hepatic encephalopathy and is also used for treatment of traveller's diarrhea.

Recent Advances

Rifamycin: It is a drug named on the class rifamycin, has been recently approved for treatment of traveller's diarrhea.

Mechanism of Action and Resistance

- Rifampicin inhibits **RNA polymerase** and has bactericidal effect against both intra and extracellular organisms. Rifampicin is the **most bactericidal drug with maximum sterilizing effect as well**. It is the only bactericidal drug **effective against dormant bacilli (persisters)** usually present in the caseous lesions.
- Resistance can be seen due to **mutation of beta subunit RNA polymerase (rpo B) gene**.

Uses of Rifampicin

- Rifampicin is the most important first line drug for treatment of tuberculosis as well as leprosy. It has a good spectrum against both gram-positives and negatives.
- It is also effective for prophylaxis in contacts of **meningococcal meningitis, H. influenza meningitis and staphylococcal infections**.

Side Effects of Rifampicin

- Most common side effect is **nausea and vomiting followed by rash**, fever etc. Rash caused by anti TB drugs are **non-petechial rash**.
- At intermittent doses it can cause **flu like symptoms**, respiratory syndrome (shortness of breath), cutaneous reactions (flushing and itching), thrombocytopenic purpura and abdominal reactions (pain and nausea).
- In case of **thrombocytopenic purpura and respiratory syndrome** rifampicin is never restarted. For other side effects it can be restarted but only after 3 weeks of stoppage to avoid hypersensitivity.
- **Reddish orange discolouration** of urine, saliva, contact lenses, tears etc. can be seen and is also known as "Red man syndrome".
- All bone marrow lineage might decrease causing **thrombocytopenia**, anaemia and leucopenia.

Drug Interactions of Rifampicin

- Rifampicin being an enzyme inducer can cause OCP failure, warfarin failure and failure of antiretroviral drugs of **protease inhibitor and NNRTI group (except efavirenz and etravirine)**.
- Hence in a patient of HIV on protease inhibitors and having TB, rifampicin should be changed to rifabutin. In case rifabutin is not available dose of protease inhibitors should be doubled for the duration of TB treatment. In case patient is on nevirapine and rifampicin, nevirapine should be changed to efavirenz.
- PAS decreases absorption of rifampicin and hence these drugs should not be taken together.

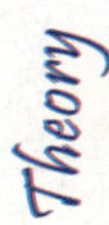

Mnemonics

Rifampicin Important Points

R : RNA Polymerase Inhibitor, Reddish orange discoloration
I : Interstitial nephritis
F : Flu like symptoms
A : Anaemia
M : Maximum cidal and sterilizing effect
P : Platelet count decreases
I : Inducer of enzyme
C : Contraceptive failure
I : INR deranged with warfarin
N : NNRTI and PI failure

Pyrazinamide

- Pyrazinamide is a nicotinamide analog.
- It is metabolized by liver and excreted by kidney.

Mechanism of Action and Resistance

- Pyrazinamide is a prodrug that is activated by mycobacterial pyrazinamidase into pyrazinoic acid, which inhibits **fatty acid synthase I** and this inhibits **mycolic acid synthesis.**
- Pyrazinamide is active in acidic environment present inside the **phagocytes** and **granulomas** and hence is effective **against intracellular, slow growing organisms**.
- It is a bactericidal drug and augments the sterilizing effect of rifampicin and hence used in short course chemotherapy regimen along with rifampicin.
- Resistance is seen due to mutation in pyrazinamidase gene (pncA) which makes pyrazinamidase that does not activate pyrazinamide.

Uses of Pyrazinamide

Pyrazinamide is effective only against *mycobacterium tuberculosis* and is combined with other first line drugs or treatment of tuberculosis. It is well concentrated in CSF and hence preferred in tubercular meningitis.

Side Effects

- Pyrazinamide is **most hepatotoxic** of all first line drugs. Its toxic metabolites are excreted by kidney and hence dose reduction is required in renal failure. The order of hepatotoxicity of first line drugs is **pyrazinamide** > **isoniazid** > **rifampicin**.
- It can also cause asymptomatic hyperuricemia and **arthralgia**.

Ethambutol

- Only 20% of ethambutol is metabolized by alcohol dehydrogenase, whereas **80% is excreted unchanged by kidney.**
- Hence it is the **most unsafe drug in renal failure** among first line drugs.

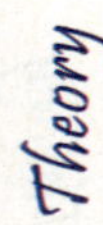

Mechanism of Action and Resistance

- Arabinosyltransferase in mycobacterium synthesizes arabinogalactan and lipoarabinomannan, which are integral component of cell wall.
- **Ethambutol inhibits cell wall synthesis by inhibiting arabinosyltransferase**.
- Resistance can be seen by mutation in arabinosyltransferase (embB) gene.

Uses of Ethambutol

- Ethambutol is a **static drug** effective against only extracellular mycobacterium. It is the **least potent** drug of all in first line.
- It is used for treatment of TB in continuous phase, MAC and *Mycobacterium kansasii* infection.

Side Effects of Ethambutol

- Ethambutol can cause **optic neuritis** and **red-green colour blindness (green > red)**. That is why it is **avoided in children. Vitamin B-12** supplementation might decrease severity of ocular toxicity.
- Other side effects like hyperuricemia (lesser than pyrazinamide) can also be seen.
- As ethambutol is excreted by kidney, its dose should be decreased in renal failure.

Second Line Drugs

- The second line drugs are reserved for treatment of drug resistant tuberculosis.
- **Multi drug resistant (MDR) TB** is a case of TB that is resistant to both **isoniazid and rifampicin.**
- **Extremely drug resistant (XDR) TB** is a case of **MDR** with additional resistance to a **fluoroquinolone** and to at least one of the **injectable second line drugs like amikacin, kanamycin or capreomycin.**

Ethionamide

- Ethionamide inhibits acyl protein carrier reductase (Inh A) and hence inhibits **mycolic acid synthesis.** It is effective against both intra and extracellular mycobacterium.
- Because of same reason Inh A gene over expression confers **cross resistance of isoniazid to ethionamide.**
- It is used for treatment of resistant tuberculosis and associated with side effects like **hypothyroidism**, nausea and vomiting (most common), neurologic symptoms, postural hypotension, eye toxicity (diplopia, blurring of vision) hepatitis, impotence and gynecomastia.

Mnemonics

Side Effects of Ethionamide

E : Elevated ALT/AST
T : Taste change (metallic)
H : Hypothyroidism
I : Impotence
O : Ocular toxicity
N : Nausea and vomiting

Thioacetazone

- Thioacetazone is a bacteriostatic prodrug activated by monooxygenase encoded by EthA gene; since this enzyme also activates ethionamide, mutation of this gene can cause cross resistance. The mechanism of activated thioacetazone is not completely understood but according to available data it seems to inhibit mycolic acid synthesis.

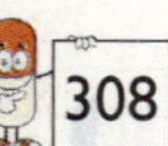

- It is associated with side effects like Steven Johnson's syndrome (hence contraindicated in HIV), blurred vision, agranulocytosis and hemolytic anemia.

Para Aminosalicylic Acid (PAS)

- PAS inhibits folic acid synthesis and is a bacteriostatic drug.
- It is associated with side effects like GIT disturbances, hepatotoxicity, hypokalemia and hypothyroidism.

Bedaquiline

Bedaquiline is a diarylquinoline which acts by inhibiting mycobacterial **ATP synthase**. It is a strong bactericidal and sterilizing drug that dramatically affects time to culture conversion in patients with MDR TB. It has been approved by FDA for treatment of MDR TB along with other drugs in 2012. In India it has been incorporated into the RNTCP.

Pharmacokinetics

- It has good oral absorption (oral route) and since **food increases absorption**, it should be taken with food.
- It is highly distributed into tissues (except CNS) as it is amphiphilic in nature and binds to tissue phospholipids following which it is slowly released and hence has an extended long half-life of 165 days (5.5 months). The plasma half-life though is 24 hours. It is given at intermittent doses 200 mg three times a week followed by a two weeks of loading phase of 400 mg to avoid accumulation of drug in plasma and tissue.
- It has a high plasma protein binding.
- 75% of Bedaquiline is excreted unchanged by liver, whereas 25% is metabolized in liver by CYP3A4 into active metabolites M2 and M3 which are less active than Bedaquiline.
- It has a concentration-time dependent killing and the AUC decides its efficacy.

Contraindications

- Bedaquiline can cause QT prolongation and hence is contraindicated in patients having prolonged QT interval (>450 ms), cardiac arrhythmia and along with other drugs that can prolong QT. It is also contraindicated in patients with high risk of torsades like CHF, hypokalemia and family history of long QT syndrome.
- It is contraindicated in age group less than 18 years of age.
- It is also contraindicated in pregnancy and the female should be on non-hormonal contraceptives or has passed 2 years of post-menopausal period during drug therapy.

Delamanid

- Delamanid is a nitroimidazole, which primarily acts by inhibiting mycolic acid synthesis (methoxy and keto mycolic acid); isoniazid inhibits synthesis of alpha mycolic acid. During the course of its metabolism nitric oxide is released, which is toxic to the mycobacterium. By inhibiting mycolic acid, it inhibits cell wall synthesis and hence is a **bactericidal** drug. Its sterilizing/bactericidal effect is as good as rifampicin.
- It is a prodrug activated by mycobacterial F420 coenzyme system. It has a **high plasma protein binding (>99%)** and is primarily **metabolized by plasma albumin** into secondary metabolites. The secondary metabolites are metabolized by CYP3A4. Half-life is approximately **36 hours**. It is not excreted by kidney.
- In India it is currently available in 7 states under conditional access program of RNTCP for treatment of MDR and XDR TB. The age group for which it is currently indicated in India is ≥18 years of age. Though it is safe in patients >6 years of age according to WHO and with due course of time the same age condition will be updated by RNTCP as well.
- It can cause QT prolongation and hence is contraindicated in patients with **long QT interval (>500 ms)**, **cardiac arrhythmia** and **with any other drug that can cause QT prolongation**. It is also contraindicated in patients with high risk of torsades like CHF, hypokalemia, hypocalcemia, hypomagnesemia and family history of long QT syndrome. It is also contraindicated in patients with **hypoalbuminemia** (albumin <2.8 g/dL) as there is increased risk of toxicity, because it is metabolized by albumin. Thus, plasma calcium, magnesium, potassium and albumin level must be checked before starting delamanid.
- It is also contraindicated in **pregnant females** and **patients less than 6 years** of age. It is contraindicated with milk, as calcium inhibits its absorption.
- The tablet to delamanid contains lactose and hence can be problematic in patients with hereditary galactose intolerance.

Bedaquiline Vs Delamanid

- **Mycobacterium with Rv0678 mutations can cause resistance to both clofazimine and bedaquiline by drug efflux.** Hence, if patient had prior exposure to clofazimine, then delamanid is preferred.
- Anti-HIV drugs like NNRTI and protease inhibitors have lesser interaction with delamanid. Hence, in case of TB with HIV, delamanid is preferred.
- Delamanid can cause hypoalbuminemia and hence in case of TB with hypoalbuminemia, bedaquiline is preferred.

Other Drugs

Other second line drugs used in tuberculosis are given in the mnemonic box given below.

Mnemonics

Second Line Antitubercular Drugs

Two : Thioacetazone
P : PAS, Prothionamide
E : Ethionamide
A : Amikacin
C : Capreomycin, Cycloserine
O : Ofloxacin
C : Clofazimine, Clarithromycin
K : Kanamycin
S : Streptomycin
Making : Moxifloxacin, Meropenem
Blind : Bedaquiline
Love : Linezolid
On
Date : Delamanid

ADR of Anti-TB Drugs

Nausea/Vomiting	Eto, Pto, PAS, Z, E, Bdq	Advise to take drugs embedded in a banana or hight snack before drugs. Use antiemetics like metoclopramide or domperidone
Gastritis and abdominal pain	PAS, Eto, Pto, Cfz, FQs, H, E, and Z	Use H2 blockers or PPI but avoid antacids as they decrease absorption of FQ
Diarrhea and flatulence	PAS, Eto/Pto	Use loperamide in case of uncomplicated diarrhea, i.e. without blood in stool and no fever
Hepatitis	Z, H, R, Pto/Eto, PAS, FQ, Bdq	In cases where patient is very sick i.e., meningitis, sputum smear grade 3+, give ATT e. g. Streptomycin, FQ and Cs. Where patient is not seriously ill and one can wait, introduction of ATT can be done once enzyme levels are near normal
Bone marrow suppression	Lzd	Start Lzd at lower doses after it resolves, if Lzd is important to continue
Hypothyroidism	Eto/Pto, PAS	Take opinion of endocrinologist
Arthralgia	Z, FQ, Bdq	Use NSAIDs like paracetamol or indomethacin
Peripheral neuropathy	Cs, Lzd, H, S, K_m, Amk, Cm, FQ, rarely Pto/Eto, E	Lzd is most common cause; decrease dose of Lzd and use amitriptyline. Pyridoxine is routinely given; it does not prevent Lzd induced peripheral neuropathy
Headache	Bdq, Cs	Use NSAIDs like paracetamol or ibuprofen
Depression	Cs, FQ, H, Eto/Pto	Discontinue drug if regimen is not compromised or add antidepressants like TCA or SSRI
Psychosis	**Cs** > H > FQ	Use antipsychotics like haloperidol
Suicidal tendency	CS, H, Eto/Pto	Hold Cs, if does not resolve hold other drugs as well
Seizure	Cs, H, FQ	Stop all drugs and start antiepileptics. Restart drugs once seizure is resolved
Optic neuritis	E, Lzd, Eto/Pto, Cfz, Rifabutin, H, S	E and Lzd are most common cause; stop both and never restart
Metallic taste	Eto/Pto, FQs	Reversible after drug stoppage
QT prolongation	Bdq, Dlm, FQ, clarithromycin, Cfz	Patient found to have a QTc value greater than 500 ms, stop all suspected QT prolonging drugs
Gynecomastia	Eto/Pto	Reversible on drug stoppage
Alopecia	H, Eto/Pto	Ask patient to tolerate

RNTCP 2016 Guidelines

The short forms used for the drugs in regimens is given below:

Drugs	Short forms used
Rifampicin	R
Isoniazid	H
Pyrazinamide	Z
Ethambutol	E
Streptomycin	S
Kanamycin	Km
Amikacin	Am
Capreomycin	Cm
Ciprofloxacin	Cfx
Ofloxacin	Ofx
Levofloxacin	Lfx
Moxifloxacin	Mfx
Ethionamide	Eto
Cycloserine	Cs
Para aminosalicylic acid	PAS
Clofazimine	Cfz
Linezolid	Lzd
Amoxicillin/Clavulanic acid	Amx/Clv
Thioacetazone	Thz
Imipenam/cilastatin	Ipm/Cln
Clarithromycin	Clr
Prothionamide	Pto
Terizidone	Trd
Meropenem	Mpm
Bedaquiline	Bdq
Delamanid	Dlm

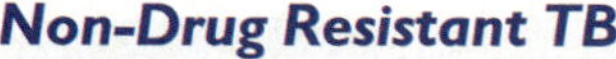

Non-Drug Resistant TB

In case there is no resistance at all to TB drugs an intensive phase (IP) of 2 months and continuous phase (CP) of 4 months is advised as given below:

Type of TB case	Treatment regimen in IP	Treatment regimen CP
New	(2) HRZE	(4) HRE
Previously treated	(2) HRZES + (1) HRZE	(5) HRE

Note: 2, 4 and 5 here represent months of treatment.

MDR TB and RR TB (Conventional Regimen)

In case of multiple drug resistant (MDR) and rifampicin resistance (RR) TB the intensive phase (IP) is of 6–9 months and continuous phase (CP) is of 18 months as given below:

Type of TB case	Treatment regimen in IP	Treatment regimen CP
Rifampicin resistant + Isoniazid sensitive or unknown Or MDR TB	(6–9) km Lfx Eto Cs Z E	(18) Lfx Eto Cs E

MDR TB and RR TB (Shorter Regimen)

A shorter regimen for MDR/RR TB has been advocated by WHO, which is associated with a better outcome, i.e. lesser treatment failure, relapse and death. It is indicated in patients with confirmed MDR/RR TB, who are sensitive to both fluoroquinolones and second line injectables (SLI). A combination of 7 drugs is given for 4-6 months of IP and 4 drugs for 5 months of CP. It is not used in pregnancy and extrapulmonary TB.

Type of TB case	Treatment regimen in IP	Treatment regimen CP
Rifampicin resisatant + Isoniazid sensitive/ unknown Or MDR TB	(4-6) Mfx Km Eto Cfz Z H E	(5) Mfx Cfz Z E

MDR TB and RR TB with Additional Resistance

In case of additional resistance in a patient of MDR or RR TB the following changes are to be made in the regimen as given below.

- In case of resistance to ethambutol it is to be omitted
- In case of resistance to pyrazinamide, it is to be omitted
- In case of resistance to both ethambutol and PZA, PAS to be added in IP and CP
- In case or resistance to levofloxacin or moxifloxacin, the sensitive one is to be used along with PAS and clofazimine.
- In case of resistance to both levofloxacin and moxifloxacin, these drugs are to be replaced with clofazimine, linezolid and PAS in IP CP. The duration of IP will be from 6 to 12 months.
- In case or resistance to any second line injectable (kanamycin or capreomycin), use one of the sensitive injectables.
- In case of resistance to all second line injectable, replace them with clofazimine, linezolid and PAS in IP and CP. The duration of IP will be from 6 to 12 months.

XDR TB

In case of extremely drug resistant tuberculosis (XDR) the intensive phase is for 6 – 12 months and continuous phase for 18 months as given below:

Type of TB case	Treatment regimen in IP	Treatment regimen CP
XDR	(6-12) Mfx Cm Eto Cs Z Lzd Cfz E	(18) Mfx Eto Cs Lzd Cfz E

Mono/Poly Drug Resistant TB

In case patient is resistant to one or more drugs but sensitive to rifampicin the following regimen is used.

Type of TB case	Treatment regimen in IP	Treatment regimen CP
Rifampicin sensitive INH Resistant TB and DST of SEZ not known	(3–6) km Lfz R E Z (modify treatment based on baseline DST report to E, Z, KM, CM, Lfx, Mfx)	(6) Lfx R E Z

MDR TB with Mixed Pattern of Resistance

- In mixed pattern resistance i.e. MDR/RR TB with FQ or SLI resistance the following regimens are to be used:

Type of TB case	Treatment regimen in IP	Treatment regimen CP
MDR/RR TB + resistance to FQ	(6-9) Mfx Km Eto Cs Z Lzd Cfz	(18) Mfx Eto Cs Lzd Cfz
MDR/RR TB + resistance to SLI	(6-9) Lfx Cm Eto Cs Z Lzd Cfz	(18) Lfx Eto Cs Lzd

- In mixed pattern resistance, i.e. MDR/RR TB + resistance to FQ/SLI + LZD or others then conventional XDR regimen or XDR regimen with new drugs (Bdq, Dlm) can be used with certain modifications as given below.

- If only Km resistant (at eis mutation), then add Cm in IP upfront in the regimen design.
- In patients with MDR/RR + FQ class resistance, XDR-TB and mixed pattern resistance where a new drug is not considered in the regimen for any reason, Mfx would be added upfront in the regimen design and the decision to continue or replace it would be taken based on LC-DST results to Mfx (2.0) by NDR-TBC; and
- Lzd to be replaced with a suitable drug if found to be resistant on LC-DST. In such situation the patient must be reclassified as mixed pattern DR-TB.

Bedaquiline Containing Regimens

- Bedaquiline is used in case second line drugs cannot be used due to resistance, intolerance, contraindications or unavailability of drugs. The Bedaquiline containing regimen for MDR and XDR TB are given below:

Resistance pattern	Treatment regimen in IP	Treatment regimen CP
Regimen with bedaquiline for MDR-TB + FQ/SLI resistance		
MDR/RR + resistance to all FQ	(6) Bdq + (6-9) Km Eto Cs Z Lzd Cfz	(18) Eto Cs Lzd Cfz
MDR/RR + resistance to all SLI	(6) Bdq + (6-9) Lfx Cm Eto Cs Z Lzd Cfz	(18) Lfx Eto Cs Lzd
Regimen with bedaquiline for XDR-TB		
XDR TB with resistance to both FQ and SLI	(6) Bdq + (6-12) Cm Eto Cs Z Lzd Cfz E	(18) Eto Cs Lzd Cfz E

- The patients which can be given bedaquiline are as follows:
  - MDR/RR-TB with resistance to all FQ
  - MDR/RR-TB with resistance to all SLI
  - XDR-TB with resistance to both FQ and SLI
  - Treatment failures of MDR-TB + FQ/SLI resistance
  - Treatment failures of XDR-TB
- The doses at which bedaquiline is prescribed is given below.
  - **Week 0–2:** BDQ 400 mg (4 tablets of 100 mg) daily (7 days per week) + OBR
  - **Week 3–24:** BDQ 200 mg (2 tablets of 100 mg) 3 times per week (with at least 48 hours between doses) for a total doses of 600 mg per week + OBR.
  - **Week 25 (start or month 7) to end of treatment:** Continue other second-line anti-TB drugs only as per RNTCP recommendations.

Delamanid Containing Regimens

- Bedaquiline is used in case second line drugs cannot be used due to resistance, intolerance, contraindications or unavailability of drugs. The Bedaquiline containing regimen for MDR and XDR TB is given below:

Resistance pattern	Treatment regimen in IP	Treatment regimen CP
Regimen with delamanid for MDR-TB + FQ/SLI resistance		
MDR/RR + resistance to all FQ	(6) Dlm + (6-9) Km Eto Cs Z Lzd Cfz	(18) Eto Cs Lzd Cfz
MDR/RR + resistance to all SLI	(6) Dlm + (6-9) Lfx Cm Eto Cs Z Lzd Cfz	(18) Lfx Eto Cs Lzd
Regimen with delamanid for XDR-TB		
XDR TB with resistance to both FQ and SLI	(6) Bdq + (6-12) Cm Eto Cs Z Lzd Cfz E	(18) Eto Cs Lzd Cfz E

- It is currently indicated in India in adults (≥18 yrs), including people living with HIV (PLHIV), not eligible for a shorter MDR-TB regimen for reasons of resistance, contraindication or tolerability like:
  - MDR/RR-TB with resistance to any/all FQ or any/all SLI
  - XDR-TB
  - Mixed Pattern DR-TB including patients who are failing any DR-TB regimen or have drug intolerance or contraindications or who return after interruption or emergence of any exclusion criteria for shorter MDR-TB regimen or with extensive or advanced disease and others deemed at higher baseline risk for poor outcomes.
- The dose of delamanid in adults is 100 mg BD every day for 6 months along with the optimized background regimen (OBR). After 6 months the OBR is continued for the rest of the period.

0-24 weeks	Delamanid 100 mg (two 50 mg tab.) BD + OBR
Week 25 till end	OBR

Treatment of TB in Special Conditions

TB in Pregnancy and Lactation

- All first line TB drugs can be safely used in pregnancy. However, pregnancy is discouraged during treatment of TB and female should be on contraceptives like barrier method (condoms/diaphragms), IUCD or depot-medroxyprogesterone. Oral contraceptives should be avoided as drugs like rifampicin can decrease their efficacy.
- During lactation breastfeeding should be continued along with anti-TB drugs in female and prophylactic isoniazid in the neonate for 6 months followed by BCG vaccination. The mother should be taught about hygiene measures like covering nose and mouth while coughing and sneezing to prevent infection via sputum droplets.
- Many of the second line drugs are not safe in pregnancy and hence management of drug resistant TB in pregnancy is complicated.
- In case the patient becomes pregnant with less than 20 weeks of gestation at time of diagnosis, she should be counselled for medical termination of pregnancy (MTP) to avoid risk to both mother and fetus.

- If she decides to continue pregnancy or in case TB is diagnosed in 20th week of gestation or more a modified regimen of TB is given as given in the table below:

Drug Resistant TB and Pregnancy

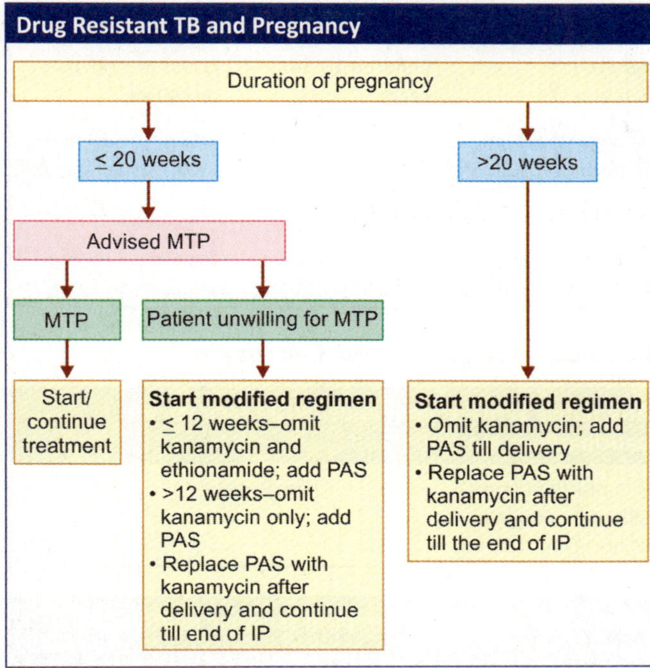

TB in Liver Disorders

- In case of nonresistant tuberculosis three regimens can be used in case the ALT/AST level is 3 times more than normal levels. The order of hepatotoxicity of first line drugs is pyrazinamide > isoniazid > rifampicin.

Regimen containing 2 hepatotoxic drugs	• 9 months of isoniazid and rifampicin along with ethambutol • 2 months of isoniazid, rifampicin, streptomycin and ethambutol followed by 7 months of isoniazid and rifampicin • 6–9 months of rifampicin, isoniazid and ethambutol
Regimen containing 1 hepatotoxic drug	• 2 months of isoniazid, ethambutol and streptomycin followed by 10 months of isoniazid and ethambutol
Regimen containing no hepatotoxic drug	• 18–24 months of streptomycin, ethambutol and a fluoroquinolone

- In case of drug resistant tuberculosis, hepatotoxic second line drugs like PAS and ethionamide should be avoided.

TB in Renal Failure

- In case of nonresistant TB, pyrazinamide, ethambutol need dose adjustment in renal failure and the dosing interval should be increased to three times weekly. The dose of pyrazinamide should be 25 mg/kg and with ethambutol should be 15 mg/kg. Streptomycin is contraindicated in patients of renal failure, however, if its use is unavoidable the dose is 15 mg/kg.
- If patient is on hemodialysis drugs can be given immediately after the procedure to avoid early removal of drug or can be given 4–6 hours after dialysis.
- In case of drug resistant TB, second line drugs like quinolones, PAS and Cycloserine also require dose adjustment.

Drugs that can be Safely Given in Renal Failure
Rifampicin
Isoniazid
Rifabutin
Rifapentine
Moxifloxacin
Ethionamide
Prothionamide
Linezolid
Clofazimine
Bedaquiline (Only in mild to moderate renal failure)

TB in Seizures and Psychosis

- Anti TB drugs that can cause seizure and hence avoided in seizure disorder are isoniazid, Cycloserine, ethionamide and fluoroquinolones.
- Pyridoxine can be used to prevent seizure with cycloserine and isoniazid.
- Fluoroquinolones, ethionamide, isoniazid and cycloserine can cause psychosis and hence should be avoided in such patients.

TB in HIV Patients

- The regimen for treatment of TB in HIV positive patients is same as other patients. Rifampicin is an enzyme inducer and hence if patient is on nevirapine, then change nevirapine to efavirenz; if patient is on protease inhibitors, then change rifampicinto rifabutin; if patient is on integrase inhibitors, then change rifampicinto rifabutin or double the dose of integrase inhibitor.
- First anti TB drugs are started and once the patients have tolerated these drugs anti-HIV drugs are started within 8 weeks of starting TB treatment. If the patient has severe immunosuppression (CD 4 count <50 cells/mm^2), anti-HIV drugs should be started along with ATT.
- When patients of HIV are started on anti TB drugs, they might develop a transient flaring up of TB symptoms called as immune reconstitution inflammatory syndrome (IRIS). The drug of choice for treatment of same is prednisolone.

Extrapulmonary TB

- In case of extrapulmonary TB including meningitis, bone and joint, spinal cord and brain, the same regimens are used as in pulmonary TB, the duration of continuation phase may be increased by 3–6 months.
- Corticosteroids are added in case of tubercular meningitis and pericarditis.
- In case of tubercular meningitis ethambutol should be changes to streptomycin.

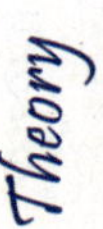

MYCOBACTERIUM LEPROSY

Mycobacterium leprae is an acid fast obligate intracellular organism responsible for leprosy.

Dapsone

- Dapsone like sulfonamides is an analog of PABA, which causes **competitive and reversible inhibition of dihydropteroate synthase.**
- It is a bacteriostatic drug given by oral route for treatment of **leprosy and malaria and prophylaxis of pneumocystis and toxoplasma.**
- It has **anti-inflammatory effect** also and hence used in **dermatitis herpetiformis**, pemphigoid and relapsing chondritis.
- Most common side effect is **hemolysis in G6PD deficiency**. Others are **peripheral neuropathy, methemoglobinemia and neuropsychiatric side effects.**

Clofazimine

- Clofazimine causes **free radical damage** to the mycobacterial cell membrane.
- It is also used by **oral route** for treatment of leprosy and TB. It is bactericidal against *M. tuberculosis* and bacteriostatic against *M. leprae.*
- Most common side effects are GIT upset like **nausea, vomiting and diarrhea**. It can also cause **reddish black or orange brown discolouration of skin and secretions, ichthyosis and QT prolongation**. Crystals of drug deposits can be seen in various tissues.

Clofazimine Induced Ichthyosis

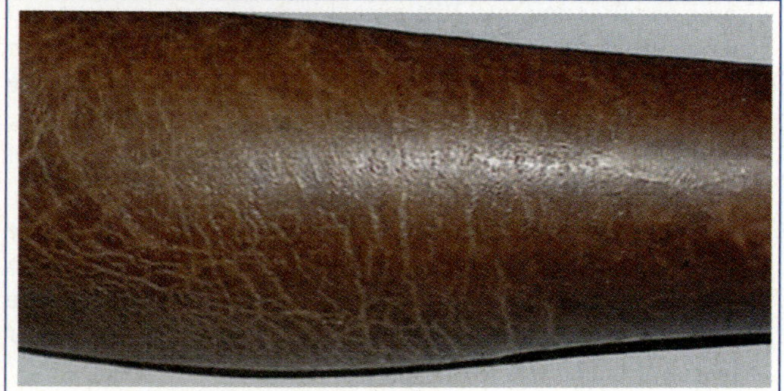

Rifampicin

Rifampicin is the most bactericidal drug used in leprosy. The other facts regarding this drug have been discussed in section of tuberculosis.

WHO Guidelines 2018

Standard Regimens

- According to the recent guidelines the number of drugs used, and doses are similar for treatment of both paucibacillary and multibacillary leprosy. The only difference is the duration of therapy, which is 12 months for multibacillary and 6 months for paucibacillary. Some drugs are given under supervision i.e. once a month and some without supervision, i.e. once a day as given below in the table:

Supervised (Once a month)		
Adults	Children 10-14 years	Children <14 years or <40 kg
Rifampicin 600 mg Clofazimine 300 mg	Rifampicin 450 mg Clofazimine 150 mg	Rifampicin 10 mg/kg Clofazimine 6 mg/kg
Nonsupervised (Once a day)		
Dapsone 100 mg Clofazimine 50 mg	Dapsone 50 mg Clofazimine 50 mg	Dapsone 2 mg/kg Clofazimine 1 mg/kg

Alternative Regimens for Leprosy

Alternative WHO recommended ROM regimen for paucibacillary leprosy	
Rifampicin 600 mg Ofloxacin 400 mg Minocycline 100 mg	Single dose

Alternative regimen in rifampicin sensitive multibacillary leprosy	
Rifapentine 900 mg Moxifloxacin 400 mg Clarithromycin 1000 mg Or Minocycline 200 mg	Once/Month for 12 months

Drug Resistant Leprosy

Currently resistance can be seen to three drugs used in leprosy, i.e. rifampicin, dapsone and ofloxacin. In case of resistance to only ofloxacin or dapsone the regimen in NLEP guidelines is to be used. In case of rifampicin resistance or resistance to both rifampicin or dapsone other drugs are to be used like ofloxacin, moxifloxacin, minocycline and clarithromycin. Moxifloxacin is more bactericidal than ofloxacin and is as good as rifampicin. Clofazimine resistance is usually not seen and it is used in rifampicin resistance.

Mechanism of Drug Resistance

Drug	Mechanism of resistance
Rifampicin	rpo B gene mutation
Dapsone	Folp1 gene mutation
Ofloxacin	gyr A gene mutation

WHO Recommended Regimens in Rifampicin Resistance

In case of rifampicin resistance ofloxacin, minocycline, clofazimine and clarithromycin are used in regimens as given below:

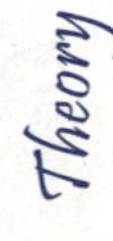

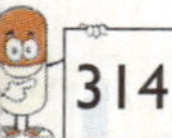

Resistance type	Treatment	
	First 6 months (daily)	Next 18 months (daily)
Rifampicin resistance	Ofloxacin 400 mg* + minocycline 100 mg + clofazimine 50 mg	Ofloxacin 400 mg* OR minocycline 100 mg + clofazimine 50 mg
	Ofloxacin 400 mg* + clarithromycin 500 mg + clofazimine 50 mg	Ofloxacin 400 mg* + clofazimine 50 mg
Rifampicin and ofloxacin resistance	Clarithromycin 500 mg + minocycline 100 mg + clofazimine 50 mg	Clarithromycin 500 mg OR minocycline 100 mg + clofazimine 50 mg

**Ofloxacin 400 mg can be replaced by levofloxacin 500 mg OR moxifloxacin 400 mg*

Postexposure Prophylaxis of Leprosy

- A person is eligible for postexposure prophylaxis if he/she hs been living/working/having social activities for more than three months and 20 hours/week with a newly detected case of leprosy in last one year. The age group eligible for postexposure prophylaxis is 2 years and above.
- Single dose rifampicin is the drug of choice for postexposure prophylaxis of leprosy and the dose given is based on weight as given below.

Age/weight	Rifampicin single dose
15 years and above	600 mg
10–14 years	450 mg
Children 6–9 years (weight ≥20 kg)	300 mg
Children <20 kg (≥2 years)	10–15 mg/kg

Treatment of Lepra Reaction

- Steroids are the drug of choice for type 1 lepra reaction.
- Steroids are drug of choice for type 2 lepra reaction (ENL) as well. In resistant cases thalidomide is the drug of choice and overall thalidomide is the best drug for ENL. Clofazimine at high doses can also be used.

Recent Advances

Anti-leprosy Vaccines

- Anti-leprosy vaccines are of utmost importance and the first-generation vaccines that were developed are not much efficacious and do not have many trials in their support.

First Generation Vaccines	
Non-cultivable Mycobacterium	**Cultivable Mycobacterium**
Killed M. leprae Acetoacetylated M. leprae	BCG M. vaccae M. habana M. welchii M. gordonae ICRC

Contd...

Recent Advances

Currently the second-generation vaccines which are under trial are **subunit vaccine** and **shuttle plasmid vaccine**.

- Various protein subunits of M. leprae like 10 Kd, 18 Kd, 31 Kd, 35 Kd, 65 Kd and 70 Kd have been identified. These subunits are being developed as vaccines for leprosy.
- In shuttle plasmid vaccine the genes coding for protective antigens are introduced into BCG and it might give protection against both TB and leprosy.

NONTUBERCULOUS MYCOBACTERIA

Type of nontuberculous mycobacteria	Treatment regimen IP regimen CP	Treatment
MAC and *M. kansasii*	(3) Clr 500 mg BD + E 800-1200 mg OD + R 45-600 mg OD + Inj. Am 750 mg-1 g thrice weekly	(12) Clr 500 mg BD + E 800-1200 mg OD + R 45-600 mg OD

- The guidelines for treatment of nontuberculous mycobacterium are based on recommendations for more commonly encountered pathogens like MAC and *M. kansasii*.
- An intensive phase of 3 months includes combination of a macrolide (clarithromycin/azithromycin), a rifamycin (rifampicin/rifabutin), ethambutol and an aminoglycoside (amikacin). If required it can be extended to a maximum duration of 6 months.
- A continuous phase of 12 months includes all the drugs of intensive phase except the aminoglycosides. It is started after the sputum culture conversion.
- Other drugs with activity against MAC are fluoroquinolones and clofazimine.

ANTIFUNGAL DRUGS

- A fungus is a two layered structure made up of a cell wall and a cell membrane.
- The cell wall is made up of **chitins, proteins and beta glucans**.
- The cell membrane is made up of lipids called as **ergosterol** and contains an enzyme called as **beta glucan synthase** that synthesizes beta glucans for the cell wall.
- Ergosterol is synthesized from **squalene,** which gets converted into **squalene epoxide** and squalene epoxide to **lanosterol**. Lanosterol in multiple steps gets converted into **ergosterol** with the help of enzyme **14-α sterol demethylase**.
- Many parts of the fungus are targets for drugs which is discussed in the following segments:

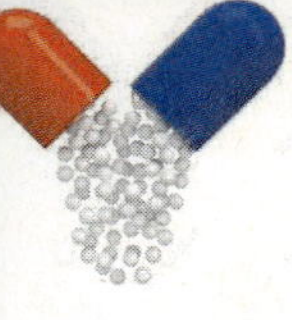

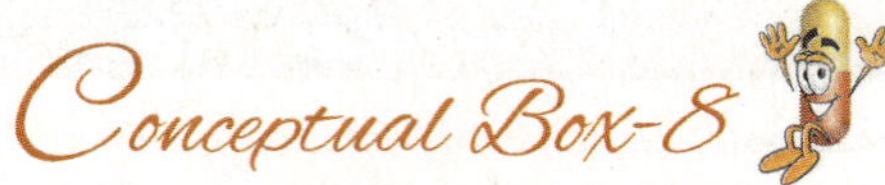

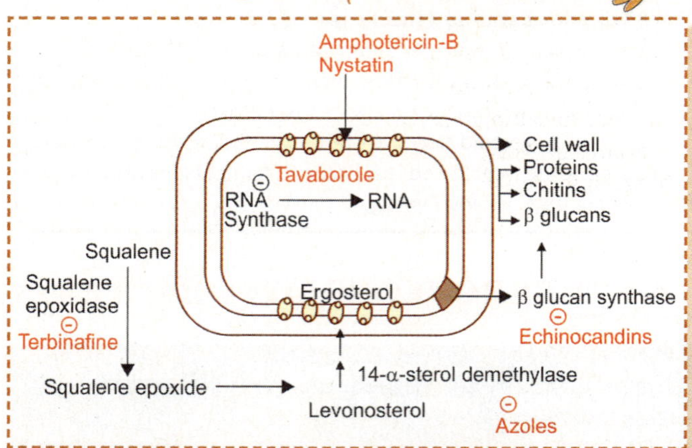

AMPHOTERICIN B

Mechanism of Action

- Amphotericin B is an amphipathic drug with a lipid and water soluble side. The water soluble side binds to **ergosterol in cell membrane** and forms **pore in the fungus** that is lined by water soluble side.
- These pores let in water and solute, which causes **fungicidal effect**.

Uses of Amphotericin B

- Amphotericin B has poor oral absorption and is given by intravenous route in 5% dextrose as a carrier.
- It is the drug of choice for **systemic fungal infections, mucormycosis, kala-azar and cryptococcal meningitis.**

Side Effects

- It is a very potent nephrotoxic drug and to prevent it the patient is preloaded with **1-2 litres of normal saline** before giving amphotericin B. To prevent nephrotoxicity amphotericin B is combined with **liposomes, lipids or colloids**.
- **Hypokalemia and hypomagnesemia** can be seen; hypokalemia being more common potassium chloride is routinely given and serum potassium is used as a marker of amphotericin B toxicity.
- Other side effects like infusion reaction, anemia, hypotension and thrombocytopenia can also be seen.

Flucytosine

- Flucytosine is a prodrug of anticancer drug **5-FU**. It is not used as a single agent due to resistance.
- It is given by IV route along with amphotericin B for induction therapy in **cryptococcal meningitis.**
- It can be given till a maximum duration of only 2 weeks because of risk of bone marrow suppression and colitis.

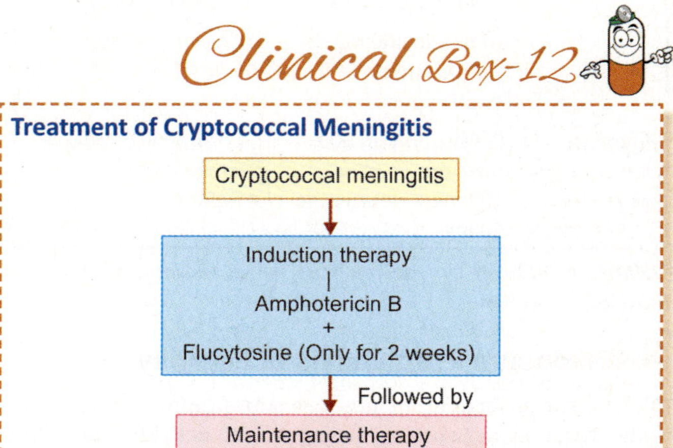

AZOLES

Mechanism of Action

- Azoles inhibit **ergosterol synthesis** by inhibiting **14-α sterol demethylase**.
- These are **broad spectrum** antifungals covering **candida, dermatophytes, cryptococcus and endemic mycoses.**
- The older azoles like **ketoconazole and clotrimazole are imidazoles** which have high blocking effect on human sterol synthesis. Hence, new class called as **triazoles** was synthesized which has drugs like **fluconazole, itraconazole, posaconazole, voriconazole and isavuconazle**, which have lesser effect on human sterol synthesis.

Uses of Azoles

- **Fluconazole** is the drug of choice for treatment of **candidiasis (only *C. albicans*) and coccidioidal meningitis.**
- **Itraconazole** is the drug of choice for treatment of **endemic mycoses, sporotrichosis and is antifungal of choice in allergic bronchopulmonary aspergillosis (ABPA)** to decrease steroid dose. Since it is an allergic phenomenon the **drug of choice for ABPA is prednisolone**.
- **Voriconazole** is the drug of choice for treatment of **invasive aspergillosis, scedosporium and trichosporon**.
- Ketoconazole can have spectrum similar to but less wide than itraconazole. It inhibits steroid synthesis and hence is used for treatment of Cushing's disease.

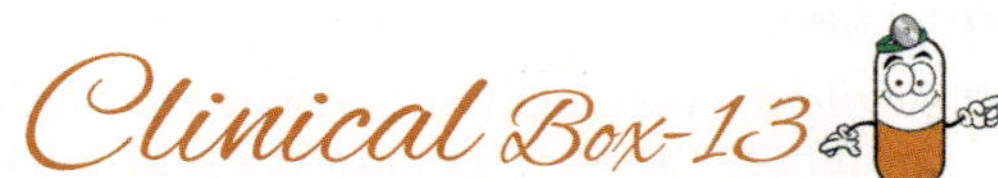

Aspergillosis Treatment

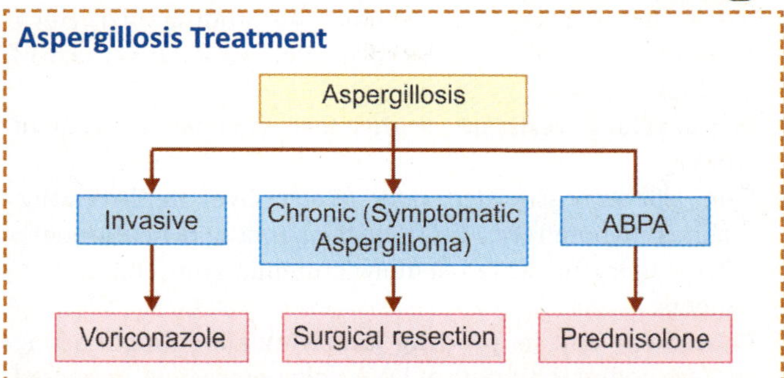

- **Posaconazole** is effective for treatment of **mucormycosis**. It is approved for treatment of voriconazole resistant invasive aspergillosis and is drug of choice for prophylaxis of aspergillosis. Prophylactically it is preferred to prevent fungal infection in patients receiving immunosuppressive therapy in **graft versus host disease (GVHD)** and patients receiving induction chemotherapy for leukemia.
- Econazole, miconazole, clotrimazole and tioconazole are topical azoles used for treatment of mucocutaneous fungal infections.

Recent Advances

Isavuconazole: Isavuconazole is a recent azole approved for treatment of mucormycosis and aspergillosis.
Efinaconazole: Efinaconazole is a recent azole approved for treatment of fungal toe nail infection.

Side Effects

- Itraconazole, fluconazole and voriconazole can cause hepatotoxicity.
- Itraconazole can cause CHF, hypokalemia and edema, whereas voriconazole can cause visual disturbances, peripheral neuropathy, periostitis due to fluoride excess, **skin cancer (squamous cell variant)** and hallucination.
- Voriconazole and posaconazole can cause QT prolongation.
- Ketoconazole has **antiandrogenic action** and can cause **gynaecomastia**.
- Fluconazole can cause alopecia.

ECHINOCANDINS

- Echinocandins inhibit beta **glucan synthase** and hence break the fungal cell wall causing **fungicidal effect**.
- The drugs in this class **caspofungin, micafungin and anidulafungin** have poor oral absorption and hence administered by intravenous route.
- These drugs have a very favourable side effect profile; caspofungin though can cause phlebitis. Caspofungin is contraindicated along with cyclosporine due to possible hepatotoxicity.
- These are second line drugs for treatment of **Candida albicans and aspergillus** resistant to the standard drugs and for empirical treatment of febrile neutropenia. These are drug of choice for Candida parapsilosis, krusei and glabrata, which are universally resistant to fluconazole.
- Caspofungin is approved for both candidiasis and aspergillosis whereas micafungin and anidulafungin are approved only for candidiasis. Micafungin is also approved for prevention of fungal infection in bone marrow transplant patients.

TERBINAFINE

- Terbinafine inhibits **ergosterol synthesis** by inhibiting squalene epoxidase.
- It is administered by **oral route** and following which it accumulates in the skin, nail and fats and hence is the **drug of choice for dermatophytes**. It can also be applied by topical route for dermatophytes.
- It can cause SJS and hepatotoxicity.

GRISEOFULVIN

- Griseofulvin **inhibits microtubules** in fungus and it has a **fungistatic effect**.
- It is given by **oral route** and then is maximum concentrated in **stratum corneum** and hence used for treatment of **dermatophytes**. It is the drug of choice for treatment of **tinea capitis** in children.
- **Fatty meal increases absorption of griseofulvin**.
- Side effects associated are hepatotoxicity, neurologic and neutropenia.

TOPICAL ANTIFUNGALS

- **Nystatin** is used only for the treatment of **candidiasis**. Azoles used for the treatment of only vaginal candidiasis are tioconazole, terconazole, butoconazole.
- Tolnaftate, undecylenic acid and Whitefield's ointment are effective only against dermatophytes. Azolos used for dermatophytes only are oxiconazole, sertaconazole and sulconazole.
- Rest are effective against both dermatophytes and Candida.
- Natamycin is the drug of choice for treatment of fungal corneal ulcers.

Mnemonics

Topical Antifungals
B : Butenafine
H : Haloprogin
U : Undecylenic acid
T : Tolnaftate, Terbinafine
A : Azoles
N : Nystatin, Naftifine

NONRETROVIRAL DRUGS

Nonretroviral drugs are discussed in three segments, i.e. anti-herpes virus drugs, anti-influenza drugs and anti-hepatitis drugs.

ANTIHERPES VIRUS DRUGS

Herpes Virus Replication

- Herpes virus is a DNA virus and like any other virus it needs a host cell for replication. It has tropism of epithelial cells. First it attaches to host cell and enters, after which it loses nucleocapsid and the DNA is exposed.
- **DNA polymerase** α by acting on the DNA synthesizes RNA primer, which is the base for DNA replication. The last phosphate in the RNA primer is known as **pyrophosphate**.
- **RNA polymerase** by acting on DNA synthesizes RNA, which further makes enzymes like **thymidylate kinase (TK).**
- TK phosphorylates nucleosides to form nucleoside triphosphate or nucleotide which are required for DNA synthesis.
- **DNA polymerase** δ **and** ε binds to nucleotides and attaches them to the pyrophosphate gradually increasing the DNA length.
- All these steps can be targeted by antiviral drugs as given in the conceptual box.

Conceptual Box-9

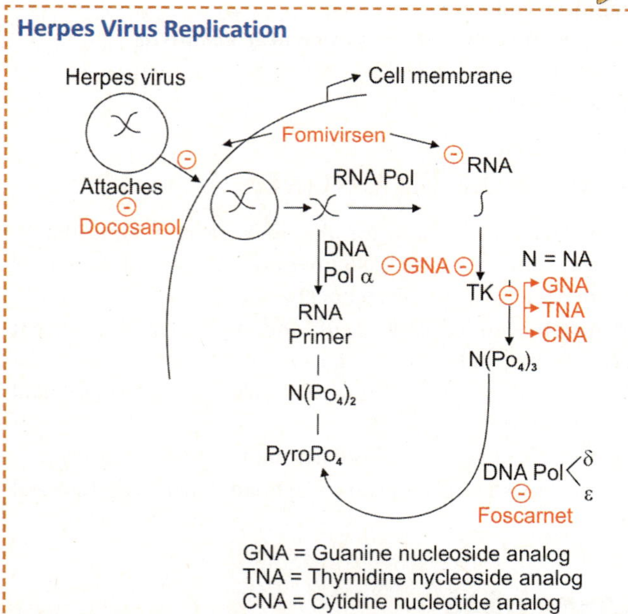

Guanine Nucleoside Analogs

- GNA act by inhibiting both **DNA polymerase** α **and TK.**
- Resistance can be seen due to impaired TK production or mutation in TK or DNA polymerase α gene. **Impaired TK production** being the most common mechanism of resistance.

Acyclovir

- Acyclovir is the drug of choice for treatment of **varicella zoster virus (VZV) and herpes simplex virus (HSV).**
- Since it has **poor oral bioavailability** its prodrug valacyclovir is more preferred. Valacyclovir is effective for treatment of CMV also.
- **For acyclovir resistant strains foscarnet is the drug of choice.**
- Side effects associated are **obstructive nephropathy**, seizures, hypotension, thrombocytopenia and neutropenia. Valacyclovir can cause haemolytic uremic syndrome in HIV patients.
- **Penciclovir** and **its prodrug famciclovir** are longer acting but less potent inhibitors of DNA polymerase α as compared to acyclovir. Penciclovir has poor oral absorption but prodrug famciclovir has good oral absorption. Penciclovir is mutagenic but as such **cancer has not been reported even in animals**.

Ganciclovir

- Ganciclovir is the drug of choice for treatment of **CMV** (cytomegalo virus) **retinitis**. It also has poor oral bioavailability and hence its prodrug valganciclovir is more preferred.
- In case of resistant cases foscarnet and fomivirsen can be used.
- It is associated with **bone marrow suppression**, which is the dose limiting toxicity.

Recent Advances

Letermovir

- It inhibits cytomegalovirus DNA terminase required for viral DNA processing and packaging, which results in improper virion maturation
- It has been recently approved for prevention of CMV infection in allogenic hematopoietic stem cell transplantation in CMV seropositive recipients

Cytidine Nucleotide Analog

- Cidofovir acts by inhibiting only TK.
- It is used for treatment of **resistant herpes (HSV, VZV, CMV), BK virus, molluscum contagiosum, respiratory papillomatosis, anogenital warts and adenovirus infection in transplant recipients.**
- Side effects associated are nephrotoxicity, Fanconi syndrome, neutropenia and anterior uveitis.

Thymidine Analog

- Idoxuridine acts by inhibiting only TK.
- It is not used by systemic route due to cardiotoxicity.
- Topic idoxuridine is used for treatment of HSV keratitis, herpes zoster and orolabial and genital herpes.

Pyrimidine Nucleoside Analog

- Trifluridine also acts by inhibiting only TK.
- It is used by topical route for treatment of HSV keratitis.
- It can cause punctate keratopathy.

Foscarnet

- Foscarnet acts by inhibiting the **pyrophosphate binding site of DNA polymerase δ and ε**.
- Since it acts at the lowest level it is effective in any type of resistance and hence is the **drug of choice for resistance to acyclovir and ganciclovir**.
- Metabolic side effects associated are **hypo/hyper calcemia, hypo/hyper phosphatemia, hypokalemia and hypomagnesemia.** It can also cause nephrotoxicity, thrombophlebitis and genital ulcers.

Fomivirsen

- Fomivirsen acts by inhibiting viral entry and viral RNA.
- It is used by intravitreal route for treatment of multidrug resistant CMV.
- Ocular side effects like iritis, vitreitis and cataract can be seen.

Docosanol

- Docosanol is an alcohol derivative and acts by inhibiting attachment of virus.
- It is used by topical route for treatment of recurrent orolabial herpes.

ANTI-INFLUENZA DRUGS

Influenza Virus Replication

- Influenza virus is an RNA virus which has tropism for respiratory epithelial cells.
- The **hemagglutinin** present in virus binds to the **sialic acid receptor (SAR)** of the respiratory epithelial cells and then it enters.

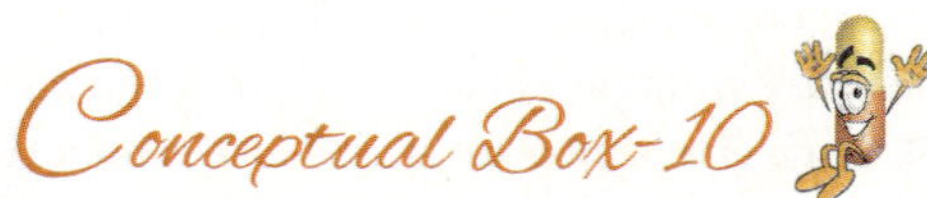

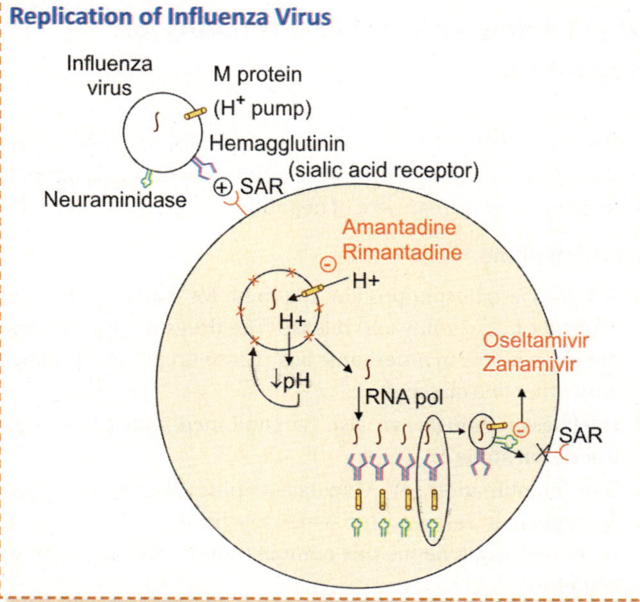

- Once inside the cell the M protein which are proton pumps, pump protons into the virus and decrease intraviral pH. This acidic pH dissolves the nucleocapsid and RNA is exposed.
- **RNA polymerase** acts on RNA and multiple copies of RNA as well as proteins like hemagglutinin, M protein and neuraminidase is synthesized. There is assortment of all these products, which gives rise to new viruses.
- **Neuraminidase** of these viruses damages the SAR and break the cell membrane, which leads to their release and propagation of infection.
- These steps can be inhibited at two levels as given in the Conceptual box below.

M Protein Inhibitors

M protein inhibitors like amantadine and rimantadine block viral uncoating.

Amantadine

- **Amantadine has good oral absorption** and is excreted unchanged by kidney; hence dose is halved in elderly.
- It can be used for **treatment and prophylaxis of influenza A only in sensitive cases**. For treatment it is best if started within **2 days** of infection and for prophylaxis it is given for **4–8 weeks** after the first case in the community.
- Side effects associated are **ankle edema, livedo reticularis**, nausea, vomiting and insomnia.

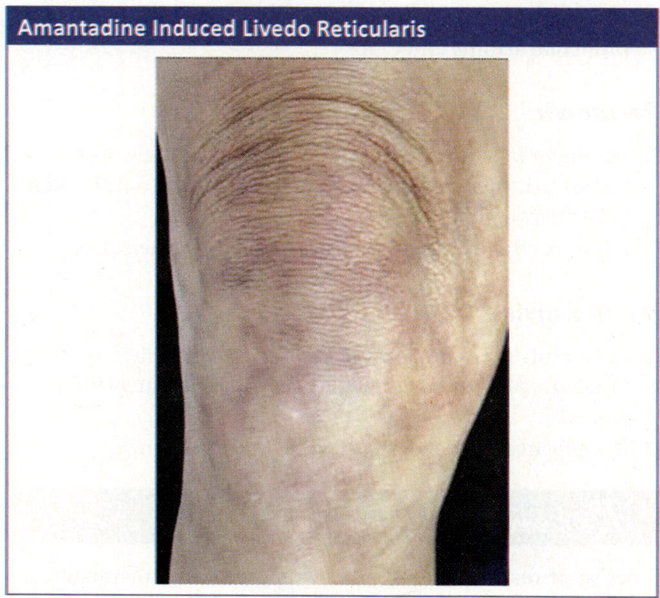
Amantadine Induced Livedo Reticularis

Rimantadine

Rimantadine is metabolized by liver and then excreted by kidney. It is **longer acting than amantadine.**

Neuraminidase Inhibitors

The neuraminidase inhibitors are sialic acid analogs and they inhibit release of virus.

Oseltamivir

- **Oseltamivir has good oral absorption** and is the drug of choice for treatment and prophylaxis of influenza A, **influenza B and bird flu.** It is most effective for treatment and prophylaxis when started **within 48 hours** of symptoms. **75 mg BD dose** is given for 5 days for treatment and **75 mg OD dose** given for prophylaxis for 7 days.
- It is approved in **all age group children for treatment** and for **prophylaxis only in children above 3 months of age**. The dose for treatment and prophylaxis in **children less than 1 year is 3 mg/kg BD**, whereas for children above 1 year age dose is decided based upon weight.
- **Oseltamivir phosphate is a prodrug** activated by esterase in intestine and liver to active compound **oseltamivir carboxylate.** It is primarily excreted unchanged by urine.
- Side effects associated are nausea and vomiting and hence it is given with food.

Zanamivir

- **Zanamivir has low oral bioavailability** and is given by inhalational route in the form of powder and by intravenous route.
- It is the drug of choice for treatment of **oseltamivir resistant influenza A and B and bird flu.** By inhalational route it is given at a dose of **10 mg BD** for 5 days for treatment and **10 mg OD** for 7 days for prophylaxis.
- It is approved for **treatment in children ≥7 years** of age and **prophylaxis in children ≥5 years** of age at doses like adults.
- It is contraindicated in bronchospastic disorders like bronchial asthma and COPD.

Peramivir

- Peramivir by intravenous route is given as a single dose of 600 mg for treatment for spectrum like oseltamivir only in **adults (>18 years)**.
- It is not active against oseltamivir resistant influenza.

Laninamivir

- Laninamivir is the longest acting in this class given by inhalational route 40 mg single dose for treatment of influenza A and B.
- It is effective against oseltamivir resistant influenza.

Recent Advances

Baloxavir marboxil: It is a prodrug approved for treatment of acute uncomplicated influenza within 48 hours of symptom onset. It inhibits viral replication by inhibiting endonuclease activity of polymerase acidic protein (present in viral RNA polymerase complex) required for viral gene transcription.

ANTIHEPATITIS DRUGS

In hepatitis C both acute and chronic stages are treated as, treatment in acute stage can prevent chronicity. In **hepatitis B, only chronic stage is treated** that is in active stage, i.e. markers for active inflammation or viral replications are positive.

Antihepatitis C Virus Drugs

Hepatitis C virus is an RNA virus. For a long time, the mainstay of therapy had been interferon α along with ribavirin, but the current treatment trend is changing due to availability of various oral drugs like NS3/4 A (protease) inhibitors, NS5B (RNA polymerase) inhibitors and NS5A inhibitors.

Interferon α

- Interferon α increases production of enzymes that **break down viral RNA and inhibit protein synthesis.**
- **Interferon α 2A and 2B** are commercially available for therapeutic use.
- It is given by IM or SC route for treatment of **acute and chronic hepatitis C, hepatitis B, papilloma virus, acyclovir resistant herpes, hairy cell leukemia and HIV associated thrombocytopenia**.
- Since it is the only drug active against hepatitis D, it is **drug of choice for cases of hepatitis B associated with hepatitis D**.
- The problem with interferon is side effects like flu like syndrome, bone marrow suppression, neurotoxicity, hypothyroidism etc.

Ribavirin

- Ribavirin acts by inhibiting vital m RNA synthesis.
- It is used by **oral route** along with interferon and recent oral drugs for treatment of chronic hepatitis C infection.
- Ribavirin by aerosol is the drug of choice for treatment of **RSV**. **Palivizumab** an anti-RSV monoclonal antibody once in a month injection is drug of choice for prophylaxis of RSV. It can cause symptoms of upper respiratory tract infections.
- Intravenous ribavirin is used for treatment of severe influenza.

Direct Acting Antiviral Agents (DAA) for Hepatitis C

The latest oral drugs contain drugs like NS3/4 A (protease) inhibitors, NS5B (RNA polymerase) inhibitors and NS5A inhibitors. These oral drugs are combined with each other to make regimens for treatment of hepatitis C.

NS5A Inhibitors

- NS5A is a phosphoprotein required for hepatitis C virus replication, assembly and release. The drugs inhibiting NS5A are given below in mnemonic box. These drugs are combined with other two classes.
- Daclatasvir though can also be combined with ribavirin or interferon alpha.
- The combination of Velpatasvir plus Voxilaprevir plus Sofosbuvir is reserved for patients who do not respond to other regimens; hence this combination is known as **rescue regimen**.

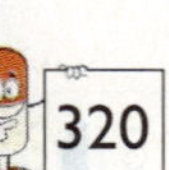

Mnemonics

Ns5a inhibitors	Protease inhibitor combined	RNA polymerase inhibitor combined
Orange: Ombitasvir	Paritaprevir	Dasabuvir
L: Ledipasvir		Sofosbuvir
E: Elbasvir	Grazoprevir	
D: Daclatasvir	Asunaprevir	Sofosbuvir or Beclabuvir
Penetrates: Pibrentasvir	Glecaprevir	
Virus: Velpatasvir	Voxilaprevir	Sofosbuvir

NS3/4 A (Protease) Inhibitors

- Protease is an enzyme required for viral maturation.
- Some protease inhibitors used with NS5A inhibitors have been discussed above.
- Simeprevir is used along with interferon α and ribavirin or sofosbuvir.
- Boceprevir, telaprevir can be used with interferon α and ribavirin whereas paritaprevir and glecaprevir can be used with ribavirin.
- Paritaprevir is boosted with ritonavir and the combination used in Paritaprevir + ritonavir plus Ombitasvir plus dasabuvir. This combination as well as simeprevir is contraindicated with protease inhibitors, efavirenz and nevirapine due to drug interactions described in section of anti-HIV drugs.
- The drugs in DAA class preferred along with anti-HIV drugs are sofosbuvir and ledipasvir.

NS5B (RNA Polymerase) Inhibitors

- Some RNA polymerase inhibitors combined with NS5A inhibitors and protease inhibitors have been discussed above.
- Sofosbuvir is a nucleoside RNA polymerase inhibitor that can also be used with interferon α and ribavirin apart from combinations discussed above. Sofosbuvir has invitro activity against Zika virus as well. This is the weakest class of drug against hepatitis C due to more chances of resistance.
- Dasabuvir and Beclabuvir are non-nucleoside RNA polymerase inhibitors used in combinations as discussed above.

Antihepatitis B Virus Drugs

Entecavir and tenofovir are the current first line drugs for treatment of hepatitis B. Interferon α is an alternative to the oral agents. In case of coinfection of hepatitis B with HIV, tenofovir is used along with lamivudine or emtricitabine.

Specific Drugs

The specific antihepatitis B virus drugs act by inhibiting the DNA polymerase α.

- **Adefovir** has low oral bioavailability and hence its prodrug adefovir dipivoxil is preferred. Though adefovir is effective in lamivudine resistant strains, it is the least potent drug. Side effect associated is nephrotoxicity.
- **Entecavir** has good oral absorption and is the drug of choice for treatment of hepatitis B. Food decreases absorption and hence given on empty stomach. Acute exacerbation can be seen on drug discontinuation.

Nonspecific Drugs

The nonspecific drugs are anti-HIV drugs secondarily used in hepatitis B. The nonspecific oral drugs used are **lamivudine, emtricitabine, tenofovir, clevudine and telbivudine**.

ANTIRETROVIRAL DRUGS

The first antiretroviral drug developed was **zidovudine**. Though it was developed as an anticancer drug, later anti-HIV effect was confirmed.

RETROVIRUS REPLICATION

- Retrovirus is a RNA virus that requires **CD-4 cells** for its replication. For entry the **glycoproteins 41 and 120** of virus attach to **CD-4 and CCR-5 receptors** on CD-4 cells respectively.
- Once it enters, the nucleocapsid is lost and RNA is exposed. This RNA is then converted to DNA by enzyme **reverse transcriptase (RT)**, which then integrates into CD-4 DNA with the help of enzyme **integrase**.
- After integration transcription of DNA leads to multiple copies of viral RNA formation and synthesis of its various proteins.
- Since the proteins are of inappropriate size and shape, they are broken down to normal size and shape by enzyme **protease; a process called as maturation.** Further protease is responsible for **assembly of these proteins**. This follows release of virus and subsequent infection of other CD-4 cells.
- With this continuous process the CD-4 count keeps on decreasing and leads to opportunistic infections.
- Various drugs targeting retrovirus replication are given in the Conceptual box below:

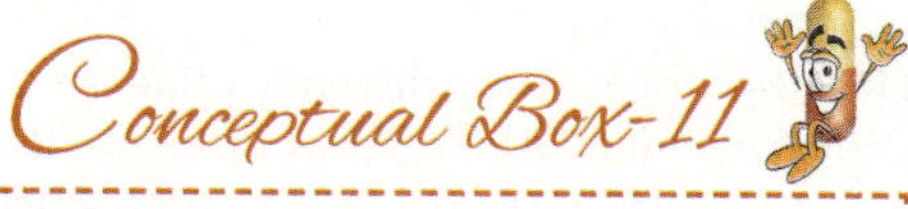

Retrovirus Replication

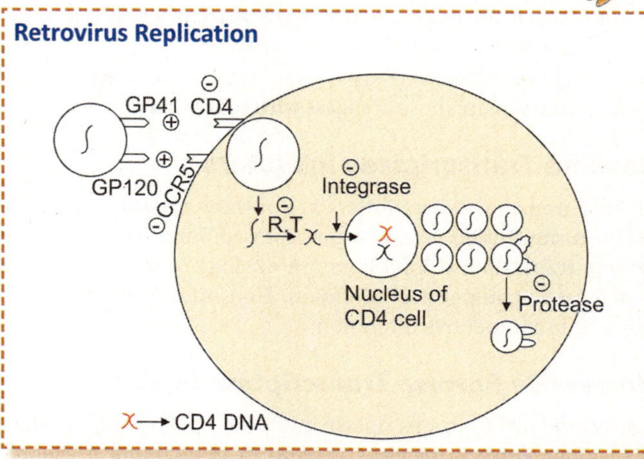

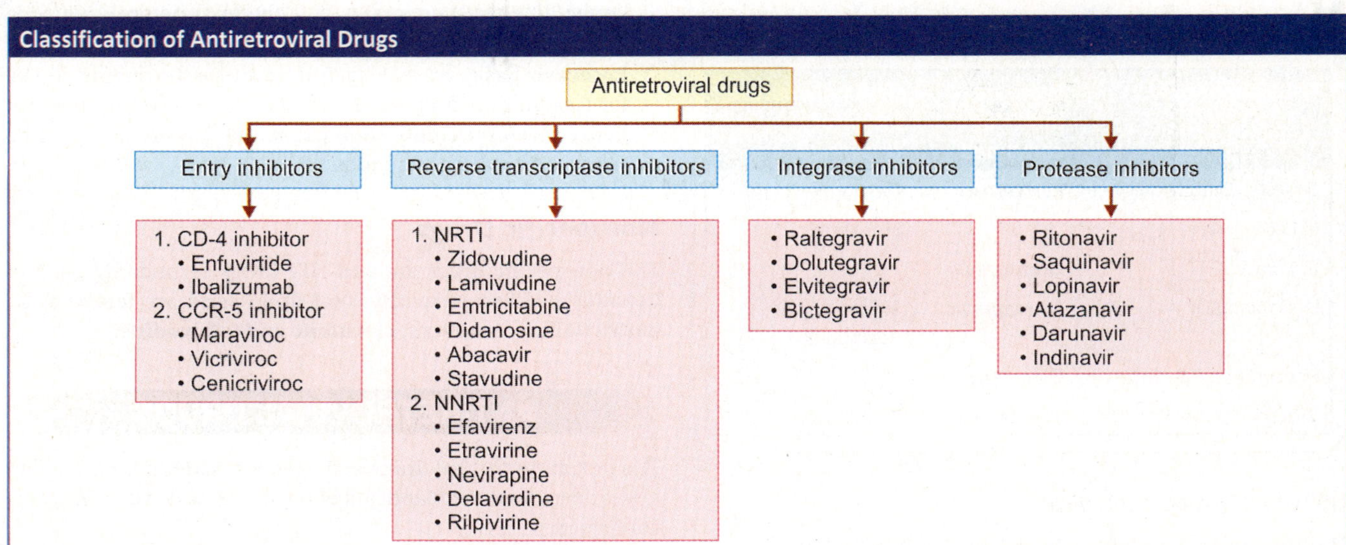

Classification of Antiretroviral Drugs

Note: Tenofovir is a nucleotide reverse transcriptase inhibitor.

Entry Inhibitors

CD-4 Receptor Inhibitor

- Enfuvirtide, a **fusion inhibitor** was synthesized as a subcutaneous vaccine against glycoprotein 41 of virus. The vaccine misfired and rather inhibited CD-4 receptor, the target of glycoprotein 41. Hence, it is used for treatment of HIV now.
- **Enfuvirtide** is a parenteral drug used in HIV used by subcutaneous route. It can cause pain on injection.

Recent Advances

Ibalizumab: It is anti-CD-4 monoclonal antibody recently approved for treatment of multi drug resistant HIV.

CCR-5 Receptor Inhibitor

- The drugs in this class are **maraviroc, vicriviroc and cenicriviroc**.
- These drugs along with enfuvirtide are used as add on drugs for treatment of HIV. These drugs are more effective early in the disease due to CCR-5 tropism by virus, whereas as disease progresses virus uses CXCR-4 for entry.
- Side effects associated are cough, fever, rash, dizziness and abdominal pain; these are **least with maraviroc.**

Reverse Transcriptase Inhibitors

Reverse transcriptase inhibitors are of three classes nucleoside and non-nucleoside reverse transcriptase inhibitors. Nucleoside reverse transcriptase inhibitors are analogs of nucleoside and hence cause competitive inhibition. Non-nucleoside inhibitors cause non-competitive inhibition.

Nucleoside Reverse Transcriptase Inhibitors

Nucleoside reverse transcriptase inhibitors (NRTI) block human DNA polymerase γ, which is present in mitochondria. Hence, mitochondrial toxicity can be seen, which causes **lactic acidosis, myopathy, peripheral neuropathy and pancreatitis**. All NRTIs are excreted by kidney except **zidovudine and abacavir**. NRTIs are not metabolized by CYP_{450} enzymes and hence can be used along with enzyme inducers like rifampicin.

Zidovudine

- **Zidovudine** is a thymidine analog used as a first line drug in children <10 years and second line drug in adults and adolescents for treatment of HIV. It is also used to prevent **perinatal HIV transmission**.
- Side effects associated are bone marrow suppression **(anemia and neutropenia – dose limiting side effects)**, hepatotoxicity, myopathy, fatigue, malaise, **insomnia** and anorexia. Anemia is most common with zidovudine, whereas neutropenia is common with both zidovudine and didanosine. Thus, zidovudine is not used in patients with hemoglobin levels of **<9 g/dL**.
- Resistance is seen due to **mutation of reverse transcriptase** and it can confer cross resistance to other thymidine analogs like **stavudine, tenofovir and abacavir**; zidovudine should be avoided with these drugs.

Stavudine

- Stavudine has more affinity for nerves and hence causes **maximum peripheral neuropathy**. Zalcitabine has been discontinued because of peripheral neuropathy.
- It also causes **maximum lipoatrophy** among NRTIs.

Lamivudine, Emtricitabine and Tenofovir

- These three drugs are **least potent inhibitors of human DNA polymerase** γ and hence cause **least peripheral neuropathy, lactic acidosis and myopathy**. All these drugs have activity against hepatitis B.
- **Tenofovir** is a **nucleoside monophosphate analog** also known as a **nucleotide reverse transcriptase inhibitor**. It is used for both **treatment and postexposure prophylaxis of HIV**. It is also used as a first line drug for the treatment

of **hepatitis B**. It can cause flatulence, **bone resorption (decreased bone density)**, **acute renal failure** and Fanconi's syndrome. Tenofovir is contraindicated in patients with GFR < 50 mL/min, uncontrolled hypertension, untreated diabetes and renal failure.

- **Lamivudine and emtricitabine** are never combined with each other due to risk of cross resistance. Both are used for treatment of HIV and hepatitis B. Emtricitabine can cause **skin discolouration.**
- In case of coinfection of HIV with hepatitis B, tenofovir is used along with lamivudine or emtricitabine.

Abacavir

- **Abacavir** is used only for treatment of **HIV-1** infection along with lamivudine or zidovudine.
- Its use is associated with side effects like hypersensitivity and myocardial infarction. It should be given only in **HLA-B 5701** negative patients as in positive patients the risk of hypersensitivity is higher. If patient once develops hypersensitivity, rechallenge should never be given.

Didanosine

- Didanosine can be used for treatment of HIV.
- It is associated with side effects like **pancreatitis**, peripheral neuropathy, dry mouth, hepatotoxicity and hyperuricemia.

Non-Nucleoside Reverse Transcriptase Inhibitor

The NNRTI are noncompetitive inhibitor of HIV-1 reverse transcriptase and hence these drugs are **not effective for treatment of HIV-2**. These drugs also do not block human DNA polymerase γ and hence related side effects are not seen.

Mnemonics

NNRTI

N : Nevirapine, **E** : Efavirenz, **E** : Etravirine — Enzyme Inducers
D : Delavirdine – Enzyme Inhibitor
Doravirine

- NNRTIs are used in combination with NRTIs for treatment of HIV, but **never used as single agents** due to risk of resistance.
- **Nevirapine is the drug of choice to prevent perinatal HIV transmission**, as single dose to mother and baby is associated with lesser toxicity and a better compliance.
- NNRTI like **nevirapine**, **delavirdine** and **doravirine** are metabolized by CYP3A4 in liver and its inducer like **rifampicin** are contraindicated. Others like **efavirenz and etravirine** can be used along with **rifampicin**, as these are primarily metabolized by CYP2B6.
- Efavirenz absorption is increased with fatty food and hence chances of neurotoxicity, hence it is taken on empty stomach.
- Rilpivirine is taken with fatty food and should be avoided with proton pump inhibitors.
- Delavirdine is not used commonly due to its short half-life, which requires TDS dosing.
- Resistance can be seen to all first generation NNRTIs except the second generation drug **etravirine**; hence it is preferred in case patient is resistant to other drugs in this class.
- Most common side effect associated with this class is **rash.** Nevirapine can cause fatal **hepatotoxicity**. Etravirine can cause peripheral neuropathy. Efavirenz is **teratogenic** (CNS defects) and hence absolutely contraindicated in pregnancy; It can also cause neuropsychiatric side effects (delusions, seizures, mania and suicidal tendency) and gynecomastia.

Recent Advances

Doravirine: It is a non-nucleoside reverse transcriptase inhibitor (NNRTI) approved for treatment of HIV.

Integrase Inhibitors

- **Raltegravir, elvitegravir, dolutegravir** and **bictegravir** are integrase inhibitors used as add on drugs in resistant HIV or intolerance to other classes.
- Elvitegravir is metabolized by CYP3A4 and hence is boosted with **cobicistat**, an inhibitor of CYP3A4. Cobicistat inhibits tubular creatinine secretion.
- Fatty food increases absorption of raltegravir. These drugs should not be taken with **antacids** as cations like aluminium, magnesium, iron and calcium chelate the drug and decrease absorption.
- Dolutegravir and raltegravir can cause hepatotoxicity and hypersensitivity reaction (e.g. Steven Johnson's syndrome).
- Raltegravir can cause **rhabdomyolysis** and myopathy, and hence should be avoided with other drugs causing myopathy like statins.

Recent Advances

Dolutegravir and **rilpivirine** combination has been recently approved for treatment of HIV.

Bictegravir: It is an integrase inhibitor recently approved for treatment of HIV in a fixed dose combination along with emtricitabine and tenofovir.

Protease Inhibitors

Inhibition of enzyme protease inhibits **maturation and assembly** of virus. These drugs are commonly used along with NRTIs and NNRTIs for treatment and post exposure prophylaxis of HIV. These are effective for treatment of both **HIV 1 and 2**.

- All protease inhibitors are **metabolized by CYP3A4** in liver **except nelfinavir**, which is metabolized by CYP2C19 primarily; all of them are hepatotoxic.
- All protease inhibitors are **enzyme inhibitor of CYP3A4**. All protease inhibitors can cause metabolic abnormalities like **dyslipidemia, diabetes mellitus and fat deposition (abdominal obesity and buffalo hump) except atazanavir**. Plasma lipid levels should be checked every year at least once.

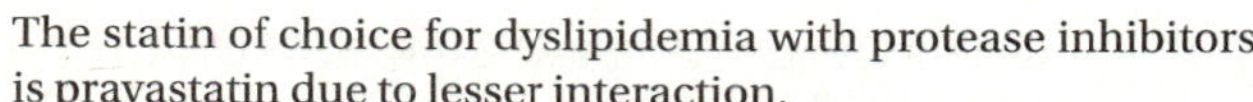

The statin of choice for dyslipidemia with protease inhibitors is pravastatin due to lesser interaction.

- All protease inhibitors are **substrate for p glycoprotein**.
- All protease inhibitors can cause **QT and PR prolongation** due to inhibition of hERG and hence should be avoided with other drugs or conditions that can precipitate torsades (hypokalemia, terfenadine etc.)
- All protease inhibitors can cause variable hepatotoxicity and the risk being maximum with tipranavir.
- **Ritonavir is the most potent enzyme inhibitor** and hence is used as a booster. It is combined with other protease inhibitors like darunavir, lopinavir, saquinavir etc. to increase their duration of action. **Ritonavir boosting is not done for nelfinavir**, as it is primarily not metabolized by CYP3A4.

Recent Advances

Cobicistat: Cobicistat is an enzyme inhibitor approved recently to be combined with atazanavir and darunavir.

- **Saquinavir** is the least potent enzyme inhibitor. Boosting of saquinavir with ritonavir decreases dyslipidemia and GIT toxicity whereas there is an increased risk of **QT and PR prolongation**.
- **Fosamprenavir and atazanavir** can cause **hyperglycemia**. Amprenavir and fosamprenavir concentration is decreased by ethynyl estradiol and hence should not be used in transgender patients on high estrogen doses.
- **Indinavir and atazanavir** can cause **unconjugated hyperbilirubinemia** and is most common side effect of atazanavir. The risk of jaundice is higher in patients with **UGT1A1 28** allele.
- PPI are contraindicated with atazanavir.
- **Indinavir** is taken on empty stomach as **fatty food decreases absorption**. It has least plasma protein binding and is associated with crystalluria and **nephrolithiasis** due to its poor solubility. It can also cause mild hyperbilirubinemia. Nephrolithiasis can also be seen with atazanavir.
- **Tipranavir** is the only nonpeptidic protease inhibitor used. It has anticoagulant effect and can cause intracranial haemorrhage; this effect is increased by vitamin E.
- **Tipranavir and darunavir** contain a sulfa group and hence patient should be monitored for allergy.
- **Darunavir** is taken with food as its absorption is increased. It can cause hypersensitivity reactions like Steven Johnson's syndrome.
- Nelfinavir and lopinavir are most commonly associated with diarrhea. Lopinavir can cause pancreatitis as well.

Drug Interactions with Anti-HIV Drugs

Anti-HIV drugs	Drug interactions	Recommendation
Zidovudine	Ribavirin and pegylated interferon alpha-2a increase risk of anemia and hepatotoxicity	Substitute zidovudine with tenofovir
Protease inhibitors	Rifampicin can induce metabolism and cause protease inhibitor failure	• Substitute rifampicin with rifabutin (Preferred) • Double dose of protease inhibitors in case rifabutin is not available • Substitute with three NRTIs (for children)
	Halofantrine and lumefantrine can cause QT prolongation Astemizole and terfenadine can cause QT prolongation Protease inhibitors can also cause QT prolongation	Choose another antimalarial agent and antihistaminic drugs
	Lovastatin and simvastatin are metabolized by microsomal enzymes and hence protease inhibitor can inhibit their metabolism and increase toxicity	Choose another hypolipidemic drug
	OCP and protease inhibitors combination can decrease effect of both	Choose another or additional contraception
	Methadone and buprenorphine concentration can be increased by protease inhibitors	Adjust dose of methadone and buprenorphine accordingly
	Tenofovir plasma concentration is increased by protease inhibitors by inhibition of p-glycoprotein induced efflux of tenofovir. Hence tenofovir induced nephrotoxicity is increased.	Monitor renal function
	Simeprevir plasma concentration is increased by protease inhibitors due to inhibition of CYP3A4	Choose another DAA
Efavirenz	Ombitasvir plus paritaprevir + ritonavir plus dasabuvir combination has multiple drug interactions if combined with additional protease inhibitors	Choose another DAA
	Methadone plasma concentration is decreased by efavirenz due to enzyme induction of CYP3A4	Adjust dose of methadone accordingly

Contd...

Anti-HIV drugs	Drug interactions	Recommendation
	OCP effect is decreased due to enzyme induction of CYP3A4	Choose or add another contraception
	Astemizole and terfenadine can cause QT prolongation Efavirenz can also cause QT prolongation	Choose another antihistaminic
	Simeprevir plasma concentration is decreased by efavirenz due to induction of CYP3A4	Choose another DAA
	Ombitasvir plus paritaprevir + ritonavir plus dasabuvir combination increases hepatotoxicity of efavirenz	Choose another DAA
Nevirapine	Nevirapine plasma concentration is decreased by rifampicin due to enzyme induction	Change nevirapine to efavirenz
	Methadone plasma concentration is decreased by nevirapine due to enzyme induction	Adjust plasma concentration of methadone accordingly
	Astemizole and terfenadine can cause QT prolongation Since both these drugs and nevirapine is metabolized by CYP3A4 there can be competitive inhibition	Choose another antihistaminic
	Ketoconazole and itraconazole plasma concentration is decreased by nevirapine	Choose another antifungal drug
	Simeprevir plasma concentration is decreased by nevirapine due to induction of CYP3A4	Choose another DAA
	Ombitasvir plus paritaprevir + ritonavir plus dasabuvir combination increases hepatotoxicity of efavirenz	Choose another DAA
Dolutegravir	Phenytoin, phenobarbital and carbamazepine can induce metabolism of dolutegravir and decrease its effect	Choose another antiepileptic agent
	Polyvalent cation products like vitamins and antacids containing Mg, Al, Fe, Ca and Zn chelate and decrease absorption of dolutegravir	Advise patient to take dolutegravir 2 hours before or 6 hours after taking these drugs

Note: DAA is Direct Acting Antiviral agent

NACO Guidelines 2018

The short form used for the drugs used for treatment of HIV in regimens is given below:

Drug	Short form
Tenofovir	TDF
Lamivudine	3 TC
Zidovudine	AZT
Abacavir	ABC
Stavudine	d4T
Efavirenz	EFV
Nevirapine	NVP
Lopinavir/ritonavir	LPV/r

Postexposure Prophylaxis

- Post exposure prophylaxis is best if started within 2 hours and can be given until 72 hours after exposure.
- Postexposure prophylaxis is given in case a person is exposed to body fluids associated with high risk of transmission like blood, saliva, breast milk, genital secretions and cerebrospinal, amniotic, peritoneal, synovial, pericardial and pleural fluid.
- However, in case patient is exposed to body fluids with low risk of transmission like tears, non-blood stained saliva, urine and sweat, post exposure prophylaxis is not required.
- The recommended regimens in adults for 28 days by NACO are given below:

First line	TDF + 3TC + LPV/r
Alternative	TDF + 3TC + EFV

- In children less than or equal to 10 years, the only change in the regimen is replacement of TDF by AZT. If AZT is contraindicated, then ABC can be used.

Treatment

- The aim of treatment is to combine at least 3 drugs from 2 different groups to produce synergism and reduce toxicity and chances of resistance. Start treatment of HIV in all age groups and population including pregnancy and lactation and associated comorbidities like TB, irrespective of CD4 count and clinical stage of HIV.
- In adults, adolescents, pregnancy and lactation a TDF based regimen is preferred.
- In children use of AZT and protease inhibitor-based regimen is preferred for reasons described ahead. Protease inhibitors are

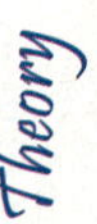

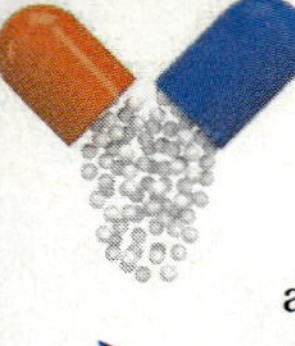

associated with better out come as compared to nevirapine in children. The safety of TDF is not well established in children till 10 years of age and patients (children + adults) less than 30 kg. Thus, in children till 10 years of age or adolescents with weight <30 kg AZT is preferred, whereas in adults with weight <30 kg ABC is preferred.

- Some changes are made in the regimen in case of associated comorbidities like renal failure and anemia. These changes are:
  - TDF is nephrotoxic and hence in case of renal failure ABC is used in place of TDF.
  - AZT can cause anemia and hence in case hemoglobin level is less than 9 g/dL, ABC is used in place of AZT. In case of intolerance to both AZT and ABC, d4T can be used in children.
  - The regimens given below are for more commonly encountered HIV-1. In case of HIV-2 NNRTI like EFV is not effective and hence LPV/r is used in place of EFV.

Population		Preferred first-line regimens
Adults and adolescents (>10–19 years) weight ≥30 kg		TDF + 3TC + EFV
Adults weight <30 kg		ABC + 3TC + EFV
Adolescents (>10-19 years) weight <30 kg		AZT + 3TC + EFV
Children 3 years to 10 years		AZT + 3TC + EFV
Children less than 3 years		AZT + 3TC + LPV/r
Pregnancy or Lactation	**Not on any ART**	TDF + 3TC + EFV
	Already on ART	Continue same ART
	Exposure to NVP in previous pregnancy	TDF + 3TC + LPV/r

Infant Prophylaxis

All pregnant and lactating women should be immediately started on standard anti-HIV regimen even if diagnosed late in pregnancy, as this is the best way to prevent perinatal transmission. The standard duration of therapy is for 6 weeks. However if <4 weeks ART is received by mother and baby is on breast feeding, then the duration should be 12 weeks.

Category	Drugs used
Standard	NVP for 6 weeks
Mother with prior exposure to NVP or Mother with HIV-2 infection	AZT for 6 weeks

Treatment Failure

- Viral load is the preferred approach to diagnose treatment failure as it is most sensitive indicator.
- If viral load is not available, then clinical monitoring or CD4 levels can be used.

Failure	Definition	Comments
Virological failure	Plasma viral load above 1000 copies/mL	An individual must be taking ART for at least 6 months before it can be determined that a regimen has failed.
Immuno-logical failure	CD4 count falls to the baseline (or below) or Persistent CD4 levels below 100 cells/cm or 50% fall from "on treatment" peak level	Concomitant or recent infection may cause a transient decline in the CD4 cell count. Some experts consider persistent CD4 counts of below 50 cells/cm after 12 months of ART to be more appropriate.
Clinical failure	New or recurrent clinical event indicating severe immunodeficiency (WHO clinical stage 4 condition) after 6 months of effective treatment	The condition must be differentiated from IRIS. Some WHO clinical stage 4 conditions (lymph node TB, uncomplicated TB pleural disease, esophageal candidiasis, recurrent bacterial pneumonia) may not indicate treatment failure. For adults, certain WHO clinical stage 3 conditions (pulmonary TB and severe bacterial infections) may also indicate treatment failure.

HIV with Coinfections

HIV with TB

- The regimen for treatment of TB in HIV positive patients is same as other patients. Rifampicin is an enzyme inducer and hence if patient is on nevirapine, then change nevirapine to efavirenz; if patient is on protease inhibitors, then change rifampicinto rifabutin; if patient is on integrase inhibitors, then change rifampicinto rifabutin or double the dose of integrase inhibitor.
- First anti TB drugs are started and once the patients have tolerated these drugs anti-HIV drugs are started within 8 weeks of starting TB treatment. If the patient has severe immunosuppression (CD 4 count <50 cells/mm^3), anti-HIV drugs should be started within 2 weeks.
- When patients of HIV are started on anti TB drugs, they might develop a transient flaring up of TB symptoms called as immune reconstitution inflammatory syndrome (IRIS). The drug of choice for treatment of same is prednisolone.

HIV with Hepatitis

- **HIV with Hepatitis B:** The first line regimen for HIV remains same, i.e. TDF + 3TC + EFV; TDF and 3TC are effective against hepatitis B as well and hence no other drug needs to be used.

However, if patient cannot tolerate TDF, then replace it with AZT. Since AZT is not active against hepatitis B, another anti-hepatitis B drug like entecavir needs to be started.

HIV with Hepatitis B	TDF + 3TC + EFV
HIV with Hepatitis B plus TDF intolerance or contraindication	AZT + 3TC + EFV + Entecavir

- **HIV with Hepatitis C:** The first line regimen for HIV remains same, i.e. TDF + 3TC + EFV; since none of these are effective against hepatitis C, the direct acting antivirals (DAA) like sofosbuvir, daclatasvir, Velpatasvir etc. are added to ART. ART is started first and only after adequate HIV suppression, DAA are started. The preferred combination of DAA depends if the patient has developed cirrhosis or not.

HCV infection with cirrhosis	Sofosbuvir + velpatasvir
HCV infection without cirrhosis	Sofosbuvir + daclatasvir

Opportunistic Infections

Opportunistic infections are quite commonly seen along with HIV and hence drugs should be given for prevention of same. In case patient already has opportunistic infection at the time of diagnosis of HIV then opportunistic infection should be treated first, stabilized and only then ART is started. The only cases where ART is started first are in case of progressive multifocal leukoencephalopathy (PML) and mycobacterium avium complex (MAC) infection.

Cotrimoxazole Preventive Therapy (CPT)

- Cotrimoxazole prevents not only pneumocystis jiroveci pneumonia and toxoplasmosis but also few other bacterial pneumonia, nocardiosis and isosporiasis.
- It is started at a dose of 160 mg trimethoprim + 800 mg sulfamethoxazole OD; in case of intolerance, cotrimoxazole desensitization can be done or dapsone 100 mg OD can be used.
- **Primary CPT indication:** A patient of HIV who has CD4 count less than 350 cells/mm3 or WHO clinical stage 3 or 4 HIV.
- **Secondary CPT indication:** A patient after successful treatment of pneumocyctis pneumonia is given cotrimoxazole until CD4 count increases more than 350 cells/mm^3 on at least two occasions, 6 months apart.
- During pregnancy it is started irrespective of the trimester.
- In case of a newborn of a HIV positive mother it is started at a dose of 5 mg/kg/day from 6 weeks of age until HIV is excluded in the infant. In case the infant is positive for HIV, it is continued till 5 years of age and after 5 years the management is same as adults.

Isoniazid Preventive Therapy (IPT)

- Isoniazid 300 mg plus pyridoxine 50 mg for 6 months is given in adults and adolescents with HIV to prevent progression of latent TB infection to disease.
- IPT is not given in case of active TB disease, active hepatitis, peripheral neuropathy, poor adherence to cotrimoxazole, poor understanding of IPT by guardian, in a contact of MDR TB case or patients treated for drug resistant TB.
- In case of a baby born to HIV positive mother, IPT is started after 12 months of age and dosing based on weight.

Cryptococcosis Prevention

- Primary prophylaxis for cryptococcal infection is not given as the incidence of infection is low and there is no definite survival benefit data.
- Secondary prophylaxis is given in patients with history of cryptococcal meningitis. Fluconazole 200 mg/day is given until CD4 count remains more than 200 cells/mm^3 for 6 months in a patient on ART.

Recent Advances

Anti-HIV Vaccines

- Many vaccines are currently under trial for prevention of HIV and approval of these vaccines might change the way we look at HIV today.
- The first ever positive result of HIV vaccine trial was **RV144**, which consists of the canary pox-vectored ALVAC-HIV prime and AIDSVAX gp120 B/E subunit vaccine boost.
- Currently viral vector (Adeno/CMV/Pox) based vaccines are under trial. One example is **RhCMV** based vaccine expressing SIV antigens.
- **BG505 SOSIP** and **engineered gp120** variants are vaccines that stimulate formation of broadly neutralizing antibodies (bnAbs) against HIV virus.
- Preformed antibodies against HIV: **VRC01** is an antibody under trial for prevention of HIV.

ANTIMALARIAL DRUGS

PLASMODIUM REPLICATION

- When a mosquito bites a human being, it injects **sporozoites** which find its way to liver via systemic circulation.
- In the liver either it can go dormant in the **hypnozoite stage**, which can reactivate later and cause **relapse of malaria**. This is seen only with **ovale and vivax**. Hypnozoite cidal drug **primaquine** is always used in case of vivax and ovale infection.
- Sporozoite can multiply inside hepatocyte to form a **hepatic schizont** and grows until hepatocyte ruptures and **merozoites** are released into blood.
- These merozoites can form **gametocytes**, which are the infective form for a mosquito and are responsible for **transmission of malaria**. **Gametocidal drugs** like **primaquine and artemisinin group** drugs prevent transmission of malaria.
- Merozoites can also enter into RBC and multiply to form a **RBC schizont**, which grows until RBC ruptures and this coincides with rise in temperature and chills, i.e. **symptoms of malaria**. Thus, RBC schizontocidal drugs are used for clinical cure of malaria. They can be either **slow acting or fast acting schizontocidal drugs** and are combined with each other to make a regimen for treatment of malaria.

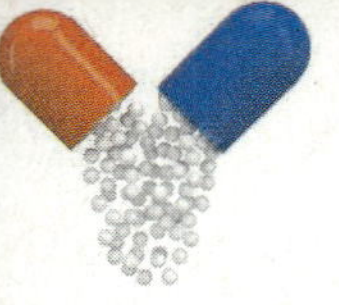

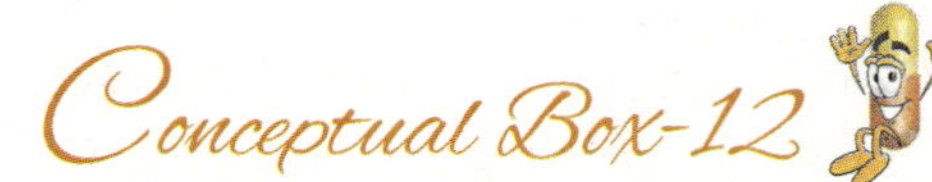

Plasmodium Replication

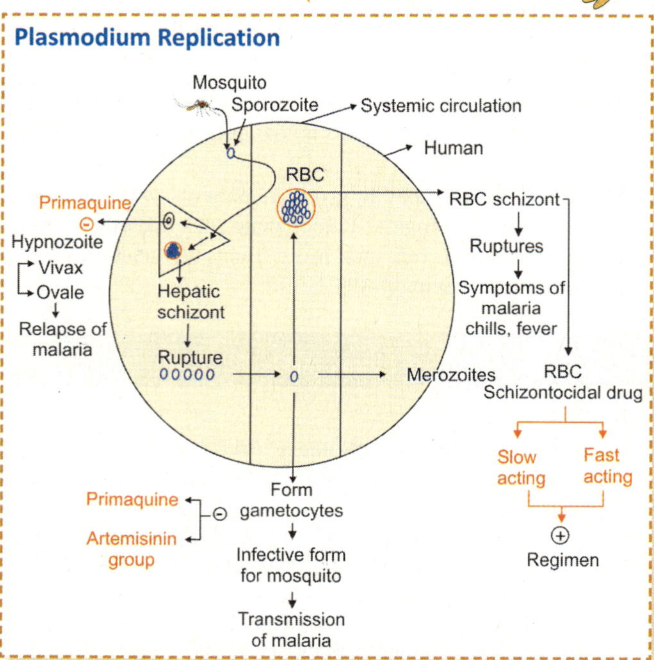

Classification of antimalarial drugs		
Hypnozoite cidal	**Gametocidal**	**Erythrocytic schizontocidal**
Primaquine atovaquone + proguanil tafenoquine	Primaquine artemisinin group	Artemisinin group Atovaquone + proguanil Chloroquine Quinine Mefloquine Sulfadoxine + pyrimethamine Lumefantrine Halofantrine Doxycycline Tetracycline Clindamycin Pyronaridine
Used in radical cure and terminal prophylaxis of malaria to prevent relapse	Used to prevent transmission of malaria	Used in clinical cure of malaria for symptomatic relief

Artemisinin Group Drugs

- **Artemisinin group drugs** are **most potent and fastest acting schizontocidal** drugs but never used as single agents as they **cannot completely clear all parasites** due to their short duration of action. Hence, they are combined with other slow acting schizontocidal drugs.
- They act by producing free radicals and toxic haem products that kills the plasmodium. Since free radicals can cause teratogenicity, these are **absolutely contraindicated in first trimester of pregnancy**. In second and third trimester however, they are used as benefit is more than risk.
- Oral and IM drugs are artesunate, artemether and dihydroartemisinin, whereas only **artesunate can be given by intravenous route**.
- **Intravenous artesunate is the drug of choice for the treatment of severe falciparum malaria**.
- Oral artesunate at dose of **200 mg OD for 3 days** is preferred for the treatment of chloroquine resistant malaria in artesunate combination therapy (ACT). Other oral drugs like artemether or dihydroartemisinin can also be used.
- These drugs are **not used for prophylaxis** of malaria due to their **short half-life**.
- GIT side effects like nausea, vomiting and diarrhea are most commonly seen.

Chloroquine

- Chloroquine enters into the vacuole of plasmodium, where hemoglobin is being digested. Chloroquine binds to haemoglobin and produces toxic haem compounds which are cidal for the plasmodium.
- Resistance is seen because of active **efflux of chloroquine** from the vacuole.
- Chloroquine is the drug of choice for **treatment and prophylaxis of malaria except *P. falciparum* malaria**. As it has a high volume of distribution, **loading dose** is required.
- Other uses of chloroquine are **amebiasis, giardiasis, infectious mononucleosis, PCT, SLE, DLE and rheumatoid arthritis**. Chloroquine is concentrated in lysosomes and can give anti-inflammatory effect.
- Side effects associated are **convulsions, bull's eye retinopathy, hypotension**, hemolysis in G6PD deficiency, myopathy and QRS and T wave abnormalities in ECG.

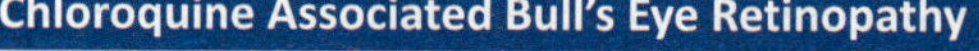

Chloroquine Associated Bull's Eye Retinopathy

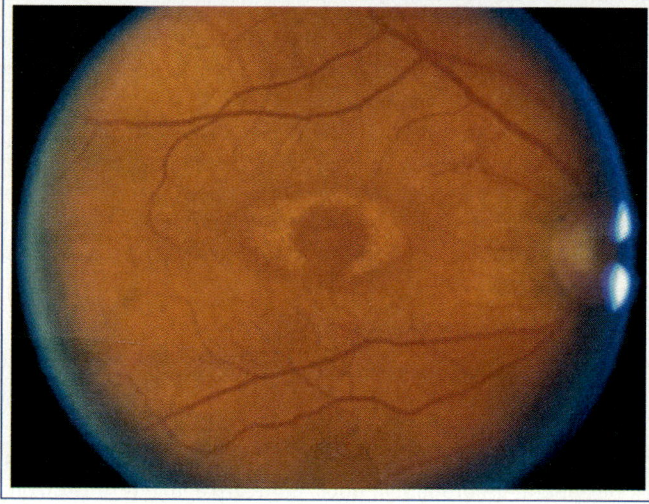

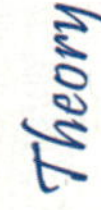

Mnemonics

Side Effects of Chloroquine

- **C :** Convulsions
- **H :** Hemolysis in G6PD deficiency
- **L :** Low blood pressure
- **O :** Ocular – Bull's eye retinopathy
- **R :** qRs and T wave abnormality in ECG

Quinine and Quinidine

- Quinine and quinidine are fast acting schizontocidal and were used in place of artemisinin group for treatment of **severe falciparum malaria and chloroquine resistant malaria.** They are combined with slow acting drugs like tetracycline, doxycycline and clindamycin.
- Quinine is the drug of choice for treatment of chloroquine resistant and falciparum malaria in pregnancy.
- Side effects associated, and causes are given below:

Side effects	Cause
Cinchonism • Tinnitus • Headache • Visual disturbances	Derived from bark of plant cinchona
Hypotension	α_1 receptor block
Hypoglycemia (Given with dextrose)	Insulin release
Black water fever	Inadequate quinine therapy causes hypersensitivity
QT prolongation	Potassium channel block

Mefloquine

- Mefloquine is used for both treatment and prophylaxis of malaria including chloroquine resistant strains. It is used along with artesunate for treatment of severe falciparum malaria.
- Side effects associated are **neuropsychiatric** in nature like seizures and psychosis. It alters cardiac conduction and hence is not used with quinine and quinidine.
- It is contraindicated to be used with quinine, quinidine and halofantrine.

Atovaquone and Proguanil

- Atovaquone inhibits electron transport in mitochondria and proguanil (DHFR inhibitor) causes direct mitochondrial toxicity and hence both are combined for synergistic effect.
- This combination is used for both treatment and prophylaxis of chloroquine resistant malaria and severe falciparum malaria along with artesunate. This combination is also effective against the hypnozoite stage in liver seen with vivax and ovale.
- Atovaquone is also used for the treatment of pneumocystis, babesiosis and toxoplasma.
- **Proguanil** acts on **oocytes of mosquitoes** and inhibits development of sporozoites.

Pyrimethamine

- **Pyrimethamine** inhibits DHFR and is a **slow acting schizontocidal** drug.
- Pyrimethamine along with sulfadoxine and artesunate called as artesunate combination therapy is used for treatment of chloroquine resistant malaria.

Primaquine

- Primaquine acts on the hypnozoite stage, i.e. exoerythrocytic tissue stage and prevents relapse of malaria in vivax and ovale. It is **gametocidal against all species of plasmodium**.
- It is used for **terminal prophylaxis,** i.e. given with chloroquine in patient travelling to an area endemic with vivax or ovale.
- It is always used for the treatment of vivax and ovale along with chloroquine for **radical cure**.
- **It is contraindicated in pregnancy and lactation and infants**.
- Side effects like **methemoglobinemia, anemia, leukocytosis and hemolysis in G6PD deficiency** can be seen. Among all antimalarials **most definitive evidence of hemolysis in G6PD deficiency is against primaquine**. In G6PD deficient individuals' **weekly therapy** can be given for 8 weeks with close monitoring of hematological status.

Tafenoquine

- Tafenoquine also acts on hypnozoite stage, i.e. exoerythrocytic tissue stage and prevents relapse of malaria in vivax and ovale.
- It is used for radical cure of malaria caused by vivax and ovale. Unlike primaquine which needs to be given for 14 days, 300 mg of tafenoquine is given once on the first or second day of therapy with other drugs like chloroquine.
- Side effects associated are hemolysis in G6PD deficiency, methemoglobinemia, and neuropsychiatric side effects.
- Pregnancy, lactation and age group less than 16 years are absolute contraindication.

Halofantrine and Lumefantrine

- Halofantrine is a phenanthrene methanol and lumefantrine is an amino alcohol.
- Both are used for the treatment of chloroquine resistant malaria; lumefantrine is used along with artemether.
- Halofantrine can cause QT prolongation and hence not used nowadays.

Pyronaridine

- Pyronaridine is a mannich-base schizontocidal used by oral route for treatment of chloroquine resistant malaria along with artesunate.

Antibiotics

- Tetracycline, doxycycline and clindamycin are slow acting schizontocidal used for the treatment of chloroquine resistant malaria in regimens.

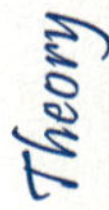

- Doxycycline is also used for short term (<6 weeks) prophylaxis of malaria.
- Sulfadoxine + pyrimethamine is used along with artesunate for the treatment of chloroquine resistant malaria. It can cause cutaneous skin reactions like **erythema multiforme** and Steven Johnson's syndrome and hence is not preferred for prophylaxis of malaria.

Malaria Guidelines by NVBDCP (National Vector Born Disease Control Program) India

Treatment of Malaria

Vivax	Falciparum			Mixed infection
Chloroquine 3 d + Primaquine 14 d	For all states	Artemether 3d + Lumefantrine 3d + Primaquine single dose on day 2	North-east	Add primaquine for 14 days to falciparum regimen for North East
d = days		Artesunate 3d + Sulfadoxine 3d + Pyrimethamine 3d + Primaquine single dose on day 2	Other state	Add primaquine for 14 days to falciparum regimen for other states

Note: Primaquine is contraindicated in pregnant and infants.

Severe Falciparum Malaria

Parenteral therapy for 48 hours	Oral therapy after 48 hours
Artesunate: Dug of choice Artemether Arteether	ACT as described for Northeast and other states
Quinine	Quinine + doxycycline or clindamycin (Pregnancy)

Prophylaxis of Malaria

Prophylaxis is given only if patient is travelling to falciparum endemic area.

Travel duration <6 weeks	Travel duration >6 weeks
Drug of choice is Doxycycline 100 mg OD started 2 days before travel and continued for 4 weeks after leaving the endemic area.	Drug of choice is **Mefloquine 250 mg weekly** started two weeks before travel and continued for 4 weeks after leaving endemic area.

Malaria in Pregnancy

Treatment of vivax, falciparum and mixed infection	Severe falciparum malaria	Prophylaxis
Everything remains same except • Primaquine is contraindicated and given postpartum • ACT contraindicated in first trimester **1st trimester:** Quinine **2nd and 3rd trimester:** ACT as described earlier	Quinine followed by quinine plus clindamycin	Mefloquine

Recent Advances

Anti-malaria Vaccines

RTS, S/ AS01 (Mosquirix TM): It is a genetically engineered vaccine synthesized from repeat region and T cell epitope (RT) of the circumsporozoite protein of *P. falciparum* carried by HBs Ag (S) and coexpressed within Saccharomyces cerevisiae (S). ASO1 is the adjuvant used to increase efficacy of vaccine. It provides humoral immunity to surface exposed sporozoite proteins and TH1 type cell mediated immunity to free sporozoites of *P. falciparum* in blood.

RTS, S-AS01/ ChAd63-TRAP/MVA-TRAP: The RTS, S-AS01 vaccine is combined with viral vectors like ChAd63-TRAP or MVA-TRAP which are modified so that they cannot multiply. However, these viruses have DNA and hence they can make malaria proteins against which both cell mediated, and humoral immunity is developed.

RTS, S-AS01 delayed fractional dose: Repetition using large fractional booster dose to determine the high level of efficacy.

Multivalent ChAd63/MVA: Multiple antigens of plasmodium in viral vectors like Chimpanzee Adenovirus 63 and Modified Vaccinia virus Ankara help in developing humoral and cell mediated immunity.

Multivalent pDNA/adenovirus: Multiple antigens of plasmodium from all stages are incorporated into adenovirus and plasmid DNA. The aim of plasmid DNA is to prime and recombinant adenovirus to boost the production of these antigens.

PvDBPII: Antibodies to *P. vivax* Duffy Binding Protein II prevents entry of *P. vivax* into red blood cell and thus prevent or reduce clinical disease.

Pfs25-VLP: It is an antibody against Pre-fertilization antigen (Pfs25) expressed in gametocytes which blocks transmission of the parasite from humans to mosquitoes by preventing the parasite from developing in the mosquito.

Contd...

> **Recent Advances**
>
> **PfSPZ:** A whole parasite vaccine against *P. falciparum* called as *P. falciparum* Sporozoite (PfSPZ) vaccine is being developed that is given by intravenous route.
>
> **VMP001/AS01B:** Vivax Malaria Protein 1 vaccine is a vaccine against some regions of circumsporozoite protein of *P. falciparum*. It provides protection against all strains.

ANTIPROTOZOAL DRUGS

AMEBIASIS

Amebiasis is an infectious disease caused by protozoa Entamoeba histolytica. Infection can be intestinal (asymptomatic or symptomatic) or extraintestinal (liver and other tissues).

Asymptomatic Intestinal Amebiasis

In case of asymptomatic intestinal infection luminal amoebicidal agents like paromomycin, diloxanide furoate and iodoquinol are used.

Paromomycin

- Paromomycin is an aminoglycoside which is most effective luminal amoebicidal drug and hence is drug of choice for treatment of asymptomatic intestinal amebiasis. It is also used for the treatment of other infections as alternatives.

Paromomycin route	Uses
Oral	Asymptomatic intestinal amebiasis Giardiasis Cryptosporidiosis
Intravenous	Visceral leishmaniasis (Kala-azar)
Topical	Cutaneous leishmaniasis Trichomoniasis

Asymptomatic intestinal	Symptomatic intestinal; extra-intestinal
Paromomycin (DOC) Diloxanide furoate Iodoquinol	**Metronidazole (DOC)** Tinidazole Nitazoxanide Emetine Dihydroemetine Chloroquine

- As it is not absorbed, side effects are limited to GIT like nausea, vomiting and diarrhea. It can be safely used in pregnancy due to no systemic absorption.

Diloxanide Furoate

- Diloxanide furoate breaks down in intestine into diloxanide and furoic acid; diloxanide produces intestinal amoebicidal effect.
- Side effects are limited to GIT like nausea, vomiting and diarrhea. It is contraindicated in pregnancy as diloxanide undergoes systemic absorption and cause teratogenicity.

Iodoquinol

- Iodoquinol is also a good luminal amoebicidal agent but is less preferred due to toxicity. It is **drug of choice for treatment of dientamoeba fragilis.**
- At normal doses side effects are limited to GIT like nausea, vomiting and diarrhea. But at high doses It is associated with neurotoxicity that can present as optic atrophy (blindness) and peripheral neuropathy. It is contraindicated in patients with iodine intolerance.

Symptomatic Intestinal or Extraintestinal Amebiasis

- In extraintestinal infection or symptomatic intestinal infection drugs active on tissue form of amoeba, i.e. trophozoites, like metronidazole, tinidazole, chloroquine, nitazoxanide, emetine and dehydroemetine are used. But since these are not effective against the luminal amoeba, a luminal amoebicidal drug should be added.
- For symptomatic intestinal infection, i.e. colitis tetracycline or erythromycin can also be used, but these are not effective in extraintestinal cases.

Nitroimidazoles

- **Metronidazole, benznidazole, satranidazole and tinidazole** are nitroimidazoles that acts by free radical production.
- **Metronidazole** is the drug of choice for treatment of **bacteroides (infradiaphragmatic anaerobic infections), symptomatic intestinal amebiasis, extra intestinal amebiasis, giardiasis, bacterial vaginosis, trichomoniasis (strawberry vagina) and tetanus.** It can also be used for treatment of mild/moderate pseudomembranous enterocolitis.
- Tinidazole can be used for the treatment of amebiasis and giardiasis. **Benznidazole** is the drug of choice for **Chagas's disease**. **Secnidazole** is recent nitroimidazole approved for treatment of bacterial vaginosis.
- Side effects associated with metronidazole are **reddish brown discolouration of urine, dysgeusia, neurologic symptoms and cystitis**. It can **sensitize tumor cells to radiation**. Metronidazole can cause toxicity of warfarin and lithium. Pregnancy is an absolute contraindication to use of metronidazole.
- All drugs in this class can cause disulfiram like reaction when consumed with alcohol except satranidazole.

Nitazoxanide

Nitazoxanide is primarily used for treatment if cryptosporidiosis and is discussed in detail ahead.

Emetine/Dihydroemetine

- Emetine and dihydroemetine are used by subcutaneous or intramuscular route.
- Both are rarely used due to toxicity like injection site reactions, GIT upset and cardiovascular toxicity (heart failure, arrhythmia and hypotension).

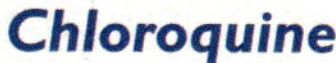

Chloroquine

Chloroquine is an antimalarial drug with activity against amebiasis as well. It is particularly used for treatment of metronidazole resistant amoebic liver abscess.

TRYPANOSOMIASIS

African Trypansomiasis (Sleeping Sickness)

African trypanasomiasis can be broadly classified as east and west African, which can be further subclassified as early and late stage trypansomiasis. The drugs of choice for all are different because strains are different in east and west African sleeping sickness. The drugs of choice are different even in early and late stage because CNS is not involved in early stage and involved in late stage. Hence, CNS penetration is crucial in late stage and most lipid soluble drug is preferred.

- **Eflornithine** acts by inhibiting ornithine decarboxylase, enzyme required for synthesis of polyamines required for cell division. It has poor oral bioavailability and hence is used by intravenous route. It is drug of choice for late stage west African sleeping sickness and it is combined with nifurtimox. In humans it can block cell proliferation and give anticancer effect and side effects like bone marrow suppression and GIT toxicity (nausea, vomiting, diarrhea). It can also cause seizures and hearing loss.
- **Melarsoprol** is an arsenic containing drug given by intravenous route. It is drug of choice for treatment of late stage east African sleeping sickness and is a second line drug for late stage west African sleeping sickness. It is associated with side effects like encephalopathy (prednisolone given to prevent it), myocardial toxicity, renal toxicity, fever, arsenic induced neuropathy. Overall it is the most lethal drug in this class.

Mnemonics

Side Effects of Melarsoprol

M : Myocardial toxicity
E : Encephalopathy
L : Lethal drug
A : Arsenic induced neuropathy
R : Renal toxicity

- **Pentamidine** inhibits topoisomerase II and is given by intravenous routes for treatment of sleeping sickness, leishmaniasis and resistant pneumosyctis infection. By inhalational route it is used for prophylaxis of resistant **pneumocystis infection**. It is associated with side effects like hypotension, prolonged hypoglycemia followed by hyperglycemia, tachycardia and hypertension.

Mnemonics

Side Effects of Pentamidine

H : Hypotension, Hypoglycemia
T : Tachycardia
N : Nephrotoxicity

- **Suramin** acts by inhibiting serine oligopeptidase and is given by intravenous route. It is drug of choice for treatment of early stage east African sleeping sickness and can be used as a second line drug for early stage west African sleeping sickness. Side effects are early onset (nausea, vomiting, seizure, shock) and late onset (fever, nephrotoxicity, neuropathy, agranulocytosis, anemia).

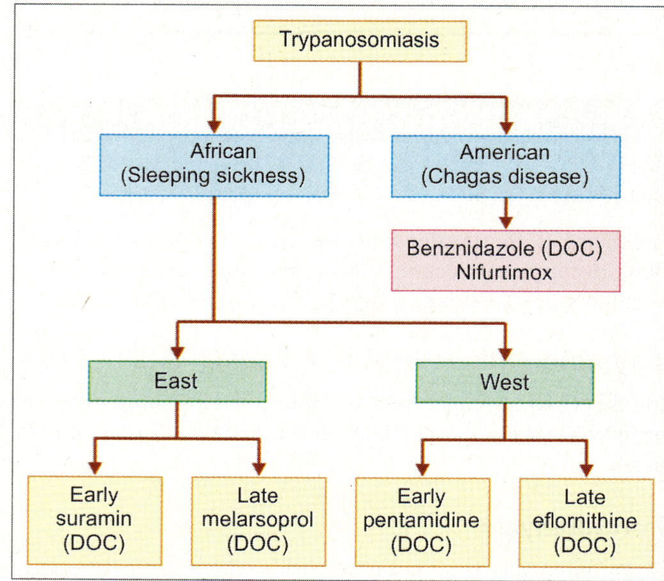

American Trypanosomiasis (Chagas Disease)

In Chagas disease oral drugs like benznidazole and nifurtimox are commonly used drugs. Both these drugs act by free radical production and have cidal effect on the protozoa.

- **Benznidazole** is a nitroimidazole, which is drug of choice for treatment of Chagas disease because it is less toxic than nifurtimox.
- **Nifurtimox** acts by producing free radicals and can be used in Chagas disease as well as late stage west African sleeping sickness. It is a very toxic drug and hence frequently associated with incompliance.

LEISHMANIASIS

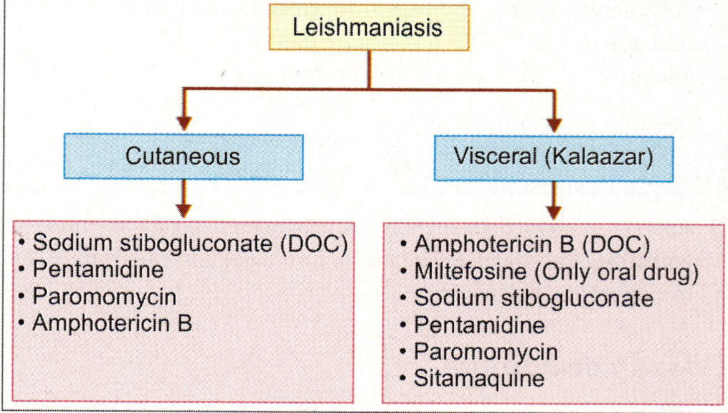

- **Intravenous liposomal amphotericin B** is the drug of choice for the treatment of visceral leishmaniasis (kala-azar). It can also be used for the treatment of cutaneous leishmaniasis. The mechanism of action is like its antifungal effect, i.e. sequesters ergosterol in the cell membrane (new mechanism) or forms pores in the cell membrane by getting into ergosterol (old mechanism). Other details about amphotericin B has been discusses in the topic of antifungal drugs.

- **Sodium stibogluconate** acts by producing free radicals. It is given by intravenous or intramuscular route (painful) for Kala-azar but not preferred in India due to resistance. Topical sodium stibogluconate is still drug of choice for cutaneous leishmaniasis. Most common side effect is pancreatitis and it can also cause QT prolongation and bone marrow suppression.
- **Miltefosine** acts by disrupting lipid metabolism. It is the **only oral drug** available for the treatment of Kala-azar. Dose limiting side effect is **vomiting and diarrhea**. It has a half-life of one week. It is a teratogenic drug and hence contraindicated in pregnancy. Thus, contraception must be used by females not only during drug intake but also for 5 months after completion of drug therapy.
- **Intravenous paromomycin** and **pentamidine** are second line drugs for treatment of both visceral and cutaneous leishmaniasis.
- **Sitamaquine** is an oral drug for treatment of visceral leishmaniasis. Its development was stopped due to nephrotoxicity.

COCCIDIOSIS

Cryptosporidiosis

- **Nitazoxanide** is the drug of choice for the treatment of **cryptosporidiosis and resistant giardiasis.** It is a wide spectrum drug with **antiparasitic, antihelminthic, antibacterial and antiviral effect.** Nitazoxanide has been synthesized from an antihelminthic drug **niclosamide**. It acts by inhibiting an enzyme for electron transport, i.e. **PFOR (Pyruvate Ferredoxin Oxido Reductase)** in the protozoas. It can cause **green discolouration of urine**.
- **Oral paromomycin** is equally effective in treatment of cryptosporidiosis.

Isosporiasis, Cyclosporiasis and Sarcocystosis

- **Cotrimoxazole** is the drug of choice for isosporiasis, cyclosporiasis and sarcocystosis.
- Pyrimethamine along with folinic acid for isosporiasis, ciprofloxacin for cyclosporiasis and albendazole for sarcocystosis are other alternatives.

MICROSPORIDIOSIS

- Albendazole is the drug of choice for the treatment of microsporidiosis.
- Fumagillin can be used as an alternate in resistant cases. It is associated with thrombocytopenia, which is reversible on drug discontinuation.

BABESIOSIS

- In mild to moderate cases **atovaquone + azithromycin** is preferred due to lesser side effects.
- **Quinine + clindamycin** is reserved for treatment of severe cases, as this combination is more toxic.

TOXOPLASMOSIS

- **Sulfadiazine + pyrimethamine** combination is the treatment of choice for toxoplasmosis. Alternatives are **clindamycin + pyrimethamine** and **cotrimoxazole + pyrimethamine**. To prevent bone marrow suppression caused by pyrimethamine, folinic acid is also added.
- Pyrimethamine is teratogenic and hence **spiramycin** is the drug of choice for toxoplasmosis in **pregnancy**.

ANTIHELMINTHIC DRUGS

Nematodes: Drug of choice			
Soil transmitted helminths Round worm Hook worm Whip worm Trichinella spiralis Enterovirus vermicularis	Albendazole	Thread worm Onchocerca Volvulus	Ivermectin
		Filariasis Loa Loa	DEC
		Dracunculiasis	Metronidazole
Cestodes: Drug of choice			
Neurocysticercosis Echinococcus	Albendazole	Intestinal T. solium T. saginata H. nana D. latum	Praziquantel
Trematodes: Drug of choice			
Liver Fluke	Triclabendazole	Lung fluke Schistosoma	Praziquantel

BENZIMIDAZOLES

- Benzimidazoles inhibit β tubulin which leads to decreased polymerization of **microtubules** in the cytoplasm. Cytoplasmic microtubules are required for glucose uptake in intestine of helminth. Thus, there is a decreased glucose uptake, which subsequently decreases ATP and mobility of helminth. These causes a delayed response of this class and hence are slower acting than other antihelminthics which directly act on ion channels.
- The drugs that belong to this class are **albendazole, mebendazole, triclabendazole and thiabendazole.**
- These drugs have poor oral absorption and high first pass metabolism; however **absorption is increased by fatty food**. First pass metabolism inactivates these drugs except albendazole which is converted into an active metabolite albendazole sulfoxide. Albendazole sulfoxide has high distribution into tissues and hence is the most effective benzimidazole against tissue form of helminths. Excretion of these drugs is primarily by **kidney**.
- These are the widest spectrum drugs active against all three classes of helminths. Albendazole is also drug of choice for treatment of **microsporidiosis**.
- Most common side effect is **hepatotoxicity**; others are nausea and vomiting, leucopenia and thrombocytopenia. Thiabendazole is most toxic drug in this class and hence is less preferred.
- The safety of these drugs is not established in **pregnancy** and **children less than 2 years**; however they can be used if the benefit outweighs the risk.

IVERMECTIN

- Ivermectin acts by stimulating **glutamate sensitive chloride channels in the helminth**, which causes hyperpolarization and induces a **flaccid paralysis**.
- These channels are only present in nematodes and hence **ivermectin is not active against cestodes and trematodes.**
- Ivermectin is drug of choice for **thread worm and Onchocerca volvulus** and for remaining nematodes it is a second line drug.
- It is the only oral drug used for the treatment of **ectoparasite like scabies**.
- When given for the treatment of filariasis, the dying filarial parasite can cause a hypersensitivity reaction called as **Mazzotti like reaction**. Hence, it is contraindicated in coinfection of filariasis and Onchocerca volvulus as the reaction can worsen ocular symptoms.
- It is also contraindicated in pregnancy and children less than 5 years.

Recent Advances

Moxidectin: It is a new antihelminthic drug approved for treatment of *O. volvulus*. It acts by stimulating glutamate sensitive chloride channels, which leads to flaccid paralysis.

DIETHYL CARBAMAZINE (DEC)

- The mechanism of action of DEC is not known, however is the drug of choice in **filariasis and Loa loa.** Doxycycline can be used as an alternative for the treatment of filariasis.
- It causes ocular side effects like uveitis, punctate keratitis and retinal atrophy.

PRAZIQUANTEL

- Praziquantel stimulates calcium influx and causes **spastic paralysis** in the helminth.
- It is drug of choice for some cestodes and trematodes discussed in the box.
- Side effects associated are impaired alertness, nausea and vomiting, arthralgia and myalgia.
- It is **contraindicated in ocular cysticercosis** as there can be irreversible ocular damage.

MISCELLANEOUS DRUGS

Metrifonate

- Metrifonate is an organophosphate that inhibits ACHE. This increases acetylcholine, which causes persistent depolarization of N_M receptors and induces a **spastic paralysis**.
- It is a prodrug that is converted into dichlorovos.
- Use is restricted to ***Schistosoma haematobium***.

Pyrantel Pamoate

- Pyrantel pamoate is a depolarizing neuromuscular blocking agent, which causes **spastic paralysis.**
- It is a second line drug for treatment of round worm, enterobius vermicularis and hook worm.

Piperazine

- Piperazine is a $GABA_A$ agonist and hence causes **flaccid paralysis** in the helminths.
- It is used as a second line drug for the treatment of round worm and enterobius vermicularis.
- Its use is associated with **seizure**, lethargy (most common) and hemolysis in patients with G6PD deficiency. It can cause asthma in workers handling piperazine.

Niclosamide

- Niclosamide acts by inhibiting oxidative phosphorylation in helminths.
- It is a second line drug for all cestodes, but not used in NCC, due to risk of ova release from gravid worms that can form larvae and cause cysticercosis.

Oxamniquine

- Oxamniquine by unknown mechanism induces a spastic paralysis in the helminths.
- It is a second line drug for the treatment of *Schistosoma mansoni*.

Bithionol

- Bithionol is used as a second line drug for treatment of lung and liver flukes.
- Side effects associated are GIT upset, rash and headache.

Tribendimidine

- Tribendimidine acts by stimulating the nicotinic acetylcholine receptors, which causes spastic paralysis.
- It is used for the treatment of soil transmitted helminths like round worm, whip worm and hook worm.

Levamisole

- Levamisole acts by stimulating nicotinic acetylcholine receptors, which causes spastic paralysis. It is used for the treatment of soil transmitted helminths like round worm, whip worm and hook worm. It is also used as an immunomodulator.
- Side effects associated are GIT upset and agranulocytosis.

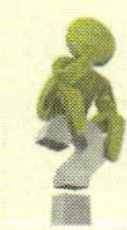

Image-based Questions

1. **Resistance to methicillin in the microorganisms given in the picture is seen because of:**

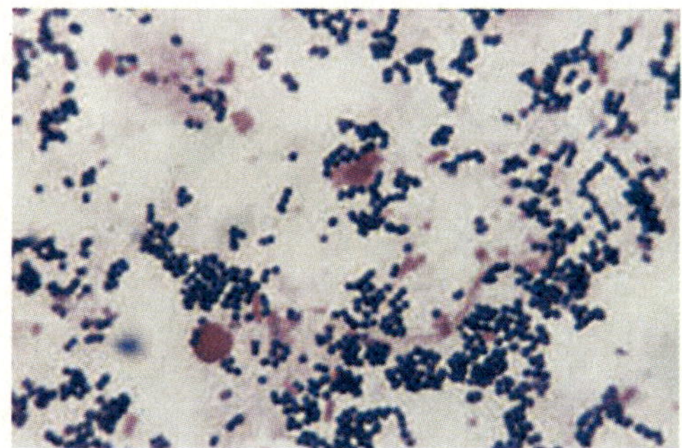

a. Beta lactamase
b. Efflux
c. Altered PBP
d. Mec A gene

2. **Which of the following is the drug of choice for the patient with severe headache and the following finding in the extremities?**

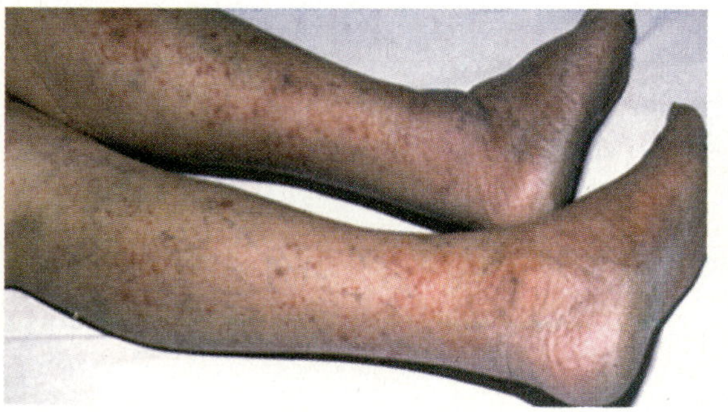

a. Ceftriaxone
b. Rifampicin
c. Penicillin-G
d. Ciprofloxacin

3. **Which of the following is the drug of choice for the condition given in the picture?**

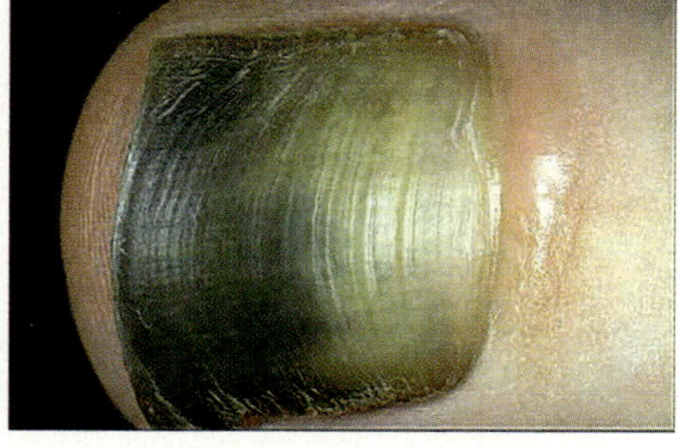

a. Piperacillin
b. Ceftriaxone
c. Carbapenams
d. Ceftazidime

4. **A 35-year-old man after 24 hours of one night stand developed discharge as given in the picture. What is the most preferred drug for this condition?**

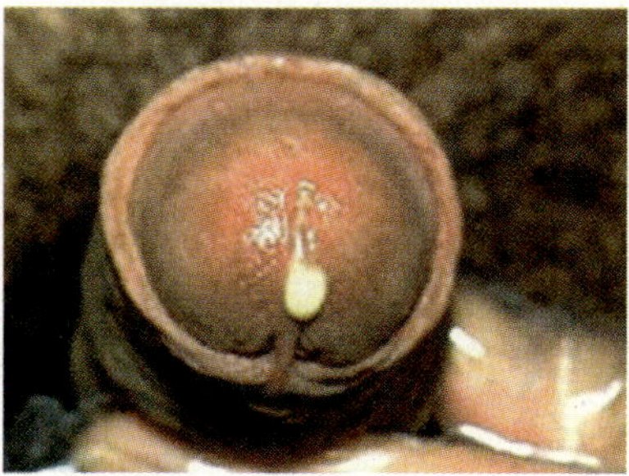

a. Gentamicin
b. Doxycycline
c. Penicillin G
d. Ceftriaxone

5. **The group encircled in the picture is present with which of the following cephalosporin:**

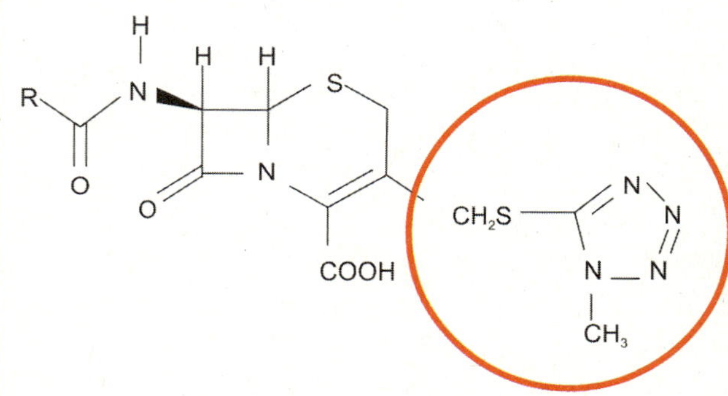

a. Ceftriaxone
b. Cefazoline
c. Cefotetan
d. Cefoxitin

6. **Which of the following antibiotic is not used in the condition given in the picture?**

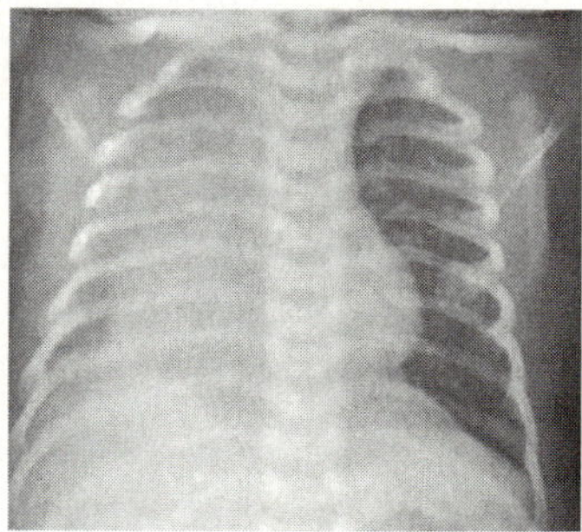

a. Vancomycin
b. Piperacillin
c. Meropenem
d. Daptomycin

7. **Which of the following drug is preferred for the procedure given in the picture?**

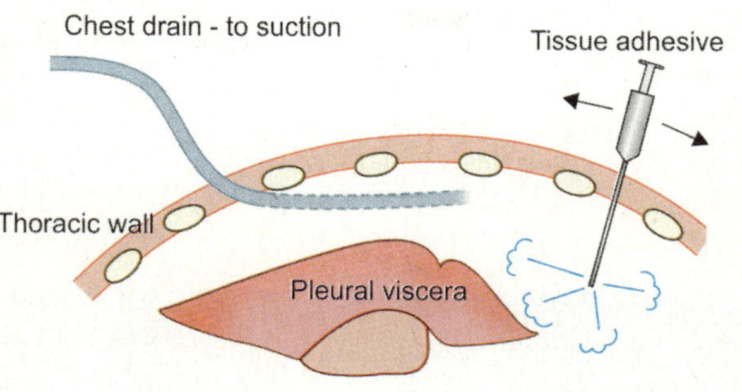

a. Talc
b. Mitomycin
c. Streptomycin
d. Doxycycline

8. **Which of the following is the drug of choice for treatment of the condition given in the picture?**

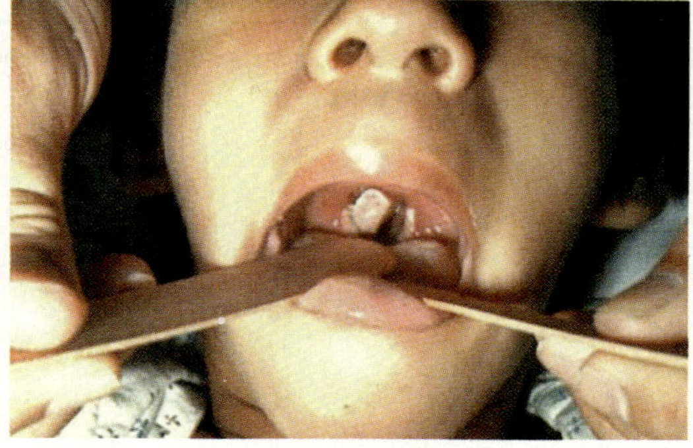

a. Doxycycline
b. Gentamycin
c. Penicillin G
d. Erythromycin

9. **A gardener had an accidental wound while working and that was followed by infection of the leg with multiple draining tracks as given in the picture. Which of the following is the preferred drug for treatment?**

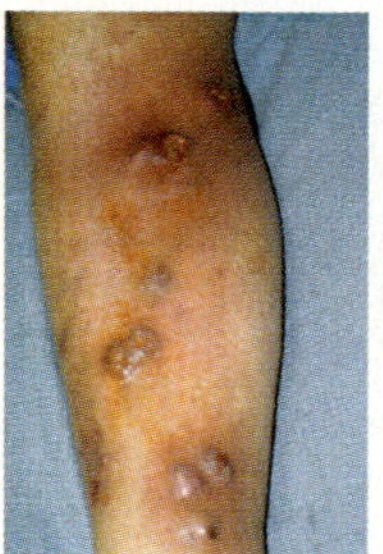

a. Doxycycline
b. Gentamicin
c. Ceftriaxone
d. Cotrimoxazole

10. **The blister packet of drugs given in the picture is used in**

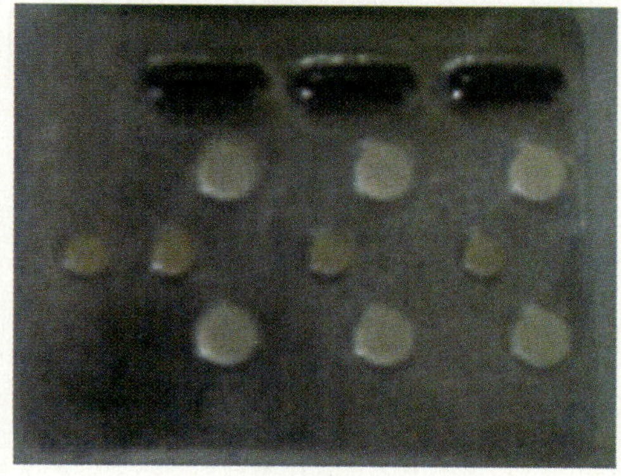

a. Leprosy
b. HIV
c. Chlamydia
d. Tuberculosis

11. **The structure given in the picture is targeted by:**

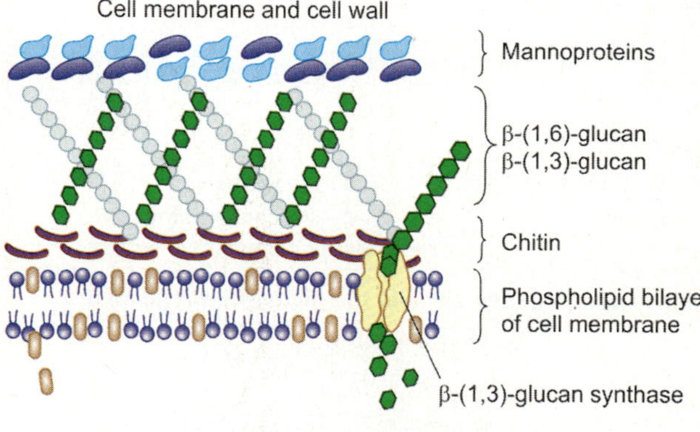

a. Azoles
b. Amphotericin B
c. Echinocandins
d. Griseofulvin

12. **What is the drug of choice for treatment of the organism given in the picture?**

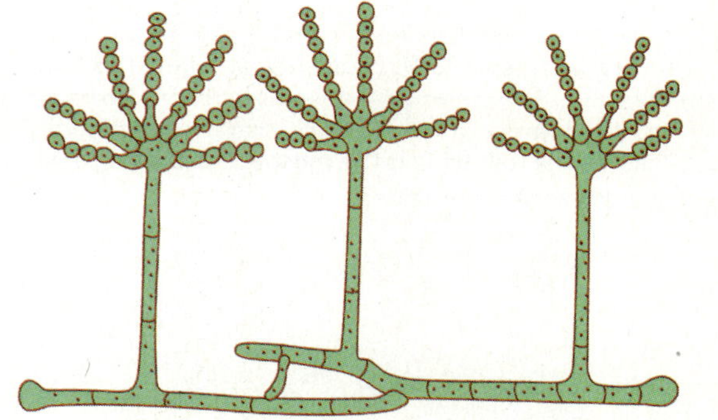

a. Amphotericin B
b. Fluconazole
c. Voriconazole
d. Posaconazole

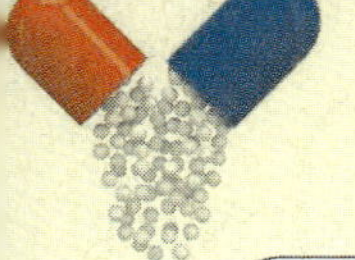

13. The part of treatment education chart given in the pic is for

If you have:	Do the following:
Nausea	Take the pill with food.
Diarrhea	Keep drinking and eating

If Nausea or diarrhea persist of get worse, or you have any of the following, report to the health worker **AT THE NEXT VISIT.**

- Tingling, number or painful feet or legs or hands.
- Arms, legs, buttock, and cheeks become THIN.
- Breasts, body, back of neck become FAT

a. Hepatitis B b. HIV
c. Tuberculosis d. Leprosy

14. Which of the following is the drug of choice for treatment of the condition given in the picture?

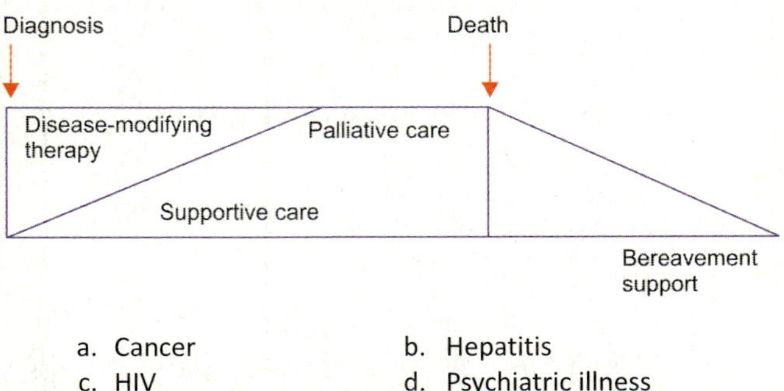

a. Cancer b. Hepatitis
c. HIV d. Psychiatric illness

15. The drug regimen given in the picture is not given if:

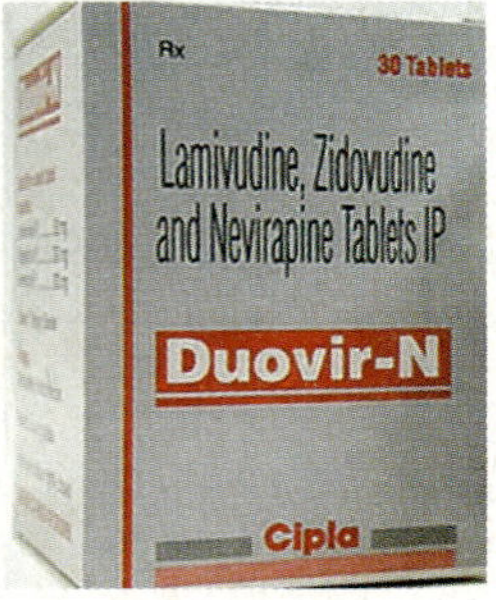

a. Patient on Rifampicin b. Hb >8 mg/dL
c. HIV with hepatitis B d. HIV with hepatitis C

16. Which of the following is the most active drug against the organism seen in the slide?

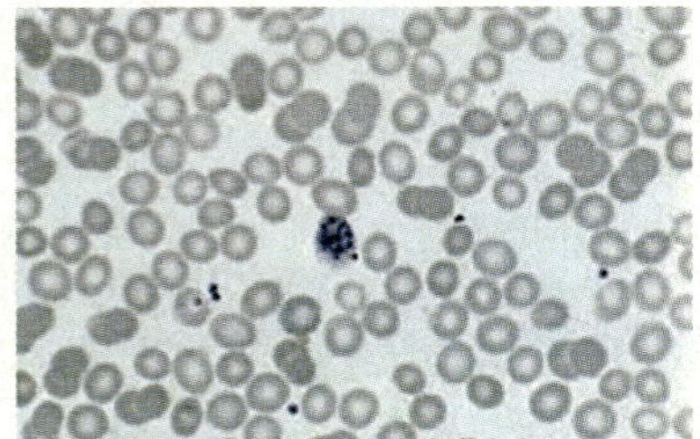

a. Chloroquine b. Quinine
c. Mefloquine d. Artesunate

17. The coloured package blisters given in the picture are used for treatment of:

Age group (Years)	1st day		2nd day		3rd day
	AS	SP	AS	PQ	AS
0-1 Pink Blister	1 (25 mg)	1 (250+12.5 mg)	1 (25 mg)	Nil	1 (25 mg)
1-4 Yellow Blister	1 (50 mg)	1 (500+25 mg each)	1 (50 mg)	1 (7.5 mg base)	1 (50 mg)
5–8 Green Blister	1 (100 mg)	1 (750+37.5 mg each)	1 (100 mg)	2 (7.5 mg base each)	1 (100 mg)
9–14 Red Blister	1 (150 mg)	2 (500+25 mg each)	1 (150 mg)	4 (7.5 mg base each)	1 (150 mg)
15 & Above White Blister	1 (200 mg)	2 (750+37.5 mg each)	1 (200 mg)	6 (7.5 mg base each)	1 (200 mg)

a. Tuberculosis b. Leprosy
c. HIV d. Malaria

18. Which of the following is the preferred drug for treatment of organism given in the picture?

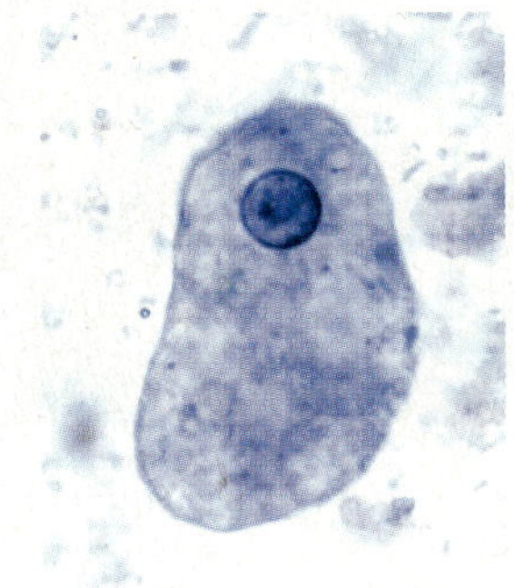

a. Metronidazole b. Albendazole
c. Tinidazole d. Mebendazole

19. The organism in the picture responds best to:

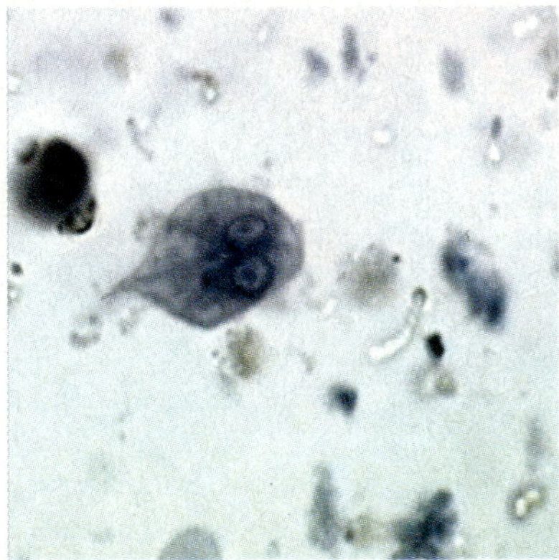

a. Metronidazole b. Albendazole
c. Tinidazole d. Mebendazole

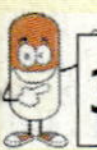
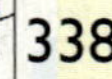

Answers with Explanations to Image-based Questions

1. Ans. (d) Mec A gene

(Ref: Goodman Gilman 12th E/P 1479)

- The grape like clusters in the gram stain are staphylococcus aureus, in which resistance is seen by penicillinase production.
- But in penicillinase resistant penicillin like methicillin resistance is due to altered penicillin binding protein.

2. Ans. (a) Ceftriaxone

(Ref: Goodman Gilman 12th E/P1484)

3. Ans. (d) Ceftazidime

(Ref: Goodman Gilman 12th E/P1498)

- The condition given in the picture is known as green nail syndrome, caused by pseudomonas.
- Ceftazidime is the antibiotic of choice for pseudomonas infection.

4. Ans. (d) Ceftriaxone

(Ref: Goodman Gilman 12th E/P1498)

- The white coloured discharge seen in the picture is specific for gonorrhoea.
- Ceftriaxone is the drug of choice for gonorrhoea.

5. Ans. (d) Cefoxitin

(Ref: Goodman Gilman 12th E/P1494)

- The extra group present in the cefalosporin, which is encircled is methylthiotetrazole group present in cefamandole, cefotetan, moxalactam and cefoperazone.

6. Ans. (d) Daptomycin

(Ref: Goodman Gilman 12th E/P1543)

- The X-ray given is a case of lobar pneumonia caused by staphylococcus.
- Daptomycin is not used in pneumonia as it is inactivated by surfactant.

7. Ans. (d) Doxycycline

(Ref: Harrison 19th E/P474)

- The procedure given in the picture is called as pleurodesis, done for recurrent pneumothorax and cardiac tamponade.
- The drug of choice for this procedure is doxycycline.

8. Ans. (d) Erythromycin

(Ref: Goodman Gilman 12th E/P1532)

- The condition given in the picture is diphtheria.
- The drug of choice in diphtheria is erythromycin.

9. Ans. (d) Cotrimoxazole

(Ref: Goodman Gilman 12th E/P1470)

- Multiple draining tracks are present in nocardiosis.
- The drug of choice for same is cotrimoxazole.

10. Ans. (d) Tuberculosis

(Ref: RNTCP guidelines)

- The blister packet given in the picture is used for category III tuberculosis.
- It contains three drugs Isoniazid, Rifampicin and Pyrazinamide.

11. Ans. (c) Echinocandins

(Ref: Goodman Gilman 12th E/P1582)

- The structure given in the picture i.e. beta glucan synthase is targeted by antifungal drugs called as echinocandins.

12. Ans. (c) Voriconazole

(Ref: Goodman Gilman 12th E/P1581)

- The organism given in the picture is aspergillus.
- Voriconazole is the drug of choice for aspergillosis.

13. Ans. (b) HIV

(Ref: NACO Guidelines 2011)

14. Ans. (c) HIV

(Ref: NACO Guidelines 2011)

- The approach of disease modifying therapy along with palliative and supportive care has been recommended by WHO and also by NACO for HIV patients.

15. Ans. (a) Patient on Riampicin

(Ref: NACO Guidelines 2011)

- Patient on rifampicin should not be given nevirapine as it is metabolized by CYP3A4.
- Rather efavirenz is substituted in its place in case of tuberculosis.

16. Ans. (d) Artesunate

(Ref: Goodman Gilman 12th E/P1395)

- This is the ring stage of falciparum with schizont seen at center.
- The most effective drug against falciparum currently is artesunate.

17. Ans. (d) Malaria

(Ref: NVDCP Guidelines 2013, Malaria India)

- The different coloured blister packages have been made for different age groups for treatment of falciparum malaria with ACT.

18. Ans. (a) Metronidazole

(Ref: Goodman Gilman 12th E/P1429)

- The organism given in the picture is Entamoeba Histolytica, for which metronidazole is the drug of choice.

19. Ans. (c) Tinidazole

(Ref: Goodman Gilman 12th E/P1429)

- The organism with tennis racket appearance is giardia.
- Drug of choice for giardiasis is tinidazole.

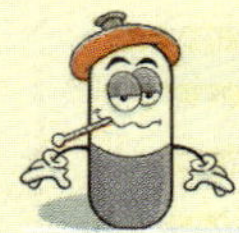

Annexures

Drug of Choice

Condition	Drug of Choice
Acinetobacter ESBL organisms Serratia Enterobacter	Carbapenams
Actinomycosis Anthrax Gas gangrene Leptospira Rat Bite Fever Streptococcus Syphilis Yaws	Penicillin G
Amoeba	• Extraintestinal/Intestinal symptomatic– Metronidazole • Intestinal asymptomatic – Paromomycin
Anaerobes	• Supradiaphragmatic Infections e.g. Prevotella ▪ Clindamycin • Infradiaphragmatic infections e.g. Bacteroides ▪ Metronidazole
Aspergillus Scedosporium Trichosporon	Voriconazole
Amebiasis (Extraintestinal/ Intestinal Symptomatic) Bacterial Vaginosis Bacteroides Tetanus Trichomoniasis Giardiasis	**Metronidazole**
Borerllia Brucella (+Rifampin) Bartonella Chlamydia Cholera Granuloma inguinale Lymphogranuloma venereum Mycoplasma hominis Inflammatory acne Rickettsia Pleurodesis Pericardiodesis	**Doxycycline**
Babesiosis	• Atovaquone Plus • Azithromycin
Chancroid Legionella Mycoplasma pneumonie Chlamydia and cholera in pregnancy Campylobacter	Azithromycin
Burn Infection	Silver Sulfadiazine
Diphtheria Pertussis	Erythromycin
Candida Coccidioidal Meningitis	Fluconazole
Cestodes	• Albendazole ▪ T. solium (NCC) ▪ Echinococcus • Praziquantel ▪ T. saginata ▪ H. nana ▪ D. latum ▪ T. solium (Intestinal)
Chagas disease (American Trypansomiasis)	Benznidazole
Clostridium difficile	Oral vancomycin
Cryptococcus Kala-azar Mucormycosis Primary amoebic meningoencephalitis Systemic fungal infections	Amphotericin B
Cryptosporidium	Nitazoxanide
Dermatophytes	• Terbinafine except for T. capitis • T. capitis – Griseofulvin
Diarrhea (Empirical Therapy)	Fluoroquinolones

E. coli Gonococcus HACEK organisms H. influenza meningitis Meningococcal meningitis Klebsiella Providencia Typhoid Salmonella Acute bacterial meningitis (Empirical treatment) Meningitis with basilar skull fracture Brain abscess Subdural empyema	Ceftriaxone
Endemic Mycoses Sporotrichosis	Itraconazole
Enterococcus	• Enterococcus faecalis – Ampicillin + Aminoglycoside • Enterococcus faecium – Vancomycin + Aminoglycoside • Aminoglycoside toxicity – Ampicillin or Vancomycin + Ceftriaxone • Vancomycin or Ampicillin resistance – Linezolid
Gonococcus	• Ceftriaxone • Spectinomycin for beta lactam resistance
Hepatitis B	Entecavir
Hepatitis C	Direct acting antivirals
Herpes Virus	• HSV and VZV – Acyclovir • CMV – Ganciclovir • Resistant herpes – Foscarnet
H. influenza Treatment	• Meningitis – Ceftriaxone • Pneumonia or Otitis – Ampicillin + Sulbactam
H. influenza Prophylaxis	Rifampicin
H. pylori	Amoxicillin + Clarithromycin + PPI
Influenza A Influenza B Bird flu	• Oseltamivir • Oseltamivir resistance - Zanamivir
Legionella	• Azithromycin • Transplant recipients – Fluoroquinolones (Macrolides can interact with calcineurin inhibitors)

Leishmania	• Cutaneous – Sodium Stibogluconate • Visceral (Kala Azar) – Amphotericin B
Listeria monocytogenes	Ampicillin
Listeria monocytogenes associated with penicillin allergy	Cotrimoxazole

• Malaria	• Treatment and Prophylaxis – Chloroquine (Except for P. falciparum)
	• P. falciparum – ACT (Artesunate Combination Therapy), Oral Artesunate 200 mgs OD for 3 days
	• Chloroquine Resistant malaria
	  ■ Treatment – ACT
	  ■ Prophylaxis – Mefloquine
	• Severe Falciparum Malaria – I/V Artesunate
	• Presumptive Self-treatment – Atovaquone + Proguanil

Melioidosis	Ceftazidime
Meningococcus	• Case – Ceftriaxone • Contact – Ciprofloxacin
Moraxella	Fluoroquinolone
Nocardia Pneumocystis-Jirovecii Cystitis Isosporiasis Cyclosporiasis Sarcocystosis Burkholderia cepacia	Cotrimoxazole

Nematodes	• Albendazole
	• Soil Transmitted Helminths
	  ■ Round Worm (Ascaris Lumbricoides)
	  ■ Whip Worm (Trichuris trichiura)
	  ■ Hook Worm (Necator americanus, Ancylostoma duodenale)
	    ♦ Trichinella Spiralis
	    ♦ Enterobius Vermicularis
	    ♦ Dracunculus Medinensis
	• Ivermectin
	  ■ Thread Worm (Strongyloides stercoralis)
	  ■ Onchocerca Volvulus
	(Also includes Scabies, cutaneous larva migrans and Streptocerciasis)
	• Diethyl Carbamazine (DEC)
	  ■ Loa loa
	  ■ Lymphatic filariasis

Plague Tularemia	Gentamicin
Pneumococcal meningitis Rhodococcus	Vancomycin
Pseudomonas	• Ceftazidime • Resistant strains – Ceftazidime + Aminoglycoside • Multidrug resistant - Colistin
RSV	• Treatment – Ribavirin • Prophylaxis – Palivizumab
Sleeping Sickness (African Trypanosomiasis)	• East African ▪ Early – Suramin ▪ Late – Melarsoprol • West African ▪ Early – Pentamidine ▪ Late – Eflornithine
Scabies	Permethrin cream (5%)
Staphylococcus	• Non-Penicillinase Producing – Penicillin G • Penicillinase Producing – Penicillinase Resistant Penicillin • MRSA – Vancomycin • VRSA – Daptomycin
Syphilis	• All stages (Except CNS involvement) - Benzathine Penicillin G • CNS involvement – Aqueous Penicillin G
Toxoplasma	• Sulfadiazine + Pyrimethamine • Pregnancy – Spiramycin
Trematodes	• Triclabendazole ▪ Liver Fluke (Fasciola Hepatica) • Praziquantel ▪ Lung Fluke (Paragonimus) ▪ Schistosoma
Typhoid	• Ceftriaxone • Oral DOC - Cefixime
Whipple disease (Tropheryma whippelei)	Ceftriaxone or Carbepenams

Treatment of Specific Infections

Antifungal prophylaxis	
Induction chemotherapy of acute leukemia	Posaconazole
Post allo bone marrow transplant	Pre-engraftment – Voriconazole Post-engraftment – Posaconazole

Asymptomatic bacteriuria	Nitrofurantoin Or Amoxicillin
Biliary tract infections (Cholangitis or cholecystitis caused by E. coli, klebsiella etc.)	Ceftriaxone Or Piperacillin – Tazobactam
Brain abscess Subdural empyema	Ceftriaxone or cefotaxime + Metronidazole
Cervicitis Urethritis	Ceftriaxone + Azithromycin

ENT Infections	
Malignant otitis externa	Piperacillin + Tazobactam
Acute otitis media	Amoxicillin + Clavulanate
Mastoiditis	Acute – Cefotaxime or Ceftriaxone Chronic – Piperacillin + Tazobactam
Epiglottitis	Ceftriaxone or Cefotaxime

Febrile neutropenia	Stable patient – Ceftazidime Unstable patient – Piperacillin – Tazobactam Or Cefoperazone – Sulbactam
Neonatal meningitis Neonatal sepsis	Ampicillin + Gentamycin

Ocular infections	
Bacterial conjunctivitis	Gatifloxacin/Levofloxacin/ Moxifloxacin ophthalmological solution
Bacterial keratitis	Moxifloxacin solution
Bacterial keratitis in contact lens users (pseudomonas)	Tobramycin or Gentamycin solution + Piperacillin or Ticarcillin solution
Fungal keratitis	Natamycin
Acanthamoeba keratitis	Chlorhexidine or Polyhexamethylenebiguanide + Hexamidine solution
Orbital cellulitis	Cloxacillin + Ceftriaxone + Metronidazole

Osteomyelitis (Acute)	Ceftriaxone
Prostatitis	Doxycycline Or Cotrimoxazole
Prosthetic joint infection	Ceftriaxone + Vancomycin

Pyelonephritis	Uncomplicated – Gentamicin or Amikacin Complicated – Piperacillin – Tazobactam Or Amikacin Or Cefoperazone – Sulbactam
Septic abortion	Ampicillin + Metronidazole
Diverticulitis	Mild – Amoxycillin + Clavulanate Moderate – Ceftriaxone + Metronidazole Severe – Meropenem
Infective endocarditis: Streptococcal or Enterococcal	Penicillin G or Ampicillin + Gentamycin
Infective endocarditis: Staphylococcal	Vancomycin
Liver Abscess	Amoxycillin – Clavulanate or Ceftriaxone + Metronidazole
Ludwig's angina Vincent's angina	Clindamycin Or Amoxicillin – Clavulanate
Lung abscess Empyema	Piperacillin – Tazobactam Or Cefoperazone – Sulbactam
Meningitis	Acute bacterial – Ceftriaxone Post neurosurgery – Meropenem + Vancomycin With basilar skull fracture – Ceftriaxone
Postnecrotizing pancreatitis: infected pseudocyst or pancreatic abscess	Piperacillin – Tazobactam Or Cefoperazone – Sulbactam
Rhinosinusitis (Acute bacterial)	Amoxicillin – Clavulanate
Skin and soft tissue infection	
Cellulitis Furunculosis	Amoxicillin – Clavulanate Or Ceftriaxone
Necrotizing fasciitis	Piperacillin – Tazobactam Or Cefoperazone – Sulbactam + Clindamycin
Spontaneous bacterial peritonitis	Cefotaxime Or Piperacillin – Tazobactam Or Cefoperazone – Sulbactam
Secondary bacterial peritonitis due to intra-abdominal abscess or GI perforation	Piperacillin – Tazobactam Or Cefoperazone – Sulbactam

New Drugs

Drugs	Mechanism of action	Uses
Baloxavir marboxil	Inhibits endonuclease activity of polymerase acidic protein (present in viral RNA polymerase complex) required for viral gene transcription	Acute uncomplicated influenza within 48 hours of symptom onset
Bictegravir	Integrase inhibitor	HIV
Ibalizumab	Anti-CD-4 receptor monoclonal antibody	Multidrug resistant HIV
Moxidectin	Stimulates glutamate sensitive chloride channels, which leads to flaccid paralysis in helminths	O. volvulus
Plazomicin	Aminoglycoside	Complicated UTI including pyelonephritis caused by gram-negative organisms
Tecovirimat	Inhibits orthopoxvirus VP37 envelope wrapping protein	Smallpox
Tafenoquine	Hypnozoite cidal drug	Radical cure of malaria caused by P. vivax
Eravacycline	Tetracycline	Complicated abdominal infections
Sarecycline	Tetracycline	Inflammatory non-nodular acne in age group > 9 years
Omadacy-cline	Tetracycline	Community acquired pneumonia and acute bacterial skin infection
Doravirine	Non-nucleoside Reverse Transcriptase Inhibitor (NNRTI)	HIV
Rifamycin	RNA polymerase inhibitor	Traveller's diarrhea caused by E. coli

Antibiotics safe in renal failure	
Tetracyclines	T: Tigecycline D: Doxycycline M: Minocycline
Cephalosporins	Cefoperazone Cefpiramide
Fluoroquinolones	Moxifloxacin Pefloxacin
Macrolides	Erythromycin Clarithromycin Azithromycin
Lincosamides	Clindamycin
Streptogramins	Quinupristin + Dalfopristin
Oxazolidinones	Linezolid

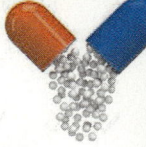

Multiple Choice Questions

ANTIBIOTICS

1. **Dose reduction is required in renal failure with all except** ***(AIIMS Nov 2018)***
   a. Amphotericin B b. Vancomycin
   c. Doxycycline d. Gentamicin
2. **Pediatrician attended infant with unconjugated serum bilirubin level of 33 mg/dL. Which drug mother might have taken in 3rd trimester** ***(AIIMS Nov 2018)***
   a. Azithromycin b. Chloroquine
   c. Ampicillin d. Cotrimoxazole
3. **Which of the following drugs is not used in typhoid?** ***(AIIMS May 2018)***
   a. Amikacin b. Ciprofloxacin
   c. Cefepime d. Azithromycin
4. **Which of the following drugs is commonly used for community acquired pneumonia caused *by S. aureus*?** ***(AIIMS May 2018)***
   a. Vancomycin b. Ceftriaxone
   c. Azithromycin d. Streptomycin
5. **Treatment of choice for late cardiovascular syphilis is?** ***(AIIMS May 2018)***
   a. Benzathine penicillin 7.2 million units in three divided doses
   b. Benzathine penicillin 2.4 million units single dose
   c. Benzyl penicillin 12-24 million units for 21 days
   d. Tetracycline 2g daily
6. **Drug of choice for gonococcal plus non-gonococcal mucopurulent cervicitis:** ***(AIIMS Nov 2017)***
   a. Azithromycin 2 g oral single dose
   b. Ciprofloxacin 500 mg oral single dose
   c. Ceftriaxone 250 mg IM single dose
   d. Cefixime 400 mg oral single dose
7. **Mechanism of action of vancomycin is:** ***(AIIMS Nov 2017)***
   a. Cell wall synthesis inhibition
   b. Cell membrane inhibition
   c. Peptide synthesis inhibition
   d. 30S ribosome inhibition
8. **A patient with 5 episodes of loose stools after eating in a hotel. He is afebrile, has tachycardia and mild dehydration. What is treatment?** ***(AIIMS Nov 2017)***
   a. Ciprofloxacin and tinidazole
   b. Because it may not be giardia give only ciprofloxacin
   c. Ciprofloxacin, tinidazole and ORS
   d. Only ORS
9. **Biofilm mechanism of resistance to antibiotics all except?** ***(AIIMS Nov 2017)***
   a. Mechanical barrier
   b. Increased excretion of antibiotics
   c. Slow metabolism
   d. Adherence
10. **Drug of choice for scrub typhus is:** ***(AIIMS May 2018, Nov 2017)***
    a. Doxycycline b. Azithromycin
    c. Ciprofloxacin d. Chloramphenicol
11. **Empirical drug of choice for treatment of meningococcal meningitis is:** ***(AIIMS May 2017)***
    a. Ceftriaxone
    b. Cefotetan
    c. Gentamicin
    d. Cefoxitin
12. **Drug of choice for prophylaxis of pneumosystis jiroveci in an immunocompropromised patient is:**
    a. Cotrimoxazole ***(AIIMS May 2017)***
    b. Amoxycillin
    c. Dexamethasone
    d. Cephalosporin
13. **What is the treatment of choice for Burkholderia Cepacia?** ***(AIIMS May 2017)***
    a. Carbepenems and 3rd generation cephalosporins
    b. Aminoglycosides and colistin
    c. Cefepime and Tigecycline
    d. Cotrimoxazole
14. **All are false about tigecycline except:**
    a. Dose reduction in renal failure ***(Recent Question 2017)***
    b. 90% pseudomonas strains are sensitive
    c. Oral and parenteral bioavailability is same
    d. Not preferred in UTI
15. **Drug not effective in mycoplasma is:** ***(Recent Question 2017)***
    a. Ceftriaxone b. Tetracycline
    c. Gentamycin d. Chloramphenicol
16. **Drug which lacks intrinsic activity against anaerobes is:** ***(Recent Question 2017)***
    a. Aminoglycosides b. Beta lactams
    c. Chloramphenicol d. Metronidazole
17. **Which of the following is not bacteriostatic:** ***(Recent Question 2017)***
    a. Linezolid b. Clindamycin
    c. Vancomycin d. Erythromycin
18. **Burkholderia cepacia is resistant to:** ***(Recent Question 2017)***
    a. Cotrimoxazole b. Polymyxin B
    c. Ceftazidime d. Ciprofloxacin
19. **A bed ridden female patient with catheter related UTI by beta lactamase producing klebsiella pneumoniae. Which of the following drug will you choose?**
    a. Ampicillin ***(Recent Question 2017)***
    b. Beta lactams and beta lactamase inhibitors
    c. 2nd generation cephalosporins
    d. 3rd generation cephalosporins

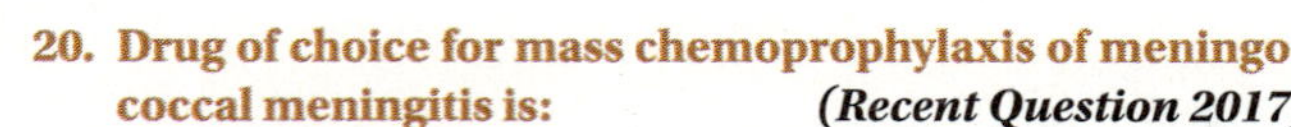

20. Drug of choice for mass chemoprophylaxis of meningococcal meningitis is: ***(Recent Question 2017)***
a. Rifampicin b. Ciprofloxacin
c. Chloramphenicol d. Doxycycline

21. Penicillinase acts on which bond of penicillin? ***(AIIMS Nov 2015)***

a. 1 b. 2
c. 3 d. 4

22. Drug which doesn't inhibit nucleic acid synthesis? ***(AIIMS Nov 2015)***
a. Rifampicin b. Fluoroquinolone
c. Nitrofurantoin d. Linezolid

23. All are ototoxic drug except: ***(AIIMS May 2015)***
a. Metronidazole, b. Vancomycin,
c. Kanamycin, d. Quinine

24. In a child admitted with H. influenza cefotaxime is preferred over ampicillin because ***(AIIMS May 2015)***
a. H. influenza has a plasmid for activity against beta lactams
b. H. influenza has altered penicillin binding protein leading to resistance against ampicillin
c. H. influenza causes ampicillin efflux
d. H. influenza decreases porins

25. Which of the following is a 5th generation cephalosporin with anti MRSA activity: ***(AIIMS Nov 2014)***
a. Ceftriaxone b. Aztreonam
c. Cefazoline d. Ceftobiprole

26. Drug used for fungal keratomycosis? ***(AIIMS Nov 2014)***
a. Vancomycin
b. Linezolid
c. Silver sulfadiazine
d. Penicillin

27. Antibiotic with time dependent killing with prolonged post antibiotic effect ***(AIIMS Nov 2014, May 2014, May 2013)***
a. Clindamycin b. Erythromycin
c. Beta lactam d. Fluoroquinolone

28. TOC for C. *difficile* infection is - ***(AIIMS Nov 2014)***
a. Oral Vancomycin
b. Metronidazole
c. Ceftriaxone
d. Clindamycin

29. Which of the following is true about penicillin G? ***(AIIMS Nov 2014, Nov 2012)***
a. It is effective orally
b. It has a wide spectrum
c. It is used in rat bite fever
d. Probenecid given along with Penicillin G decreases its duration of action

30. Which of the following drugs is useful against pseudomonas? ***(AIIMS Nov-2014)***
a. Piperacillin-tazobactam b. Cefotaxime
c. Streptomycin d. Cephalexin

31. Treatment of choice for extended spectrum beta-lactamase producing enterococci: ***(AIIMS Nov 2012)***
a. Amoxicillin-clavulanic acid
b. Piperacillin-Tazobactam
c. Cefepime
d. Ampicillin + Sulbactam

32. Cotrimoxazole can be used for the treatment of all of the following except: ***(AIIMS May 2011)***
a. Chancroid
b. Lower urinary tract infections
c. Prostatitis
d. Typhoid

33. A patient develops an infection of methicillin resistant Staphylococcus aureus. All of the following can be used to treat this infection except: ***(AI 2012) (AIIMS Nov 2011, May 2007)***
a. Cotrimoxazole b. Cefaclor
c. Ciprofloxacin d. Vancomycin

34. Which of the following statement is false about extended spectrum beta-lactamases (ESBL)? ***(AIIMS May 2011)***
a. These can hydrolyze penicillins, cephalosporins as well as monobactams
b. Carbapenems are sensitive to ESBL
c. Amber classification of ESBL is based on structural differences
d. Third and fourth generation cephalosporins are used for detection of ESBL

35. A patient diagnosed as having ventilator associated pneumonia, is on treatment with ceftriaxone and amikacin. Culture and sensitivity turned out to be positive for ESBL producing Klebsiella infection. The most appropriate next action should be: ***(AIIMS Nov 2010)***
a. Continue same antibiotic but at higher dose
b. Replace ceftazidime for ceftriaxone
c. Remove amikacin and add quinolone
d. Change over to imipenem

36. True about aminoglycosides is all except: ***(AIIMS May 2008)***
a. Are bacteriostatic
b. Distributed only extracellularly
c. Excreted unchanged in urine
d. Teratogenic

37. Erythromycin is given in intestinal hypomotility because: ***(AIIMS Nov 2009)***
a. It increases bacterial count
b. It decreases bacterial count
c. It binds to adenylyl cyclase
d. It binds to motilin receptors

38. All are true about cephalosporins, except: ***(AIIMS May 2009)***
a. Ceftazidime is a 3rd generation cephalosporin
b. Cefoperazone has got antipseudomonal effect
c. Cefoxitin has got no activity against anaerobes
d. Cephalosporins act by inhibiting cell wall synthesis

39. **A girl on sulphonamides developed abdominal pain and presented to emergency with seizure. What is the probable cause?** ***(AIIMS Nov 2008)***
   a. Acute intermittent porphyria
   b. Congenital erythropoietic porphyria
   c. Infectious mononucleosis
   d. Kawasaki's disease

40. **Cephalosporin that does not require dose reduction in patient with any degree of renal impairment is:** ***(AIIMS Nov 2008)***
   a. Cefuroxime b. Cefoperazone
   c. Ceftazidime d. Cefotaxime

41. **For which of the following drugs, dosage interval should be maximum in a patient with creatinine clearance less than 10?** ***(AIIMS Nov 2006)***
   a. Amikacin b. Rifampicin
   c. Vancomycin d. Amphotericin B

42. **Antimicrobial agent acting by inhibition of cell wall synthesis is:** ***(AI 2007; AIIMS Nov 2006)***
   a. Erythromycin b. Tetracycline
   c. Lomefloxacin d. Cefepime

43. **Fluoroquinolone with maximum bioavailability is** ***(Recent Question 2019)***
   a. Ciprofloxacin b. Levofloxacin
   c. Moxifloxacin d. Norfloxacin

44. **What is the treatment of diarrhea in a patient with immunosuppression caused by the organism in the picture?** ***(Recent Question 2019)***

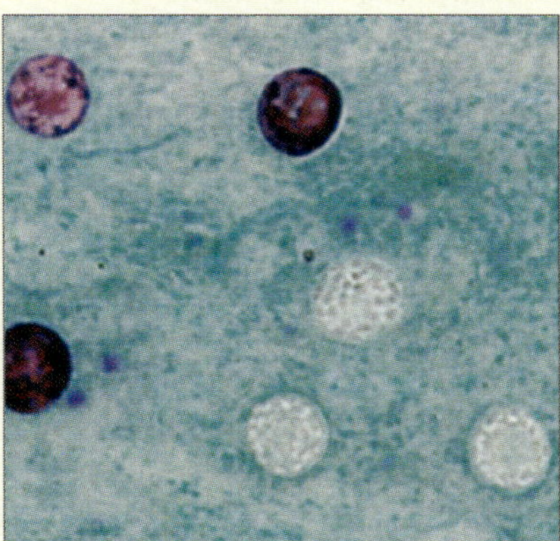

   a. Metronidazole b. TMP-SMX
   c. Paromomycin d. Nitazoxanide

45. **Drug of choice in diphtheria carrier is:** ***(Recent Question 2019)***
   a. Erythromycin b. Rifampicin
   c. Ampicillin d. Amoxicillin

46. **Imipenem given with cilastatin because of:** ***(Recent Question 2019)***
   a. Synergism
   b. Decrease side effect
   c. Increase duration of action
   d. Increase potency

47. **Carbapenem causing max seizure is:** ***(Recent Question 2019)***
   a. Imipenem b. Meropenem
   c. Doripenem d. Ertapenem

48. **Drug of choice for treatment of mastitis:** ***(Recent Question 2019)***
   a. Ampicillin b. Cloxacillin
   c. Metronidazole d. Cefuroxime axetil

49. **Eye defect by anti Tb drug:** ***(Recent Question 2018)***
   a. Ethambutol b. Pyrazinamide
   c. Rifampicin d. Isoniazid

50. **The drug of choice for treatment of meningococcal meningitis is:** ***(Recent Question 2018)***
   a. Piperacillin b. Ceftriaxone
   c. Ampicillin d. Meropenem

51. **Topical antibiotic of choice for MRSA is:** ***(Recent Question 2018)***
   a. Erythromycin b. Polymyxin B
   c. Mupirocin d. Ampicillin

52. **Drug active against new Delhi beta lactamase producing strain:** ***(Recent Question 2018)***
   a. Meropenem b. Colistin
   c. Cephalosporins d. Penicillins

53. **TOC for methicillin resistant *Staph aureus*?** ***(Recent Question Dec 2016)***
   a. Gentamycin b. Cefotaxime
   c. Penicillinase d. Ceftobiprole

54. **Which of the following antibiotic is contraindicated in children?** ***(Recent Question Dec 2016)***
   a. Fluoroquinolones b. Chloramphenicol
   c. Macrolides d. Beta lactams

55. **Which of the following is most nephrotoxic cephalosporin?** ***(Recent Question Dec 2016)***
   a. Cephaloridine b. Cefphalothin
   c. Cefoperazone d. Ceftriaxone

56. **Which cephalosporin causes thrombocytopenia?** ***(Recent Question Dec 2016)***
   a. Ceftriaxone b. Cetazidime
   c. Cefoperazone d. Cefaclor

57. **Drug of Choice for enterococcal endocarditis?** ***(Recent Question Dec 2016)***
   a. Ampicillin b. Vancomycin
   c. Linezolid d. Daptomycin

58. **Empirical treatment for a >60 year old patient with signs of meningitis?** ***(Recent Question Dec 2016)***
   a. Ampicillin
   b. Vancomycin
   c. Ampicillin + Ceftobiprole
   d. Ampicillin + Vancomycin + Ceftobiprole

59. **Which of the following cephalosporin is the oral drug of choice for typhoid?** ***(Recent Question Dec 2016)***
   a. Cefixime b. Ceftriaxone
   c. Cefoperazone d. Moxalactam

60. **Most effective antibiotic for acne.** ***(Recent Question)***
   a. Minocycline b. Gentamycin
   c. Bacitracin d. Sulfadiazine

61. **Drug not used for chemoprophylaxis of meningococcal carrier is** ***(Recent Question Dec 2016)***
   a. Rifampicin b. Minocycline
   c. Ciprofloxacin d. Ceftriaxone

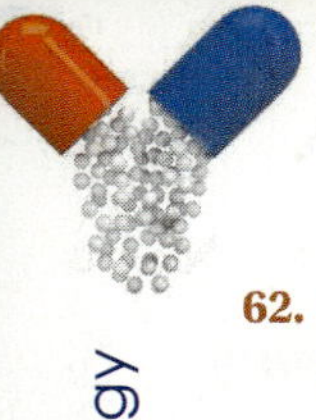

62. Ophthalmia neonatorum due to gonorrhea is prevented by using all except ***(Recent Question Dec 2016)***
a. 1% silver nitrate b. Erythromycin
c. Ceftriaxone d. Tetracyline

63. Best drug for diplococci bacteria is ***(Recent Question Dec 2016)***
a. Vancomycin b. Erythromycin
c. Ceftriaxone d. Penicillin

64. Which of the following most often causes cholestatic jaundice? ***(Recent Question 2016)***
a. INH b. Erythromycin
c. Pyrazinamide d. Ethionamide

65. What is the mechanism of action of fluoroquinolones? ***(Recent Question 2016)***
a. Block translocation of peptide chain from A to P site
b. Inhibit peptidyl transferase
c. Inhibit binding of aminoacyl-t-RNA to A site
d. Inhibit DNA gyrase

66. Antibiotic of choice in campylobacter gastroenteritis is: ***(Recent Question 2016)***
a. Erythromycin b. Ampicillin
c. Ciprofloxacin d. Amoxicillin

67. Which of the following cephalosporins can be used in patient with low GFR? ***(Recent Question 2016)***
a. Cefuroxime b. Cefixime
c. Ceftazidime d. Cefoperazone

68. Which of the following statements are true regarding cefepime? ***(Recent Question 2016)***
a. It is a 4th generation cephalosporin
b. Once day dose is sufficient
c. It has no antipseudomonal activity
d. It is a prodrug

69. Drugs used in treatment of MRSA are all except: ***(Recent Question 2016)***
a. Quinupristin/dalfopristin
b. Linezolid
c. Teicoplanin
d. Penicillin

70. Which of the following statements about drugs associated with deafness are true: ***(Recent Question 2016)***
a. Streptomycin is mostly vestibulotoxic
b. Frusemide causes irreversible deafness
c. Cisplatin causes reversible deafness
d. Amikacin causes reversible deafness

71. Multiple drug resistance is transferred through? ***(Recent Question 2016)***
a. Transduction b. Transformation
c. Conjugation d. Mutation

72. This inhibitor of bacterial protein synthesis has a narrow spectrum of antibacterial activity. It has been used in the management of abdominal abscess caused by bacteroides fragilis, but antibiotic associated colitis has occurred, which of the following drugs is being described? ***(Recent Question 2016)***
a. Clarithromycin b. Clindamycin
c. Minocycline d. Ticarcillin

73. This drug depolarizes cell membrane of aerobic gram-positive bacteria. It is effective against vancomycin resistant enterococcal infections. It may cause myopathy especially in patients taking statins. It is: ***(Recent Question 2016)***
a. Teicoplanin b. Daptomycin
c. Linezolid d. Streptogramin

74. Which of the following is a fourth generation cephalosporin? ***(Recent Question 2016)***
a. Ceftazidime b. Cefepime
c. Cephaloridine d. Cefixime

75. Which of the following is a Ketolide antibiotic? ***(Recent Question 2016)***
a. Erythromycin b. Azithromycin
c. Telithromycin d. Clarithromycin

76. Drug of choice for chemoprophylaxis of whooping cough is? ***(Recent Question 2016)***
a. Azithromycin b. Amoxycillin
c. Erythromycin d. Tetracycline

77. Fluoroquinolone with least oral bioavailability ***(Recent Question 2016)***
a. Norfloxacin b. Ofloxacin
c. Ciprofloxacin d. Levofloxacin

78. Which of the following drugs is contraindicated in liver dysfunction? ***(Recent Question 2016)***
a. Pefloxacin b. Vancomycin
c. Amikacin d. Hydralazine

79. Irreversible hearing loss caused by: ***(Recent Question 2016)***
a. Gentamycin b. Clarithromycin
c. Both of the above d. None of the above

80. Drug of choice for MRSA infection ***(Recent Question 2016)***
a. Ciprofloxacin b. Oxacillin
c. Vancomycin d. Clindamycin

81. Colistin is obtained from ***(Recent Question 2016)***
a. Bacteria b. Fungi
c. Actinomycetes d. Herbs

82. Treatment agent for scarlet fever is: ***(Recent Question 2016)***
a. Penicillin b. Ciprofloxacin
c. Erythromycin d. Chloramphenicol

83. Which of the following can prolong QT interval ***(Recent Question 2016)***
a. Nalidixic acid b. Ofloxacin
c. Gatifloxacin d. Pefloxacin

84. Treatment for impetigo ***(Recent Question 2016)***
a. Dicloxacillin
b. Ciprofloxacin
c. Gentamycin
d. Amoxicillin and clavulanic acid

85. Which of these is not used for the treatment of typhoid ***(Recent Question 2016)***
a. Chloramphenicol b. Ciprofloxacin
c. Ceftriaxone d. Cefixime

86. Bacteria not affected by streptogramins is *(Recent Question 2016)*

a. *E. coli* b. *Staphylococcus aureus*
c. Legionella d. *M. pneumonia*

87. Drug not affecting pseudomonas aeruginosa *(Recent Question 2016)*

a. Levofloxacin b. Ampicillin
c. Norfloxacin d. Ciprofloxacin

88. Cephalosporin causing thrombocytopenia is *(Recent Question 2016)*

a. Cefixime b. Ceftazidime
c. Ceftriaxone d. Cefdinir

89. Which of the following antibiotics is a cell wall synthesis inhibitor? *(Recent Question 2016)*

a. Streptomycin b. Penicillin G
c. Erythromycin d. Chloramphenicol

90. Which among the following is the longest acting sulphonamide? *(Recent Question 2016)*

a. Sulfisoxazole b. Sulfamethoxazole
c. Sulfadiazine d. Sulfadoxine

91. Pseudomonas is best treated with a penicillin with adequate coverage or a combination of penicillin with aminoglycoside. Which of the following is an antipseudomonal penicillin? *(Recent Question 2016)*

a. Piperacillin b. Methicillin
c. Oxacillin d. Cloxacillin

92. Drug of choice for syphilis in a pregnant lady is *(Recent Question 2016)*

a. Penicillin b. Azithromycin
c. Tetracycline d. Ceftriaxone

93. Fluoroquinolone having longest half-life is: *(Recent Question 2016)*

a. Levofloxacin b. Lomefloxacin
c. Ciprofloxacin d. Moxifloxacin

94. All of the following drugs are bactericidal except *(Recent Question 2016)*

a. Isoniazid b. Tigecycline
c. Daptomycin d. Ciprofloxacin

95. Drug resistance transmitting factor present in bacteria is: *(Recent Question 2016)*

a. Plasmid b. Chromosome
c. Introns d. Centromere

96. Highly vestibulotoxic drug is *(Recent Question 2016)*

a. Cisplatin
b. Streptomycin
c. Dihydrostreptomycin
d. Quinine

97. Tetracycline is used for the prophylaxis of *(Recent Question 2016)*

a. Cholera b. Brucellosis
c. Leptospirosis d. Meningitis

98. Which of the following beta-lactam antibiotics can be safety used in a patient with a history of allergy to penicillins? *(Recent Question 2016)*

a. Aztreonam b. Monobactam
c. Loracarbef d. Ceftriaxone

99. Enzyme inactivation is the main mode of resistance to *(Recent Question 2016)*

a. Aminoglycosides b. Quinolones
c. Rifamycins d. Glycopeptides

100. Which of the following drug should not be used to treat klebsiella infection? *(Recent Question 2016)*

a. Ampicillin b. Amikacin
c. Imipenem d. Tigecycline

101. Drug of choice for chlamydial infection in pregnancy is *(Recent Question 2016)*

a. Doxycycline b. Tetracycline
c. Erythromycin d. Ciprofloxacin

102. Which of the following should be monitored if linezolid is given for more than 14 days? *(Recent Question 2016)*

a. Liver function tests b. Kidney function tests
c. Platelet count d. Audiometry

103. Which of the following drugs is effective against pseudomonas infection? *(Recent Question 2016)*

a. Ampicillin b. Ceftriaxone
c. Colistin d. Cefixime

104. Drug resistance in *Staphylococcus aureus* is most commonly acquired by *(Recent Question 2016)*

a. Mutation b. Transformation
c. Transduction d. Conjugation

105. Drug of choice for methicillin resistant *Staphylococcus aureus* is *(Recent Question 2016)*

a. Macrolides
b. Third generation cephalosporins
c. Carbapenems
d. Glycopeptides

106. Methicillin resistant *Staphylococcus aureus* is not expected to respond to *(Recent Question 2016)*

a. Aminoglycoside b. Lincosamide
c. Oxazolidinone d. Carbapenem

107. Drug of choice for prophylaxis of diphtheria is *(Recent Question 2016)*

a. Tetracycline b. Erythromycin
c. Ciprofloxacin d. Amikacin

108. Which of the following is least nephrotoxic? *(Recent Question 2016)*

a. Streptomycin b. Gentamycin
c. Polymyxin B d. Doxycycline

109. Which of the following is an antipseudomonal antibiotic? *(Recent Question 2016)*

a. Ciprofloxacin b. Vancomycin
c. Cefaclor d. Tetracycline

110. All of the following antibacterial agents act by inhibiting cell wall synthesis except *(Recent Question 2016)*

a. Carbapenems
b. Monobactams
c. Cephalosporins
d. Nitrofurantoin

111. Therapeutic uses of penicillin G-all except *(Recent Question 2016)*

a. Bacterial meningitis b. Rickettsial infection
c. Syphilis d. Anthrax

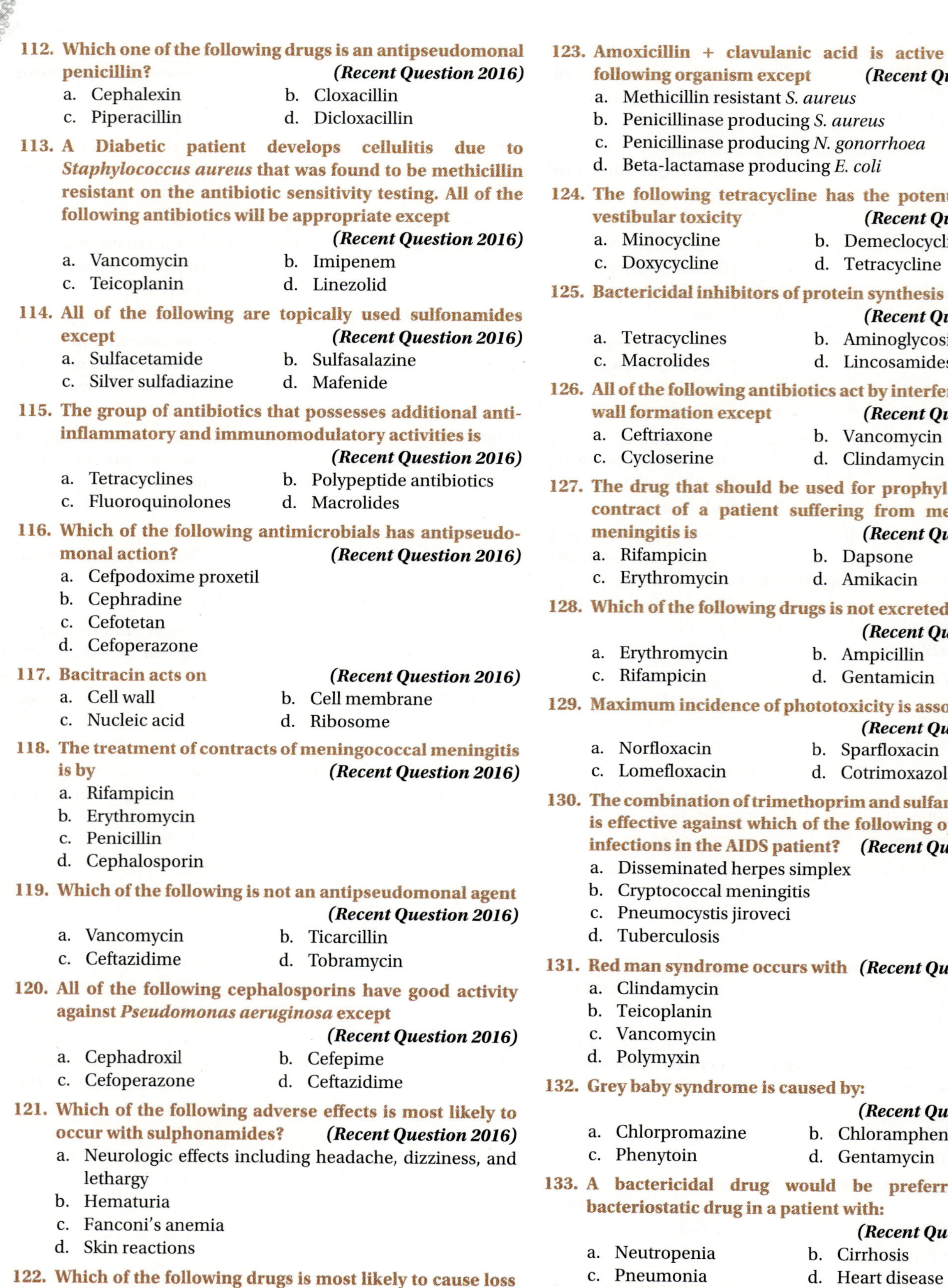

112. Which one of the following drugs is an antipseudomonal penicillin? ***(Recent Question 2016)***

a. Cephalexin
b. Cloxacillin
c. Piperacillin
d. Dicloxacillin

113. A Diabetic patient develops cellulitis due to *Staphylococcus aureus* that was found to be methicillin resistant on the antibiotic sensitivity testing. All of the following antibiotics will be appropriate except ***(Recent Question 2016)***

a. Vancomycin
b. Imipenem
c. Teicoplanin
d. Linezolid

114. All of the following are topically used sulfonamides except ***(Recent Question 2016)***

a. Sulfacetamide
b. Sulfasalazine
c. Silver sulfadiazine
d. Mafenide

115. The group of antibiotics that possesses additional anti-inflammatory and immunomodulatory activities is ***(Recent Question 2016)***

a. Tetracyclines
b. Polypeptide antibiotics
c. Fluoroquinolones
d. Macrolides

116. Which of the following antimicrobials has antipseudomonal action? ***(Recent Question 2016)***

a. Cefpodoxime proxetil
b. Cephradine
c. Cefotetan
d. Cefoperazone

117. Bacitracin acts on ***(Recent Question 2016)***

a. Cell wall
b. Cell membrane
c. Nucleic acid
d. Ribosome

118. The treatment of contracts of meningococcal meningitis is by ***(Recent Question 2016)***

a. Rifampicin
b. Erythromycin
c. Penicillin
d. Cephalosporin

119. Which of the following is not an antipseudomonal agent ***(Recent Question 2016)***

a. Vancomycin
b. Ticarcillin
c. Ceftazidime
d. Tobramycin

120. All of the following cephalosporins have good activity against *Pseudomonas aeruginosa* except ***(Recent Question 2016)***

a. Cephadroxil
b. Cefepime
c. Cefoperazone
d. Ceftazidime

121. Which of the following adverse effects is most likely to occur with sulphonamides? ***(Recent Question 2016)***

a. Neurologic effects including headache, dizziness, and lethargy
b. Hematuria
c. Fanconi's anemia
d. Skin reactions

122. Which of the following drugs is most likely to cause loss of equilibrium and auditory damage? ***(Recent Question 2016)***

a. Amikacin
b. Ethambutol
c. Isoniazid
d. Rifabutin

123. Amoxicillin + clavulanic acid is active against the following organism except ***(Recent Question 2016)***

a. Methicillin resistant *S. aureus*
b. Penicillinase producing *S. aureus*
c. Penicillinase producing *N. gonorrhoea*
d. Beta-lactamase producing *E. coli*

124. The following tetracycline has the potential to cause vestibular toxicity ***(Recent Question 2016)***

a. Minocycline
b. Demeclocycline
c. Doxycycline
d. Tetracycline

125. Bactericidal inhibitors of protein synthesis are ***(Recent Question 2016)***

a. Tetracyclines
b. Aminoglycosides
c. Macrolides
d. Lincosamides

126. All of the following antibiotics act by interfering with cell wall formation except ***(Recent Question 2016)***

a. Ceftriaxone
b. Vancomycin
c. Cycloserine
d. Clindamycin

127. The drug that should be used for prophylaxis of close contract of a patient suffering from meningococcal meningitis is ***(Recent Question 2016)***

a. Rifampicin
b. Dapsone
c. Erythromycin
d. Amikacin

128. Which of the following drugs is not excreted in bile ***(Recent Question 2016)***

a. Erythromycin
b. Ampicillin
c. Rifampicin
d. Gentamicin

129. Maximum incidence of phototoxicity is associated with ***(Recent Question 2016)***

a. Norfloxacin
b. Sparfloxacin
c. Lomefloxacin
d. Cotrimoxazole

130. The combination of trimethoprim and sulfamethoxazole is effective against which of the following opportunistic infections in the AIDS patient? ***(Recent Question 2016)***

a. Disseminated herpes simplex
b. Cryptococcal meningitis
c. Pneumocystis jiroveci
d. Tuberculosis

131. Red man syndrome occurs with ***(Recent Question 2016)***

a. Clindamycin
b. Teicoplanin
c. Vancomycin
d. Polymyxin

132. Grey baby syndrome is caused by: ***(Recent Question 2016)***

a. Chlorpromazine
b. Chloramphenicol
c. Phenytoin
d. Gentamycin

133. A bactericidal drug would be preferred over a bacteriostatic drug in a patient with: ***(Recent Question 2016)***

a. Neutropenia
b. Cirrhosis
c. Pneumonia
d. Heart disease

134. Antipseudomonals are all except: ***(Recent Question 2016)***

a. Cephalexin
b. Carbenicillin
c. Piperacillin
d. Ceftazidime

135. **Drug resistance due to drug destroying enzymes is seen in all of the following except:** ***(Recent Question 2016)***
a. Tobramycin b. Aminoglycosides
c. Chloramphenicol d. Quinolones

136. **Dose of which of the following antibiotic does not require alteration in renal failure?** ***(Recent Question 2016)***
a. Vancomycin b. Ethambutol
c. Erythromycin d. Metronidazole

137. **Cilastatin is given along with** ***(Recent Question 2016)***
a. Imipenem b. Amoxicillin
c. Erythromycin d. Ampicillin

138. **Drug acting by inhibiting cell wall synthesis** ***(Recent Question 2016)***
a. Erythromycin b. Cephalosporins
c. Chloramphenicol d. Sulphonamides

139. **Drug which should not be given in renal disease is** ***(Recent Question 2016)***
a. Gentamicin b. Nitroprusside
c. Doxycycline d. Ceftriaxone

140. **Drug causing megaloblastic anemia is** ***(Recent Question 2016)***
a. INH b. Chloramphenicol
c. Pyrimethamine d. Methyldopa

141. **Carbenicillin** ***(Recent Question 2016)***
a. Is effective in pseudomonas infection
b. Has no effect in proteus infection
c. Is a macrolide antibiotic
d. Is administered orally

142. **A potent inhibitor of beta-lactamase is:** ***(Recent Question 2016)***
a. Carbenicillin b. Clavulanic acid
c. Cefamandole d. Idoxuridine

143. **Drug which acts by binding to P site in prokaryotes is** ***(Recent Question 2016)***
a. Actinomycin D b. Chloramphenicol
c. Puromycin d. Penicillin

144. **Drug used in the treatment of resistant gonorrhoe is** ***(Recent Question 2016)***
a. Penicillin b. Cotrimoxazole
c. Spectinomycin d. Erythromycin

145. **Antibiotic causing pseudomembranous colitis is:** ***(Recent Question 2016)***
a. Clindamycin b. Garamycin
c. Erythromycin d. Vancomycin

146. **Most phototoxic quinolone is** ***(Recent Question 2016)***
a. Ciprofloxacin b. Ofloxacin
c. Norfloxacin d. Sparfloxacin

147. **All are hepatotoxic drug except** ***(Recent Question 2016)***
a. Erythromycin estolate b. Rifampicin
c. Tetracycline d. None

148. **Mechanism of action of penicillins and cephalosporins is to inhibit** ***(Recent Question 2016)***
a. Cell wall synthesis
b. Leakage from cell membrane
c. Protein synthesis
d. DNA gyrase

149. **Jarisch-Herxheimer reaction is seen in syphilis with** ***(Recent Question 2016)***
a. Tetracyclines b. Penicillins
c. Co-trimoxazole d. Sulphonamides

150. **Which of the following drugs is bactericidal?** ***(Recent Question 2016)***
a. Sulphonamides b. Erythromycin
c. Chloramphenicol d. Cotrimoxazole

151. **Red cell aplasia can be caused by** ***(Recent Question 2016)***
a. Aminoglycosides b. Chloramphenicol
c. Penicillins d. Ciprofloxacin

152. **The following organisms are known to develop resistance to develop resistance to penicillin except** ***(Recent Question 2016)***
a. Staphylococcus b. Streptococcus
c. Pneumococcus d. Treponema

153. **Which one of the following is primarily bacteriostatic?** ***(Recent Question 2016)***
a. Ciprofloxacin b. Chloramphenicol
c. Vancomycin d. Rifampicin

154. **Drug with high degree of photosensitivity is** ***(Recent Question 2016)***
a. Tetracycline b. Doxycycline
c. Minocycline d. Methacycline

155. **Drug of choice in pertussis is** ***(Recent Question 2016)***
a. Penicillin b. Doxycycline
c. Erythromycin d. Ciprofloxacin

156. **Acid susceptible penicillin is** ***(Recent Question 2016)***
a. Methicillin b. Ampicillin
c. Amoxicillin d. Cloxacillin

157. **Broad spectrum antibiotic is** ***(Recent Question 2016)***
a. Erythromycin b. Streptomycin
c. Tetracycline d. All

158. **All are aminoglycosides except** ***(Recent Question 2016)***
a. Netilmicin b. Streptomycin
c. Kanamycin d. Azithromycin

159. **Drug effective against pseudomonas is:** ***(Recent Question 2016)***
a. Penicillin b. Gentamycin
c. Tetracycline d. Chloramphenicol

160. **Pseudomembranous colitis is associated mostly with which drug?** ***(Recent Question 2016)***
a. Erythromycin b. Ampicillin
c. Vancomycin d. Ciprofloxacin

161. **Which of the following aminoglycoside has highest nephrotoxicity?** ***(Recent Question 2016)***
a. Paromomycin b. Streptomycin
c. Amikacin d. Neomycin

162. **Second generation cephalosporin that can be used orally is** ***(Recent Question 2016)***
a. Cefepime b. Cephalothin
c. Cefaclor d. Cefadroxil

163. **Which of the following antibiotic does not act by inhibiting protein synthesis?** ***(Recent Question 2016)***
a. Vancomycin b. Tetracycline
c. Streptomycin d. Azithromycin

164. Ampicillin is not given in EBV infection due to *(Recent Question 2016)*

a. Increased toxicity b. Skin rash
c. Blindness d. Convulsions

165. Microbial killing by an antibiotic below its "minimum inhibitory concentration" is known as *(Recent Question 2016)*

a. Concentration dependent killing
b. Time dependent killing
c. Sequential blockade
d. Postantibiotic effect

166. Drug of choice for nocardiosis? *(Recent Question 2016)*

a. Trimethoprim + SMX b. Penicillins
c. Amikacin d. Rifampicin

167. Eosinophilia is caused by *(Recent Question 2016)*

a. Penicillins b. Salicylates
c. Cephalosporins d. All of the above

168. Drug withdrawn in India is *(Recent Question 2016)*

a. Levofloxacin b. Gatifloxacin
c. Moxifloxacin d. Ofloxacin

169. Drug that inhibits cell wall synthesis is *(Recent Question 2016)*

a. Tetracyclines b. Penicillins
c. Aminoglycosides d. Chloramphenicol

170. Which drug is not given in renal failure? *(Recent Question 2016)*

a. Rifampicin b. Pyrazinamide
c. Penicillin G d. Cephalothin

171. Sulphonamide injection causes decrease in folic acid by *(Recent Question 2016)*

a. Competitive inhibition
b. Noncompetitive inhibition
c. Uncompetitive inhibition
d. Allosteric inhibition

172. Long postantibiotic effect is seen in *(Recent Question 2016)*

a. Quinolones b. Macrolides
c. Panicillin d. Cephalosporin

173. Which among the following is not a beta lactamase resistant penicillin? *(Recent Question 2016)*

a. Methicillin
b. Carbenicillin
c. Nafcillin
d. Oxacillin

174. Mechanism of action of quinolones is *(Recent Question 2016)*

a. DNA gyrase inhibitors
b. Bind to 30S unit
c. Bind to bacterial cell membrane
d. Bind to tetrahydrofolate reductase

175. True about imipenem is *(Recent Question 2016)*

a. It is a narrow spectrum antibiotic
b. it is easily broke by beta lactam
c. It can be used with cilastatin
d. It is used with sulbactam

176. All have beta lactam ring except *(Recent Question 2016)*

a. Penicillin b. Linezolid
c. Cefotaxime d. Imipenem

177. All are third generation cephalosporin except *(Recent Question 2016)*

a. Cefixime b. Ceftazidime
c. Cefuroxime d. Cefoperazone

178. Not a mechanism of resistance to erythromycin? *(Recent Question 2016)*

a. Alteration in ribosomal binding site
b. Plasmid mediated
c. Erythromycin esterase production
d. Efflux proteins

179. Drug of choice for *Treponema pallidum* is *(Recent Question 2016)*

a. Penicillin G b. Tetracycline
c. Azithromycin d. Doxycycline

180. Treatment for clostridial myonecrosis is *(Recent Question 2016)*

a. Amikacin b. Penicillin
c. Ampicillin d. Gentamicin

181. Drug to prevent staphylococcus colonization of nose in patient of recurrent staphylococcus pyoderma is? *(Recent Question 2016)*

a. Rifampicin b. Amoxycillin
c. Tetracycline d. Mupirocin

182. True about cefuroxime is *(Recent Question 2016)*

a. Active against B. fragilis
b. Superior to ceftriaxone for treatment of meningitis
c. Poor CSF penetration
d. Excreted rapidly by kidney

183. Most enzyme resistant aminoglycoside is *(Recent Question 2016)*

a. Gentamycin b. Amikacin
c. Kanamycin d. Tobramycin

184. Chloramphenicol does not increase the blood level of which drug? *(Recent Question 2016)*

a. Phenytoin b. Tolbutamide
c. Phenylbutazone d. Cyclophosphamide

185. Timing of antibiotic therapy for surgical prophylaxis *(Recent Question 2016)*

a. At the time of skin incision
b. At the time of induction
c. One hour later
d. Along with preanesthetic medication

186. Linezolid-mechanism of resistance *(Recent Question 2016)*

a. Efflux mechanism
b. Mutation of linezolid binding site
c. Development of lytic enzymes
d. All of the above

187. Not a semi synthetic penicillin *(Recent Question 2016)*

a. Penicillin V b. Penicillin G
c. Methicillin d. Amoxicillin

188. Streptomycin is a *(Recent Question 2016)*

a. Peptide b. Glycoside
c. Phospholipid d. Glycoprotein

189. Composition of double strength septra *(Recent Question 2016)*

a. 80 mg trimethoprim + 400 mg
b. Sulfamethoxazole
c. 160 mg trimethoprim + 800 mg sulfamethoxazole
d. 800 mg trimethoprim + 160 mg sulfamethoxazole

190. The toxicity of depolarizing skeletal muscle relaxants are enhanced by ***(Recent Question 2016)***

a. Daptomycin b. Vancomycin
c. Streptomycin d. Azithromycin

191. Drug of choice for rickettsia is ***(Recent Question 2016)***

a. Erythromycin b. Tetracycline
c. Chloramphenicol d. Penicillins

192. Pseudomembranous colitis false is

a. Treated by tetracycline ***(Recent Question 2016)***
b. Most common antibiotic associated with pseudo membranous colitis is clindamycin
c. Life-threatening complication
d. Presents with severe diarrhea, fever, and stools containing mucous membrane neutrophils

193. Drug of choice in chlamydia ***(Recent Question 2016)***

a. Doxycycline b. Penicillin
c. Cephalosporin d. Aminoglycoside

194. Antibiotic not effective for rickettsia is ***(Recent Question 2016)***

a. Sulfonamide b. Tetracycline
c. Ofloxacin d. Chloramphenicol

195. Mechanism of action of sulphonamides

a. Inhibition of cell wall synthesis ***(Recent Question 2016)***
b. Inhibition of formation of folic acid
c. Inhibition of protein synthesis
d. Altered DNA gyrase with reduced affinity

196. Drug causing macular toxicity on intra ocular administration ***(Recent Question 2016)***

a. Gentamicin b. Penicillin
c. Amoxicillin d. Metronidazole

197. Drug causing disulfiram reaction are A/E ***(Recent Question 2016)***

a. Cefoxitin b. Cefamandole
c. Cefotetan d. Moxalactam

198. Drug not used in typhoid ***(Recent Question 2016)***

a. Clindamycin b. Ciprofloxacin
c. Ofloxacin d. Ceftriaxone

199. True regarding aztreonam are all except

a. Is a monobactam group ***(Recent Question 2016)***
b. Has activity against gram-positive bacteria
c. Active against pseudomonas
d. Can be given to a patient who develops sever hypersensitivity reaction to a penicillin

200. True regarding vancomycin resistance in VRE

a. It is plasmid mediated ***(Recent Question 2016)***
b. It is due to inactivating enzyme
c. 3rd generation cephalosporins are effective
d. It causes community acquired epidemic throughout the world

201. Gyrase inhibitors are ***(Recent Question 2016)***

a. Fluoroquinolones b. Penicillins
c. Aminoglycosides d. Azoles

202. Mechanism of action of streptomycin

a. Freezing of initiation ***(Recent Question 2016)***
b. Inhibits translocation
c. Inhibits peptidyl transferase
d. Inhibits cell wall synthesis

203. Child presenting with diarrhea was treated successfully with erythromycin. The causative agent is ***(Recent Question 2016)***

a. *Giardia lamblia* b. *Vibrio cholera*
c. *Staphylococcus aureus* d. *C. jejuni*

204. Aminoglycosides toxicity first affects

a. Outer hair cell and basal turn of cochlea
b. Apex ***(Recent Question 2016)***
c. Cochlear nerve
d. Vestibular nerve

205. Generation of cephalosporins which has least activity against gram-positive? ***(Recent Question 2016)***

a. I b. II
c. III d. IV

206. Treatment of listeria ***(Recent Question 2016)***

a. Vancomycin b. Ampicillin
c. Ceftriaxone d. Imipenem

207. Anti-pseudomonal penicillin is ***(Recent Question 2016)***

a. Methicillin b. Ampicillin
c. Piperacillin d. Penicillin-G

208. Tigecycline is a/an ***(Recent Question 2016)***

a. Tetracyclines b. Erythromycin
c. Penicillin d. Rifampicin

209. Drug of choice for anaerobic cocci is ***(Recent Question 2016)***

a. Clindamycin b. Aztreonam
c. Metronidazole d. Erythromycin

210. Treatment of legionella ***(Recent Question 2016)***

a. Tetracyclines b. Erythromycin
c. Penicillin d. Rifampicin

211. Most commonly used drug in community acquired pneumonia is ***(Recent Question 2016)***

a. Ofloxacin b. Ciprofloxacin
c. Moxifloxacin d. Sparfloxacin

212. True statement regarding penicillin G is

a. Orally active drug ***(Recent Question 2016)***
b. Ototoxicity is the major limiting side effect
c. Broad spectrum
d. DOC in rat bite fever

213. Linezolid is a ***(Recent Question 2016)***

a. DNA gyrase inhibitors
b. Bind to 30S unit
c. Binds to 23S fraction of 50S ribosomes
d. Bind to tetrahydrofolate reductase

214. Drug used for prophylaxis of plague ***(Recent Question 2016)***

a. Tetracycline b. Penicillin
c. Erythromycin d. Cephalosporins

215. Drug of choice for antimicrobial prophylaxis before surgery is ***(Recent Question 2016)***

a. Ampicillin b. Cefazolin
c. Ceftazidime d. Ceftriaxone

216. Time dependent killing is seen with ***(Recent Question 2016)***

a. Metronidazole b. β lactam antibiotics
c. Vancomycin d. Erythromycin

217. Amikacin-mechanism of action *(Recent Question 2016)*
a. Protein synthesis inhibitors
b. Inhibits DNA synthesis
c. Inhibits cell wall synthesis
d. Antimetabolite

218. Not an ototoxic drug *(Recent Question 2016)*
a. Aminoglycosides b. Vancomycin
c. Furosemide d. Acetaminophen

219. Streptomycin is a *(Recent Question 2016)*
a. Peptide b. Aminoglycoside
c. Phospholipid d. Glycolipid

220. Drug which can cause photosensitivity reaction is *(Recent Question 2016)*
a. Streptomycin b. Demeclocycline
c. Clindamycin d. Clofibrate

221. Which of the following is a side effect of sulfonamide? *(Recent Question 2016)*
a. Constipation b. Joint pain
c. Crystalluria d. Hyperkalemia

ANTIMYCOBACTERIAL AGENTS

222. A known case of TB is now resistant to Rifampicin and Isoniazid. Which of the following would be most appropriate in treating this patient? *(AIIMS Nov 2018)*
a. 6 drugs for 4 months; 4 drugs for 12 months
b. 6 drugs for 6 months; 4 drugs for 18 months
c. 4 drugs for 4 months, 6 drugs for 12 months
d. 5 drugs 2 months; 4 drugs 1 month; 3 drug 5 months

223. Dapsone is used as antibacterial, antifungal and as an immunomodulator. What is the mechanism behind all these actions? *(AIIMS Nov 2018)*
a. Inhibition of cell wall synthesis
b. Inhibition of sterol of the cell wall
c. Inhibition of protein synthesis in ribosomes
d. Competes with PABA in folic acid synthesis

224. Antitubercular drug causing ophthalmic toxicity is: *(AIIMS Nov 2018)*
a. Isoniazid b. Rifampicin
c. Ethambutol d. None of above

225. A patient in ATT develops tingling on lower limb. Which of the following drugs should be used? *(AIIMS Nov 2017)*
a. Pyridoxine b. Thiamine
c. Folic acid d. Vitamin B-12

226. A 12-year-old child presents with four lesions of leprosy on back and four lesions on left arm. What should be the treatment of this child? *(AIIMS May 2017)*
a. Rifampicin 600 mg once a month + dapsone 100 mg daily + clofazimine 300 mg once a month and 50 mg daily
b. Rifampicin 600 mg once a month + dapsone 100 mg daily
c. Rifampicin 450 mg once a month + dapsone 50 mg daily + clofazimine 150 mg once a month + 50 mg alternate days
d. Rifampicin 450 mg once a month + dapsone 50 mg daily + clofazimine 150 mg once a month + 50 mg daily

227. Which of the following is a bactericidal antileprotic drug? *(AIIMS May 2017)*
a. Amoxicillin
b. Ciprofloxacin
c. Erythromycin
d. Ofloxacin

228. Which of the following is not true for rifabutin when compared to rifampicin *(AIIMS Nov 2016)*
a. Rifabutin has a longer half-life than rifampicin
b. Rifabutin is more effective for newly diagnosed TB
c. Rifabutin has lesser incidence of drug interactions.
d. Rifampicin is more effective against MAC as compared to rifabutin

229. Anti TB drug associated with max ocular side effects is *(Recent Question Dec 2016)*
a. Rifampicin b. Isoniazid
c. Ethambutol d. Pyrazinamide

230. Which of the following anti TB drug causes iridocyclitis? *(Recent Question Dec 2016)*
a. Rifabutin b. Ethambutol
c. Pyrazinamide d. Ethionamide

231. Which anti tubercular drug causes hyperuricemia? *(Recent Question Dec 2016)*
a. Isoniazid b. Rifampicin
c. Pyrazinamide d. Ethambutol

232. Which ATT is not given to a HIV +ve patient? *(Recent Question Dec 2016)*
a. Rifampicin b. Pyrazinamide
c. Ethambutol d. Isoniazid

233. Antitubercular drug acting on intracellular mycobacterium *(Recent Question Dec 2016)*
a. Rifampicin
b. Ethambutol
c. Isoniazid
d. Pyrazinamide

234. Which side effect seen in Rifampicin warrants that, it should be stopped immediately and never used again *(Recent Question Dec 2016)*
a. Thrombocytopenia
b. Hepatotoxicity
c. Peripheral neuropathy
d. Flu like symptoms

235. Antituberculous drug causing sideroblastic anemia: *(Recent Question Dec 2016)*
a. Isoniazid b. Rifampicin
c. Pyrazinamide d. Ethambutol

236. Which gene is responsible for Rifampicin resistance? *(Recent Question Dec 2016)*
a. epoA b. epoRf
c. rpoA d. rpoB

237. Which of the following is a latest drug approved for MDR TB? *(AIIMS Nov 2015)*
a. Bedaquiline
b. Tipranavir
c. Levofloxacin
d. Linezolid

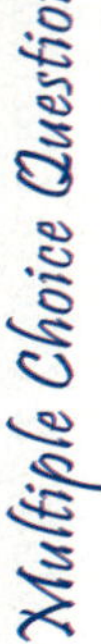

238. **The kit in the picture is used for treatment of** ***(AIIMS Nov 2018, Nov 2015)***

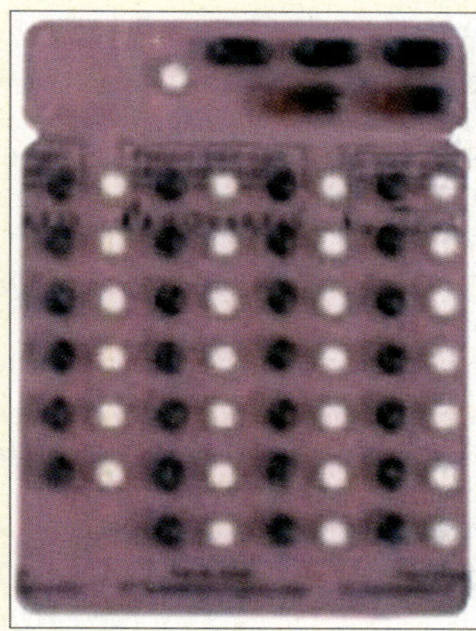

a. HIV b. Leprosy
c. Urethral discharge d. TB

239. **Which of the following antitubercular drugs is associated with hypothyroidism?** ***(AIIMS May 2014)***
a. Rifampicin b. PZA
c. Ethionamide d. Streptomycin

240. **Cross resistance of isoniazid is seen with:** ***(AIIMS May 2008)***
a. Rifampicin b. Ethionamide
c. Cycloserine d. Ethambutol

241. **All the following are administered under supervision in India except:** ***(AIIMS Nov 2009)***
a. Dapsone b. Clofazimine
c. Pyrazinamide d. Rifampicin

242. **One of the antitubercular drugs is contraindicated in children below 6 years of age, because they may be unable to appreciate and report visual field defects or changes in vision, which is a known side effect of that drug. Which among the following is that drug?** ***(Recent Question 2016)***
a. Ethambutol b. INH
c. Rifampicin d. Pyrazinamide

243. **Which fluoroquinolone is highly active against mycobacterium leprae and is being used in alternative multidrug therapy regimens?** ***(Recent Question 2016)***
a. Norfloxacin
b. Ofloxacin
c. Ciprofloxacin
d. Lomefloxacin

244. **The tetracycline with highest antileprotic activity is** ***(Recent Question 2016)***
a. Minocycline b. Doxycycline
c. Demeclocycline d. Oxytetracycline

245. **Which of the following drugs was initially developed as an antitubercular drug, but later found to have mood elevating properties?** ***(Recent Question 2016)***
a. Isoniazid b. Selegiline
c. Fluoxetine d. Lithium

246. **A patent suffering from AIDS is on zidovudine, lamivudine and indinavir therapy. He develops pulmonary TB for which treatment is started. Which of the following should be avoided in him?** ***(Recent Question 2016)***
a. INH b. Ethambutol
c. Pyrazinamide d. Rifampicin

247. **Drug used in prophylaxis of H. influenzae is:** ***(Recent Question 2016)***
a. Doxycycline b. Rifampicin
c. Erythromycin d. None

248. **Which of the following antimicrobials need dose reduction even in mild renal failure?** ***(Recent Question 2016)***
a. Ciprofloxacin b. Carbenicillin
c. Cefotaxime d. Ethambutol

249. **Which of the following ATT is not hepatotoxic?** ***(Recent Question 2016)***
a. Isoniazid b. Rifampicin
c. Pyrazinamide d. Streptomycin

250. **Arthralgia is commonly caused by which anti tuberculous drug?** ***(Recent Question 2016)***
a. INH b. Rifampicin
c. Pyrazinamide d. Ethambutol

251. **Which of the following anti leprosy drugs cause skin ichthyosis?** ***(Recent Question 2016)***
a. Rifampicin b. Dapsone
c. Clofazimine d. Ethionamide

252. **Which ATT drug is implicated in causing transient memory loss?** ***(Recent Question 2016)***
a. Ethionamide b. Isoniazid
c. Ethambutol d. Pyrazinamide

253. **A 30-year-old pregnant woman develops tuberculosis. Which of the following ATT drugs should not be used?** ***(Recent Question 2016)***
a. INH b. Rifampicin
c. Streptomycin d. Ethambutol

254. **Which Anti tubercular drug cause pneumonia like syndrome?** ***(Recent Question 2016)***
a. INH b. Rifampicin
c. Ethambutol d. Pyrazinamide

255. **Maximum sterilising action is shown by which anti TB drug** ***(Recent Question 2016)***
a. Rifampicin b. INH
c. Pyrazinamide d. Streptomycin

256. **Neuropsychiatry symptoms are seen with which anti TB drug** ***(Recent Question 2016)***
a. INH b. Rifampicin
c. Pyrazinamide d. Streptomycin

257. **Flu like symptoms is side effect of which anti TB drug** ***(Recent Question 2016)***
a. INH b. Rifampicin
c. Pyrazinamide d. Streptomycin

258. **Which anti TB drug is avoided in HIV patient** ***(Recent Question 2016)***
a. INH b. Rifampicin
c. Pyrazinamide d. Streptomycin

259. Bacteriostatic anti TB drug ***(Recent Question 2016)***
a. INH b. Rifampicin
c. Ethambutol d. Pyrazinamide

260. Pyridoxine should be given when treating with ***(Recent Question 2016)***
a. Isoniazid b. Rifampicin
c. Pyrazinamide d. Streptomycin

261. Pigmentation and ichthyosis are side effects of ***(Recent Question 2016)***
a. Clofazimine b. Rifampicin
c. Dapsone d. Ethionamide

262. XDR TB is resistance to ***(Recent Question 2016)***
a. Isoniazid
b. Isoniazid + Rifampicin
c. Isoniazid + Rifampicin + Ethambutol
d. Isoniazid + Rifampicin + Kanamycin

263. Hepatotoxic drug used in tuberculosis is ***(Recent Question 2016)***
a. Isoniazid b. Streptomycin
c. Kanamycin d. Ethambutol

264. Maximum liver toxicity is seen with which anti-TB drug? ***(Recent Question 2016)***
a. Isoniazid b. Rifampicin
c. Pyrazinamide d. Streptomycin

265. Which anti-tubercular drug is implicated in the causation of transient memory loss? ***(Recent Question 2016)***
a. Ethionamide b. Isoniazid
c. Ethambutol d. Pyrazinamide

266. Patients suffering from multidrug resistant tuberculosis can be treated with all the following drugs except ***(Recent Question 2016)***
a. Tobramycin b. Amikacin
c. Ciprofloxacin d. Clarithromycin

267. Ethambutol causes ***(Recent Question 2016)***
a. Retrobulbar neuritis b. Deafness
c. Red urine d. Peripheral neuritis

268. The most common side effect of dapsone is ***(Recent Question 2016)***
a. Hemolytic anemia
b. Thrombocytopenia
c. Cyanosis
d. Bone marrow depression

269. Slow acetylators of isoniazid are more prone to develop ***(Recent Question 2016)***
a. Failure of therapy b. Peripheral neuropathy
c. Hepatotoxicity d. Allergic reactions

270. In leprosy, the best bactericidal agents is ***(Recent Question 2016)***
a. Clofazimine b. Dapsone
c. Rifampicin d. Ethionamide

271. The adverse reaction that absolutely contraindicates further use of rifampicin in the treatment of tuberculosis ***(Recent Question 2016)***
a. Respiratory syndrome b. Cutaneous syndrome
c. Flu like syndrome d. Abdominal syndrome

272. Most common drug used in leprosy is ***(Recent Question 2016)***
a. Dapsone b. Clofazimine
c. Ethionamide d. Ofloxacin

273. The bacterial drug resistance in tuberculosis is via ***(Recent Question 2016)***
a. Transduction b. Transformation
c. Plasmid mediated d. Mutation

274. ATT with maximum CSF penetration: ***(Recent Question 2016)***
a. Streptomycin b. INH
c. Rifampicin d. Pyrazinamide

275. The following is not a hepatotoxic antitubercular drug: ***(Recent Question 2016)***
a. Ethambutol b. Isoniazid
c. Rifampicin d. Pyrazinamide

276. DNA dependent RNA synthesis is inhibited by: ***(Recent Question 2016)***
a. Rifampicin b. Ethambutol
c. Colchicine d. Chloromycetin

277. Peripheral neuropathy is caused by ***(Recent Question 2016)***
a. Rifampicin b. Pyrazinamide
c. INH d. Ethambutol

278. Rifampicin act by ***(Recent Question 2016)***
a. Inhibiting DNA dependent RNA polymerase
b. Inhibiting RNA dependent DNA polymerase
c. Mycolic acid inhibition
d. Mycolic acid incorporation defects

279. Drug of choice for prophylaxis of TB is ***(Recent Question 2016)***
a. Rifampicin b. Isoniazid
c. Pyrazinamide d. Streptomycin

280. ATT drug causing contact lens staining ***(Recent Question 2016)***
a. INH b. Rifampicin
c. Pyrazinamide d. Thioacetazone

281. Hepatitis d/t isoniazid is due to formation of ***(Recent Question 2016)***
a. Hydrazine complex b. Isobutene complex
c. Isoazoic complex d. Hydralazine complex

282. Antitubercular drug which reaches the interior of caseous material is ***(Recent Question 2016)***
a. Isoniazid b. Rifampicin
c. Pyrazinamide d. Ethambutol

283. Side effects of isoniazid are all except: ***(Recent Question 2016)***
a. Hepatitis b. Optic neuritis
c. Peripheral neuropathy d. Thrombocytopenia

284. All are true about rifampicin except: ***(Recent Question 2016)***
a. Microsomal enzyme inducer
b. Used in treatment of meningococcal meningitis
c. May cause OCP failure
d. Bactericidal in nature

285. **Antitubercular drug associated with psychosis is:** *(Recent Question 2016)*
a. INH b. Rifampicin
c. Ethambutol d. Streptomycin

286. **Pregnant lady on ATT develops hearing abnormality and tinnitus. Causative drug is** *(Recent Question 2016)*
a. INH b. Rifampicin
c. Ethambutol d. Streptomycin

287. **Not a use of dapsone** *(Recent Question 2016)*
a. Malaria b. G6PD deficiency
c. Dermatitis herpetiformis d. Leprosy

288. **MDR-TB is defined as a strain resistant to** *(Recent Question 2016)*
a. Isoniazid and pyrazinamide
b. Isoniazid and rifampicin
c. Rifampicin and streptomycin
d. Pyrazinamide and rifampicin

289. **XDR-TB is defined as** *(Recent Question 2016)*
a. Resistance isoniazid and rifampicin + quinolone
b. Resistance isoniazid+ quinolone + injectable aminoglycoside
c. Resistance isoniazid and rifampicin and quinolone + injectable aminoglycoside
d. Resistance rifampicin + quinolone + injectable aminoglycoside Anti-Viral

ANTIVIRAL AGENTS

290. **A patient is on indinavir, zidovudine, lamivudine and ketoconazole. He developed breast hypertrophy, nephrolithiasis, hyperlipidemia and central obesity; identify the drug causing these side effects amongst all:** *(AIIMS Nov 2018)*
a. Lamivudine b. Indinavir
c Ketoconazole d. Zidovudine

291. **Mechanism of action of oseltamivir is:** *(AIIMS May 2017)*
a. Neuraminidase inhibitor
b. RNA dependent RNA Polymerase inhibition
c. Viral M2 ion channel protein inhibition
d. Fusion inhibitor

292. **Mechanism of action of protease inhibitors is:** *(AIIMS May 2017)*
a. Inhibits proviral RNA synthesis
b. Inhibits assembly of viral proteins
c. Inhibits conversion of RNA to DNA
d. Cell death (apoptosis) of the infected cell

293. **Mechanism of action of Tamiflu is** *(Recent Question 2019)*
a. Neuraminidase inhibition
b. Protein synthesis inhibition
c. Thymidylate kinase inhibition
d. RNA polymerase inhibition

294. **H1N1 influenza prophylaxis** *(Recent Question 2018)*
a. Oseltamivir b. Zanamivir
c. Amantadine d. Rimantadine

295. **Which antiviral drug is used in both HIV and hepatitis B:** *(Recent Question 2017)*
a. Acyclovir b. Abacavir
c. Emtricitabine d. Enfuvirtide

296. **What is the next step when you diagnose a pregnant woman as HIV patient in first trimester?** *(Recent Question 2017)*
a. Start regimen immediately and continue till puerperium
b. Start regimen after first trimester
c. Terminate pregnancy
d. Start regimen before delivery

297. **Which of the following is drug of choice for prophylaxis of Influenza A?** *(Recent Question Dec 2016)*
a. Oseltamivir b. Zanamivir
c. Amantadine d. Rimantadine

298. **Regarding oseltamivir FDA approved true statement:** *(Recent Question Dec 2016)*
a. Hemagglutinin inhibitor
b. Intranasal prophylaxis for influenza
c. Effective if given less than 72 hour of flu symptom
d. Given at a dose of 75 mg

299. **Mechanism of action of acyclovir is on** *(Recent Question Dec 2016)*
a. Viral polymerase b. Proteolytic
c. Capping of m RNA d. Attachment inhibition

300. **Protease inhibitor not metabolized by CYP3A4?** *(Recent Question Dec 2016)*
a. Saquinavir b. Nelfinavir
c. Ritonavir d. Atazanavir

301. **Dose of Oseltamivir in a 6month old baby?** *(Recent Question Dec 2016)*
a. 20 mg OD b. 20 mg BD
c. 20 mg/kg body weight d. 20 mg TID

302. **Which is an oral drug for hepatitis C treatment?** *(AIIMS Nov 2015)*
a. Lamivudine b. Ribamivir
c. Ledipasvir d. Peg IFN α

303. **Drug of choice for bird flu:** *(AIIMS Nov 2015)*
a. Oseltamivir b. Ribavirin
c. Entecavir d. Acyclovir

304. **All are used in influenza B except** *(AIIMS Nov 2015)*
a. Oseltamivir b. Zanamivir
c. Peramivir d. Ribavirin

305. **Which of the following drug is topically used for treatment of recurrent respiratory papillomatosis?** *(AIIMS May 2015)*
a. Acyclovir b. Cidofovir
c. Zinc d. Ranitidine

306. **Which of the following is a protease inhibitor:** *(AIIMS May 2015)*
a. Abacavir b. Saquinavir
c. Zidovudine d. Lamivudine

307. **Which of the following is not used in chronic hep b:** *(AIIMS Nov 2014)*
a. Zidovudine b. Lamivudine
c. Telbivudine d. Entecavir

308. **Nonnucleoside reverse transcriptase inhibitors (NNRTIs) include all of the following except:** *(AIIMS May 2014)*
a. Nevirapine b. Delavirdine
c. Etravirine d. Lamivudine

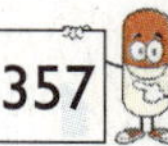

309. Which of the following is an ocular side effect of HAART therapy? ***(AIIMS Nov 2012)***
a. Retinitis b. Uveitis
c. Optic neuritis d. Scleritis

310. Efavirenz is used for treatment of HIV infections. It acts: ***(AIIMS Nov 2011)***
a. As protease inhibitor
b. As reverse transcriptase inhibitor
c. As integrase inhibitor
d. By inhibiting the HIV entry into the cell

311. Which of the following drugs is used to prevent HIV transmission from an HIV positive pregnant mother to child? ***(AIIMS Nov 2011)***
a. Lamivudine b. Stavudine
c. Nevirapine d. Didanosine

312. True about protease inhibitors are all except: ***(AIIMS Nov 2007)***
a. Acts as a substrate for P-glycoprotein and action is mediated by mdr-1 gene
b. Undergo hepatic oxidative metabolism
c. Protease inhibitors interfere with metabolism of several drugs
d. Saquinavir causes maximum induction of CYP3A4

313. Ritonavir, a potent inhibitor of cytochrome P540 3A4 (CYP3P4) and CYP2D6, can cause clinically significant increases in serum levels of other protease inhibitors. This is the basis for "boosted protease inhibitor regimes" which combine ritonavir (in low doses 100-200 mg) with a second, 'boosted' protease inhibitor to enhance patient exposure to the latter agent, thereby preventing or overcoming resistance and allowing less frequent dosing. Which is the protease inhibitor drug that is not recommended for boosting with ritonavir? ***(Recent Question 2016)***
a. Indinavir b. Saquinavir
c. Nelfinavir d. Lopinavir

314. Which is the integrase inhibitor used in treatment of HIV? ***(Recent Question 2016)***
a. Raltegravir b. Indinavir
c. Lopinavir d. Fosamprenavir

315. Drug causing maximum peripheral neuropathy is: ***(Recent Question 2016)***
a. Zidovudine b. Lamivudine
c. Stavudine d. Didanosine

316. Drug used for the Rx of chorioretinitis in HIV is: ***(Recent Question 2016)***
a. Valacyclovir b. Ganciclovir
c. Rivavirin d. Amantadine

317. ART drug which is entry inhibitor ***(Recent Question 2016)***
a. Enfuvirtide b. Abacavir
c. Efavirenz d. Amprenavir

318. Oseltamivir is ***(Recent Question 2016)***
a. Neuraminidase inhibitor b. Neuraminidase activator
c. Carboxylase inhibitor d. Carboxylase activator

319. HIV integrase inhibitor is ***(Recent Question 2016)***
a. Elvitegravir b. Abacavir
c. Maraviroc d. Tenofovir

320. Anti-HIV drug used for prevention of transmission ***(Recent Question 2016)***
a. Nevirapine b. Lamivudine
c. Efavirenz d. Tenofovir

321. Ganciclovir is preferred over acyclovir in the following condition ***(Recent Question 2016)***
a. Herpes simplex keratitis
b. Herpes zoster
c. Chicken pox
d. Cytomegalovirus retinitis in AIDS patients

322. Drug that is active against both HIV and hepatitis B virus ***(Recent Question 2016)***
a. Lamivudine b. Indinavir
c. Didanosine d. Efavirenz

323. The basis of combining ritonavir with lopinavir
a. Pharmaceutical compatibility ***(Recent Question 2016)***
b. CYP3A4 inhibition by ritonavir
c. Long elimination half-life of ritonavir
d. Ability to counteract side effect of lopinavir

324. Efavirenz used for treatment of HIV infections is a
a. Protease inhibitor ***(Recent Question 2016)***
b. Reverse transcriptase inhibitor
c. Integrase inhibitor
d. Inhibitor of the HIV entry into the cell

325. Integrase inhibitor used in treatment of HIV ***(Recent Question 2016)***
a. Raltegravir b. Indinavir
c. Lopinavir d. Fosamprenavir

326. All of the following cause inhibition of CYP3A except ***(Recent Question 2016)***
a. Saquinavir b. Ritonavir
c. Itraconazole d. Erythromycin

327. Which of the following drug is a reverse transcriptase inhibitor? ***(Recent Question 2016)***
a. Indinavir b. Ritonavir
c. Nelfinavir d. Abacavir

328. Nevirapine is ***(Recent Question 2016)***
a. Non-nucleoside reverse transcriptase inhibitor (NNRTI)
b. Nucleoside reverse transcriptase inhibitor (NRTI)
c. Protease inhibitor
d. Fusion inhibitor

329. Drug causing maximum peripheral neuropathy is ***(Recent Question 2016)***
a. Zidovudine b. Lamivudine
c. Stavudine d. Didanosine

330. Which of the following anti-retroviral drugs does not cause peripheral neuropathy? ***(Recent Question 2016)***
a. Lamivudine b. Stavudine
c. Didanosine d. Zalcitabine

331. Zidovudine causes ***(Recent Question 2016)***
a. Neurotoxicity
b. Nephrotoxicity
c. Neutropenia
d. Ototoxicity

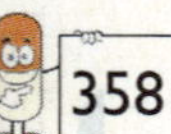

332. Enfuvirtide belongs to the class of
a. Fusion inhibitors *(Recent Question 2016)*
b. Protease inhibitors
c. Gp 120 inhibitors
d. Nucleotide reverse transcriptase inhibitors

333. In antiretroviral therapy, zidovudine should not be combined with *(Recent Question 2016)*
a. Lamivudine b. Nevirapine
c. Didanosine d. Stavudine

334. All the following antiretroviral drugs produce lipodystrophy except *(Recent Question 2016)*
a. Atazanavir
b. Saquinavir
c. Amprenavir
d. Nelfinavir

335. Drug of choice for herpes simplex encephalitis is *(Recent Question 2016)*
a. Mepacrine b. Albendazole
c. Niclosamide d. None of the above

336. Side effect of NRTI is *(Recent Question 2016)*
a. Pneumonia
b. Hyperglycemia
c. Steven Johnson's syndrome
d. Lactic acidosis

337. Reverse transcriptase inhibitor is *(Recent Question 2016)*
a. Didanosine b. Acyclovir
c. Enfuvirtide d. Maraviroc

338. Reverse transcriptase inhibitor *(Recent Question 2016)*
a. Ritonavir b. Saquinavir
c. Amprenavir d. Tenofovir

339. Cidofovir can be used for *(Recent Question 2016)*
a. Respiratory papillomatosis
b. Herpes simplex
c. Herpes zoster
d. All of the above

340. Which of the following has poorest oral bioavailability? *(Recent Question 2016)*
a. Oseltamivir b. Zanamivir
c. Rimantadine d. Amantadine

341. Drug of choice for H1N1 *(Recent Question 2016)*
a. Oseltamivir b. Tenofovir
c. Abacavir d. Acyclovir

342. Drug of choice for acyclovir resistant herpes is *(Recent Question 2016)*
a. Cidofovir b. Ganciclovir
c. Valacyclovir d. Foscarnet

343. Drug of choice for herpes simplex is *(Recent Question 2016)*
a. Acyclovir b. Valacyclovir
c. Ganciclovir d. Foscarnet

344. HAART drug causing insomnia and bad dreams *(Recent Question 2016)*
a. Efavirenz b. Nevirapine
c. Lamivudine d. Zidovudine

345. Ritonavir is an *(Recent Question 2016)*
a. Non-nucleoside reverse transcriptase inhibitor (NN-RTI)
b. Nucleoside reverse transcriptase inhibitor (NRTI)
c. Protease inhibitor
d. Fusion inhibitor

346. Drug not used in HBV *(Recent Question 2016)*
a. Lamivudine b. Telbivudine
c. Entecavir d. Zidovudine

ANTIFUNGAL AGENTS

347. Which of the following antifungal drug is developing drug resistance and has not been prescribed for tinea cruris and tinea corporis since last 2 years? *(AIIMS May 2018)*
a. Terbinafine b. Griseofulvin
c. Voriconazole d. Itraconazole

348. Which of the following is wrongly matched regarding mechanism of action of antifungal drugs? *(AIIMS May 2018)*
a. Azoles: Inhibit 14 alpha sterol demethylase thereby preventing ergosterol synthesis
b. Flucytosine: Inhibit microtubule thereby preventing mitosis
c. Echinocandins: Inhibit glycan synthesis by inhibiting beta 1,3 glycan synthase
d. Amphotericin B: Impair barrier mechanism in cell membrane

349. Amphotericin B acts on: *(Recent Question 2017)*
a. Cell membrane b. Cell wall
c. Nucleus d. Cytoplasm

350. Local antifungal agent used in corneal fungal ulcer: *(AIIMS Nov. 2016)*
a. Silver sulfadiazine b. Neomycin
c. Griseofulvin d. Natamycin

351. Only topically used antifungal? *(Recent Question Dec 2016)*
a. Clotrimazole b. Griseofulvin
c. Terbinafine d. Fluconazole

352. Treatment of choice for boggy swelling on scalp/kerion? *(Recent Question Dec 2016)*
a. Oral betamethasone b. Topical ketoconazole
c. Oral griseofulvin d. Oral terbinafine

353. Drug whose absorption is increased in fatty meal? *(AIIMS Nov 2015)*
a. Griseofulvin b. Amphotericin-B
c. Nimesulide d. Azoles

354. Mucormycosis, drug of choice is: *(AIIMS May 2013)*
a. Amphotericin B b. Itraconazole
c. Voriconazole d. Griseofulvin

355. Voriconazole is not effective against: *(AIIMS Nov 2009)*
a. Candida albicans
b. Mucormycosis
c. Candida tropicalis
d. Aspergillosis

356. Triazole acts by inhibiting ***(Recent Question 2019)***
a. Ergosterol synthesis b. Cell wall inhibition
c. DNA synthesis d. Microtubules

357. The antimicrobial agent which inhibits the ergosterol biosynthesis: ***(Recent Question 2016)***
a. Ketoconazole b. Amphotericin B
c. 5-Flucytosine d. Griseofulvin

358. A fungicidal drug that can be used orally for the treatment of onychomycosis: ***(Recent Question 2016)***
a. Griseofulvin b. Amphotericin B
c. Clotrimazole d. Terbinafine

359. Antifungal which can be used orally but not iv is- ***(Recent Question 2016)***
a. Voriconazole b. Amphoterecin B
c. Terbinafine d. None of the above

360. Amphotericin B causes deficiency of ***(Recent Question 2016)***
a. Sodium b. Calcium
c. Potassium d. Chloride

361. Which of the following is not an antifungal drug? ***(Recent Question 2016)***
a. Ketoconazole b. Undecylenic acid
c. Ciclopirox d. Clofazimine

362. All are used in systemic fungal infections except ***(Recent Question 2016)***
a. Ketoconazole b. Fluconazole
c. Amphotericin B d. Griseofulvin

363. Broad spectrum antifungal agent is ***(Recent Question 2016)***
a. Econazole b. Miconazole
c. Ketoconazole d. Clotrimazole

364. Topically used antifungal agent is ***(Recent Question 2016)***
a. Ketoconazole b. Clotrimazole
c. Amphotericin B d. Voriconazole

365. Induction of treatment in serious fungal infections is mostly done by ***(Recent Question 2016)***
a. IV amphotericin B b. Ketoconazole
c. 5-flucytosine d. Fluconazole

366. Topical antifungal agent that inhibits saprophytic fungi is ***(Recent Question 2016)***
a. Nystatin b. Amphotericin
c. Fluconazole d. Itraconazole

367. Drug of choice for systemic aspergillosis is ***(Recent Question 2016)***
a. Itraconazole b. Amphotericin B
c. Voriconazole d. Caspofungin

368. Amphotericin B toxicity is monitored by
a. Serum sodium measurement ***(Recent Question 2016)***
b. Serum potassium measurement
c. Liver function test
d. Blood sugar

369. Topical antifungal agent used for dermatophytes ***(Recent Question 2016)***
a. Hamycin b. Natamycin
c. Nystatin d. Tolnaftate

370. Drug not effective in Candidial infection ***(Recent Question 2016)***
a. Fluconazole b. Ketoconazole
c. Terbinafine d. Griseofulvin

371. Amphotericin-B is not useful in ***(Recent Question 2016)***
a. Fungal meningitis b. Fungal keratitis
c. Dermatophytes d. Candidiasis

ANTIMALARIALS

372. Which is gametocidal for all species ***(AIIMS Nov 2018)***
a. Quinine b. Chloroquine
c. Primaquine d. None

373. Treatment of chloroquine resistant malaria for a patient from NE? ***(AIIMS May 2018)***
a. Artemether lumefantrine
b. Sulfadoxine Pyrimethamine
c. Chloroquine
d. Mefloquine

374. Artemisinin is not used as chemoprophylaxis in malaria because? ***(Recent Question Dec 2016)***
a. Ion trapping b. Short plasma half-life
c. Toxicity d. Cost

375. What is the dose of Mefloquine in prophylaxis of malaria? ***(Recent Question Dec 2016)***
a. 100 mg b. 150 mg
c. 200 mg d. 250 mg

376. Which of the following drugs can cause bull's eye retinopathy? ***(Recent Question Dec 2016)***
a. Chloroquine b. Amiodarone
c. Ethambutol d. Vigabatrin

377. Drug of choice for uncomplicated falciparum malaria in pregnancy ***(Recent Question Dec 2016)***
a. Chloroquine b. Quinine
c. ACT d. Primaquine

378. Lorry driver after long travel got fever, chills and rigor for 5 days. The drug of choice is:
a. IV artesunate ***(Recent Question Nov/Dec 2016)***
b. Oral artesunate
c. Chloroquine 600+300+150
d. Chloroquine + Primaquine for 14 days

379. Which is true regarding Malaria 2013 recommendation? ***(AIIMS Nov 2015)***
a. Primaquine is contraindicated in pregnancy and infants.
b. Presumptive treatment with chloroquine is recommended.
c. *P. falciparum* is treated with ACT and Primaquine is not given in them.
d. *P. vivax* is treated with chloroquine for 3 days and Primaquine for 7 days.

380. Most effective drug in severe falciparum malaria ***(AIIMS Nov 2014)***
a. Quinine b. Chloroquine
c. Artesunate d. Mefloquine

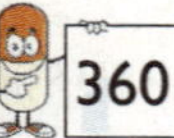

381. Erythema multiforme is caused by *(Recent Question 2019)*
a. Antimalarials b. Antidepressants
c. Antipsychotics d. Antifungals

382. The fastest acting schizonticidal drug among the following is: *(Recent Question 2016)*
a. Artemether b. Mefloquine
c. Chloroquine d. Proguanil

383. Drug causing megaloblastic anemia is: *(Recent Question 2016)*
a. INH b. Chloramphenicol
c. Pyrimethamine d. Methyl dopa

384. Not a drug recommended for P. falciparum is *(Recent Question 2016)*
a. Quinine b. Ciprofloxacin
c. Artemether d. Doxycycline

385. Why quinine is unsafe in pregnancy? *(Recent Question 2016)*
a. It causes hemolysis
b. It causes hypokalemia
c. It causes hyponatremia
d. It causes smooth muscle contraction

386. Which antimalarial Drug can be safely administered in baby with glucose-6-phosphate dehydrogenase deficiency? *(Recent Question 2016)*
a. Chloroquine b. Quinine
c. Mefloquine d. Primaquine

387. Drug of choice in a patient with severe complicated falciparum malaria is *(Recent Question 2016)*
a. Chloroquine b. Quinine
c. Artesunate d. Artemether

388. Lumefantrine is an *(Recent Question 2016)*
a. Antimycobacterial b. Antifungal
c. Antimalarial d. Antiamoebic

389. Pyronaridine is *(Recent Question 2016)*
a. Antimalarial b. Anti-HIV
c. Antifungal d. Antibacterial

390. Drug of choice for treatment of malaria due to *P. vivax* in a 25-year-old pregnant female *(Recent Question 2016)*
a. Chloroquine
b. Primaquine
c. Sulfadoxine-pyrimethamine
d. Quinine

391. Which of the following antimalarial agents is most commonly associated with acute hemolytic reaction in patients with glucose-6-phosphate dehydrogenase deficiency? *(Recent Question 2016*
a. Chloroquine b. Clindamycin
c. Mefloquine d. Primaquine

392. Drug of choice for treatment of chloroquine resistant falciparum malaria is *(Recent Question 2016)*
a. Quinine b. Chloroquine
c. Pyrimethamine d. Primaquine

393. Drug deposited in retina *(Recent Question 2016)*
a. Isoniazid b. Chloroquine
c. Rifampicin d. Pyrazinamide

ANTIHELMINTHIC AND ANTIPROTOZOAL AGENTS

394. Treatment of choice for the organism in the picture is *(AIIMS May 2018)*
a. Praziquantel b. Mebendazole
c. Albendazole d. Pyrantel pamoate

395. The drug of choice for H. nana is praziquantel. Drug of choice for strawberry vagina is: *(AIIMS May 2017)*
a. Metronidazole b. Doxycycline
c. Fluconazole d. Amoxycillin

396. If a patient is resistant to septran in PCP pneumonia other drug that can be used is? *(Recent Question Dec 2016)*
a. Pentamidine b. Melarsoprol
c. Eflornithine d. Suramin

397. Which of the following is least likely to be associated with disulfiram like reaction?? *(Recent Question Dec 2016)*
a. Metronidazole b. Tinidazole
c. Satranidazole d. Benznidazole

398. All of these are used in the treatment of visceral leishmaniasis except: *(AIIMS Nov 2009)*
a. Sitamaquine b. Paromomycin
c. Miltefosine d. Hydroxychloroquine

399. Which of the following drugs is not used in scabies? *(AIIMS May 2008)*
a. Benzene hexachloride b. Permethrin
c. Ciclopirox olamine d. Crotamiton

400. Wrong statement about albendazole is: *(Recent Question 2016)*
a. Poor CSF penetration
b. Contraindicated in pregnancy
c. Useful in neurocysticercosis
d. Can cause hepatotoxicity

401. Drug of choice for schistosomiasis is: *(Recent Question 2016)*
a. Albendazole b. Metronidazole
c. Praziquantel d. Triclabendazole

402. Most common side effect of miltefosine is? *(Recent Question 2016)*
a. Vomiting and diarrhea b. Dermatitis
c. Hepatotoxicity d. Nephrotoxicity

403. Which of the following drugs has both antihelminthic and antiprotozoal activity *(Recent Question 2016)*
a. Nitazoxanide b. Emetine
c. Chloroquine d. Diloxanide furoate

404. All of these are used in the treatment of visceral leishmaniasis except *(Recent Question 2016)*
a. Amphotericin b. Paromomycin
c. Miltefosine d. Hydroxychloroquine

405. Choose the most effective drug for mild intestinal amoebiasis and asymptomatic cyst passers *(Recent Question 2016)*
a. Metronidazole b. Emetine
c. Quiniodochlor d. Diloxanide furoate

406. The drug of choice for Kala-azar is ***(Recent Question 2016)***

a. Pentamidine b. Suramin
c. Sodium stibogluconate d. Ketoconazole

407. What is true of ivermectin? ***(Recent Question 2016)***

a. It is the most effective drug for strongyloidiasis
b. It is the drug of choice for onchocerciasis
c. It can be sued to treat scabies
d. All of the above

408. Which of the following drug is least effective luminal amebicide ***(Recent Question 2016)***

a. Metronidazole b. Diloxanide furoate
c. Iodoquinol d. Paromomycin

409. An antihelminthic drug that is effective against blood fluke, liver fluke, lung fluke and cysticercosis is: ***(Recent Question 2016)***

a. Albendazole b. Praziquantel
c. Ivermectin d. Thiabendazole

410. Drug of choice for treatment of infestation due to onchocerca volvulus is: ***(Recent Question 2016)***

a. Albendazole b. Ivermectin
c. Praziquantel d. Suramin

411. Treatment of neurocysticercosis includes all of the following except: ***(Recent Question 2016)***

a. Albendazole b. Prednisolone
c. Niclosamide d. Praziquantel

412. Metrifonate is effective against: ***(Recent Question 2016)***

a. Amoebiasis b. Leishmaniasis
c. Schistosomiasis d. Giardiasis

413. Round worm infection is best treated with: ***(Recent Question 2016)***

a. Metronidazole b. Mebendazole
c. Albendazole d. Pyrantel pamoate

414. Drug of choice for bacterial vaginosis is: ***(Recent Question 2016)***

a. Metronidazole b. Ampicillin
c. Ciprofloxacin d. Fluconazole

415. Mebendazole cannot be used for ***(Recent Question 2016)***

a. Ascariasis b. Enterobius vermicularis
c. Onchocercosis d. Hydatid cyst disease

416. Which of the following drug acts by inhibiting protein synthesis: ***(PGI May 2018)***

a. Penicillin b. Chloramphenicol
c. Fluoroquinolones d. Vancomycin
e. Aminoglycosides

417. Which of the following is/are indications of use of antibiotics in diarrhea: ***(PGI May 2018)***

a. Cholera b. Traveller's diarrhea
c. Dysentery caused by Shiga toxin producing E. coli
d. Bacillary dysentery
e. All of above

418. Which of the following drugs is/are used in treatment of mucormycosis: ***(PGI May 2018)***

a. Fluconazole b. Amphotericin B
c. Voriconazole d. Posaconazole
e. 5-flurocysteine

419. Which of the following anti-viral drug is/are prodrug: ***(PGI May 2018)***

a. Acyclovir b. Oseltamivir
c. Valganciclovir d. Valaciclovir
e. Ganciclovir

420. A tuberculosis patient was sputum positive even 5 months after treatment with isoniazid, rifampicin, kanamycin, moxifloxacin and streptomycin. He belongs to which drug resistance category: ***(PGI May 2018)***

a. Multidrug resistance (MDR-TB)
b. Poly-drug resistance TB
c. Extensively drug resistance (XDR-TB)
d. Pro-extensively drug resistance
e. Mono-resistance TB

421. WHO updated new treatment for MDR-TB in 2016. It includes 4-6 months intensive phase and 5 month continuation phase for short regimen. Which of the following drugs are included in the intensive phase regimen apart from pyrizinamide + ethambutol + kanamycin + moxifloxacin: ***(PGI May 2018)***

a. Delamanid b. Bedaquiline
c. High dose isoniazid d. Clofazimine
e. Linezolid

422. Which of the following drugs should not be used in myasthenia gravis: ***(PGI May 2018)***

a. Neostigmine b. Paracetamol
c. Amikacin d. Edrophonium
e. Atropine

423. IFN α is used in ***(PGI Nov 2017)***

a. Hep. B b. Hep C
c. Hairy cell leukemia d. Multiple sclerosis

424. Drugs used in XDR TB ***(PGI Nov 2017)***

a. Amikacin b. Fluoroquinolone
c. Pyrazinamide d. Streptomycin
e. Ethionamide

425. Bedaquiline ***(PGI Nov 2017)***

a. New antibacterial class
b. MOA is ATP synthase inhibitor
c. Not given for more than 12 months
d. Not given as single drug but is given as add-on drug

426. Drug of choice for Strongyloides stercoralis: ***(PGI May 2017)***

a. Mebendazole
b. Albendazole c. Ivermectin
d. Levamisole e. Diethylcarbamazine

427. Which of the following drugs can be used in rifampicin-resistance Leprosy: ***(PGI May 2017)***

a. Rifapentine b. Moxifloxacin
c. Clofazimine d. Minocycline
e. Clarithromycin

428. DOC for mycoplasma is/are: ***(PGI May 2017)***

a. Doxycycline
b. Ceftriaxone
c. Azithromycin
d. Penicillin
e. Gentamycin

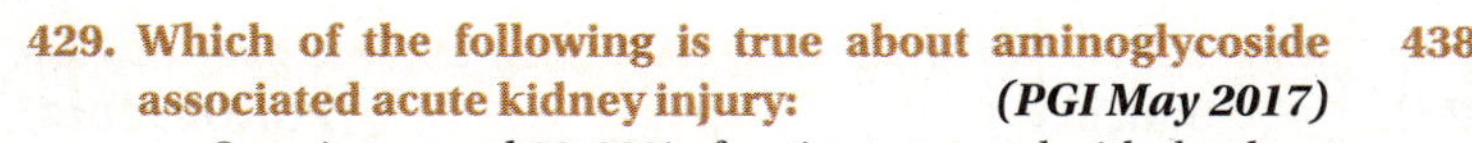

429. Which of the following is true about aminoglycoside associated acute kidney injury: ***(PGI May 2017)***
- a. Seen in around 10-20% of patients treated with the drug
- b. May occur within 1 week of initiation of treatment
- c. Occur only after 3 weeks of treatment
- d. Interstitial nephritis occurs
- e. Usually develops within 72 hours of initiation of treatment

430. Which of the following is true about antifungal drugs: ***(PGI May 2017)***
- a. Echinocandins have very less side effects
- b. Fluconozole is first line drug for invasive aspergillosis
- c. Oral fluconazole has 100 % bioavailability
- d. Amphotericin B is fungistatic
- e. Nephrotoxicity is dose limiting side effect of amphotericin B

431. Which of the following is/are not 5th generation Cephalosporin: ***(PGI May 2017)***
- a. Cefoxitin
- b. Cefoperazone
- c. Ceftolozane
- d. Ceftaroline
- e. Ceftobiprole

432. Which of the following drugs is excreted mainly by kidney: ***(PGI May 2017)***
- a. Tetracycline
- b. Rifampicin
- c. Digoxin
- d. Penicillin
- e. Lithium

433. True statement(s) about albendazole: ***(PGI May 2017)***
- a. Undergoes first-pass metabolism in the liver
- b. Active against both larva and adult of Nematodes
- c. Absorption increases with fatty meal
- d. Excreted in the urine
- e. Thiabendazole is less toxic than albendazole

434. Which of the following dyad of anti-HIV drug and mechanism of action is/are correctly matched: ***(PGI May 2017)***
- a. Maraviroc - Entry inhibitor
- b. Raltegravir - Integrase inhibitor
- c. Indinavir - Protease inhibitor
- d. Nevirapine - Nonnucleoside reverse transcriptase inhibitor
- e. Darunavir- Fusion inhibitor

435. Anti-influenza drug which is/are given through inhalation route: ***(PGI May 2017)***
- a. Amantadine
- b. Oseltamivir
- c. Zanamivir
- d. Rimantadine

436. Which of the following is/are newer drugs for TB: ***(PGI Nov. 2016)***
- a. Bedaquiline
- b. Clofazimine
- c. Ceftaroline
- d. Rifapentine
- e. Etanercept

437. True about Mafenide: ***(PGI Nov. 2016)***
- a. Can penetrate eschars
- b. Doesn't cause burning sensation when applied to raw surface
- c. Can be used orally
- d. May cause metabolic acidosis

438. Which of the following drugs show clinically significant drug interactions: ***(PGI Nov. 2016)***
- a. Vancomycin—Amphotericin B
- b. Ranitidine—Atorvastatin
- c. Warfarin—Aspirin
- d. Allopurinol—Azathioprine
- e. Aminoglycoside + Vancomycin

439. True about Jarisch-Herxheimer reaction: ***(PGI June 2015)***
- a. Occur within hours after giving penicillin
- b. Develop only after 1 week of Penicillin therapy
- c. Aggravation of signs and symptoms of syphilis
- d. It occur due to allergy to penicillin
- e. Most common in secondary syphilis

440. For which of the following drug bacteria acquire drug resistance by inactivation or degradation by enzyme: ***(PGI June 2015)***
- a. Quinolones
- b. Aminoglycosides
- c. Vancomycin
- d. Ampicillin
- e. Chloramphenicol

441. Which of the following drug is mainly excreted by kidney: ***(PGI June 2015)***
- a. Tetracyclines
- b. Doxycyclines
- c. Ampicillin
- d. Acyclovir
- e. Rifampicin

442. All are true about acyclovir except: ***(PGI June 2015)***
- a. Guanosine analogue
- b. Inhibit viral DNA gyrase
- c. Inhibit viral DNA polymerase
- d. Requires phosphorylation for activation
- e. Excreted mainly in urine

443. S/E of clofazimine includes: ***(PGI June 2015)***
- a. Ichthyosis
- b. Thrombocytosis
- c. Skin pigmentation
- d. Gastrointestinal disturbances
- e. Weight gain

444. ATT drug with significant renal excretion is/are: ***(PGI Nov 2014)***
- a. INH
- b. Rifampicin
- c. Pyrazinamide
- d. Amikacin
- e. Streptomycin

445. True about amphotericin B: ***(PGI Nov 2014)***
- a. Liposomal preparation is available
- b. Orally absorbed
- c. Used only in intravenous form
- d. Protein synthesis inhibitor

446. Antibiotic which acts through cell wall inhibition: ***(PGI Nov 2014)***
- a. Penicillin
- b. Daptomycin
- c. Aminoglycoside
- d. Cephalosporin
- e. Imipenem

447. Not indicated for anaerobic colitis treatment: ***(PGI Nov 2014)***
- a. Metronidazole
- b. Aminoglycoside
- c. Amikacin
- d. Piperacillin-tazobactam
- e. Imipenem

448. Treatment of nocardia infection includes: *(PGI May 2014)*
a. Ampicillin b. Fluoroquinolones
c. Azithromycin d. Cotrimoxazole
e. Amikacin

449. Drugs active against MRSA: *(PGI May 2014)*
a. Vancomycin b. Ceftriaxone
c. Linezolid d. Piperacillin-tazobactam
e. Meropenem

450. True about daptomycin: *(PGI May 2014)*
a. Causes diarrhea as side effect
b. It is a glycopeptide antibiotic
c. Cause myopathy
d. It can be used orally
e. Excretion through kidney

451. Drug used in MRSA are all except: *(PGI Nov 2013)*
a. Vancomycin
b. 3rd generation cephalosporin
c. Amphotericin B
d. Meropenem
e. Linezolid

452. Isoniazid is metabolised in body by: *(PGI May 2013)*
a. Acetylation b. Sulfation
c. Hydroxylation d. Methylation
e. First metabolized in liver and then excreted in urine

453. ATT drug which is not bacteriostatic: *(PGI May 2013)*
a. INH b. Rifampicin
c. Pyrazinamide d. PAS
e. Ethambutol

454. Antibiotics acting through cell wall inhibition: *(PGI May 2013)*
a. Cephalosporin b. Vancomycin
c. Penicillin d. Aminoglycosides
e. Sulfonamides

455. Antagonistic drug combination(s) is/are: *(PGI May 2013)*
a. Penicillin + Aminoglycosides
b. Penicillin + Tetracycline
c. Vancomycin + Ceftriaxone
d. Ceftriaxone+ Tazobactam
e. Amphotericin B + Flucytosine

456. Antifungal not act by inhibiting cell wall formation: *(PGI Nov 2012)*
a. Caspofungin b. Itraconazole
c. Amphotericin B d. Echinocandins

457. Bacteriostatic drug(s) among ATT drugs used in initiation phase: *(PGI May 2012)*
a. INH
b. Pyrazinamide
c. Streptomycin
d. Rifampicin
e. Ethambutol

458. As per WHO protocol ATT drug C/I in pregnancy: *(PGI May 2012)*
a. Rifampicin b. Pyrazinamide
c. Ethambutol d. Streptomycin
e. INH

459. Which ATT drug(s) is/are safe in chronic liver disease patients: *(PGI May 2012)*
a. INH b. Rifampicin
c. Pyrazinamide d. Ethambutol
e. Streptomycin

460. Anti-methicillin-Resistance Staphylococcus aureus (MRSA) drugs are: *(PGI May 2012)*
a. Linezolid
b. Vancomycin
c. Daptomycin
d. Cefepime
e. Piperacillin-tazobactam

461. True about Ganciclovir: *(PGI May 2012)*
a. Inhibits viral DNA polymerase
b. Used in cytomegalovirus (CMV) infection
c. Used in Herpes Simplex virus (HSV) infection
d. Active against Kaposi's sarcoma-associated herpesvirus

462. Gonorrhoea become resistant to following during in last decade: *(PGI Nov 2011)*
a. Penicillin G b. Azithromycin
c. Tetracycline d. Ciprofloxacin
e. 3rd generation cephalosporins

463. True statement about β lactam antibiotics: *(PGI Nov 2011)*
a. Aztreonam is cross allergic with benzyl Penicillin
b. Meropenem not require concurrent cilastatin administration
c. Methicillin cause interstitial nephritis
d. Moxalactam can cause disulfiram like action

464. Metronidazole cause: *(PGI May 2011)*
a. Disulfiram-like effect
b. Antagonise warfarin
c. It has metallic taste

465. Drugs used in pseudomonas treatment: *(PGI May 2011)*
a. Cefixime b. Ceftazidime
c. Ceftriaxone d. Colistin
e. Ampicillin

466. False statement regarding tetracyclines: *(PGI May 2011)*
a. Bind 30S
b. Hepatotoxic
c. Cause pseudotumor cerebri
d. Cause vestibular toxicity
e. Used in malignant pleural effusion

467. Correct statement about aminoglycosides: *(PGI May 2011)*
a. Streptomycin- least nephrotoxic
b. Ca salt reverse neuromuscular blockade by aminoglycoside
c. Bind 50S
d. Do not show post antibiotic effect
e. Gentamycin is more vestibulotoxic

468. Drugs used in treatment of Aspergillosis: *(PGI May 2011)*
a. Itraconazole b. Voriconazole
c. Clotrimazole d. Amphotericin B
e. Ketoconazole

469. **True about ATT:** ***(PGI Nov 2010)***
a. Ethambutol readily cross BBB
b. Pyrazinamide is bactericidal for intracellular bacteria
c. NH does not has cross-resistance with other antitubercular drugs
d. Resistance to rifampin is difficult to develop

470. **Drugs not used in MRSA:** ***(PGI Nov 2010)***
a. Vancomycin b. Teicoplanin
c. Imipenem d. Cloxacillin
e. Amoxiclav

471. **Drugs not used in Gram -ve infections:** ***(PGI Nov 2010)***
a. Imipenem b. Ceftazidime
c. Vancomycin d. Ciprofloxacin
e. Amikacin

472. **Drugs not effective in pseudomonas infection:** ***(PGI May 2010)***
a. Ciprofloxacin b. Norfloxacin
c. Aminoglycosides d. Ampicillin
e. Piperacillin

473. **Aminoglycosides are used against following organisms except:** ***(PGI May 2010)***
a. *S. aureus* b. Streptococci
c. *E. coli* d. Anaerobes
e. *Salmonella typhi*

474. **Correctly matched pairs are:** ***(PGI May 2010)***
a. Rifampicin - inhibit bacterial DNA polymerase
b. Terbinafine- inhibit fungal DNA polymerase
c. Acyclovir- inhibit viral DNA polymerase
d. Cytarabine- inhibit human DNA polymerase

475. **Drugs that crosses blood brain barrier:** ***(PGI May 2010)***
a. Erythromycin b. Cotrimoxazole
c. Ampicillin d. Aminoglycosides
e. Ceftriaxone

476. **Amphotericin B toxicity is ↑ed by:** ***(PGI May 2010)***
a. Normal saline b. Cardiac failure
c. Lipid formulations d. Aminoglycosides

477. **Which of the following combination (s) is/are false** ***(PGI Nov 2009)***
a. Oral valacyclovir -DOC for herpes zoster
b. Cidifovir-CMV retinitis
c. Ribavarin-Chronic HBV infection
d. Valganciclovir->90% oral bioavailability
e. Fomivirsen-An antisense oligonucleotide for treatment of CMV retinitis

478. **Adverse effect (s) of Foscarnet includes all except:** ***(PGI Nov 2009)***
a. Hypercalcemia b. Hyperkalemia
c. Hypocalcemia d. Hypokalemia
e. Penile ulcer

479. **Most common side effect of artemisinin is:**
a. Nausea b. Vomiting ***(PGI Nov 2009)***
c. Diarrhea d. Bone marrow suppression
e. Pigmentation

480. **Adverse effect of dapsone includes:** ***(PGI Nov 2009)***
a. Peripheral neuropathy b. Hemolytic anemia
c. Agranulocytosis d. Hepatitis
e. Methemoglobinemia

481. **Cephalosporin having renal excretion (or renal failure) is/are** ***(PGI Nov 2009)***
a. Cefazolin b. Ceftriaxone
c. Ceftazidime d. Cefuroxime
e. Cefoperazone

482. **Mutational drug resistance is/are seen in:**
a. Rifampicin – *Staphylococcus aureus* ***(PGI May 2009)***
b. Multidrug resistant – *Mycobacteria*
c. Fluoroquinolones – *S. typhi*
d. Tetracyclin – *Vibrio chloreae*
e. β lactam – Enterococcus

483. **Peripheral neuropathy is limiting factor in use of:** ***(PGI May 2009)***
a. Zidovudine b. Stavudine
c. Efavirenz d. Zalcitabine
e. Nevirapine

484. **True about Methicillin-resistance staphylococcus aureus (MRSA):** ***(PGI May 2009)***
a. Isoxazolyl penicillin is highly effective
b. All MRSA are multidrug resistance
c. Vancomycin is effective
d. MRSA are more virulent than sensitive strains
e. Resistance develop due to altered binding protein

485. **Synergistic action is used in:** ***(PGI May 2009)***
a. Enterococcal endocarditis
b. Viridans streptococcal endocarditis
c. Penicillin + Erythromycin: Gr. A Streptococci
d. Carbenicillin/ticarcillin + gentamicin: Pseudomonas infection
e. Penicillin + Tetracycline/ chloramphenicol: Pneumococci

486. **Which of the following HIV drug inhibit drug metabolizing enzymes:** ***(PGI Dec 2008)***
a. Ritonavir b. Lamivudine
c. Nevirapine d. Delavirdine
e. Enfuvirtide

487. **About silver sulfadiazine which of the following is true**
a. Penetrate sore ***(PGI Dec 2008)***
b. Bacteriostatic
c. Thrombocytopenia occur as a S/E
d. Adverse reactions are frequent
e. Systemic absorption may occur

488. **Extended spectrum β lactamase inhibitors are:** ***(PGI June 2007)***
a. Imipenem b. Ceftazidime
c. Cefoperazone d. Ceftriaxone
e. Aztreonam

489. **Drugs used in MRSA:** ***(PGI June 2006)***
a. Quinupristin/dalfopristin
b. Linezolid
c. Teicoplanin
d. Penicillin
e. Piperacillin (Tazobactam)

490. **In antibiotic associated colitis, organism involved is:** ***(PGI June 2006)***
a. *Clostridium difficile* b. *Pseudomonas*
c. *Staphylococcus* d. *Enterococcus*

491. **NRTI** *(PGI Dec 2005)*
a. Lamivudine b. Zalcitabine
c. Nevirapine d. Delavirdine
e. Ticlopidine

492. **A person's creatinine clearance is < 10 mL/min. Which of the following drugs dose reduction is needed:** *(PGI June 2005)*
a. Amikacin b. Ketoconazole
c. Lithium d. Budesonide
e. Theophylline

493. **Which of the following drugs combination shows antimicrobial synergism** *(PGI June 2005)*
a. Penicillin+streptomycin in SABE
b. Ampicillin + tetracycline in endocarditis
c. Sulphamethoxazole + trimethoprim in UTI
d. Amphotericin B + flucytosine in cryptoccocal meaninings

494. **Time dependent PK all except** *(JIPMER Nov 2018)*
a. Linezolid
b. Daptomycin
c. Lincosamide
d. Meropenem

495. **Concentration dependent PK all except** *(JIPMER Nov 2018)*
a. Amikacin b. Metronidazole
c. Linezolid d. Daptomycin

496. **Which of the following drugs should not be given with midazolam** *(JIPMER Nov 2018)*
a. Ritonavir b. Indinavir
c. Zidovudine d. Lamivudine

497. **Which is not a mechanism of bacterial resistance** *(JIPMER Nov 2018)*
a. By synthesizing enzymes against antibiotics
b. By altering the permeability of porin channels in cell wall
c. By active efflux of the drug after entering into the cell
d. By altering the binding site (DNA gyrase, topoisomerase) of the antibiotic

498. **False about Bedaquiline is:** *(JIPMER May 2018)*
a. Mycobacterial ATP synthase inhibitor
b. Food intake increases bioavailability
c. It should be given alone
d. It has cross resistance with clofazimine

499. **The drug having higher concentration in the bone:** *(JIPMER May 2018)*
a. Piperacillin b. Vancomycin
c. Clindamycin d. Paromomycin

500. **Treatment of ventilator associated pneumonia (VAP) caused by MDR Acinetobacter baumannii is:** *(JIPMER May 2018)*
a. Quinupristin and dalfopristin
b. Colistimethate sodium
c. Lavendamycin
d. Tedizolid

501. **Antibiotic of choice for toxic shock syndrome:** *(JIPMER 2018, 2017)*
a. Linezolid b. Clindamycin
c. Rifampicin d. Penicillin

502. **Ritonavir given along with which drug causes prolonged QT interval** *(JIPMER 2017)*
a. Atazanavir b. Saquinavir
c. Indinavir d. Nelfinavir

503. **Cobicistat is used to boost effect of** *(JIPMER 2017)*
a. Indinavir b. Elvitegravir
c. Lamivudine d. Enfuvirtide

504. **TDK (Time Dependent Killing) is seen with all except** *(JIPMER 2017)*
a. Clindamycin b. Meropenem
c. Erythromycin d. Linezolid

505. **Antifungal used in GVHD is** *(JIPMER 2017)*
a. Posaconazole b. Fluconazole
c. Itraconazole d. Voriconazole

506. **Famciclovir is a prodrug of** *(JIPMER 2017)*
a. Valacyclovir b. Ganciclovir
c. Acyclovir d. Penciclovir

507. **Which anti-TB drug can cause uveitis?** *(JIPMER 2017)*
a. Ethambutol b. Rifabutin
c. Ethionamide d. Cycloserine

508. **A 23-years-old woman complaints of recurrent acne over her face. History revealed that she had taken topical antibiotics for her acne without any significant improvement. Which one of the following tetracyclines is mot preferred for her acne?** *(JIPMER 2016)*
a. Oxytetracycline b. Demeclocycline
c. Doxycycline d. Minocycline

509. **The drug that acts by inhibiting bacterial RNA polymerase is** *(JIPMER 2016)*
a. Cephalosporins b. Rifampicin
c. Macrolides d. Aminoglycosides

510. **Mechanism of action of azoles:** *(JIPMER 2014)*
a. Inhibition ergosterol synthesis
b. Squalene epoxidase inhibitor
c. Mitotic inhibitor
d. Micropore formation

511. **Fusion inhibitor approved for use in HIV is:** *(JIPMER 2014)*
a. Enfuvirtide b. Efavirenz
c. Emtricitabine d. Atazanavir

512. **Which of the following drugs is not used for the treatment of anaerobic infections?** *(JIPMER 2009)*
a. Penicillin
b. Clindamycin
c. Chloramphenicol
d. Gentamicin

513. **Which of the following impairs GI motility?** *(JIPMER 2013)*
a. Erythromycin b. Verapamil
c. Botulinum d. Nitroglycerine

514. **All are true regarding Mechanism of action except:** *(JIPMER 2013)*
a. Chloramphenicol-Protein synthesis
b. Tetracycline-Cell wall synthesis
c. Metronidazole - DNA
d. Penicillin - cell wall synthesis

515. Which drug acts by inhibiting protein synthesis? *(JIPMER 2012)*

a. Ciprofloxacin b. Penicillin
c. Erythromycin d. Nalidixic acid

516. Which of the following drug causes interstitial nephritis? *(JIPMER 2012)*

a. Methicillin b. Cloxacillin
c. Amoxycillin d. Piperacillin

517. All are true except: *(JIPMER 2012)*

a. Famciclovir is the prodrug of penciclovir
b. Penciclovir does not cause chain termination
c. Penciclovir triphosphate has lower affinity for the viral DNA polymerase than acyclovir triphosphate
d. Incidence of mammary adenocarcinoma increased in female rats

518. Which of the following antibiotic is a glycopeptides? *(JIPMER 2012)*

a. Clindamycin b. Vancomycin
c. Azithromycin d. Linezolid

519. Which group of drugs potentiates the action of Neuromuscular blockers? *(JIPMER 2011)*

a. Aminoglycosides b. Cephalosporins
c. Ampicillin d. Penicillin

520. Antihelminthic contraindicated in seizure disorder is: *(JIPMER 2011, 2008)*

a. DEC b. Albendazole
c. Piperazine d. Pyrantel Pamoate

521. All the following can occur with tetracycline therapy during pregnancy except: *(JIPMER 2011)*

a. Teeth discoloration b. Gingival hyperplasia
c. Raised ICT d. Reduced bone growth

522. Linezolid belongs to which class of Drugs? *(JIPMER 2011)*

a. Macrolide b. Aminoglycoside
c. Oxazolidinones d. Streptogramins

523. Which of the following antibiotics has a Nonspecific MAO Inhibitor activity? *(JIPMER 2011)*

a. Tazobactam b. Ampicillin
c. Spectinomycin d. Linezolid

524. Drug most active against for Bacteroides fragilis is? *(JIPMER 2011)*

a. Cefepime b. Ceftazidime
c. Cefoxitin d. Cefotetan

525. Drug not acting on cell membrane is: *(JIPMER 2010)*

a. Daptomycin b. Cycloserine
c. Amoxicillin d. Bacitracin

526. Ivermectin is indicated in all of the following except: *(JIPMER 2010)*

a. Ascaris b. Filariasis
c. Malaria d. Onchocerciasis

527. Grey colour and yellow fluorescence in infant teeth is caused by: *(JIPMER 2010)*

a. Phenytoin
b. Porphyria
c. Tetracycline
d. Barbiturate

528. Dyslipedaemia is least commonly seen with: *(JIPMER 2010)*

a. Amprenavir b. Atazanavir
c. Saquinavir d. Nelfinavir

529. Which of the following drugs is used to treat Chlamydia infection in pregnancy? *(JIPMER 2009)*

a. Doxycycline b. Erythromycin
c. Meropenem d. Tetracycline

530. Side effect of acute pancreatitis is due to following anti-HIV drugs: *(JIPMER 2009)*

a. Lamivudine b. Zidovudine
c. Didanosine d. Zalcitabine

531. Following are third generation cephalosporins except: *(JIPMER 2009)*

a. Cefuroxime b. Ceftriaxone
c. Ceftazidime d. Cefotaxime

532. The mechanism of action of cephalosporin is:

a. Interferes with cell wall synthesis *(JIPMER 2009)*
b. Inhibition of DNA gyrase
c. Inhibition of protein synthesis
d. Inhibition of DNA polymerase

533. Which of the following is not an example an NNRTI? *(JIPMER 2008)*

a. Efavirenz b. Etravirine
c. Emtricitabine d. Delavirdine

534. Which of the following drugs will not cause hypo-thyroidism? *(JIPMER 2007)*

a. Ethambutol b. Lithium
c. Amiodarone d. Pyrazinamide

535. Aztreonam differs from imipenem in: *(JIPMER 2006)*

a. Not active against enterobacteriaceae
b. Aztreonam is effective against ESBL whereas imipenem is not
c. In penicillin allergy, aztreonam tolerated but not imipenem
d. Aztreonam does not penetrate CSF in contrast to imipenem

536. All of the following are useful against MRSA except: *(JIPMER 2006)*

a. Vancomycin b. Linezolid
c. Retapamulin d. Streptogramin

537. Drug of choice for treating extended spectrum beta lactamase (ESBL) organism is: *(JIPMER 2006)*

a. Aztreonam b. Imipenem
c. Cefepime d. Ceftazidime

538. All of the following antitubercular drugs can cause hepatic toxicity EXCEPT *(NIMHANS 2014)*

a. Rifampicin
b. Isoniazid
c. Pyraizinamide
d. Ethambutol

539. The HIV fusion inhibitor, Enfuvirtide, acts at the site of *(NIMHANS 2014)*

a. Gp120 b. Gp41
c. P24 d. CXCR4

540. **The mechanism of action of Enfuvirtide includes** *(NIMHANS 2014)*
   a. Fusion/entry inhibitor
   b. Reverse transcriptase inhibitor
   c. Integrase inhibitor
   d. Protease inhibitors

541. **NOT an NRTI drug is** *(NIMHANS 2013)*
   a. Efavirenz b. Zidovudine
   c. Stavudine d. Abacavir

542. **The antifungal drug which is NOT an Azole** *(NIMHANS 2013)*
   a. Ketoconazole b. Mebendazole
   c. Miconazole d. Voriconazole

543. **Which of the following doesn't belong to Triazole?** *(NIMHANS 2013)*
   a. Posconazole b. Voriconazole
   c. Ketoconazole d. Itraconazole

544. **Which one of the following does NOT increase neuromuscular blockade?** *(NIMHANS 2012)*
   a. Clindamycin
   b. Lincomycin
   c. Streptomycin
   d. Erythromycin

545. **Excess pyridoxine is given along with Isoniazid because (How does INH cause pyridoxine deficiency)?** *(NIMHANS 2011)*
   a. INH increase pyridoxine excretion
   b. INH increase pyridoxine secretion
   c. INH inhibits the enzyme pyridoxine phosphokinase
   d. INH stimulates the enzyme pyridoxine phosphokinase

546. **Mechanism of action of Acyclovir is** *(NIMHANS 2011)*
   a. Inhibitor of viral DNA polymerase
   b. Inhibitor of viral thymidine kinase
   c. Inhibitor of viral reverse transcriptase
   d. Inhibitor of HSV polymerase

547. **Mechanisms of action of the following drug is FALSE** *(NIMHANS 2010)*
   a. Amphotericin B-Ergosterol inhibition
   b. Capsofungin-3, 4 glucans
   c. Fluconazole-Mitosis inhibition
   d. Flucytosine-Pyrimidine metabolism inhibition

548. **Pyridoxine is given with which antitubercular drug?** *(NIMHANS 2010)*
   a. Rifampicin b. Isoniagid
   c. Pyrazinamide d. Ethambutol

549. **All of the following are nucleoside reverse transcriptase inhibitors (RTIS), except** *(NIMHANS 2007)*
   a. Zidovudine b. Lamivudine
   c. Nevirapine d. Didanosine

550. **Drug of choice for MRSA is** *(NIMHANS 2009)*
   a. Streptogramin
   b. Vancomycin
   c. Quinupristin
   d. Linezolid

551. **Which one of the following is a nucleoside analog reverse transcriptase inhibitor?** *(NIMHANS 2009)*
   a. Efavirenz b. Nevirapine
   c. Zidovudine d. Saquinavir

Answers with Explanations to Multiple Choice Questions

1. Ans. (c) Doxycycline

(Ref: Goodman Gilman 13th E/P1052)

2. Ans. (d) Cotrimoxazole

(Ref: Goodman Gilman 13th E/P1014)

- In this infant there is a significant increase in the serum unconjugated bilirubin level.
- Among the given options clotrimazole has sulfamethoxazole, which has a high plasma protein binding, which can displace bilirubin from its binding site in albumin and cause unconjugated hyperbilirubinemia.

Drugs causing hyperbilirubinemia	Mechanism of hyperbilirubinemia
Sulfonamides	Displace bilirubin from albumin binding sites
Rifampicin Probenecid Novobiocin	Inhibit bilirubin uptake by liver
Chloramphenicol Gentamicin Pregnanediol Novobiocin	Inhibit UGT1A1
Ribavirin	Hemolysis

3. Ans. (a) Amikacin

(Ref: Goodman Gilman 13th E/P1053)

4. Ans. (a) Vancomycin

(Ref: National Antibiotic Guidelines of India, Harrison 20th E/P1631)

- In case of community acquired pneumonia beta lactams like amoxycillin and ceftriaxone are first line drugs.
- In case of staphylococcal pneumonia there might be MRSA infection and in that case linezolid or vancomycin is also used.

Note: Beta lactams are not effective against MRSA.

5. Ans. (a) Benzathine penicillin 7.2 million units in three divided doses

(Ref: Harrison 20th E/P1820)

6. Ans. (a) Azithromycin 2 g oral single dose

(Ref: CMDT 2017/P1486)

- There is growing resistance to cephalosporins and hence currently dual therapy is recommended for gonorrhoea:
  - Ceftriaxone 250 mg IM + Azithromycin 1 g oral: Both single dose

- Cefixime 400 mg oral + Azithromycin 1 g oral: Both single dose, in case patient does not want to take injectable drug.
- An alternative is azithromycin 2 g oral as single dose, which is less preferred as discussed.
- For non-gonococcal cervicitis which is most commonly caused by chlamydia doxycycline 100 mg for 7 days or Azithromycin 1 g single dose is preferred.
- In case of coinfection dual therapy is preferred and treatment is similar to gonorrhoea.
- However if a single drug is to be used in coinfection, only azithromycin 2 g single dose can be used, as it is effective against both gonorrhoea and chlamydia.

7. Ans. (a) Cell wall synthesis inhibition

(Ref: Goodman Gilman 12th E/P1540)

Vancomycin inhibits cell wall synthesis by inhibiting d-alanine of cell wall subunit.

8. Ans. (d) Only ORS

(Ref: CMDT 2017/P1305)

- It is a case of acute diarrhea which can be managed by just ORS in stable patients.
- If patient is afebrile antibiotics are not given.
- Patients with mild to moderate symptoms of dehydration are treated with ORS. In case of severe dehydration IV fluids are given.
- In a febrile patient antibiotics are used empirically; in Asian countries ciprofloxacin is used. In countries like Russia, giardia is common and hence metronidazole or tinidazole is also recommended. However if giardia infection is suspected in India the same may be added.
- Since patient is afebrile in this case, we can use only ORS.

9. Ans. (d) Adherence

(Ref: Journals)

Biofilm Mediated Drug Resistance

A biofilm is a population of bacteria enclosed in a exopolysaccharide matrix, growing on a surface of a medical device like catheter. Quorum sensing is a bacterium to bacterium signaling to coordinate among themselves for contribution in biofilm synthesis. This biofilm contributes to resistance to antibiotics by various mechanisms.

- **Mechanical barrier:** The exopolysaccharide matrix serves as a mechanical barrier to diffusion of antibiotics through the biofilm.
- **Efflux pumps:** Biofilms develop efflux pumps that can actively pump the drug out of the biofilm.
- **Enzymatic inactivation:** Biofilms can produce drug inactivating enzymes like pseudomonas biofilms producing beta lactamase.
- **Decreased growth rate:** Decreased oxygen and nutrients passage through the biofilms slows down the metabolism of bacteria and growth rate. As antibiotics are most effective against rapidly growing bacteria, a decreased growth rate decreases efficacy of antibiotics.
- **Persisters:** Some bacteria undergo phenotypic modification into dormant, spore like structure and survive antibiotic insult. These are called as persisters which are activated later.

Note: Adherence is a mechanism of bacteria to attach to host cell for penetration. It's not a mechanism of resistance.

10. Ans. (a) Doxycycline

(Ref: CMDT 2017/P1313)

- Doxycycline is the drug of choice for all rickettsial infections like
  - **Scrub typhus**
  - Murine typhus
  - Rocky mountain spotted fever
  - Recrudescent epidemic typhus (Brill disease)
  - Rickettsial pox
  - Q fever
- Azithromycin, fluoroquinolones and chloramphenicol are other alternatives.

11. Ans. (a) Ceftriaxone

(Ref: Harrison 19th E/P767)

- Ceftriaxone is the empirical drug of choice for treatment of meningitis. It is frequently combined with vancomycin.

12. Ans. (a) Cotrimoxazole

(Ref: CMDT 2018/P1565)

- DOC for prophylaxis and treatment of pneumocystis infection in both immunocompetent as well as immunocompromised is cotrimoxazole.
- Other drugs used are
  - Dapsone + Pyrimethamine
  - Clindamycin + Primaquine
  - Pentamidine
  - Atovaquone
  - Prednisolone is given only in immunocompromised along with antimicrobials in case they present with PaO_2 less than 70 mm Hg or oxygen saturation less than 90%.

13. Ans. (a) Carbepenams and 3rd generation cephalosporins

(Ref: Harrison 19th E/P1048)

- First line drugs for B. Cepecia
  - Cotrimoxazole
  - Meropenem
  - Doxycycline
- Second line drugs
  - 3rd generation cephalosporins
  - Fluoroquinolones
- Combination therapy like meropenem plus a 3rd generation cephalosporin is used in case of serious pulmonary infection. However meropenem should be never combined with cotrimoxazole due to their antagonizing effect.

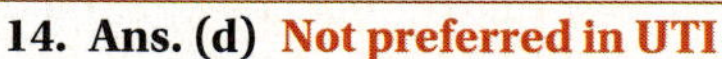

14. Ans. (d) Not preferred in UTI

(Ref: Goodman Gilman 12th E/P1523)

- Tigecycline, doxycycline and minocycline are safe in renal failure.
- Tigecycline is active against gram-negatives with the exception of pseudomonas, providencia, morganella and proteus.
- Tigecycline has poor bioavailability and hence is given only by parenteral route.
- Tigecycline is poorly concentrated in urine and hence should be avoided in treatment of urinary tract infection.

15. Ans. (a) Ceftriaxone

(Ref: Harrison 19th E/P1164)

Drugs active against mycoplasma are

- Doxycycline (More preferred than tetracycline)
- Azithromycin
- Fluoroquinolones
- Chloramphenicol
- Gentamicin
- Clindamycin: Only against M. hominis

Note: Since mycoplasma does not have a cell wall and beta lactam drugs like ceftriaxone inhibit cell wall synthesis, these drugs are not effective against mycoplasma.

16. Ans. (a) Aminoglycosides

(Ref: Goodman Gilman 12th E/P1515)

Aminoglycosides require oxygen and ATP for entry into the bacteria and hence are ineffective against anaerobes.

17. Ans. (c) Vancomycin

(Ref: Goodman Gilman 12th E/P1539)

Bactericidal Drugs

- Cell wall synthesis inhibitors: Beta lactams, vancomycin, cycloserine, Fosfomycin, Bacitracin
- Drugs acting on cell membranes: Daptomycin, Polymyxins
- DNA gyrase inhibitors: Fluoroquinolones
- Cotrimoxazole

18. Ans. (b) Polymixin B

(Ref: Harrison 19th E/P1048)

Burkholderia cepacia is sensitive to

- Cotrimoxazole
- Carbepenems
- Doxycycline
- 3rd generation cephalosporins
- Fluoroquinolones

Note: Polymyxin B is intrinsically resistant to polymyxins and aminoglycosides.

19. Ans. (b) Beta lactams and beta lactamase inhibitor

(Ref: Harrison 19th E/P1033)

- Since it is a case of beta lactamase producing klebsiella it will break down beta lactams like ampicillin and cephalosporins.
- Hence a combination of beta lactams with beta lactamase inhibitor should be used.
- In case of ESBL producing organisms carbepenems are the drug of choice.
- In case the organism produces carbapenamese, tigecycline or polymyxins can be used.

20. Ans. (b) Ciprofloxacin

(Ref: Park's PSM 24th E/P176)

Drugs preferred in mass chemoprophylaxis of meningococcal meningitis are:

- Ciprofloxacin
- Minocycline
- Spiramycin
- Ceftriaxone

21. Ans. (c) 3

(Ref: Goodman Gilman 12th E/P1478)

22. Ans. (d) Linezolid

(Ref: Goodman Gilman 12th E/P1537)

- Linezolid acts by inhibiting translocation and protein synthesis.

23. Ans. (a) Metronidazole

(Ref: Goodman Gilman 12th E/P1512)

24. Ans. (a) H.influenza has plasmid for activity against beta lactams

(Ref: Harrison 19th E/P1012)

- Resistance to ampicillin in H. influenzae can be seen due to both beta lactamase production (penicillinase) and alteration in PBP.
- Alteration in PBP is rare and has been seen only recently.

25. Ans. (d) Ceftobiprole

(Ref: Harrison 19th E/P962)

- The only anti MRSA cephalosporins are the fifth-generation ones like ceftobiprole and ceftaroline.

26. Ans. (c) Silver sulfadiazine

(Ref: Goodman and Gilman 12th E/P1466)

- Silver sulfadiazine is a sulfonamide active against most of the pathogenic bacteria and fungi.
- It can be applied topically for treatment of fungal keratomycosis.
- It is used as a topical antibiotic for prevention of bacterial infections in burn patients.

27. Ans. (d) Fluoroquinolones

(Ref: Goodman and Gilman 12th E/P1372-73)

- The efficacy of antibiotics depends on the relationship of MIC (Minimum Inhibitory concentration) to various pharmacokinetic parameters e.g. Cmax (Max plasma concentration achieved), AUC and T (Time for which the concentration of antibiotic remains more than MIC).

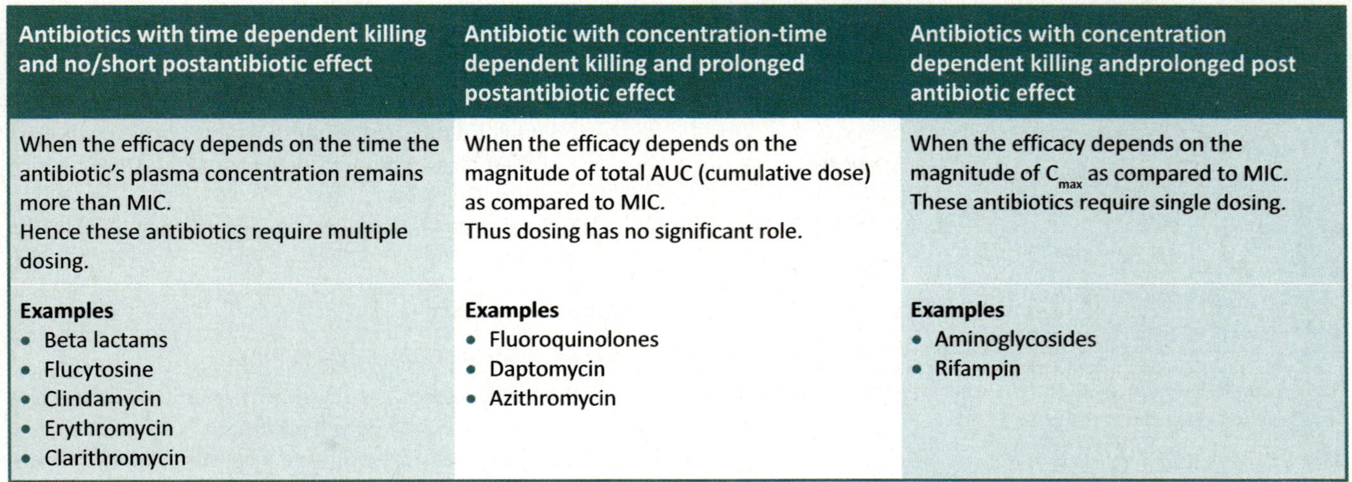

Antibiotics with time dependent killing and no/short postantibiotic effect	Antibiotic with concentration-time dependent killing and prolonged postantibiotic effect	Antibiotics with concentration dependent killing andprolonged post antibiotic effect
When the efficacy depends on the time the antibiotic's plasma concentration remains more than MIC. Hence these antibiotics require multiple dosing.	When the efficacy depends on the magnitude of total AUC (cumulative dose) as compared to MIC. Thus dosing has no significant role.	When the efficacy depends on the magnitude of C_{max} as compared to MIC. These antibiotics require single dosing.
Examples • Beta lactams • Flucytosine • Clindamycin • Erythromycin • Clarithromycin	**Examples** • Fluoroquinolones • Daptomycin • Azithromycin	**Examples** • Aminoglycosides • Rifampin

28. Ans. (a) Oral Vancomycin

(Ref: Goodman and Gilman 12th E/P1540-41)

Drugs used in Clostridium Difficile Infection

FDA Approved	Non-FDA Approved
Oral vancomycin - DOC Oral Fidaxomicin	Oral metronidazole Parenteral metronidazole

29. Ans. (c) It is used in rat bite fever

(Ref: Goodman Gilman 12th E/P1485)

Uses of Penicillin-G

Mnemonics

Penicillin G is Drug of Choice for Following Infections

B : Bacillus (Anthrax)
L : Leptospira (Rat bite fever)
A : Actinomyces
S : Streptococcus
T : Treponema Pallidum (Syphilis)
Penicillin : Pertunae (Yaws), Pasteurella multocida
G : Gas gangrene

30. Ans. (a) Piperacillin-tazobactam

(Ref: Goodman Gilman 12th E/P1485)

Antipseudomonal Penicillins

- Piperacillin
- Mezlocillin
- Carbenicillin
- Ticarcillin

31. Ans. (d) Ampicillin + Sulbactam

(Ref: Harrison 19th E/P975)

Harrison 19th E/P975

"In rare cases, β-lactamase-producing isolates may be found. Because these isolates are not detected by conventional minimal inhibitory concentration determination, additional tests (e.g., the nitrocefin disk) are recommended for isolates from endocarditis. The use of **ampicillin/sulbactam** (12–24 g/d) is suggested in these cases."

32. Ans. (a) Chancroid

(Ref: Goodman Gilman 12th E/P1537)

33. Ans. (b) Cefaclor

(Ref: Harrison 19th E/P962)

Conceptual Box-13

Treatment of *Staphylococcus Aureus*

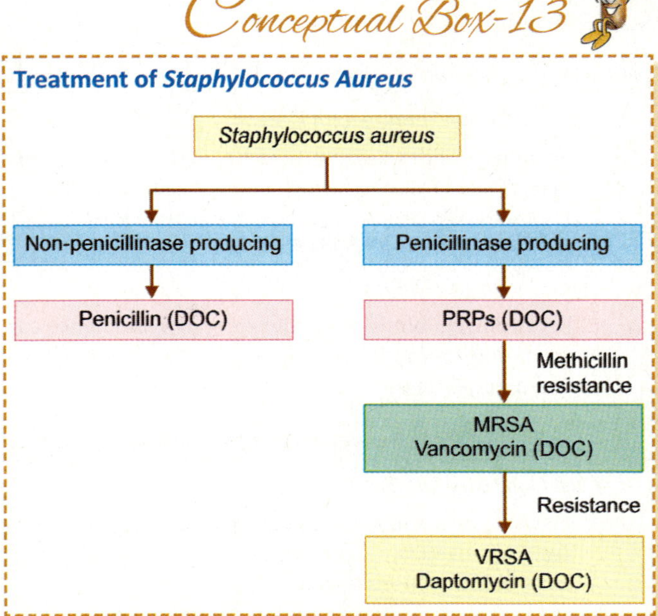

Alternative antibiotics for MRSA and VRSA	
MRSA and VRSA	**MRSA**
Linezolid	Clindamycin
Tedizolid	Minocycline
Streptogramins	Doxycycline
Tigecycline	Cotrimoxazole
5th generation	cephalosporins
Other glycopeptides	
(dalbavancin, telavancin, oritavancin)	

34. Ans. (d) Third and fourth generation cephalosporins are used for detection of ESBL

(Ref: Goodman Gilman 12th E/P1481)

- ESBL can break down penicillins, cephalosporins and monobactams but usually not carbepenems.
- However, recently some ESBL strains are capable of producing carbepenemase, which possess a major therapeutic challenge.
- Ambler's molecular classification is based on **structure**, i.e. protein sequence of enzymes; class A, C and D use serine for beta lactam hydrolysis, whereas class B are metalloenzymes which use zinc ion for beta lactam hydrolysis.
- ESBL production is detected by the ability of the micro-organisms to hydrolyse 3rd generation cephalosporins.

35. Ans. (d) Change over to imipenem

(Ref: Goodman Gilman 12th E/P1500)

- Since this is an ESBL producing strain of klebsiella, carbepenems which are the drug of choice for ESBL producing strains is used.
- Hence, option d is the best answer.

36. Ans. (a) Are bacteriostatic

(Ref: Goodman Gilman 12th E/P1507)

- Aminoglycosides cause misreading of t-RNA and cause toxic protein synthesis which has cidal effect.

37. Ans. (d) It binds to motilin receptors

(Ref: Goodman Gilman 12th E/P1533)

- Erythromycin binds to motilin receptors and hence can cause diarrhea and is used for treatment of gastroparesis and paralytic ileus.

38. Ans. (c) Cefoxitin has got no activity against anaerobes

(Ref: Goodman Gilman 12th E/P1497)

- Cefoxitin is a second generation cephalosporin active against anaerobes and is used for prophylaxis of anaerobic infections in colorectal surgery.

39. Ans. (a) Acute intermittent porphyria

(Ref: Goodman Gilman 12th E/P1468)

40. Ans. (b) Cefoperazone

(Ref: Goodman Gilman 12th E/P1481)

- Nephrotoxicity can be seen with most cephalosporins (cephaloridine > cephalothin) except ceftriaxone (50%), Cefpiramide (100%) and **cefoperazone (100%)** which are excreted by liver.
- Cefoperazone is the safest cephalosporin in renal failure patients.

41. Ans. (a) Amikacin

(Ref: Goodman Gilman 12th E/P1514)

- Aminoglycosides are the most nephrotoxic drugs and hence are given by once daily dosing.
- This produces maximum effect because of their concentration dependent killing and causes lesser side effect as well.

42. Ans. (d) Cefepime

(Ref: Goodman Gilman 12th E/P1496)

- Cefepime is a 4th generation cephalosporin and cephalosporins are beta lactams which act by inhibiting cell wall synthesis.

43. Ans. (b) Levofloxacin

(Ref: Katzung 13th E/P812)

- Among the given options levofloxacin has maximum bioavailability.
- The order of bioavailability of fluoroquinolones is gatifloxacin > levofloxacin/ofloxacin > Moxifloxacin > Norfloxacin > Ciprofloxacin/Gemifloxacin.

44. Ans. (b) TMP-SMX

(Ref: Goodman Gilman 13th E/P990)

- The picture shows oocysts of Cyclospora.
- Cyclosporiasis causes diarrhea in both normal as well as immunocompromised patients.
- The drug of choice is cotrimoxazole (TMP-SMX).

45. Ans. (a) Erythromycin

(Ref: Goodman Gilman 13th E/P1055)

- Macrolides like erythromycin is more effective than penicillins in carriers and hence is the drug of choice.

46. Ans. (c) Increased duration of action

(Ref: Goodman Gilman 13th/P1035)

- Imipenem is metabolized by renal dehydropeptidase and hence is short acting.
- Thus, it is combined with cilastatin (inhibitor of renal dehydropeptidase) to increase duration of action.
- Other carbapenems are not substrate for renal dehydropeptidase and hence do not require cilastatin addition.

47. Ans. (a) Imipenem

(Ref: Goodman Gilman 13th E/P1035)

- Seizures can be seen with imipenem > meropenem.

48. Ans. (b) Cloxacillin

(Ref: Bailey and Love 25th E/ P832)

- Antibiotics preferred for mastitis are cloxacillin and amoxicillin.

49. Ans. (a) Ethambutol

(Ref: Goodman Gilman 13th E/P1074)

50. Ans. (b) Ceftriaxone

(Ref: Goodman Gilman 13th E/P1035)

- Ceftriaxone is the drug of choice for treatment of meningitis caused by *H. influenza, N. meningitidis* (meningococcal meningitis) and *S. pneumoniae.*
- Ampicillin is the drug of choice for treatment of meningitis caused by *L. monocytogenes.*
- Meningitis seen in post neurosurgery or penetrating head trauma patients caused by staphylococcus, Propionibacterium, pseudomonas or acinetobacter is treated by meropenem + vancomycin.

Note: For prophylaxis of meningococcal meningitis (contacts or mass chemoprophylaxis) ciprofloxacin is the drug of choice. Ceftriaxone though us the best drug for prophylaxis is not the drug of choice as it is a parenteral drug.

51. Ans. (c) Mupirocin

(Ref: Goodman Gilman 13th E/P1062)

- Mupirocin is a protein synthesis inhibitor which acts by inhibiting t-RNA synthase.
- It is used only by topical route in the form of cream and ointment for application on skin and nasal cavity.
- It is used for treatment of skin infection caused by *Staphylococcus aureus* (methicillin sensitive as well as resistant) and *Streptococcus pyogenes.*
- It is the drug of choice for treatment of staphylococcal nasal carriage.

52. Ans. (b) Colistin

(Ref: Harrison 19th E/P918)

53. Ans. (d) Ceftobiprole

(Ref: Harrison 19th E/P962)

54. Ans. (a) Fluoroquinolones

(Ref: Goodman Gilman 12th E/P1472)

- **Fluoroquinolones can cause cartilage growth defect and hence are absolutely contraindicated in children and pregnancy.**

55. Ans. (a) Cephaloridine (Goodman Gilman 12th E/ P1498)

- **Nephrotoxicity can be seen with most cephalosporins (cephaloridine > cephalothin)** except ceftriaxone (50%), cefpiramide (100%) and cefoperazone (100%) which are excreted by liver.
- Cefoperazone and cefpiramide are the safest cephalosporins in renal failure patients.

56. Ans. (a) Ceftriaxone

(Ref: Harrison 19th E/P727)

Drug Induced Thrombocytopenia

- **Most common cause is heparin.**
- **Cephalosporins like ceftriaxone and cephamandole are associated.**
- **Quinine and quinidine are also common cause after heparin.**
- **GP IIB/IIIa inhibitors are also common cause.**

57. Ans. (a) Ampicillin

(Ref: AMDT 2017/P1462)

Enterococcal Endocarditis

- **Drug of choice – Ampicillin**
- **Treatment of choice – Ampicillin + Gentamycin**

58. Ans. (d) Ampicillin+Vancomycin+Ceftobiprole

(Ref: Harrison 19th E/P887)

Empirical treatment of meningitis	
age	Drugs used
0 – 3 months	Ampicillin + Cefotaxime
3 months – 55 years	Vancomycin + Cefotaxime/ Ceftriaxone/Cefepime
>55 years	**Vancomycin + Cefotaxime/ Ceftriaxone/Cefepime + Ampicillin**

59. Ans. (a) Cefixime

(Ref: National Treatment Guidelines for Antimicrobial Use in Infectious Disease/P11)

Drug of Choice in Typhoid

- **Outpatients:**
  Cefixime 20 mg/kg/day for 14 days or Azithromycin 500 mg BD for 7 days.
- **Inpatients:**
  Ceftriaxone 2 g IV BD for 2 weeks +/–Azithromycin 500 mg BD for 7 days

60. Ans. (a) Minocycline

(Ref: Harrison 19th E/P352)

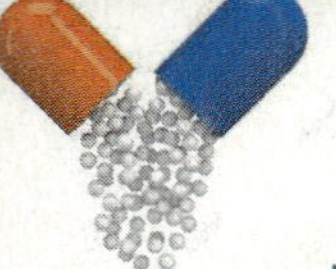

Treatment of acne	
Topical drugs	**Systemic drugs**
Retinoic Acid Benzyl peroxide Salicylic acid Azelaic acid Erythromycin Clindamycin Dapsone	Tetracycline Doxycycline **Minocycline**

61. Ans. (b) Minocycline

(Ref: CMDT 2017/P1465)

62. Ans. (c) Ceftriaxone

(Ref: William's Obstetrics 20th E/P631)

Prevention of opthalmia neonatorum	
Silver nitrate solution	1%
Erythromycin	0.5%
Tetracycline	1%

63. Ans. (c) Ceftriaxone

(Ref: Goodman Gilman 12th E/P1499)

- **Ceftriaxone is the best drug for treatment of diplococci like streptococcus and gonococcus.**

64. Ans. (b) Erythromycin

(Ref: Goodman Gilman 12th E/P 1533)

65. Ans. (d) Inhibit DNA gyrase

(Ref: Goodman Gilman 12th E/P 1472)

66. Ans. (a) Erythromycin

(Ref: Harrison 19th E/P 1061)

Treatment of choice – Fluid and electrolyte replacement
Antibiotic of choice – Erythromycin
Indications for antibiotic therapy are
- High fever
- Bloody diarrhea
- Severe diarrhea, persistence for >1 week
- Worsening of symptoms

67. Ans. (d) Cefoperazone

(Ref: Goodman Gilman 12th E/P 1499)

68. Ans. (a) It is a 4th generation cephalosporin

(Ref: Goodman Gilman 12th E/P 1498)

Fourth generation cephalosporins	Fifth-generation cephalosporins
Cefepime Cefpirome	Ceftobiprole Ceftaroline

69. Ans. (d) Penicillin

(Ref: Harrison 19th E/P 962)

70. Ans. (a) Streptomycin is mostly vestibulotoxic

(Ref: Harrison 19th E/P 205e-5)

- Streptomycin is most vestibulotoxic aminoglycoside.
- Cisplatin and aminoglycoside cause irreversible deafness due to hair cell damage.
- Loop diuretics cause reversible deafness due to change in ions of endolymph. As drug is discontinued ion concentration becomes normal and ototoxicity is reversed.

71. Ans. (c) Conjugation

(Ref: Goodman Gilman 12th E/P 1376)

- Conjugation and then transfer of plasmid causes resistance to multiple drugs.
- Mutation in genes causes resistance to one drug

72. Ans. (b) Clindamycin

(Ref: Goodman Gilman 12th E/P 1535-36)

73. Ans. (b) Daptomycin

(Ref: Goodman Gilman 12th E/P 1543)

- Daptomycin depolarizes the cell membrane and the bacteria dies due to potassium efflux.
- It is the drug of choice for treatment of VRSA and VRE.
- It can cause myopathy.

74. Ans. (b) Cefepime

(Ref: Goodman Gilman 12th E/P 1498)

75. Ans. (c) Telithromycin

(Ref: Goodman Gilman 12th E/P 1529)

76. Ans. (c) Erythromycin

(Ref: Harrison 19th E/P 1024)

Pertussis Treatment and Prophylaxis

Drug of choice	Erythromycin
Drug used in macrolide allergy	Cotrimoxazole

77. Ans. (a) Norfloxacin

(Ref: Goodman Gilman 12th E/P1472)

Oral Bioavailability with Fluoroquinolones

- Maximum – Gatifloxacin
- Minimum – Gemifloxacin < Norfloxacin

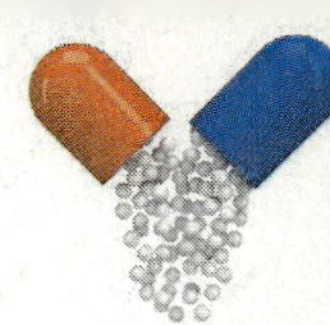

78. Ans. (a) Pefloxacin

(Ref: Goodman Gilman 12th E/P1473)

- Pefloxacin and moxifloxacin are metabolized by liver and hence are contraindicated in liver failure.

79. Ans. (a) Gentamicin

(Ref: Goodman Gilman 12th E/P1512)

80. Ans. (c) Vancomycin

(Ref: Harrison 19th E/P 962)

Drug of Choice for MRSA and VRSA

MRSA	Vancomycin
VRSA	Daptomycin

81. Ans. (a) Bacteria

(Ref: Goodman Gilman 12th E/P1538)

- Colistin or Polymyxin E is derived from Bacillus colistinus.

82. Ans. (a) Penicillin

(Ref: Goodman Gilman 12th E/P1484)

Rheumatic Fever

Treatment and prophylaxis	Benzathine Penicillin G
Penicillin allergy	Erythromycin

83. Ans. (c) Gatifloxacin

(Ref: Goodman Gilman 12th E/P1474)

84. Ans. (a) Dicloxacillin

(Ref: Harrison 19th E/P349)

85. Ans. (d) Cefixime

(Ref: CMDT 2016/P1444)

86. Ans. (a) E. coli

(Ref: Goodman Gilman 12th E/P1536)

87. Ans. (b) Ampicillin

(Ref: Goodman Gilman 12th E/P1490)

88. Ans. (c) Ceftriaxone

(Ref: Goodman Gilman 12th E/P1499)

89. Ans. (b) Penicillin G

(Ref: Goodman Gilman 12th E/P 1482)

90. Ans. (d) Sulfadoxine

(Ref: Goodman Gilman 12th E/P 1465)

Sulfonamides

Longest acting	Sulfadoxine
Shortest acting	Sulfacytine
Most water soluble	Sulfisoxazole

91. Ans. (a) Piperacillin

(Ref: Goodman Gilman 12th E/P 1482)

Anti Pseudomonal Drugs

Drug of Choice – Ceftazidime
Treatment of Choice – Ceftazidime Plus Aminoglycosides

Other Drugs
- Cephalosporins
  - Cefoperazone
  - Cefepime
  - Cefpirome
  - Ceftobiprole
  - Ceftaroline
- Penicillins
  - Piperccillin
  - Azlocillin
  - Mezlocillin
  - Carbenicillin
  - Ticarcillin
- Carbepenems
- Fluoroquinolones

92. Ans. (a) Penicillin

(Ref: Goodman Gilman 12th E/P 1485)

Syphilis Treatment in Pregnancy

Drug of choice	Penicillin
Penicillin Allergy	Penicillin desensitization and then give penicillin

93. Ans. (d) Moxifloxacin

(Ref: Katzung 12th E/P836)

94. Ans. (b) Tigecycline

(Ref: Goodman Gilman 12th E/P1523)

95. Ans. (a) Plasmid

(Ref: Goodman Gilman 12th E/P1376)

96. Ans. (b) Streptomycin

(Ref: Goodman Gilman 12th E/P1512)

97. Ans. (a) Cholera

(Ref: Goodman Gilman 12th E/P1525)

- Prophylactic antimicrobial drugs are not used in cholera.

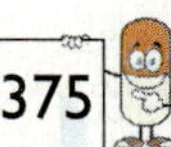

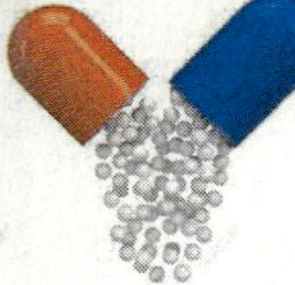

- But among the options the best possible answer is tetracycline, which can be used for treatment of cholera.

98. Ans. (a) Aztreonam

(Ref: Goodman Gilman 12th E/P1500)

- Penicillin does not produce cross sensitivity to monobactams, i.e. aztreonam.
- Hence aztreonam can be safely used in penicillin allergic patient.

99. Ans. (a) Aminoglycosides

(Ref: Goodman Gilman 12th E/P1508)

100. Ans. (a) Ampicillin

(Ref: Goodman Gilman 12th E/P1489)

- Ampicillin is effective against listeria, enterococcus, E.coli and pneumococcus but not against klebsiella.
- Klebsiella is a Gram-negative organism against which only penicillin which are active are piperacillin and mezlocillin.

101. Ans. (c) Erythromycin

(Ref: Goodman Gilman 12th E/P1533)

- Doxycycline is the drug of choice for treatment of chlamydia.
- But since doxycycline is contraindicated in pregnancy, azithromycin is the current drug of choice for chlamydia in pregnancy.
- Erythromycin can also be used and hence is the answer here.

102. Ans. (c) Platelet count

(Ref: Goodman Gilman 12th E/P1538)

- Linezolid can cause bone marrow suppression and thrombocytopenia and hence platelet count monitoring is mandatory.

103. Ans. (c) Colistin

(Ref: Goodman Gilman 12th E/P1539)

- Polymyxin B and E (colistin) are used as topical antibiotics for Gram-negative infections **(pseudomonas)** of skin and mucous membranes.
- Colistin can be given by oral and intravenous route for treatment of multidrug resistant gram-negative organisms like **pseudomonas**, klebsiella, acinetobacter etc.

104. Ans. (d) Conjugation

(Ref: Harrison 19th E/P961)

- Most common mechanism of resistance to Staphylococcus is by penicillinase production, that is acquired from plasmid by conjugation.

105. Ans. (d) Glycopeptide

(Ref: Harrison 19th E/P962)

- Vancomycin is a glycopeptide, which is drug of choice for treatment of MRSA infection.

106. Ans. (d) Carbepenem

(Ref: Harrison 19th E/P962)

107. Ans. (b) Erythromycin

(Ref: Goodman Gilman 12th E/P1533)

- Erythromycin is the drug of choice both for treatment and prophylaxis of diphtheria.

108. Ans. (d) Doxycycline

(Ref: Goodman Gilman 12th E/P1526)

- Nephrotoxicity is lesser with tetracyclines like tigecycline, doxycycline and minocycline.

109. Ans. (a) Ciprofloxacin

(Ref: Goodman Gilman 12th E/P1473)

110. Ans. (d) Nitrofurantoin

(Ref: Goodman Gilman 12th E/P1537)

111. Ans. (b) Rickettsial infection

(Ref: Goodman Gilman 12th E/P1484-85)

112. Ans. (c) Piperacillin

(Ref: Goodman Gilman 12th E/P1490)

113. Ans. (b) Imipenem

(Ref: Harrison 19th E/P692)

114. Ans. (b) Sulfasalazine

(Ref: Goodman Gilman 12th E/P1466)

115. Ans. (d) Macrolides

(Ref: Goodman Gilman 12th E/P1531)

116. Ans. (d) Cefoperazone

(Ref: Goodman Gilman 12th E/P1498)

117. Ans. (a) Cell wall

(Ref: Goodman Gilman 12th E/P1543)

118. Ans. (a) Rifampicin

(Ref: Harrison 19th E/P1002)

Meningococcal Meningitis in Contacts

Rifampicin	High resistance and hence not preferred
Ciprofloxacin	DOC
Ceftriaxone	Best drug

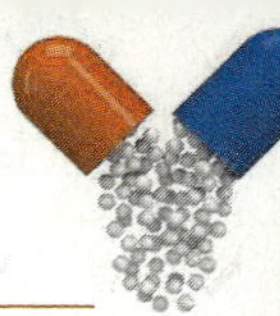

119. Ans. (a) Vancomycin

(Ref: Goodman Gilman 12th E/P1539)

120. Ans. (a) Cephadroxil

(Ref: Goodman Gilman 12th E/P1498)

Cephaosporins Active Against Pseudomonas

3rd generation	Ceftazidime Cefoperazone
4th generation	Cefepime Cefpirome
5th generation	Ceftobiprole Ceftaroline

121. Ans. (d) Skin reactions

(Ref: Goodman Gilman 12th E/P1468)

122. Ans. (a) Amikacin

(Ref: Goodman Gilman 12th E/P1512)

Mnemonics

Auditory Toxicity
- K : Kanamycin
- A : Amikacin
- N : Neomycin

123. Ans. (a) Methicillin resistant s. aureus

(Ref: Goodman Gilman 12th E/P1479)

- Clavulanic acid increases spectrum of ampicillin against beta lactamase producing strains.
- But in MRSA resistance is because of altered penicillin binding protein and hence addition of clavulanic acid is not effective.

124. Ans. (a) Minocycline

(Ref: Goodman Gilman 12th E/P1526)

125. Ans. (b) Aminoglycosides

(Ref: Goodman Gilman 12th E/P1507)

126. Ans. (d) Clindamycin

(Ref: Goodman Gilman 12th E/P1534)

- Clindamycin is a protein synthesis inhibitor.

127. Ans. (a) Rifampicin

(Ref: Harrison 19th E/P1002)

128. Ans. (d) Gentamicin

(Ref: Goodman Gilman 12th E/P1510)

129. Ans. (b) Sparfloxacin

(Ref: Goodman Gilman 12th E/P1474)

130. Ans. (c) Pneumocystis jiroveci

(Ref: Goodman Gilman 12th E/P1469)

131. Ans. (c) Vancomycin

(Ref: Goodman Gilman 12th E/P542)

132. Ans. (b) Chloramphenicol

(Ref: Goodman Gilman 12th E/P1528)

133. Ans. (a) Neutropenia

(Ref: Goodman Gilman 12th E/P1375)

- Bactericidal drugs are preferred in neutropenia due to inability of the body to kill the microorganism.

134. Ans. (a) Cephalexin

(Ref: Goodman Gilman 12th E/P1496)

- Cephalexin is a first generation cephalosporin not active against pseudomonas.

135. Ans. (d) Quinolones

(Ref: Goodman Gilman 12th E/P1472)

- Drug inactivating enzymes: Drug inactivating enzymes are produced against **beta lactams, chloramphenicol, aminoglycosides and tetracyclines**.
- In quinolones resistance is seen due to DNA gyrase mutation or drug efflux.

136. Ans. (c) Erythromycin

(Ref: Goodman Gilman 12th E/P1531)

137. Ans. (a) Imipenem

(Ref: Goodman Gilman 12th E/P1500)

- Imipenem is short acting due to rapid degradation by renal dehydropeptidase.
- Hence an inhibitor of this enzyme, i.e. cilastatin is combined.

138. Ans. (b) Cephalosporins

(Ref: Goodman Gilman 12th E/P1493)

139. Ans. (a) Gentamicin

(Ref: Goodman Gilman 12th E/P1513)

140. Ans. (c) Pyrimethamine

(Ref: Goodman Gilman 12th E/P1468)

141. Ans. (a) Is effective in pseudomonas infection

(Ref: Goodman Gilman 12th E/P1490)

142. Ans. (b) Clavulanic acid

(Ref: Goodman Gilman 12th E/P1501)

143. Ans. (b) Chloramphenicol

(Ref: Goodman Gilman 12th E/P1527)

- Chloramphenicol binds to P site and prevents transpeptidation.

144. Ans. (c) Spectinomycin

(Ref: Goodman Gilman 12th E/P1538)

145. Ans. (a) Clindamycin

(Ref: Goodman Gilman 12th E/P1535)

146. Ans. (d) Sparfloxacin

(Ref: Goodman Gilman 12th E/P1470)

147. Ans. (d) None

(Ref: Goodman Gilman 12th E/P1533)

148. Ans. (a) Cell wall synthesis

(Ref: Goodman Gilman 12th E/P1477)

149. Ans. (b) Penicillins

(Ref: Goodman Gilman 12th E/P1485)

- In patients of secondary syphilis, penicillin associated release of spirochetal antigen can cause hypersensitivity reaction known as **Jarisch-Herxheimer reaction**, characterized by fever, arthralgia, myalgia and worsening of cutaneous lesions.

150. Ans. (d) Cotrimoxazole

(Ref: Goodman Gilman 12th E/P1468)

151. Ans. (b) Chloramphenicol

(Ref: Goodman Gilman 12th E/P1528)

152. Ans. (d) Treponema

(Ref: Goodman Gilman 12th E/P1485)

- Resistance due to penicillinase production can be seen in both staphylococcus and streptococcus.
- Treponema does not produce penicillinase and hence penicillin G is still the drug of choice.

153. Ans. (b) Chloramphenicol

(Ref: Goodman Gilman 12th E/P1527)

154. Ans. (b) Doxycycline

(Ref: Goodman Gilman 12th E/P1526)

- Maximum photosensitivity with fluoroquinolones is seen with demeclocycline > doxycycline.

155. Ans. (c) Erythromycin

(Ref: Goodman Gilman 12th E/P1533)

156. Ans. (a) Methicillin

(Ref: Goodman Gilman 12th E/P1486)

- Oxacillin, cloxacillin and dicloxacillin are structurally similar, acid stable penicillins and hence are given by oral route.
- Nafcillin and methicillin are acid labile and hence given by parenteral route.

157. Ans. (c) Tetracycline

(Ref: Goodman Gilman 12th E/P1521)

158. Ans. (d) Azithromycin

(Ref: Goodman Gilman 12th E/P1505)

159. Ans. (b) Gentamicin

(Ref: Goodman Gilman 12th E/P1515)

160. Ans. (b) Ampicillin

(Ref: Harrison 19th E/P858)

> "Clindamycin, **ampicillin**, and cephalosporins were the first antibiotics associated with CDI. The second- and third-generation cephalosporins, particularly cefotaxime, ceftriaxone, cefuroxime, and ceftazidime, are frequently responsible for this condition, and the fluoroquinolones (ciprofloxacin, levofloxacin, and moxifloxacin) are the most recent drug class to be implicated in hospital outbreaks."

161. Ans. (d) Neomycin

(Ref: Goodman Gilman 12th E/P1514)

- Most nephrotoxic aminoglycoside is neomycin and least nephrotoxic is streptomycin.

162. Ans. (c) Cefaclor

(Ref: Goodman Gilman 12th E/P1494)

Oral 2nd Generation Cephalosporins

- Cefaclor
- Cefprozil

163. Ans. (a) Vancomycin

(Ref: Goodman Gilman 12th E/P1539)

164. Ans. (b) Skin rash

(Ref: Goodman Gilman 12th E/P1187)

165. Ans. (d) Postantibiotic effect

(Ref: Goodman Gilman 12th E/P1372)

166. Ans. (a) Trimethoprim + SMX

(Ref: Goodman Gilman 12th E/P1469)

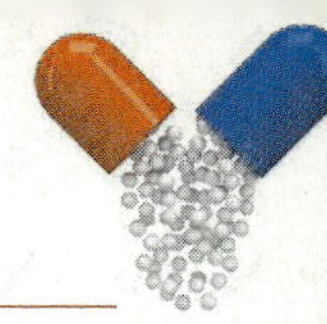

167. Ans. (d) All of the above

(Ref: Harrison 19th E/P422)

> "A common cause of eosinophilia is allergic reaction to drugs (iodides, aspirin, sulfonamides, nitrofurantoin, penicillins, and cephalosporins)."

168. Ans. (b) Gatifloxacin

(Ref: Goodman Gilman 12th E/P1493)

169. Ans. (b) Penicillins

(Ref: Goodman Gilman 12th E/P1477)

170. Ans. (d) Cephalothin

(Ref: Goodman Gilman 12th E/P1499)

Nephrotoxicity can be seen with most cephalosporins (cephaloridine > cephalothin) except ceftriaxone (50%), Cefpiramide (100%) and cefoperazone (100%) which are excreted by liver.

171. Ans. (a) Competitive inhibition

(Ref: Goodman Gilman 12th E/P1464)

172. Ans. (a) Quinolones

(Ref: Goodman Gilman 12th E/P1372)

Antibiotics with Prolonged Postantibiotic Effect

- Aminoglycoside
- Rifampicin
- **Fluoroquinolones**
- Azithromycin
- Clarithromycin

173. Ans. (b) Carbenicillin

(Ref: Goodman Gilman 12th E/P1486)

174. Ans. (a) DNA gyrase inhibitors

(Ref: Goodman Gilman 12th E/P1470)

175. Ans. (c) It can be used with cilastatin

(Ref: Goodman Gilman 12th E/P1500)

176. Ans. (b) Linezolid

(Ref: Goodman Gilman 12th E/P1477)

177. Ans. (c) Cefuroxime

(Ref: Goodman Gilman 12th E/P1494)

178. Ans. (b) Plasmid mediated

(Ref: Goodman Gilman 12th E/P1530)

179. Ans. (a) Penicillin G

(Ref: Goodman Gilman 12th E/P1485)

180. Ans. (b) Penicillin

(Ref: Goodman Gilman 12th E/P1485)

181. Ans. (d) Mupirocin

(Ref: Harrison 19th E/P166e-3)

182. Ans. (d) Excreted rapidly by kidney

(Ref: Goodman Gilman 12th E/P1497)

- Unlike other second-generation drugs cefuroxime is not active against bacteroides.
- It is effective against gram-negatives and used in meningitis due to good CSF penetration, but is less effective than ceftriaxone.

183. Ans. (b) Amikacin

(Ref: Goodman Gilman 12th E/P1508)

- Amikacin and netilmicin are resistant to enzymatic inactivation.

184. Ans. (c) Phenylbutazone

(Ref: Goodman Gilman 12th E/P1529)

- Chloramphenicol is an enzyme inhibitor and can increase blood level of drugs metabolized by CYP_{450} enzymes.
- All drugs in options are metabolized by CYP_{450} enzymes except phenylbutazone.

185. Ans. (d) along with preanesthetic medication

(Ref: Goodman Gilman 12th E/P1374)

- Antibiotics are given 60 minutes before incision and continued at least 24 hours after surgery.

186. Ans. (b) Mutation of linezolid binding site

(Ref: Goodman Gilman 12th E/P1537)

187. Ans. (b) Penicillin G

(Ref: Goodman Gilman 12th E/P1477)

188. Ans. (b) Glycoside

(Ref: Goodman Gilman 12th E/P1505)

189. Ans. (c) 160 mg trimethoprim + 800 mg sulfamethoxazole

(Ref: KDT 7th E/P707)

190. Ans. (c) Streptomycin

(Ref: Goodman Gilman 12th E/P1514)

191. Ans. (b) Tetracycline

(Ref: Goodman Gilman 12th E/P1525)

- The current drug of choice for rickettsia is doxycycline.
- Since doxycycline is not in option, tetracycline is answer.

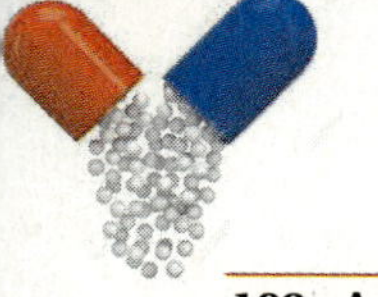

192. Ans. (a) Treated by tetracycline

(Ref: Harrison 19th E/P858)

- Vancomycin, fidaxomicin and metronidazole are used for treatment of pseudomembranous enterocolitis.

193. Ans. (a) Doxycycline

(Ref: Goodman Gilman 12th E/P1525)

194. Ans. (a) Sulfonamide

(Ref: Harrison 19th E/P1155)

195. Ans. (b) Inhibition of formation of folic acid

(Ref: Goodman Gilman 12th E/P1464)

196. Ans. (a) Gentamicin

(Ref: Goodman Gilman 12th E/P1515)

- Accidental intraocular administration of gentamicin can cause macular toxicity and blindness.

197. Ans. (a) Cefoxitin

(Ref: Goodman Gilman 12th E/P1499)

198. Ans. (a) Clindamycin

(Ref: Goodman Gilman 12th E/P1534)

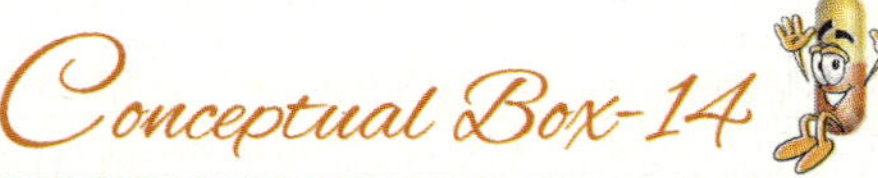

Conceptual Box-14

Drugs used in Typhoid

- **Ciprofloxacin:** Drug of choice
- **Ceftriaxone:** Empirical drug of choice and drug of choice in MDR strains
- Amoxicillin
- Azithromycin
- Cotrimoxazole

199. Ans. (b) Has activity against gram-positive bacteria

(Ref: Goodman Gilman 12th E/P1500)

Monobactams

- Aztreonam is a narrow spectrum drug that is active **against only gram-negative organisms**.
- As it has no cross reactivity with other beta lactams, it is used for treatment of gram-negatives in penicillin allergic patients. It can be used for treatment of enterobacter and pseudomonas as well.

200. Ans. (a) It is plasmid mediated

(Ref: Goodman Gilman 12th E/P1541)

201. Ans. (a) Fluoroquinolones

(Ref: Goodman Gilman 12th E/P1470)

202. Ans. (d) Freezing of initiation

(Ref: Goodman Gilman 12th E/P1470)

- Aminoglycosides cause misreading of t-RNA and freeze normal protein synthesis and facilitate toxic protein synthesis.

203. Ans. (d) C. jejuni

(Ref: Goodman Gilman 12th E/P1533)

204. Ans. (a) Outer hair cell and basal turn of cochlea

(Ref: Goodman Gilman 12th E/P1512)

205. Ans. (c) III

(Ref: Goodman Gilman 12th E/P1541)

- As we move from first to third generation cephalosporins activity increases against gram-negative and decreases against gram-positive.

206. Ans. (b) Ampicillin

(Ref: Goodman Gilman 12th E/P1485)

207. Ans. (c) Piperacillin

(Ref: Goodman Gilman 12th E/P1490)

208. Ans. (a) Tetracycline

(Ref: Goodman Gilman 12th E/P1521)

- Tigecycline is a glycycline, which is structurally similar to tetracycline.
- It spectrum is similar to tetracycline but is effective also in resistant cases as, it is resistant to drug efflux.

209. Ans. (c) Metronidazole

(Ref: Goodman Gilman 12th E/P1428)

210. Ans. (b) Erythromycin

(Ref: Goodman Gilman 12th E/P1533)

- The current drug of choice for legionella is azithromycin.
- Erythromycin was earlier drug of choice and is answer here.

211. Ans. (c) Moxifloxacin

(Ref: Goodman Gilman 12th E/P1473)

- Moxifloxacin is a respiratory quinolone and is a first-line drug for empirical treatment of pneumonia.

212. Ans. (d) DOC in rat bite fever

(Ref: Goodman Gilman 12th E/P1485)

213. Ans. (c) Binds to 23S fraction of 50S ribosome

(Ref: Goodman Gilman 12th E/P1537)

214. Ans. (a) Tetracycline

(Ref: Goodman Gilman 12th E/P1450)

- The current drug of choice for prophylaxis of plague is doxycycline.
- Since doxycycline is not in the options, tetracycline is a better option.

215. Ans. (b) Cefazolin

(Ref: Goodman Gilman 12th E/P1497)

- Cefazolin is the drug of choice for surgical prophylaxis.

216. Ans. (b) β lactam antibiotics

(Ref: Goodman Gilman 12th E/P1372)

217. Ans. (a) Protein synthesis inhibitors

(Ref: Goodman Gilman 12th E/P1507)

218. Ans. (d) Acetaminophen

(Ref: Goodman Gilman 12th E/P1512)

219. Ans. (b) Aminoglycoside

(Ref: Goodman Gilman 12th E/P1517)

220. Ans. (b) Demeclocycline

(Ref: Goodman Gilman 12th E/P1526)

221. Ans. (c) Crystalluria

(Ref: Goodman Gilman 12th E/P1467)

222. Ans. (b) 6 drugs for 6 months; 4 drugs for 18 months

(Ref: RNTCP guidelines)

- Resistance to rifampicin and isoniazid is termed as multiple drug resistance TB (MDR TB). In such a case 6 drugs are used for 6-9 months in intensive phase followed by 4 drugs for 18 months in continuous phase. Hence option b is the answer here.

Type of TB	Number of drugs used
Non-drug resistant – New case	4 drugs for 2 months + 3 drugs for 4 months
Non-drug resistant – Previously treated	5 drugs for 2 months + 4 drugs for 1 month + 3 drugs for 5 months
Rifampicin resistance + Isoniazid sensitive	7 drugs for 6-9 months + 5 drugs for 18 months
MDR TB	6 drugs for 6-9 months + 4 drugs for 18 months
XDR TB	7 drugs for 6-12 months + 6 drugs for 18 months

223. Ans. (d) Competes with PABA in folic acid synthesis

(Ref: Goodman Gilman 13th E/P1078)

- Dapsone is an analog of para amino benzoic acid (PABA) and hence competitively inhibits dihydropteroate synthase (DHPS) required for folic acid synthesis.

224. Ans. (c) Ethambutol

(Ref: Goodman Gilman 13th E/P1074)

225. Ans. (a) Pyridoxine

(Ref: Goodman Gilman 12th E/P1557)

- Most common ATT causing neuropathy is isoniazid by depleting active form of pyridoxine.
- Hence pyridoxine is the answer here.

226. Ans. (c) Rifampicin 450 mg once a month + dapsone 50 mg daily + clofazimine 150 mg once a month + 50 mg alternate days

(Ref: NLEP guidelines)

227. Ans. (d) Ofloxacin

(Ref: Goodman Gilman 12th E/P1470)

- **Among the drugs used in standard regimens for pauci and multibacillary leprosy, Rifampicin is cidal.**
- **In another regimen for paucibacillary i.e. ROM therapy, Rifampicin and Ofloxacin are cidal.**

228. Ans. (d) Rifampicin is more effective against MAC as compared to rifabutin

(Ref; Goodman Gilman 12th E/P1552)

- **Rifabutin is more effective against MAC as compared to rifampicin. The most effective first-line drug against MAC is ethambutol.**
- **Rifabutin is more effective in a newly diagnosed case as compared to when given in resistant cases.**
- **Among rifamycin's rifabutin has the longest half-life and least potent enzyme induction. Hence it is associated with lesser drug interaction.**

229. Ans. (c) Ethambutol

(Ref: Goodman Gilman 12th E/P1559)

230. Ans. (a) Rifabutin

(Ref: Harrison 19th E/P205-e5)

231. Ans. (c) Pyrazinamide

(Ref: Goodman Gilman 12th E/P1554)

- **Asymptomatic hyperuricemia is seen with pyrazinamide > ethambutol.**

232. Ans. (a) Rifampicin

(Ref: Goodman Gilman 12th E/P1554)

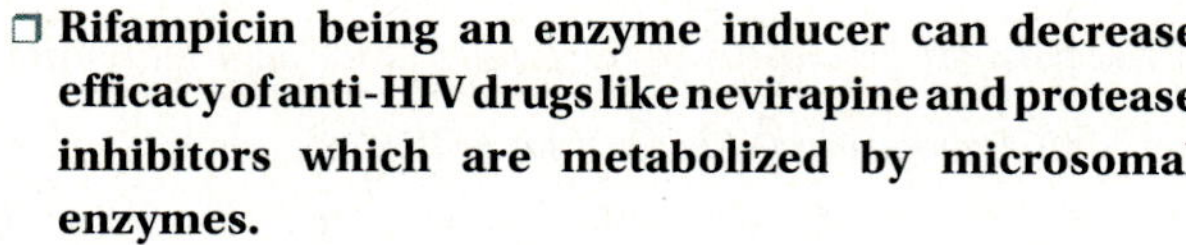

- Rifampicin being an enzyme inducer can decrease efficacy of anti-HIV drugs like nevirapine and protease inhibitors which are metabolized by microsomal enzymes.

233. Ans. (d) Pyrazinamide

(Ref: Goodman Gilman 12th E/P1554)

234. Ans. (a) Thrombocytopenia

(Ref: Goodman Gilman 12th E/P1553)

- **Rifampicin if causes respiratory syndrome and thrombocytopenia should be stopped and never started again.**
- **In case of hepatotoxicity it should be stopped and started once ALT/AST is normalized.**

235. Ans. (a) Isoniazid

(Ref: Goodman Gilman 12th E/P1558)

236. Ans. (d) rpoB

(Ref: Goodman Gilman 12th E/P1550)

237. Ans. (a) Bedaquiline

(Ref: Harrison 19th E/P205e-7)

- Bedaquiline, a mycobacterial ATP synthase inhibitor was approved by FDA in 2013 for treatment of tuberculosis.
- Another promising drug delamanid, an inhibitor of mycolic acid synthesis is under trial for treatment of tuberculosis.

238. Ans. (b) Leprosy,

(Ref: National Leprosy Eradication Program Guidelines, India)

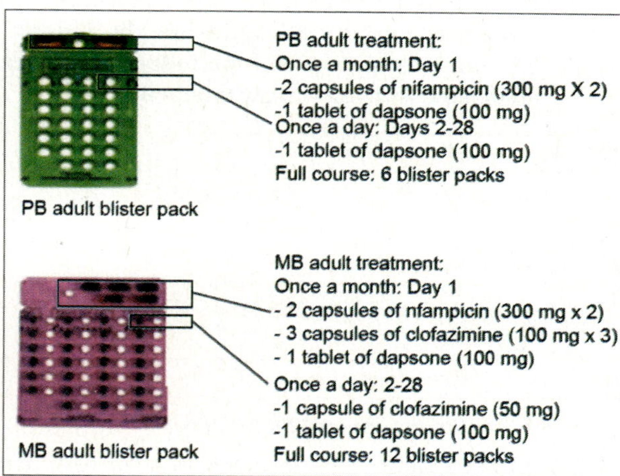

PB adult treatment:
Once a month: Day 1
-2 capsules of nifampicin (300 mg X 2)
-1 tablet of dapsone (100 mg)
Once a day: Days 2-28
-1 tablet of dapsone (100 mg)
Full course: 6 blister packs
PB adult blister pack
MB adult treatment:
Once a month: Day 1
- 2 capsules of nfampicin (300 mg x 2)
- 3 capsules of clofazimine (100 mg x 3)
- 1 tablet of dapsone (100 mg)
Once a day: 2-28
-1 capsule of clofazimine (50 mg)
-1 tablet of dapsone (100 mg)
Full course: 12 blister packs
MB adult blister pack

239. Ans. (c) Ethionamide

(Ref: Goodman Gilman 12th E/P1562)

Mnemonics

Side Effects of Ethionamide

E : Elevated ALT/AST
T : Taste change (metallic)
H : Hypothyroidism
I : Impotence
O : Ocular toxicity
N : Nausea and vomiting

240. Ans. (b) Ethionamide

(Ref: Goodman Gilman 12th E/P1562)

Resistance to Isoniazid

Kat G gene mutation	Severest resistance
Kas A mutation	Moderate resistance
Inh A overexpression	Moderate resistance Cross resistance to ethionamide

241. Ans. (d) Rifampicin

(Ref: National Leprosy Control Program, India)

- Rifampicin and clofazimine are given under supervision for leprosy and pyrazinamide for tuberculosis.
- Dapsone in leprosy is given at daily doses and hence supervision is not possible.

242. Ans. (a) Ethambutol

(Ref: Goodman Gilman 12th E/P1559)

Ethambutol can cause optic neuritis which presents as

- Reduced visual acuity
- Scotoma
- Green>Red Colour blindness

243. Ans. (b) Ofloxacin

(Ref: Harrison 19th E/P1127)

Alternative WHO recommended ROM regimen for paucibacillary leprosy	
Rifampicin 600 mg **Ofloxacin** 400 mg **Minocycline** 100 mg	Single dose

244. Ans. (a) Minocycline

(Ref: Harrison 19th E/P1127)

245. Ans. (a) Isoniazid

(Ref: Goodman Gilman 12th E/P 1558)

Neuropsychiatric Side effects of Isoniazid

- Euphoria
- Transient memory loss
- Psychosis

246. Ans. (d) Rifampicin

(Ref: Harrison 19th E/P 205-e4)

- Rifampicin being an enzyme inducer can decrease effect of protease inhibitors and NNRTI like nevirapine and delavirdine.
- Hence rifampicin should not be used with these drugs.

247. Ans. (b) Rifampicin

(Ref: Harrison 19th E/P 205-e4)

248. Ans. (d) Ethambutol

(Ref: Goodman Gilman 12th E/P1559)

249. Ans. (d) Streptomycin

(Ref: Harrison 19th E/P 205e-5)

- Pyrazinamide > Isoniazid > Rifampicin are hepatotoxic.
- Streptomycin and ethambutol are nephrotoxic.

250. Ans. (c) Pyrazinamide

(Ref: Harrison 19th E/P 250e-3)

251. Ans. (c) Clofazimine

(Ref: Goodman Gilman 12th E/P1560)

252. Ans. (b) Isoniazid

(Ref: Goodman Gilman 12th E/P1558)

253. Ans. (c) Streptomycin

(Ref: Goodman Gilman 12th E/P1512-14)

254. Ans. (b) Rifampicin

(Ref: Harrison 19th E/P 205e-4)

255. Ans. (a) Rifampicin

(Ref: Goodman Gilman 12th E/P1550)

- Rifampicin has maximum sterilizing and cidal action.

256. Ans. (a) INH

(Ref: Goodman Gilman 12th E/P1557)

257. Ans. (b) Rifampicin

(Ref: Goodman Gilman 12th E/P1552)

- Rifampicin can cause flu like or pneumonia like symptoms on intermittent dosing.

258. Ans. (b) Rifampicin

(Ref: Goodman Gilman 12th E/P1554)

259. Ans. (c) Ethambutol

(Ref: Goodman Gilman 12th E/P1559)

260. Ans. (a) Isoniazid

(Ref: Goodman Gilman 12th E/P1558)

- Pyridoxine replacement with isoniazid can improve symptoms of peripheral neuropathy, neuropsychiatric side effects and anemia as well.

261. Ans. (a) Clofazimine

(Ref: Goodman Gilman 12th E/P1560)

262. Ans. (d) Isoniazid + Rifampicin + Kanamycin

(Ref: Goodman Gilman 12th E/P1565)

- Multidrug resistant (MDR) TB is a case of TB that is resistant to both isoniazid and rifampicin.
- Extremely drug resistant (XDR) TB is a case of MDR with additional resistance to a Fluoroquinolone and to at least one of the injectable second-line drugs like amikacin, kanamycin or capreomycin.

263. Ans. (a) Isoniazid

(Ref: Goodman Gilman 12th E/P1556)

264. Ans. (c) Pyrazinamide

(Ref: Goodman Gilman 12th E/P1554)

- **Order of hepatotoxicity in first-line TB drugs is Pyrazinamide > Isoniazid > Rifampicin.**

265. Ans. (b) Isoniazid

(Ref: Goodman Gilman 12th E/P1556)

266. Ans. (a) Tobramycin

(Ref: Goodman Gilman 12th E/P1559)

267. Ans. (a) Retrobulbar neuritis

(Ref: Goodman Gilman 12th E/P1559)

268. Ans. (a) Hemolytic anemia

(Ref: Goodman Gilman 12th E/P1562)

269. Ans. (b) Peripheral neuropathy

(Ref: Goodman Gilman 12th E/P1556)

- In slow acetylators peripheral neuropathy is more common, whereas in fast acetylators hepatotoxicity is more common.
- Rifampicin can increase hepatotoxicity of isoniazid by enzyme induction and increase in production of hepatotoxic metabolite.

270. Ans. (c) Rifampicin

(Ref: Goodman Gilman 12th E/P1552)

271. Ans. (a) Respiratory syndrome

(Ref: J.D.Williams Chemotherapy Vol 3/P10)

- At intermittent doses rifampicin can cause flu like symptoms, respiratory syndrome (shortness of breath), cutaneous reactions (flushing and itching), thrombocytopenic purpura and abdominal reactions (pain and nausea).
- In case of **purpura and respiratory syndrome** rifampicin is never restarted.

272. Ans. (a) Dapsone

(Ref: Goodman Gilman 12th E/P1563)

- Dapsone is used in both pauci and multibacillary leprosy.
- Clofazimine is used only in multibacillary leprosy.

273. Ans. (d) Mutation

(Ref: Goodman Gilman 12th E/P1550)

274. Ans. (b) INH

(Ref: Goodman Gilman 12th E/P1558)

275. Ans. (a) Ethambutol

(Ref: Goodman Gilman 12th E/P1559)

276. Ans. (a) Rifampicin

(Ref: Goodman Gilman 12th E/P1550)

277. Ans. (c) INH

(Ref: Goodman Gilman 12th E/P1556)

278. Ans. (a) Inhibiting DNA dependent RNA polymerase

(Ref: Goodman Gilman 12th E/P1550)

279. Ans. (b) Isoniazid

(Ref: Harrison 19th E/P1120)

280. Ans. (b) Rifampicin

(Ref: Goodman Gilman 12th E/P1553)

281. Ans. (a) Hydrazine complex

(Ref: Goodman Gilman 12th E/P1556)

282. Ans. (c) Pyrazinamide

(Ref: Goodman Gilman 12th E/P1554)

- Pyrazinamide is active in acidic environment present inside the phagocytes and granulomas and hence is effective against intracellular, slow growing organisms.

283. Ans. (b) Optic neuritis

(Ref: Goodman Gilman 12th E/P1556)

284. Ans. (b) Used in treatment of meningococcal meningitis

(Ref: Goodman Gilman 12th E/P1552)

- Rifampicin is used for prophylaxis of meningococcal meningitis in contacts.
- It is not used for treatment.

285. Ans. (a) INH

(Ref: Goodman Gilman 12th E/P1556)

286. Ans. (d) Streptomycin

(Ref: Goodman Gilman 12th E/P1512)

287. Ans. (b) G6PD deficiency

(Ref: Goodman Gilman 12th E/P1562)

288. Ans. (b) Isoniazid and rifampicin

(Ref: Goodman Gilman 12th E/P1565)

289. Ans. (c) Resistance isoniazid and rifampicin and quinolone + injectable aminoglycoside

(Ref: Goodman Gilman 12th E/P1565)

290. Ans. (b) Indinavir

(Ref: Goodman Gilman 13th E/P1147)

- Protease inhibitors like indinavir and atazanavir can cause nephrolithiasis and among the given options only indinavir causes it.
- Apart from this dyslipidemia, obesity and gynecomastia/breast hypertrophy are common with protease inhibitors.
- Ketoconazole can cause gynecomastia/breast hypertrophy, but other side effects mentioned are not seen.
- NRTI like zidovudine and stavudine rather cause lipodystrophy and not obesity.

291. Ans. (a) Neuraminidase inhibitor

(Ref: Goodman Gilman 12th E/P1607)

Neuraminidase Inhibitors

- Oseltamivir
- Zanamivir
- Peramivir
- Laninamivir

292. Ans. (b) Inhibits assembly of viral proteins

(Ref: Goodman Gilman 12th E/P1645)

- During the final stages of viral assembly protease cuts Gag pol precursor protein into smaller proteins and enzymes required by the virus. This step is required for maturation of the virus as well.
- Hence protease inhibitors block both assembly and maturation of virus.

293. Ans. (a) Neuraminidase inhibition

(Ref: Goodman Gilman 13th E/P1114)

- Tamiflu or oseltamivir inhibits neuraminidase, which leads to block of viral release from the respiratory epithelial cells.
- It is the drug of choice for treatment of influenza A and B, and bird flu.

294. Ans. (a) Oseltamivir

(Ref: Goodman Gilman 12th E/P1114)

295. Ans. (c) Emtricitabine

(Ref: Goodman Gilman 12th E/P1640)

Drugs active against both HIV and hepatitis B are

- Lamivudine
- Emtricitabine
- Tenofovir
- Clevudine
- Telbivudine

296. Ans. (a) Start regimen immediately and continue till puerperium

(Ref: Park's PSM 24th E/P370)

ART regimen should be started immediately after diagnosis of HIV in pregnant females or breast feeding mothers irrespective of CD4 count and clinical staging.

297. Ans. (a) Oseltamivir

(Ref: Goodman Gilman 12th E/P1608)

298. Ans. (d) Given at a dose of 75 mg

(Ref: Goodman Gilman 12th E/P1608)

- **Oseltamivir is given only by oral route at dose of 75 mg BD and OD for treatment and prophylaxis respectively.**
- **It is a neuraminidase inhibitor.**
- **It is effective if given till 48 hours after symptoms onset.**

299. Ans. (a) Viral polymerase

(Ref: Goodman Gilman 12th E/P1594)

Acyclovir Acts by Inhibiting

- **Viral DNA polymerase**
- **Viral thymidine kinase**

300. Ans. (b) Nelfinavir

(Ref: Goodman Gilman 12th E/P1645)

- **All protease inhibitors are metabolized by CYP3A4 except nelfinavir, which is metabolizd by CYP2C19.**
- **Hence, ritonavir boosting cannot be used with nelfinavir.**

301. Ans. (b) 20 mg BD

(Ref: CDC)

- Oseltamivir has good oral absorption **and is the drug of choice for treatment and prophylaxis of influenza A,** influenza B and bird flu. **It is most effective for treatment and prophylaxis when started** within 48 hours **of symptoms.** 75 mg BD dose **is given for 5 days for treatment and** 75 mg OD dose **given for prophylaxis for 7 days.**
- **It is approved in** all age group children for treatment **and for** prophylaxis only in children above 3 months of age**. The dose for treatment and prophylaxis in** children less than 1 year is 3 mg/kg BD**, whereas for children above 1 year age dose is decided based upon weight.**
- **Now weight of 6 months child will be around 7 kg and hence 20 mg/kg BD is best option.**

302. Ans. (c) Ledipasvir

(Ref: CMDT 2016/P678)

Recent Advances

Latest Oral Direct Acting Drugs for Hepatitis C

The latest oral drugs contains drugs like NS3/4 A (protease) inhibitors, NS5B (RNA polymerase) inhibitors and NS5A inhibitors. These oral drugs are combined with each other to make regimens for treatment of hepatitis C.

NS5A Inhibitors

NS5A is a phosphoprotein required for hepatitis C virus replication, assembly and release. The drugs inhibiting NS5A are given below in mnemonic box. These drugs are combined with other two classes.

NS5A inhibitors	Protease inhibitor combined	RNA polymerase inhibitor combined
Orange: Ombitasvir	Paritepревir	Dasabuvir
L : Ledipasvir		Sofosbuvir
E : Elbasvir	Grazoprevir	
D : Daclatasvir	Asunaprevir	Sofosbuvir or Beclabuvir

NS3/4 A (Protease) Inhibitors

- Protease is an enzyme required for viral maturation.
- Some protease inhibitors used with NS5A inhibitors have been discussed above.
- Simeprivir is used along with IFN α and ribavirin or sofosbuvir.

NS5B (RNA Polymerase) Inhibitors

- Some RNA polymerase inhibitors combined with NS5A inhibitors have been discussed above.

303. Ans. (a) Oseltamivir

(Ref: Goodman Gilman 12th E/P1608)

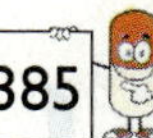

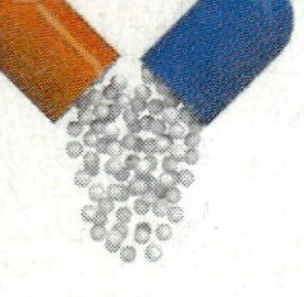

Influenza A	Amantidine rimantidine
Influenza B Bird flu Amantadine resistant influenza A	Oseltamivir Zanamivir Peramivir

304. Ans. (d) Ribavirin

(Ref: Goodman Gilman 12th E/P1608)

305. Ans. (b) Cidofovir

(Ref: Goodman Gilman 12th E/P1601)

Uses of Cidofovir

- CMV retinitis
- Resistant herpes
- BK virus
- Molluscum contagiosum
- Respiratory papillomatosis
- Anogenital warts
- Adenovirus infection in transplant recipients.

306. Ans. (b) Saquinavir

(Ref: Goodman Gilman 12th E/P1648)

307. Ans. (a) Zidovudine

(Ref: Goodman Gilman 12th E/P1616-18)

Hepatitis B Drugs

Specific drugs	Non specific drugs
Entecavir Adefovir	Tenofovir Lamivudine Clevudine Telbivudine

308. Ans. (d) Lamivudine

(Ref: Goodman Gilman 12th E/P1641)

Mnemonics

NNRTI

- **N** : Nevirapine }
- **E** : Efavirenz } Enzyme Inducers
- **E** : Etravirine }
- **D** : Delavirdine – Enzyme Inhibitor
  Doravirine

309. Ans. (c) Optic neuritis

(Ref: Fredrick's Drug Induced Ocular side effects 7th E/P289)

Ocular Side effects of HAART

Probable	Possible
Ptosis EOM palsy (Diplopia)	Uveitis Ocular icterus

310. Ans. (b) As reverse transcriptase inhibitor

(Ref: Goodman Gilman 12th E/P1641)

311. Ans. (c) Nevirapine

(Ref: NACO Guidelines 2011)

- Zidovudine and nevirapine can be used to prevent perinatal HIV transmission.
- In India, nevirapine is preferred because of single dosing, which decreases toxicity and improves compliance.

312. Ans. (d) Saquinavir causes maximum induction of CYP3A4

(Ref: Goodman Gilman 12th E/P1641)

- All protease inhibitors are enzyme inhibitors.

313. Ans. (c) Nelfinavir

(Ref: Goodman Gilman 12th E/P 1650)

> Nelfinavir is metabolized primarily by CYP2C19 and hence Ritonavir which is an inhibitor of CYP3A4 cannot be combined to increase half-life of nelfinavir.

314. Ans. (a) Raltegravir

(Ref: Goodman Gilman 12th E/P 1659)

315. Ans. (c) Stavudine

(Ref: Goodman Gilman 12th E/P 1635)

Maximum peripheral neuropathy	Stavudine
Least peripheral neuropathy	Lamivudine

316. Ans. (b) Ganciclovir

(Ref: Harrison 19th E/P 1193)

317. Ans. (a) Enfuvirtide

(Ref: Goodman Gilman 12th E/P1657)

318. Ans. (a) Neuraminidase inhibitor

(Ref: Goodman Gilman 12th E/P1608)

319. Ans. (a) Elvitegravir

(Ref: Goodman Gilman 12th E/P1658)

320. Ans. (a) Nevirapine

(Ref: Goodman Gilman 12th E/P1642)

321. Ans. (d) Cytomegalovirus retinitis in AIDS patients

(Ref: Goodman Gilman 12th E/P1603)

Antiherpes Virus Drug Preference

HSV VZV	Acyclovir
CMV	Ganciclovir

322. Ans. (a) Lamivudine

(Ref: Goodman Gilman 12th E/P1635)

323. Ans. (b) CYP3A4 inhibition by ritonavir

(Ref: Goodman Gilman 12th E/P1645)

324. Ans. (b) Reverse transcriptase inhibitor

(Ref: Goodman Gilman 12th E/P1643)

325. Ans. (a) Raltegravir

(Ref: Goodman Gilman 12th E/P1658)

326. Ans. (a) Saquinavir

(Ref: Goodman Gilman 12th E/P1647)

- All the drugs in the option are enzyme inhibitors.
- Saquinavir is best answer as it is a very less potent enzyme inhibitor.

327. Ans. (d) Abacavir

(Ref: Goodman Gilman 12th E/P1635)

328. Ans. (a) Non-nucleoside reverse transcriptase inhibitor (NN-RTI)

(Ref: Goodman Gilman 12th E/P1642)

329. Ans. (c) Stavudine

(Ref: Goodman Gilman 12th E/P1634)

330. Ans. (a) Lamivudine

(Ref: Goodman Gilman 12th E/P1634)

- Lamivudine, emtricitabine and tenofovir are least potent inhibitors of human DNA polymerase gamma and hence associated side effects like peripheral neuropathy is negligible.

331. Ans. (c) Neutropenia

(Ref: Goodman Gilman 12th E/P1633)

332. Ans. (a) Fusion inhibitor

(Ref: Goodman Gilman 12th E/P1656)

333. Ans. (d) Stavudine

(Ref: Goodman Gilman 12th E/P1633)

- Resistance to zidovudine is seen due to mutation of reverse transcriptase and it can confer cross resistance to other thymidine analogs like **stavudine, tenofovir and abacavir**; zidovudine should be avoided with these drugs.

334. Ans. (a) Atazanavir

(Ref: Goodman Gilman 12th E/P1652)

335. Ans. (d) None of the above

(Ref: Goodman Gilman 12th E/P1599)

- Acyclovir is the drug of choice for herpes simplex encephalitis.

336. Ans. (d) Lactic acidosis

(Ref: Goodman Gilman 12th E/P1631)

337. Ans. (a) Didanosine

(Ref: Goodman Gilman 12th E/P1638)

338. Ans. (d) Tenofovir

(Ref: Goodman Gilman 12th E/P1637)

339. Ans. (d) All of the above

(Ref: Goodman Gilman 12th E/P1600)

340. Ans. (b) Zanamivir

(Ref: Goodman Gilman 12th E/P1609)

341. Ans. (a) Oseltamivir

(Ref: Goodman Gilman 12th E/P1608)

342. Ans. (d) Foscarnet

(Ref: Goodman Gilman 12th E/P1603)

343. Ans. (a) Acyclovir

(Ref: Goodman Gilman 12th E/P1599)

344. Ans. (d) Zidovudine

(Ref: Goodman Gilman 12th E/P1633)

345. Ans. (c) Protease inhibitor

(Ref: Goodman Gilman 12th E/P1648)

346. Ans. (d) Zidovudine

(Ref: Goodman Gilman 12th E/P1615)

347. Ans. (a) Terbinafine

(Ref: Goodman Gilman 13th E/P1098)

- Terbinafine is primarily used for treatment of dermatophytes (onychomycosis).
- In the last 2 years it is not being used in tinea cruris and corporis due to resistance.

348. Ans. (b) Flucytosine: Inhibit microtubule thereby preventing mitosis

(Ref: Goodman Gilman 13th E/P1098)

- Flucytosine being a prodrug of anticancer drug 5-FU, inhibits DNA replication of fungus in S phase.

349. Ans. (a) Cell membrane

(Ref: Goodman Gilman 12th E/P1572)

Amphotericin B binds to ergosterol in cell membrane and forms pores in the fungus.

350. Ans. (d) Natamycin

(Ref: Goodman Gilman 12th E/P1783)

351. Ans. (a) Clotrimazole

(Ref: Goodman Gilman 12th E/P1587)

352. Ans. (c) Oral Griseofulvin

(Ref: Goodman Gilman 12th E/P1585)

353. Ans. (a) Griseofulvin

(Ref: Goodman Gilman 12th E/P1585)

Drugs whose Absorption is Increased by Fatty food

Mnemonics

PLAGuE

- **P :** Posaconazole
- **L :** Lumefantrine
- **A :** Albendazole, Atovaquone
- **Gu :** Griseofulvin
- **E :** Efavirenz

354. Ans. (a) Amphotericin B

(Ref: Goodman Gilman 12th E/P1574)

Amphotericin B is DOC for

- Systemic fungal infections
- Mucormycosis
- Kala azar
- Cryptococcal meningitis.

355. Ans. (b) Mucormycosis

(Ref: Goodman Gilman 12th E/P1581)

Only azoles effective against mucormycosis are

- Posaconazole
- Isuvaconazole

356. Ans. (a) Ergosterol synthesis

(Ref: Goodman Gilman 13th E/P1091)

357. Ans. (a) Ketoconazole

(Ref: Goodman Gilman 12th E/P 1572)

Antifungals Inhibiting Ergosterol Synthesis	Antifungals Acting on Ergosterol
Terbinafine Azoles	Amphotericin B Nystatin

358. Ans. (d) Terbinafine

(Ref: Harrison 19th E/P350)

359. Ans. (c) Terbinafine

(Ref: Goodman Gilman 12th E/P1586)

360. Ans. (c) Potassium

(Ref: Goodman Gilman 12th E/P1574)

Amphotericin B causes deficiency of

- Potassium
- Magnesium

361. Ans. (d) Clofazimine

(Ref: Goodman Gilman 12th E/P1589)

362. Ans. (d) Griseofulvin

(Ref: Goodman Gilman 12th E/P1585)

- Griseofulvin is used only for treatment of dermatophytes.

363. Ans. (c) Ketoconazole

(Ref: Goodman Gilman 12th E/P1587)

364. Ans. (b) Clotrimazole

(Ref: Goodman Gilman 12th E/P1587)

365. Ans. (a) IV amphotericin B

(Ref: Goodman Gilman 12th E/P1575)

366. Ans. (a) Nystatin

(Ref: Goodman Gilman 12th E/P1589)

Mnemonics

Topical Antifungals

- **B :** Butenafine
- **H :** Haloprogin
- **U :** Undecylenic acid
- **T :** Tolnaftate, Terbinafine
- **A :** Azoles
- **N :** Nystatin, Naftifine

367. Ans. (c) Voriconazole

(Ref: Goodman Gilman 12th E/P1573)

368. Ans. (b) Serum potassium measurement

(Ref: Goodman Gilman 12th E/P1574)

369. Ans. (d) Tolnaftate

(Ref: Goodman Gilman 12th E/P1558)

- Nystatin is used only for treatment of candidiasis.

- Tolnaftate, undecylenic acid and Whitefield's ointment are effective only against dermatophytes.

370. Ans. (d) Griseofulvin

(Ref: Goodman Gilman 12th E/P1585)

371. Ans. (c) Dermatophytes

(Ref: Goodman Gilman 12th E/P1574)

372. Ans. (c) Primaquine

(Ref: Goodman Gilman 13th E/P980, NVBD guidelines)

373. Ans. (a) Artemether lumefantrine

(Ref: NVBD malaria guidelines)

374. Ans. (b) Short plasma half-life

(Ref: Goodman Gilman 12th E/P1396)

375. Ans. (d) 250 mg

(Ref: NBVD Guideline India)

376. Ans. (a) Chloroquine

(Ref: Goodman Gilman 12th E/P1405)

377. Ans. (b) Quinine

(Ref: NBVD Guideline India)

378. Ans. (b) Oral artesunate

(Ref: NBVD Guideline India)

379. Ans. (a) Primaquine is contraindicated in pregnancy and infants

(Ref: NVBDP 2013, India)

Vivax		Falciparum		Mixed Infection
Chloroquine 3 d + Primaquine 14 d d = days	For all states	Artemether 3d + Lumefantrine 3d + Primaquine single dose on day 2	North East	Add primaquine for 14 days to falciparum regimen for North East
		Artesunate 3d + Sulfadoxine 3d + Pyrimethamine 3d + Primaquine single dose on day 2	Other state	Add primaquine for 14 days to falciparum regimen for other states

Note: Primaquine is contraindicated in pregnant and infants.

380. Ans. (c) Artesunate

(Ref: Goodman and Gilman 12th E/P 1395-96)

- Artemisinin group drugs are the most potent and fastest acting schizontocidal drugs. I/V artesunate is considered as the drug of choice for severe falciparum malaria.

381. Ans. (a) Antimalarials

(Ref: Katzung 13th E/P897)

- Antimalarial drug sulfadoxine + pyrimethamine can cause cutaneous skin reactions like erythema multiforme and Steven Johnson's syndrome and hence is not preferred for prophylaxis of malaria.
- Most commonly it is caused by sulfonamides; other drugs that can cause erythema multiforme are antiepileptics (carbamazepine, phenytoin), OCPs, delavirdine, unithiol and salicylates.

382. Ans. (a) Artemether

(Ref: Goodman Gilman 12th E/P 1395)

> Artemisinin group of drugs are the fastest acting schizontocidal drugs and hence are preferred for severe falciparum malaria.

383. Ans. (c) Pyrimethamine

(Ref: Goodman Gilman 12th E/P 1400)

384. Ans. (b) Ciprofloxacin

(Ref: NVBDP 2013, India)

385. Ans. (a) It causes hemolysis

(Ref: Goodman Gilman 12th E/P1407)

386. Ans. (c) Mefloquine

(Ref: Harrison 19th E/P656)

Antimalarials implicated in causing hemolysis in G6PD deficiency
Primaquine – Maximum risk
Proguanil
Chloroquine
Quinine

387. Ans. (c) Artesunate

(Ref: Goodman Gilman 12th E/P1396)

388. Ans. (c) Antimalarial

(Ref: CMDT 2016/P1495)

389. Ans. (a) Antimalarial

(Ref: CMDT 2016/P1491)

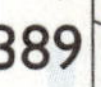

390. Ans. (a) Chloroquine

(Ref: NBVD 2013, India)

391. Ans. (d) Primaquine

(Ref: Harrison 19th E/P656)

392. Ans. (a) Quinine

(Ref: Goodman Gilman 12th E/P1406)

- The drug of choice for chloroquine resistant falciparum malaria, though is artesunate, quinine can also be used.

393. Ans. (b) Chloroquine

(Ref: Goodman Gilman 12th E/P1405)

394. Ans. (a) Praziquantel

(Ref: Goodman Gilman 13th E/P1005)

- The image in the question is egg of helminth H. nana, which can be guessed by the hooklets (finger like projections) present in the centre.

395. Ans. (a) Metronidazole

(Ref: Katzung 13th E/P865)

- Strawberry vagina is seen with trichomoniasis for which the drug of choice is meteonidazole 2 grams single oral dose. In case of intolerance to single dose 500 mg BD is given for 7 days.
- In resistant cases tinidazole is used at 2 grams as single oral dose.

Strawberry Vagina seen in trichomoniasis:

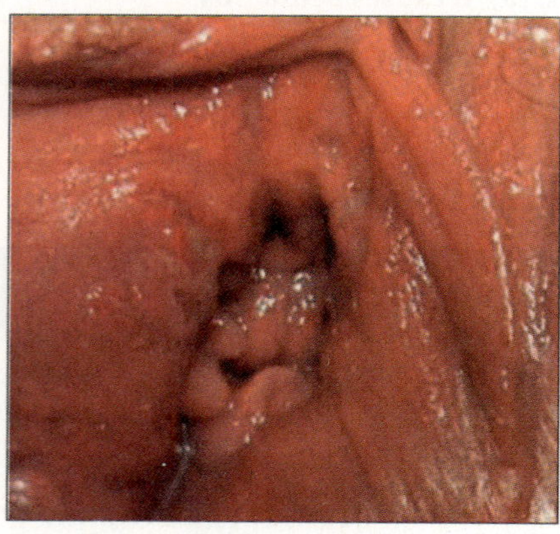

396. Ans. (a) Pentamidine

(Ref: Goodman Gilman 12th E/P

397. Ans. (c) Satranidazole

(Ref: Goodman Gilman 12th E/P1429)

398. Ans. (d) Hydroxychloroquine

(Ref: Goodman Gilman 12th E/P1423)

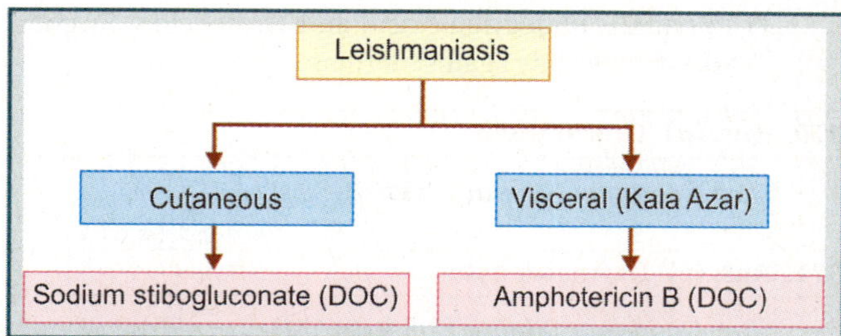

399. Ans. (c) Ciclopirox olamine

(Ref: Goodman Gilman 12th E/P 1588)

- Ciclopirox olamine is an antifungal drug.
- 5% permethrin is the drug of choice for scabies.
- Only oral drug used in scabies is ivermectin.

400. Ans. (a) Poor CSF penetration

(Ref: Goodman Gilman 12th E/P 1451)

> Albendazole is a highly lipid soluble drug with good blood brain penetration.

401. Ans. (c) Praziquantel

(Ref: Harrison 19th E/P 428)

402. Ans. (a) Vomiting and diarrhea

(Ref: Goodman Gilman 12th E/P 1431)

403. Ans. (a) Nitazoxanide

(Ref: Goodman Gilman 12th E/P 1433)

Effects of nitazoxanide
Antiparasitic
Antihelminthic
Antibacterial
Antiviral

404. Ans. (d) Hydroxychloroquine

(Ref: Goodman Gilman 12th E/P1423)

405. Ans. (d) Diloxanide furoate

(Ref: Goodman Gilman 12th E/P1420)

406. Ans. (c) Sodium stibogluconate

(Ref: Goodman Gilman 12th E/P1423)

- The current drug of choice for kala azar is amphotericin B.
- Sodium stibogluconate was the previous drug of choice and hence is the better answer.

407. Ans. (d) All of the above

(Ref: Goodman Gilman 12th E/P1455)

408. Ans. (a) Metronidazole

(Ref: Goodman Gilman 12th E/P1420)

Asymptomatic intestinal	Symptomatic intestinal; extra-intestinal
Paromomycin (DOC) Diloxanide furoate Iodoquinol	Metronidazole (DOC) Chloroquine Nitazoxanide Emetine Dihydroemetine

409. Ans. (b) Praziquantel

(Ref: Goodman Gilman 12th E/P1457)

410. Ans. (b) Ivermectin

(Ref: Goodman Gilman 12th E/P1455)

411. Ans. (c) Niclosamide

(Ref: Goodman Gilman 12th E/P1458)

- Niclosamide is not used in NCC, due to risk of ova release from gravid worms that can form larvae and cause cysticercosis.

412. Ans. (c) Schistosomiasis

(Ref: Goodman Gilman 12th E/P1458)

413. Ans. (c) Albendazole

(Ref: Goodman Gilman 12th E/P1450)

414. Ans. (a) Metronidazole

(Ref: Goodman Gilman 12th E/P1429)

415. Ans. (c) Onchocercosis

(Ref: Goodman Gilman 12th E/P1429)

416. Ans. (b, e) (b) Chloramphenicol, (e) Aminoglycosides

(Ref: Goodman Gilman 13th E/P1049)

417. Ans. (a, b, d) (a) Cholera; (b) Traveller's diarrhea; (d) Bacillary dysentery

(Ref: CMDT 2019/P1476)

- All cases of diarrhea caused by bacteria must be treated with appropriate antibiotics.
- Antibiotics however are avoided in shiga toxin producing *E. coli* because, death or lysis of bacteria releases stored toxins that can worsen the condition.

418. Ans. (b, d) (b) Amphotericin B; (d) Posaconazole

(Ref: Goodman Gilman 13th E/P1089)

Antifungal drugs effective against mucormycosis are

- Amphotericin B
- Posaconazole
- Isavuconazole

419. Ans. (b, c, d) (b) Oseltemivir; (c) Valganciclovir; (d) Valaciclovir

(Ref: Goodman Gilman 13th E/P1111)

- Acyclovir and ganciclovir are prodrugs and hence prodrugs like valaciclovir and valganciclovir were made.
- There are two compounds related to oseltamivir. Oseltamivir phosphate is a prodrug that lacks antiviral effect. Oseltamivir carboxylate is not a prodrug and it has antiviral effect.

420. Ans. (c) Extensively drug resistance (XDR-TB)

(Ref: RNTCP 2016)

- Since in this case there is resistance to both isoniazid and rifampicin + one fluoroquinolone + injectables i.e. aminoglycosides, it ios to be labelled as a case of XDR TB.
- In case of MDR TB there is resistance to only isoniazid and rifampicin.

421. Ans. (c, d) (c) High dose isoniazid; (d) Clofazimine

(Ref: WHO TB guidelines)

- Kindly refer to text for details on the short course regimen for MDR TB.

422. Ans. (c) Amikacin

(Ref: Goodman Gilman 13th E/P1044)

- Aminoglycosides can cause neuromuscular blockade and hence worsen symptoms of myasthenia gravis.

423. Ans. (a) Hepatitis B, (b) Hepatitis C, (c) Hairy cell leukemia

(Ref: Goodman Gilman 12th E/P1612)

Uses of IFN alpha:

- Hepatitis B
- Hepatitis C
- Hepatitis D
- Hairy cell leukemia
- HIV induced thrombocytopenia
- Papilloma virus
- Acyclovir resistant herpes

424. Ans. (a) Amikacin (b) Fluoroquinolone

(Ref: Park's PSM 24th E/P199)

Drugs used in MDR and XDR TB are given below in box:

MDR TB	XDR TB
Kanamycin Levofloxacin Ethambutol Pyrazinamide Ethionamide Cycloserine	Capreomycin Moxifloxacin Linezolid PAS Clofazimine High dose INH Amoxicillin + Clavulinic acid

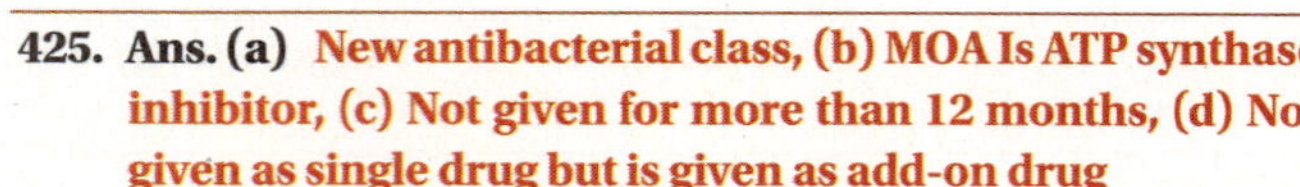

425. Ans. (a) New antibacterial class, (b) MOA Is ATP synthase inhibitor, (c) Not given for more than 12 months, (d) Not given as single drug but is given as add-on drug

(Ref: Park's PSM 24th E/P197,200)

- Bedaquiline is a new antimycobacterial drug that acts by inhibiting ATP synthase.
- It is indicated currently in the following cases
  - MDR TB or rifampicin resistant TB with resistance to all fluoroquinolones or all second line injectables
  - XDR TB with resistance to all fluoroquinolones and second line injectables
  - XDR TB with resistance to all fluoroquinolones and any second line injectables
  - XDR TB with resistance to all second line injectables and any fluoroquinolone
  - Treatment failure of MDR TB with fluoroquinolone or second line injectables resistance
  - Treatment failure of XDR TB
- Bedaquiline is combined with other drugs depending on the resistance pattern. It is given for 6 months with the dose being 400 mg OD for first two weeks, followed by 600 mg per week (200 mg three times with 48 hours gape between two doses) for 22 weeks.
- Bedaquiline is contraindicated in
  - Age < 18 years
  - Pregnant
  - Cardiac arrhythmia – As it can cause QT prolongation.

426. Ans. (c) Ivermectin

(Ref: Goodman Gilman 12th E/P1445)

427. Ans. (b) Moxifloxacin, (c) Clofazimine, (d) Minocycline, (e) Clarithromycin

(Ref: WHO)

WHO Recommended Regimens in Rifampicin Resistance

Ofloxacin 400 mg Minocycline 100 mg Clofazimine 50 mg	Once a day for 6 months	Moxifloxacin 400 mg Minocycline 100 mg Clarithromycin 500 mg Clofazimine 50 mg	Once a day for 6 months
↓		↓	
Followed by Ofloxacin 400 mg Or Minocycline 100 mg Clofazimine 50 mg	Once a day for 18 months	Followed by Moxifloxacin 400 mg Clarithromycin 1000 mg Minocycline 200 mg	Once a month for 18 months

Note: Rifapentine can be used only in rifampicin sensitive cases as both these drugs have same mechanism of action.

428. Ans. (a) Doxycycline, (c) Azithromycin

(Ref: CMDT 2018/P1323)

- The current drug of choice for treatment of mycoplasma is either doxycycline or azithromycin as given below:
  - Mycoplasma genitalium – Doxycycline
  - Mycoplasma pneumoniae - Azithromycin
- Fluoroquinolones are an alternative.

429. Ans. (a) Seen in around 10-20% of patients treated with the drug, (b) May occur within 1 week of initiation of treatment

(Ref: Katzung 13th E/P802, Goodman Gilman 12th E/P1514)

- Nephrotoxicity and ototoxicity are seen with aminoglycosides only after 5 days of therapy.
- Out of all patients who receive aminoglycosides nearly 8-26% develop nephrotoxicity.
- Aminoglycosides get concentrated in and damage the proximal tubular cells of nephron. Since these cells can regenerate, nephrotoxicity is reversible.
- The most common finding is a mild rise in serum creatinine level.
- To prevent nephrotoxicity aminoglycosides should be given as once a day dosing, as multiple dosing or continuous infusion is associated with more nephrotoxicity.
- The most nephrotoxic aminoglycoside is neomycin and the least nephrotoxic is streptomycin.

430. Ans. (a) Echinocandins have very less side effects, (e) Nephrotoxicity is the dose limiting side effect of amphotericin B

(Ref: Goodman Gilman 12th E/P1571-80)

- Echinocandins have a very favorable side effect profile.
- Voriconazole is the first line drug for invasive aspergillosis.
- The bioavailability of oral fluconazole is near 100% but not 100%.
- Amphotericin B disrupts the cell membrane and is a fungicidal drug.
- The most common dose limiting side effect of amphotericin is nephrotoxicity and hence to prevent it patient is preloaded with 1-2 liters of normal saline. For same purpose liposomal amphotericin b is preferred now a days, though it is more costlier.

431. Ans. (a) Cefoxitin, (b) Cefoperazone, (c) Ceftolozane

(Ref: Katzung 13th E/P779)

5th Generation Cephalosporins

- Ceftobiprole
- Ceftaroline

432. Ans. (a) Tetracycline (c) Digoxin, (d) Penicillin, (e) Lithium

(Ref: Goodman Gilman 12th E)

- All the drugs mentioned in options are mainly excreted by kidney except rifampicin.
- Rifampicin is metabolized and excreted by liver and only a very small part is excreted unchanged in kidney. Hence it is the safest first line TB drug in patients of renal failure.

433. Ans. (a) Undergoes first-pass metabolism in the liver, (b) Active against both larva and adult of Nematodes, (c) Absorption increases with fatty meal, (d) Excreted in the urine

(Ref: Goodman Gilman 12th E/P1450-51)

- Albendazole has unpredictable oral absorption and it also undergoes first pass metabolism and is metabolized into active compound albendazole sulfoxide. This active compound makes it more effective than mebendazole.
- Its absorption is increased by fatty food and bile acid.
- It is excreted in urine.
- It is effective against both adult and larval stages of nematodes.
- Thiabendazole the first drug in this group is not preferred now a days due to toxicity of CNS, liver, hypersensitivity etc.

434. Ans. (a) Maraviroc - Entry inhibitor, (b) Raltegravir - Integrase inhibitor, (c) Indinavir - Protease inhibitor, (d) Nevirapine - Nonnucleoside reverse transcriptase inhibitor

(Ref: Goodman Gilman 12th E/P1624)

435. Ans. (c) Zanamivir

(Ref: Goodman Gilman 12th E/P1607)

Anti Influenza drugs given by inhalational route are
- Zanamivir
- Peramivir

436. Ans. (a) Bedaquiline

(Ref: Park's PSM 24th E/P197)

New drugs approved for TB are
- Bedaquiline: Inhibits ATP synthase
- Delamanid: Inhibits mycolic acid synthesis

437. Ans. (d) May cause metabolic acidosis

(Ref: Goodman Gilman 12th E/P1466)

Mafenide inhibits carbonic anhydrase and hence causes metabolic acidosis.

438. Ans. (a) Vancomycin—Amphotericin B, (c) Warfarin—Aspirin, (d) Allopurinol— Azathioprine (e) Aminoglycoside + Vancomycin

(Ref: Goodman Gilman 12th E/P1542, 1574)

- Vancomycin increases risk of nephrotoxicity with drugs like amphotericin b, aminoglycosides and colistin.
- Aspirin increases risk of bleeding if given with warfarin.
- Allopurinol inhibits metabolism of azathioprine and 6 mercaptopurine and increases their toxicity.

439. Ans. (a) Occur within hours after giving penicillin, (c) Aggravation of signs and symptoms of syphilis, (e) Most common in secondary syphilis

(Ref: Goodman Gilman 12th E/P1485)

- In syphilis benzathine penicillin G is drug of choice for all stages except CNS stage, where aqueous penicillin G is more preferred.
- In pregnancy as there are no alternatives, in case of penicillin allergy the female is desensitized to penicillin and then administered.
- In patients of **secondary syphilis**, penicillin associated release of spirochetal antigen can cause hypersensitivity reaction known as **Jarisch-Herxheimer reaction**, characterized by fever, arthralgia, myalgia and **worsening of cutaneous lesions**.

440. Ans. (b) Aminoglycosides, (e) Chloramphenicol

(Ref: Goodman Gilman 12th E/P1528)

441. Ans. (a) Tetracyclines, (c) Ampicillin, (d) Acyclovir

(Ref: Goodman Gilman 12th E/P1524)

442. Ans. (b) Inhibits viral DNA gyrase

(Ref: Goodman Gilman 12th E/P1594)

443. Ans. (a) Ichthyosis, (c) Skin pigmentation, (d) Gastrointestinal disturbances

(Ref: Goodman Gilman 12th E/P1560)

444. Ans. (a) INH, (c) Pyrazinamide, (d) Amikacin, (e) Streptomycin

(Ref: Goodman Gilman 12th E/P1554,56,59)

445. Ans. (a) Liposomal preparation is available, (c) Used only in intravenous form

(Ref: Goodman Gilman 12th E/P1572)

446. Ans. (a) Penicillin, (d) Cephalosporin

(Ref: Goodman Gilman 12th E/P1477)

447. Ans. (b) Aminoglycosides

(Ref: Goodman Gilman 12th E/P1507)

448. Ans. (b) Fluoroquinolones, (d) Cotrimoxazole, (e) Amikacin

(Ref: CMDT 2016/P1456)

Drugs Used in Nocardiosis
- **Cotrimoxazole – DOC**
- **Amikacin**
- **Imipenem**
- **Minocycline**

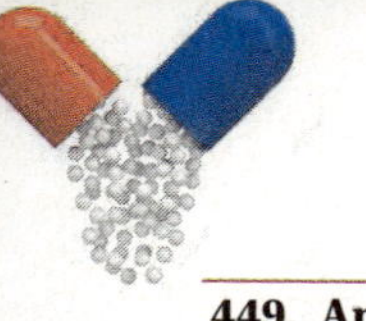

449. Ans. (a) Vancomycin, (c) Linezolid

(Ref: Harrison 19th E/P692)

450. Ans. (c) Cause myopathy, (e) Excretion through kidney

(Ref: Goodman Gilman 12th E/P1543)

451. Ans. (b) 3rd generation cephalosporin, (c) Amphotericin B, (d) Meropenem

(Ref: Harrison 19th E/P692)

452. Ans. (a) Acetylation

(Ref: Goodman Gilman 12th E/P1556)

453. Ans. (a) INH, (b) Rifampicin, (c) Pyrazinamide

(Ref: Goodman Gilman 12th E/P1556)

454. Ans. (a) Cephalosporin, (b) Vancomycin, (c) Penicillin

(Ref: Goodman Gilman 12th E/P1477)

455. Ans. (a) Penicillin + Aminoglycoside, (b) Penicillin + Tetracycline

(Ref: Goodman Gilman 12th E/P1511)

- In a solution **penicillins can inactivate aminoglycosides** and hence should not be mixed together.

456. Ans. (b) Itraconazole, (c) Amphotericin B

(Ref: Goodman Gilman 12th E/P1582)

- Echinocandins like caspofungin inhibit cell wall synthesis by inhibiting beta glucan synthesis.

457. Ans. (e) Ethambutol

(Ref: Goodman Gilman 12th E/P1559)

458. Ans. (d) Streptomycin

(Ref: Goodman Gilman 12th E/P1559)

459. Ans. (d) Ethambutol, (e) Streptomycin

(Ref: Goodman Gilman 12th E/P1559)

460. Ans. (a) Linezolid, (b) Vancomycin, (c) Daptimycin

(Ref: Harrison 19th E/P692)

461. Ans. (a) Inhibits viral DNA polymerase, (b) Used in cytomegalovirus (CMV) infection, (c) Used in Herpes Simplex virus (HSV) infection

(Ref: Goodman Gilman 12th E/P1638)

462. Ans. (a) Penicillin G, (c) Tetracycline, (d) Ciprofloxacin

(Ref: Harrison 19th E/P1008)

463. Ans. (b) Meropenem not require concurrent cilastatin administration, (c) Methicillin cause interstitial nephritis, (d) Moxalactam can cause disulfiram like action

(Ref: Goodman Gilman 12th E/P1491,1500)

464. Ans. (a) Disulfiram-like effect, (c) It has metallic taste

(Ref: Goodman Gilman 12th E/P1429)

465. Ans. (b) Ceftazidime, (d) Colistin

(Ref: Goodman Gilman 12th E/P1498, 1538)

466. None

(Ref: Goodman Gilman 12th E/P1521-26)

467. Ans. (a) Streptomycin-least nephrotoxic

(Ref: Goodman Gilman 12th E/P1514)

- Aminoglycosides bind t0 30 S subunit of ribosome.
- They have prolonged post antibiotic effect.
- Streptomycin is most vestibulotoxic.

468. Ans. (a) Itraconazole, (b) Voriconazole, (d) Amphotericin B

(Ref: Goodman Gilman 12th E/P1573)

469. Ans. (b) Pyrazinamide is bactericidal for intracellular bacteria

(Ref: Goodman Gilman 12th E/P1559)

470. Ans. (c) Imipenem, (d) Cloxacillin, (e) Amoxiclav

(Ref: Harrison 19th E/P692)

- Because of large molecular size, vancomycin is unable to penetrate porins of gram-negatives.

471. Ans (c) Vancomycin

(Ref: Goodman Gilman 12th E/P1540)

- Because of large molecular size, vancomycin is unable to penetrate porins of Gram-negatives.

472. Ans. (b) Norfloxacin, (d) Ampicillin

(Ref: Goodman Gilman 12th E/P1490)

473. Ans. (a) S. aureus, (b) Streptococci, (d) Anaerobes, (e) Salmonella typhi

(Ref: Goodman Gilman 12th E/P1509)

- Aminoglycosides are narrow spectrum drugs with effect only against Gram-negative organisms like pseudomonas, E. coli and klebsiella.

474. Ans. (c) Acyclovir-inhibit viral DNA polymerase, (d) Cytarabine-inhibit human DNA polymerase

(Ref: Goodman Gilman 12th E/P1594)

475. Ans. (b) Cotrimoxazole, (c) Ampicillin, (e) Ceftriaxone

(Ref: Goodman Gilman 12th E/P1487, 1497)

- **Cotrimoxazole, ampicillin and ceftriaxone can cross blood brain barrier and hence are used for treatment of meningitis.**

476. Ans. (b) Cardiac failure, (d) Aminoglycosides

(Ref: Goodman Gilman 12th E/P1574)

- Lipid formulation and normal saline are used to decrease toxicity of amphotericin B.
- Cardiac failure can decrease GFR and Amphotericin B clearance and cause toxicity.
- Aminoglycosides are also nephrotoxic and thus can increase amphotericin B toxicity.

477. Ans. (c) Ribavirin-Chronic HBV infection, (d) Valganciclovir->90% oral bioavailability

(Ref: Goodman Gilman 12th E/P1604, 1613)

- Valganciclivir has a bioavailability of 61%.
- Ribavirin is used for treatment of chronic hepatitis C infection.

478. Ans. (b) Hyperkalemia

(Ref: Goodman Gilman 12th E/P1603)

479. Ans. (a) Nausea, (b) Vomiting, (c) Diarrhea

(Ref: CMDT 2016/P1494)

480. Ans. (a) Peripheral neuropathy, (b) Hemolytic anemia, (e) Methemoglobinemia

(Ref: Goodman Gilman 12th E/P1564)

481. Ans. (a) Cefazolin, (b) Ceftriaxone, (c) Ceftazidime, (d) Cefuroxime

(Ref: Goodman Gilman 12th E/P1496)

- All cephalosporins are excreted by kidney except cefoperazone and cefpiramide.
- Ceftriaxone is 50% excreted by kidney and 50% by liver.

482. Ans. (a) Rifampin – Staphylococcus aureus, (b) Multidrugresistant-Mycobacteria, (c) Fluoroquinolones – S. typhi, (d) Tetracycline – Vibrio cholerae

(Ref: Goodman Gilman 12th E/P1550)

483. Ans. (b) Stavudine, (d) Zalcitabine

(Ref: Goodman Gilman 12th E/P1640, 1634)

484. Ans. (b) All MRSA are multidrug resistance, (c) Vancomycin is effective, (d) MRSA are more virulent than sensitive strains, (e) Resistance develop due to altered binding protein

(Ref: Goodman Gilman 12th E/P1479)

485. Ans. (a) Enterococcal endocarditis, (b) Viridans streptococcal endocarditis, (d) Carbenicillin/ticarcillin + gentamicin: Pseudomonas infection

(Ref: Katzung 12th E/P910)

486. Ans. (a) Ritonavir, (d) Delavirdine

(Ref: Goodman Gilman 12th E/P1648)

487. Ans. (b) Bacteriostatic, (c) Thrombocytopenia occur as a S/E, (e) Systemic absorption may occur

(Ref: Goodman Gilman 12th E/P1466)

- Inhibition of DHPS gives bacteriostatic effect.
- Systemic absorption occurs and achieves significant plasma concentration if applied on a large surface area.
- Thus, systemic side effects like bone marrow suppression and thrombocytopenia can be seen.

488. None

(Ref: Goodman Gilman 12th E/P1501)

- None of these is a beta lactamase inhibitor.

489. Ans. (a) Quinupristin/dalfopristin, (b) Linezolid

(Ref: Harrison 19th E/P692)

490. Ans. (a) Clostridium difficile

(Ref: Goodman Gilman 12th E/P1493)

491. Ans. (a) Lamivudine, (c) Zalcitabine

(Ref: Goodman Gilman 12th E/P1634, 1640)

492. Ans. (a) Amikacin, (c) Lithium

(Ref: Goodman Gilman 12th E/P1513)

493. Ans. (a) Penicillin + streptomycin in SABE, (c) Sulphamethoxazole + trimethoprim in UTI, (d) Amphotericin B + flucytosine in cryptococcal meaninings

(Ref: Katzung 12th E/P910)

494. Ans. (b) Daptomycin

(Ref: Charles's Antimicrobial Pharmacodynamics in theory and clinical practice)

495. Ans. (c) Linezolid

(Ref: Charles's Antimicrobial Pharmacodynamics in theory and clinical practice)

496. Ans. (a) Ritonavir

(Ref: Goodman Gilman 13th E/P342)

- Midazolam is metabolized by CYP3A4 cytochrome P450 enzyme.

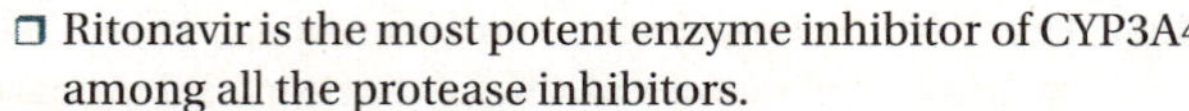

- Ritonavir is the most potent enzyme inhibitor of CYP3A4 among all the protease inhibitors.
- Hence ritonavir can inhibit metabolism of midazolam and precipitate toxicity.

497. Ans. None

(Ref: Goodman GILMAN 13th E/P965)

- All the mechanisms mentioned in the options can contribute to bacterial resistance.
- Please look into the theory section; it has been covered in detail.

498. Ans. (c) It should be given alone

(Ref: Goodman Gilman 13th E/P1076)

- New drugs like Bedaquiline and delamanid are used in combination with other drugs for treatment of MDR and XDR TB. In fact, no drug is used as monotherapy for mycobacterium due to risk of resistance.
- Bedaquiline is an inhibitor of ATP synthase.
- Mycobacterium with Rv0678 mutations can cause resistance to both clofazimine and bedaquiline by drug efflux.
- Food increases absorption and bioavailability of bedaquiline.

499. Ans. (c) Clindamycin

(Ref: Goodman Gilman 13th E/P1057)

- Clindamycin has good penetration into bones and has good activity against staphylococcus. Hence, it is one of the preferred agents for osteomyelitis.
- The drug of choice for osteomyelitis is ceftriaxone.

500. Ans. (b) Colistimethate sodium

(Ref: Goodman Gilman 13th E/P1059)

Colistin can be given by intravenous route for treatment of multidrug resistant gram-negative organisms like

- Pseudomonas
- Klebsiella
- Acinetobacter

501. Ans. (b) Clindamycin

(Ref: Netter's OBG 3rd E/P791)

- Toxic Shock syndrome (TSS) is usually caused by staphylococcus or streptococcus and hence suitable antibiotics must be given.
- Clindamycin inhibits toxin synthesis in staphylococcus and streptococcus and hence is the drug of choice for treatment of toxic shock syndrome (TSS); for complete antimicrobial coverage vancomycin is also added.

502. Ans. (b) Saquinavir

(Ref: Katzung 12th E/P880)

Boosting of saquinavir with ritonavir decreases dyslipidemia and GIT toxicity whereas there is an increased risk of QT and PR prolongation.

503. Ans. (b) Elvitegravir

(Ref: CMDT 2018/P1372)

- Elvitegravir 125 mg is combined with cobicistat 150 mg in a fixed dose combination, where cobicistat is used as a boosting agent.
- Cobicistat boosting is also used along with atazanavir and darunavir.

504. Ans. (d) Linezolid

(Ref: Goodman Gilman 12th E/P1372)

- Time dependent killing is seen with drugs like beta-lactams (penicillins, cephalosporins, carbepenems and monobactams), vancomycin, clindamycin, erythromycin and flucytosine.
- Linezolid on the other hand follows concentration time dependent killing as its affect correlates with the area under the curve (AUC).

505. Ans. (a) Posaconazole

(Ref: Katzung 12th E/P855)

Posaconazole is currently approved for

- Invasive aspergillosis
- Prophylaxis of fungal infections in graft versus host disease and induction chemotherapy for leukemia.

506. Ans. (d) Penciclovir

(Ref: Goodman Gilman 12th E/P1601)

507. Ans. (b) Rifabutin

(Ref: Harrison 19th E/P205-e5)

508. Ans. (d) Minocycline

(Ref: Harrison 19th E/P352)

509. Ans. (b) Rifampicin

(Ref: Goodman Gilman 12th E/P1550)

510. Ans. (a) Inhibition of ergosterol synthesis

(Ref: Goodman Gilman 12th E/P1576)

- **Azoles inhibit ergosterol synthesis by inhibiting rate limiting enzyme 14-alpha sterol demethylase.**
- **Terbinafine can also inhibit ergosterol synthesis by inhibiting squalene epoxidase.**

511. Ans. (a) Enfuvirtide

(Ref: Goodman Gilman 12th E/P1657)

512. Ans. (d) Gentamicin

(Ref: Goodman Gilman 12th E/P1507)

- **Aminoglycosides need oxygen to enter into the bacteria and hence are not effective against anaerobes.**

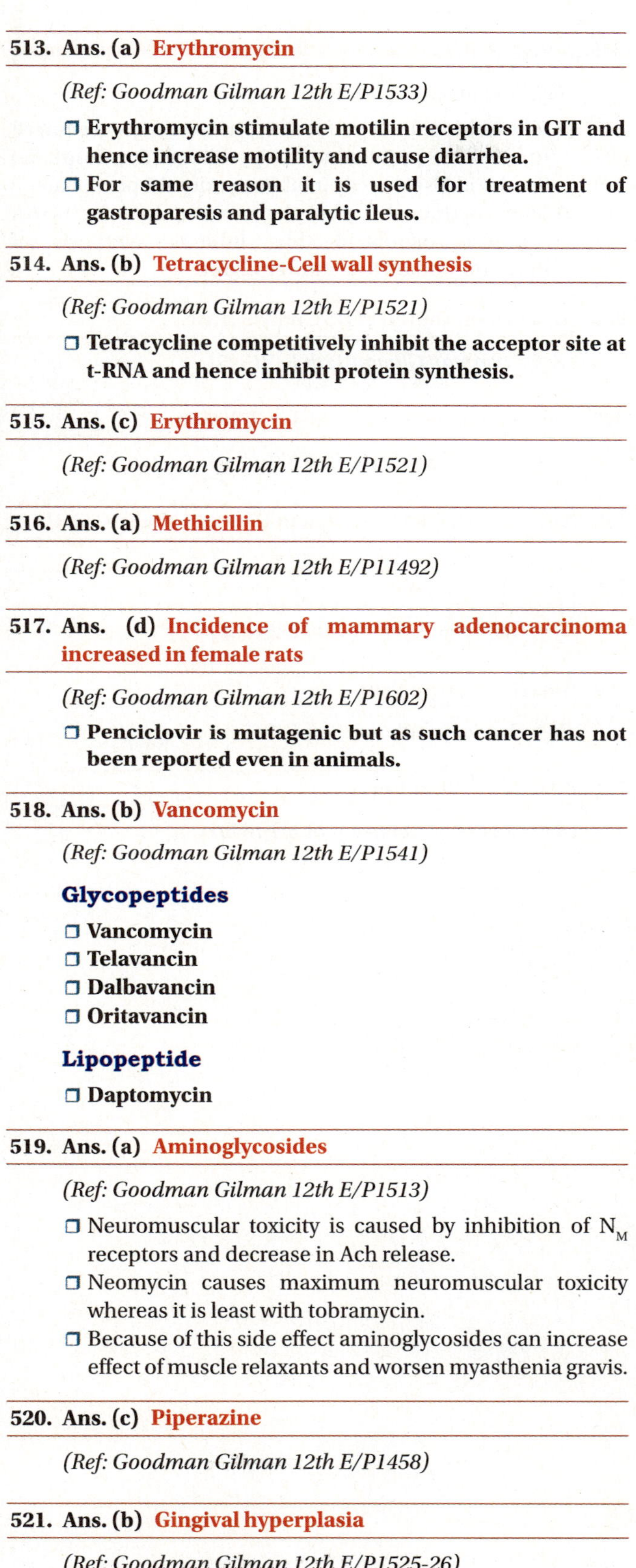

513. Ans. (a) Erythromycin

(Ref: Goodman Gilman 12th E/P1533)

- **Erythromycin stimulate motilin receptors in GIT and hence increase motility and cause diarrhea.**
- **For same reason it is used for treatment of gastroparesis and paralytic ileus.**

514. Ans. (b) Tetracycline-Cell wall synthesis

(Ref: Goodman Gilman 12th E/P1521)

- **Tetracycline competitively inhibit the acceptor site at t-RNA and hence inhibit protein synthesis.**

515. Ans. (c) Erythromycin

(Ref: Goodman Gilman 12th E/P1521)

516. Ans. (a) Methicillin

(Ref: Goodman Gilman 12th E/P11492)

517. Ans. (d) Incidence of mammary adenocarcinoma increased in female rats

(Ref: Goodman Gilman 12th E/P1602)

- **Penciclovir is mutagenic but as such cancer has not been reported even in animals.**

518. Ans. (b) Vancomycin

(Ref: Goodman Gilman 12th E/P1541)

Glycopeptides

- **Vancomycin**
- **Telavancin**
- **Dalbavancin**
- **Oritavancin**

Lipopeptide

- **Daptomycin**

519. Ans. (a) Aminoglycosides

(Ref: Goodman Gilman 12th E/P1513)

- Neuromuscular toxicity is caused by inhibition of N_M receptors and decrease in Ach release.
- Neomycin causes maximum neuromuscular toxicity whereas it is least with tobramycin.
- Because of this side effect aminoglycosides can increase effect of muscle relaxants and worsen myasthenia gravis.

520. Ans. (c) Piperazine

(Ref: Goodman Gilman 12th E/P1458)

521. Ans. (b) Gingival hyperplasia

(Ref: Goodman Gilman 12th E/P1525-26)

522. Ans. (c) Oxazolidinidiones

(Ref: Goodman Gilman 12th E/P1537)

523. Ans. (d) Linezolid

(Ref: Goodman Gilman 12th E/P1537)

524. Ans. (d) Cefotetan

(Ref: Goodman Gilman 12th E/P1493)

525. Ans. (a) Daptomycin

(Ref: Goodman Gilman 12th E/P1543)

- **Daptomycin depolarizes cell membrane and causes death of bacteria due to loss of membrane potential.**

526. Ans. (c) Malaria

(Ref: Goodman Gilman 12th E/P1455-56)

527. Ans. (c) Tetracycline

(Ref: Goodman Gilman 12th E/P1533)

528. Ans. (b) Atazanavir

(Ref: Goodman Gilman 12th E/P1652)

529. Ans. (b) Erythromycin

(Ref: Goodman Gilman 12th E/P1533)

530. Ans. (c) Didanosine

(Ref: Goodman Gilman 12th E/P1639)

531. Ans. (a) Cefuroxime

(Ref: Goodman Gilman 12th E/P1495)

532. Ans. (a) Interferes cell wall synthesis

(Ref: Goodman Gilman 12th E/P1493)

533. Ans. (c) Emtricitabine

(Ref: Goodman Gilman 12th E/P1638)

534. Ans. (a) Ethambutol

(Ref: Goodman Gilman 12th E/P1559)

Hypothyroidism is caused by ethionamide and not ethambutol.

535. Ans. (c) In penicillin allergy, aztreonam tolerated but not imipenem

536. Ans. (c) Retapamulin

(Ref: Harrison 19th E/P962)

537. Ans. (b) Imipenem

(Ref: Goodman Gilman 12th E/P1500)

538. Ans. (d) **Ethambutol**

(Ref: Goodman Gilman 12th E/P1559)

539. Ans. (b) **Gp41**

(Ref: Goodman Gilman 12th E/P1657)

540. Ans. (a) **Fusion/entry inhibitor**

(Ref: Goodman Gilman 12th E/P1657)

541. Ans. (a) **Efavirenz**

(Ref: Goodman Gilman 12th E/P1642)

542. Ans. (b) **Mebendazole**

(Ref: Goodman Gilman 12th E/P1576)

- **Mebendazole is a benzimidazole used for helminths.**

543. Ans. (c) **Ketoconazole**

(Ref: Goodman Gilman 12th E/P1576)

Imidazoles	Triazoles
Clotrimazole	Fluconazole
Ketoconazole	Itraconazole
Butoconazole	Voriconazole
Sertaconazole	Posaconazole
Sulconazole	Isavuconazole

544. Ans. (d) **Erythromycin**

(Ref: Goodman Gilman 12th E/P1513)

545. Ans. (c) **INH inhibits the enzyme pyridoxine phosphokinase**

(Ref: Goodman Gilman 12th E/P1558)

- **Isoniazid** inhibits pyridoxine phosphokinase **required to convert pyridoxine to pyridoxal 5 phosphate; isoniazid also** directly inhibits pyridoxal 5 phosphate.
- **Since pyridoxal 5 phosphate is required for GABA synthesis, isoniazid thus inhibits synthesis of inhibitory neurotransmitter GABA.**

546. Ans. (d) **Inhibition of HSV polymerase**

(Ref: Goodman Gilman 12th E/P1595)

547. Ans. (c) **Fluconazole-Mitosis inhibition**

(Ref: Goodman Gilman 12th E/P1576)

548. Ans. (b) **Isoniazid (Goodman Gilman 12th E/P1558)**

549. Ans. (c) **Nevirapine**

(Ref: Goodman Gilman 12th E/P1632)

550. Ans. (b) **Vancomycin**

(Ref: Goodman Gilman 12th E/P1540)

551. Ans. (b) **Nevirapine**

(Ref: Goodman Gilman 12th E/P1640)

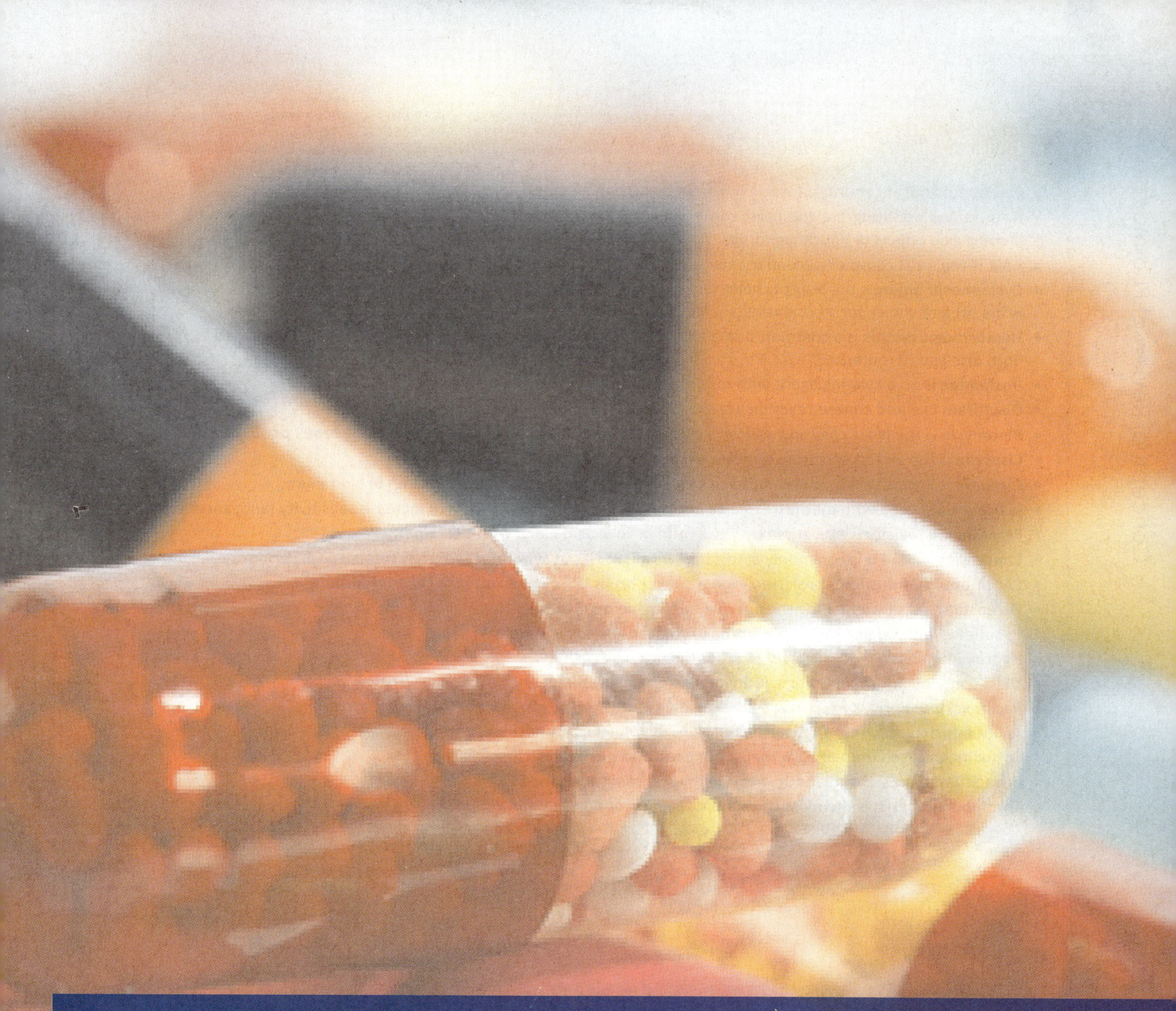

Anticancer Drugs

One Liners

- Parenteral anticancer drugs are administered by **CODAN IV set**.
- **Nausea** and **vomiting** are the most common side effects, whereas **bone marrow suppression** is the most common dose limiting side effects of anticancer drugs.
- **AML** is the most common secondary malignancy associated with anticancer drugs.
- **Cyclophosphamide** is the drug of choice for steroid dependent Nephrotic syndrome (frequent relapsers), whereas **cyclosporine** is the drug of choice for steroid resistant Nephrotic syndrome.
- **Hemorrhagic cystitis** is a common side effect of **ifosfamide > cyclophosphamide**, which can be prevented by **mesna** given by both **oral** and IV route.
- **Ifosfamide** is an alkylating agent with maximum neurotoxicity, caused by chloracetyldehyde.
- **Disulfiram like and cheese reaction** are side effects associated with procarbazine.
- **Bleomycin** is the most common anticancer drug causing pulmonary fibrosis by damaging **type I pneumocytes**.
- **Cisplatin** is the widest spectrum anticancer drug.
- **Cisplatin** is inactivated by **aluminum** and hence not used with equipment made up of aluminum.
- **Leucovorin** is used with **methotrexate** to ameliorate toxicity and with **5-FU** to increase sensitivity (anticancer effect).
- **Pemetrexed toxicity** is prevented by **leucovorin** or **folic acid** along with **vitamin B_{12}**.
- **Capecitabine > 5-FU** is commonly associated with **Hand-Foot syndrome**, which is treated with pyridoxine.
- **Continuous IV infusion** is preferred for anticancer drugs like **cytarabine (ara-c)** and **cladribine**.
- **Pentostatin** acts by inhibiting the enzyme **adenosine deaminase**.
- In patients with **Crigler-Najjar syndrome irinotecan** toxicity is increased.
- **Hydroxyurea** has a bioavailability of 80–100%.
- Most common anticancer drug causing **peripheral neuropathy** and **SIADH** is **vincristine**.
- **Paclitaxel** was derived from yew tree, but now synthesized by genetic engineering in ***E. coli***.
- **Acute infusion reaction** is the most common side effect of **monoclonal antibodies**.
- **Cetuximab** is used for palliative therapy in **head and neck cancer**.
- **Bevacizumab** is used in **diabetic retinopathy** and **renal cell cancer**.
- **Thrombocytopenia** is the most common side effect of **bortezomib**.

INTRODUCTION

Neoplasia is an abnormal and rapid proliferation of cells that gives rise to unwanted tissue mass or tumor. Since the tumor cells also require the cell cycle for proliferation, it can be said that an increase in frequency of cell cycle causes neoplasia. The cause is almost always targeted in chemotherapy and hence cell cycle is inhibited by various chemicals, either in a specific phase (cell-cycle specific) or in all phases (noncell-cycle specific). This is the broad classification of anticancer drugs into:

- **Noncell-cycle specific anticancer drugs**
- **Cell-cycle specific anticancer drugs**

CLASSIFICATION OF ANTICANCER DRUGS

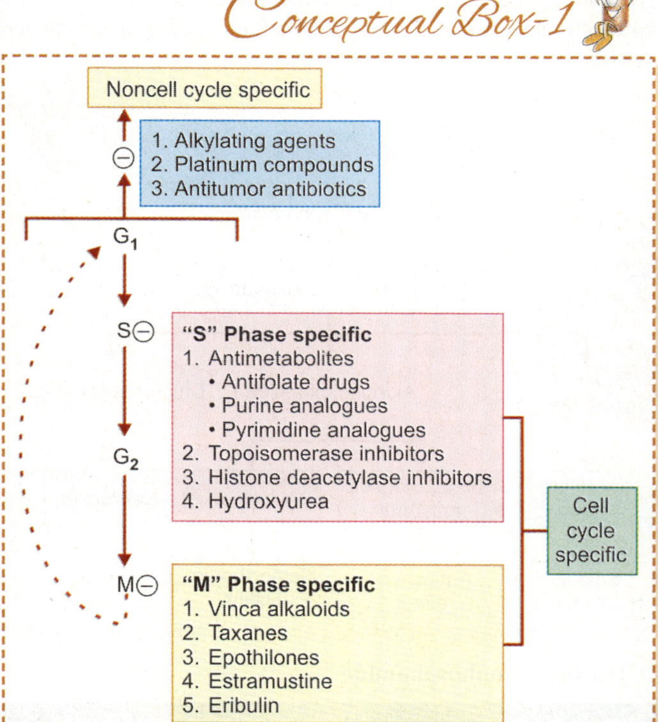

Note: Bleomycin is relatively cell cycle specific for G1-S phase.

GENERAL SIDE EFFECTS OF ANTICANCER DRUGS

When anticancer drugs are introduced into the human body, they not only inhibit proliferation of tumor cells, but also normal cells which are rapidly proliferating. Inhibition of proliferation of gastrointestinal tract (GIT) epithelial cells, hair follicles, gonadal cells and bone marrow cells can present as following side effects.

- GIT epithelium depletion causes mucositis and diarrhea.
  - Mucositis is common with anticancer drugs like **alkylating agents, 5-FU**, **methotrexate** and **cytarabine**.
  - Diarrhea is common with 5-FU, capecitabine, irinotecan and tyrosine kinase inhibitors (imatinib, sunitinib, sorafenib etc.)
- Hair follicle depletion causes alopecia. Maximum alopecia is seen with alkylating agents, **anthracyclines** and topoisomerase inhibitors (etoposide and irinotecan).
- Gonadal dysfunction can cause anovulation and oligospermia.
- Bone marrow suppression is the most common **dose limiting toxicity**. It is not seen with cisplatin, bleomycin and vincristine. Maximum bone marrow suppression and agranulocytosis is seen with alkylating agents.
- Nausea and vomiting are the most common side effects associated with anticancer drugs.
  - Nausia and vomiting are maximum with **cisplatin (most emetogenic),** carmustine, anthracyclines, high dose cyclophosphamide, dacarbazine, mechlorethamine and minimum with **chlorambucil**, busulfan, bleomycin, fludarabine, vinca alkaloids and monoclonal antibodies.
  - Toxic drugs stimulate the vomiting center causing nausea and vomiting. They also stimulate enterochromaffin cells in GIT that releases serotonin and substance P, which by acting on 5-HT3 receptors and Neurokinin-1 (NK1) receptors respectively cause nausea and vomiting. Hence inhibitors of these receptors are best drugs used to prevent chemotherapy induced nausea and vomiting.
  - Drugs used for prevention of chemotherapy induced nausea and vomiting.

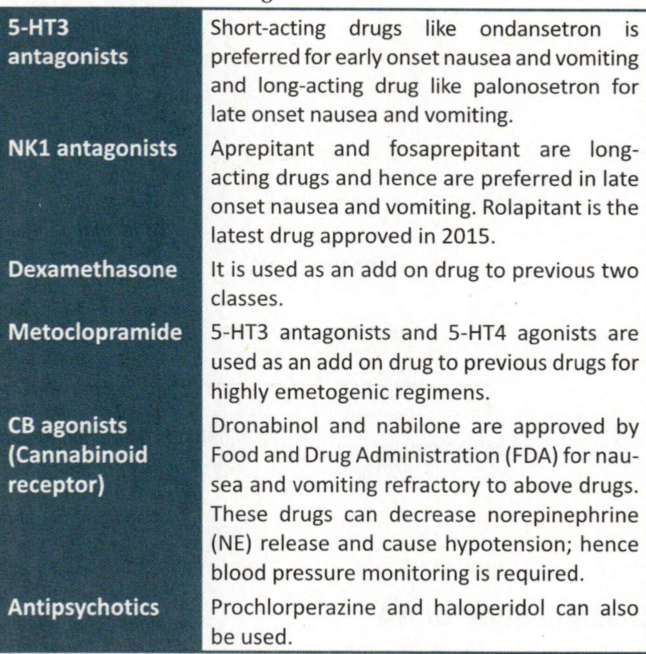

5-HT3 antagonists	Short-acting drugs like ondansetron is preferred for early onset nausea and vomiting and long-acting drug like palonosetron for late onset nausea and vomiting.
NK1 antagonists	Aprepitant and fosaprepitant are long-acting drugs and hence are preferred in late onset nausea and vomiting. Rolapitant is the latest drug approved in 2015.
Dexamethasone	It is used as an add on drug to previous two classes.
Metoclopramide	5-HT3 antagonists and 5-HT4 agonists are used as an add on drug to previous drugs for highly emetogenic regimens.
CB agonists (Cannabinoid receptor)	Dronabinol and nabilone are approved by Food and Drug Administration (FDA) for nausea and vomiting refractory to above drugs. These drugs can decrease norepinephrine (NE) release and cause hypotension; hence blood pressure monitoring is required.
Antipsychotics	Prochlorperazine and haloperidol can also be used.

NON-CELL CYCLE SPECIFIC ANTICANCER DRUGS

ALKYLATING AGENTS

- Alkylating agents (AA) have an alkyl group, which is devoid of a hydrogen (H) atom. Thus, when this class is introduced into human body it binds to H atoms of DNA at N-7 position of guanine in all phases of cell cycle, however this class is most effective on G1-S phase. This causes mispairing of guanine with thymine and an attempt to repair leads to DNA breakage. Cell cycle check gate detects this abnormal DNA

and stimulates apoptotic pathway that, leads to death of tumor cells.

- However, in some cases the cells can escape the check gate with an abnormal DNA with deletions of chromosome 5 or 7 and in such case, neoplasia can be seen, which is secondary leukemia acute myeloid leukemia (AML). Secondary leukemia is maximum with **melphalan (most leukemogenic)**, nitrosoureas and procarbazine; least with **cyclophosphamide**.
- Secondary leukemia can be seen with other drugs also like cisplatin and topoisomerase II inhibitors.

I	Leukemia type	Duration after which leukemia is seen
Alkylating agents	AML due to deletions in chromosome 5 or 7	4 years
Cisplatin	AML	4 years
Topoisomerase II inhibitors	AML due to translocations of mixed lineage leukemia (MLL) gene in 11q23	2–3 years

Mechanism of Action of AA

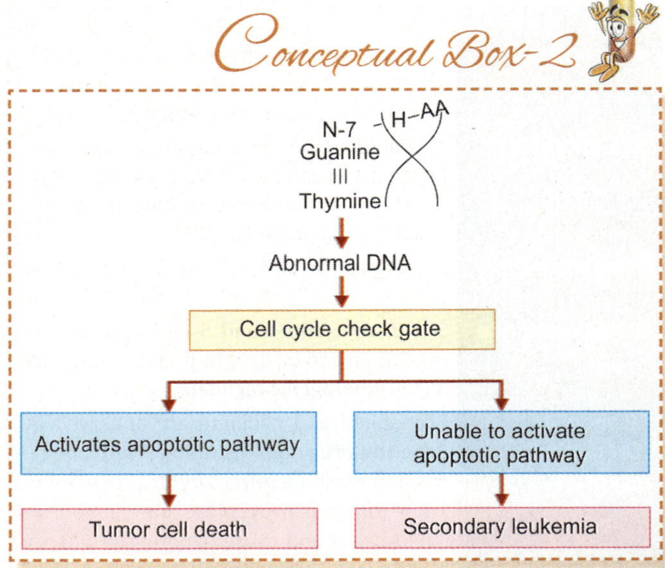

Classification of AA

- AA can be broadly classified as **nitrogen mustards, nitrosoureas, AA acting by methylation** and **miscellaneous**.
- **Most alkylating agents are bifunctional**, i.e. they have two reactive groups, that can bind to both strands of DNA and can cause DNA cross linking. Cross linking of DNA gives these drugs a very high cytotoxic effect.
- However, **alkylating agents acting by methylation, i.e. procarbazine, dacarbazine and temozolomide are monofunctional**. They have only one reactive group and can bind to one strand of DNA; hence there is no cross linking of DNA. These drugs have relatively lesser cytotoxic effect and hence if a cell survives with a mutation, the risk of secondary cancer is higher.
- Other drugs that can crosslink DNA are platinum compounds and mitomycin C.

Nitrogen Mustards

The anticancer effect of nitrogen mustard originated from use of mustard gas in World War 1, which caused depletion of rapidly proliferating cells in the victims. Then Goodman and Gilman established the anticancer effect of nitrogen mustards. This class contains drugs like cyclophosphamide, ifosfamide, mechlorethamine, melphalan and chlorambucil.

Cyclophosphamide

Cyclophosphamide is a prodrug with good oral absorption. It is metabolized in the liver by CYP2B6 to 4-Hydroxycyclophosphamide, which further cleaves into aldophosphamide, chloroacetaldehyde and inactive metabolites excreted by liver. Aldophosphamide breaks into phosphoramide mustard which gives anticancer effect, chloroacetaldehyde causes neurotoxicity and acrolein which is toxic to bladder causes hemorrhagic cystitis.

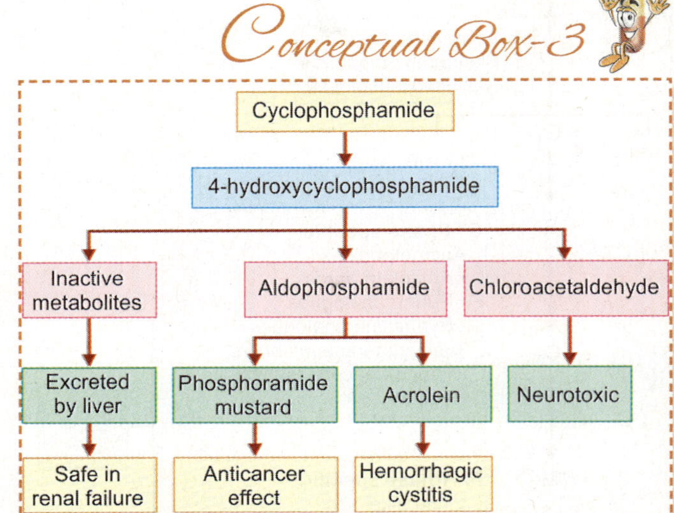

- **Uses of cyclophosphamide**

Neoplastic uses	Non-neoplastic uses (Due to immunosuppressive effects)
• Non-Hodgkin's lymphoma • Breast cancer • Ovarian cancer • Paediatric solid tumors	• Wegener's granulomatosis: Drug of choice • Rheumatoid arthritis • Steroid dependent nephrotic syndrome: Drug of choice

- ***Side effects of cyclophosphamide***
    - Cyclophosphamide causes **hemorrhagic cystitis (ifosfamide > cyclophosphamide) at high doses**, which can be prevented by coadministration of **mesna** (2-mercaptoethane sulfonate) by initial bolus IV dose followed by subsequent doses by IV or **oral route** and vigorous hydration. The usual dose of mesna is 60% of the dose of cyclophosphamide and ifosfamide.
    - Neurotoxicity manifests in the form of SIADH followed by hyponatremia.

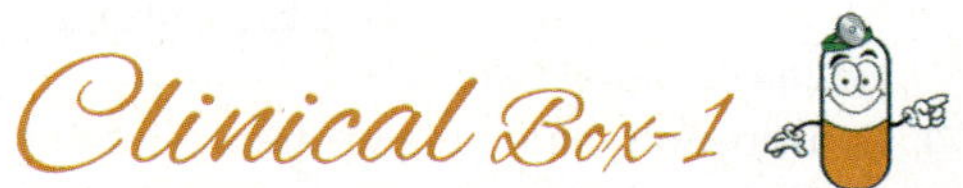

Nephrotic Syndrome in Children

Most common cause is MCD (minimal change disease)
Drug of choice is prednisolone, 60 mg/m²/day

- Steroid dependence/ Frequent relapsers → Drug of choice is cyclophosphamide
- Steroid resistance, Most common cause is FSGS → Drug of choice is cyclosporine

Other drugs used in NS: Mycophenolate mofetil, Tacrolimus, Levamisole, Rituximab and ACEI/ARB.

- Bone marrow suppression with relative sparing of platelets can be seen.
- Cardiotoxicity is observed only at high doses only.
- Since it is metabolized by liver, dose should be reduced in liver dysfunction; it is safe though in patients with renal dysfunction.

Ifosfamide

Ifosfamide is an analog of cyclophosphamide, which is much slowly activated by CYP 450 enzymes as compared to cyclophosphamide. Hence, the toxic metabolites like acrolein and chloroacetaldehyde accumulate for a longer period and cause **more toxicity than cyclophosphamide**.

- ***Uses of ifosfamide:***
  - **Testicular cancer:** It can be used with BEP (Bleomycin + Etoposide + Platinum compound, i.e. Cisplatin) regimen.
  - **Sarcoma:** It is one of the preferred drugs in the regimen for treatment of osteosarcoma.
- ***Side effects of ifosfamide:***
  - It is more toxic than cyclophosphamide due to reason mentioned above.
  - Hemorrhagic cystitis is seen at normal doses and hence **mesna is routinely given**.
  - Chloroacetaldehyde is responsible for neurotoxicity like GTCS, ataxia and even coma. Hence, it is the **most neurotoxic alkylating agent**. Methylene blue can be used for treatment of neurotoxicity.

Cyclophosphamide/Ifosfamide Induced Hemorrhagic Cystitis

Mechlorethamine

- Mechlorethamine was the first nitrogen mustard used clinically and was used in MOPP regimen for Hodgkin's disease. However, now another alkylating agent dacarbazine has replaced it for the same in ABVD regimen. It is still used topically for cutaneous T-cell lymphoma.
  - It is the most reactive nitrogen mustard and can cause **vesication** (blister formation), which can be treated by injecting **thiosulfate** into the site. Thrombophlebitis and hypersensitivity can also be seen.
- Like other vesicants (doxorubicin) it is also given by rapidly flowing IV line to prevent vesication.

Melphalan

- Melphalan is a second line drug for treatment of multiple myeloma, which can be combined with prednisolone and bortezomib/lenalidomide/thalidomide for induction. It is contraindicated in patients eligible for stem cell transplants, as it can destroy the stem cells.
- It is least reactive in this group and does not cause vesication.
- It has high plasma protein binding, both to albumin and α_1-acidic glycoprotein.

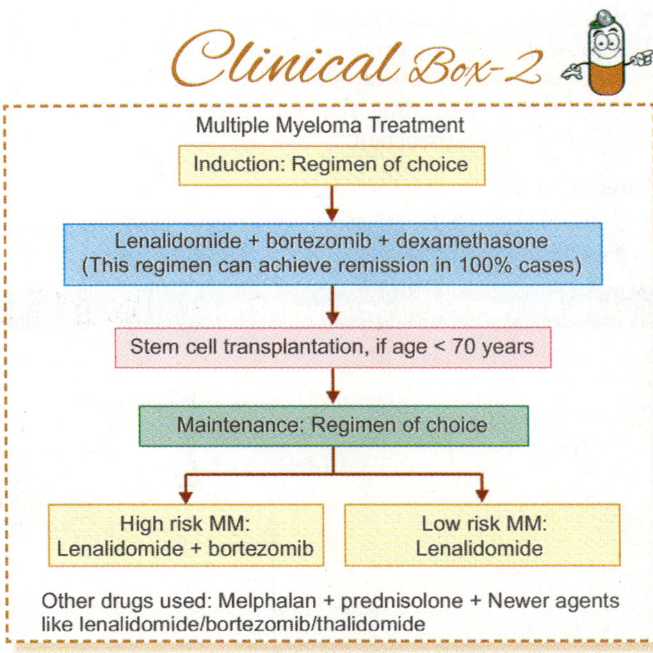

Clinical Box-2
Multiple Myeloma Treatment
Induction: Regimen of choice
Lenalidomide + bortezomib + dexamethasone
(This regimen can achieve remission in 100% cases)
Stem cell transplantation, if age < 70 years
Maintenance: Regimen of choice
High risk MM: Lenalidomide + bortezomib
Low risk MM: Lenalidomide
Other drugs used: Melphalan + prednisolone + Newer agents like lenalidomide/bortezomib/thalidomide

Chlorambucil

- Chlorambucil was used for treatment of chronic lymphocytic leukemia (CLL).
- It has been replaced by better drugs like fludarabine, cyclophosphamide and rituximab.

Bendamustine

- Bendamustine is a nitrogen mustard derivative similar in structure to chlorambucil.
- It is used for treatment of CLL and Hodgkin's lymphoma.

Nitrosoureas

Carmustine (BCNU), Lomustine (CCNU) and Somustine (methyl-CCNU)

- Both carmustine and lomustine can easily cross blood brain barrier due to high lipid solubility. Hence, they are used for treatment of brain tumors.
- Semustine on long term use causes renal failure and hence is not used.
- All the three drugs can cause **sustained neutropenia** due to profound and delayed myelosuppression

Streptozocin

- Streptozocin is an antibiotic with high affinity for pancreatic beta islet cells.
- Thus, it is used for treatment of **pancreatic islet cell carcinoma** and **malignant carcinoid tumors**.

Alkylating Agents Acting by Methylation

Procarbazine and Dacarbazine

- Procarbazine was earlier used for treatment of Hodgkin's disease in the MOPP regimen. Currently dacarbazine is preferred for Hodgkin's disease in ABVD regimen. Dacarbazine can also be used in malignant melanoma and sarcoma.
- Procarbazine can cause **disulfiram like reaction** if consumed with alcohol. Bone marrow suppression and neurotoxicity are more common with procarbazine than dacarbazine.
- Procarbazine has MAO inhibitor action and hence can precipitate cheese reaction.

Temozolomide

- Temozolomide is an alkylating agent structurally similar to dacarbazine.
- It is the drug of choice for treatment of brain tumors (malignant glioma and astrocytoma).
- Constipation and fatigue are commonly seen, but it is relatively bone marrow sparing.

Miscellaneous Alkylating Agents

Busulfan

- Busulfan was used for treatment of chronic myelogenous leukemia (CML) but has been replaced by imatinib as the drug of choice.
- It can cause **pulmonary fibrosis**, myelosuppression (spares lymphocytes), cataract and veno-occlusive disease (VOD) of liver.

Altretamine

- Altretamine is used for treatment of ovarian cancer resistant to cisplatin.
- Neurotoxicity in the form of mood swings and neuropathy are major limitations.

Thiotepa

Thiotepa is used in high dose regimens for treatment of breast, ovary and bladder cancer.

Trabectedin

- Trabectedin acts by alkylating DNA at N2 position of guanine. It is used for treatment of soft tissue sarcoma and ovarian cancer.
- Hepatotoxicity is the most common side effect which can be prevented by steroids.

Classification of Noncell-cycle Specific Drugs

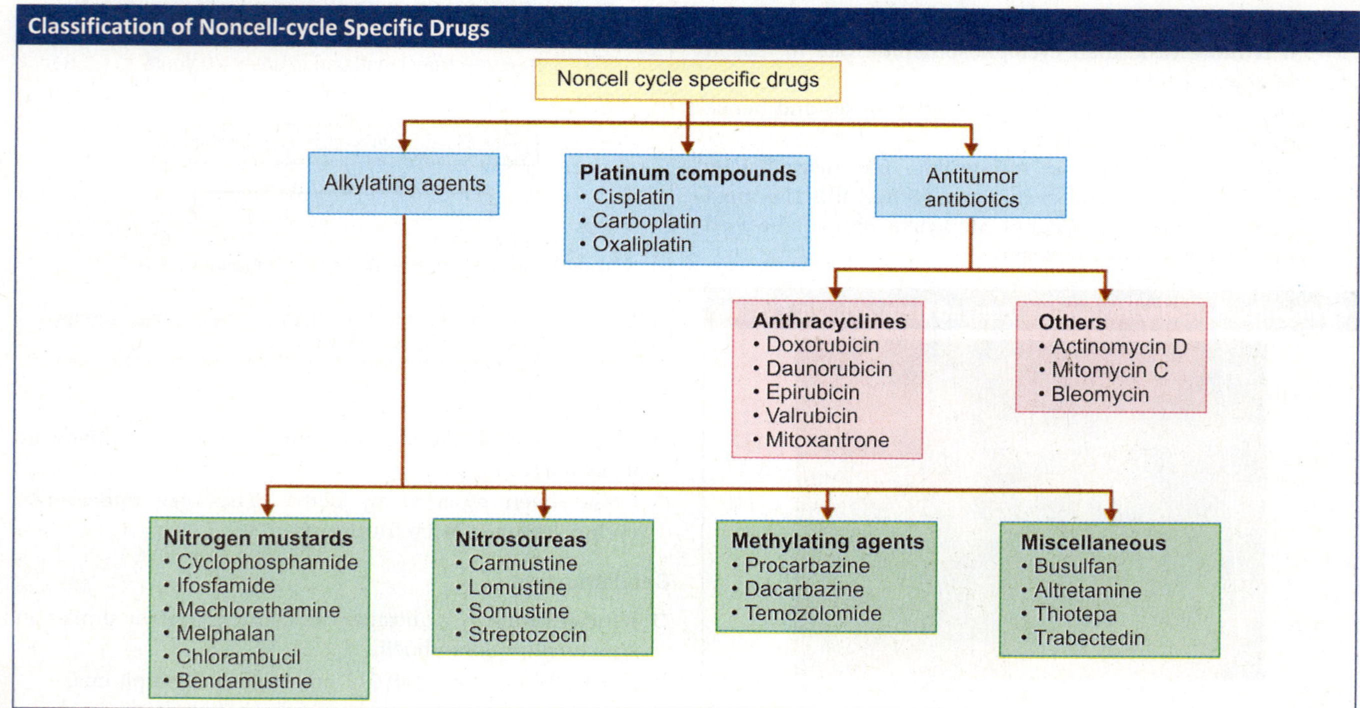

PLATINUM COMPOUNDS

Platinum compounds (PC) have free electrons in their outer orbit of atoms. Compounds with two free electrons (cisplatin and carboplatin) are called as bivalent PC and four free electrons (oxaliplatin) are called as quadrivalent PC. These free electrons form covalent bonds at the N-7 position of guanine in DNA and forms platinum based cross links. This leads to anticancer effect and secondary leukemia (AML) just like alkylating agents.

Cisplatin

Cisplatin, when administered by IV route combines with chloride ions and becomes inactive. Once cisplatin enters the cells by Cu2+ transporter, chloride ion is replaced by water molecule, which activates cisplatin. Aluminum also inactivates cisplatin, hence should be avoided with needles made up of aluminum.

Uses of Cisplatin

Cisplatin is the widest spectrum anticancer drug and used for treatment of lung, GIT, urogenital, head and neck cancer. The standard dose of cisplatin is 20 mg/m^2/day for 5 days in a week and given for 3–4 weeks. Alternatively, it can be given 100 mg/m2 once in a month.

- **Lung cancer:** Cisplatin is first line drug for treatment of small cell and non-small cell lung cancer along with other drugs like etoposide, pemetrexed and gemcitabine. **Double platin based therapy** containing cisplatin and carboplatin is used for lung cancer as well.
- **GIT cancer:** Cisplatin is the drug of choice for **esophageal** and gastric cancer, however regimens of cisplatin along with 5-FU or taxanes are preferred.
- **Urogenital cancer:** Cisplatin is first line drug and used along with **taxanes (paclitaxel)** for **ovarian cancer**, gemcitabine for bladder cancer and bleomycin + etoposide for testicular cancer. It is the drug of choice for cervical cancer.
- **Head and neck cancer:** Cisplatin is used along with 5-FU.
- **Osteosarcoma:** Cisplatin is one of the preferred drugs for treatment of osteosarcoma.

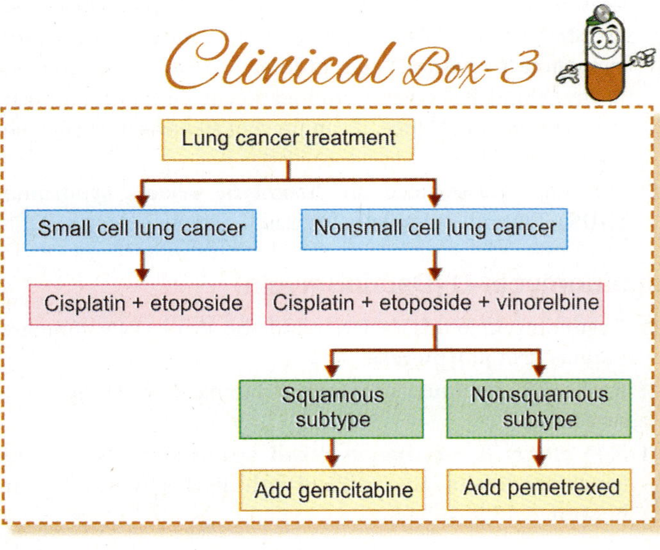

Side Effects of Cisplatin

- **Nephrotoxicity:** Cisplatin is a highly nephrotoxic drug and hence to prevent the same, the patient is preloaded with 1–2 L of NaCl, which causes **chloride diuresis**. As discussed earlier chloride inactivates cisplatin and thus nephrotoxicity is decreased. The patient is also given mannitol, which removes inactivated cisplatin by forced diuresis. **Amifostine** a radioprotectant can be used to prevent both nephrotoxicity and neurotoxicity.
- **Ototoxicity:** High frequency **irreversible hearing loss** which is mostly bilateral, and tinnitus is seen in half of the patients at normal doses. Children are more prone to ototoxicity.
- **Neurotoxicity:** Stock and glove sensorimotor **peripheral neuropathy** are seen. The symptoms of neuropathy can worsen transiently on drug discontinuation; this phenomenon is known as **coasting effect**.
- **Emesis:** Cisplatin is **most emetogenic** anticancer drug and requires premedication with combination of various drugs mentioned in the beginning of chapter. Since emesis is an early onset, the single best drug of choice is ondansetron which is short acting.
- Other side effects seen are **Raynaud's phenomenon**, hypomagnesemia, hypocalcemia and tetany.

Carboplatin

- Carboplatin is less toxic than cisplatin in all aspects, except bone marrow suppression (predominantly thrombocytopenia) which is the dose limiting toxicity.
- Being less toxic, it is an alternative to cisplatin for treatment of same spectrum disorders.

Oxaliplatin

- Oxaliplatin being quadrivalent PC forms four covalent bonds with DNA as compared to two with cisplatin and carboplatin. Hence, it is the most effective PC.
- It is highly effective in colorectal cancer.
- Since oxaliplatin inhibits thymidylate synthase (target of 5-FU), synergistic effect can be seen with 5-FU. Thus, oxaliplatin along with 5-FU is used in colorectal cancer.
- Neurotoxicity is the prominent side effect that presents as neuropathy identical to cisplatin but resolves sooner. In fact, peripheral neuropathy is the dose-limiting side effect.

ANTITUMOR ANTIBIOTICS

Antitumor antibiotics are substances derived from microorganisms that have inhibitory effect on tumor cells. These antibiotics by binding to DNA inhibit topoisomerase II and generate free radicals due to electron transfer. This causes DNA damage in all the phases, but the cell cycle arrest is seen particularly in G2 or S phase. Most of the toxicities caused by this class are related to the free radicals that can cause damage to organs like heart (cardiomyopathy) and lungs (pulmonary fibrosis).

Anthracycline Group

This class is derived from a fungus Streptomyces peucetius. Free radical production by this group requires Fe atoms for electron transport. Since these free radicals lead to toxicity, Fe chelating agent **dexrazoxane** is the antidote of choice for anthracycline toxicity.

Uses

- Doxorubicin is used for treatment of ovarian cancer, sarcoma **(osteosarcoma)**, lymphoma and multiple myeloma. Doxorubicin and daunorubicin are the drug of choice for treatment of Kaposi sarcoma.
- Daunorubicin/Idarubicin along with cytarabine (Ara-c) is the treatment of choice for acute myelogenous leukemia (AML).
- Epirubicin and valrubicin are used for breast cancer and bladder cancer respectively.
- Mitoxantrone is a doxorubicin derivative which is less cardiotoxic, however it causes secondary leukemia (PML). It is used for treatment of AML, prostate cancer and multiple sclerosis.

Side Effects

- **Cardiotoxicity:** It is maximum with doxorubicin and daunorubicin. Acute toxicity presents as **pericarditis-myocarditis syndrome** followed by arrhythmia. Chronic toxicity on long term use precipitates congestive heart failure due to **dilated cardiomyopathy**. Myocardial damage can be seen in the form of **vacuolar myofibril degeneration** and mitochondrial changes in electron microscopy. Cardiotoxicity can be potentiated by high dose cyclophosphamide, trastuzumab and cardiac irradiation.

Anthracyclines Induce Vacuolar Myofibril Degeneration

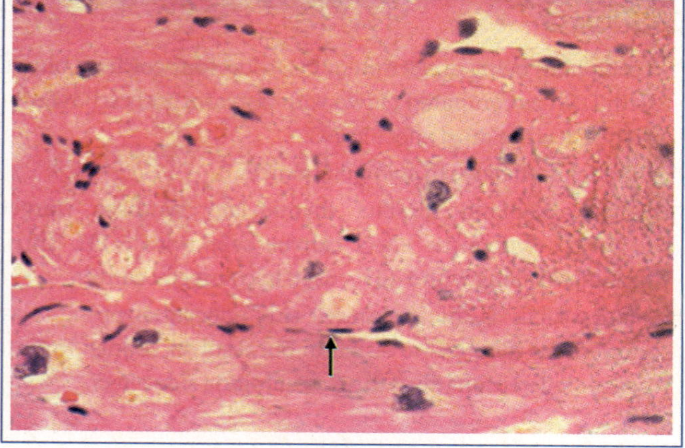

- **Vesication:** Doxorubicin is a powerful vesicant and hence is given by rapid flowing IV line.
- Red discoloration of urine is seen with doxorubicin and daunorubicin.
- **Radiation recall syndrome:** Radiotherapy causes local changes like desquamation, erythema, etc., which subsides with time. After this if chemotherapy is started and the same local changes reappear, it is called as radiation recall. This can be seen with **doxorubicin, daunorubicin** and another antibiotic **actinomycin-D**.

Clinical Box-4

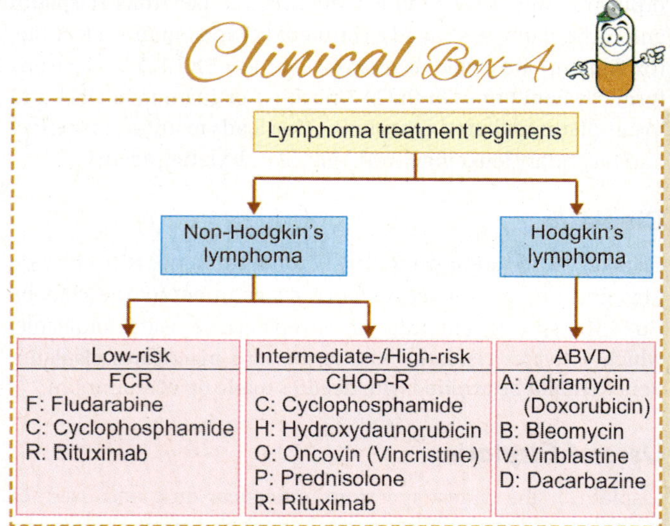

Bleomycin

- Bleomycin is used for treatment of testicular cancer in BEP regimen and Hodgkin's lymphoma in ABVD regimen.
- It is metabolized by bleomycin hydrolase, which is scant in lungs and skin. Thus, free radical damage is maximum at these organs and leads to **pulmonary fibrosis** and **flagellate dermatitis (streaks of hyperpigmentation)**. Free radicals damage **type I pneumocyte**, which leads to type II pneumocyte hyperplasia. Oxygen increases free radical production and hence can augment these toxicities.
- Other side effects seen are **Raynaud's phenomenon** and acute hypertension after rapid infusion.

Mitomycin-C

- Mitomycin has an alkylating agent like activity and is a potent **radiosensitizer**.
- It is used along with 5-FU for treatment of anal cancer. Other uses are bladder cancer, prevention of **laryngotracheal and esophageal stenosis** and prevention of **postnasal surgery synechiae formation**. Being an anticancer drug when applied to any wound, it decreases proliferation of fibroblasts and scar tissue formation. Hence, it can prevent stenosis or synechiae formation.
- Side effects associated are **hemolytic uremic syndrome (HUS)**, TTP and pulmonary fibrosis.

Actinomycin-D (Dactinomycin)

- Dactinomycin binds to DNA and the drug DNA complex inhibits **RNA polymerase**.
- It is used for treatment of choriocarcinoma, Wilms' tumor and sarcoma.
- Side effects like **radiation recall syndrome**, GIT toxicity (proctitis, glossitis, cheilitis) and early myelosuppression can be seen.

CELL CYCLE SPECIFIC ANTICANCER DRUGS

S PHASE SPECIFIC DRUGS

S phase is characterized by DNA synthesis, which can be inhibited by various drug classes like antimetabolites (antifolate drugs, pyrimidine and purine analogs), TI inhibitors, histone deacetylase inhibitors (HDI) and hydroxyurea.

Antimetabolites

- Antimetabolites are drugs that are structurally like purines and pyrimidines or drugs that inhibit purine or pyrimidine synthesis. The antimetabolite class has three groups namely **antifolate drugs** (inhibit purine and pyrimidine synthesis), **purine analogs** and **pyrimidine analogs**.
- They have common side effects like mucositis, diarrhea and bone marrow suppression, though secondary leukemia is never seen.

Antifolate Anticancer Drugs

Dihydrofolic acid (DHFA) is activated by dihydrofolic acid reductase (DHFR) to tetrahydrofolate (THF). Thymidylate synthase (TS) is activated by methyl group from THF, which then activates dUMP to TMP. TMP is required for DNA synthesis and THF for purine synthesis. Hence inhibition of this pathway inhibits DNA synthesis (S phase) and purine synthesis.

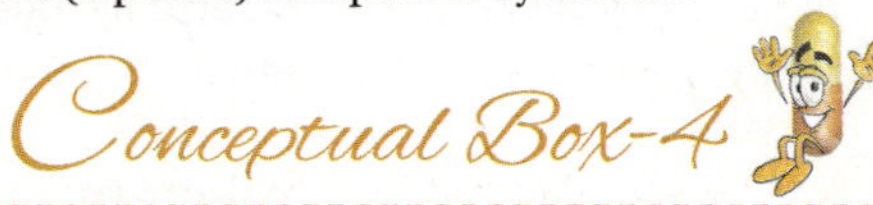

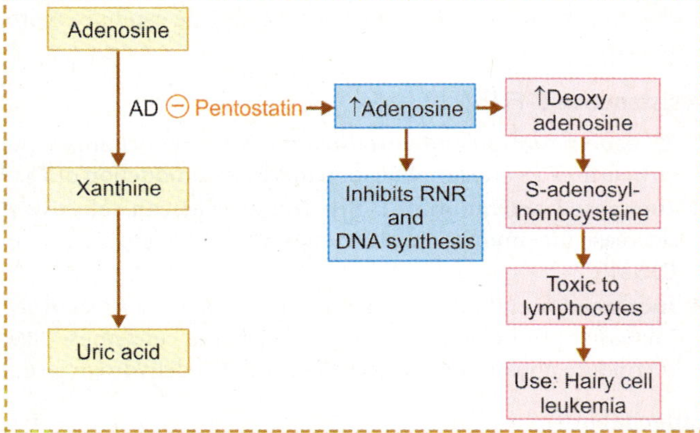

Methotrexate

Methotrexate is an inhibitor of DHFR and its metabolite methotrexate polyglutamate also inhibits TS. Inhibition of DNA synthesis gives anticancer effects, whereas inhibition of purine synthesis gives anti-inflammatory and immunomodulatory effect. Purine synthesis inhibition selectively depletes lymphocytes as they have only de-novo pathway but no salvage pathway for purine synthesis.

Uses of Methotrexate

- Methotrexate is drug of choice for **choriocarcinoma** and one of the preferred first line drug for **osteosarcoma**. Other neoplastic uses are NHL and ALL.
- It is the DMARD of choice for **rheumatoid arthritis**. Other non-neoplastic uses are **ectopic pregnancy, GVHD**, psoriasis, multiple sclerosis, Wegener's granulomatosis and Crohn's disease.

Mnemonics

Uses of Methotrexate: METOTRECAT

- **M :** Multiple sclerosis
- **E :** Ectopic pregnancy
- **T :** Transplant rejection (GVHD)
- **O :** Osteosarcoma
- **T :** Topically for psoriasis
- **R :** Rheumatoid arthritis
- **E :** wegener's granulomatosis
- **C :** Crohn's disease
- **A :** ALL
- **T :** Trophoblastic disease, choriocarcinoma

Side Effects of Methotrexate

- Myelosuppression and mucositis are common side effects seen due to inhibition of DNA synthesis. These side effects can be prevented by **leucovorin** (folinic acid, active form of folic acid) or folic acid. **Leucovorin or folinic acid is more preferred as compared to folic acid**.
- Methotrexate metabolites are excreted by kidney. **Glucarpidase** is an enzyme which metabolizes methotrexate into inactive metabolites excreted by liver and hence is given to patients with impaired renal function. Since glucarpidase also degrades leucovorin, it should not be given 2 hours before or after intake of leucovorin.
- **Hepatotoxicity** and **cirrhosis** are seen on **low dose, long-term use** as in case of psoriasis and rheumatoid arthritis.
- Methotrexate can crystallize in renal tubules and cause renal failure. Adequate hydration and alkalization of urine with **bicarbonate loading** is ensured to prevent this nephrotoxicity. Since methotrexate is an acidic drug, alkalization of urine makes it water soluble.
- Methotrexate is collected in body spaces like abdominal and pleural cavity (third space), from where it can diffuse back for longer period and cause prolonged myelosuppression.
- Intrathecal administration can cause neurotoxicity in the form of arachnoiditis, **meningismus** and seizures.

Mechanisms of Resistance to Methotrexate

- Resistance to anticancer drugs or antimicrobials is mostly associated with its mechanism of action, which is inhibition of DHFR in this case
- **DHFR:** Changes in DHFR can take place either at the level of enzyme itself or gene. DHFR **enzyme induction** is seen within 24 hours of drug use (acute resistance). DHFR gene amplification **(increased intracellular DHFR)** or mutation (altered DHFR structure) is seen after 24 hours of drug use (chronic resistance).
- Methotrexate is taken into tumor cells by transporters, following which it is metabolized by tumor cell enzymes into methotrexate polyglutamate (active metabolite). The tumor cells can decrease uptake and activation of methotrexate and increase efflux of methotrexate.

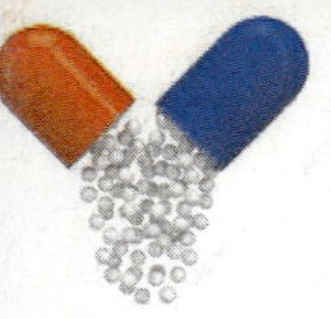

Conceptual Box-5

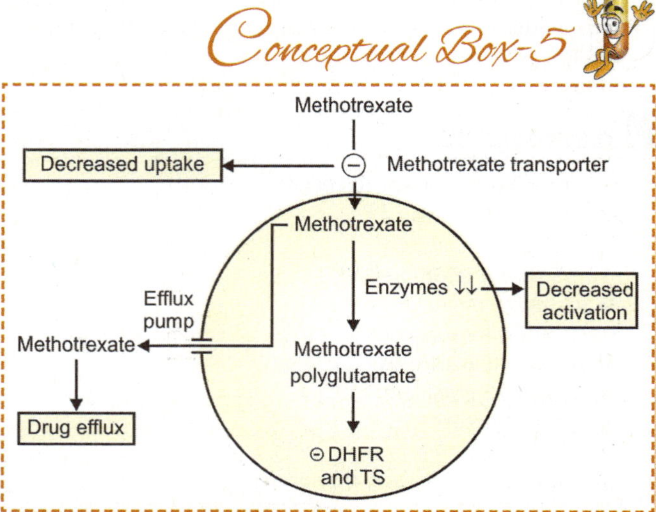

Pemetrexed

- Pemetrexed is a less potent inhibitor of DHFR than methotrexate but has also inhibitory action on TS and glycinamide ribonucleotide formyl transferase or GART also. Thus, it inhibits synthesis of both purines and pyrimidines.
- It is used for treatment of non-small cell, nonsquamous type lung cancer along with cisplatin and for treatment of mesothelioma.
- Side effects are like methotrexate, but since it is a less potent inhibitor of DHFR, low dose **folinic acid or folic acid** is used to ameliorate toxicity. Due to its multiplicity in mechanism of action, it can cause severe bone marrow suppression and hence injections of **vitamin B-12 (1 mg)** is also given with the first dose of pemetrexed

Pralatrexate

- Pralatrexate is approved by FDA for treatment of cutaneous T-cell lymphoma.
- Side effect profile is like methotrexate.

Raltitrexed

- Raltitrexed is approved in Canada and EU for treatment of colorectal cancer in case of 5-FU intolerance due to toxicity. It can also be used for treatment of breast cancer, gastroesophageal cancer and mesothelioma.
- Like 5-FU, raltitrexed is also a potent TS inhibitor and hence can be used as a substitute.

Pyrimidine Analogs

5-Fluoro Uracil (5-FU)

Mechanism of Action

- 5-FU is metabolized by the tumor cells enzymes into fluoro Deoxyuridine Monophosphate (fDUMP), which is similar in structure to dUMP. Both fDUMP and dUMP are metabolized by same enzyme, i.e. TS and hence 5-FU is a competitive inhibitor of TS.
- **Leucovorin increases the anticancer effect or sensitivity of 5-FU,** by forming a ternary complex with fDUMP and TS, that stabilizes TS inhibition.
- 5-FU is also a potent radiosensitizer.

Uses of 5-FU

- 5-FU has poor oral absorption and hence is administered by IV route for systemic uses.
- **Colorectal cancer:** 5-FU is the first line drug for treatment of colorectal cancer, which is combined with leucovorin (folinic acid) and oxaliplatin or irinotecan, to form two regimens namely **FOLFOX** (**FOL**inic acid + 5-**FU** + **OX**aliplatin), **FOLFIRI** (**FOL**inic acid + 5-**FU** + **IRI**notecan) and **FOLFIRINOX** (**FOL**inic acid + 5-**FU** + **IRI**notecan + Oxaliplatin). These regimens are also used for treatment of pancreatic cancer.
- **Anal cancer:** 5-FU is the first line drug for anal cancer, which is combined with mitomycin-c, applied by topical route.
- **Head and neck cancer:** 5-FU is combined with cisplatin for treatment of head and neck cancer.

Side Effects of 5-FU

- **Hand and foot syndrome:** Also known as palmar plantar dysesthesia, in characterized by desquamation and erythema of palms and soles. It is seen with 5-FU, capecitabine, doxorubicin, gemcitabine and VEGFR TK inhibitors like sorafenib, sunitinib and pazopanib.
- **Pulmonary toxicity:** 5-FU is metabolized in liver, but the metabolites are primarily excreted by lungs as CO2.
- **Acute coronary vasospasm:** It is seen shortly after 5-FU infusion.
- 5-FU is metabolized by **dihydropyrimidine dehydrogenase** and in patients with deficiency of this enzyme can have more toxicity.

Resistance to 5-FU

- **TS gene mutation and amplification:** Mutation changes the structure of TS and amplification increases production of TS.
- **Decreased activation of 5-FU:** Tumor cells can selectively decrease the production of enzymes which activate 5-FU in to fDUMP.
- **Increased metabolism of 5-FU:** Tumor cells can selectively increase production of 5-FU degrading enzymes like thymidine phosphorylase and dihydrouracil dehydrogenase.

Capecitabine

- Capecitabine is a prodrug of 5-FU, which has better oral absorption.
- It is administered by oral route for treatment of metastatic colorectal cancer and drug resistant metastatic breast cancer.
- The side effect profile is like 5-FU, except **hand and foot syndrome which is more commonly seen with capecitabine.**

Cytarabine (Ara-C) or Cytosine Arabinoside

- Ara-C is phosphorylated by cytidine kinase into Ara cytidine triphosphate, which when incorporated in to DNA, inhibits DNA polymerase. Since it has a very short half-life of ten minutes, it is administered by **continuous IV infusion** for 5–7 days for effective inhibition of 'S' phase.

- Cytarabine along with daunorubicin or idarubicin is the treatment of choice for AML. It can be used in other leukemia like ALL, CML and high-grade lymphoma. Intrathecal liposomal cytarabine is used for treatment of lymphomatous meningitis.
- Myelosuppression is the dose limiting toxicity. At high systemic doses or intrathecal use is associated with **cerebellar (ataxia, dysarthria)** and cerebral toxicity (seizures, dementia). After infusion, the patient can have flu like symptoms. **Noncardiogenic pulmonary edema** is a rare side effect that can also be seen.

Gemcitabine

- Gemcitabine's effect on DNA is like cytarabine with some exception, i.e. it also inhibits RNR (Ribonucleotide diphosphate reductase). Like 5-FU it is also a potent **radiosensitizer** and hence dose should be decreased with radiotherapy.
- It is the drug of choice for **pancreatic cancer** and used in regimens for treatment of nonsmall cell squamous lung cancer, bladder cancer and ovary cancer.
- Most important limiting factor of gemcitabine is myelosuppression. Other side effects associated are hepatotoxicity, **HUS**, interstitial pneumonitis and posterior leucoencephalopathy syndrome.

Azacytidine and Decitabine

- Azacytidine and decitabine inhibit DNA cytosine methyltransferase and hence cause **demethylation of DNA**.
- DNA methylation inhibits differentiation of myelocytes and is the most important cause of myelodysplasia. Azacitidine and decitabine act on pathophysiology of **myelodysplasia**, and hence they are the **drugs of choice**. Azacitidine though is more potent drug than decitabine.
- **Myelodysplasia with 5q syndrome** (anemia) does not respond well to these drugs and hence **lenalidomide** is the drug of choice.

Purine Analogs

Purines are synthesized by De nova and salvage pathways in all cells, except lymphocytes which completely depend on De nova pathway. Thus, if purine synthesis is interfered with, there is selective depletion of lymphocytes. Hence this class of drugs are used for leukemia. Most of the drugs of this class also inhibit ribonucleotide diphosphate reductase (RNR).

6-Thiopurine Analogs

- This class has drugs like 6-Mercaptopurine (6-MP) and 6-Thioguanine (6-TG). Azathioprine is an analog of 6-MP and used as an immunomodulator.
- 6-MP and 6-TG are metabolized by HGPRT into abnormal substrates 6-ITP and 6-GTP respectively, which inhibit De nova purine synthesis and are also incorporated into DNA.

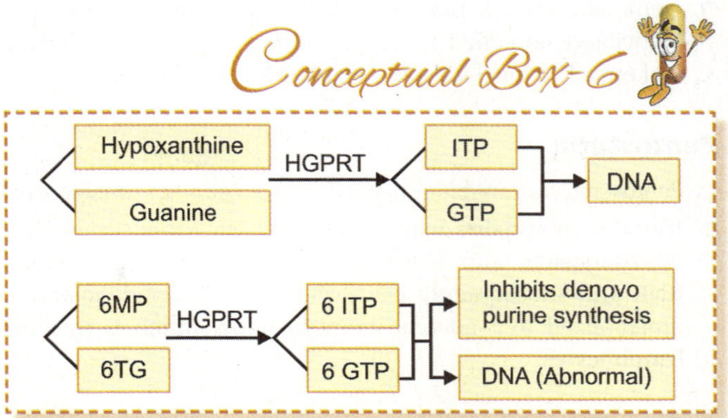

- The use of these drugs is limited to treatment of **ALL** and **AML**.
- Most important side effects are bone marrow suppression and hepatotoxicity. Since they can cause lymphocyte depletion, opportunistic infections and squamous cell cancer of skin (T-cells are protective) can also be seen. Long-term use of 6-MP can cause secondary leukemia, i.e. AML. 6-MP and azathioprine are metabolized by an enzyme **thiopurine methyltransferase (TPMT)** and hence a deficiency of this enzyme increases risk of toxicity.
- 6-MP is metabolized by xanthine oxidase (XO) and hence **allopurinol** (XO inhibitor) can inhibit 6-MP metabolism and precipitate toxicity. Thus, when allopurinol is used along with 6-MP to decrease chances of gout, the **dose of 6-MP is reduced by 75%.**
- Phosphoribosylpyrophosphate (PRPP) activates 6-MP and PRPP concentration is increased by **methotrexate**. Hence both drugs have synergistic action that can be beneficial for treatment of ALL.

Fludarabine

- Fludarabine is an analog of antiviral drug vidarabine, which acts by inhibiting DNA polymerase, DNA primase, DNA ligase and RNR (ribonucleotide diphosphate reductase).
- Fludarabine is the **drug of choice for CLL** and combined with **C**yclophosphamide and **R**ituximab that gives the regimen of choice **FCR**. Fludarabine blocks repair of DNA damage caused by AA and hence it has synergistic effect with cyclophosphamide.

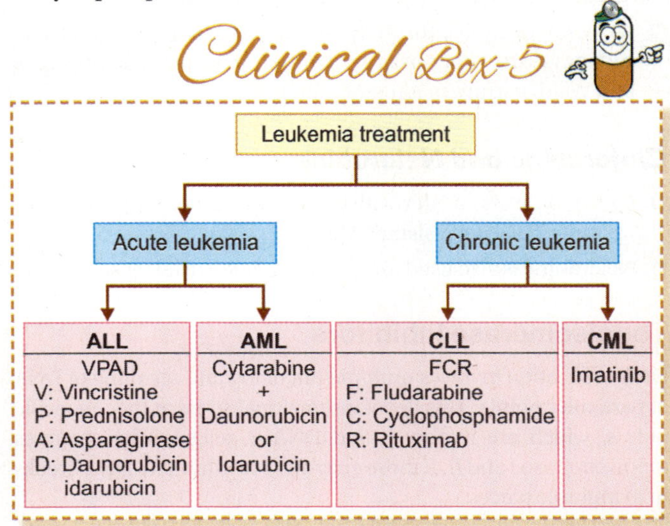

- Hemolytic anemia, pure red cell aplasia and pneumonitis are associated side effects. Long term use can cause secondary leukemia like myelodysplasia and AML.

Pentostatin

- Pentostatin is an antibiotic derived from *Streptomyces antibioticus*.
- It inhibits **adenosine deaminase**, which leads to accumulation of adenosine and deoxyadenosine. Adenosine inhibits RNR and subsequently DNA synthesis. Deoxyadenosine is metabolized to S-adenosylhomocysteine, which is toxic to lymphocytes.

Conceptual Box-7

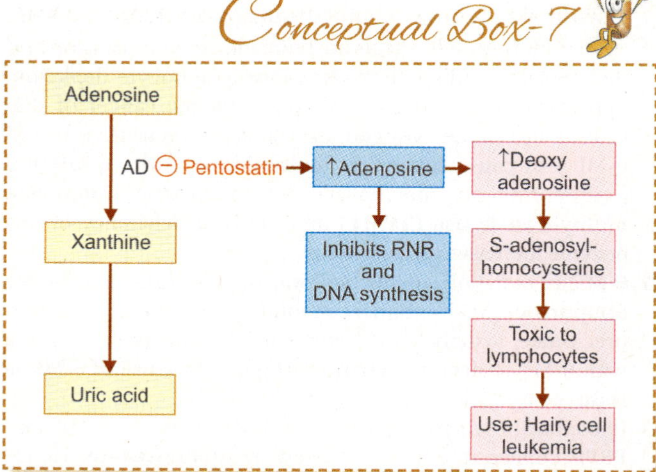

- Pentostatin was the first drug ever approved for treatment of **hairy cell leukemia**.
- Long-term immunosuppression can be seen even after drug discontinuation. It can augment the pulmonary toxicity of fludarabine.

Cladribine

- Cladribine causes DNA strand breaks by incorporation and inhibits RNR. Like cytarabine, it is also given by continuous IV infusion for 7 days.
- It is drug of choice for treatment of **hairy cell leukemia** and **histiocytosis**. Other uses are lymphomas, mycosis fungoides and Waldenstrom macroglobulinemia.

Clofarabine and Nelarabine

- Clofarabine is a derivative of cladribine, approved for treatment of drug resistant ALL.
- Nelarabine is also used for the treatment of drug resistant ALL.

Topoisomerase Inhibitors

DNA replication involves multiple uncoiling and recoiling of DNA at particular points. This develops torsional stress at these specific points, which are removed, and DNA is religated by enzymes topoisomerase I and II. If these enzymes are inhibited, DNA breaks in to multiple pieces.

Topoisomerase I Inhibitors

The drugs in this class are derived from a Chinese tree *Camptotheca acuminata* and hence are also known as camptothecin analogs.

Irinotecan

- Irinotecan is used as a first line drug for colorectal cancer along with 5-FU and leucovorin (FOLFIRI), as discussed earlier. It has been approved by FDA in 2015 for the treatment of pancreatic cancer and FOLFIRI regimen can be used for pancreatic cancer progressive on gemcitabine.
- **Delayed secretory diarrhea** due to a metabolite SN-38, is the most common side effect followed by myelosuppression (neutropenia). For treatment of diarrhea, high dose loperamide is used. It inhibits ACHE and cholinergic side effects can be seen, usually till 24 hours after starting irinotecan.
- It is metabolized by glucunoridation and excreted by liver. Hence in patients of **Crigler-Najjar syndrome** (glucunoryl transferase deficiency or absence) increased toxicity can be seen.

Topotecan

- Topotecan is used for treatment of ovarian cancer and small cell lung cancer.
- Myelosuppression (neutropenia) is the most common side effect associated.
- It is primarily excreted by kidney.

Topoisomerase II Inhibitors

The drugs in this class are derived from podophyllotoxin and hence are also called as epipodophyllotoxins. They can cause secondary leukemia, i.e. AML with translocations of mixed lineage leukemia (MLL) gene in 11_q23. Secondary leukemia associated with this class develops after 2–3 years and is associated with poor prognosis.

Etoposide

- Etoposide is first line drug for treatment of testicular cancer (**BEP** regimen: **B**leomycin + **E**toposide + **P**latinum compound, i.e. Cisplatin) and both small and nonsmall cell lung cancer. It is also used for treatment of NHL and Kaposi sarcoma.
- Myelosuppression is the dose limiting side effect. It is also a mild vesicant.

Teniposide

- Teniposide is used for treatment of refractory acute lymphoblastic leukemia (ALL) in children.
- It has synergistic effect with cladribine.

Histone Deacetylase Inhibitors

Histone is a negatively charged protein that attracts the negatively charged strands of DNA and maintains the structure. Prior to DNA replication for unwinding, histone acetyltransferase is activated with acetylates histone and makes it negatively charged. The DNA strands repel due to this negative charge and after DNA replication is complete, histone deacetylase is activated which removes acetyl and again makes histone positively charged.

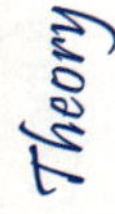

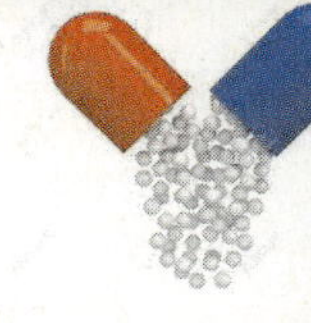

Conceptual Box-8

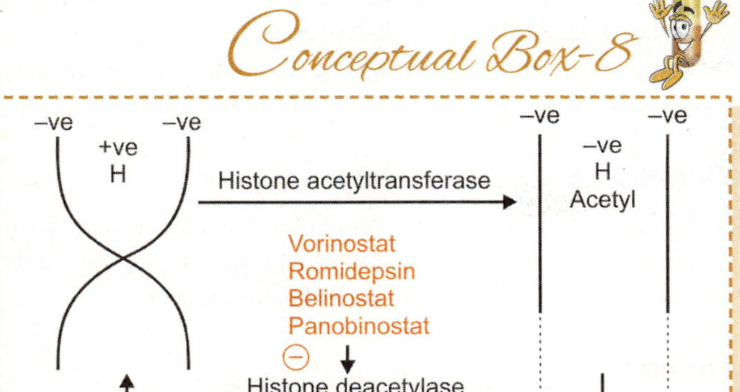

Vorinostat, Romidepsin and Belinostat

- All these drugs are used for treatment of refractory cutaneous T-cell lymphoma. Belinostat is the latest one approved in 2014.
- QT prolongation is a common side effect seen with this class, though serious clinical adversaries not associated.

Panobinostat

- Panobinostat is the recently approved (2015) drug in this class for treatment of multiple myeloma.

Hydroxyurea

- Hydroxyurea has **good oral absorption** and a bioavailability of 80–100%. It acts by inhibiting **ribonucleotide diphosphate reductase (RNR)**, which converts ribose nucleotides into deoxyribose nucleotides, required for DNA synthesis. Hence inhibition of this enzyme inhibits DNA synthesis, i.e. S phase. It is also a **radiosensitizer**.
- It is drug of choice for **sickle cell anemia** and **essential thrombocythemia**. It increases fetal hemoglobin production which is resistant to sickling. In essential thrombocythemia hydroxyurea is used along with antiaggregant aspirin.
- **CML** and **polycythemia vera (PCV)** are other indications of hydroxyurea, but **anagrelide** is more preferred for PCV.
- Bone marrow suppression is the most common side effect encountered. Other side effects like **painful leg ulcers**, skin and nail hyperpigmentation and interstitial pneumonitis can also be seen.

Mnemonics

Uses of Hydroxyurea: PACE

P : PCV
A : Anemia (sickle cell)
C : CML
E : Essential thrombocytosis

Classification of Cell-cycle Specific Drugs

- Cell cycle specific drugs
  - S phase specific drugs
    - Antimetabolites
      - **Antifolates**: Methothrexate, Pemetrexed, Pralatrexate, Raltitrexed
      - **Pyrimidine analogs**: 5-fluorouracil, Capecitabine, Gemcitabine, Azacytidine, Decitabine, Cytarabine
      - **Purine analogs**: 6-mercaptopurine, 6-thioguanine, Fludarabine, Cladribine, Clofarabine, Nelarabine, Pentostatin
    - Hydroxyurea
    - **Histone deacetylase inhibitors**: Vorinostat, Romidepsin, Belinostat, Panobinostat
    - Topoisomerase inhibitors
      - **Topoisomerase-I inhibitors**: Irinotecan, Topotecan
      - **Topoisomerase-II inhibitors**: Etoposide, Teniposide
  - M phase specific drugs
    - Eribulin
    - Estramustine
    - **Epothilones**: Ixabepilone, Patupilone, Sagopilone
    - **Taxanes**: Paclitaxel, Docetaxel, Cabazitaxel
    - **Vinca alkaloids**: Vincristine, Vinblastine, Vinorelbine

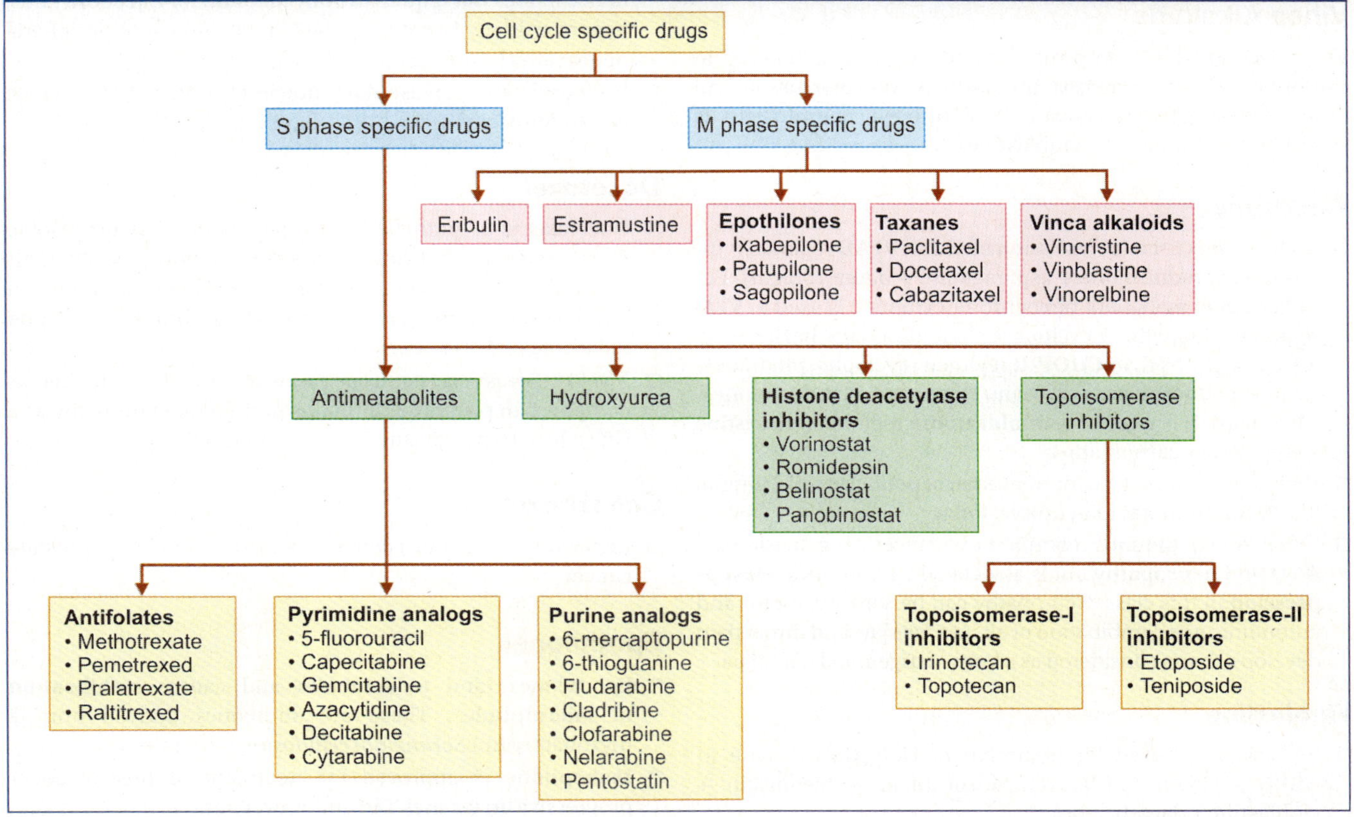

M PHASE SPECIFIC DRUGS

- M phase is characterized by mitosis, for which centrioles appear in the equator of cell first.
- These centrioles synthesize microtubules by polymerization of two proteins α-tubulin and β-tubulin, which are required for physiological functions (phagocytosis, axonal transport) in CNS and PNS.
- The β-tubulin is the target for all drugs of this class, i.e. vinca alkaloids, taxanes, epothilones, estramustine and eribulin.
- These drugs also inhibit the physiological functions in CNS and PNS, which presents as neurotoxicity in the form of peripheral neuropathy

Conceptual Box-9

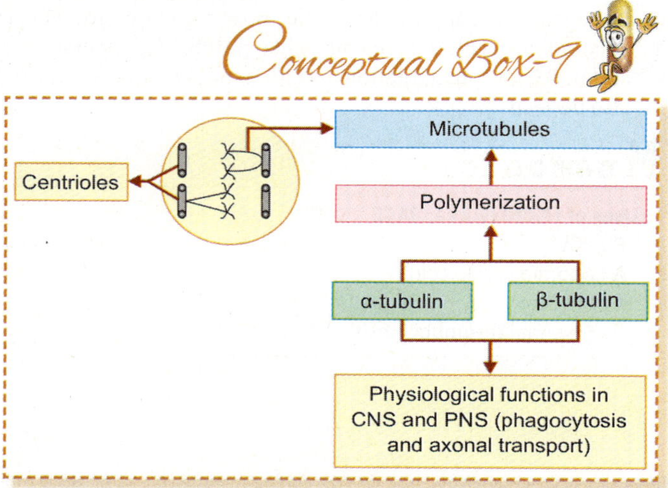

Vinca Alkaloids

Vinca alkaloids binds to β-tubulin and prevents its binding to α-tubulin, which decreases microtubule polymerization. All drugs in this class are vesicants. The order of neurotoxicity is vincristine > vinorelbine > vinblastine.

Vincristine

- Vincristine is used for remission of ALL in **VPAD** regimen (vincristine + prednisolone + asparaginase + daunorubicin). For treatment of malignant pheochromocytoma it is used in **VCD** regimen (vincristine + cyclophosphamide + dacarbazine). It is also used for NHL in **CHOP-R** regimen (cyclophosphamide + hydroxydaunorubicin + oncovin/vincristine + prednisolone + rituximab). It is used in **retinoblastoma** regimen (vincristine + etoposide + carboplatin).
- Vincristine is also used for treatment of pediatric solid tumors like Wilms' tumor and neuroblastoma.
- Vincristine is the most common anticancer drug causing **SIADH** and **neuropathy** but is associated with **least myelosuppression** in this class. Neuropathy can be sensory, motor and autonomic or a combination of all. At times jaw and throat pain develops, that is considered as a form of trigeminal neuralgia.

Vinblastine

- Vinblastine is used for treatment of Hodgkin's disease in **ABVD** regimen (adriamycin/doxorubicin + bleomycin + vinblastine + dacarbazine).
- It is also used for treatment of bladder cancer and testicular cancer in **BEP** regimen as discussed earlier.
- Vinblastine is the least neurotoxic vinca alkaloid, however it is associated with hypertension and **Raynaud's disease**.

Vinorelbine

- Vinorelbine is used for treatment of nonsmall cell lung cancer of nonsquamous subtype, along with cisplatin and etoposide.
- It can also be used for treatment of breast cancer.

Taxanes

Taxanes bind to β-tubulin and stimulate its binding to α-tubulin, which **increases microtubule polymerization**. They are used for treatment of head and neck cancer, urogenital cancers (ovarian and prostate cancer), GIT cancers and breast cancer.

Paclitaxel

- Paclitaxel is a natural drug that was derived from yew tree, but as the source is limited it is now synthesized by genetic engineering in ***E. coli***.
- It has low water solubility and hence injected with equal amounts of ethanol and castor oil (cremophor containing vehicle). This medium is responsible for the most common side effect of paclitaxel, i.e. **hypersensitivity** and to prevent it the patient is premedicated with steroids and antihistaminics. Peripheral sensory neuropathy is the second most common side effect.
- Nab-paclitaxel is a water-soluble form of paclitaxel and hence it does not require the oily medium for injection. Thus, hypersensitivity is not seen, but the incidence of peripheral neuropathy is more than paclitaxel.
- Paclitaxel can decrease doxorubicin clearance and enhance its cardiotoxicity.

Docetaxel

- Docetaxel is a synthetic taxane that is more water soluble than paclitaxel and administered in polysorbate 80. This polysorbate 80 medium causes fluid retention that can develop into peripheral edema, ascites, pleural effusions and pulmonary edema.
- Myelosuppression (neutropenia) is more commonly seen as compared to paclitaxel. It retains peripheral neuropathy as a side effect. Hypersensitivity is less commonly seen.

Cabazitaxel

- Cabazitaxel is the most active taxane for treatment of prostate cancer.

Epothilones

- Epothilones bind to β-tubulin and causes **stabilization of microtubules**. These are antibiotics derived from a myxobacterium *Sorangium cellulosum*.
- **Ixabepilone** is approved for treatment of breast cancer progressive on taxanes and anthracyclines.

- Other drugs in this class like **patupilone** and **sagopilone** are under trial for treatment of ovarian cancer and recurrent glioblastoma respectively.

Eribulin

- Eribulin acts like vinca alkaloids by inhibiting microtubule polymerization.
- Like ixabepilone it is also used for treatment of breast cancer resistant to taxanes and anthracyclines.

Estramustine

- Estramustine is a compound synthesized from estradiol and alkylating agent (normustine). It also binds to β-tubulin and prevents its binding to α-tubulin, which decreases microtubule polymerization.
- It is indicated for treatment of advanced hormone resistant prostate cancer.
- Congestive heart failure (CHF), thrombosis and gynecomastia are specific side effects that can be seen.

MISCELLANEOUS ANTICANCER DRUGS

L–ASPARAGINASE

- L-asparaginase is an anticancer enzyme, when given by IV route depletes systemic asparagine. Lymphocytes cannot synthesize asparagine, but other cells can and hence L-asparaginase causes selective death of lymphocytes by cutting off systemic supply of asparagine.
- Since lymphocytes are depleted, L-asparaginase is used for treatment of leukemia and lymphoma. It is used in VPAD regimen for treatment of **ALL**, as discussed earlier.
- Side effects are related to asparagine depletion, which leads to selective protein synthesis inhibition. Decrease in insulin production causes **hyperglycemia**. Coagulation and anticoagulation factors, both can be decreased and hence **hemorrhage** or **thrombosis** can be seen, that varies from patient to patient. Overall decrease in proteins increase free lipids and cause **hyperlipidemia** which is a cause for **pancreatitis**. Finally, since it is an exogenous protein, **hypersensitivity** can also be seen.

Mnemonics

Side Effects of L-Asparginase: H
- **H :** Hyperglycemia
- **H :** Hemorrhage or thrombosis
- **H :** Hyperlipidemia induced pancreatitis
- **H :** Hypersensitivity
- **H :** Hepatotoxicity

RETINOIC ACID

- Retinoic acid (RA) induces differentiation of myelocytes by acting on retinoic acid receptor (RAR) in the nucleus. RAR is produced by RAR gene in chromosome 17.
- In case of t (15;17), promyelocytic leukemia protein (PML) gene from chromosome 15 translocates near RAR gene and RAR is produced by both genes. This results in a weak form of RAR, which cannot differentiate all immature myelocytes into mature ones and accumulates immature myelocytes causing promyelocytic leukemia (PML).
- Thus, **retinoic acid is the drug of choice for PML**, which at supraphysiological concentrations maturate myelocytes by acting even on weak RAR.
- Adhesion of differentiated myelocytes to pulmonary blood vessels can cause a side effect known as **pulmonary syndrome** characterized by pulmonary infiltrates, pleural effusion, chest pain, fluid retention and fever. If patient develops pulmonary syndrome, the drug of choice for same is **dexamethasone**.
- RA resistant PML is treated by **arsenic trioxide**, which acts by free radical formation. It causes hypokalemia and QT prolongation.

MONOCLONAL ANTIBODIES AND TYROSINE KINASE INHIBITORS

Monoclonal antibodies (MABs) are produced by hybridoma technique.

Conceptual Box-10

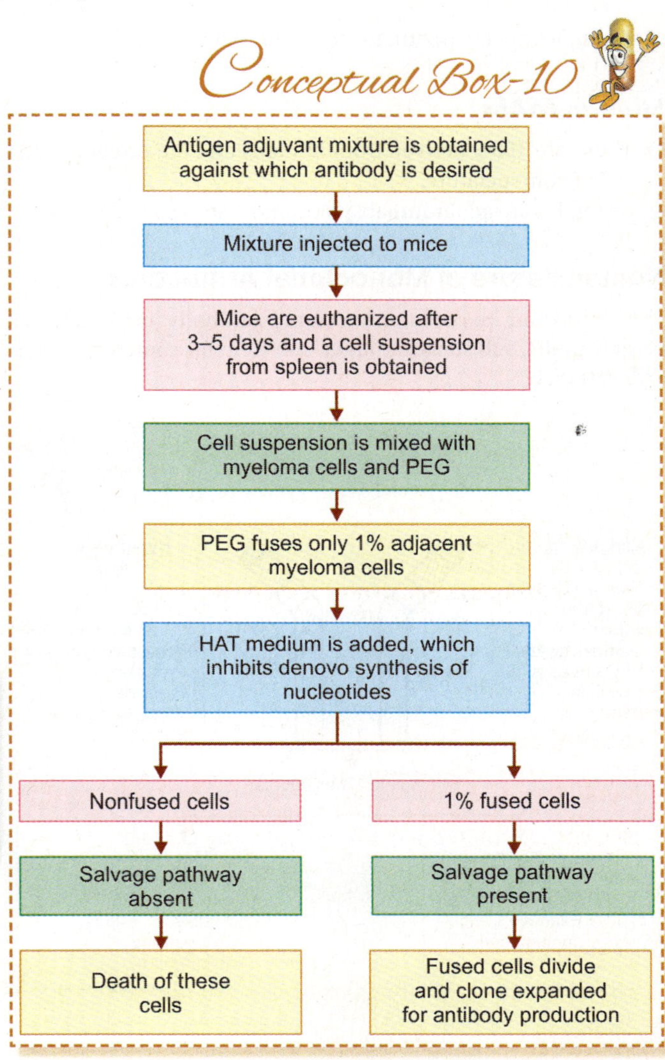
Antigen adjuvant mixture is obtained against which antibody is desired
Mixture injected to mice
Mice are euthanized after 3–5 days and a cell suspension from spleen is obtained
Cell suspension is mixed with myeloma cells and PEG
PEG fuses only 1% adjacent myeloma cells
HAT medium is added, which inhibits denovo synthesis of nucleotides
Nonfused cells
1% fused cells
Salvage pathway absent
Salvage pathway present
Death of these cells
Fused cells divide and clone expanded for antibody production

Classification of Monoclonal Antibodies

Murine MAbs

- These are 100% derived from mouse and are designated as "o" in the nomenclature.
- The drawbacks of these antibodies are higher hypersensitivity reaction, shorter half-life and their inability to activate human compliments. This leads to development of MAbs with gradually increasing human part.
- Examples are ibritumomab, tositumomab etc.

Chimeric MAbs

- These are derived both from mouse and human, but only variable region is from mouse. They are designated as **"xi"** in nomenclature.
- Examples are ritu**xi**mab, cetu**xi**mab, infli**xi**mab etc.

Humanized MAbs

- These are also derived both from mouse and human, but only hypervariable region from mouse. They are designated as "**zu**" in nomenclature.
- Examples are trastu**zu**mab, bevaci**zu**mab, eculi**zu**mab etc.

Human MAbs

- These are 100% derived from humans and are designated as "**u**" in nomenclature.
- Examples are adalim**u**mab, panitum**u**mab, ipilim**u**mab etc.

Nomenclature of Monoclonal Antibodies

There are four parts in monoclonal antibody nomenclature namely prefix, sub stem for target, sub stem for source and stem called as mab.

Conceptual Box-11

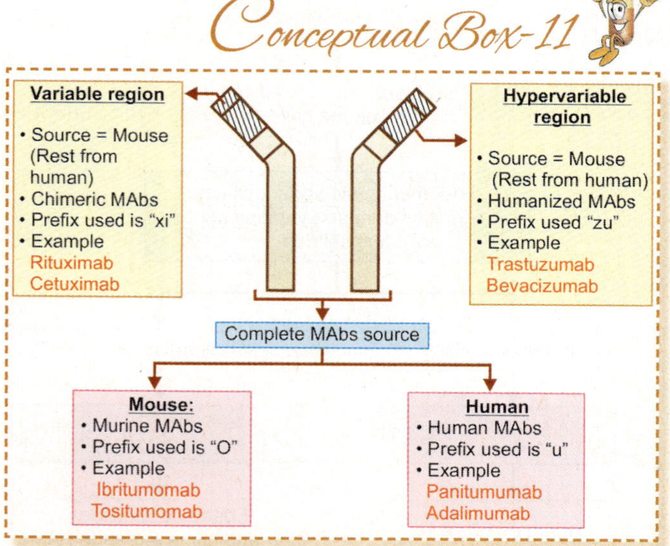

Pharmacokinetics of Monoclonal Antibodies

Absorption

- MAbs have poor oral absorption and most of them are administered by intravenous (IV) route.
- Some are given by subcutaneous (SC) route like adalimumab and omalizumab, some by intramuscular (IM) route like palivizumab and by intravitreous route like ranibizumab.

Distribution

Distribution is variable, and it depends on the location of receptors which is targeted by the antibodies.

Metabolism and Elimination

- Most of the MABs are eliminated by receptor mediated endocytosis (intracellular uptake by the receptors on which they act) followed by intracellular catabolism. Hence as the dose will increase receptor saturation will gradually decrease uptake of drug and elimination, which is known as nonlinear/first order/**dose dependent elimination kinetics**. For example, **Rituximab**, trastuzumab, gemtuzumab, panitumumab etc.
- However, only few MAbs are removed by phagocytosis and hence they display linear/zero order/dose independent elimination kinetics. For example, omalizumab and denosumab.

Side Effects of Monoclonal Antibodies

- **Acute infusion reaction** is the most common side effect of monoclonal antibodies. Mild reaction presents as fever, rash, abdominal pain, diarrhea and rashes. Hence patients are commonly premedicated with antihistaminics and NSAIDs. Occasionally the most severe form can be seen, i.e. anaphylaxis.
- Specific side effects are seen due to the effect of the antibodies on a specific receptor on target organ.

Monoclonal Antibodies and TK Inhibitors Against Specific TK Receptors

Conceptual Box-12

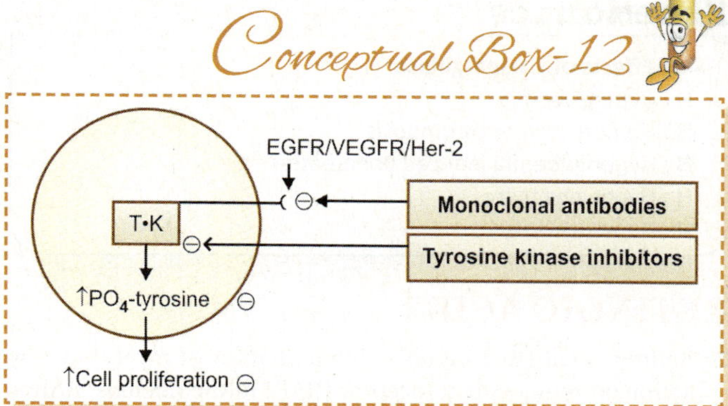

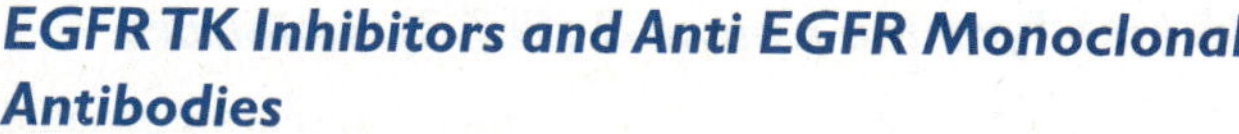

EGFR TK Inhibitors and Anti EGFR Monoclonal Antibodies

Epithelial growth factor receptor (EGFR) also known as **Her-1 receptor** is an enzyme linked receptor, attached to an intracellular TK enzyme. Whenever receptor is stimulated, it increases TK activity which phosphorylates intracellular tyrosine. Phosphorylated tyrosine increases cell proliferation. Thus, for similar anticancer effect, receptor can be inhibited by monoclonal antibodies or inhibitors of tyrosine kinase enzymes can be used.

- Anti-EGFR monoclonal antibodies like **cetuximab** and **panitumumab** are approved for treatment of **head and neck cancer** and metastatic colon cancer. **Necitumumab** has been recently approved for treatment of metastatic squamous non-small cell cancer of lung along with cisplatin and gemcitabine.
- EGFR TK inhibitors like **gefitinib, erlotinib** and **afatinib** are used for treatment of non-small cell cancer of lung. Erlotinib is also approved for treatment of pancreatic cancer. **Osimertinib** and **dacomitinib** are used for treatment of **L858R mutation** positive nonsmall cell lung cancer, which is resistant to other drugs in this class.

VEGFR TK Inhibitors and Anti-VEGFR Monoclonal Antibodies

- **VEGFR TK inhibitors** like **sunitinib** and **axitinib** are the drugs of choice for RCC along with **bevacizumab**.

Drugs	Uses
Sunitinib	• Renal cell cancer • GIST resistant to imatinib • Pancreatic cancer
Sorafenib	Drug of choice for hepatocellular carcinoma (HCC)
Pazopanib	Drug resistant soft tissue sarcoma
Axitinib	Renal cell cancer
Vandetanib	Medullary thyroid cancer
Lenvatinib	• Medullary thyroid cancer • Renal cell cancer

- **Anti-VEGFR monoclonal antibodies**

Drugs	Uses
Bevacizumab	• **RCC (Renal cell cancer)** • **Diabetic retinopathy** • Colorectal cancer • Nonsmall cell lung cancer • Ovary cancer • Glioblastoma
Ranibizumab	• Macular degeneration • Choroidal neovascularization
Ramucirumab (Approved in 2014)	• Gastric cancer treatment along with cisplatin • Colorectal cancer

- These drugs can cause delayed wound healing and more bleeding during surgery. Hence, they should be discontinued four weeks before surgery. Other side effects like hypertension (due to decrease Nitric oxide synthesis), proteinuria and thromboembolism can be seen.

Human Epidermal Growth Factor Receptor 2 (HER-2) Tyrosine Kinase (TK) Inhibitors and Anti-HER-2 Monoclonal Antibodies

- Anti HER-2 monoclonal antibodies like **trastuzumab (herceptin)** and **pertuzumab** are the drugs of choice for treatment of HER-2 positive breast cancer. They are also used for treatment of HER-2 positive gastric cancer. Resistance to these drugs is achieved by the tumor cells due to loss of the external receptor part, but the intracellular TK persists.
- Hence HER-2 tyrosine kinase inhibitor **lapatinib** is the drug of choice for trastuzumab resistant breast cancer. Lapatinib is a dual TK inhibitor, i.e. it inhibits both **HER-1 (EGFR)** and **HER-2 TK**. It is used along with capecitabine for treatment of trastuzumab resistant HER-2 positive metastatic breast cancer. It can cause QT prolongation.
- **Neratinib** is an inhibitor of HER-1, HER-2 and HER-4 tyrosine kinase recently approved for treatment of trastuzumab resistant breast cancer.
- **Trastuzumab emtansine or T-DM1** is a targeted chemotherapy recently approved for treatment of HER-2 positive breast cancer. Emtansine (DM1) is a derivative of maytensine, which inhibits microtubules and inhibits M phase of cell cycle. Development of maytensine was stopped due to side effects like neuropathy. However, now its derivative emtansine can be safely used as it is delivered specifically only to cells positive for HER-2 receptors by trastuzumab.
- Trastuzumab can cause **cardiotoxicity** due to HER-2 antigen present in heart, because it is an antibody produced against HER-2 by **injecting HER-2 antigen**.

Other Tyrosine Kinase Inhibitors

BCR-ABL Tyrosine Kinase Inhibitors

- **Imatinib**, the first generation a BCR-ABL tyrosine kinase inhibitor, is the drug of choice for treatment of CML and gastrointestinal stromal tumour **(GIST)**. **Imatinib is the least potent** whereas **ponatinib is most potent** BCR-ABL tyrosine kinase inhibitor.
- Ponatinib is the only BCR-ABL TK inhibitor active against **T315I mutant resistant CML**, which does not respond to any other TKI.
- Dasatinib and bosutinib are dual SRC-ABL tyrosine kinas inhibitors.
- Omacetaxine is a semisynthetic derivative of homoharringtonine which inhibits BCR-ABL protein synthesis and is approved for treatment of multidrug resistant CML. Interferon alpha can also be used for treatment of resistant CML.
- Tyrosine kinase inhibitors failure is characterized by either cytogenetic relapse or intolerable side effects. Dasatinib causes myelosuppression (thrombocytopenia), nilotinib causes hyperglycemia and pancreatitis and bosutinib causes diarrhea. Nilotinib and bosutinib can cause QT prolongation as well.

BCR-ABL Tyrosine Kinase Inhibitors		
First generation	**Second generation**	**Third generation**
Imatinib	• Bosutinib • Dasatinib • Nilotinib	Ponatinib

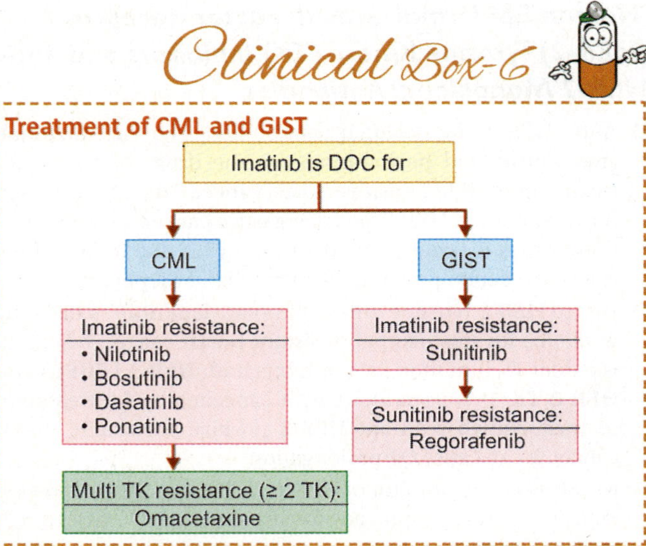

Clinical Box-6
Treatment of CML and GIST
Imatinb is DOC for
CML
GIST
Imatinib resistance:
• Nilotinib
• Bosutinib
• Dasatinib
• Ponatinib
Imatinib resistance:
Sunitinib
Sunitinib resistance:
Regorafenib
Multi TK resistance (≥ 2 TK):
Omacetaxine

Bruton's Tyrosine Kinase Inhibitors

Bruton's tyrosine kinase promotes maturation and prevents apoptosis of B lymphocytes. Hence, inhibition of this tyrosine kinase leads to death of B cells and these drugs can be used for treatment of B cell neoplasm.

- **Ibrutinib**, the first generation Bruton's tyrosine kinase inhibitor is approved for treatment of **CLL** and **Waldenstrom macroglobulinemia**. Other possible uses are **mantle cell lymphoma and marginal zone lymphoma**. Ibrutinib can cause thrombocytopenia and life-threatening bleeding when used with warfarin and hence is contraindicated with warfarin.
- **Acalabrutinib** is a second generation Bruton's tyrosine kinase inhibitor developed to overcome ibrutinib resistance. It is FDA approved for treatment of resistant mantle cell lymphoma.

Anaplastic Lymphoma Tyrosine Kinase (ALK) Inhibitors

Lymphoma tyrosine kinase is expressed in embryogenesis for development of brain and neurons; later it becomes dormant. In some patients ALK can undergo mutation and become active to increase cell proliferation, which leads to cancer like non-small cell cancer of lungs. These cancers do not respond to other drugs like cisplatin and gefitinib/erlotinib used in non-small cell lung cancer.

- **Crizotinib**, a first generation drug approved for the treatment of ALK positive non-small cell cancer of lung. It also inhibits ROS1 tyrosine kinase and hence is effective against ROS1 positive non-small cell lung cancer as well. The drawback however is development of resistance within 1–2 years of beginning therapy.
- **Ceritinib, brigatinib** and **alectinib** are second generation drugs of this class used for treatment of crizotinib resistant ALK positive non-small cell cancer of lungs.
- **Lorlatinib** is a third generation drug which is more potent and is approved for treatment of ALK positive non-small cell cancer of lungs, resistant to second generation drugs.

FMS Like Tyrosine Kinase-3 (FLT-3) Inhibitors

- FLT-3 ligand binding to FLT-3 receptors present in myeloid cells mediates proliferation and differentiation. Mutation of FLT-3 gene leads to increased activity of FLT-3 receptors which results in hematological neoplasms myeloid cells.
- **Midostaurin** is an multityrosine kinase inhibitor including FLT-3 and is approved for the treatment of:
  - FLT-3 mutation positive AML along with cytarabine and daunorubicin
  - Mastocytosis
  - Mast cell leukemia
- **Gilteritinib** is a specific FLT-3 inhibitor approved for treatment of FLT-3 mutation positive AML

Mitogen Activated Protein Kinase (MAPK) Pathway Inhibitors

In MAPK pathway activation of a tyrosine kinase receptor stimulates RAS, which further activates BRAF. Activated BRAF increases MEK 1/2, which stimulates ERK 1/2. The final product ERK 1/2 is responsible for transcription of genes responsible for cell proliferation. Hence, inhibitors of MAPK pathways have been developed for treatment of malignant melanoma.

- BRAF inhibitors **vemurafenib, dabrafenib** and **encorafenib** are drugs of choice for the treatment of unresectable or metastatic melanoma with V600E BRAF mutation.
- MEK 1/2 inhibitors **trametinib, cobimetinib** and **binimetinib** are approved for treatment of unresectable or metastatic melanoma with V600E or V600K BRAF mutations. These drugs are combined with BRAF inhibitors to make regimens.

Conceptual Box-13

MAPK Pathway

(+) Tyrosine kinase receptor
↓
RAS
↓
BRAF ⊖ Encorafenib, Vemurafenib, Dabrafenib
↓
MEK1/2 ⊖ Trametinib, Cobimetinib, Binimetinib
↓
ERK1/2
↓
Gene transcription cell proliferation
↓
Malignant melanoma

Phosphoinositide-3 Kinase (PI3K) Inhibitors

- PI3K is a kinase involved in cell proliferation and implicated in etiogenesis of bone marrow cancers.
- **Idelalisib** and **duvelisib** are PI3K inhibitors used for treatment of CLL, NHL and small lymphocytic lymphoma (SLL).

Kinase Inhibitors List

Kinase inhibitors	Targeted kinase	Uses
• Abemaciclib • Rivociclib • Palbociclib	Cyclin dependent kinase 4 and 6	ER/PR positive breast cancer
Acalabrutinib	Bruton's tyrosine kinase	Ibrutinib resistant mantle cell lymphoma
Afatinib	EGFR > HER 2 tyrosine kinase	Non-small cell cancer of lungs
Axitinib	VEGFR tyrosine kinase	Renal cell cancer
Imatinib – 1st generation	BCR-ABL tyrosine kinase	Drug of choice for CML GIST
Bosutinib Dasatinib 2nd generation Nilotinib Ponatinib – 3rd generation	BCR-ABL tyrosine kinase	Used for treatment of Imatinib resistant CML
Baricitinib	Janus Kinase 1 and 2	Rheumatoid arthritis not responding to TNF alpha inhibitors
Crizotinib	Anaplastic Lymphoma tyrosine Kinase (ALK)	ALK positive non-small cell cancer of lung
• Ceritinib • Brigatinib • Alectinib	Anaplastic Lymphoma tyrosine Kinase (ALK)	Crizotinib resistant ALK positive non-small cell cancer of lung
Lorlatinib	Anaplastic Lymphoma tyrosine Kinase (ALK)	Ceritinib and alectinib resistant ALK positive non-small cell cancer of lung
Cabozantinib	PAN tyrosine kinase	Medullary thyroid cancer RCC
Erlotinib	EGFR tyrosine kinase	Non-small cell cancer of lungs Pancreatic cancer
Fostamatinib	Spleen tyrosine kinase	Immune thrombocytopenic purpura
• Gefitinib • Dacomitinib	EGFR tyrosine kinase	Non-small cell cancer of lungs
Ibrutinib	Bruton's tyrosine kinase	• CLL • Waldenström macroglobulinemia (WM) • Mantle cell lymphoma • Marginal zone lymphoma
Idelalisib Duvelisib	Phosphoinositide-3 Kinase (PI3K)	• Relapsed CLL • Follicular B cell NHL • Small lymphocytic lymphoma
Lapatinib	Her-2 tyrosine kinase	Trastuzumab resistant breast cancer
Lenvatinib	VEGFR tyrosine kinase	• Renal cell carcinoma • Medullary thyroid cancer
Midostaurin	FMS like tyrosine kinase-3 (FLT-3)	• FLT-3 mutation positive AML along with cytarabine and daunorubicin • Mastocytosis • Mast cell leukemia
Gilteritinib	FMS Like Tyrosine kinase-3 (FLT-3)	FLT-3 mutation positive AML
Larotrectinib	Tropomyosin receptor kinases (TRK)	Solid tumors in children and adults caused by neurotropic receptor kinase (NTRK) gene fusion. NTRK gene codes for TRK
Neratinib	HER 1, 2 and 4 tyrosine kinase	Trastuzumab resistant breast cancer
Osimertinib	EGFR tyrosine kinase	Non-small cell cancer of lung positive for EGFR T790M mutation
Pazopanib	VEGFR tyrosine kinase	Soft tissue sarcoma
Regorafenib	PAN tyrosine kinase	GIST
Ruxilotinib	Janus kinase	Myelofibrosis
Sunitinib	VEGFR tyrosine kinase	Renal cell cancer GIST

Contd...

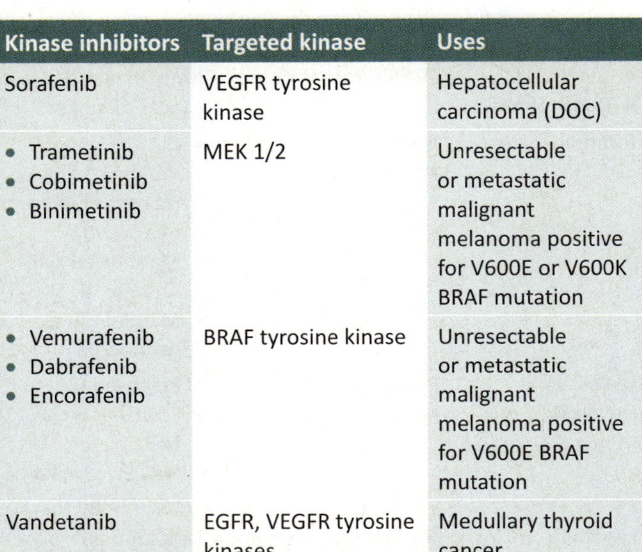

Kinase inhibitors	Targeted kinase	Uses
Sorafenib	VEGFR tyrosine kinase	Hepatocellular carcinoma (DOC)
• Trametinib • Cobimetinib • Binimetinib	MEK 1/2	Unresectable or metastatic malignant melanoma positive for V600E or V600K BRAF mutation
• Vemurafenib • Dabrafenib • Encorafenib	BRAF tyrosine kinase	Unresectable or metastatic malignant melanoma positive for V600E BRAF mutation
Vandetanib	EGFR, VEGFR tyrosine kinases	Medullary thyroid cancer

Other Monoclonal Antibodies

Monoclonal antibodies	Target	Uses
Actoxumab	Clostridium diffi cile toxin A	Prevention of C. *difficile* infection
Aducanumab	Beta-amyloid	Alzheimer's disease
Alemtuzumab	CD52	• Low-grade lymphoma • Multiple sclerosis
• Alirocumab • Evolocumab	PCSK-9 receptor – degrades LDL receptor	Familial hypercholesterolemia
Atezolizumab	PDL-1 (Programmed death ligand)	• Urothelial carcinoma – Locally advanced or metastatic • Non-small cell lung cancer – Metastatic
Avelumab	PDL-1 (Programmed death ligand)	Metastatic Merkel cell carcinoma
Burosumab	Fibroblast growth factor 23	X linked hypophosphatemia
• Basiliximab • Daclizumab	CD-25/IL-2 receptor	• Acute graft rejection • Multiple sclerosis
Belimumab	B Lymphocyte	SLE
Bezlotoxumab	*C. difficile* toxin B	Prophylaxis of pseudomembranous enterocolitis
Blinatumomab	Bispecific T cell Engager (BiTE)	Relapsed/Refractory ALL (Philadelphia chromosome negative)
• Bolosozumab • Romosozum-ab	Sclerostin	Osteoporosis

Contd...

Monoclonal antibodies	Target	Uses
Brodalumab	IL-17 A receptor	Plaque psoriasis
Brentuximab vedotin	CD 30	CLL
Bevacizumab	VEGFR	• Renal cell cancer • Diabetic retinopathy
• Cetuximab • Panitumumab	EGFR	• Head and neck cancer • Colorectal cancer
Cemiplimab	PD-1	Metastatic or advanced cutaneous squamous cell carcinoma
Dartaumumab	CD 38	Multiple myeloma resistant to bortezomib plus lenalidomide
Denosumab	RANK ligand	• Metastatic osteolytic lesions • Postmenopausal osteoporosis
Dinutuximab	GD-2 glycolipid	High-risk neuroblastoma
Diridivumab	Hemagglutinin	Influenza
Dupilumab	IL-4	Atopic dermatitis
Durvalumab	PDL-1	Urothelial carcinoma – Locally advanced or metastatic
• Eculizumab • Ravulizumab	Complement-5	PNH
Efungumab	Heat shock protein (HSP) of Candida	Invasive candidiasis treatment along with amphotericin B
Elotuzumab	SLAMF 7 (Signalling lymphocytic activation molecule family member 7)	Multiple myeloma treatment in combination with lenalidomide and dexamethasone who received prior 1–3 therapies
Emapalumab	Interferon gamma	Primary hemophagocytic lymphohistiocytosis (HLH)
Emicizumab	Bispecific antifactor IX a and factor X antibody	Hemophilia A
Erenumab	CGRP-receptor	Migraine prophylaxis
• Fremanezum-ab Galcane-zumab	CGRP ligand	Migraine prophylaxis
Gemtuzumab ozogamicin	CD 33	CD 33 positive AML
Girentuximab	Carbonic anhydrase 9 or G250 antigen expressed in clear cell RCC	Clear cell RCC

Contd...

Monoclonal antibodies	Target	Uses
Guselkumab	IL-23	Plaque psoriasis
Ibalizumab	CD-4 receptor	Multidrug resistant HIV
Idarucizumab	Dabigatran	Reversal of dabigatran's anticoagulant effect
Ipilimumab	CTLA-4	Malignant melanoma
Inotuzumab ozogamicin	CD 22	Relapsed or refractory B cell ALL
Mogamulizumab	CCR4 receptor	Relapsed or refractory mycosis fungoides or Sezary syndrome
Necitumumab	EGFR	Metastatic squamous non-small cell cancer of lung
• Nivolumab • Pembrolizum-ab	PD1 (Programmed death 1) receptor	Malignant melanoma
Obiltoxaximab	Bacillus anthrax	Anthrax
Ocrelizumab	CD20	Multiple sclerosis – RRMS and PPMS
• Ofatumumab • Obinutuzum-ab	CD20	Rituximab resistant CLL
Olaratumab	PDGFR-alpha	Soft tissue sarcoma
Omalizumab	Ig E	Bronchial asthma
• Otelixizumab • Teplizumab	CD-3	Type I DM in children
Palivizumab	RSV	RSV prophylaxis
Rafivirumab	Rabies virus	Prophylaxis of rabies
Ramucirumab	VEGFR	Gastric cancer
Ranibizumab	VEGFR	• Choroidal neovascularization • Macular edema • Deafness associated with NF-II
Reslizumab	IL-5	Severe asthma
Rituximab	CD20	Mnemonic: CANT MIS Ritu C: CLL A: Autoimmune haemolytic anemia N: NHL T: TTP M: Multiple sclerosis I: ITP S: SLE Ritu: Rheumatic arthritis
• Sarilumab • Tocilizumab		Rheumatoid arthritis
• Secukinumab • Ixekizumab	IL-17	Psoriasis
Siltuximab	IL-6	Multicentric Castleman's disease
Tildrakizumab	IL-23	Plaque psoriasis
• Trastuzumab • Pertuzumab	HER-2	HER-2 positive breast cancer
Ustekinumab	IL 12,23	Psoriasis
Vedolizumab	α4β7 integrin	• Inflammatory bowel disease • Ulcerative colitis • Crohn's disease
Ziv-aflibercept VEGFR, PLGFR	VEGFR, PLGFR	Colorectal cancer

Recent Advances

Bispecific Monoclonal Antibodies

Bispecific antibodies (BsAbs) are specially designed antibodies that can simultaneously bind to two targets. This can be helpful in many ways like redirecting T cells to tumor cells, inhibiting two different pathways involved in a disease etc. The most developed and approved by FDA currently are the ones which redirect immune cells to cancer cells and are discussed below.

Bispecific Antibodies Redirecting Immune cells to Cancer cells

- **Triomab antibodies** are trifunctional antibodies with three binding sites, i.e. tumor associated antigen, CD3 on T cells and different receptors for accessory cells like macrophages and natural killer cells. By binding to these sites, these antibodies mediate tumor cell killing by the immune cells.
  - **Catumaxomab:** It binds to epithelial cell adhesion molecule (EpCAM) in tumor cells and other two sites as mentioned above. It is currently under trial for treatment of malignant ascites in patients with EpCAM positive carcinomas.
  - **Ertumaxomab:** It binds to HER-2 receptors in tumor cells and other two sites as mentioned above. It is under trial for the treatment of metastatic HER-2 positive breast cancer progressive on trastuzumab.
- **Bispecific T cell engager (BiTE) antibodies** have two binding sites, i.e. tumor associated antigen and CD3 on T cells.
  - **Blinatumomab:** It binds to CD19 expressing B cell malignancies and to CD3 on T cells and facilitates killing of CD-19 positive tumor cells. It is currently approved for treatment of **Philadelphia chromosome negative refractory/relapsed acute lymphoblastic leukemia (ALL)** in adults and under trial for ALL in children, diffuse large B cell lymphoma and non-Hodgkin's lymphoma.
  - **Solitomab:** It binds to EpCAM on tumor cells and CD3 on T cells and is under trial for treatment of solid tumors.

Contd...

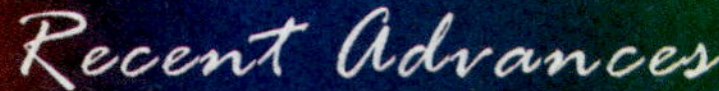

- Other types of antibodies in this class like dual-affinity retargeting molecules (DARTs) for AML and colorectal cancer, bispecific natural killer cell engager (BiKE), tandem antibodies (TandAbs) Hodgkin's and non-Hodgkin's lymphoma are currently under development.

Other Biphasic Antibodies Under Development

- **Duligotuzumab:** It is a two in one or dual actin Fab (DAF) antibody that binds to both HER-1 (EGFR) and HER-3. It is under trial for the treatment of head and neck cancer.
- **Ozoralizumab:** It is a nanobody that consists of only a heavy chain, which binds to TNF-α and human serum albumin (HAS). The albumin binding increases its half-life. It is under trial for the treatment of rheumatoid arthritis.

PROTEASOME INHIBITORS

- Proteasome is responsible for stimulating cell survival mechanisms by increasing NF-kβ activity. Hence, proteasome inhibitors decrease NF-kβ which leads to cell apoptosis.
- **Bortezomib** is indicated for the treatment of drug resistant multiple myeloma and mantle cell lymphoma.
- **Carfilzomib** and **ixazomib** are used for treatment of drug resistant multiple myeloma.
- Most common side effect is **thrombocytopenia** followed by peripheral neuropathy and fatigue.

IMMUNOTOXINS

Immunotoxins are made up of two parts, an immune part and a toxin part. The immune part is carrier and toxin is cell killer. The aim of developing this class is to selectively target tumor cells, that decreases toxicity associated with chemotherapy.

- **Denileukin difitox**
  - The immune part, i.e. denileukin is IL-2 which targets CD-8 cells and the killer is diphtheria toxin.
  - There is selective toxicity to CD-8 cells and hence it is used for the treatment of cutaneous T-cell lymphoma.
- **Gemtuzumab Ozogamycin**
  - The immune part, i.e. gemtuzumab is anti-CD33 monoclonal antibody, which carries toxin ozogamycin.
  - Hence, it is used for treatment of CD33 positive acute myelogenous leukemia (AML).
- **Brentuximab Vedotin**
  - The immune part, i.e. brentuximab is anti-CD30 monoclonal antibody, which carries toxin vedotin.
  - It is approved for the treatment of chronic lymphocytic leukemia (CLL).
- **Inotuzumab ozogamycin**
  - The immune part, i.e. inotuzumab is anti-CD-22 monoclonal antibody, which carries toxin ozogamycin.
  - It is approved for the treatment of relapsed or refractory B cell precursor acute lymphoblastic leukemia (ALL).
- **Moxetumomab pasudotox**
  - The immune part, i.e. moxetumomab is anti-CD-22 monoclonal antibody, which carries pseudomonas exotoxin (PE-38).
  - It is approved for the treatment of resistant hairy cell leukemia.
- **Tagraxofusp**
  - The immune part is IL-3, which carries diphtheria toxin.
  - It is approved for the treatment of blastic plasmacytoid dendritic cell neoplasm (BPDCN).

MITOTANE

- Mitotane is a structural analog of DDT and it acts by selectively destroying adrenal cortex.
- Hence, it is used for the treatment of symptomatic adrenocortical carcinoma.

CYCLIN DEPENDENT KINASE 4/6 INHIBITORS

- Cyclin dependent kinase 4/6 is required for proliferation of cells in the G1-S phase. Hence, inhibitions of these kinases inhibit cell proliferation in G1-S phase.
- **Palbociclib, abemaciclib** and **rivociclib** are the drugs in this class approved for the treatment of ER/PR positive breast cancer.
- Antiestrogen drugs increase the efficacy of these drugs and hence these drugs are combined with fluvestrant or letrozole.

IMMUNE CHECKPOINT INHIBITORS

PD-1 and PDL-1 Inhibitors

Immune checkpoints prevent immune cells from targeting normal cells in the body. Programmed death cell (PD-1) receptor is present on T cells; normal cells produce programmed death ligand (PDL-1) protein which binds to PD-1 and prevents death. Some cancer cells produce a huge amount of PDL-1 to evade destruction by Tcells and hence inhibitors of PD-1 and PDL-1 have been developed as anticancer drugs. The drugs in this class are given below:

PD-1 receptor inhibitors	Uses
• Pembrolizumab • Nivolumab	Drug of choice for BRAF negative malignant melanoma

PDL-1 inhibitors	Uses
Atezolizumab	• Urothelial carcinoma – Locally advanced or metastatic • Non-small cell lung cancer – Metastatic
Avelumab	Metastatic Merkel cell carcinoma
Durvalumab	Urothelial carcinoma – Locally advanced or metastatic
Cemiplimab	Squamous cell cancer of skin – Advanced or metastatic

CTLA-4 Inhibitors

CTLA-4 also acts like PD-1 on Tcells and keeps a check on their activity. Inhibition of CTLA-4 increases activity of Tcells against cancer cells. **Ipilimumab** is an anti-CTLA-4 monoclonal antibody approved for the treatment of malignant melanoma. **Tremelimumab** is currently under trial.

POLY ADP RIBOSE POLYMERASE (PARP) INHIBITORS

The PARP and BRCA are responsible for repair of single stranded DNA break. In some cancers like ovarian, BRCA can be mutated and hence the cancer cells cannot repair DNA. An addition of PARP inhibitor further compromises DNA repair and increases activity of drugs that break DNA like cisplatin.

- Olaparib and niraparib can be used for the treatment of BRCA positive ovarian, fallopian tube and primary peritoneal cancer resistant to cisplatin.
- Talazoparib is approved for the treatment of BRCA positive, HER-2 negative breast cancer.
- Rucaparib and veliparib are other drugs currently under trial.

IMMUNOMODULATORS

IL-2 Analogue

- **Aldesleukin** acts on IL-2 receptors of resting CD-8 cells and stimulates proliferation. These T cells are responsible for anticancer effect by killing tumor cells.
- It is approved for the treatment of metastatic renal cell cancer (RCC) and metastatic melanoma.
- Side effects associated are capillary leak syndrome, thrombocytopenia and hypothyroidism.

M-tor Inhibitor

- M-tor is a protein that mediates the G1-S transition in cell cycle of proliferation. Hence, inhibition of this protein produces anticancer effect.
- **Everolimus** is a m-tor inhibitor approved for the treatment of pancreatic cancer and renal angiomyolipoma associated with tuberous sclerosis.

Thalidomide

- **Thalidomide** is an old drug that can be used for the treatment of CLL, pancreatic cancer and multiple myeloma, however it is less preferred due to toxicity.
- The analogs of thalidomide like **lenalidomide** and **pomalidomide** are preferred for the treatment of multiple myeloma.

HEDGEHOG PATHWAY INHIBITORS

- Hedgehog pathway is involved in cell proliferation in embryo and abnormal activity in adults can cause cancers.
- **Sonidegib** is used for the treatment of basal cell carcinoma and **glasdegib** for AML.

Recent Advances

Anticancer Vaccines

- **Sipuleucel-T:** It is a vaccine approved for the treatment of metastatic prostate cancer. It acts by generating an immune response against prostatic acid phosphatase (PAP).
- **T-VEC:** It is approved for the treatment of malignant melanoma. It is talimogene laherparepvec in oncolytic virus, which kills the melanoma cells.

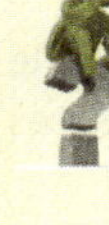

Image-based Questions

1. A 25-year-old patient presented with a swelling near distal interphalangeal joint associated with pain on movement. What is the recent drug approved for this condition seen in the picture?

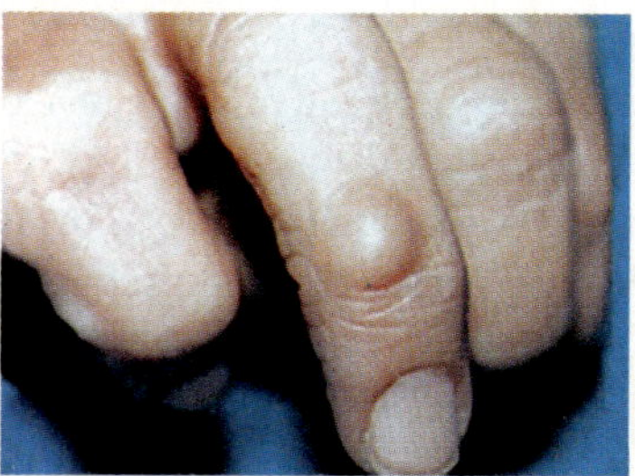

a. Doxorubicin b. Zoledronic acid
c. Denosumab d. Teriparatide

2. A male presented with a dark colored lesion with irregular borders on his back as seen in the picture. All of the following are part of non-surgical management, except:

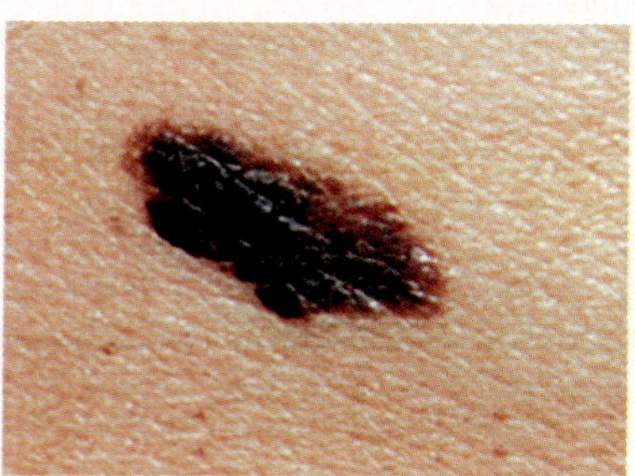

a. Ipilimumab b. Vemurafenib
c. Denileukin diftitox d. Aldesleukin

3. A patient presented with deep and boring pain in the hip area, but on examination no mass was detected. An X-ray was advised which came out as the picture given. Which of the following drug is used for treatment of this condition?

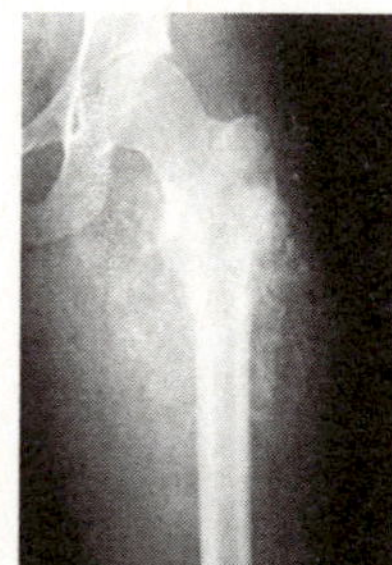

a. Paclitaxel b. Doxorubicin
c. Etoposide d. Asparginase

4. The procedure in the diagram given below is used for synthesis of:

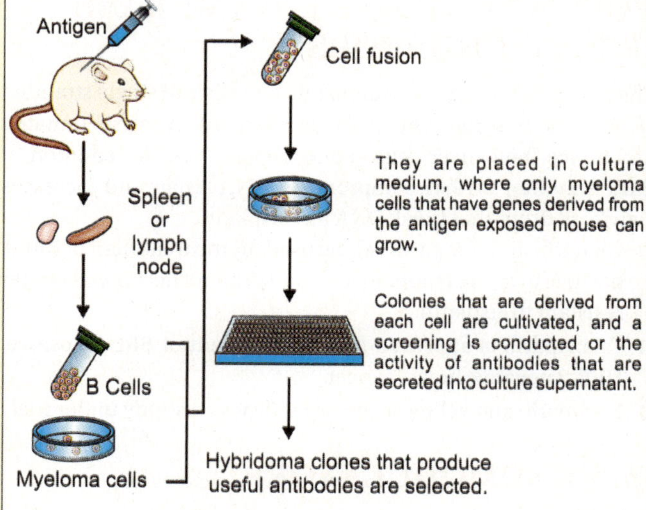
Antigen
Cell fusion
Spleen or lymph node
They are placed in culture medium, where only myeloma cells that have genes derived from the antigen exposed mouse can grow.
Colonies that are derived from each cell are cultivated, and a screening is conducted or the activity of antibodies that are secreted into culture supernatant.
B Cells
Myeloma cells
Hybridoma clones that produce useful antibodies are selected.

a. Tyrosine kinase inhibitors
b. Monoclonal antibodies
c. Both
d. None

5. A patient presented with the streaks of hyperpigmentation after starting a chemotherapeutic agent. Which of the following drugs might have done it?

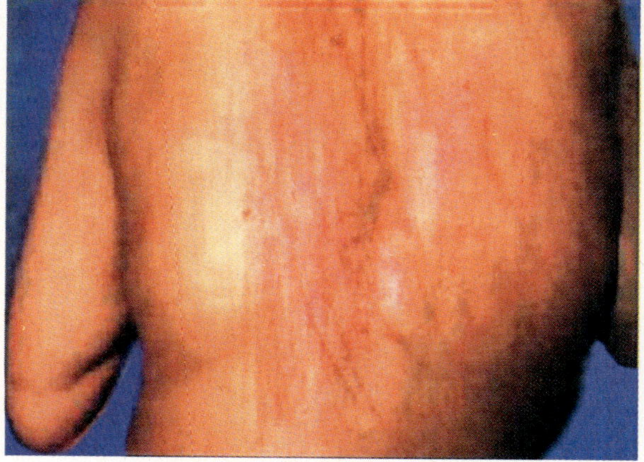

a. Hydroxyurea
b. Cisplatin
c. Bleomycin
d. Methotrexate

6. Which of the following anticancer drug is not given with the equipment in the picture?

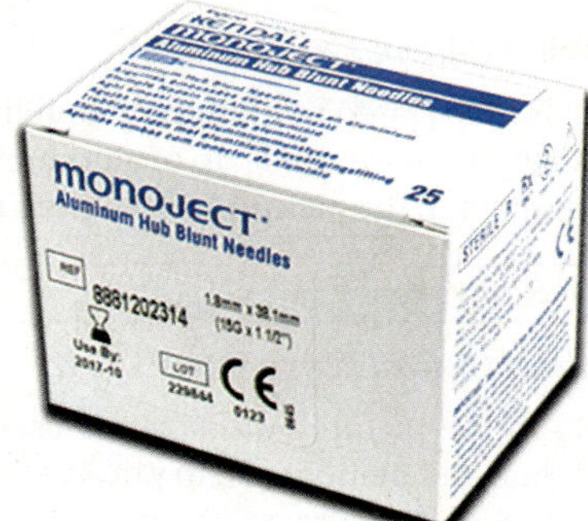

a. Hydroxyurea
b. Cyclophosphamide
c. Cladribine
d. Cisplatin

7. The drug in the picture is used with all anticancer drugs in the options, except:

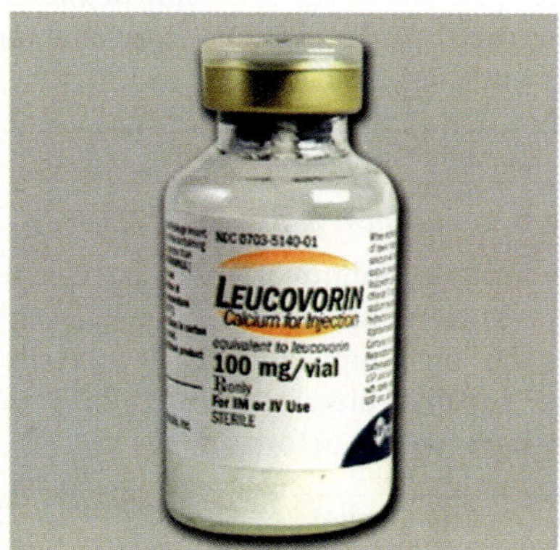

a. Methotrexate
b. 5-FU
c. Pemetrexed
d. Hydroxyurea

8. A patient presented with the side effect given in the picture. Which of the following anticancer was prescribed to the patient?

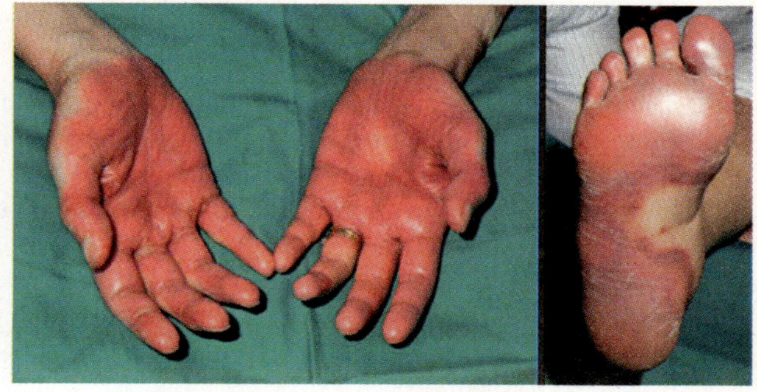

a. Capecitabine
b. Methotrexate
c. Cisplatin
d. Etoposide

9. A patient presented with complaints of exertional dyspnea and nonproductive cough. History confirmed use of a drug for the treatment of Hodgkin's disease before one year. Which of the following drug might have caused the finding seen on X-ray given?

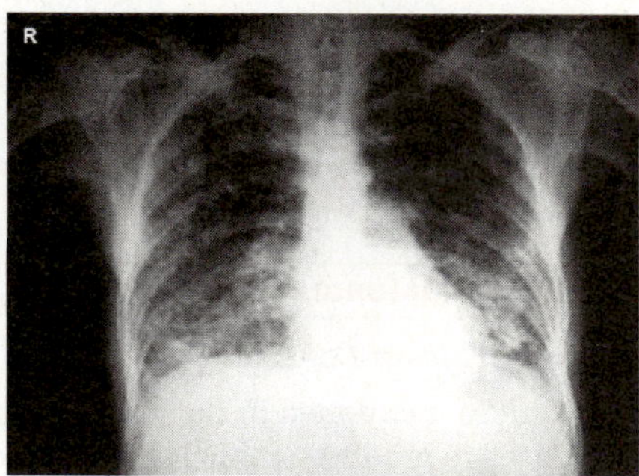

a. Doxorubicin
b. Bleomycin
c. Vinvlastine
d. Dacarbazine

10. The drug in the picture is used to prevent chemotherapy induced:

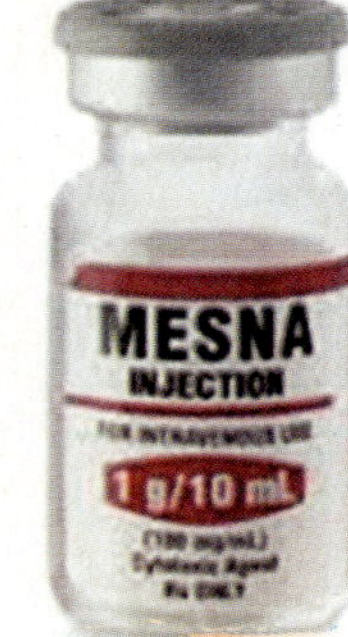

a. Pulmonary fibrosis
b. Bone marrow suppression
c. Nephrotoxicity
d. Cystitis

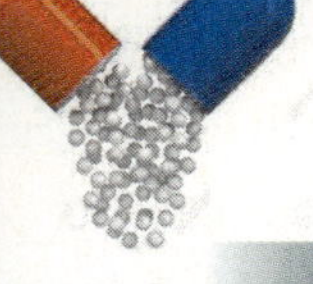

Answers with Explanations to Image-based Questions

1. Ans. (c) Denosumab

(Ref: http://www.fda.gov/ NewsEvents/ Newsroom/Press Announcements/ucm356528.htm)

- The picture depicts a patient of giant cell tumor, which presents as swelling near the joints with movement restrictions.
- Denosumab has been approved in 2013 for treatment of giant cell tumor by FDA.

2. Ans. (c) Denileukin diftitox

(Ref: CMDT 2015/P2599)

- This is a case of malignant melanoma, which is most commonly located on upper back side of males and lower limbs in females.
- Ipilimumab, vemurafenib and high dose aldesleukin are first-line drugs for treatment of malignant melanoma.
- Denileukin diftitox is used for treatment of cutaneous T-cell lymphoma.

3. Ans. (b) Doxorubicin

(Ref: CMDT 2015/P1599)

- This is a classic case of osteosarcoma with sunray appearance and Codman triangle.
- First-line drugs for osteosarcoma are ifosfamide, doxorubicin, cisplatin and methotrexate.

4. Ans. (b) Monoclonal antibodies

(Ref: Goodman Gilman 12th E/P1745)

- The procedure mentioned in the picture is hybridoma, which is used to produce monoclonal antibodies.

5. Ans. (c) Bleomycin

(Ref: Goodman Gilman 12th E/P1717)

- The streaks of hyperpigmentation seen on the back is called as flagellate dermatitis.
- It is a common complication associated with bleomycin, as the enzyme bleomycin hydrolase to metabolize bleomycin is sparse in skin.

6. Ans. (d) Cisplatin

(Ref: Goodman Gilman 12th E/P1689)

- Cisplatin is inactivated by aluminum and hence it is not used with equipments made up of aluminum.
- The equipment in the picture is aluminum needle.

7. Ans. (d) Hydroxyurea

(Ref: Goodman Gilman 12th E/P1691, 1697)

- The drug in the picture leucovorin is used along with methotrexate and pemetrexed to prevent toxicity.
- It is used to 5-FU to increase its sensitivity or anticancer effect.

8. Ans. (a) Capecitabine

(Ref: Goodman Gilman 12th E/P1698)

- This is a case of hand and foot syndrome, which presents with desquamation and erythema of palms and soles.
- Among the drugs in options, capecitabine commonly causes this side effect.

9. Ans. (b) Bleomycin

(Ref: Goodman Gilman 12th E/P1717)

- This is a case of pulmonary fibrosis, that can be seen up to two years after discontinuation of bleomycin.
- It is a common complication associated with bleomycin, as the enzyme bleomycin hydrolase to metabolize bleomycin is sparse in lungs also.

10. Ans. (d) Cystitis

(Ref: Goodman Gilman 12th E/P1684)

- The drug in the picture, mesna is used to prevent hemorrhagic cystitis associated with ifosfamide and cyclophosphamide.

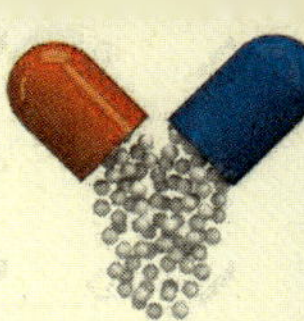

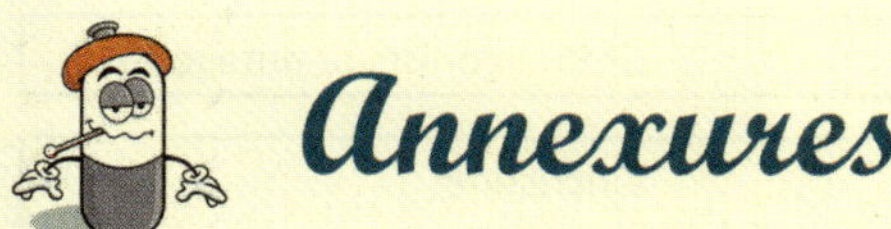

Annexures

Drug of Choice

ALL	**Regimen of choice:** VPAD V: Vincristine P: Prednisolone A: Asparginase D: Daunorubicin
AML	Daunorubicin or Idarubicin (+) Cytarabine (Ara C)
Anal ca	5 FU (+) Mitomycin
Bladder cancer	Cisplatin (+) Gemcitabine
Brain tumor	Temozolomide
Breast cancer	• ER/PR Positive ▪ **Premenopausal:** Tamoxifen ▪ **Postmenopausal:** Aromatase inhibitors • **Her 2 positive:** Trastuzumab • **Tamoxifen or Aromatase inhibitor resistant:** Fluvestrant • **Metastatic:** Aromatase inhibitors
Carcinoid tumors	Octreotide
Carcinomatous Meningitis	Methotrexate (Intrathecal)
Cervical cancer	Cisplatin
Choriocarcinoma	Methotrexate
CLL	**Regimen of choice:** FCR F: Fludarabine C: Cyclophosphamide R: Rituximab **Monotherapy:** Drug of Choice Ibrutinib Or Obinutuzumab Or Chlorambucil
CML • GIST • Hypereosinophilic syndrome • Dermatofibrosarcoma protuberans	Imatinib
CML resistant to imatinib	• Ponatinib • Nilotinib • Bosutinib • Dasatinib
Multi TK resistant (≥2) CML	Omacetaxine
Colorectal ca	• Drug of choice: 5 FU • Regimen of choice: ▪ FOLFOX – Folinic acid + 5 FU + Oxaliplatin ▪ FOLFIRI – Folinic acid + 5 FU + Irinotecan
Esophageal Ca	Cisplatin + 5 FU or Carboplatin + paclitaxel
Gastric ca	5FU or docetaxel Plus Cisplatin or oxaliplatin
Hairy cell leukemia	Cladribine
Hepatocellular carcinoma	Sorafenib
Hodgkin's disease	**Regimen of choice:** ABVD A: Adriamycin (Doxorubicin) B: Bleomycin V: Vincristine D: Dacarbazine
Kaposi sarcoma	Doxorubicin or Daunorubicin
Lung cancer	Non-small cell • Cisplatin plus vinorelbine Plus etoposide or gemcitabine (squamous) or pemetrexed (Non-squamous) Small cell • Cisplatin plus Etoposide

Malignant Melanoma	**BRAF Negative:** PD-1 Inhibitors like Pembrolizumab/Nivolumab **BRAF Positive:** BRAF inhibitors like vemurafenib/dabrafenib
Mesothelioma	Pemetrexed
Multiple myeloma	Lenalidomide plus Dexamethasone
Myelodysplasia	Azacitidine
Myelodysplasia with 5q syndrome (Anemia)	Lenalidomide
Non-Hodgkin's lymphoma	• **Drug of choice:** Rituximab • TOC for high/intermediate grade NHL: CHOP – R C – Cyclophosphamide H – Hydroxy doxorubicin O – Oncovin (Vincristine) P – Prednisolone R – Rituximab • **TOC for low grade NLH:** FCR F – Fludarabine C – Cyclophosphamide R – Rituximab
Neuroblastoma	C – Cyclophosphamide and Cisplatin plus D – Doxorubicin plus E - Etoposide
Osteosarcoma	A combination of two drugs given below High dose methotrexate with leucovorin Cisplatin Doxorubicin Ifosfamide
Ovarian cancer	Platinum compound (Cisplatin or carboplatin) Plus Taxane (Paclitaxel or docetaxel)
Paget's disease	Zoledronic acid
Pancreatic cancer	Gemcitabine
Pheochromocytoma (Malignant)	**Averbuch's Protocol:** VCD V – Vincristine C – Cyclophosphamide D – Dacarbazine
Prostate cancer	GnRH agonists or antagonists
Retinoblastoma	Vincristine Plus Etoposide plus Carboplatin
Renal cell cancer	Anti VEGFR drugs (Bevacizumab, sunitinib, sorafenib) Or Mtor inhibitors (Temsirolimus)
• Testicular cancer • Dysgerminoma	**Regimen of choice:** BEP B: Bleomycin E: Etoposide P: Platinum compound (Cisplatin)
Thyroid cancer	I^{131} or VEGFR inhibitors like Sunitinib/Sorafenib/Lenvatinib
Waldenström macroglobulinemia (WM)	Rituximab

MISCELLANEOUS DRUGS

Drugs	Mechanism of action	Uses
Ivosidenib	Inhibitor of mutant isocitrate dehydrogenase 1 (IDH1)	Relapsed or refractory AML positive for isocitrate dehydrogenase 1 (IDH1) mutation
Venetoclax	Antiapoptotic protein bcl-2 inhibitor	CLL with 17-p deletion
Sonidegib	Hedgehog pathway inhibitor	Locally advanced basal cell carcinoma
Glasdegib	Hedgehog pathway inhibitor	AML along with cytarabine in patients > 75 years or in patients with comorbidities that are contraindication for intensive induction chemotherapy
Axicabtagene ciloleucel	CD 19 directed genetically modified autologous T cell immunotherapy	Large B cell lymphoma

ANTICANCER DRUGS SIDE EFFECTS

Hemorrhagic cystitis	Ifosfamide > cyclophosphamide
Nephrotoxicity	Cisplatin
Hepatotoxicity	• 6-MP, 6-TG • Methotrexate on long term use • BCR-ABL TK inhibitors (Imatinib, dasatinib, nilotinib) • Dacarbazine
Cardiotoxicity	Mnemonic: **FAT** Cardio **F:** 5-FU causes coronary vasospasm and precipitates ischemia **A:** Anthracyclines, maximum with doxorubicin and daunorubicin **T:** Trastuzumab Cardio: Cyclophosphamide at high doses
Pulmonary fibrosis	**Bleomycin:** Most common cause Busulfan and other alkylating agents
Neuropathy	Mnemonic: **PCMB** **P:** Pyrimidine analogs: Fludarabine and Nelarabine **C:** Cisplatin and oxaliplatin (sensory and motor) **M:** M phase specific drugs Vinca alkaloids (Vincristine > Vinorelbine > Vinblastine): Sensory, motor and autonomic or mixed Taxanes (Nab paclitaxel > Paclitaxel): Sensory Epothilones (Ixabepilone): Sensory **B:** Bortezomib
SIADH	Vincristine: Most common cause cyclophosphamide
Raynaud's disease	Mnemonic: **B**lood **V**essels **C**an **N**ot **P**ass blood **B**lood: Bleomycin **V**essels: Vinblastine **C**an: Cisplatin **N**ot: Nilotinib **P**ass blood: Ponatinib
Hand and foot syndrome	Capecitabine > 5FU Doxorubicin Gemcitabine VEGFR TK inhibitors: Sunitinib, sorafenib, pazopanib
Vesication	• Mechlorethamine • Nitrosoureas • Dactinomycin • Doxorubicin and daunorubicin • Vinca alkaloids
Mucositis	Mnemonic: **HAD** **M**ucositis **H**: Hydroxyurea **A**: Alkylating agents **D**: Dactinomycin, Doxorubicin and Daunorubicin **M**ucositis: Metabolites antagonists like 5-FU, Cytarabine and Methotrexate
Diarrhe	• 5-FU • Capecitabine • Irinotecan • Tyrosine kinase inhibitors (Imatinib, sunitinib, sorafenib etc.)
Flu like symptoms	• Dacarbazine • Gemcitabine
Alopecia	• Anthracyclines • Dactinomycin • Topoisomerase inhibitors (Etoposide and irinotecan) • Alkylating agents
Radiation recall syndrome	Mnemonic: **D** **D**: Dactinomycin **D**: Doxorubicin **D**: Daunorubicin
Radiation toxicity due to radiosensitization	Mnemonic: **C**ount **FGHI** **C**ount: **C**isplatin and oxaliplatin Mitomycin-**C** **F**: 5-**FU** **G**: **G**emcitabine **H**: **H**ydroxyurea **I**: **I**rinotecan
Secondary leukemia: **AML** is the most common type seen with all, except mitoxantrone which causes **PML**. Drug induced leukemia has poorer prognosis as compared to de-novo leukemia.	Alkylating agents Platinum compounds Topoisomerase II inhibitors (Etoposide) Mitoxantrone 6-MP Fludarabine
Hemolytic uremic syndrome	• Mitomycin • Gemcitabine

Contd...

ANTIDOTES FOR ANTICANCER DRUGS ASSOCIATED TOXICITY

Toxicity	Antidote
Hand and foot syndrome	Pyridoxine
Methotrexate associated mucositis and bone marrow suppression	Leucovorin (Folinic acid) or Folic acid
Pemetrexed associated mucositis and bone marrow suppression	Leucovorin (Folinic acid) or Folic acid + Vitamin B_{12}
Anthracyclines induced cardiotoxicity and vesication	Dexrazoxane
Cyclophosphamide and ifosfamide induced hemorrhagic cystitis	Mesna

Contd...

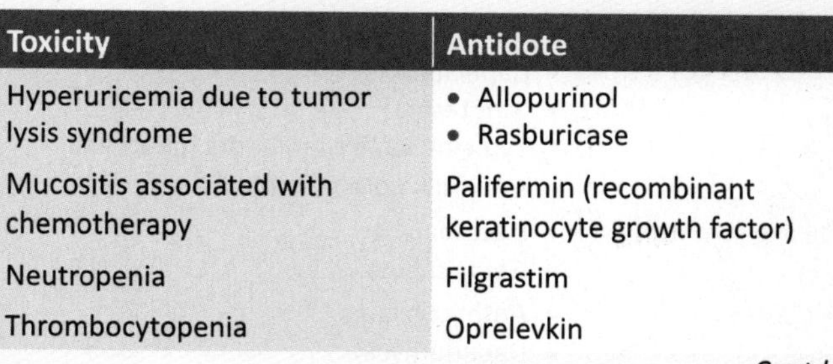

Toxicity	Antidote
Hyperuricemia due to tumor lysis syndrome	• Allopurinol • Rasburicase
Mucositis associated with chemotherapy	Palifermin (recombinant keratinocyte growth factor)
Neutropenia	Filgrastim
Thrombocytopenia	Oprelevkin
Anemia	• Epoetin alfa • Darbepoetin alfa
Irinotecan induced delayed diarrhea	High-dose loperamide
Mechlorethamine associated vesication	Thiosulfate

Contd...

Note: Denosumab and zoledronic acid can be used for treatment of osteolytic bone metastasis.

Multiple Choice Questions

NONCELL CYCLE SPECIFIC ANTICANCER DRUGS

1. **Most common agent associated with agranulocytosis is:** ***(Recent Question 2017)***
   a. Steroids b. Alkylating agents
   c. Paracetamol d. Endotoxemia

2. **The most common side effect of cancer chemotherapy is nausea with or without vomiting. The anticancer drugs vary in their ability to cause nausea and vomiting. Which of the following anti-cancer drugs is least likely to cause nausea and vomiting?** ***(AIIMS May 2014)***
   a. Chlorambucil b. Cisplatin
   c. Doxorubicin d. Daunorubicin

3. **All of the following are true regarding ifosfamide except:** ***(AIIMS May 2011)***
   a. Metabolised by cytochrome p450 enzymes
   b. Less neurotoxic than cyclophosphamide
   c. Chloracetaldehyde is the metabolite of ifosfamide
   d. It is a nitrogen mustard

4. **Hemorrhagic cystitis is caused by:** ***(AIIMS Nov 2010, Recent Question 2016)***
   a. Cyclophosphamide b. 6 Mercaptopurine
   c. 5 Fluorouracil d. Busulfan

5. **Which of the following can be given orally:** ***(AIIMS May 2009)***
   a. Cytosine arabinoside b. Cisplatin
   c. Doxorubicin d. Mesna

6. **Most emetogenic anticancer drug is:** ***(AIIMS May 2009)***
   a. Cisplatin
   b. Carboplatin
   c. High dose cyclophosphamide
   d. High dose methotrexate

7. **Ifosfamide belongs to which group of anticancer drugs?** ***(AIIMS Nov 2008; AI 2009; DNB 2008)***
   a. Alkylating agents b. Antimetabolites
   c. Mitotic inhibitors d. Topoisomerase inhibitors

8. **Which of the following chemotherapeutic agents is associated with secondary leukemia?** ***(AIIMS May 2006)***
   a. Vinblastine b. Paclitaxel
   c. Cisplatin d. Bleomycin

9. **Which of the following drugs is associated with untoward side effect of renal tubular damage?** ***(AIIMS May; 2006)***
   a. Cisplatin b. Streptozocin
   c. Methysergide d. Cyclophosphamide

10. **Sustained neutropenia is seen with:** ***(AIIMS May 2008)***
    a. Vinblastine
    b. Cisplatin
    c. Carmustine
    d. Cyclophosphamide

11. **Dose of cisplatin in head and neck squamous cell carcinoma is---- mg/m^2** ***(Recent Question Dec 2016)***
    a. 100 b. 200
    c. 300 d. 400

12. **Double Platin based therapy is used for:** ***(Recent Question Dec 2016)***
    a. Wilm's tumor
    b. Hodgkin's lymphoma
    c. Non-hodgkin's lymphoma
    d. Lung cancer

13. **Secondary leukemia associated with anticancer drugs develop at:** ***(Recent Question Dec 2016)***
    a. 3 months b. 1 year
    c. <7 years d. <10 years

14. **Anticancer drug leading to HUS as a toxicity is:** ***(Recent Question Dec 2016)***
    a. Paclitaxel b. Vinorelbine
    c. Mitomycin C d. Cyclophosphamide

15. **Mechanism of action of actinomycin D is:** ***(Recent Question 2016)***
    a. Inhibits DNA-dependent RNA synthesis
    b. Activates DNA-dependent RNA synthesis
    c. Inhibits RNA-dependent DNA synthesis
    d. Activates RNA-dependent DNA synthesis

16. **Histopathology of doxorubicin toxicity shows?** ***(Recent Question 2016)***
    a. Vacuolar degeneration of the myofibrils
    b. Muscle spindle whorls
    c. Hyalinization of the bundles of muscles
    d. Apoptosis of muscles

17. **Sunder, a young male was diagnosed as suffering from a/c myeloid leukemia. He was started on induction chemotherapy with doxorubicin based regimen. Induction was successful. Two months later, he presents to OPD with swelling of both feet and breathlessness on climbing stairs. He also complains that he had to wake up many times because of breathlessness. Which of the following is most likely responsible for the patient's symptoms?** ***(Recent Question 2016)***
    a. Restrictive cardiomyopathy
    b. Hypertrophic cardiomyopathy
    c. Dilated cardiomyopathy
    d. Pericardial fibrosis

18. **Most emetogenic anticancer drug is:** ***(Recent Question 2016)***
    a. Cisplatin
    b. Carboplatin
    c. High dose cyclophosphamide
    d. High dose methotrexate

19. **A 35-year-old patient is having carcinoma lung with a past history of lung disease. Which of the following drugs should not be given?** ***(Recent Question 2016)***
    a. Vinblastine b. Bleomycin
    c. Mithramycin d. Adriamycin

20. Which of the following antineoplastic drugs should not be administered to a chronic alcoholic patient due to risk of development of disulfiram like reaction? ***(Recent Question 2016)***

a. Dacarbazine b. Procarbazine
c. Melphalan d. Hydroxyurea

21. Alkylating agents are all except: ***(Recent Question 2016)***

a. Buslfan b. Carmustine
c. Dacarbazine d. Etoposide

22. Nitrosoureas used in the treatment of cancer are: ***(Recent Question 2016)***

a. Carmustine b. 5FU
c. Methotrexate d. Cisplatin

23. An antibiotic not acting on tubulin is: ***(Recent Question 2016)***

a. Bleomycin b. Colchicine
c. Paclitaxel d. Vincristine

24. Which antineoplastic drug has a very high cardiac toxicity? ***(Recent Question 2016)***

a. Bleomycin b. Actinomycin-D
c. Doxorubicin d. Mitomycin-C

25. Cyclophosphamide is: ***(Recent Question 2016)***

a. Alkylating agent b. Antitumor antibiotic
c. Monoclonal antibody d. Antimet abolites

26. Most characteristic side effect of adriamycin is: ***(Recent Question 2016)***

a. Nephrotoxicity b. Neurotoxicity
c. Cardiotoxicity d. Hemorrhagic cystitis

27. Antineoplastic which is not an antibiotic: ***(Recent Question 2016)***

a. Azathioprine b. Bleomycin
c. Mitomycin d. Doxorubicin

28. All are alkylating agents used in chemotherapy except: ***(Recent Question 2016)***

a. Melphalan b. Busulfan
c. Cladribine d. Cyclophosphamide

29. All are examples of alkylating agents except: ***(Recent Question 2016)***

a. Bleomycin b. Busulfan
c. Procarbazine d. Melphalan

30. Alkylating agent used in chemotherapy: ***(Recent Question 2016)***

a. Mechlorethamine b. Procarbazine
c. Cyclophosphamide d. All of the above

31. True about cyclophosphamide: ***(Recent Question 2016)***

a. Antimetabolites b. Alkylating agent
c. Platinum compound
d. Topoisomerase inhibitors

32. First-line chemotherapy for cancer cervix: ***(Recent Question 2016)***

a. Cyclophosphamide b. Lomustine
c. Vincristine d. Cisplastin

33. Most widely used anti CA drug: ***(Recent Question 2016)***

a. 5 FU b. Methotrexate
c. Cisplatin d. All

34. Which of the following anticancer drug causes hemolytic uremic syndrome: ***(Recent Question 2016)***

a. Vincristine b. Vinblastine
c. Cisplatin d. Mitomycin

35. Pulmonary fibrosis is a complication of: ***(Recent Question 2016)***

a. Methotrexate b. Doxorubicin
c. Cisplatin d. Busulfan

36. Anticancer drug causing nephrotoxicity: ***(Recent Question 2016)***

a. Imitanib b. Irinotecan
c. fosfestrol d. Cisplatin

CELL CYCLE SPECIFIC ANTICANCER DRUGS

37. Which of the following drugs can cause flagellate hyperpigmentation? ***(AIIMS May 2018)***

a. Bleomycin b. Minocycline
c. Doxorubicin d. Vincristine

38. Regimen of choice for retinoblastoma is: ***(Recent Question 2019)***

a. Vincristine + etoposide + carboplatin
b. Carboplatin + etoposide + cyclophosphamide
c. Vincristine + etoposide + chlorambucil
d. Etoposide + vinblastine + carboplatin

39. Which enzyme deficiency leads to serious side effects with 5FU ***(Recent Question 2018)***

a. CYPD29
b. Dihydropyrimidine dehydrogenase
c. Uridine di phosphate
d. Purine

40. All of the following are G2 phase inhibitors except: ***(AIIMS May 2016)***

a. Paclitaxel b. Etoposide
c. Topotecan d. Daunorubicin

41. Wrong about paclitaxel: ***(AIIMS Nov 2014)***

a. Derived from E.coli
b. Causes stabilization of microtubules
c. Most important toxicity is bone marrow suppression
d. Used in breast, ovarian & other genital malignancy

42. Which of the following medications is essential for ameliorating the toxicity of pemetrexed? ***(AIIMS May 2014)***

a. Folinic acid and vitamin B6
b. Folic acid and vitamin B12
c. Vitamin B6 and Vitamin B12
d. Folic acid and dexamethasone

43. Methotrexate is used for the management of all of these conditions except: ***(AIIMS May 2011)***

a. Rheumatoid arthritis b. Psoriasis
c. Sickle cell anemia d. Organ transplantation

44. Which of the following drug is used for the treatment of sickle cell anemia? ***(AIIMS May 2011)***

a. Hydroxyurea b. Cisplatin
c. Paclitaxel d. Carboplatin

45. **Methotrexate resistance is due to:** ***(AIIMS Nov 2010, Recent Question 2016)***
   a. Depletion of folate
   b. Overproduction of DHFRase
   c. Overproduction of Thymidylate kinase
   d. Decreased DHFRase

46. **A pregnant woman of >35 weeks gestation has SLE. All of the following drugs are used in treatment except:** ***(AIIMS May 2010)***
   a. Methotrexate b. Sulfasalazine
   c. Prednisolone d. Chloroquine

47. **Cerebellar toxicity is seen with:** ***(AIIMS May 2009)***
   a. Cisplatin b. Cytarabine
   c. Bleomycin d. Actinomycin D

48. **Which of the following anticancer drug is excreted by lungs?** ***(AIIMS Nov 2008)***
   a. 5-Fluorouracil b. Cyclophosphamide
   c. Doxorubicin d. Cisplatin

49. **Which of the following is an antimetabolite?** ***(AIIMS May, 2007)***
   a. Methotrexate b. Cyclosporine
   c. Etoposide d. Vinblastine

50. **The new drug pemetrexed useful in breast cancer belongs to which of the following category of the drugs?** ***(AIIMS Nov 2005)***
   a. Antitumor agent b. Alkylating agent
   c. Hormonal agent d. Antimetabolite

51. **Pemetrexed is drug of choice for:** ***(Recent Question Dec 2016)***
   a. Small cell carcinoma b. Mesothelioma
   c. Non small cell carcinomad. Breast cancer

52. **Most common chemo used in epithelial ovarian cancers:** ***(Recent Question Dec 2016)***
   a. Paclitaxel b. Dactinomycin
   c. Cyclophosphamide d. Methotrexate

53. **Which antineoplastic is cell cycle phase inhibitor?** ***(Recent Question Dec 2016)***
   a. Vincristine b. 5FU
   c. Paclitaxel d. Cyclophosphamide

54. **Antidote for methotrexate poisoning is:** ***(Recent Question Dec 2016)***
   a. Folic acid b. Folinic acid
   c. Pyridoxine d. Vitamin B-12

55. **The antimetabolite 'X' inhibits DNA polymerase and is one of the most active drugs in the treatment of leukemia. Although myelosuppression is dose limiting, the drug may also cause cerebellar dysfunction including ataxia and dysarthria:** ***(Recent Question 2016)***
   a. Blemycin b. Cytarabine
   c. Meracptopurine d. Methotrxate

56. **Hydroxyurea mechanism of action in cancer is by inhibiting the enzyme:** ***(Recent Question 2016)***
   a. Ribonucleoside diphosphate reductase
   b. Ribonucleotide oxidase
   c. DNA lyase
   d. DNA synthetase

57. **Gemcitabine is used mainly in which cancer?** ***(Recent Question 2016)***
   a. Colorectal b. Breast
   c. Pancreatic d. Cranipharyngioma

58. **Microtubule formation is inhibited by:** ***(Recent Question 2016)***
   a. Paclitaxel b. Vincristine
   c. Etoposide d. Irinotectan

59. **Methotrexate resistance is due to?**
   a. Increased concentrations of intracellular DHFR through gene amplification ***(Recent Question 2016)***
   b. Failure of efflux pumps
   c. Bacterial modification
   d. Increased synthesis of poly glutamates

60. **Which is not an antimetabolite?** ***(Recent Question 2016)***
   a. Methotrexate b. 5 Fluorouracil
   c. Gemcitabine d. Vinca alkaloids

61. **All of the following anticancer drugs are cell-cycle nonspecific except:** ***(Recent Question 2016)***
   a. Doxorubacin b. Vincristine
   c. Mitomycin-C d. Cyclophosphamide

62. **Mechanism of action of 5-FU is:** ***(Recent Question 2016)***
   a. Antimetabolite b. Direct DNA chelating agent
   c. Anti-mitotic d. Topoisomerase inhibitor

63. **Which is a purine antagonist?** ***(Recent Question 2016)***
   a. 5 FU b. Methotrexate
   c. Allopurinol d. Mercaptopurine

64. **Which antineoplastic agent is an antifolate drug?** ***(Recent Question 2016)***
   a. Methotrexate b. Adriamycin
   c. Vincristine d. Cyclophosphamide

65. **Drug used to counteract methotrexate toxicity?** ***(Recent Question 2016)***
   a. Folinic acid b. Folic acid
   c. VitBu d. Mesna

66. **The drug of choice in choriocarcinoma is:** ***(Recent Question 2016)***
   a. Methotrexate b. Actinomycin-D
   c. Vincristine d. 6-thioguanine

67. **Which of the following drug is not a purine analogue?** ***(Recent Question 2016)***
   a. 6-Mercaptopurine b. Cladribine
   c. Cytarabine d. Fludarabine

68. **Methotrexate mechanism of action:** ***(Recent Question 2016)***
   a. Inhibit dihydrofolate Reductase
   b. Stimulate dihydrofolate Reductase
   c. Inhibit tetrahydrofolate reductse
   d. Stimulate tetrahydrofolate reductse

69. **Which of the following antineoplastic drug causes hepatotoxicity?** ***(Recent Question 2016)***
   a. 6-mercaptopurine b. 5-flurouracil
   c. Doxorubicin d. Etoposide

70. **Not used in treatment protocol of Hodgkin's lymphoma:** ***(Recent Question 2016)***
   a. Vincristine b. Vinblastine
   c. Bleomycin d. Adriamycin

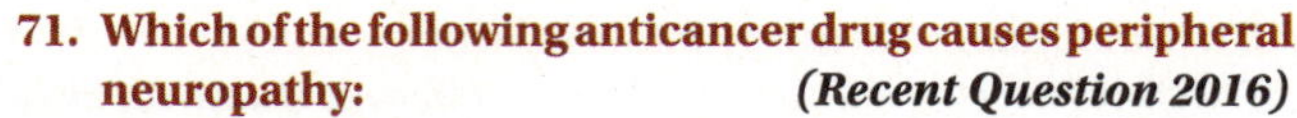

71. **Which of the following anticancer drug causes peripheral neuropathy:** ***(Recent Question 2016)***
    a. Methotrexate b. Vincristine
    c. Cytarabine d. Etoposide

MISCELLANEOUS ANTICANCER DRUGS AND MCQS

72. **The technique given in the picture is used for:** ***(AIIMS Nov 2018)***
    a. Synthesis of monoclonal antibodies
    b. Preparing cell lines for viral culture
    c. Synthesis of vaccine
    d. Process of genetic engineering

73. **A girl with APML was treated and during treatment she developed tachypnea, fever, pulmonary infiltrate. What is the treatment of choice?** ***(AIIMS May 2017)***
    a. Dexamethosone
    b. Cytarabine
    c. Doxorubicin
    d. Methotrexate

74. **All are true about rituximab except:** ***(AIIMS Nov-2014)***
    a. Has dose independent pharmacokinetics
    b. Most common side effect is infusion reaction
    c. First FDA drug approved for resistant lymphomas
    d. Chimeric monoclonal antibody against CD-20 B cell antigen

75. **Most common dose-limiting toxicity of cancer chemotherapy is:** ***(AIIMS May 2010)***
    a. Gastrointestinal toxicity b. Neurotoxicity
    c. Bone marrow suppression
    d. Nephrotoxicity

76. **Cetuximab (an EGFR antagonist) can be used in:**
    a. Palliation in head and neck cancer ***(AIIMS May 2009)***
    b. Anal canal carcinoma
    c. Gastric carcinoma
    d. Lung carcinoma

77. **Imatinib is used in the treatment of:** ***(AIIMS May 2008)***
    a. Chronic myelomonocytic leukemia
    b. Myelodysplastic syndrome
    c. Acute lymphoid leukemia
    d. Gastrointestinal stromal tumors

78. **Rituximab is used in all except:** ***(AIIMS May 2008)***
    a. Non-Hodgkin lymphoma
    b. Paroxysmal nocturnal hemoglobinurea
    c. Rheumatoid arthritis
    d. Systemic lupus erythematosis

79. **A 56-year-old female presented with breast carcinoma and she was prescribed herceptin (trastuzumab). Which of the following statements regarding this drug is true?**
    a. It is an antibody produced entirely from mouse containing no human component ***(AIIMS Nov 2008)***
    b. It is a monoclonal antibody produced by injecting her-2 antigen
    c. It is a polyclonal antibody
    d. It is a monoclonal antibody containing only human component

80. **Mechanism of action of imatinib mesylate is:** ***(AIIMS May 2007)***
    a. Increase in metabolism of P glycoprotein
    b. Blocking the action of P glycoprotein
    c. Blocks the action of chimeric fusion protein of bcr-abl
    d. Noncompetitive inhibition of ATP binding site

81. **The drug imatinib acts by the inhibition of:** ***(AIIMS May 2006)***
    a. Tyrosine kinase b. Glutathione reductase
    c. Thymidylate synthetase d. Protein kinase

82. **Drug of choice for chemotherapy induced early and late onset nausea and vomiting is:** ***(Recent Question Dec 2016)***
    a. Aprepitant b. CB receptor agonist
    c. Promethazine d. TCA

83. **Doc for HER-2 positive breast carcinoma is:** ***(Recent Question 2018)***
    a. Trastuzumab b. Tamoxifen
    c. Exemestane d. Fluvestrant

84. **The dose of human series rabies Immunoglobulin is:** ***(Recent Question Dec 2016)***
    a. 20 IU/kg b. 40 IU/kg
    c. 60 IU/kg d. 80 IU/kg

85. **Drugs not used for Imatinib resistant CML?** ***(Recent Question Dec 2016)***
    a. Bosutinib b. Ponatinib
    c. Omacetaxine d. Bortezomib

86. **Dronabinol is an orally active cannabinoid, which is used in management of chemotherapy induced nausea and vomiting. Which of the following parameters is to be monitored in a patient taking dronabinol?** ***(Recent Question 2016)***
    a. Blood pressure b. Respiratory rate
    c. Temperature d. Urine output

87. **Drug of choice for CML is:** ***(Recent Question 2016)***
    a. Imatinib b. Rituximab
    c. Vincristine d. Bleomycin

88. **Which of the following drugs act by inhibiting tyrosine Kinase activated by EGF receptor as well as HER-2?** ***(Recent Question 2016)***
    a. Imatinib b. Gefitinib
    c. Erlotinib d. Lapatinib

89. **Drug that is radioprotective is:** ***(Recent Question 2016)***
    a. Paclitaxel b. Vincristine
    c. Etoposide d. Amifostine

90. **Bevacizumab is used in:** ***(Recent Question 2016)***
    a. Carcinoma colon b. Liver carcinoma
    c. Renal cell carcinoma d. Pancreatic carcinoma

91. **Bevacizumab is:** ***(Recent Question 2016)***
    a. Anti-VEGF antibody
    b. Histone decyclase inhibitor
    c. Proteosome inhibitor d. Her-2 neu inhibitor

92. **Which of the following anticancer drugs are competitive inhibitors of tyrosine kinase?** ***(Recent Question 2016)***
    a. Imatinib and suntinib b. Letrozole
    c. Bicalutamide d. Fulvestrant

93. Tocilizumab is antibody against: ***(Recent Question 2016)***
a. IL 2
b. IL 4
c. IL 6
d. IL 8

94. Cardiomyopathy is caused by which monoclonal antibody? ***(Recent Question 2016)***
a. Tratuzumab
b. Infliximab
c. Eternacept
d. Adalimumab

95. Drug of choice for neutropenia due to cancer chemotherapy is: ***(Recent Question 2016)***
a. Vitamin B12
b. IL11
c. Filgrastim
d. Erythropoietin

96. Trastuzumab all are true except: ***(Recent Question 2016)***
a. Shows better response in combination with paclitaxel
b. Used in metastatic breast cancer
c. Causes upregulation of HER2/neu
d. Do not causes bone marrow toxicity

97. Rituximab is antibody against: ***(Recent Question 2016)***
a. CD20
b. VEGF
c. EGFR
d. IL-2

98. Which of the following is not used in treatment for multiple myeloma: ***(Recent Question 2016)***
a. Melphalan
b. Thalidomide
c. Zolendronic acid
d. Methotrexate

99. Drugs which do not suppress bone marrow: ***(PGI Nov 2017)***
a. 5FU
b. Cisplatin
c. Chlorambucil
d. Vincristine
e. Vinblastine

100. Drugs affecting purine synthesis: ***(PGI May 2017)***
a. Azathioprine
b. Methotrexate
c. Fludarabine
d. 6-Mercaptopurine
e. Capecitabine

101. Methotrexate affects: ***(PGI May 2017)***
a. Purine synthesis
b. Pyrimidine synthesis
c. Conversion of DHFA to THFA
d. Polymerization of mitotic tubule

102. Which of the following anti-tumor drugs have high risk of gonadotoxicity: ***(PGI May 2017)***
a. Dactinomycin
b. Cyclophosphamide
c. Busulfan
d. Vinblastine
e. Ifosfamide

103. A person was on chemotherapy for 2 weeks for some mediastinal tumor. Now he develops high frequency hearing loss. Most probable cause of this condition is use of: ***(PGI June 2015)***
a. Cisplatin
b. Etoposite
c. Doxorubicin
d. Methotrexate

104. All of the following are true about hydroxyurea except: ***(PGI Nov 2014)***
a. Cause myelosuppression
b. Oral bioavailability is very less
c. Used in CML
d. Act as radiosensitizer
e. Used in sickle cell anaemia

105. True about doxorubicin: ***(PGI May 2014)***
a. Antineoplastic drug
b. Alkylating agent
c. Topoisomerase III inhibitor
d. Anthracycline antibiotic
e. Cardiotoxic

106. Side effect of cisplatin is/are: ***(PGI May 2014)***
a. Ototoxic
b. Nephrotoxic
c. Cardiotoxic
d. Neurotoxic
e. Retinopathy

107. Which of the following is/are small molecule tyrosine kinase inhibitor: ***(PGI Nov 2013)***
a. Sirolimus
b. Imatinib
c. Erlotinib
d. Nilotinib
e. Bevaclizumab

108. Alkylating agent(s) is/are: ***(PGI May 2012)***
a. Methotrexate
b. Busulfan
c. Doxorubicin
d. Daunorubicin
e. Chlorambucil

109. Toxicity of MOPP regimen for Hodgkin's disease includes: ***(PGI Nov 2011)***
a. Sterility
b. Bone hyperplasia
c. Sensory & motor neuropathy
d. Cardiotoxicity
e. Secondary malignancy

110. True statement regarding anticancer drugs: ***(PGI Nov 2011)***
a. Bleomycin chelate Zn
b. Doxorubicin- nephrotoxicity is main adverse effect
c. Vincristine is more myelotoxic while vinblastine is more neurotoxic
d. Acrolein is toxic form of Cyclophosphamide
e. Pentostatin- inhibit adenosine deaminase

111. Drugs used in chemotherapy induced nausea and vomiting: ***(PGI Nov 2010)***
a. Dexamethasone
b. Ondansetron
c. Palonosetrone
d. Mitoxantrone
e. Metoclopramide

112. Epilation agents are: ***(PGI Nov 2010)***
a. Methotrexate
b. Vincristine
c. 5-FU
d. Cisplatin
e. Adriamycin

113. Antifolate cancer drugs are: ***(PGI Nov 2009)***
a. Methotrexate
b. Azathioprine
c. Cyclosporin
d. Vincristne
e. Cisplatin

114. Which of the following statement(s) is/are true regarding anticancer drugs: ***(PGI Nov 2009)***
a. Cell cycle non specific agents- can act on any phase of cycle including G0
b. Mitosis during cell division – devoted to DNA replication
c. No mitotic activity –G0 phase
d. Cytarbine act on S phase of cell cycle
e. Cyclophosphamide is cell cycle specific

115. Alkylating agent(s) is/are: ***(PGI June 2009)***
a. Isosfamide
b. Chlorambucil
c. Paclitaxel
d. Nitrosoureas
e. Cytarabine

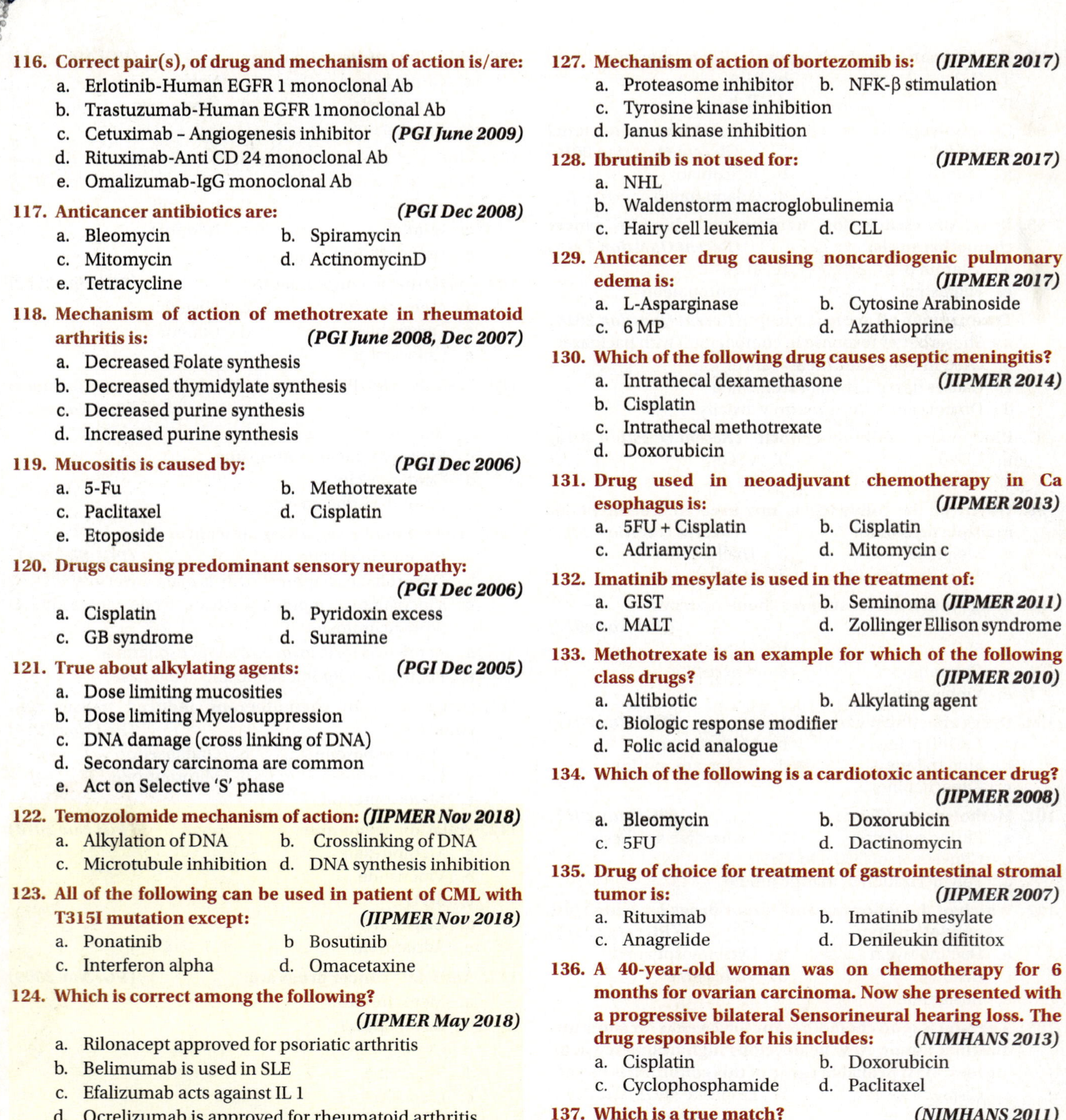

116. Correct pair(s), of drug and mechanism of action is/are: *(PGI June 2009)*
a. Erlotinib-Human EGFR 1 monoclonal Ab
b. Trastuzumab-Human EGFR 1monoclonal Ab
c. Cetuximab – Angiogenesis inhibitor
d. Rituximab-Anti CD 24 monoclonal Ab
e. Omalizumab-IgG monoclonal Ab

117. Anticancer antibiotics are: *(PGI Dec 2008)*
a. Bleomycin b. Spiramycin
c. Mitomycin d. ActinomycinD
e. Tetracycline

118. Mechanism of action of methotrexate in rheumatoid arthritis is: *(PGI June 2008, Dec 2007)*
a. Decreased Folate synthesis
b. Decreased thymidylate synthesis
c. Decreased purine synthesis
d. Increased purine synthesis

119. Mucositis is caused by: *(PGI Dec 2006)*
a. 5-Fu b. Methotrexate
c. Paclitaxel d. Cisplatin
e. Etoposide

120. Drugs causing predominant sensory neuropathy: *(PGI Dec 2006)*
a. Cisplatin b. Pyridoxin excess
c. GB syndrome d. Suramine

121. True about alkylating agents: *(PGI Dec 2005)*
a. Dose limiting mucosities
b. Dose limiting Myelosuppression
c. DNA damage (cross linking of DNA)
d. Secondary carcinoma are common
e. Act on Selective 'S' phase

122. Temozolomide mechanism of action: *(JIPMER Nov 2018)*
a. Alkylation of DNA b. Crosslinking of DNA
c. Microtubule inhibition d. DNA synthesis inhibition

123. All of the following can be used in patient of CML with T315I mutation except: *(JIPMER Nov 2018)*
a. Ponatinib b Bosutinib
c. Interferon alpha d. Omacetaxine

124. Which is correct among the following? *(JIPMER May 2018)*
a. Rilonacept approved for psoriatic arthritis
b. Belimumab is used in SLE
c. Efalizumab acts against IL 1
d. Ocrelizumab is approved for rheumatoid arthritis

125. Axicabtagene ciloleucel is used in: *(JIPMER May 2018)*
a. Relapsed myeloma b. T cell lymphoma
c. Diffuse large B cell lymphoma
d. Small cell lung Ca

126. A new drug approved for treatment of FLT-3 mutation AML is: *(JIPMER 2017)*
a. Midostaurin b. Nivolumab
c. Cabozantinib d. Dupilumab

127. Mechanism of action of bortezomib is: *(JIPMER 2017)*
a. Proteasome inhibitor b. NFK-β stimulation
c. Tyrosine kinase inhibition
d. Janus kinase inhibition

128. Ibrutinib is not used for: *(JIPMER 2017)*
a. NHL
b. Waldenstorm macroglobulinemia
c. Hairy cell leukemia d. CLL

129. Anticancer drug causing noncardiogenic pulmonary edema is: *(JIPMER 2017)*
a. L-Asparginase b. Cytosine Arabinoside
c. 6 MP d. Azathioprine

130. Which of the following drug causes aseptic meningitis? *(JIPMER 2014)*
a. Intrathecal dexamethasone
b. Cisplatin
c. Intrathecal methotrexate
d. Doxorubicin

131. Drug used in neoadjuvant chemotherapy in Ca esophagus is: *(JIPMER 2013)*
a. 5FU + Cisplatin b. Cisplatin
c. Adriamycin d. Mitomycin c

132. Imatinib mesylate is used in the treatment of: *(JIPMER 2011)*
a. GIST b. Seminoma
c. MALT d. Zollinger Ellison syndrome

133. Methotrexate is an example for which of the following class drugs? *(JIPMER 2010)*
a. Altibiotic b. Alkylating agent
c. Biologic response modifier
d. Folic acid analogue

134. Which of the following is a cardiotoxic anticancer drug? *(JIPMER 2008)*
a. Bleomycin b. Doxorubicin
c. 5FU d. Dactinomycin

135. Drug of choice for treatment of gastrointestinal stromal tumor is: *(JIPMER 2007)*
a. Rituximab b. Imatinib mesylate
c. Anagrelide d. Denileukin difititox

136. A 40-year-old woman was on chemotherapy for 6 months for ovarian carcinoma. Now she presented with a progressive bilateral Sensorineural hearing loss. The drug responsible for his includes: *(NIMHANS 2013)*
a. Cisplatin b. Doxorubicin
c. Cyclophosphamide d. Paclitaxel

137. Which is a true match? *(NIMHANS 2011)*
a. Carmustine-Alkylator
b. Etoposide-Anitumor antibiotic
c. Vincristine-Alkylator d. Cisplatin-Antimetabolite

138. Which one of the following is not correct about adverse effects of anticancer drugs? *(NIMHANS 2010)*
a. Daunorubicin-Cardiotoxicity
b. Bleomycin-Pulmonar fibrosis
c. Cisplatin-Hepatotoxicity
d. Vincristine-Neuropathy

Practice Questions & Answers from 139 to 168 are given at the end of the chapter.

Answers with Explanations to Multiple Choice Questions

1. Ans. (b) Alkylating agents

(Ref: Harrison 19th E/P417)

- Most common cause of agranulocytosis is iatrogenic i.e. drug induced.
- Most common drugs causing agranulocytosis are anticancer drugs which inhibit cell cycle like alkylating agents and antimetabolites like methotrexate, 5-FU and 6-MP.

2. Ans. (a) Chlorambucil

(Ref: Goodman Gilman 12th E/P1684

Severity of nausea and vomiting with anticancer drugs

Maximum	Minimum
Cisplatin (most emetogenic)	**Chlorambucil**
Carmustine	Busulfan
Anthracyclines	Bleomycin
High dose cyclophosphamide	Fludarabine
Dacarbazine	Vinka alkaloids
Mechlorethamine	Monoclonal antibodies

3. Ans. (b) Less neurotoxic than cyclophosphamide

(Ref: Goodman Gilman 12th E/P1682

- Ifosfamide is the most neurotoxic alkylating agent, which is caused by the metabolite chloracetyldehyde.
- Neurotoxicity presents as seizures, ataxia and coma.

4. Ans. (a) Cyclophosphamide

(Ref: Goodman Gilman 12th E/P1683)

- Hemorrhagic cystitis is caused by ifosfamide (at normal doses) > Cyclophosphamide(at high doses only).
- Mesna is used for prophylaxis of hemorrhagic cystitis.

5. Ans. (d) Mesna

(Ref: Goodman Gilman 12th E/P1684)

Mesna for prophylaxis of hemorrhagic cystitis

- The dose of mesna is 60% of ifosfamide dose (if ifosfamide dose is 100 mg, then cyclophosphamide dose will be 60 mg), given in 3 divided doses.
- First 20% dose is given along with ifosfamide by bolus IV route.
- Second and third 20% dose can be given by IV route (after 4 and 8 hours) or oral route (after 2 and 6 hours) only if ifosfamide dose is ≤ 2 g/m².

6. Ans. (a) Cisplatin

(Ref: Goodman Gilman 12th E/P1689

7. Ans. (a) Alkylating agents

(Ref: Goodman Gilman 12th E/P1683

Alkylating Agents			
Nitrogen Mustards	**Nitrosoureas**	**Methylating Agents**	**Miscellaneous**
Cyclophosphamide Ifosfamide Mechlorethamine Chlorambucil Melphalan Bendamustine	Carmustine Lemustine Semustine Streptozocin	Procarbazine Dacarbazine Temozolomide	Busulfan Altretamine Thiotepa Trabectedin

8. Ans. (c) Cisplatin

(Ref: Goodman Gilman 12th E/P1689

Drugs Causing Secondary Leukemia

Alkylating agents
Platinum compounds
Topoisomerase II inhibitors (Etoposide)
Mitoxantrone
6-MP
Fludarabine

9. Ans. (a) Cisplatin

(Ref: Goodman Gilman 12th E/P1689

Cisplatin Toxicity

- Nephrotoxicity
- Ototoxicity
- Neurotoxicity\
- Most emetogenic

10. Ans. (c) Carmustine

(Ref: Goodman Gilman 12th E/P1686

Sustained neutropenia is seen with:

- Carmustine
- Lemustine
- Semustine

11. Ans. (a) 100

(Ref: Goodman Gilman 12th E/P1689)

12. Ans. (d) Lung cancer

(Ref: Goodman Gilman 12th E/P1689)

13. Ans. (c) < 7 years

(Ref: Goodman Gilman 12th E/P1682)

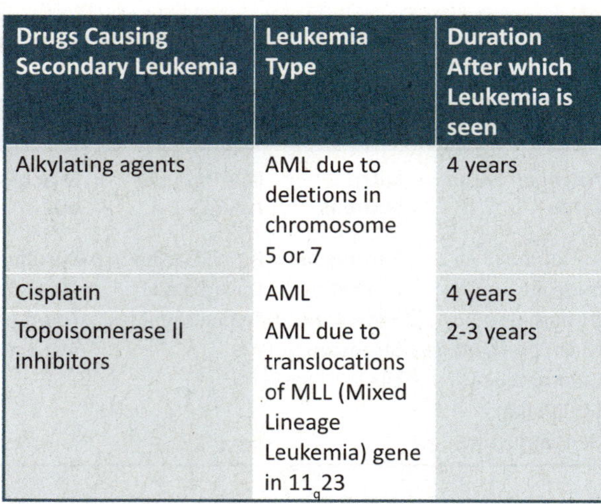

Drugs Causing Secondary Leukemia	Leukemia Type	Duration After which Leukemia is seen
Alkylating agents	AML due to deletions in chromosome 5 or 7	4 years
Cisplatin	AML	4 years
Topoisomerase II inhibitors	AML due to translocations of MLL (Mixed Lineage Leukemia) gene in 11_q23	2-3 years

14. Ans. (c) Mitomycin C

(Ref: Goodman Gilman 12th E/P1718)

Hemolytic uremic syndrome
- Mitomycin-C
- Gemcitabine

15. Ans. (a) Inhibits DNA-dependent RNA synthesis

(Ref: Goodman Gilman 12th E/P1712

- Actinomycin binds with DNA and drug DNA complex inhibits DNA polymerase.
- Thus it inhibits DNA dependent RNA synthesis.

16. Ans. (a) Vacuolar degeneration of the myofibrils

(Ref: Goodman Gilman 12th E/P1714

Electron microscopy features of doxorubicin cardiotoxicity
- Vacuolar degeneration of myofibrils
- Mitochondrial changes

17. Ans. (c) Dilated cardiomyopathy

(Ref: Goodman Gilman 12th E/P1714

Doxorubicin cardiotoxicity
- **Acute:** Pericarditis-myocarditis syndrome, arrhythmia and ST and T wave changes in ECG.
- **Chronic:** Dilated cardiomyopathy

18. Ans. (a) Cisplatin

(Ref: Goodman Gilman 12th E/P1689

19. Ans. (b) Bleomycin

(Ref: Goodman Gilman 12th E/P1717

Anticancer drugs causing pulmonary fibrosis
- Bleomycin
- Busulfan
- Other alkylating agents like temozolomide

20. Ans. (b) Procarbazine

(Ref: Goodman Gilman 12th E/P1687

Side Effects of procarbazine
- Disulfiram like reaction
- Neurotoxicity
- Bone marrow suppression
- Cheese reaction

21. Ans. (d) Etoposide

(Ref: Goodman Gilman 12th E/P1682

22. Ans. (a) Carmustine

(Ref: Goodman Gilman 12th E/P1686

Nitrosoureas
Carmustine
Lemustine
Semustine
Streptozocin

23. Ans. (a) Bleomycin

(Ref: Goodman Gilman 12th E/P1717)

- Colchicine inhibits microtubules and is used for treatment of acute gout due to its anti-inflammatory effect.
- Paclitaxel and vincristine are Ans. (M) phase specific drugs which act on microtubules.

24. Ans. (c) Doxorubicin

(Ref: Goodman Gilman 12th E/P1714)

Cardiotoxic anticancer drugs
- Anthracyclines (Maximum with doxorubicin and daunorubicin)
- Trastuzumab
- High dose cyclophosphamide

25. Ans. (a) Alkylating agent

(Ref: Goodman Gilman 12th E/P1682)

26. Ans. (c) Cardiotoxicity

(Ref: Goodman Gilman 12th E/P1714)

27. Ans. (a) Azathioprine

(Ref: Goodman Gilman 12th E/P1712-16)

- Azathioprine is a prodrug of anticancer drug 6-MP used as an immunodmodulator.

28. Ans. (c) Cladribine

(Ref: Goodman Gilman 12th E/P1682)

29. Ans. (a) Bleomycin

(Ref: Goodman Gilman 12th E/P1682)

30. Ans. (d) All of the above

(Ref: Goodman Gilman 12th E/P1682)

31. Ans. (b) Akylating agent

(Ref: Goodman Gilman 12th E/P1682)

32. Ans. (d) Cisplatin

(Ref: Goodman Gilman 12th E/P1689)

Cisplatin is first-line drug in urogenital cancers:

- Bladder cancer
- Ovary cancer
- Testicular cancer
- Cervical cancer

33. Ans. (c) Cisplatin

(Ref: Goodman Gilman 12th E/P1689)

Cisplatin is most widely used anticancer drug because of its huge spectrum of activity. It is first-line drug in

- GIT cancers
- Lung cancer
- Urogenital cancers
- Head and neck cancer

34. Ans. (d) Mitomycin

(Ref: Goodman Gilman 12th E/P1718)

Hemolytic uremic syndrome is seen with:

- Mitomycin
- Gemcitabine

35. Ans. (d) Busulfan

(Ref: Goodman Gilman 12th E/P1685)

Anticancer drugs causing pulmonary fibrosis:

- Bleomycin: Most common cause
- Alkylating agents like busulfan and temozolomide

36. Ans. (d) Cisplatin

(Ref: Goodman Gilman 12th E/P1689)

Cell cycle specific anticancer drugs

37. Ans. (a) Bleomycin

(Ref: Goodman Gilman 13th E/P1193)

- Bleomycin is metabolized by bleomycin hydrolase in human body. This enzyme is present in lesser quantity in lungs and skin, which causes more toxicity in these organs.
- This presents as flagellate dermatitis and pulmonary fibrosis.

38. Ans. (a) Vincristine + etoposide + carboplatin

(Ref: Nelson 19th E/P1769)

39. Ans. (b) Dihydropyrimidine dehydrogenase

(Ref: Goodman Gilman 13th E/P1182)

- 5FU is metabolized by dihydropyrimidine dehydrogenase in liver and other tissues including tumor cells.
- Deficiency of this enzyme in patients can lead to a decreased metabolism and increased toxicity of 5FU like severe diarrhoea and shock leading to death as well.
- Deficiency of this enzyme can be diagnosed in lymphocytes by assays or by comparing ratio of 5FU to its metabolite in plasms.

40. Ans. (a) Paclitaxel

(Ref: Goodman Gilman 12th E/P1707)

- Paclitaxel acts on microtubules and hence is an M phase specific drug.
- Daunorubicin an antitumor antibitotic inhibits G2 and S phase.
- Etoposide and topotecan are S phase inhibitors and hence automatically G2 phase is inhibited which comes after S phase.

41. Ans. (b) Causes stabilization of microtubules

(Ref: Goodman Gilman 12th E/P1707)

- Paclitaxel stimulates β-tubulin and promotes microtubule polymerization.
- The source of paclitaxel was yew tree, but as the source is limited, now a days paclitaxel is synthesized by genetic engineering in E.coli.

42. Ans. (b) Folic acid and vitamin B12

(Ref: Goodman Gilman 12th E/P1689)

- Bone marrow suppression is more severe with pemetrexed and hence apart from leucovorin or folic acid, an injection of vitamin B12 is given with the first dose of pemetrexed.

43. Ans. (c) Sickle cell anemia

(Ref: Goodman Gilman 12th E/P1693)

Uses of Methotrexate

Neoplastic Uses (Due to Inhibition of DNA Synthesis)	Non Neoplastic Uses (Due to Inhibition of Purine Synthesis)
Choriocarcinoma: Drug of choice **Osteosarcoma**: High doses of methotrexate with leucovorin rescue Non-Hodgkin) s lymphoma ALL: For remission and consolidation	**Rheumatoid arthritis**: DMARD of choice **Ectopic pregnancy**: Used with misoprostol **GVHD** Psoriasis Multiple sclerosis Wegener) s granulomatosis Crohn) s disease

44. Ans. (a) Hydroxyurea

(Ref: Goodman Gilman 12th E/P1721)

Uses of hydroxyurea

- Sickle cell anemia
- Essential thrombocythemia
- Polycythemia vera
- CML

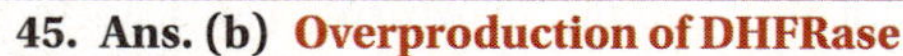

45. Ans. (b) Overproduction of DHFRase

(Ref: Goodman Gilman 12th E/P1692)

Resistance mechanisms of methotrexate related to DHFR

- DHFR enzyme induction
- DHFR gene amplification: Increases DHFR synthesis
- DHFR gene mutation: Alters structure of DHFR

46. Ans. (a) Methotrexate

(Ref: Goodman Gilman 12th E/P1694)

- Methotrexate is absolutely contraindicated in pregnancy due to teratogenic effects.

47. Ans. (b) Cytarabine

(Ref: Goodman Gilman 12th E/P1694)

Neurotoxicity with cytarabine

- Cerebellar toxicity: Ataxia and dysarthria
- Cerebral toxicity: Seizure, dementia and coma

48. Ans. (a) 5-Fluorouracil

(Ref: Goodman Gilman 12th E/P1694)

- 5-FU is metabolized by liver, but mainly excreted by lungs as CO_2.

49. Ans. (a) Methotrexate

(Ref: Goodman Gilman 12th E/P1690)

Antimetabolites

- Antifolate drugs: Methotrexate and Pemetrexed
- Pyrimidine analogs
- Purine analogs

50. Ans. (d) Antimetabolite

(Ref: Goodman Gilman 12th E/P1692)

51. Ans. (b) Mesothelioma

(Ref: Goodman Gilman 12th E/P1691)

52. Ans. (a) Paclitaxel

(Ref: CMDT 2017/P1623)

53. Ans. (b) 5FU

(Ref: Goodman Gilman 12th E/P1695)

54. Ans. (b) Folinic acid

(Ref: Goodman Gilman 12th E/P1694)

- Myelosuppression and mucositis are common side effects seen due to inhibition of DNA synthesis.
- These side effects can be prevented by leucovorin (folinic acid, active form of folic acid) or folic acid.
- Leucovorin or folinic acid is more preferred as compared to folic acid.

55. Ans. (b) Cytarabine

(Ref: Goodman Gilman 12th E/P1700)

- The drug in the question is cytarabine which is metabolized into Ara-CTP, which competitively inhibits DNA polymerase.
- Cerebellar dysfunction including ataxia and dysarthria are seen with cytarabine at high doses or intrathecal use.
- Myelosuppression is the dose limiting t.

56. Ans. (a) Ribonucleotide diphosphate reductase

(Ref: Goodman Gilman 12th E/P1721)

Drugs inhibiting RNR (Ribonucleotide diphosphate reductase)

- Hydroxyurea
- Gemcitabine
- Purine analogues: Fludarabine, cladribine, clofarabine and pentostatin

57. Ans. (c) Pancreatic

(Ref: Goodman Gilman 12th E/P1700)

Drugs used for treatment of pancreatic cancer

- Gemcitabine: Drug of choice
- Streptozocin
- Erlotinib
- Sunitinib
- Everolimus

58. Ans. (b) Vincristine

(Ref: Goodman Gilman 12th E/P1705)

Drugs acting on microtubules

- Vinka alkaloids: Inhibit microtubule polymerization
- Taxanes: Stimulate microtubule polymerization
- Epothilones: Stabilize microtubules
- Estramustine: Inhibits microtubule polymerization

59. Ans. (a) Increased concentrations of intracellular DHFR through gene amplification

(Ref: Goodman Gilman 12th E/P1692)

60. Ans. (d) Vinca alkaloids

(Ref: Goodman Gilman 12th E/P1690)

61. Ans. (b) Vincristine

(Ref: Goodman Gilman 12th E/P1672)

- Vincristine is an Ans. (M) phase specific anticancer drug.

62. Ans. (a) Antimetabolite

(Ref: Goodman Gilman 12th E/P1695)

63. Ans. (d) Mercaptopurine

(Ref: Goodman Gilman 12th E/P1701)

Purine analogs/antagonists:
- 6-MP and 6-TG
- Fludarabine
- Pentostatin
- Cladribine
- Clofarabine

64. Ans. (a) Methotrexate

(Ref: Goodman Gilman 12th E/P1691)

65. Ans. (a) Folinic acid

(Ref: Goodman Gilman 12th E/P1691)

- Folic acid or Folinic acid (leucovorin) can be used to prevent toxicity of antifolate drugs like bone marrow suppression and mucositis.
- Glucarpidase is used with methotrexate in case of renal impairement, as it metabolizes methotrexate into inactive metabolites excreted by liver.

66. Ans. (a) Methotrexate

(Ref: Goodman Gilman 12th E/P1693)

Drugs used for choriocarcinoma
- Methotrexate: Drug of choice
- Actinomycin D

67. Ans. (c) Cytarabine

(Ref: Goodman Gilman 12th E/P1701-04)

- Cytarabine is a pyrimidine analogue.

68. Ans. (a) Inhibit dihydrofolate reductase

(Ref: Goodman Gilman 12th E/P1690)

69. Ans. (a) 6-mercaptopurine

(Ref: Goodman Gilman 12th E/P1702)

Hepatotoxic anticancer drugs
- 6-MP, 6-TG
- Methotrexate
- BCR-ABL TK inhibitors (Imatinib, dasatinib, nilotinib)
- Dacarbazine
- Busulfan

70. Ans. (a) Vincristine

(Ref: Goodman Gilman 12th E/P1706)

ABVD regimen for Hodgkin) s disease

A: Adriamycin

B: Bleomycin

V: Vinblastine

D: Dacarbazine

71. Ans. (b) Vincristine

(Ref: Goodman Gilman 12th E/P1706)

Anticancer drugs causing neuropathy
- M phase specific drugs
  - Vinka alkaloids: Vincristine > Vinorelbine > Vinblastine
  - Taxanes: Nab paclitaxel > Paclitaxel
  - Epothilones: Ixabepilone
- Platinum compounds: Cisplatin and Oxaliplatin
- Pyrimidine analogs: Fludarabine and Nelarabine

72. Ans. (a) Synthesis of monoclonal antibodies

(Ref: Manfred's Pharmacology 3rd E/P306)

- The given diagram is known as hybridoma technique for development of monoclonal antibodies.
- An antigen is injected to mouse against which B-lymphocytes in spleen produces antibodies.
- These B lymphocyte cells (spleen cells in diagram) are collected and fused with myeloma cells; the fused cells being known as hybridomas.
- These hybridomas are allowed to divide and produce antibodies.

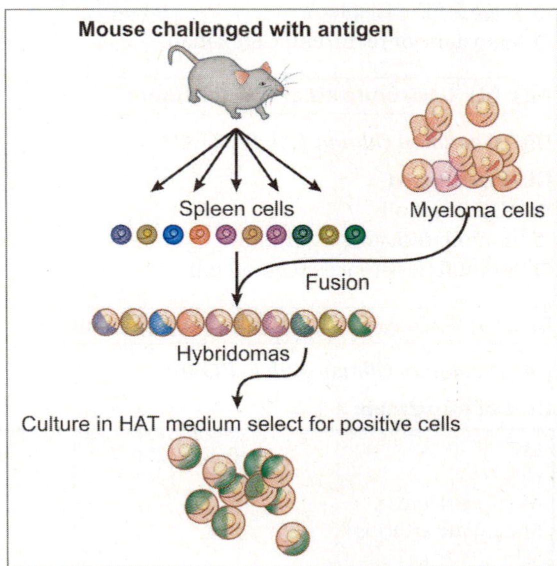

73. Ans. (a) Dexamethasone

(Ref: Harrison 19th E/1686-87)

- Patient of APML when treated with retinoic acid can develop pulmonary syndrome charcetrized by fever, dyspnea, pulmonary infiltrates, chest pain, fluid retention and hypoxemia.
- The treatment of choice for same is dexamethasone.

74. Ans. (a) Has dose-independent pharmacokinetics

(Ref: Goodman Gilman 12th E/P1746, Monoclonal Antibodies Pharmacokinetics and Pharmacodynamics: Wang W, Wang EQ, Balthasar JP)

Metabolism and elimination of monoclonal antibodies
- Most of the MABs are eliminated by receptor mediated endocytosis (intracellular uptake by the receptors on which they act) followed by intracellular catabolism. Hence as the dose will increase receptor saturation will gradually decrease uptake of drug and elimination, which

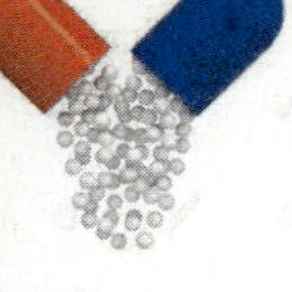

is known as non-linear/first order/dose dependent elimination kinetics. E.g. Rituximab, trastuzumab, gemtuzumab, panitumumab etc.

- However only few MAbs are removed by phagocytosis and hence they display linear/zero order/dose independent elimination kinetics. E.g. Omalizumab and denosumab.

75. Ans. (c) Bone marrow suppression

(Ref: Harrison 19th E/103e-23)

- Most common side effect: Nausea and vomiting.
- Most common dose limiting toxicity: Bone marrow suppression.

76. Ans. (a) Palliation in head and neck cancer

(Ref: Goodman Gilman 12th E/P1736)

Head and neck cancer treatment

- TOC: 5-FU + Cisplatin
- Metastatic or recurrent: Cetuximab

77. Ans. (d) Gastrointestinal stromal tumor

(Ref: Goodman Gilman 12th E/P1732)

GIST treatment

- DOC: Imatinib
- Imatinib resistance: Sunitinib
- Sunitinib resistance: Regorafenib

78. Ans. (b) Paroxysmal nocturnal hemoglobinuria

(Ref: Goodman Gilman 12th E/P1746)

Uses of Rituximab:

CLL
NHL
Multiple sclerosis
Rheumatic arthritis
SLE
Autoimmune haemolytic anemia

79. Ans. (b) It is a monoclonal antibody produced by injecting her-2 antigen

(Ref: Goodman Gilman 12th E/P1737)

- Trastuzumab and pertuzumab are anti Her-2 monoclonal antibodies produced by injecting Her-2 antigen.

80. Ans. (c) Blocks chimeric fusion of bcr-abl

(Ref: Goodman Gilman 12th E/P1732)

- Imatinib is a bcr-abl tyrosine kinase inhibitor.
- It is drug of choice for treatment of CML and GIST.

81. Ans. (a) Tyrosine kinase

(Ref: Goodman Gilman 12th E/P1732)

82. Ans. (a) Aprepitant

(Ref: Goodman Gilman 12th E/P1814)

83. Ans. (a) Trastuzumab

(Ref: Goodman Gilman 13th E/P1209)

84. Ans. (b) 40 IU/Kg

(Ref: WHO)

Dose of immunogobuin in rabies

- Human series – 40 IU/Kg
- Equine series - 20 IU/Kg

85. Ans. (d) Bortezomib

(Ref: CMDT 2017/P1622)

86. Ans. (a) Blood pressure

(Ref: Goodman Gilman 12th E/P1345)

Dronabinol has central sympathomimetic action which causes

- Tachycardia
- Hypotension: BP should be monitored.

87. Ans. (a) Imatinib

(Ref: Goodman Gilman 12th E/P1732)

CML treatment

- DOC: Imatinib
- Imatinib resistance: Nilotinib, Bosutinib, Ponatinib, Dasatinib
- Multi TK resistance: Omacetaxine

88. Ans. (d) Lapatinib

(Ref: Goodman Gilman 12th E/P1737)

- Lapatinib is a dual TK inhibitor i.e. Her-1 (EGFR) and Her-2.

89. Ans. (d) Amifostine

(Ref: Harrison 19th E/P622)

- Amifostine is primarily a radioprotectant, that acts by scavenging free radicals and by protecting and repairing DNA.
- Apart from radioprotective indication it is also approved by FDA to prevent nephrotoxicity associated with cisplatin.

90. Ans. (c) Renal cell carcinoma

(Ref: Goodman Gilman 12th E/P1739)

DOC for renal cell cancer

- Bevacizumab

  Or
- Sunitinib

91. Ans. (a) Anti-VEGF antibody

(Ref: Goodman Gilman 12th E/P1732)

Anti VEGFR antibodies:

- Bevacizumab
- Ranibizumab
- Ramucirumab

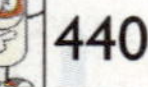

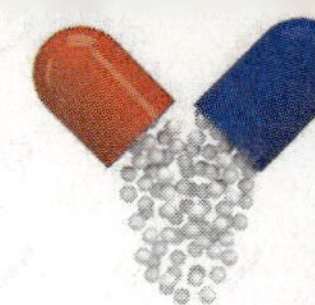

92. Ans. (a) Imatinib and sunitinib

(Ref: Goodman Gilman 12th E/P1732)

93. Ans. (c) IL-6

(Ref: Harrison 19th E/P2147)

- Lapatinib is IL-6 antagonist approved for treatment of rheumatoid arthritis.

94. Ans. (a) Trastuzumab

(Ref: Goodman Gilman 12th E/P1737)

95. Ans. (c) Filgrastim

(Ref: CMDT 2015/P1647)

- Neutropenia and opportunistic infections can be commonly associated with anticancer therapy.
- Drug of choice to prevent neutropenia is filgrastim.

96. Ans. (c) Causes upregulation of Her2/neu

(Ref: Goodman Gilman 12th E/P1737)

97. Ans. (a) CD20

(Ref: Goodman Gilman 12th E/P1745)

98. Ans. (d) Methotrexate

(Ref: Harrison 19th E/P716)

Drugs used in multiple myeloma:

- Lenalidomide along with dexamethasone is the treatment of choice for multiple myeloma. Thalidomide though can be used, is less preferred than lenalidomide.
- Bortezomib is used in case of resistant cases.
- Melphalan is less preferred now a days, though it can be used in combination with dexamethasone and newer agents like bortezomib and lenalidomide.

99. Ans. (b) Cisplatin, (d) Vincristine

(Ref: CMDT 2018/P1677-84)

- Most anticancer drugs which act on cell cycle cause bone marrow suppression and it is the most common dose limiting toxicity of anticancer drugs.
- However some anticancer drugs which are bone marrow sparing are
  - Cisplatin
  - Vincristine
  - Bleomycin

100. Ans. (a) Azathioprine, (b) Methotrexate, (c) Fludarabine, (d) 6-Mercaptopurine

(Ref: Goodman Gilman 12th E/P1701-05)

- Purine synthesis is inhibited by purine analog anticancer drugs like
  - 6-Mercaptopurine
  - 6-Thioguanine
  - **Fludarabine**
  - Cladribine
  - Pentostatin
- **Azathioprine** is an immunomodulator, which is a prodrug of 6-Mercaptopurine and hence also inhibits purine synthesis.
- **Methotrexate** inhibits activation of folic acid in to DHFA which is required for purine synthesis and hence it also inhibits purine synthesis.
- Mycophenolate mofetil is an immunomodulator which inhibits purine synthesis by inhibiting inosine monophosphate dehydrogenase.

101. Ans. (a) Purine synthesis, (c) Conversion of DHFA to THFA

Ref: Goodman Gilman 12th E/P1692

- Methotrexate inhibits dihydrofolate reductase (DHFR) and thereby inhibits conversion of DHFA to THFA.
- Since THFA is required for synthesis of purine, methotrexate also inhibits purine synthesis.

102. Ans. (b) Cyclophosphamide, (c) Busulfan, (e) Ifosfamide

(Ref: Goodman Gilman 12th E/P1683)

Gonadotoxicity is maximum with alkylating agents and hence options a, c and e are answers as these are only alkylating agents in options.

103. Ans. (a) Cisplatin

(Ref: Goodman Gilman 12th E/P1689)

104. Ans. (b) Oral bioavailability is less

(Ref: Goodman Gilman 12th E/P1721)

105. Ans. (a) Antineoplastic drug, (d) Anthracycline antibiotic, (e) Cardiotoxic

(Ref: Goodman Gilman 12th E/P1714)

106. Ans. (a) Ototoxic, (b) Nephrotoxic, (d) Neurotoxic

(Ref: Goodman Gilman 12th E/P1689)

107. Ans. (b) Imatinib, (c) Erlotinib, (d) Nilotinib

(Ref: Goodman Gilman 12th E/P1732)

108. Ans. (b) Bususlfan, (e) Chlorambucil

(Ref: Goodman Gilman 12th E/P1682)

109. Ans. (a) Sterility, (c) Sensory & motor neuropathy, (e) Secondary malignancy

(Ref: Goodman Gilman 12th E/P1687)

MOPP regimen

- MOPP is an older regimen used for treatment of Hodgkin)slymphoma, which has been replaced by ABVD regimen.

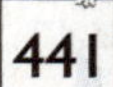

- The drugs in MOPP regimen and their toxicities are
  - Mechlorethamine: Secondary leukemia, sterility
  - Oncovin (Vincristine): Peripheral neuropathy, SIADH
  - Procarbazine: Disulfiram like reaction
  - Prednisolone: Steroid related side effects

110. Ans. (d) Acrolein is toxic form of Cyclophosphamide, (e) Pentostatin-inhibit adenosine deaminase

(Ref: Goodman Gilman 12th E/P1683 and 1704)

111. Ans. (a) Dexamethasone, (b) Ondansetron, (c) Palonosetron, (e) Metoclopramide

(Ref: Goodman Gilman 12th E/P1689)

112. Ans. (e) Adriamycin

(Ref: Harrison 19th E/P103e-25)

Anticancer drugs causing maximum alopecia

- Anthracyclines
- Alkylating agents
- Topoisomerase inhibitors

113. Ans. (a) Methotrexate

(Ref: Goodman Gilman 12th E/P1692)

114. Ans. (a) Cell cycle non specific agents- can act on any phase of cycle including G0, (b) Mitosis during cell division - devoted to DNA replication, (c) No mitotic activity -G0 phase, (d) Cytarbine act on S phase of cell cycle

(Ref: Goodman Gilman 12th E/P1672)

115. Ans. (a) Isosfamide, (b) Chlorambucil, (d) Nitrosoureas

(Ref: Goodman Gilman 12th E/P1682)

116. None

(Ref: Goodman Gilman 12th E/P1732-40)

- Erlotinib: Anti EGFR TK inhibitor
- Trastuzumab: Anti Her-2 MAb
- Cetuximab: Anti EGFR MAb
- Rituximab: Anti CD20 MAb
- Omalizumab: Anti Ig E MAb

117. Ans. (a) Bleomycin, (c) Mitomycin, (d) Actinomycind

(Ref: Goodman Gilman 12th E/P1712)

118. Ans. (c) Decreased purine synthesis

(Ref: Goodman Gilman 12th E/P1693)

Uses of methotrexate

Neoplastic uses (Due to inhibition of DNA Synthesis)	Non neoplastic uses (Due to Inhibition of Purine Synthesis)
Choriocarcinoma: Drug of choice Osteosarcoma: High doses of methotrexate with leucovorin rescue Non-Hodgkin) s lymphoma ALL: For remission and consolidation	Rheumatoid arthritis: DMARD of choice Ectopic pregnancy: Used with misoprostol GVHD Psoriasis Multiple sclerosis Wegener) s granulomatosis Crohn) s disease

119. Ans. (a) 5-Fu, (b) Methotrexate, (c) Paclitaxel

(Ref: CMDT 2015/P1647)

Anticancer Drugs Causing Mucositis

- Alkylating agents
- 5-FU
- Cytarabine
- Paclitaxel
- Methotrexate
- Dactinomycin
- Doxorubicin and daunorubicin
- Hydroxyurea

120. Ans. (a) Cisplatin, (b) Pyridoxin excess

(Ref: Goodman Gilman 12th E/P1689)

Anticancer Drugs Causing Neuropathy

M phase specific drugs
- Vinka alkaloids (Vincristine > Vinorelbine > Vinblastine): Sensory, motor and autonomic or mixed
- Taxanes (Nab paclitaxel > Paclitaxel): Sensory
- Epothilones (Ixabepilone): Sensory

Platinum compounds (Cisplatin and Oxaliplatin: Sensory and motor

Pyrimidine analogs: Fludarabine and Nelarabine

Bortezomib

121. Ans. (a) Dose limiting mucositis, (b) Dose limiting Myelosuppression, (c) DNA damage (cross linking of DNA)

122. Ans. (a) Alkylation of DNA

(Ref: Goodman Gilman 13th E/P1169)

123. Ans. (b) Bosutinib

(Ref: CMDT 2019/P535)

- Imatinib, a BCR-ABL tyrosine kinase inhibitor is the drug of choice for treatment of CML, whereas dasatinib and nilotinib are reserved for treatment of imatinib resistant cases.
- Bosutinib is used in case there is resistance to all above mentioned drugs.
- In case of T315I mutation none of the above mentioned drugs are effective. The drug of choice for such a case is ponatinib.
- Omacetaxine is an inhibitor of bcr-abl protein and is also effective in case of T135I mutation.
- Interferon alpha targets the stem cells and is also effective in case of T135I mutation. It is rarely used now a days in CML.

124. Ans. (b) Belimumab is used in SLE

(Ref: Goodman Gilman 13th E/P649)

- Belimumab is anti-B lymphocyte antibody approved for SLE.

- Rilonacept is an IL-1 approved for CAPS.
- Efalizumab is anti-CD 11a antibody, which was used for treatment of psoriasis. It has been withdrawn from the market due to risk of PML (Progressive Multifocal Leucoencephalopathy)
- Ocrelizumab is approved only for treatment of multiple sclerosis (RRMS and PPMS).

125. Ans. (c) Diffuse large B cell lymphoma

(Ref: FDA)

- Axicabtagene ciloleucel is a CD 19 directed genetically modified autologous T cell immunotherapy approved for treatment of large B cell lymphoma.

126. Ans. (a) Midostaurin

(Ref: https://www.centerwatch.com/drug-information/fda-approved-drugs/drug/100200/rydapt-midostaurin)

Midostaurin is a multikinase inhibitor approved by FDA in 2017 for treatment of four disorders.

- Acute Myelogenous Leukemia (AML) which is FLT-3 mutation positive - Midoastaurin is to be combined with the standard drugs for AML i.e. cytarabine and daunorubicin.
- Aggressive Systemic Mastocytosis (ASM)
- Mast Cell Leukemia
- Systemic mastocytosis with associated hematological neoplasm (SM-AHN)

127. Ans. (a) Proteasome inhibitor

(Ref: Goodman Gilman 12th E/P1742)

- Proteasome is responsible for stimulating cell survival mechanisms by increasing NF-kβ activity. Hence proteasome inhibitors decrease NF-kβ which leads to cell apoptosis.
- Bortezomib and carfilzomib are the drugs in this class, indicated for treatment of drug resistant multiple myeloma and mantle cell lymphoma.
- Most common side effect is thrombocytopenia followed by peripheral neuropathy and fatigue.

128. Ans. (c) Hairy cell leukemia

(Ref: CMDT 2018/P538, 546)

129. Ans. (b) Cytosine arabinoside

(Ref: Nelson's Pulmonary Manifestation of Pulmonary Diseases/P66

Noncardiogenic pulmonary edema can be seen with anticancer drugs like

- Cytarabine (Cytosine arabinoside)
- Methotrexate
- Cyclophosphamide

Uses of ibrutinib

- Chronic lymphocytic leukemia
- Waldenstorm macroglobulinemia - A form of low grade NHL.

130. Ans. (c) Intrathecal methotrexate

(Ref: Goodman Gilman 12th E/P1694)

Intrathecal administration can cause neurotoxicity in the form of

- Arachnoiditis
- Meningismus
- Seizures.

131. Ans. (a) 5FU+Cisplatin

(Ref: Goodman Gilman 12th E/P1689)

132. Ans. (a) GIST

(Ref: Goodman Gilman 12th E/P1734)

133. Ans. (d) Folic acid analogue

(Ref: Goodman Gilman 12th E/P1690)

134. Ans. (b) Doxorubicin

(Ref: Goodman Gilman 12th E/P1714)

135. Ans. (b) Imatinib mesylate

(Ref: Goodman Gilman 12th E/P1734)

136. Ans. (a) Cisplatin

(Ref: Goodman Gilman 12th E/P1689)

137. Ans. (a) Carmustine-Alkylator

(Ref: Goodman Gilman 12th E/P1686)

Carmustine is a nitrosourea group of alkylating agent.

138. Ans. (c) Cisplatin-Hepatotoxicity

(Ref: Goodman Gilman 12th E/P1689)

Practice Questions

139 Which of the following drug is given by rapid IV infusion?
a. Ara-C
b. Mechlorethamine
c. Amphotericin B
d. Cisplatin

Ans. (b) Mechlorethamine

(Ref: Harrison 19th E/P103e-8)

140. Raltitrexed can be used for treatment of:
a. Osteosarcoma
b. Mesothelioma
c. ALL
d. Cutaneous T cell lymphoma

Ans. (d) Cutaneous T cell lymphoma

(Ref: Goodman Gilman 19th E/P1691)

141. A patient of testicular cancer was prescribed ifosfamide at doses of 1200 mg/day for 5 days. What is the dose of mesna that should be given?
a. 1200 mg/day
b. 600 mg/day
c. 300 mg/day
d. 2400 mg/day

Ans. (b) 600 mg/day

(Ref: Goodman Gilman 12th E/P1684)

- Dose of mesna is 60% of the dose of ifosfamide, which comes to 720 mg in this case.
- 600 is the closest option and best answer.

142. Mesna is given for prophylaxis of hemorrhagic cystitis by:
a. Oral route
b. IV route
c. Both
d. None

Ans (c) Both

(Ref: Goodman Gilman 12th E/P1684)

143. Neurotoxicity caused by cisplatin affects:
a. Sensory fibers
b. Motor fibers
c. Autonomic fibers
d. Both a and b

Ans. (d) Both a and b

(Ref: Goodman Gilman 12th E/P1684)

144. Neurotoxicity caused by vincristine affects:
a. Sensory fibers
b. Motor fibers
c. Autonomic fibers
d. All of the above

Ans. (d) All of the above

(Ref: CMDT 2015/P1648)

145. Which of the following drugs can cause trigeminal neuralgia?
a. Cyclophosphamide
b. Methotrexate
c. Vincristine
d. Doxorubicin

Ans. (c) Vincristine

(Ref: CMDT 2015/P1648)

146. Which of the following is a specific drug to prevent chemotherapy induced mucositis?
a. Leucovorin
b. Pyridoxine
c. Palifermin
d. Cobalamin

Ans. (c) Palifermin

(Ref: CMDT 2015/P1646)

147. All of the following drugs can cause alopecia except:
a. Doxorubicin
b. Cyclophosphamide
c. Etoposide
d. Methotrexate

Ans. (d) Methotrexate

(Ref: Harrison 19th E/P103e-11)

148. Regimen of choice for low grade Non-Hodgkin's lymphoma is:
a. CHOP-R
b. MOPP
c. FCR
d. ABVD

Ans. (a) CHOP-R

(Ref: CMDT 2015/P1597)

149. All are used for prevention of chemotherapy induced nausea and vomiting except:
a. Domperidone
b. Dexamethasone
c. Haloperidol
d. Metoclopromide

Ans. (a) Domperidone

(Ref: CMDT 2015/P1645)

150. Which of the following anticancer drug can cause cheese reaction?
a. 5-FU
b. Cyclophosphamide
c. Hydroxyurea
d. Procarbazine

Ans. (d) Procarbazine

(Ref: Harrison 19th E/P103e-9)

151. Coasting effect can be seen with:
a. Methotrexate
b. Doxorubicin
c. Cisplatin
d. L-Asparginase

Ans. (c) Cisplatin

(Ref: Goodman Gilman 19th E/P1689)

152. Cisplatin can be inactivated by which metal:
a. Steel
b. Platinum
c. Aluminium
d. Copper

Ans. (c) Aluminium

(Ref: Goodman Gilman 19th E/P1689)

153. Oxaliplatin has synergism with:
a. Methotrexate b. Leucovorin
c. 5-FU d. Hydroxyurea

Ans. (c) 5-FU

(Ref: Goodman Gilman 19th E/P1690)

154. Leucovorin is given along with 5-FU to:
a. Decrease toxicity b. Increase sensitivity
c. Increase metabolism d. Decrease metabolism

Ans. (b) Increase sensitivity

(Ref: Harrison 19th E/103e-14)

155. AVBD regimen is used for treatment of:
a. NHL b. Hodgkin's disease
c. CLL d. AML

Ans. (b) Hodgkin's disease

(Ref: CMDT 2015/P1597)

156. Which of the following antibiotic can cause secondary leukemia?
a. Doxorubicin b. Daunorubicin
c. Mitoxantrone d. Epirubicin

Ans. (c) Mitoxantrone

(Ref: Harrison 19th E/P103e-13)

157. Cardiotoxicity of doxorubicin can be potentiated by all, except:
a. Trastuzumab b. Cyclophosphamide
c. Radiotherapy d. Methotrexate

Ans. (d) Methotrexate

(Ref: CMDT 2015/P1649)

158. All are used in testicular tumor except:
a. Etoposide b. Cisplatin
c. Mitoxantrone d. Bleomycin

Ans. (c) Mitoxantrone

(Ref: CMDT 2015/P1598)

159. Flagellate dermatitis is a side effect of:
a. Hydroxyurea b. Bleomycin
c. Cisplatin d. Mitoxantrone

Ans. (b) Bleomycin

(Ref: Goodman Gilman 19th E/P1717)

160. Resistance to 5-FU can be seen because of all, except:
a. Thymidilate synthase induction
b. Increased metabolism of 5FU
c. Thymidilate synthase gene amplification
d. Decreased activation of 5-FU

Ans. (a) Thymidilate synthase induction

(Ref: Goodman Gilman 19th E/P1697)

161. When given along with allopurinol, the dose of 6-MP is decreased by
a. 15% b. 25%
c. 50% d. 75%

Ans. (d) 75%

(Ref: Goodman Gilman 19th E/P1702)

162. Bone marrow suppression is not seen with:
a. Vinblastine b. Vincristine
c. Vinorelbine d. Cisplatin

Ans. (b) Vincristine

(Ref: Goodman Gilman 19th E/P1706)

163. Cremophor vehicle is used for injecting:
a. Paclitaxel b. Nab-Paclitaxel
c. Docetaxel d. Cabazitaxel

Ans. (a) Paclitaxel

(Ref: Goodman Gilman 19th E/P1707)

164. Drug of choice for imatinib resistant GIST is:
a. Regorafenib b. Sunitinib
c. Sorafenib d. Axitinib

Ans. (b) Sunitinib

(Ref: Harrison 19th E/P536)

165. Most common side effect of bortezomib is:
a. Myelosuppression b. Neuropathy
c. Mucositis d. Fatigue

Ans. (b) Neuropathy

(Ref: Goodman Gilman 19th E/P1743)

166. Mitotane has selective affinity for cells of:
a. Adrenal medulla b. Adrenal cortex
c. Both d. None

Ans. (b) Adrenal cortex

(Ref: Goodman Gilman 19th E/P1719)

167. Stevens-Johnson syndrome is a side effect of:
a. Rituximab b. Lapatinib
c. Trastuzumab d. Ofatumumab

Ans. (a) Rituximab

(Ref: Goodman Gilman 19th E/P1747)

168. Which of the following is drug of choice for Kaposi sarcoma?
a. Methotrexate
b. Doxorubicin
c. Hydroxyurea
d. IFN alpha

Ans. (b) Doxorubicin

(Ref: CMDT 2015/P1599)

NOTES

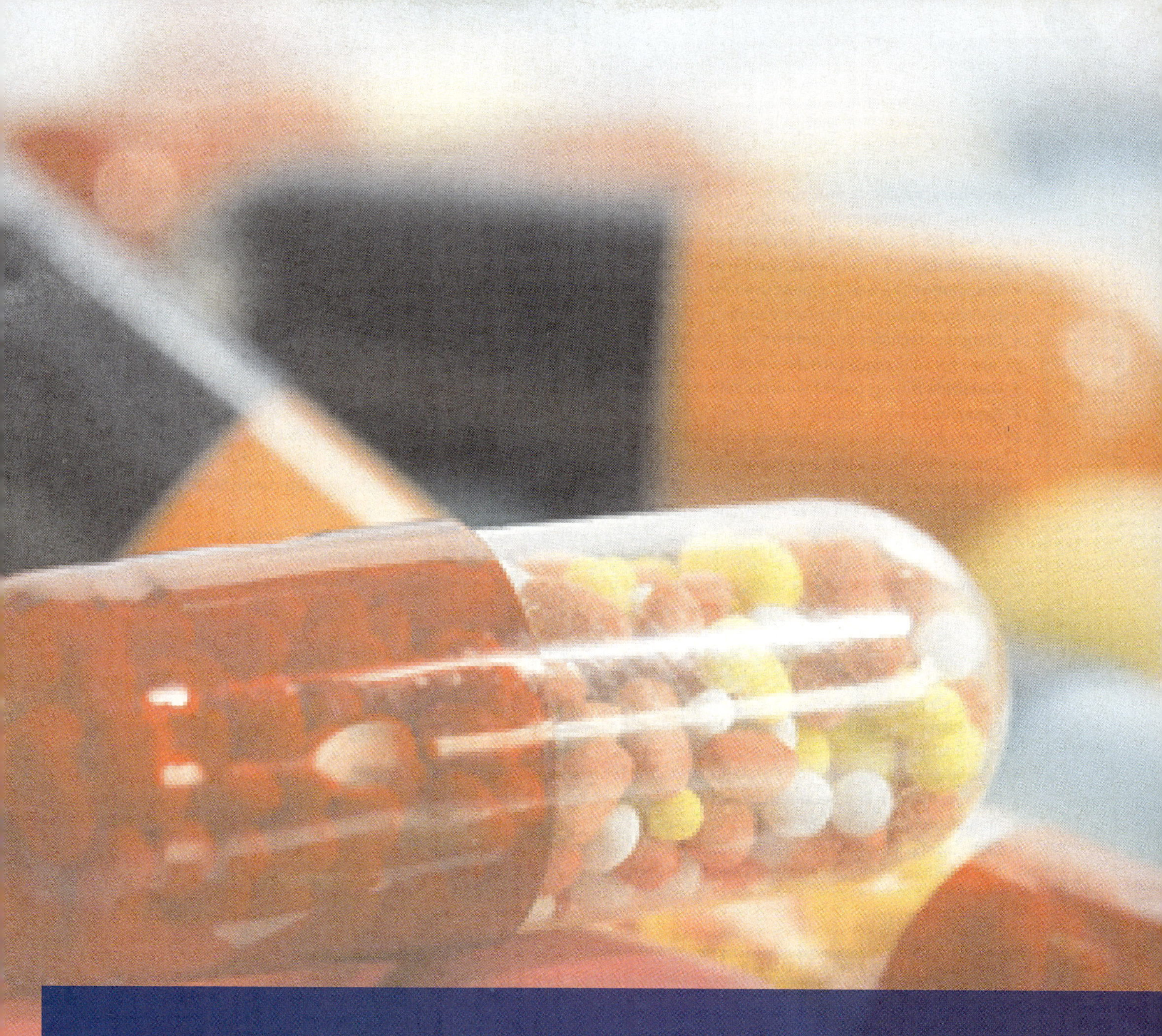

Endocrinology

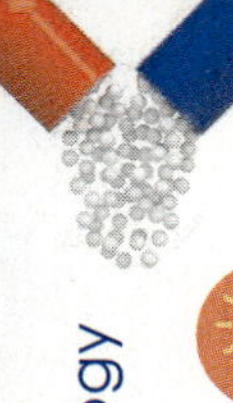

One Liners

- **Acarbose, voglibose and miglitol** are α-glucosidase inhibitors used for treatment of prandial and postprandial hyperglycemia in **type II diabetes mellitus (DM)**.
- **GLP-1 agonists** and **DPP-4 inhibitors** are used only in **type II DM**.
- **Pramlintide** is amylin analog used in both **type I and II DM**.
- **Teduglutide** is a GLP-2 agonist used for the treatment of malabsorption associated with short bowel syndrome.
- **Glulisine, aspart** and **lispro** are ultrashort acting monomeric insulins.
- **Glargine, degludec** and **detemir** are ultralong acting insulins that produce smooth peakless effect.
- Among insulin regular insulin causes maximum, whereas degludec causes minimum hypoglycemia.
- **Glyburide** is most potent whereas **tolbutamide** is least potent sulfonylurea.
- **Repaglinide** and **nateglinide** are meglitinide analogs used in **postprandial hyperglycemia**.
- **Metformin** causes **lactic acidosis** and **vitamin B12 deficiency** and is contraindicated in **renal failure**.
- **Thiazolidinediones like pioglitazone are safest OHAs in renal failure.**
- **Urinary tract infection (UTI)** and **vaginal infections** are the most common side effects associated with **SGLT-2 inhibitors.**
- **Lugol's iodine** is made up of **5% iodine** and **10% KI**.
- **Teriparatide** is the only drug to increase bone formation, whereas **strontium ranelate** is the only drug to both increase drug formation and decrease bone resorption.
- **Bisphosphonates** should be taken with a **full glass of water** and patient should remain upright for at least 30 minutes.
- Bisphosphonates can cause **osteonecrosis of jaw**.
- GNRH agonist like **goserelin** can be used for **advanced prostate cancer**.
- Oral contraceptives (OCP) increases all types of cancer risk except **colon cancer** which decreases.
- **Finasteride** and **dutasteride** are 5-α reductase inhibitors used for treatment of benign prostatic hyperplasia (BPH), hirsutism and androgenic alopecia.
- **Cyproterone, megestrol, flutamide, nilutamide** and **bicalutamide** are androgen receptor antagonists used in prostate cancer and hirsutism.
- **Levonorgestrel, ulipristal** and **IUCD** are preferred for emergency contraception.
- **Dexamethasone** and **betamethasone** are most potent systemic steroids.
- **Fluticasone** is most potent inhalational steroid.
- **Clobetasol propionate** is most potent topical steroid.
- **Dexamethasone, betamethasone** and **triamcinolone** are devoid of mineralocorticoid activity.

DIABETES MELLITUS

GLUCOSE HOMEOSTASIS

- Glucose is consumed in food either as monosaccharide or starch and disaccharide. The latter are metabolized to glucose in intestine by α-glucosidase.
- As glucose is absorbed into epithelial cells of intestine, it stimulates release of **incretin or glucagon like peptide 1 (GLP-1)** even before glucose is absorbed into systemic circulation.
- GLP-1 acts on G_s subtype of G-protein-coupled receptor (GPCR) in beta islet cells of pancreas and releases **insulin** and **amylin**. Insulin acts on insulin receptors and brings the **GLUT-4** receptors outside the cell. The release of insulin by GLP-1 is for very short period, as it is immediately metabolized in plasma by an enzyme **DPP-4**. Amylin delays gastric emptying and induces satiety.
- By this time glucose reaches systemic circulation and is taken up by GLUT-4 receptors of cells. Thus, GLP-1 and amylin prevent **postprandial hyperglycemia**.
- Glucose that is absorbed further to systemic circulation stimulates **GLUT-2** receptors in the beta islet cells and glucose taken up is metabolized to ATP. This ATP inhibits **ATP sensitive K^+ channels**, that leads to depolarization of beta islet cells and an influx of calcium leads to insulin release. As GLUT receptors cause facilitated diffusion of glucose that is concentration dependent, insulin release is proportional to the amount of glucose in systemic circulation.
- Glucose is reabsorbed from kidney by **SGLT-2 receptors** in renal tubules.
- Glycogenolysis and gluconeogenesis are endogenous sources of glucose from liver and muscles, activated in the absence of insulin.
- These steps of glucose homeostasis can be targeted by various drugs as mentioned in the conceptual box.

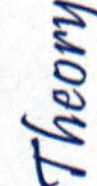

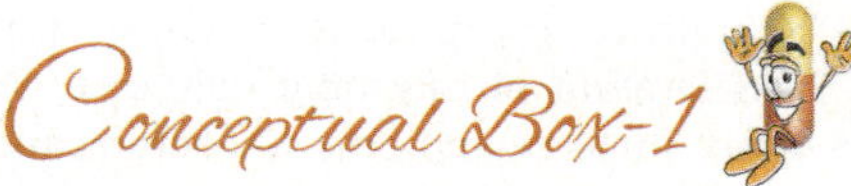

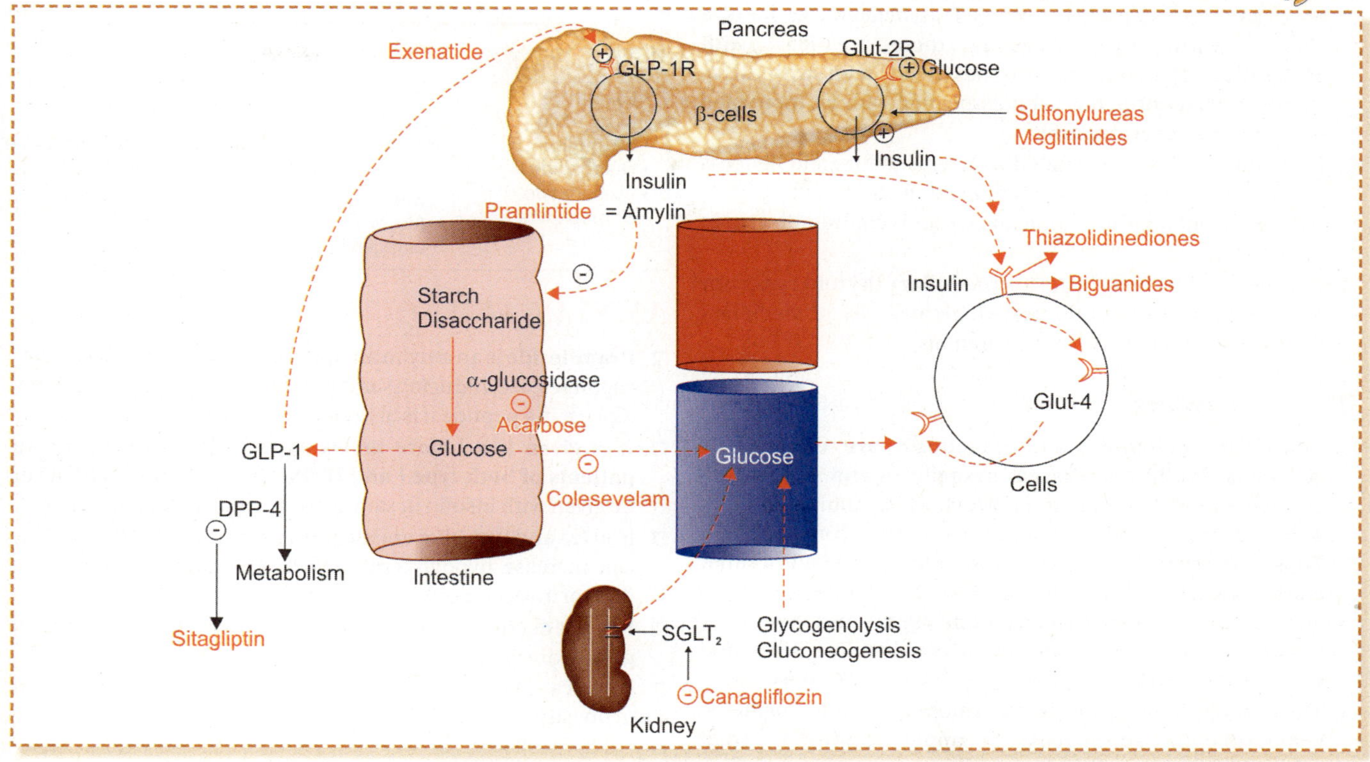

α-GLUCOSIDASE INHIBITORS

- **Acarbose, voglibose and miglitol** are α-glucosidase inhibitors derived from **bacteria**. These **are pseudo carbohydrates** which act by competitively inhibiting α-glucosidase which metabolizes starch and disaccharides in intestine into glucose. Their effect is partially due to stimulation of release of **GLP-1**. They have effect on both **prandial and postprandial hyperglycemia.** The drug is taken along with the food in the beginning of meal.
- These are approved for treatment of **type II DM** as adjunct to diet control and exercise or to other oral hypoglycemic agents.
- Starch and disaccharides upon reaching colon are metabolized by bacteria and generate gas, which causes **most common side effect, i.e. flatulence**. Starch and disaccharides are osmotic and hence can also cause **diarrhea**. These drugs usually **do not cause hypoglycemia,** but can precipitate if combined with insulin or insulin releasing drugs. Hypoglycemia **cannot be corrected by disaccharides like sucrose (table sugar)** as the enzyme α-glucosidase which breaks disaccharides is blocked. Thus, for the treatment of hypoglycemia associated with these drugs monosaccharide **glucose is used**.
- These drugs are absorbed into systemic circulation (maximum with miglitol) and hence dose is decreased in **renal failure** and contraindicated in stage-4 renal failure or creatinine level is >2 mg/dL. These drugs are also contraindicated in patients with inflammatory bowel disease and gastroparesis.
- Absorption of other drugs can be decreased if taken together and hence should be avoided. Plasma concentration of sulphonylureas can be increased by these drugs and hence there is increased risk of hypoglycemia.

GLP-1 RELATED DRUGS

GLP-1 Agonists

- **Exenatide, liraglutide, albiglutide, dulaglutide, lixisenatide** and **semaglutide** are GLP-1 agonists that act by stimulating insulin release, delaying gastric emptying, decreasing glucagon release and inducing satiety. These are approved for **monotherapy or as adjuncts to other oral hypoglycemic agents for treatment of type II DM**. Since these are peptides, they cannot be given by oral route, rather subcutaneous route is preferred.
- **Exenatide** is a natural compound **exendin-4** derived from saliva of Gila monster lizard, whereas **lixisenatide** is a longer acting **analog of exendin-4**. Other drugs in this class are GLP-1 analogs with changes made in amino acid sequence to achieve resistance to DPP-4.
- Exenatide requires BD, liraglutide and lixisenatide OD and albiglutide, dulaglutide and semaglutide are long acting and hence require once weekly dosing.
- **Liraglutide** is also approved for treatment of **obesity**. Liraglutide and semaglutide reduce risk of death associated with cardiovascular disorders, myocardial infarction and stroke.
- **Teduglutide** is a **GLP-2 agonist** used by **subcutaneous route**

to improve absorption in short bowel syndrome. It stimulates proliferation of intestinal epithelial cells. It can cause GIT upset, flu like symptoms and **colon cancer**.

- Most common side effects are GIT associated like **nausea (MC), vomiting and diarrhea**; these are **least with albiglutide**. **Pancreatitis** also has been seen with these agents. **Semaglutide** has been associated with an **increased risk of diabetic retinopathy**.
- Exenatide has been associated with renal failure and hence is contraindicated, if GFR is less than 30 mL/min. Lixisenatide has significant renal excretion and hence is contraindicated in renal failure.
- In patients with family history of **medullary thyroid cancer or MEN II** these are contraindicated, because risk of medullary thyroid cancer has been seen in animals.

DPP-4 Inhibitors

- **Sitagliptin, alogliptin and linagliptin are competitive reversible inhibitors whereas saxagliptin and vildagliptin** are noncompetitive inhibitors, which act by inhibiting DPP-4 and increasing the endogenous GLP-1 concentration. Thus, they increase insulin release, but are devoid of other effects associated with GLP-1 agonists. These are approved as adjuncts to other **oral hypoglycemic agents and insulin** for treatment of type II DM. Since these are chemicals with good oral absorption, they are given by oral route at OD doses.
- These drugs inhibit CD-26 in lymphocytes and might be responsible for an increase in **upper respiratory tract infections** seen.
- Hypersensitivity reactions are seen rarely with this class in the form of anaphylaxis, angioedema, SJS etc.
- Sitagliptin and linagliptin have been associated with **pancreatitis**, saxagliptin > alogliptin with **heart failure** and vildagliptin with **hepatitis**. Severe joint pain can also be seen with these drugs.
- Excretion is primarily by kidney and hence dose should be decreased in **renal impairment, except for linagliptin which is excreted by liver**.
- **Linagliptin** has a high plasma protein binding. **Saxagliptin** is metabolized by microsomal enzymes and can interact with enzyme inducers and inhibitors.
- These are **weight neutral drugs**.

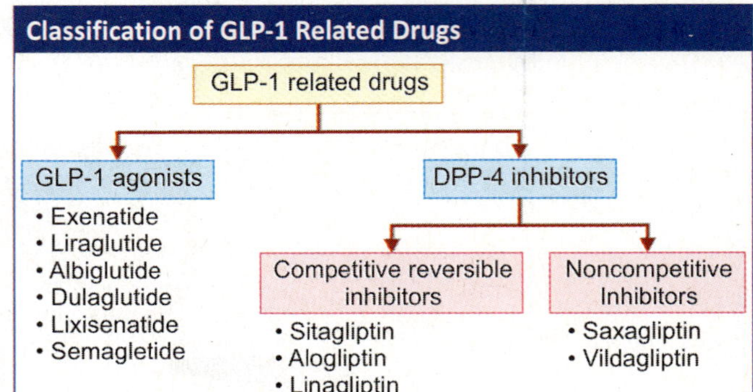

AMYLIN ANALOG

- **Pramlintide** is an amylin analog which acts by decreasing glucagon release, inducing satiety and delaying gastric emptying. Since it is a peptide it is also given by **subcutaneous route**.
- **It is given just before meals as an adjunct to insulin in patients of both type I and II DM**. However, it should never be given with insulin in same syringe, due to difference in pH.
- Nausea and vomiting are the most common side effects. They can increase hypoglycemic effect of insulin and hence the dose of insulin should be reduced by 50%.
- Since it decreases contraction of GIT, it is contraindicated in gastroparesis.
- It can cause weight loss and hence is under trial for treatment of obesity.

INSULIN

- Insulin is the drug of choice for treatment of type I DM, gestational DM and diabetic ketoacidosis. It is also used in type II DM later stages, when most of the beta islet cells have been exhausted. It is used in hyperkalemia as well, where it moves potassium into the cell along with glucose.
- Insulin can be broadly classified on their duration of action into ultrashort acting, short acting, intermediate acting and long acting. Changing the amino acid sequence in human insulin, changes the onset and duration of effect and this is done for synthesis of ultrashort and long-acting insulin. The short and ultrashort acting insulin are used for post-prandial hyperglycemia, whereas intermediate and long-acting are used for maintenance. All insulins are dispensed as clear solutions except **NPH, which is dispensed as turbid white suspension and looks cloudy or milky**.

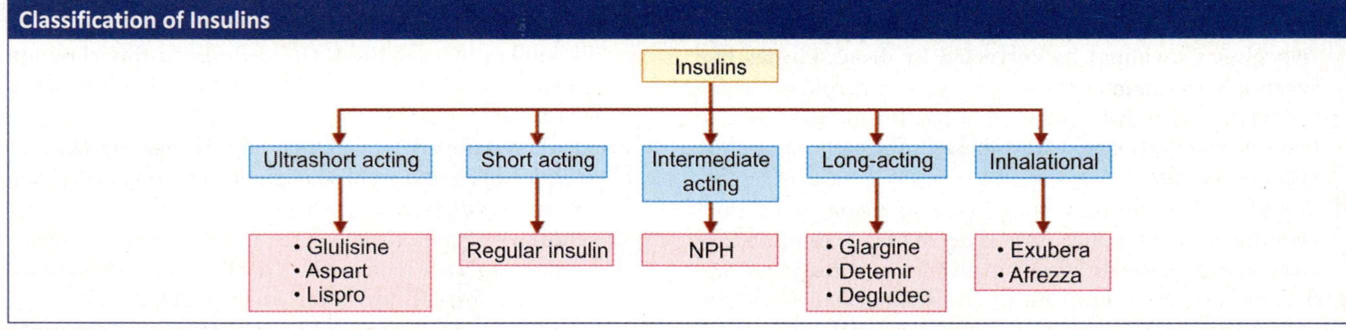

Note: In some classifications ultrashort and short-acting are mentioned as short-acting, long-acting is mentioned as intermediate acting and ultralong acting mentioned as long-acting.

Types of Insulin

Ultra-short-acting

- **Glulisine, aspart and lispro** are **ultra-short-acting insulin** with most rapid onset of action, i.e. within 20 minutes and shortest duration of action, i.e. 4 hours. Thus, these are taken just 20 minutes before meal.
- All are given by subcutaneous route, except **aspart** which can also be given by **intravenous route** for treatment of diabetic ketoacidosis. However, it does not have any advantage over intravenous regular insulin.
- After being injected subcutaneously, they immediately breakdown into monomers and hence also known as **monomeric insulins**. The duration of action does not depend on dose.

Short-acting

- **Regular human insulin** is short-acting with onset of action after 60 minutes, which persists for 6 hours. Thus, regular insulin needs to be taken 60 minutes before meal.
- It is associated with an increased risk of hypoglycemia as compared to ultra-short-acting ones. It can be used by subcutaneous, intramuscular and intravenous route. The duration of action depends on dose.

Intermediate Acting

- **Neutral protamine hagedorn (NPH) or isophane** is an intermediate acting insulin with effect lasting till maximum of 16 hours. It is synthesized by mixing regular insulin with zinc and protamine in a phosphate buffer. The amount of insulin and protamine mixed is same so that neither is present in uncomplexed form or isophane. It is used for the maintenance of blood glucose and given once or twice a day by subcutaneous route. By subcutaneous route **absorption is more from abdomen as compared to limbs**. Unrefrigerated NPH insulin can lose its activity and precipitate or cause **frosting of container** at times.
- **Lente** is intermediate acting insulin invented by Hallas-Moller by combining zinc with insulin, which lead to formation of short-acting amorphous precipitate (semilente) and **long-acting stable crystals (ultralente)**. **Lente** is made by combining 30% semilente with 70% ultralente, which is intermediate acting.

Long-acting

- **Detemir (17 hours), glargine (24 hours) and degludec (42 hours)** are **long-acting insulin**, and degludec being the longest acting. Glargine and degludec require once daily administration at any time of day, whereas detemir requires once or twice daily administration. These are given by subcutaneous route and the site of injection does not alter absorption. These have lesser risk of hypoglycemia as compared to NPH due to their smooth peakless effect. Overall **insulin with least risk of hypoglycemia is degludec** as it has slowest rate of absorption.
- **Glargine** has an acidic pH and hence precipitates in the neutral pH of our body at the injection site; then it is slowly released. Glargine has an acidic pH and hence should not be mixed with other insulin as they have neutral pH; if mixed it forms a **white cloudy precipitate**.
- **Detemir** has a fatty acid side chain that has high binding to albumin at injection site and plasma and hence is long-acting.
- **Degludec** is made by removing the last amino acid threonine from B chain of human insulin and adding hexadecanedioic fatty acid to lysine at B29 position. This causes increased albumin binding and formation of multihexamers at site of injection from which monomers are slowly released. It can be combined with ultra-short-acting insulins like aspart.

Inhalational

- **Afrezza** (technosphere) is inhalational insulin available as powders. Due to rapid onset of action it is taken just before meals for postprandial hyperglycemia. For maintenance basal insulin is also given at loading dose along with these insulins.
- Absorption is rapid with peak plasma insulin level reaching within 15 minutes and then declines to baseline after 3 hours.
- Use and throw color coded cartridges of afrezza are available with 4, 8 and 12 units of insulin.
- The most common associated side effect is cough. Lung cancer has also been reported in some patients. These are contraindicated in smokers and patients of asthma and COPD.

Color Coded Afrezza Cartridges

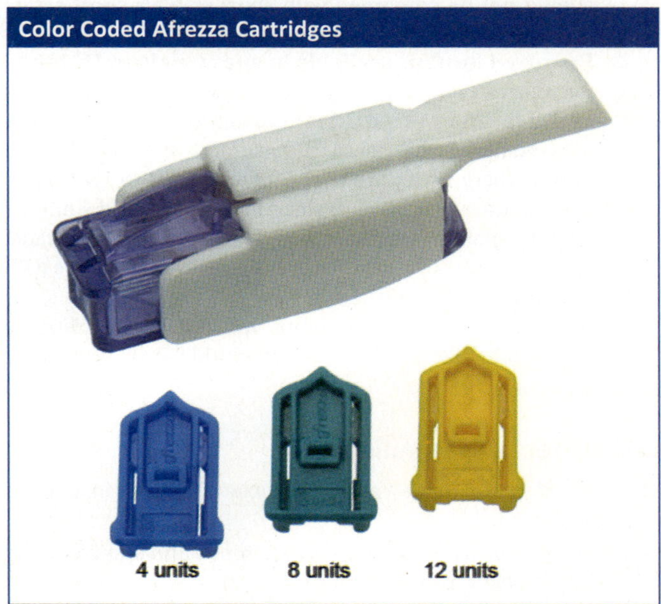

Insulin Administration

- Insulin is injected most commonly in the **abdomen, followed by other sites like anterior thigh, upper buttocks and upper arm**. Absorption for regular insulin is most rapid from abdomen followed by other sites.

Insulin Injection Sites

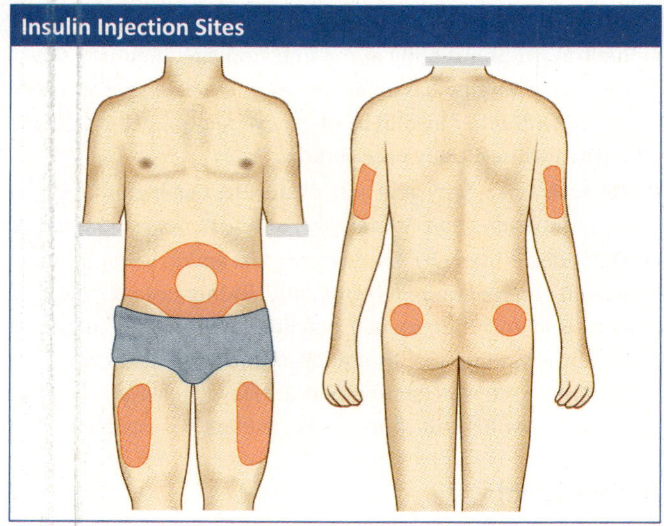

Insulin Induced Lipodystrophy

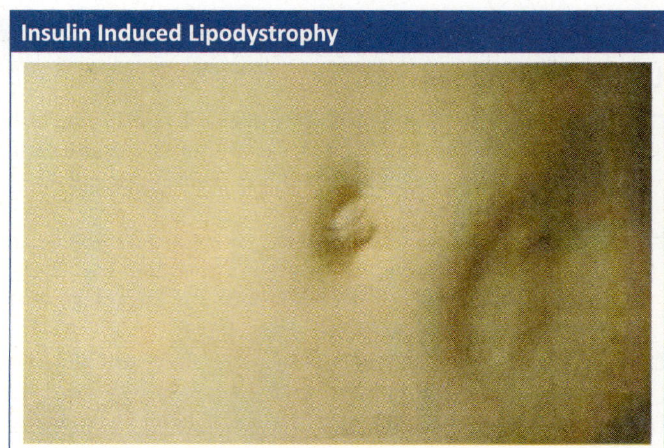

- A patient is administered short or ultra-short-acting insulin for postprandial hyperglycemia and basal insulin (intermediate or long-acting) for maintenance.
- Both these forms of insulin combined and given by three different ways:
  1. **Drawn from different containers in one syringe:** Only NPH can be combined with short and ultra-short acting insulin in one syringe. The short or ultra-short acting is drawn first and then NPH is drawn in syringe and injected.
  2. **Drawn from different containers in different syringe:** Long acting insulin like detemir, glargine and degludec should not be combined with short or ultra-short acting insulins. Hence, they are injected separately.
  3. **Premixed insulins available in one container:** Premixed formulation of 70% NPH and 30% regular insulin is available. However, if NPH and ultra-short-acting ones are premixed the solution becomes unstable. Hence, intermediate acting neutral protamine lispro (NPL) has been synthesized which is mixed with lispro and similarly insulin aspart protamine is mixed with aspart in 70:30 ratio. Among long-acting insulins only degludec is available with aspart in a 70:30 ratio.
- Long-acting insulin combinations with GLP-1 agonists are also available like degludec + liraglutide and glargine + lixisenatide.

Side Effects of Insulin

- Most common side effect associated with insulin is hypoglycemia.
- Other side effects seen are lipohypertrophy and lipodystrophy at site of injection and weight gain.

Effect of Antidiabetic Drugs on Weight

Weight loss	Weight gain	Wight neutral
Metformin	Insulin	Metformin
GLP-1 agonists	Sulfonylureas	DPP-4 Inhibitors
SGLT-2 Inhibitors	Pioglitazone	Alpha glucosidase inhibitors
Pramlintide		

Note: Metformin in some cases is weight neutral and some cases causes weight loss.

ORAL HYPOGLYCEMIC AGENT (OHAS) INCREASING INSULIN RELEASE

- Sulfonylureas and meglitinide analogs are drugs that increase insulin release by inhibiting **ATP sensitive K^+ channels.**
- **Sulfonylureas are more potent** and longer acting drugs and hence release more insulin for a longer period. Thus, they are used for **maintenance in type II DM**. Sulfonylureas cause a maximum decrease in HbA1C levels followed by biguanides.
- **Meglitinide analogs are less potent** and shorter acting and hence lesser insulin for a short period of time. Thus, they are used for **postprandial hyperglycemia in type II DM.**
- The most common side effects of these drugs are **hypoglycemia** and **weight gain.**

Sulfonylureas

- **Acetohexamide, chlorpropamide and tolbutamide** are first generation drugs, which are not preferred due to toxicity. **Tolbutamide is hepatotoxic and chlorpropamide can cause SIADH and disulfiram like reaction.**
- Glyburide (glibenclamide), glipizide, gliclazide and glimepiride are second generation drugs with better side effect profile and are more preferred. Glimepiride and glipizide are long-acting drugs and require once daily dosing; thus preferred in elderly.
- **Chlorpropamide** is the longest acting whereas **glyburide has maximum potency** and plasma protein binding. Tolbutamide is least potent and shortest acting sulfonylurea.
- Glyburide is the only sulfonylurea that is concentrated in the beta islet cells as well and its metabolite is also active; both of these contribute to longer duration of action despite its short half-life. Glyburide has high affinity for the myocardial ATP sensitive potassium channel and it blunts myocardial response to ischemia.
- Glipizide is short-acting and less potent, the risk of hypoglycemia is lesser and hence preferred in elderly and kidney disease patients.
- Glyburide can increase cardiovascular mortality due to its effect on heart and rarely causes disulfiram like reaction.
- Sulfonylureas are contraindicated in **liver and kidney**

(1st generation > 2nd generation) failure due to risk of hypoglycemia. Due its shorter duration of action, **tolbutamide** is safest sulfonylurea in renal failure. Other contraindications are **pregnancy and lactation**.

Meglitinide Analogs

- **Repaglinide, mitiglinide and nateglinide** are meglitinide analogs used for treatment of **postprandial hyperglycemia**.
- They are combined with other OHAs which are used for maintenance.
- These are metabolized by liver and some part excreted by kidney and hence **dose reduction is required in both hepatic and renal failure**.

OHA DECREASING HEPATIC GLUCOSE PRODUCTION

Biguanides

- Biguanides act by stimulating **AMPK** (adenosine monophosphate activated protein kinase), which leads to **inhibition of gluconeogenesis, decreased hepatic glucose production** and **increase in lipid oxidation (decreases LDL)**. The effect on insulin resistance is minimal.
- They also delay gastric emptying and reduce appetite. This produces weight loss in some cases and in some it is weight neutral. They also decrease microvascular complications associated with diabetes mellitus.
- Delayed gastric emptying causes the **most common side effect, i.e. GIT related nausea, vomiting, diarrhea and anorexia**. Inhibition of oxidative phosphorylation in mitochondria **causes lactic acidosis**. A decrease in calcium dependent **vitamin B-12** absorption is also seen and hence increased calcium intake might prevent it.
- Biguanides are excreted unchanged in urine and hence **contraindicated in renal failure (serum creatinine >1.5 mg/dL)**. as the chances of lactic acidosis increases. Other conditions with increased lactic acid like severe respiratory disease and liver disease, CHF, old age and chronic alcohol abuse are also contraindications.

Metformin

- **Metformin is the drug of choice for the treatment and prophylaxis (glucose intolerance) of type II DM**. It is used as monotherapy or in combination with other OHAs.
- Metformin is also used in **PCOD** to decrease insulin resistance and improve ovulation, **metabolic syndrome in HIV, non-alcoholic fatty liver disease and to reduce antipsychotics associated weight gain**.
- Metformin use is associated with a decreased risk of pancreatic cancer in DM.

> **Recent Advances**
>
> **Metformin** is currently under trial as an **antiaging agent**.

Phenformin

Phenformin has been **banned** due to high risk of **lactic acidosis**.

OHA DECREASING INSULIN RESISTANCE

Thiazolidinedione

- **Thiazolidinediones stimulate PPAR** γ, a nuclear receptor which increases transcription factors for adipocyte proliferation and **decrease insulin resistance** by direct effect on muscle and liver and indirectly via adiponectin. They are not effective in type I DM and used only in type II DM as monotherapy or along with other OHAs.
- Thiazolidinedione stimulate amiloride sensitive Na^+ channels and hence can cause **solute and water retention**. This can cause edema, dilutional anemia and congestive heart failure (CHF). Both adipocyte proliferation and water retention cause **weight gain**.
- Other side effects associated are **macular edema** and an **increased risk of bone fracture in females**.
- Thiazolidinedione are metabolized and excreted by liver and hence are **safe in renal failure**.

Pioglitazone

- **Pioglitazone** is the only thiazolidinediones in use. It can cause bladder cancer and hence a black box warning has been issued against it in India. It has effect on PPAR α, as well because of which it decreases triglycerides and increases high-density lipoprotein (HDL).

Troglitazone and Rosiglitazone

- Troglitazone has been banned due to risk of **hepatotoxicity**.
- Rosiglitazone has been banned due to risk of **myocardial infarction** and stroke.

> **Recent Advances**
>
> **Dual PPAR agonists: Saroglitazar** is an agonist at both PPAR γ and α, developed to take care of both DM and dyslipidemia. It is approved only in India.

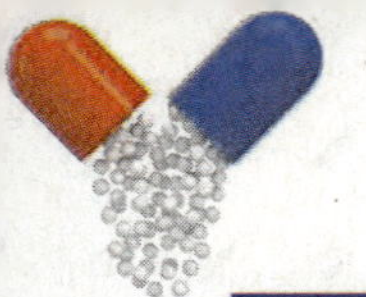

Classification of Classical Oral Hypoglycemic Agents

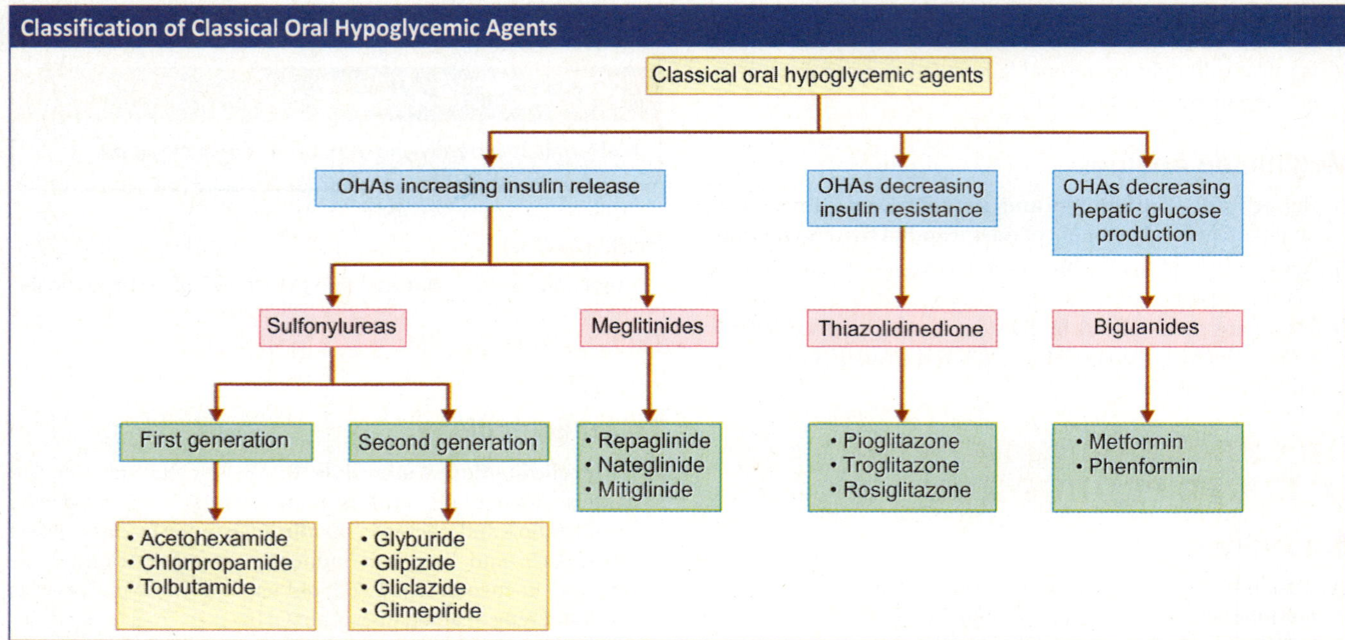

SGLT-2 INHIBITORS

- SGLT-2 receptors present in the PCT are responsible for absorption of glucose and sodium. An upregulation of SGLT- 2 is seen particularly in type II DM.
- **Canagliflozin, dapagliflozin, empagliflozin and ertugliflozin** are the drugs in this class used for treatment of **type II DM only** along with other oral hypoglycemic agents or insulin at once a day dosing (long-acting). These are available as fixed dose combinations along with metformin and DPP-4 inhibitors.
- These drugs are not used in type I DM due to increased risk of diabetic ketoacidosis.
- Glucose in urine is a medium for bacterial and fungal growth and hence **UTI and vaginal infections (mycotic) are the most common side effects. Osteoporosis and increased bone fracture** is seen. Dapagliflozin is associated with an increased risk of **breast** and **bladder cancer** and canagliflozin with increased leg amputation.
- These drugs can cause **weight loss** and a minimal **decrease in blood pressure (hypotension)**.
- Empagliflozin and canagliflozin are associated with a decrease in cardiac mortality.

Recent Advances

Sotagliflozin: It is a dual SGLT1 and 2 inhibitor under trial for treatment of type II diabetes mellitus.

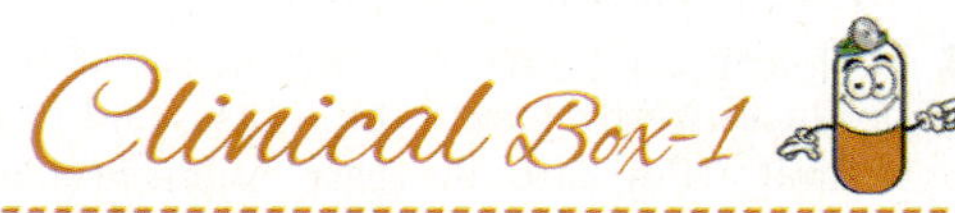

Treatment of Diabetes Mellitus

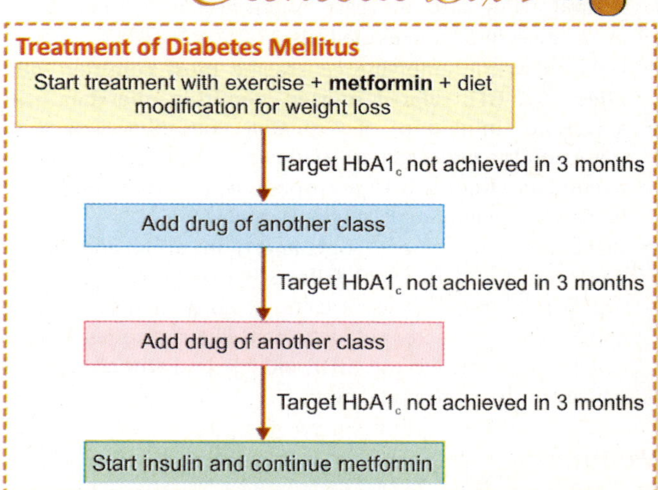

Recent Advances

Anti CD-3 monoclonal antibodies: Teplizumab and otelixizumab are currently under trial to delay type I diabetes mellitus in children. These drugs prevent T-cell mediated beta islet cell destruction.

MISCELLANEOUS DRUGS

- **Bromocriptine** is used for treatment of DM II along with other OHAs. The exact mechanism is not known, but is thought to block the hypothalamic drive for hyperglycemia.
- **Colesevelam** is a bile acid binding resin used in type II DM. It is thought to act by inhibiting glucose absorption.

THYROID

THYROID HORMONE PHYSIOLOGY

- Thyrotropin releasing hormone (TRH) released from hypothalamus acts on Gq subtype of receptors on thyrotrope

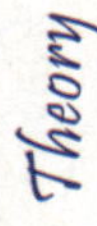

cells in pituitary; this activates protein kinase C which increases synthesis of TSH.

- Thyroid stimulating hormone (TSH) acts on TSH receptors (GPCR) on thyroid follicular cells and increase synthesis of **Na^+/I symporters, H_2O_2 or thyroid peroxidase (TP) and thiol endopeptidases (TEP).**
- Na^+/I symporters are transported to follicular cell membranes, where they increase both Na and iodine uptake. Iodine is acted upon by TP to synthesize monoiodotyrosine (MIT) and diiodotyrosine (DIT) by **organification**, followed by T_3 and T_4 by **coupling**. These thyroid hormones are packed in **thyroglobulin (TG)** and transported to the colloids for storage.
- When required, they are taken up by the follicular cells due to interaction of thyroglobulin (TG) with the TG receptors.
- In the follicular cells the TG is broken down by **TEP** and then T_3 and T_4 is released into the systemic circulation.
- Thyroid hormones act on thyroid hormone receptor α and β. T_3 and T_4 action on α receptors are responsible for the effects in the body mentioned in the clinical box. **T_3 and T_4 action on β receptors are responsible for a decrease in transcription factors for synthesis of TRH and TSH.**
- Various antithyroid drugs acting on this process are mentioned in the conceptual box.

Conceptual Box-2

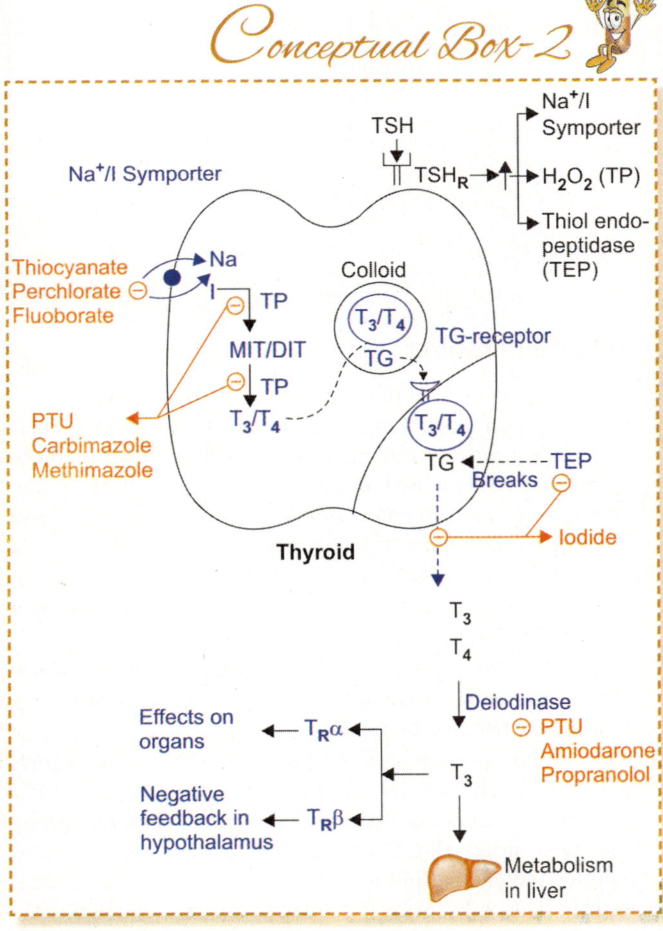

Clinical Box-2

Effects of Thyroid Hormone

- **Growth and development:** Thyroid hormones are required for growth and development including brain development. Hence deficiency can cause cretinism.
- **CVS:** There is an increase in cardiac output and heart rate. Hyperthyroidism can cause cardiac arrhythmias including atrial fibrillation.
- **Blood vessels:** An increase in nitric oxide (NO) causes vasodilation.
- **Lipids:** An increase in low-density hpoprotein (LDL) receptor synthesis decreases plasma LDL. There is an increased synthesis of bile acid from cholesterol and hence plasma cholesterol level also decreases.
- **Glucose:** There is an increase in insulin resistance, gluconeogenesis and glycogenolysis. The overall effect is hyperglycemia.
- **Thermogenesis:** Stimulation of muscle calcium dependent ATPase, increases thermogenesis. Hyperthyroidism causes heat intolerance and hypothyroidism causes cold intolerance.

ANTITHYROID DRUGS

Na^+/I Symporter Inhibitors

- The drugs in this class are **thiocyanate, perchlorate and fluoborate**. These are rarely used nowadays due to toxicity.
- Thiocyanate can cause psychosis and perchlorate can cause aplastic anemia.
- Perchlorate along with other drugs like propylthiouracil (PTU) and methimazole has immunosuppressive action and they can decrease long-acting thyroid stimulators (LATS) antibodies. Hence are additionally beneficial in Grave's disease.

Thyroid Peroxidase (TP) Inhibitors

Thyroid peroxidase inhibitors are **thioamide** drugs which act by inhibiting organification and coupling process as given in the conceptual box. These are the most preferred drugs for the treatment of hyperthyroidism currently. The common side effects seen with this class of drugs is **agranulocytosis**, GIT upset and allergic dermatitis.

Propylthiouracil

- PTU is a short-acting drug ($T_{1/2}$ = 1–2 hours) and hence requires multiple dosing; it is **hepatotoxic** as well. Because of these reasons it is not much preferred in general. Hepatotoxicity is more pronounced in pregnant females and children.
- However, being nonteratogenic it is the drug of choice for hyperthyroidism in **first trimester of pregnancy** and is also drug of choice during **breastfeeding** as it is not concentrated in breast milk. In second and third trimester the liver of baby is developed and fetal hepatotoxicity can be seen and hence methimazole is preferred.
- PTU also inhibits deiodinase and peripheral conversion of T_4 to T_3 and hence is drug of choice in **severe thyrotoxicosis and thyroid storm**.

- Side effects specific to PTU are acute hepatitis (prednisolone used for treatment), liver failure, aplastic anemia, SLE, arthritis, vasculitis (ANCA positive) and hypoprothrombinemia.

Methimazole

- Methimazole ($T_{1/2}$ = 4-6 hours) is long-acting and requires once daily dosing; it is not hepatotoxic. Hence is **more preferred in general and is drug of choice for the treatment of hyperthyroidism, amiodarone induced hyperthyroidism and Grave's disease**. It is teratogenic and can **cause aplasia cutis and choanal and esophageal atresia**; hence is contraindicated in first trimester of pregnancy. However, it is safe in **2nd and 3rd trimester and is drug of choice for hyperthyroidism in pregnancy** after organogenesis in these trimesters.
- Response to methimazole is seen usually after 1-1.5 months of starting treatment.
- Side effects specific to methimazole are teratogenicity, cholestatic jaundice, hypoglycemia, alopecia, nephrotic syndrome and taste loss.
- **Lithium** can be used for the treatment of Grave's disease in patients who are intolerant to both propylthiouracil and methimazole.

Methimazole Induced Scalp Defect

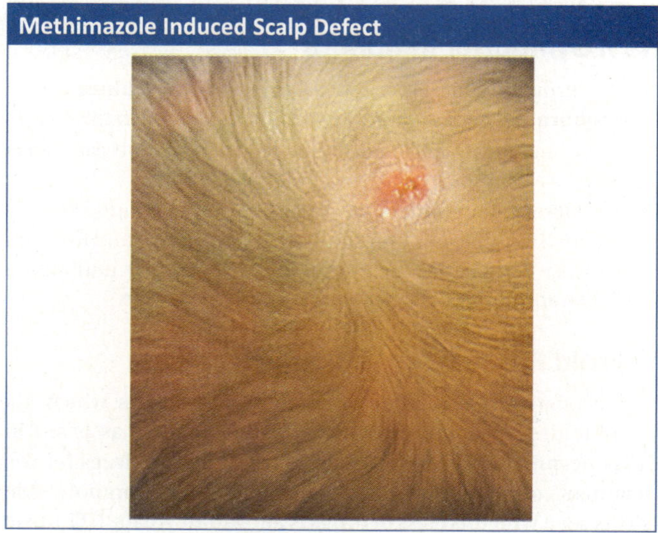

- Carbimazole is a prodrug of methimazole and is even longer acting than methimazole (**$T_{1/2}$ = 8-10 hours**) but is less preferred.

Treatment of Hyperthyroidism in Pregnancy	
First trimester	Second and third trimester
Propylthiouracil	Methimazole

Iodides

- Potassium iodide (KI) and Lugol's iodine **(5% iodine + 10% KI)** act by inhibiting TEP and subsequently release of thyroid hormones. Hence, these are **fastest acting antithyroid drugs**, but the limitation is rapid development of **tolerance**.
- Apart from this they decrease proliferation of thyroid cells (decrease size and weight of gland) and angiogenesis.
- Iodides are used to **make patients euthyroid prior to surgery to decrease risk of thyroid storm** and for treatment of thyroid storm but only after starting propylthiouracil. Secondary benefits are decreased bleeding to decrease vasculogenesis and decrease recurrent laryngeal nerve injury due to decreased size of gland.
- Iodides are also used to protect thyroid gland from radiation exposure. An increase in uptake of iodine by thyroid decrease uptake of radioactive iodine.
- Side effects of systemic iodine therapy are given in the mnemonic box below.

Mnemonics

Side effects of iodides

I: Idiosyncratic reactions (TTP, Periarteritis nodosa)
O: Oropharyngeal glands inflammation (Mimics mumps)
D: Dysgeusia
I: Iodism (Head Cold – Headache)
D: Dermatological (Acneiform rashes)
E: Edema of lungs and larynx (Angioedema)

Clinical Box-3

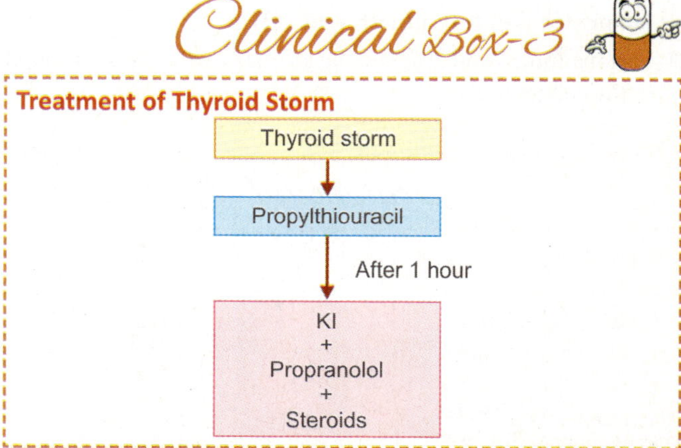

Radioactive Iodine

- I^{123} emits only γ rays and hence is used for **thyroid scan**.
- I^{131} emits both β and γ rays and hence destroys the follicular cells. It is used for treatment of hyperthyroidism in older patients or patients with heart disease, toxic nodular goiter, thyroid cancer (except medullary thyroid cancer) and recurrent Grave's disease postsurgery.
- Side effects associated are permanent hypothyroidism and secondary malignancies of GIT, kidney and breast. There is a risk of hyperparathyroidism in these patients later.
- As it can destroy fetal thyroid, **pregnancy is an absolute contraindication**. It should not be given to females within 3 months of planned pregnancy.
- Thyroid cancer cells have less affinity for iodine uptake, which is further decreased by antithyroid drugs. Hence, PTU > methimazole can cause failure of radioactive iodine therapy and these drugs should be stopped at least 4 days before planned radioactive iodine therapy. The other way to increase iodine uptake is by giving **thyrotropin alpha**, a TSH agonist.

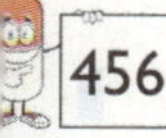

- Ocular symptoms with Grave's disease are worsened with radioactive iodine and to prevent it prophylactic prednisolone is given before 2 months of therapy. Ocular symptoms are also worsened by smoking and pioglitazone. The drugs used for treatment of ocular symptoms are steroids, rituximab (steroid resistant cases) and selenium.

Miscellaneous Drugs

- **Cholestyramine** is a bile acid binding resin that can also inhibit thyroid hormone absorption. It can be used for treatment of hyperthyroidism.
- **Rituximab** is an anti CD-20 monoclonal antibody used along with methimazole in Grave's disease treatment.
- Aspirin is drug of choice for subacute thyroiditis.
- Tamoxifen is drug of choice for treatment of Riedel thyroiditis.
- **Amiodarone, propranolol and steroids** along with **propylthiouracil** inhibit peripheral conversion of T_4 to T_3.

Drugs Causing Hyperthyroidism

- **Amiodarone** – Type 1 hyperthyroidism is caused by increased T_3/T_4 production, wheres type 2 hyperthyroidism is caused by thyroiditis.
- **Iodine (Jod-Basedow disease)**
- **Tyrosine kinase inhibitors** - Due to thyroiditis
- **Alemtuzumab:** Due to Grave's disease

THYROID HORMONE REPLACEMENT

Levothyroxine

- **Levothyroxine** is sodium salt of T_4 and hence is longer acting with a half-life of 7 days. Absorption is excellent on empty stomach.
- It is used for treatment of hypothyroidism, thyroid nodule (if TSH increased), thyroid cancer (to suppress TSH) and depression. The dose is calculated based on lean body mass.
- Thyroid hormone deficiency is caused by pregnancy and hence in case of hypothyroidism with pregnancy the dose should be increased by 30% immediately after pregnancy.
- Intravenous levothyroxine is preferred for treatment of myxedema coma as myxedema interferes with absorption of levothyroxine by oral route. Intravenous route can be used for patients unable to take oral drugs, but the dose should be decreased by 20% as this percentage of drug is not absorbed by oral route.
- It can increase risk of atrial fibrillation and hence dose should be decreased in patients of arrhythmia. Other side effects seen are the effect of thyroid hormone like osteoporosis, heat intolerance, hyperglycemia and asthenia.

Liothyronine

- **Liothyronine** is salt of T_3 and hence is short-acting with a half-life of 1 day. It is not used for replacement therapy in hypothyroidism.
- It is used for the treatment of myxedema coma and for preparation of patients of thyroid cancer for radioiodine treatment.
- It can be used by both oral and intravenous route; since its oral absorption is 100%, the doses by both routes are same.

DRUGS ACTING ON BONE

BONE HOMEOSTASIS

- Bone is made up of **minerals (Ca^{++} and PO_4^-)** and **osteoid matrix (osteoblasts)**.
- Bone resorption and formation are two continuous process important to maintain bone strength. In absence of any of these process bone becomes brittle.
- **PTH, calcitriol (Vitamin D_3)** and **interleukins** stimulate the osteoblasts to form rank ligand, which binds to the rank receptors present in osteoclasts. This leads to a conformational change in structure of osteocytes and they form spiky borders known as ruffled borders for bone resorption.
- PTH also increases sclerostin which inhibits osteoblast proliferation.
- Bone resorption causes release of factors, like—insulin like growth factor-1 (IGF-1), transformation growth factor β (TGF β) and bone morphogenic protein (BMP). These factors stimulate the **osteoblasts for bone formation**.
- Endogenous ligands inhibiting bone resorption are **calcitonin** and **estrogen** and inhibiting bone formation are corticosteroids.
- Various drugs acting on bone homeostasis are mentioned in the conceptual box.

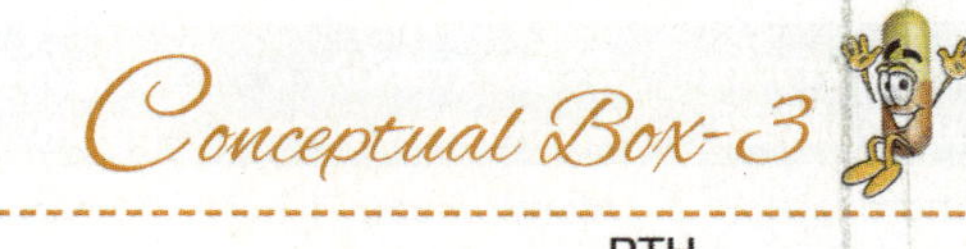

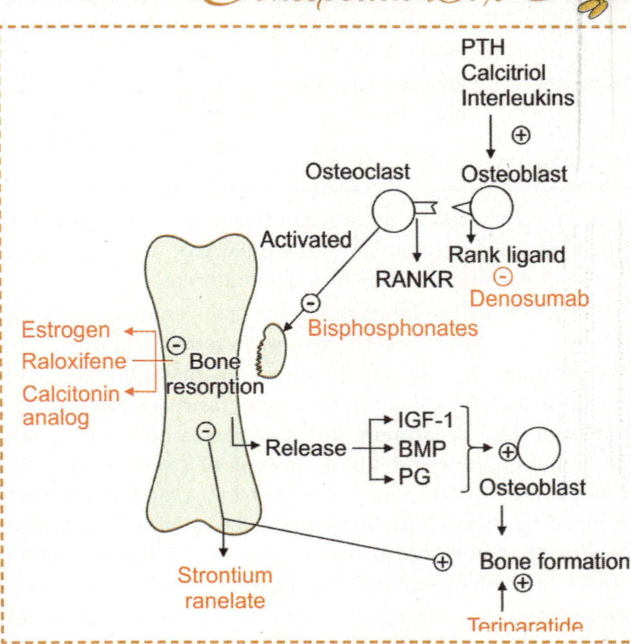

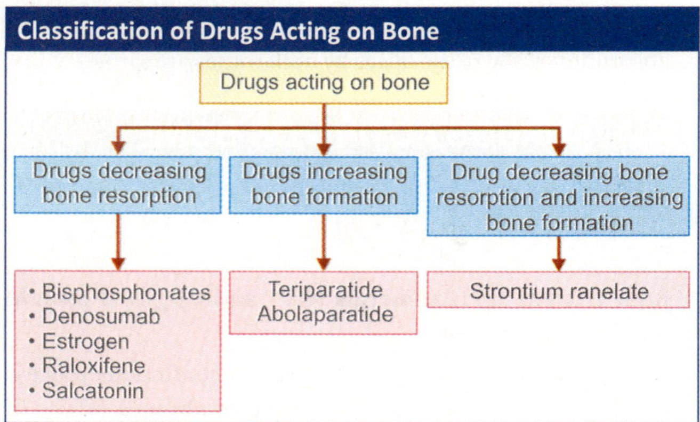

Denosumab

- **Denosumab** is an **anti-RANK ligand antibody** that acts by inhibiting stimulation of osteoclasts to form ruffled border osteoclasts.
- It is given by **subcutaneous route at dose of 60 mg every six months** for 3-5 years for treatment and prophylaxis of osteoporosis and its efficacy is comparable to bisphosphonates. Other uses are **giant cell tumor of bone, hypercalcemia associated with malignancy and hyperparathyroidism and prevention of bone metastasis in prostate cancer.**
- It can cause **osteonecrosis of jaw**, femoral fractures, flu like symptoms, dermatitis, secondary cancer and pancreatitis.
- It can be safely used in patients with renal failure.

Bisphosphonates

- Bisphosphonates act by inhibiting **osteoclast mediated bone resorption by mediating osteoclast apoptosis**. The drugs have gradually developed from 1st to 3rd generation.

1st generation: Least potent	2nd generation: Moderately potent	3rd generation: Most potent
Etidronate Clodronate Medronate	**Alendronate:** 70 mg/week **Pamidronate:** 30–60 mg/month	**Zoledronate:** 2–5 mg/year **Risedronate:** 150 mg/month **Ibandronate:** 150 mg/month

- The 1st generation drugs are very less potent and hence the 2nd and 3rd generation are more preferred. All are given by oral route except zoledronate and pamidronate.
- All drugs decrease both vertebral and nonvertebral fractures, whereas ibandronate decreases only vertebral fracture.
- **Zoledronate is the most potent bisphosphonate** and is the drug of choice for **treatment and prophylaxis of osteoporosis, treatment of hypercalcemia associated with malignancy and for treatment of Page t's disease.** It is given by intravenous route once in a year. Pamidronate is given by intravenous route every 3-6 months. Parenteral bisphosphonates are also used for treatment of hypercalcemia associated with hyperparathyroidism.
- **Alendronate** is the drug of choice for the treatment of osteoporosis caused by long-term glucocorticoid therapy.
- **Oral bisphosphonates** have poor oral absorption and hence are given empty stomach, **30 minutes before food with a full glass of water**. Since all drugs can cause **esophagitis**, the patient is asked to remain upright after drug intake.
- The half-life of bisphosphonates in bone is 10 years. The duration of therapy is for 3 years and if T score in bone densitometry is >2.5, bisphosphonates are stopped, otherwise continued for another 2 years. Thus, duration of therapy for osteoporosis is around **3–5 years**.
- **Osteonecrosis of jaw is seen with intravenous > oral bisphosphonates and mandible > maxilla is involved. Patients with C telopeptide levels of less than 100 pg/mL are at high risk for osteonecrosis.**
- **Other side effects seen are hypo and hypercalcemia, increased risk of bone fracture (femoral chalk stick fractures)** and bone pain.
- Osteonecrosis is more common in patients of cancer than osteoporosis. Zoledronate causes more osteonecrosis whereas alendronate causes more fracture.
- Zoledronate can cause seizures because of severe hypocalcemia and is associated with renal failure as well. Infusion reaction seen with zoledronate can be treated with acetaminophen.
- Since bisphosphonates are excreted unchanged by kidney, renal failure is an absolute contraindication.

Estrogen and SERM

- **Estrogen** and the SERM **raloxifene** and bazedoxifene inhibit bone resorption and are indicated for **treatment and prophylaxis of postmenopausal osteoporosis**. Raloxifene is only effective in case of vertebral fractures.
- Raloxifene also decreases incidence of breast cancer and MI, however it causes **hot flashes** which can be problematic in postmenopausal females.
- **Bazedoxifene** is available along with estrogen for prophylaxis of osteoporosis in postmenopausal females with intact uterus. It has no effect on breast cancer.

Salcatonin

- Salcatonin is a calcitonin analog that acts by inhibiting osteoclast mediated bone resorption. It is the least effective drug for osteoporosis.
- **Subcutaneous salcatonin** is used for treatment of Page t's disease, whereas **intranasal salcatonin** is used for prophylaxis of osteoporosis. It has **analgesic effect** on acute vertebral fractures caused by osteoporosis.
- It has been associated with an increased risk of liver cancer and decreased risk of breast cancer.

PTH Analogs

- **Teriparatide** is a PTH analog whereas **abolaparatide** is a PTHrP (PTH related peptide) analog that activate osteoblasts for **bone matrix** synthesis that augments bone formation in all bones except **distal radius**. However, as calcium is also required for bone formation vitamin D and calcium supplementation is also given along with these drugs.

- These are peptides and hence given by subcutaneous route in thigh or abdomen once daily, for a maximum period of 2 years for treatment of osteoporosis. The duration is limited to 2 years due to risk **of osteosarcoma**. Bisphosphonates are continued after that to retain the bone effect. The target patients are postmenopausal female and men with hypogonadal osteoporosis. These are used for treatment of severe osteoporosis where patients have a high risk of bone fracture. These can also be used for treatment of femoral chalk stick fractures seen with bisphosphonates.
- Side effects associated are hypotension, pneumonia and hypercalcemia. A **black box warning** has been issued regarding risk of osteosarcoma.
- Due to risk of osteosarcoma it is **contraindicated in patients** of **Paget's disease**, unexplained alkaline phosphatase elevation, history of osteosarcoma/chondrosarcoma, history of radiotherapy to bones and in patients with open epiphyses. These are also contraindicated with other drugs that can cause hypercalcemia like steroids and thiazides.

Strontium Ranelate

- **Strontium ranelate** is made up of two atoms of strontium and ranelic acid.
- Strontium is like calcium and hence incorporated into bone and thus increases bone formation. However, as strontium cannot be removed by osteoclasts there is also a decrease in bone resorption.
- It is the only drugs that acts on both bone formation and resorption.

Plicamycin

- **Plicamycin**, also known as mithramycin is an antibiotic used for treatment of Page t's disease and hypercalcemia.
- It acts by inhibiting bone resorption.

Calcimimetics

- When there is excess calcium in plasma it stimulates calcium sensing receptors in parathyroid gland and decreases release of PTH. **Cinacalcet and etecalcetide** in a similar way decreases PTH release.
- **Cinacalcet** is used by oral route for treatment of initial treatment of hyperparathyroidism, failed surgical parathyroid-ectomy, secondary hyperparathyroidism seen in chronic kidney disease and for treatment of parathyroid carcinoma. Zoledronate can be added to cinacalcet in patients with severe hypercalcemia and parathyroid carcinoma. It causes GIT upset and hypocalcemia.
- **Etelcalcetide** is an intravenous drug used for treatment of dialysis induced hypercalcemia.
- Calcium sensing receptor antagonists are under development for treatment of osteoporosis. They can increase PTH release which can increase bone formation.

Recent Advances

Romosozumab and blosozumab: These are antisclerostin antibodies under trial for treatment of osteoporosis. They increase bone formation by removing the sclerostin induced block of osteoblast proliferation.

HYPOTHALAMO-PITUITARY AXIS

- Hypothalamus is the source for agonists like GHRH, TRH, GNRH and CRH which act on a G_s subtype of GPCR on somatotrope, thyrotrope, gonadotrope and corticotrope cells respectively in pituitary. An increase in calcium in these pituitary cells increases release of GH, TSH, LH/FSH and ACTH respectively.
- Somatostatin is an agonist at G_i receptors in somatotrope and thyrotrope cells and hence decrease release of GH and TSH. Dopamine is an agonist at G_i receptors, i.e. D2 receptors in lactotrope cells and decrease release of prolactin.

GROWTH HORMONE AND RELATED DRUGS

Physiology of Growth Hormone

- **GHRH** from hypothalamus stimulates release of **GH** from the pituitary. GH then acts on the GH receptors sequentially on type 1 followed by type 2, which leads to an increase in linear growth.
- An increase in linear growth of bone and muscles require more glucose. This is achieved by GH mediated **insulin like growth factor-1 (IGF-1)** stimulation, which acts on insulin receptors and increases glucose uptake.
- **Somatostatin** is an antagonist at somatotrope **and thyrotrope cells and decreases release of GH and TSH**.
- **GH and somatostatin** are both insulin antagonists and cause **hyperglycemia**. IGF-1 by acting on insulin receptors cause hypoglycemia.
- Various drugs acting on the growth hormone system are mentioned in the conceptual box.

Conceptual Box-4

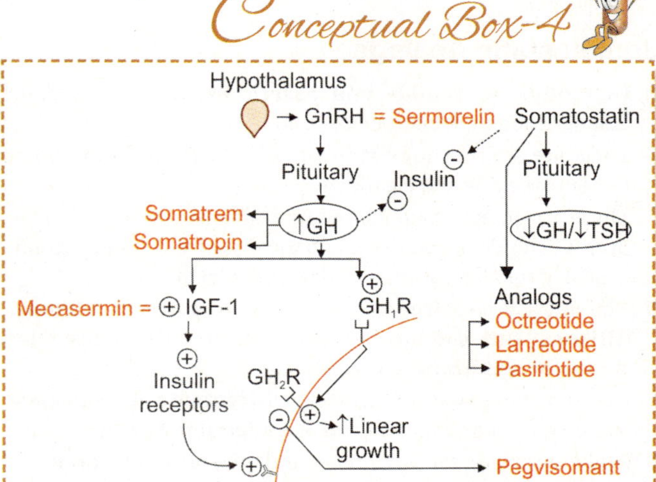

GHRH Analog

- **Sermorelin** and tesamorelin are GHRH analogs used for treatment of GH deficiency and for differential diagnosis in the cause of GH deficiency, i.e. pituitary or hypothalamic. It is however approved only for treatment of lipodystrophy in AIDS patients.

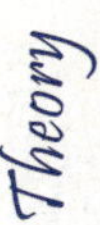

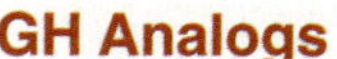

GH Analogs

- **Somatrem** and **somatropin** are growth hormone analogs administered by subcutaneous route at bedtime.
- The uses and side effects are mentioned in the mnemonic box below.

Uses of GH	Side effects and contraindication of GH	
S: SGA baby M: Malabsorption due to short bowel Syndrome A: AIDS related wasting L: Length decreased in dwarfism and genetic disorders like Prader-Willi, Turner and Noonan syndrome	C: Carpal tunnel syndrome H: Hyperglycemia I: ICT is raised L: Leukemia D: Diabetes mellitus	Side effects
	Re: Retinopathy N: Neoplasia	Contraindications

Note: The uses, side effects and contraindications can be remembered as SMAL CHILDREN.

IGF-1 Analogs

- IGF-1 in plasma is bound to IGF-1 binding protein-3 that increases its duration of action.
- **Mecasermin** is IGF-1 analog and **mecasermin rinfabate** is analog of IGF-1 + IGF-1 binding protein-3.
- These can be used for treatment of dwarfism caused by selective IGF-1 deficiency, GH receptor mutation or anti GH antibodies.
- As it can stimulate insulin receptors the side effects are hypoglycemia and lipohypertrophy at the site of subcutaneous injection.

Somatostatin Analogs

- **Octreotide, lanreotide and paseriotide** are somatostatin analogs used by subcutaneous route.
- These are drug of choice for treatment of GH excess condition like **acromegaly** and gigantism.
- These are potent vasoconstrictors and hence octreotide is the drug of choice for **acute esophageal variceal bleeding** and used in pancreatic surgery to decrease bleeding.
- Octreotide is also drug of choice for **glucagonoma, VIPoma, GRFoma and somatostatinoma**. Paseriotide is used for treatment of **Cushing's disease**.
- As somatostatin is an antagonist at thyrotrope cells, octreotide is used for treatment of **thyrotrope adenoma** as well.
- Other uses are for treatment and diagnosis of **carcinoid tumor** and pituitary adenoma and can be used in treatment of insulinoma and **secretory diarrhea**.
- Side effects associated are hyperglycemia, hypothyroidism, gall stones and GIT related like nausea and vomiting.

Recent Advances

Lutathera is a recently approved radiolabeled somatostatin analog approved for treatment of gastroenteropancreatic neuroendocrine tumors.

GH2 Receptor Antagonist

- **Pegvisomant** is a GH_2 receptor antagonist used by subcutaneous route for treatment of acromegaly in case response is not satisfactory with octreotide.
- Side effect associated is pituitary adenoma due to negative feedback mechanism, which increases release of GHRH. It can also cause lipohypertrophy at the site of injection.

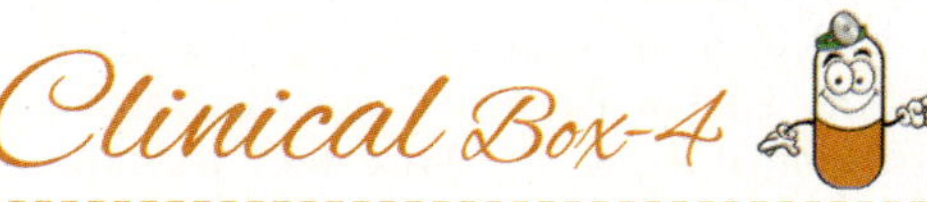

Treatment of Acromegaly

Octreotide (Subcutaneous)	Drug of choice
Pegvisomant (Subcutaneous)	Used in cases resistant to octreotide
Cabergoline (Oral)	May be used first as it is an oral drug
Tamoxifen	Used in persistent acromegaly
Surgery	Transsphenoidal pituitary microsurgery

DRUGS ACTING ON REPRODUCTIVE SYSTEM

GNRH AND RELATED DRUGS

Physiology of GNRH

- The physiological release of **GNRH** is pulsatile which acts on pituitary and increases release of luteinizing hormone (LH) and follicle-stimulating hormone (FSH).
- LH and FSH in men are responsible for spermatogenesis and testosterone production.
- LH and FSH in females are responsible for ovulation and production of estrogen and progesterone.

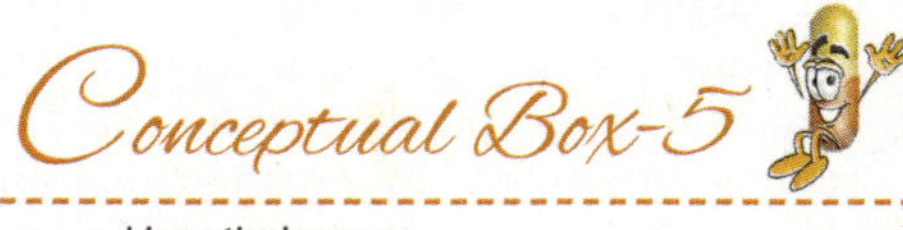

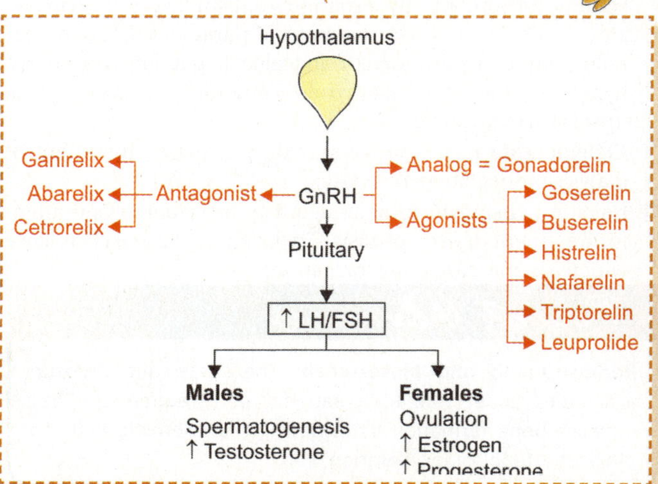

GNRH Analog

- **Gonadorelin** is GNRH analog given by subcutaneous or intravenous route.
- It was used to differentiate in between hypothalamic and pituitary causes of hypogonadotropic hypogonadism. An adequate increase in LH after gonadotropin hints at hypothalamic defect, whereas a blunted response hints at pituitary defect.
- It can be used for treatment of female infertility caused by anovulation. Unlike GNRH agonists, it is associated with lesser incidence of multiple gestation.

GNRH Agonists

- GNRH agonists can be used at pulsatile or continuous doses. At pulsatile doses, they mimic physiological effect and increases LH and FSH and hence can be used for treatment of **anovulation, oligospermia and delayed puberty**.
- At continuous doses there is an initial rise followed by decrease in LH/FSH. Hence, at continuous doses they are used for treatment of **breast cancer, fibroids and endometriosis in females and prostate cancer in males**. Other uses are **precocious puberty**, acute intermittent porphyria and priapism. At continuous doses there could be initial worsening of symptoms due to transient increase in LH/FSH.

GNRH agonist	Route
Goserelin Histrelin	Subcutaneous implant
Leuprolide	Subcutaneous or intramuscular injection
Triptorelin	Intramuscular injection
Nafarelin	Intranasal

- Side effects that can be seen are due to sex steroid synthesis inhibition like **hot flashes and vaginal atrophy in females and impotence in males. Osteoporosis** can be seen in all patients.
- These are absolutely **contraindicated in pregnancy**.

GNRH Antagonists

- GNRH antagonists are given at continuous doses and the only effect seen is a decrease in LH/FSH. Hence, there is no initial worsening as seen with agonists.
- **Ganirelix, abarelix, degarelix and cetrorelix** are used by subcutaneous injection for conditions like GNRH agonists are used. Degarelix is used in prostate cancer and cetrorelix for endometriosis and uterine fibroids. **Elagolix** has been recently approved for treatment of pain associated with endometriosis.
- The use specific to this class is to prevent premature ovulation in treatment of infertility.
- These are absolutely contraindicated in pregnancy.
- Side effects are similar to GNRH agonists and apart from that degarelix can cause QT prolongation as well.

ESTROGEN, PROGESTERONE AND RELATED DRUGS

Physiology of Estrogen and Progesterone Synthesis

- **Cholesterol** is precursor for **progesterone** which further forms androstenedione and testosterone.
- Androstenedione and testosterone with the help of enzyme **aromatase** produce oestradiol and oestrone respectively.
- Testosterone is activated into **dihydroxy testosterone by 5-α reductase**, which further acts on androgen receptors.
- Various drugs acting on this physiological process have been mentioned in the conceptual box.

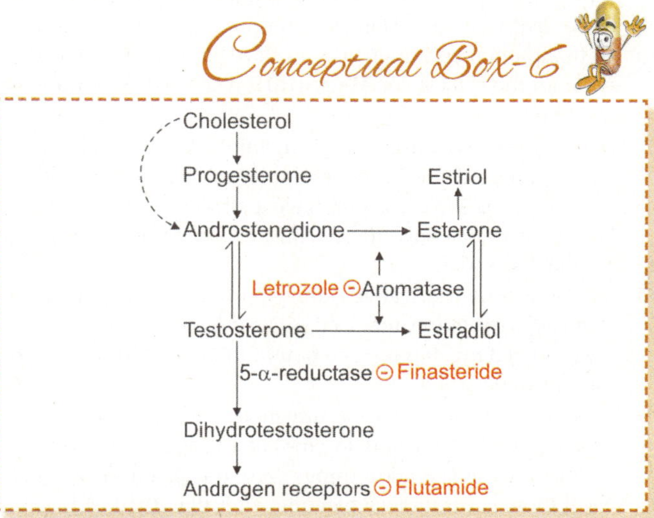

Estrogen

- Natural estrogen, estradiol is synthesized by the ovary, which gets converted into other estrogens like estrone and estriol by the liver. Estradiol is most active natural estrogen and hence synthetic drugs like **ethinyl estradiol** and **mestranol** have been synthesized from it for clinical use. Mestranol is activated into ethinyl estradiol by liver.
- These are used for **hormone replacement therapy (HRT) in primary ovarian failure (Turner's syndrome) and in postmenopausal females**. HRT improves **vaginal dryness, osteoporosis and vasomotor symptoms**.
- In contraception, estrogens are used along with progesterone; as if only estrogen is used there is risk of endometrial hypertrophy and dysfunctional uterine bleeding.
- Side effects associated are nausea and vomiting, **uterine cancer, salt** and **water retention, increased risk of GERD (also with SERM), edema, gallstones** and **thromboembolism (only by oral route and not transdermal)**; there is a **decrease in colorectal and ovarian cancer risk** though. Estrogen can worsen migraine and hypertension.
- Estrogen increases HDL and decreases LDL but has **no effect on atherosclerosis and CVS mortality**.
- **Stilbestrol** use in pregnancy is associated with increased risk of **vaginal cancer** in off-springs and hence not used.

Progesterone

- Progesterone can be broadly classified as progesterone derivatives, testosterone derivatives and spironolactone derivative.

Progesterone Derivatives	Testosterone Derivatives		Spironolactone Derivative
	Estranes	Gonanes	
Medroxyprogesterone Hydroxyprogesterone Dihydroprogesterone Megestrol	Norethindrone Lynestrenol Allylestrenol	Norgestrel Levonorgestrel Desogestrel Norgestimate Gestodene	Drospirenone

- Progesterone derivatives are poor inhibitors of ovulation and hence not preferred for contraception. But since there is no androgenic action, they are preferred for HRT (with estrogen). These drugs have good effect on endometrium and hence used for treatment if endometriosis, dysfunctional uterine bleeding and endometrial cancer. **Megestrol** is also used as an **appetite stimulant**.
- Testosterone derivatives are strong inhibitors of ovulation and hence preferred for contraception with estrogen or without estrogen (mini pill). Estranes have a strong androgenic effect, whereas gonanes have none. Thus, estranes have androgenic side effects as well.
- Spironolactone derivative, drospirenone is also a strong inhibitor of ovulation and used with estrogen for contraception at a dose of 3 mg. It has more potent mineralocorticoid action than spironolactone.
- Other uses of progesterone are in premenstrual syndrome, threatened abortion and for test of estrogen secretion. For test of estrogen secretion, progesterone is given for 5-7 days and if there is withdrawal bleeding after that, then estrogen is secreted.
- It has antiandrogenic effects as well and this part has been described in respective section.
- Side effects associated are androgenic effects like acne and atherogenesis (decreased HDL), edema (salt and fluid retention), weight gain, irregular menstrual cycle and breakthrough bleeding.

Side effects of progesterone
A – Androgenic like acne, atherogenesis
B – Breakthrough bleeding
C – Cycle is irregular
D – Depression, decreased libido
E – Edema due to salt and fluid retention

Oral Contraceptive Pills

Combined OCPs

- Combined OCPs contain 30-50 micrograms of estrogen and 0.5-1 mg of progesterone. Estrogen and progesterone inhibit release of FSH and LH respectively and thus **suppress ovulation**.
- **Monophasic pills:** A combination of estrogen and progesterone is given for 21 days following which a 7 days drug free period is given for menstruation. Since the dose is constant throughout all phases, it is called as monophasic pill.
- **Biphasic pills:** The estrogen dose is constant for 21 days, but progesterone dose is low in days 1 to 10 and high in days 11 to 21. The remaining 7 days are free.
- **Triphasic pills:** The drug is given in three phases of 1-6 days, 7-11 days and 12-21 days. Dose of estrogen is constant in first and third phase and more in second phase. The dose of progesterone keeps on increasing from first to third phase. The remaining 7 days are free.

Monophasic pill	EE 30 mcg + Norgestrel (300 mcg) or levonorgestrel (150 mcg) or desogesterel (150 mcg) for 21 days	7 days free
Biphasic pill	EE 35 mcg + norethindrone 0.5 mg for days 1 to 10 days followed by EE 35 mcg + Norethindrone 1 mg for days 11–21	7 days free
Triphasic pill	EE 30 mcg + Norgestrel 0.3 mg for 1–6 days followed by EE 40 mcg + norgestrel 0.375 mg for days 7–11 and EE 30 mcg + Norgestrel 1.25 mg for days 12–21	7 days free

- OCPs are also used for treatment of PCOS, menorrhagia, fibroids and ovarian cysts.
- Side effects associated are related to estrogen and progesterone like **thromboembolism, weight gain, acne, hepatotoxicity, nausea and vomiting and amenorrhea. There is a decreased risk of uterine and breast cancer with OCPs**.

Mini Pills

- Mini pills contain only progesterones like norethindrone and norgestrel, which increases the viscosity of **cervical mucous and makes it impermeable to sperms**. Apart from that it has **effect on blastocyst implantation as well**.
- These are preferred in females with estrogen contraindication.
- Mini pills are less effective than combined OCPs and are also associated with break through bleeding.
- The side effects are similar to progesterones as discussed above.

Emergency Contraception

- Drugs used in emergency contraception primarily act by **inhibition of blastocyst implantation**.

- **Levonorgestrel** 0.75 mg is used within 72 hours for unprotected intercourse. Another dose is repeated after 12 hours. Another option is to give 1.5 mg once within 72 hours of unprotected intercourse.
- **Ulipristal** is a selective progesterone receptor modulator can be used at a dose of 30 mg up to 5 days.
- **IUCD** is more effective than levonorgestrel and can be inserted up to 5 days of unprotected intercourse.
- **Yuzpe regimen** containing an estrogen and progesterone is less efficacious and hence not preferred.
- **Mifepristone** is not FDA approved but can be used for emergency contraception up to 72 hours at doses of 600 mg.

Dose of drugs used for emergency contraception	
Levonorgestrel	0.75 mg + 0.75 mg, 2 tablets with 12 hours gap or 1 tablet of 1.5 mg, within 72 hours of intercourse
Ulipristal	30 mg within 5 days of intercourse
Mifepristone (Not FDA approved)	600 mg mifepristone within 72 hours of intercourse

Depot and Implantable Contraceptives

- **Levonorgestrel 6 capsules (36 mg in each capsule)** are implanted subcutaneously and the effect can be seen up to 5 years.
- **Intramuscular medroxyprogesterone** depot formulation at a dose of 150 mg can be given every 3 months.

Recent Advances

Annovera: It is a toroidal shaped vaginal drug delivery system containing segesterone acetate (progesterone) and ethinyl estradiol (estrogen), approved for contraception recently. It is placed inside vagina for 21 days following a drug free interval of 7 days, when withdrawal bleeding occurs. The same device can be used for 13 such cycles; it should be cleaned and kept dry during the drug free interval.

Selective Estrogen Receptor Modulators (SERM)

- **Tamoxifen** is a partial agonist/antagonist with antagonism on estrogen receptors of breast and hence is the drug of choice for treatment and prophylaxis of premenopausal **ER positive breast cancer**. It can also be used for treatment of **persistent acromegaly** as it decreases IGF-1 levels and is drug of choice for treatment of Riedel thyroiditis. However, it has stimulatory (partial agonism) effect on **estrogen receptors of bone (decreases bone resorption), lipids (decreases LDL and cholesterol), uterus (causes uterine hyperplasia and carcinoma) and coagulation (thrombosis).** It is associated with acute side effects like **hot flashes (most common)** and nausea. Long-term side effects seen are **deep vein thrombosis (most common)**, uterine cancer and cataract.
- Toremifene can be used for treatment of tamoxifen resistant breast cancer. It can cause QT prolongation.
- **Raloxifene** has stimulatory effect on estrogen receptors of **bone** and hence used for prophylaxis and treatment of postmenopausal osteoporosis and to decrease risk of breast cancer in high risk postmenopausal females. It is also used for treatment of **gynecomastia** and is more effective than tamoxifen. It also has **stimulatory effect on lipids (increases HDL and decreases LDL) and coagulation (thrombosis), and has inhibitory effect on breast and uterus. Its use is associated with hot flashes.**
- Ospemifene is a latest SERM approved for treatment of dyspareunia.

Selective Estrogen Receptor Downregulator (SERD)

Fulvestrant

- **Fluvestrant** is a pure antiestrogenic drug that has only inhibitory effect on estrogen receptors. It is 100 times more potent inhibitor than tamoxifen and also causes proteasomal degradation of estrogen receptors.
- It is the drug of choice for **treatment of tamoxifen resistant ER positive breast cancer in postmenopausal females**. Dose is 250 mg by subcutaneous route once in a month.
- Side effects are rare and is **safer as compared to tamoxifen**.

Clomiphene

- **Clomiphene** is an estrogen partial agonist/antagonist at the **anterior pituitary** and hence by preventing negative feedback it increases release of GNRH followed by LH/FSH.
- This induces ovulation and causes spermatogenesis. Hence, clomiphene is the **drug of choice for treatment of infertility related to anovulation and oligospermia.**
- **Multiple gestation** is a side effect seen but incidence is lesser than GNRH agonists. It can also cause ovarian hyperstimulation, hot flashes, ovarian cysts and cancer, and blurring of vision. It is teratogenic and hence contraindicated in pregnancy.

Aromatase Inhibitors

- Aromatase converts testosterone into estrogen in postmenopausal females in adipocytes and hence is the main cause of breast cancer in this subset of population.
- The drugs in this class are in three generations as given below:

First Generation	Second Generation	Third Generation
Aminoglutethimide	Formestane Fadrozole Rogletimide	Exemestane Anastrozole Letrozole Vorozole

- Exemestane and formestane are steroidal analogs of androstenedione that **irreversibly inhibit aromatase**. Other drugs are nonsteroidal **reversible inhibitors** of aromatase.
- The third generation **drugs are currently more preferred and are drug of choice for treatment and prophylaxis of postmenopausal ER positive breast cancer**. These are also used in advanced breast cancer, precocious puberty, endometriosis, gynecomastia and anovulation. Aromatase inhibitors are more effective than clomiphene for treatment of infertility caused by anovulation.
- An increase in **bone fracture** rate is associated with these drugs. Nausea, thrombosis, vaginal bleeding and hot flashes can also be seen but the incidence is lesser than tamoxifen.

Drugs used for treatment of ER+ breast cancer	
Tamoxifen used for both prophylaxis and treatment of ER+ breast cancer in premenopausal (DOC) and postmenopausal females	20 mg OD for 5 years
Raloxifene used for prophylaxis of ER+ breast cancer in postmenopausal females only	60 mg OD for 5 years
Fluvestrant used in treatment of metastatic ER+ breast cancer in postmenopausal females only	500 mg IM on day 1, 15 and 29 and then once monthly
Aromatase inhibitors for prophylaxis and treatment of ER+ breast cancer in postmenopausal females only (DOC)	Anastrazole 1mg OD for 5 years Letrozole 2.5 mg OD for 5 years Exemestane 25 mg OD for 5 years

Selective Progesterone Receptor Modulators

Mifepristone (RU-486)

- **Mifepristone (RU-486)** is a **partial agonist** at progesterone receptors and hence acts as antagonist in presence of progesterone. It also blocks glucocorticoid and androgen receptors.
- It has a high plasma protein binding and hence a long half-life.
- Mifepristone causes decidual break down and detachment of blastocyst by acting on uterus, cervical softening and increases prostaglandin effect on uterus. Thus, along with another uterine stimulator like misoprostol (prostaglandin E1 analog) it is used for medical abortion until 7 weeks. 600 mg of mifepristone is given and then after 2 days 400 mg of oral misoprostol or 1 mg of gemeprost pessary for medical abortion.
- For its stimulatory effect on uterus, it can be used for induction of labour as well. By acting on hypothalamus/pituitary it decreases release of LH followed by inhibition of ovulation. Hence, it can be used in emergency contraception at a dose of 600 mg within 72 hours of unprotected intercourse, as well as for regular contraception at dose of 200 mg once a month.
- Since it causes cervical softening, it can be used prior to surgical abortion. It inhibits glucocorticoid receptors and hence can be used in Cushing's disease as well.
- Most common side effect is **vaginal bleeding** and other prostaglandins related side effects like abdominal cramps and diarrhoea can be seen.

Ulipristal

- **Ulipristal** is a is a partial agonist at progesterone receptors and **inhibits ovulation (inhibits LH release) and implantation of fertilized ovum.**
- It inhibits LH release and also inhibits LH induced follicular rupture in ovary.
- It is approved for emergency contraception and can be used at a dose of **30 mg** up to 5 days.
- Side effects associated are headache and abdominal pain.

Onapristone and Gestinone

- Onapristone is a pure progesterone receptor antagonist under trial for treatment of **prostate cancer** progressive on antiandrogenic drugs.
- Gestinone is a partial agonist at progesterone receptors and is used for treatment if **endometriosis**.

Androgens

- Testosterone is produced in response to LH by the Leydig cells. Then it is activated by 5-α reductase into dihydrotestosterone (DHT); both testosterone and DHT are agonist at androgen receptors but **DHT is more potent**.
- Testosterone has a good oral absorption but a high first pass metabolism, hence it cannot be given by oral route. Resistance to first pass metabolism was gained by alkylation of testosterone and this resulted in oral drugs like methyltestosterone, fluoxymesterone, oxandrolone, danazol and stenozol. These oral drugs while getting absorbed pass via liver and result in hepatotoxicity, which is not seen by drugs with other routes.
- Intramuscular depot formulation is made by addition of esters like enanthate, cypionate, decanoate and undecanoate to testosterone. Addition of esters increases their lipid solubility and hence these are injected in oily medium, which increases their duration of action. All of these are given every 2 weeks once, except the undecanoate formulation which is longest acting and given every 10 weeks once.
- Transdermal formulation of testosterone is given in the form of patch, gel and buccal tablets.

Transdermal testosterone	Intramuscular depot formulations	Oral formulations
Patch Gel Buccal tablets	Testosterone enanthate Testosterone cypionate Testosterone undecanoate Nandrolone decanoate	Methyl testosterone Fluoxy mesterone Oxandrolone Danazol Stenozol

- Testosterone is used for treatment of **male hypogonadism, female hypogonadism (to increase libido), aids related wasting, aplastic anemia**. Oral drugs can be used for **hereditary angioedema prophylaxis**.
- Nandrolone has maximum anabolic effect and hence is abused by athletes.
- In males benign prostate hyperplasia, prostate cancer, oligozoospermia and gynecomastia can be seen. In females hirsutism, decreased breast size and voice deepening is seen.
- In children stunting of growth is seen due to premature closure of epiphyses.
- Other side effects common to both sexes are edema (sodium and water retention), acne, precocious puberty and hepatotoxicity. Hepatotoxicity is seen with oral drugs in the form of cholestatic jaundice, dyslipidemia (decreased HDL and increased LDL) and hepatocellular carcinoma.

Antiandrogens

- **Cyproterone** and **megestrol** are progesterone derivatives whereas flutamide, nilutamide, apalutamide, enzalutamide and bicalutamide are synthetic inhibitors of androgen receptors. These are **used along with GNRH agonists or antagonists for treatment of prostate cancer** and **hirsutism**. Cyproterone and flutamide can cause hepatotoxicity. Enzalutamide can cause seizures and nilutamide can cause interstitial pneumonitis. Other common side effects associated are **impotence** and **gynecomastia**.
- **Finasteride** and **dutasteride** are 5-α reductase inhibitors used for treatment of **BPH, hirsutism and androgenic alopecia**. These drugs **decrease size of prostate** and increase urine flow. Finasteride is a selective 5-α reductase II inhibitor whereas dutasteride is a nonselective 5-α reductase I and II inhibitor. Impotence and gynecomastia are less common than androgen receptor antagonists.

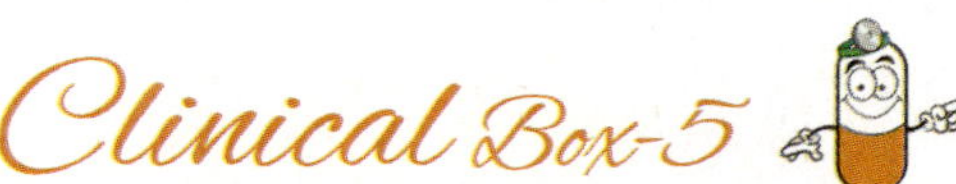

Drugs used for Treatment of Hirsutism

- Finasteride
- Flutamide
- Spironolactone
- Metformin
- Simvastatin
- Clomiphene
- GnRH agonists
- OCPs with antiandrogenic progestins (Desogestrel, Drospirenone and Norgestimate)

Danazol

- Danazol is a synthetic steroid with inhibitor effect on GNRH, which subsequently leads to decrease in LH/FSH followed by decrease in estrogen, progesterone and testosterone. It also has androgenic action and hence is discussed in the section of androgens as well.
- Uses are estrogen dependent conditions like **endometriosis, gynecomastia and fibrocystic disease of breast**. It is drug of choice for prophylaxis of hereditary angioedema. It acts by increasing synthesis of C1 esterase.
- It can cause androgenic side effects like **hirsutism** etc. in females as mentioned above.

Drugs Acting on Uterus

Uterine Stimulants

- **Oxytocin** is given by slow intravenous infusion and is drug of choice to induce labour at doses of **6 mIU/min every 40 minutes** till expected labour progression. A **maximum dose of 40 mIU/min** can be given in nonresponsive cases. It is also used for treatment of postpartum hemorrhage at a dose of **10 mIU** after labor. It can cause uterine rupture, hypotension and antidiuretic effect. It acts by stimulating G_q (OXT) subtype of GPCRs in uterus which increase calcium and thus contraction of uterus. It also increases local prostaglandin synthesis which can increase contraction by acting on **prostaglandin F_2 alpha receptors**. Progesterone can inhibit the effect of oxytocin.
- **Ergometrine** is used for treatment of postpartum hemorrhage. It can cause nausea and vomiting and vasoconstriction.

Recent Advances

Carbetocin is a long-acting derivative of oxytocin under trial for treatment of postpartum hemorrhage.

Uterine Relaxants

- Beta-2 agonists like **ritodrine** can cause uterine relaxation and is used for management of premature labor. It is associated with tachycardia, hypotension and pulmonary edema. Terbutaline is also used for same purpose though is not FDA approved.
- Calcium channel blocker like **nifedipine** is better tolerated by mother and fetus than ritodrine.
- **Atosiban** is a nonapeptide oxytocin antagonist used in preterm labor for females with cardiac problems. It can cause nausea and vomiting, hypotension and hyperglycemia.
- **Indomethacin,** an NSAID can decrease prostaglandin synthesis and hence decrease uterine contraction. Though not routinely used due to side effects in fetus like closure of ductus arteriosus.

Drugs used in Erectile Dysfunction

Mnemonics

Pyar : Phentolamine
Bhi : Bremelanotide
Nahi : Naltrexone
Kar : Ketanserine
S : Sildenafil (DOC)
Ak : Alviptadil
T : Trazadone
A : Alprostadil

STEROIDS

STEROID SYNTHESIS

- Steroid synthesis begins with cholesterol and by multiple steps and by multiple enzymes it is converted into hydrocortisone as given in the conceptual box.
- Different drugs that inhibit steroid synthesis are also mentioned.

Conceptual Box-7

Cholesterol
↓ CYP11A1 ⊖ Aminoglutethimide
Pregnenolone
↓ 17-α-hydroxylase ⊖ Ketoconazole
17-α-hydroxypregnenolone
↓ 3-β-dehydrogenase ⊖ Trilostane
17-α-hydroxyprogesterone
↓ 21-β-hydroxylase
11 deoxycortisol
↓ 11-β-hydroxylase ⊖ Metyrapone, Etomidate
Hydrocortisone (cortisol)

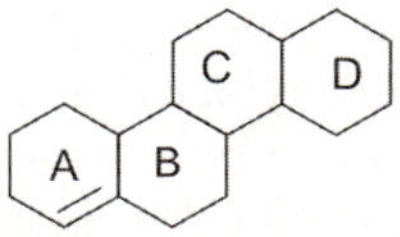

A B C D

Steroid Synthesis Inhibitors

Drug	Target	Use	Side effects
Ketoconazole	17-α hydroxylase	Cushing's disease treatment	Hepatotoxicity Gynecomastia
Abiraterone	17-α hydroxylase	Metastatic prostate cancer	
Metyrapone	11-β hydroxylase	Cushing's disease treatment and diagnosis	Hirsutism
Etomidate	11-β hydroxylase	Emergency management of Cushing's disease	Vitamin C deficiency
Aminoglutethimide	CYP11A1	Withdrawn from market	
Trilostane	3-β dehydrogenase	Not used in humans	

Note: Mitotane is an adrenolytic drug used for treatment of inoperable adrenocortical tumors.

DEVELOPMENT OF STEROIDS

The endogenous steroid **hydrocortisone** is taken as a reference steroid, which has **equal glucocorticoid and mineralocorticoid effect taken as 1**. Its duration of action is **8–12 hours**. The structure of hydrocortisone contains four rings A, B, C and D and selective changes were made to these rings to synthesize new and better steroids. Hydrocortisone primarily binds to corticosteroid binding globulin (CBG), whereas the synthetic steroids bind to albumin.

- An addition of a **double bond in ring A** increased the glucocorticoid effect by **4 times** and slightly decreased mineralocorticoid effect. There was an increased duration of action to **12–36 hours** as well. These steroids are **prednisone and prednisolone**.
- Methylation of prednisolone (Methylprednisolone) increased the glucocorticoid effect by **5 times** with duration of action unchanged i.e. **12–36 hours**.
- Addition of fluorine at ring B increased glucocorticoid effect by **15 times** and mineralocorticoid effect by 150 times. There is an increase in half-life to **24 hours**. This steroid is a mineralocorticoid called as **fludrocortisone**. **Aldosterone** has only mineralocorticoid effect which is **500 times** that of hydrocortisone. However, the affinity of mineralocorticoid receptors is higher with fludrocortisone as compared to aldosterone.
- Addition of both **double bond at ring A and fluorine at ring B** increased the glucocorticoid effect by **30 times (betamethasone and dexamethasone) and 5 times (triamcinolone)**. However, this led to **zero mineralocorticoid effect**. Hence these steroids are called as **pure glucocorticoids**. The increase in half life for dexamethasone and betamethasone was to **36–72 hours** and triamcinolone was to **12–36 hours**.
- However, the glucocorticoid with maximum affinity for glucocorticoid receptors is **dexamethasone > betamethasone**.
- Further steroids were added with functional groups like **valerate, propionate and butyrate that increased the lipid solubility**. This is essential for topical use of steroids in cream and ointment form.

- Addition of functional group like dipropionate to beclomethasone made it inactive and it is activated in lungs by esterase where they produce anti-inflammatory effect in bronchial asthma. The benefit is a lesser incidence of oropharyngeal candidiasis.

Important properties of steroids	
Most potent glucocorticoid	Dexamethasone and betamethasone
Glucocorticoid with maximum affinity for glucocorticoid receptors	Dexamethasone > Betamethasone
Longest acting glucocorticoid	Dexamethasone and betamethasone
Shortest acting glucocorticoid	Hydrocortisone
Most potent mineralocorticoid	Aldosterone
Mineralocorticoid with maximum affinity for mineralocorticoid receptors	Fludrocortisone
Pure glucocorticoids (Zero mineralocorticoid activity)	Dexamethasone Betamethasone Triamcinolone
Pure mineralocorticoid (Zero glucocorticoid activity)	Aldosterone Deoxycorticosterone acetate (DOCA)

Conceptual Box-8

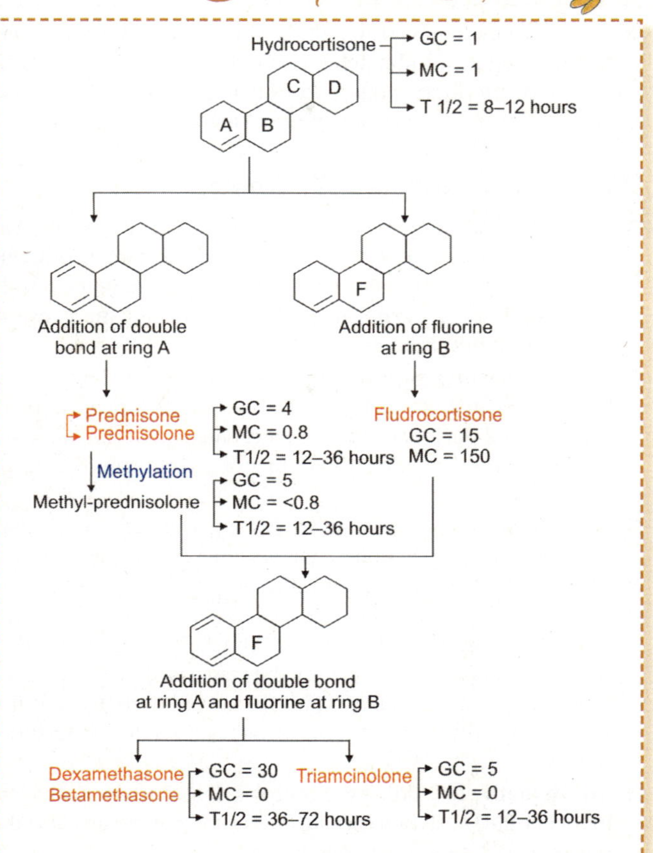

GLUCOCORTICOIDS

Effects of Glucocorticoids

- **Anti-inflammatory and immunomodulatory effect:** Anti-inflammatory and immunomodulatory effects are correlated and seen due to a decrease in inflammatory mediators like **IL-1, IL-6, TNF-α** and an increase in anti-inflammatory mediators like **IL-10 and annexin-1**. They also inhibit phospholipase A2 and cyclooxygenase, which decreases synthesis of prostaglandins. Apart from this, steroids can also cause lymphocyte apoptosis, redistribution and decrease macrophage activity.
- **Immunosuppression:** The above mentioned effects can cause immunosuppression and increase risk of infections like H. pylori, TB etc.
- **Decreased capillary permeability:** They decrease release of histamine by mast cells and basophils, which decreases capillary permeability.
- **Metabolic effects:** They stimulate gluconeogenesis and break down amino acids from muscles which are used in gluconeogenesis. They also inhibit glucose uptake by skeletal muscles by inducing insulin resistance. Thus, the overall effect is hyperglycemia. Since glucose is not utilized by skeletal muscles, there is lipolysis in the limbs which causes thinning. Hyperglycemia increases insulin release which inhibits lipolysis and stimulates lipogenesis in the trunk and neck. This causes the classical cushingoid features, i.e. moon facies, buffalo hump and central obesity with thin limbs, which gives a lemon on stick appearance.
- **Musculoskeletal effects:** Musculoskeletal effects are osteoporosis (bone resorption), growth retardation in children and muscle atrophy (myopathy).
- **Renal effects:** Glucocorticoids have some mineralocorticoid effect as well and hence cause sodium, water absorption and cause potassium, proton loss. There is also decreased calcium absorption in gut and increased excretion by kidney.
- **HPA suppression:** Hypothalamo pituitary axis suppression can lead to a decreased release of pituitary hormones like growth hormone, FH/LSH, TSH and ACTH.
- **Fetal effects:** In fetus glucocorticoids are responsible for surfactant activation in third trimester.
- **CNS effects:** Neuropsychiatric effects like insomnia, euphoria, depression and psychosis can be seen. There is also an increase in intracranial tension.
- **Permissive effects:** Glucocorticoids enhance production of catecholamine receptors (alpha and beta) and hence maintain effectiveness of catecholamines in blood vessels and bronchi. Thus, long-term glucocorticoid use can cause hypertension. For same reason glucocorticoids can increase effectiveness of beta-2 agonists in bronchial asthma.
- **Bone marrow effect:** Glucocorticoids increase RBC (polycythemia) and neutrophils. However, they decrease lymphocyte, basophils, monocytes and eosinophils.

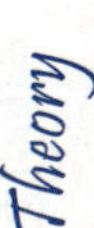

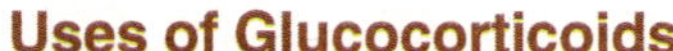

Uses of Glucocorticoids

Anti-inflammatory

- The anti-inflammatory uses are rheumatoid arthritis, giant cell arteritis, bronchial asthma, subacute thyroiditis, inflammatory skin conditions, inflammatory bowel disease and sarcoidosis. Prednisolone is the preferred drug for systemic anti-inflammatory uses.
- Topically steroids are applied for inflammatory skin disorders like psoriasis, atopic dermatitis, mycosis fungoides, lichen planus and pemphigoid. The most potent topical steroids are **clobetasol propionate, diflorasone diacetate and halobetasol propionate. Ointment is a more potent** form of topical steroid than cream form.

Immunomodulatory

- The uses are in conditions like autoimmune hemolytic anemia, multiple sclerosis, nephrotic syndrome, thrombocytopenia (Idiopathic), ITP, **Loeffler's syndrome**, GVHD and graft rejection.
- Prednisolone is again the preferred drug in immunomodulatory uses.

Neoplasia

- Steroids are commonly used in neoplastic conditions like **leukemia, lymphoma, multiple myeloma etc**. They are also effective in chemotherapy induced nausea and vomiting.
- The preferred steroid is prednisolone.

Infections

- In some infections like pneumocystis pneumonia with hypoxia in AIDS patients and *H. influenzae* meningitis, steroids are lifesaving drugs.
- Prednisone is the drug of choice for treatment of Bell's palsy.

Ocular Inflammation

- Topical glucocorticoids are used for treatment of ocular inflammation like choroiditis, optic neuritis and uveitis. However, steroids are contraindicated in **herpes simplex keratitis** due to risk of **irreversible clouding of cornea**.

Steroid Replacement

- For steroid replacement in **adrenal insufficiency (acute and chronic), congenital adrenal hyperplasia and post-adrenalectomy patients od Cushing's syndrome**, the steroid of choice is **hydrocortisone**. Fludrocortisone is given for mineralocorticoid replacement.
- The dose of steroids in chronic replacement is given below in the table.

Replacement in Chronic Adrenal Insufficiency	
Hydrocortisone replacement (Oral)	Fludrocortisone replacement (Oral)
Children: 10 mg/m²/day in three divided doses **Adults:** 15–30 mg/day in three divided doses	**Children:** 0.05–0.2 mg/day **Adults:** 0.05–0.3 mg/day

- In case of acute adrenal insufficiency only hydrocortisone is given at doses given below:

Hydrocortisone (IV) Bolus in Acute Crisis of Adrenal Insufficiency	
Infants	10 mg
Toddlers	25 mg
Older Children	50 mg
Adults	100 mg

Chrousos Syndrome

- Chrousos syndrome is characterized by glucocorticoid resistance due to mutation of glucocorticoid receptors. This increases release of ACTH, which further increases cortisol/aldosterone (hypertension and alkalosis) and androgens (hirsutism, infertility, baldness in females). Thus to normalize the production of these hormones, dexamethasone is given.

Pregnancy

- In pregnancy steroids are given in premature labor for fetal lung maturity; the preferred steroids are **dexamethasone or betamethasone**. Betamethasone is more effective in preventing mortality as compared to dexamethasone.

Dose of Steroids for Fetal Lung Maturation	
Betamethasone 12 mg 24 hourly 2 doses	Dexamethasone 6 mg 12 hourly 4 doses

- In a pregnant female with baby having CAH, **dexamethasone** is preferred to inhibit fetal androgen production. In CAH the fetus produces huge amount of androgen that causes virilization and ambiguous genitalia in female fetus.

Diagnosis of Cushing's Syndrome

- Cushing syndrome may be caused by Cushing's disease, ectopic tumors producing ACTH and tumors producing cortisol in the adrenals. The first thing in diagnosis is to confirm Cushing's syndrome and then to find the cause of Cushing's syndrome.
- **Dexamethasone suppression test** is done for diagnosis of Cushing's syndrome. 1 mg of dexamethasone is given at night (11 PM) and plasma cortisol level is checked in the morning. A plasma cortisol level of >5 mcg/dL conforms Cushing's syndrome.
- Dexamethasone is then given 0.5 mg 6 hourly for 2 days followed by 2 mg 6 hourly for another 2 days and plasma cortisol level is checked in the morning. A decrease in cortisol levels of >50% confirms Cushing's disease. If there is no decrease in cortisol levels, then ACTH is measured. If ACTH is increased, then clearly the cause is an ectopic tumor producing ACTH and if ACTH is decreased then it is a tumor producing cortisol in adrenals. This test is called as **Liddle's test**.
- An alternative to Liddle's test is giving dexamethasone 8 mg at night (11 PM) and then measuring serum cortisol levels in the morning to draw similar conclusions.

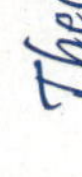

Miscellaneous Uses

Steroids are also used for various other conditions like malignant exophthalmos, hypercalcemia, mountain sickness, cerebral edema, ARDS and sepsis.

Recent Advances

Deflazacort is a steroid recently approved for treatment of Duchenne's muscular dystrophy.

Side Effects of Glucocorticoids

- Glucocorticoids by systemic route cause posterior subcapsular cataract and central serous retinopathy, but by topical route cause glaucoma. Children are more prone to cataract and despite stopping drug it may progress.
- There can be thinning of skin and hair, striae, folliculitis, hirsutism, acne and ecchymoses due to easy bruising.
- Immunosuppression can cause *H. pylori* colonization of stomach, that can cause gastric ulcers. Other infections like TB can be seen due to immunosuppression.
- Mineralocorticoid effect as well as permissive effect of catecholamines can cause hypertension. Mineralocorticoid effect can cause potassium and proton loss, leading to hypochloremic, hypokalemic alkalosis.
- Negative nitrogen, potassium and calcium balance can be seen, i.e. there is increased excretion. Thus, hypokalemia and hypocalcemia can be seen. Hence, patients on glucocorticoid therapy should be on high protein and potassium rich diet.
- Osteoporosis, femoral head necrosis and growth retardation (children) can be seen.
- Hyperglycemia and diabetes mellitus can be seen. Glucocorticoid induced diabetes is treated by insulin.
- Neuropsychiatric side effects like insomnia, euphoria, psychosis and depression are seen.
- Myopathy characterized by proximal muscle involvement is seen.
- To minimize these side effects minimum possible dose should be used or an alternate day regimen is preferred.

Mnemonics

C: Cataract
U: Ulcer of stomach
S: Skin thinning and striae
H: Hirsutism (females), Hypertension, Hypokalemia
I: Infections, Inflammation of follicles
N: Necrosis of femoral head
G: Glucose intolerance, Glaucoma
O: Osteoporosis, Obesity
I: Impaired calcium absorption
D: Depression, Diabetes mellitus
P: Psychosis, Pancreatitis
A: Acne, Alkalosis (hypochloremic, hypokalemic)
T: Telangiectasia
I: Insomnia
E: Ecchymoses due to easy bruising
N: Negative nitrogen, calcium and potassium balance
T: Thinning of hair

Withdrawal Effects of Glucocorticoids

- Glucocorticoids on stopPage can cause withdrawal symptoms like fever, postural hypotension, malaise, arthralgia, myalgia and pseudotumor cerebri.
- Thus, to decrease the severity of withdrawal symptoms steroids should not be abruptly stopped, rather tapered down.

MINERALOCORTICOIDS

- Aldosterone and deoxycorticosterone (DOC) are the mineralocorticoids produced by adrenals. Both are pure mineralocorticoids and devoid of any glucocorticoid effect. Secretion of aldosterone is controlled by ACTH, angiotensin and potassium, whereas secretion of DOC is controlled only by ACTH.
- Aldosterone acts on the mineralocorticoid receptors in the epithelial cells of collecting duct and increases expression of ENaC, which causes sodium and water absorption, and this is followed by loss of potassium and protons.
- Aldosterone is the most potent mineralocorticoid, however clinically it is not used due to low oral bioavailability.
- Deoxycorticosterone acetate (DOCA) can be used by intramuscular or sublingual route for replacement in adrenal insufficiency.
- Fludrocortisone is a synthetic mineralocorticoid, which has glucocorticoid effect as well. It is the preferred mineralocorticoid for replacement in adrenal insufficiency and CAH. It is also the drug of choice for long term management of idiopathic postural hypotension. It has a half-life of more than 24 hours and hence once a day dosing is sufficient.

GLUCOCORTICOID AND MINERALOCORTICOID ANTAGONISTS

- Mifepristone is primarily used for its partial agonistic action on progesterone receptors. However, at high doses it also inhibits glucocorticoid receptors and hence can be used for treatment of Cushing's syndrome caused by inoperable ectopic ACTH producing tumor and resistant cortisol producing tumor. It is an orphan drug for treatment of hyperglycemia caused by Cushing syndrome in diabetic patients.
- Spironolactone and drospirenone are mineralocorticoid antagonists. Spironolactone is used for diagnosis and treatment of primary hyperaldosteronism.

ACTH SECRETION INHIBITORS

- Somatostatin analog paseriotide inhibits release of growth hormone, TSH and ACTH. Hence, it is approved for treatment of Cushing's disease caused by ACTH secretion by pituitary corticotroph tumors.
- D2 agonist cabergoline can also decrease ACTH release and can be used for treatment of Cushing's disease caused by ACTH secretion by pituitary corticotroph tumors.

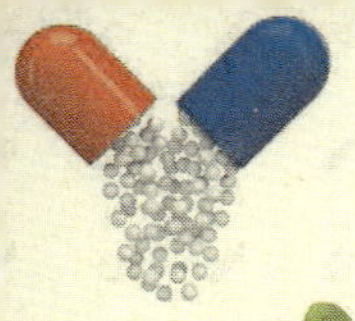

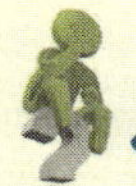

Image-based Questions

1. **Which of the following drugs might have caused the effect given in the picture?**

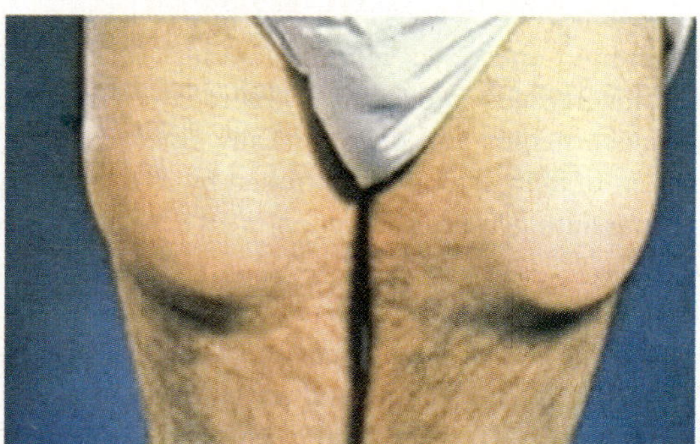

a. Somatropin b. Octreotide
c. Insulin d. Goserelin

2. **Which of the following is drug of choice in the condition given below?**

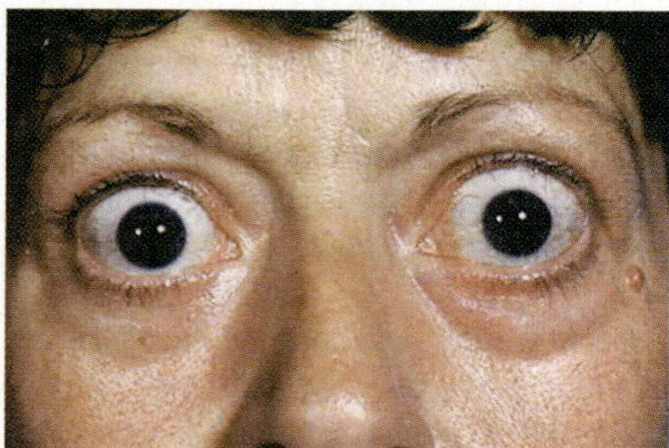

a. Propylthiouracil b. KI
c. Methimazole d. Thiocyanate

3. **Which of the following drug might have caused the side effect given in the picture?**

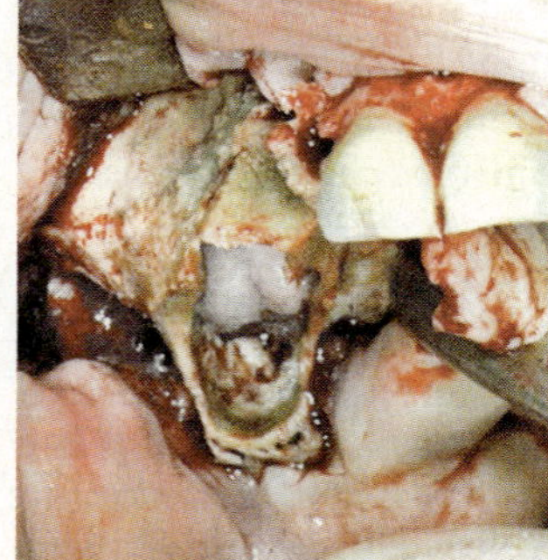

a. Inhalational steroids b. Denosumab
c. Tetracyclines d. Zolendronic acid

4. **Which of the following is used for the condition given in the picture?**

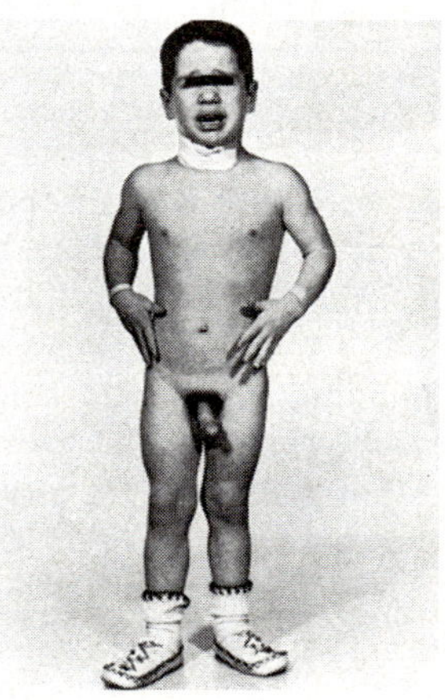

a. Intermittent dose ganirelix
b. Intermittent dose goserelin
c. Continuous dose goserelin
d. Continuous dose ganirelix

5. **The drug in the picture is used for:**

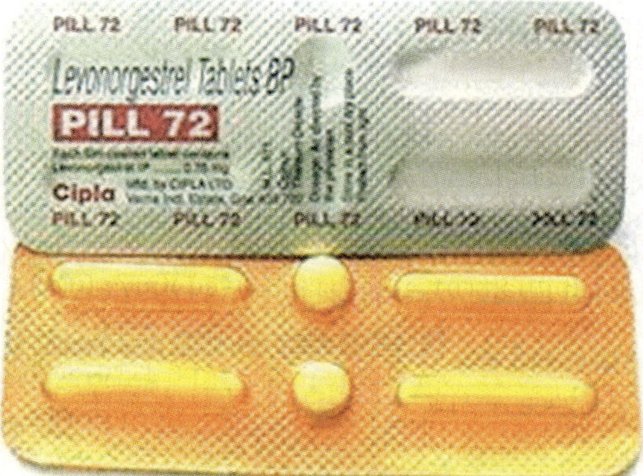

a. Breast cancer
b. Routine contraception
c. Emergency contraception
d. Abortion

Answers with Explanations to Image-based Questions

1. Ans. (c) Insulin

Lipohypertrophy at the site of injection due to inhibition of lipolysis can be seen with insulin.

2. Ans. (c) Methimazole

- Exophthalmos in the picture is suggestive of hyperthyroidism.
- Methimazole is the drug of choice for hyperthryoidism.

3. Ans. (d) Zolendronic acid

The side effect given in the picture is osteonecrosis of jaw seen with bisphosphonates like zolendronic acid.

4. Ans. (d) Continuous dose ganirelix

The picture depicts a case of precocious puberty for which GNRH agonists like goserelin is preferred by continuous administration.

5. Ans. (c) Emergency contraception

2 tablets of levonorgastral given in the picture are used 12 hours apart for emergency contraception.

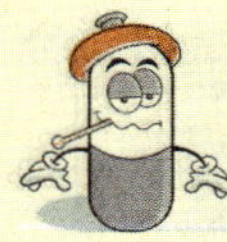

Annexures

Drug of Choice

Acromegaly	Octreotide
Addison disease Congenital adrenal hyperplasia in patient	Hydrocortisone
Anovulation PCOS	Clomiphene citrate
BPH	α1a antagonists • Tamsulosin • Silodosin
Carcinoid Syndrome GRFoma Glucagonoma Somatostatinoma VIPoma	Somatostatin analogues
Diabetes insipidus	Desmopressin
Diabetes mellitus type I Gestational diabetes Diabetic ketoacidosis	Insulin
Diabetes mellitus type II	• Treatment – Metformin • Prophylaxis – Metformin
Hypercalcemia of malignancy	Bisphosphonates
Hyperprolactinemia	Cabergoline
Hyperthyroidism	Methimazole
Hyperthyroidism in pregnancy	• 1st trimester – Propylthiouracil • 2nd and 3rd trimester – Methimazole
Hypothyroidism	Levothyroxine sodium
Insulinoma	Diazoxide
Oral contraception	Monophasic pills
Oligospermia	Clomiphene citrate
Osteoporosis	Zoledronic acid
Page t disease	Zoledronic acid
Premature labor Fetal CAH	Dexamethasone
Prolactinoma	Dopamine agonists
Riedel struma	Tamoxifen
Subacute thyroiditis	Aspirin
SIADH	Vaptans (Tolvaptan)
Thyroid storm	• Overall DOC - Propylthiouracil • Initial DOC – Propranolol
Toxic multinodular goiter Hyperfunctioning solitary Nodule	Radioiodine

New Drugs

New drugs	Mechanism of action	Uses
Lutathera	Radiolabeled somatostatin analog	Gastroenteropancreatic neuroendocrine tumors
Apalutamide	Androgen receptor antagonist	Prostate cancer
Elagolix	GnRH receptor antagonist	Endometriosis

Multiple Choice Questions

DIABETES MELLITUS

1. **A diabetic, obese patient on metformin presents with uncontrolled sugar level even after increasing dosage. He is allergic to sulphonylureas, has pancreatitis and family history of bladder cancer. He does not want to take injections, so what will you give next?** ***(AIIMS Nov 2017)***
   a. Sitagliptin b. Liraglutide
   c. Pioglitazone d. Canagliflozin
2. **Which of the following drugs is to be immediately stopped in a patient of diabetes with hypertension and serum creatinine level of 5.6 mg/dL?** ***(AIIMS Nov 2017)***
   a. Metformin b. Insulin
   c. Metoprolol d. Linagliptin
3. **Components of lente insulin are:** ***(AIIMS May 2017)***
   a. 30% amorphous + 70% crystalline
   b. 30% crystalline + 70% amorphous
   c. Same as NPH insulin
   d. Only 70% amorphous
4. **A 70-year-old patient has diabetes mellitus and hypertension. He presents with CKD stage 5 and does not want to take insulin. Which antidiabetic drug will you prefer in this patient that does not require dose modification in renal disease?** ***(AIIMS May 2017)***
   a. Linagliptin b. Vildagliptin
   c. Repaglinide d. Glimepiride
5. **Least commonly used site for insulin administration is:** ***(AIIMS Nov 2016)***
   a. Anterior thigh b. Lateral thigh
   c. Around umbilicus d. Dorsal area of arm
6. **Risk factors for increased lactic acidosis in patients on metformin are all except:** ***(AIIMS Nov 2016)***
   a. Advanced age b. Liver dysfunction
   c. Renal dysfunction d. Smoking
7. **Drug used safely in renal failure without change in dose:** ***(AIIMS Nov 2016)***
   a. Linagliptin b. Sitagliptin
   c. Vildagliptin d. Saxagliptin
8. **Which does not act by increasing insulin secretion?** ***(AIIMS May 2015)***
   a. Exenatide b. Sitagliptin
   c. Rosiglitazone d. Repaglinide
9. **True about pioglitazone are all except:**
   a. Metabolized in the liver by CYP3A4 ***(AIIMS May 2011)***
   b. Selective agonist for the nuclear peroxisome proliferator activated receptor gamma
   c. It causes transcription of gene for carbohydrate and fat metabolism in the absence of insulin
   d. It should be avoided in a patient with cardiovascular disease
10. **All of the statements about exenatide are true except:**
    a. It is a GLP-1 analogue ***(AIIMS May 2011)***
    b. It can be used for treatment of Type 1 diabetes mellitus
    c. It is given subcutaneously
    d. It decreases glucagon
11. **A patient is receiving insulin and acarbose for diabetes mellitus and developed hypoglycemia. Which of the following should be used for treatment of hypoglycemia in this patient?** ***(AIIMS May 2011)***
    a. Sucrose
    b. Maltose
    c. Glucose
12. **What will happen if insulin alone is given rapidly in diabetic ketoacidosis?** ***(AI 2009, AIIMS May 2010)***
    a. Hypokalemia b. Hypernatremia
    c. Hyperkalemia d. Hypocalcemia
13. **Insulin causes all of the following except:** ***(AIIMS May 2010)***
    a. Glycogenesis b. Glycolysis
    c. Lipogenesis d. Ketogenesis
14. **Regarding teduglutide, which is correct?**
    a. GLP-2 agonist ***(Recent Question 2019)***
    b. GLP-1 agonist
    c. Oral drug
    d. Pancreatic enzyme replacement
15. **Teduglutide is used in small bowel syndrome because of it is:** ***(Recent Question 2018)***
    a. Pancreatic lipase enzyme similarity
    b. Biliary lipase
    c. Glucagon like peptide 2
    d. Somatostatin
16. **Which of the following statements regarding acarbose is false?** ***(Recent Question 2008, AIIMS Nov 2008)***
    a. It acts by inhibiting the enzyme alpha-glucosidase
    b. It reduces both pre- and postprandial hyperglycemia
    c. It decreases the progression of impaired glucose tolerance to overt diabetes mellitus
    d. It reduces fibrinogen level
17. **Bromocriptine is used for treatment in:**
    a. DM ***(Recent Question Dec 2016)***
    b. Hypoprolactinemia
    c. Hypoglycemia
    d. Psychosis
18. **In DKA insulin of choice:** ***(Recent Question Dec 2016)***
    a. Regular b. Glargine
    c. NPH d. Lispro
19. **If a patient with severe hyperglycemia is given IV insulin, which of the following can occur?** ***(Recent Question 2016)***
    a. Hypokalemia b. Hyperkalemia
    c. Hyponatremia d. Hypernatremia

20. The most potent among antidiabetic drugs are the insulin secretagogues. Which of the following drugs is an insulin secretagogue? ***(Recent Question 2016)***
a. Metformin b. Pioglitazone
c. Tolbutamide d. Pramlintide

21. Longest acting insulin is: ***(Recent Question 2016)***
a. Global zinc suspension
b. Insulin zinc suspension
c. Neutral protamine hagedorn
d. Protamine zinc insulin

22. Exenatide is a newer drug proposed for treatment of: ***(Recent Question 2016)***
a. Osteoporosis
b. Diabetes mellitus
c. Hyperparathyroidism
d. Anovulatory infertility

23. Insulin glargine is given? ***(Recent Question 2016)***
a. Once daily before lunch
b. Once daily before breakfast
c. Once daily before dinner
d. Once daily anytime during day

24. Antidiabetic drug given subcutaneously is? ***(Recent Question 2016)***
a. Vildagliptin b. Metformin
c. Pramlintide d. Acarbose

25. Which of the following drug causes vitamin B12 deficiency? ***(Recent Question 2016)***
a. Valproate b. Azithromycin
c. Metformin d. Rifampicin

26. HbAlc is decreased most by? ***(Recent Question 2016)***
a. Biguanides b. Sulfonylureas
c. Thiazolidinediones d. Acarbose

27. If a diabetic patient being treated with an oral hypoglycemic agent develops dilutional hyponatremia, which of the following could be responsible for this effect? ***(Recent Question 2016)***
a. Chlorpropamide b. Tolbutamide
c. Glyburide d. Glimepiride

28. Adverse effect of thiazolidinediones is/are: ***(Recent Question 2016)***
a. Weight gain
b. Fractures
c. Macular edema
d. All of the above

29. Drug used in both type 1 and 2 DM ***(Recent Question 2016)***
a. Bromocriptine b. Colesevelam
c. Pramlintide d. Exenatide

30. All are true about sitagliptin except: ***(Recent Question 2016)***
a. Weight neutral
b. ↑ insulin secretion
c. Given along with insulin
d. Hypoglycemia is the major adverse effect

31. Pramlintide is: ***(Recent Question 2016)***
a. Synthetic amylin analog
b. Inhibitor of DPP 4
c. GLP 1 analogue
d. PPAR gamma

32. Rosiglitazone mechanism of action is:
a. Acts as PPAR gamma agonist ***(Recent Question 2016)***
b. Inhibitor of alpha glucosidase
c. Acts as amylin analogue
d. Acts as dipeptidyl peptidase inhibitor

33. Incretin like function is seen in: ***(Recent Question 2016)***
a. Exenatide b. Miglitol
c. Pioglitazone d. Repaglinide

34. Which is a long-acting insulin? ***(Recent Question 2016)***
a. Lispro b. Aspart
c. Glargine d. Glulisine

35. Special feature of glargine insulin is ***(Recent Question 2016)***
a. It produces a smooth peakless effect
b. It is not suitable for once daily administration
c. It remains soluble at pH 7
d. It can control meal time hyperglycemia

36. Insulin secretion increasing drug by acting on beta cells of pancreas is: ***(Recent Question 2016)***
a. Repaglinide b. Metformin
c. Pioglitazone d. Acarbose

37. Which insulin is never mixed with other insulins? ***(Recent Question 2016)***
a. Lente b. Aspart
c. Lispro d. Glargine

38. Insulin release due to closure of K^+ channel is seen with: ***(Recent Question 2016)***
a. Nateglinide b. Acarbose
c. Exenatide d. Sitagliptin

39. All are true about sitagliptin except:
a. Always given with insulin ***(Recent Question 2016)***
b. Preferentially reduce postprandial sugar
c. Less side effects
d. Lowers HbA1c

40. In diabetes mellitus with increased HbA1c, drug that is not used in treatment is: ***(Recent Question 2016)***
a. Sulfonylureas b. Acarbose
c. Biguanides d. Thiazolidinediones

41. Drug used in postprandial sugar control is:
a. Alfa glucosidase inhibitors ***(Recent Question 2016)***
b. Biguanides
c. Sulfonylurea
d. Repaglinide

42. Which is not an insulin analogue? ***(Recent Question 2016)***
a. Insulin glargine b. Insulin lispro
c. Insulin actrapid d. Insulin aspart

43. Which of the following antidiabetic drugs can cause vitamin B12 deficiency? ***(Recent Question 2016)***
a. Glipizide b. Acarbose
c. Metformin d. Pioglitazone

44. Which of the following drugs does not cause hypoglycemia: ***(Recent Question 2016)***
a. Acarbose b. Insulin
c. Glimepiride d. Nateglinide

45. All of the following preparations of insulin are rapid and short acting except: ***(Recent Question 2016)***

a. Lispro b. Aspart
c. Glargine d. NPH

46. Which of the following statements about biguanides is not true? ***(Recent Question 2016)***

a. Do not stimulate insulin release
b. Decrease hepatic glucose production
c. Renal dysfunction is not a contraindication for their use
d. Can be combined with sulfonylurea

47. Which of the following is not administered by intradermal route? ***(Recent Question 2016)***

a. BCG b. Insulin
c. Mantoux d. Drug sensitivity injection

48. Drug used in diabetes is: ***(Recent Question 2016)***

a. Salmeterol b. Acetohexamide
c. Benserazide d. Methoxamine

49. Lactic acidosis is common in: ***(Recent Question 2016)***

a. Metformin b. Phenformin
c. Repaglinide d. Rosiglitazone

50. Tolbutamide acts by increasing: ***(Recent Question 2016)***

a. Insulin receptors b. Glucose entry
c. Glucose absorption d. Insulin secretion

51. Long-acting insulin is: ***(Recent Question 2016)***

a. Lente b. Semilente
c. Ultralente d. Lispro insulin

52. 2nd generation hypoglycemic drugs are all except: ***(Recent Question 2016)***

a. Glipizide b. Gliclazide
c. Tolbutamide d. Glibenclamide

53. Alpha-glucosidase inhibitor is: ***(Recent Question 2016)***

a. Pioglitazone b. Miglitol
c. Metformin d. Nateglinide

54. Common side effect of thiazolidinediones is: ***(Recent Question 2016)***

a. Dysgeusia
b. Hypoglycemia
c. Water retention with weight gain
d. Anemia

55. Antidiabetic contraindicated in renal failure are all except: ***(Recent Question 2016)***

a. Repaglinide
b. Acarbose
c. Metformin
d. Pioglitazone

56. Stimulator of insulin release: ***(Recent Question 2016)***

a. Metformin b. Pramlintide
c. Meglitinide d. Thiazolidinedione

THYROID

57. Which of the following is correct regarding T_3 and T_4 acting on TRH? ***(AIIMS Nov 2018)***

a. It activates phospholipase A
b. It acts on transcription factor
c. It acts by increasing cAMP
d. It is a tyrosine kinase receptor

58. All of the following are rare but serious/fatal side effects of thioanamide group of antithyroid drugs except: ***(AIIMS Nov 2016)***

a. Agranulocytosis b. Aplastic anemia
c. Liver toxicity d. Lung fibrosis

59. Iodine used in thyroid disorder not true: ***(AIIMS May 2013)***

a. Causes iodism
b. Contraindicated in hyperthyroidism
c. Inhibit formation of Iodothyronine
d. Thyroxine release

60. Conversion of T_4 to T_3 is inhibited by all except: ***(AIIMS Nov 2011)***

a. Propranolol b. Propylthiouracil
c. Amiodarone d. Methimazole

61. A pregnant female is taking carbimazole. Which of the following is not seen in the neonate? ***(AIIMS May 2007)***

a. Choanal atresia b. Scalp defects
c. Cleft lip/palate d. Fetal goiter

62. The first line antithyroid drug is methimazole, and the antithyroid drug which is safest in pregnancy is Propylthiouracil. Which among the following is the fastest acting antithyroid drug? ***(Recent Question 2016)***

a. Sodium iodide b. Propylthiouracil
c. Methimazole d. Carbimazole

63. Which drug prevent peripheral conversion of T_4 to T_3: ***(Recent Question 2016)***

a. Propylthiouracil b. Propranolol
c. Iodides d. Diltiazem

64. Which of the following drug does not act on thyroid: ***(Recent Question 2016)***

a. Propranolol b. Propylthiouracil
c. Sodium iodide d. Thiocyanate

65. Fastest acting antithyroid drugs ***(Recent Question 2016)***

a. Iodides of Na/K b. Propylthiouracil
c. Methimazole d. Nitrates

66. Lugol's iodine contains ***(Recent Question 2016)***

a. 5% iodine and 10% Kl b. 10% iodine and 20% Kl
c. 10% iodine and 15% Kl d. 5% iodine and 15% Kl

67. Plasma half-life of carbimazole is: ***(Recent Question 2016)***

a. 4 hours b. 8 hours
c. 16 hours d. 24 hours

68. True about proplythiouracil: ***(Recent Question 2016)***

a. Inhibit peripheral conversion of T_4 to T_3
b. Crosses placenta and secreted in breast milk
c. Active metabolite formed inside the body
d. 5 times more potent than carbimazole

69. Thyroid storm-management all except: ***(Recent Question 2016)***

a. Propylthiouracil b. Lugol's iodine
c. Steroids d. Thyroid surgery

70. A patient on treatment with carbimazole develops sore throat. Immediate investigation to be done is: ***(Recent Question 2016)***

a. Renal function tests
b. Thyroid function test
c. Complete blood count
d. Liver function tests

71. Propylthiouracil is used in all except: *(Recent Question 2016)*
a. Thyroid storm
b. Life-threatening thyrotoxicosis
c. First trimester pregnancy
d. Agranulocytosis caused by methimazole

DRUGS ACTING ON BONE

72. All drugs act to decrease bone resorption except: *(Recent Question 2017)*
a. Teriparatide
b. Raloxifene
c. Strontium ranelate
d. Risedronate

73. Drug used in osteoporosis all except: *(AIIMS Nov 2016)*
a. PTH b. Strontium
c. Denosumab d. Milnacipran

74. What will be advices given to a bisphosphonate taking patient? *(AIIMS Nov 2015)*
a. Take tab before food with full glass of water
b. Take tab after food with full glass of water
c. Stop if gastroesophageal discomfort persists
d. Stop if consistent bone pain persists

75. Both decreased bone resorption and increased bone formation is caused by: *(AIIMS May 2010, Nov 2008)*
a. Strontium ranelate b. Ibandronate
c. Teriparatide d. Calcitonin

76. Bisphosphonates are used in all expect: *(AIIMS Nov 2007)*
a. Malignancy
b. Vitamin D excess
c. Postmenopausal osteoporosis
d. Hypercalcemia

77. Denosumab, a monoclonal antibody against rank ligand is used for the treatment of: *(AIIMS Nov 2006)*
a. Rheumatoid arthritis
b. Osteoporosis
c. Osteoarthritis
d. Systemic lupus erythematosus

78. Teriparatide acts by: *(Recent Question Dec 2016)*
a. Increasing osteoblastic activity
b. Decreasing osteoclastic activity
c. Decreasing osteoclastic and increasing osteoblastic activity
d. Increasing calcium

79. Denosumab acts by: *(Recent Question Dec 2016)*
a. Activation of osteoclasts b. Osteoclast inhibition
c. Osteoblast activation d. RANK antagonist

80. Bisphosphonates act by: *(Recent Question 2016)*
a. Increasing osteoid formation
b. Increasing mineralization of osteoid
c. Decreasing osteoclast mediated resorption of bone
d. Decreasing PTH secretion

81. Which of the following drug causes osteonecrosis by giving IV route? *(Recent Question 2016)*
a. Zoledronate b. Dalteparin
c. Calcitriol d. Zidovudine

82. Parathyroid hormone: *(Recent Question 2016)*
a. Decreases bone resorption
b. Increases bone resorption
c. Enhances phosphate reabsoption from kidney
d. Decreases calcium reabsoption from kidney

83. Intranasal calcitonin is given in: *(Recent Question 2016)*
a. Page t's disease
b. MEN syndrome
c. Hypercalcemia
d. Postmenopausal osteoporosis

84. Parathormone is useful in: *(Recent Question 2016)*
a. Hyperparathyroidism b. Page t's disease
c. Osteoporosis d. Osteomalacia

85. All of the following decrease bone resorption in osteoporosis except: *(Recent Question 2016)*
a. Alendronate b. Etidronate
c. Strontium d. Teriparatide

86. Bisphosphonate is: *(Recent Question 2016)*
a. Risedronate b. Raloxifene
c. Tamoxifen d. Teriparatide

87. Which of the following is a serious adverse effect seen with bisphosphonates? *(Recent Question 2016)*
a. Acute renal failure b. Ventricular fibrillation
c. Peptic ulcer d. Anterior uveitis

GH AND RELATED DRUGS

88. Octreotide is used in all except: *(AIIMS May 2011)*
a. Glucagonoma b. Insulinoma
c. Carcinoid syndrome d. Glioma

89. Which of the following statements about octreotide is true? *(AIIMS Nov 2011)*
a. Stimulates growth hormone
b. Used in secretory diarrhea
c. Used orally
d. Contraindicated in acromegaly

90. Octreotide is used for: *(Recent Question Dec 2016)*
a. Acromegaly b. Osteoarthritis
c. Pancreatitis d. Constipation

91. Cabergoline is used in: *(Recent Question 2016)*
a. Acromegaly
b. Hyperprolactinemia
c. Both a and b
d. None of the above

92. Pegvisomant is a: *(Recent Question 2016)*
a. Growth hormone receptor agonist
b. Growth hormone receptor antagonist
c. GHRH agonist d. GHRH analogue

93. Drug of choice for esophageal varices: *(Recent Question 2016)*
a. Demeclocycline b. Dopamine
c. Octreotide d. Adrenaline

94. Treatment for acromegaly: *(Recent Question 2016)*
a. Octreotide
b. Sermorelin
c. Hexarelin
d. Nafarelin

DRUGS ACTING ON REPRODUCTIVE SYSTEM

95. Drug that decreases size of prostate is: ***(AIIMS Nov 2017)***
a. Tamsulosin b. Sildenafil
c. Finasteride d. Flutamide

96. A 27-year-old female came for treatment of infertility to OPD; bromocriptine was prescribed. What could be the possible reason? ***(AIIMS Nov 2017)***
a. Hyperprolactinemia
b. PCOD
c. Hypogonadotropic hypogonadism
d. PID

97. Dose of ulipristal is: ***(Recent Question 2019)***
a. 30 mg b. 30 mcg
c. 2000 mcg d. 60 mg

98. Tamoxifen is an antagonist at: ***(Recent Question 2019)***
a. Estrogen receptor b. Aromatase
c. Progesterone receptor d. Androgen receptor

99. Which of the following is incorrect regarding breast cancer treatment? ***(Recent Question 2019)***
a. Aromatase inhibitors are drug of choice for premenopausal breast cancer
b. Tamoxifen is drug of choice for postmenopausal breast cancer
c. Tamoxifen dose is 20 mg OD for 5 years
d. Anastrazole dose is 10 mg OD for 5 years

100. All of the following are not seen with OCP except: ***(Recent Question 2019)***
a. Psychosis b. Thromboembolism
c. Dyslipidemia d. Osteoporosis

101. Main indication of HRT: ***(Recent Question 2017)***
a. Menstrual irregularities
b. Intolerant hot flushes
c. Deep vein thrombosis
d. Atherosclerosis

102. Drug of choice for precocious puberty: ***(AIIMS Nov 2016)***
a. Cyproterone b. Danazol
c. Medroxyprogesterone d. GnRH agonist

103. WHO recommended oral dose of misoprostol for prevention of postpartum hemorrhage is: ***(AIIMS Nov 2016)***
a. 400 mcg b. 600 mcg
c. 800 mcg d. 1000 mcg

104. Which cannot be used as emergency contraceptive? ***(AIIMS Nov 2015)***
a. IUCD b. Ulipristal
c. Levonorgestrel d. Desogestrel

105. Dose of misoprostol recommended by WHO for prophylaxis of PPH: ***(AIIMS Nov 2015)***
a. 1000 mcg b. 800 mcg
c. 700 mcg d. 600 mcg

106. Which of the following drugs is not used in PCOD? ***(AIIMS May 2015)***
a. OCP b. Tamoxifen
c. Clomiphene d. Metformin

107. Which of the following drugs is useful for the treatment of advanced prostate cancer? ***(AIIMS May 2014)***
a. Ganirelix b. Cetrorelix
c. Abarelix d. Goserelin

108. Prolonged testosterone treatment to a man results in: ***(AIIMS Nov 2010)***
a. Increased spermatogenesis
b. Increased sperm motility
c. Azoospermia
d. Increased gonadotropins

109. Which of the following drug is a SERM useful for treatment of osteoporosis? ***(AIIMS Nov 2010)***
a. Raloxifene b. Bisphosphonate
c. Strontium d. Estradiol

110. Which of the following drug is used in the treatment of estrogen dependent breast carcinoma? ***(AIIMS Nov 2010)***
a. Tamoxifen b. Methotrexate
c. Paclitaxel d. Adriamycin

111. Which of the following progesterone is used in emergency contraception? ***(AIIMS May, Nov 2009)***
a. Levonorgestrel
b. Micronized progesterone
c. Norgesterone
d. Depot medroxyprogesterone acetate

112. Hormone replacement therapy is helpful in all of the following conditions except: ***(AIIMS May 2007)***
a. Vaginal atrophy b. Flushing
c. Coronary heart disease d. Osteoporosis

113. Which of the following is an aromatase inhibitor? ***(AIIMS May 2006)***
a. Tamoxifen b. Letrozole
c. Danazol d. Taxane

114. Most common long-term side effect of tamoxifen: ***(Recent Question Dec 2016)***
a. Weight gain b. Osteoporosis
c. Venous thrombosis d. Uterine cancer

115. For treatment of hirsutism the drug not used is: ***(Recent Question Dec 2016)***
a. Spironolactone
b. Levenorgestrel
c. Finasteride d. Flutamide

116. Oxytocin acts on? ***(Recent Question Dec 2016)***
a. PGI_2 b. PGF_2 alpha
c. Endothelin d. Prostacyclin

117. Oxytocin is useful in PPH due to stimulation of: ***(Recent Question Dec 2016)***
a. PGF2 alpha
b. PGE2
c. Prostacyclin
d. Thromboxane

118. Which of the following is an SPRM? ***(Recent Question Dec 2016)***
a. Letrozole b. Raloxifene
c. Ranolazine d. Ulipristal

119. Clomiphene citrate which is given in PCOD acts on: ***(Recent Question Dec 2016)***
a. Hypothalamus b. Pituitary Gland
c. Ovary d. Primordial follicles

120. Which of the following is used for treatment of infertility with hypogonadism? ***(Recent Question Dec 2016)***
a. Clomiphene b. Testosterone
c. GnRH agonists d. Flutamide

121. Mifepristone can be used as in abortion up to which gestational age? ***(Recent Question Dec 2016)***
a. 6 weeks b. 8 weeks
c. 14 weeks d. 20 weeks

122. Fulvestrant is used in the treatment of: ***(Recent Question Dec 2016)***
a. T-ALL b. Multiple myeloma
c. Breast cancer d. Prostate Ca

123. Mifepristone (RU-486) is the most commonly used drug for medical abortion and emergency contraception. Pharmacologically the drug is a: ***(Recent Question 2016)***
a. Antiprogesterone b. Progestin analogue
c. PGE1 analogue d. PGE2 analogue

124. All of the following drugs can cause hirsutism except: ***(Recent Question 2016)***
a. Phenytoin
b. Flutamide
c. Norethindrone
d. Danazol

125. Hormone replacement therapy decreases the risk of: ***(Recent Question 2016)***
a. Carcinoma colon
b. Carcinoma breast
c. Carcinoma endometrium
d. Thromboembolism

126. Drug of choice for male type baldness in female: ***(Recent Question 2016)***
a. Flutamide b. Finasteride
c. Cyproterone acetate d. Danazol

127. Following is true about GnRH agonists except: ***(Recent Question 2016)***
a. Used in cases of precocious puberty
b. They have action similar to gonadotropin releasing hormone
c. Long-acting preparations can be used as nasal spray
d. Ganirelix is the most potent agent

128. Flutamide is used in CA: ***(Recent Question 2016)***
a. Cervix b. Prostate
c. Kidneys d. Liver

129. Tamoxifen ***(Recent Question 2016)***
a. SSRI b. SERM
c. SNRI d. DNRI

130. Letrozole belongs to which group? ***(Recent Question 2016)***
a. SERM b. SERD
c. LHRH analogues d. Aromatase inhibitors

131. DMPA is given once in: ***(Recent Question 2016)***
a. 3 months b. 6 months
c. 9 months d. 45 days

132. Reason for hepatic involvement in oral contraceptives is: ***(Recent Question 2016)***
a. Estrogen b. Progesterone
c. Estrogen + progesterone d. Mixed trace elements

133. Drug which decreases efficacy of testosterone: ***(Recent Question 2016)***
a. Isoniazid b. Ketoconazole
c. Rifampicin d. Spironolactone

134. Danazol has which of the following action: ***(Recent Question 2016)***
a. Weak androgenic b. Progestational
c. Anabolic d. All the above

135. Mechanism of action of oral contraceptive pill can be all except: ***(Recent Question 2016)***
a. Hostile to sperm penetration
b. Anovulatory cycle
c. Failure of blastocyst implantation
d. Blockade of fimbrial ostia

136. Which of the following is not an antiandrogenic drug? ***(Recent Question 2016)***
a. Flutamide b. Spironolactone
c. Finasteride d. Cyproterone

137. All are true about estrogen except: ***(Recent Question 2016)***
a. Causes cholestasis
b. Used in treatment of gynecomastia
c. Used in HRT
d. Increased risk of breast cancer

138. True about bicalutamide is: ***(Recent Question 2016)***
a. Binds to androgen receptor
b. Causes gynecomastia
c. It can be given as monotherapy in prostatic carcinoma
d. All are true

139. Finasteride acts by blocking: ***(Recent Question 2016)***
a. α-receptors b. 5-α reductase enzyme
c. Androgen receptors d. β-receptors

140. The drug not used in prostatic carcinoma is: ***(Recent Question 2016)***
a. Finasteride b. Diethylstibestrol
c. Testosterone d. Flutamide

141. The 5-α reductase inhibitor that has been found to be effective both in benign prostatic hypertrophy and male pattern baldness is: ***(Recent Question 2016)***
a. Flutamide b. Finasteride
c. Prazosin d. Minoxidil

142. Oral contraceptive pills can cause all except: ***(Recent Question 2016)***
a. Mastalgia b. Dysmenorrhea
c. Chloasma d. Breakthrough bleeding

143. Most potent androgen is: ***(Recent Question 2016)***
a. Dihydrotestosterone b. Testosterone
c. Dihydroepiandrosterone d. Piandrosterone

144. An example of antiprogesterone is: ***(Recent Question 2016)***
a. Gossypol b. Atosiban
c. Clomiphene d. Mifepristone (RU 486)

145. Which of the following is antiandrogenic drug? ***(Recent Question 2016)***
a. Bicalutamide b. Oxymetholone
c. Raloxifene d. Stanozolol

146. Which of the following is given at intervals as a pulsatile therapy? ***(Recent Question 2016)***

a. GnRH b. GH
c. FSH d. Estrogen

147. Which among the following is not a SERM? ***(Recent Question 2016)***

a. Flutamide b. Ormeloxifene
c. Tamoxifen d. Raloxifene

148. Flutamide is an: ***(Recent Question 2016)***

a. Anticonvulsant b. Antiandrogen
c. Antiprogestin d. Antioestrogen

STEROIDS

149. Hydrocortisone dosing in mg/m²/kg: ***(Recent Question 2017)***

a. 5 b. 10
c. 15 d. 20

150. Which of the following is glucocorticoid inhibitor: ***(Recent Question 2017)***

a. Metyrapone b. Mapracorat
c. Mitotane d. Miltefosine

151. Which of the following is true about antenatal use of steroids for fetal lung maturation? ***(AIIMS Nov 2016)***

a. Dexamethasone 6 mg 12 hourly 4 doses
b. Dexamethasone 12 mg 12 hourly 4 doses
c. Betamethasone 6 mg 12 hourly 4 doses
d. Betamethasone 12 mg 12 hourly 4 doses

152. Glucocorticoids are not used for: ***(AIIMS Nov 2015)***

a. CLL b. Hodgkin's lymphoma
c. Kaposi sarcoma d. Multiple myeloma

153. Glucocorticoids deficiency can cause all except: ***(AIIMS Nov 2015)***

a. Hyperkalemia
b. Fever
c. Weight loss
d. Postural hypotension

154. Drug of choice for pregnant female suspected of having a baby with congenital adrenal hyperplasia is: ***(AIIMS Nov 2011)***

a. Dexamethasone
b. Betamethasone
c. Hydrocortisone
d. Prednisolone

155. Hyperaldosteronism causes all except: ***(AI 2009, AIIMS May 2010)***

a. Hypernatremia
b. Hypokalemia
c. Hypertension
d. Metabolic acidosis

156. A girl presented with Bell's palsy on the third day. What is the ideal treatment? ***(AIIMS May 2010)***

a. Oral steroids and acyclovir
b. Oral steroids alone
c. Intratympanic steroids
d. Vitamin B and vasodilators

157. Which of the following drugs causes pharmacological adrenalectomy? ***(Recent Question 2016)***

a. Guanethidine b. Bretylium
c. Metyrapone d. Amiodarone

158. Compared to hydrocortisone maximum glucocorticoid action is found in: ***(Recent Question 2016)***

a. Dexamethasone b. Prednisolone
c. Methyl prednisolone d. Cortisone

159. Steroid with max mineralocorticoid activity: ***(Recent Question 2016)***

a. Fludrocortisone b. DOCA
c. Prednisolone d. Triamcinolone

160. Long-acting corticosteroid is: ***(Recent Question 2016)***

a. Triamcinolone b. Betamethasone
c. Hydrocortisone d. Prednisolone

161. Adrenocortical suppression causing drugs are all except ***(Recent Question 2016)***

a. Prednisone b. Ketoconazole
c. Mitotane d. Spironolactone

162. Mechanism of action trilostane: ***(Recent Question 2016)***

a. 11 beta hydroxylase inhibitor
b. 1 alpha hydroxylase inhibitor
c. 3 betahydroxysteroid dehydrogenase inhibitor
d. 7 alpha hydrolase inhibitor

163. Drug of choice for acute adrenal insufficiency is: ***(Recent Question 2016)***

a. Oral prednisone b. Hydrocortisone
c. Betamethasone d. Dexamethasone

164. All are side effects of steroids except: ***(Recent Question 2016)***

a. Skin atrophy b. Telangiectasia
c. Folliculitis d. Photosensitivity

165. Corticosteroid with the minimum potency: ***(Recent Question 2016)***

a. Hydrocortisone b. Fludrocortisone
c. Dexamethasone d. Triamcinolone

166. All of the following are topical steroids except: ***(Recent Question 2016)***

a. Hydrocortisone valerate b. Fluticasone propionate
c. Triamcinolone d. Prednisolone

167. Corticosteroid with maximum sodium retaining potential: ***(Recent Question 2016)***

a. Dexamethasone
b. Prednisolone
c. Aldosterone
d. Betamethasone

168. Steroid with equal mineralocorticoid and glucocorticoid activity is ***(Recent Question 2016)***

a. Betamethasone b. Dexamethasone
c. Hydrocortisone d. Beclomethasone

169. Which of the following is an indication for the use of corticosteroids? ***(Recent Question 2016)***

a. Psychosis b. Herpes simplex
c. Loeffler's syndrome d. Subacute thyroiditis

170. At same concentration of steroid which of the following is most potent? ***(Recent Question 2016)***

a. Ointment b. Cream
c. Lotion d. Gel

171. The most potent topical corticosteroid is: ***(Recent Question 2016)***
a. Hydrocortisone butyrate cream 0.1%
b. Betamethasone valerate cream 0.5%
c. Clobetasol propionate cream 0.5%
d. Clobetasone butyrate

172. Which of the following disorders in not aggravated by corticosteroid therapy? ***(Recent Question 2016)***
a. Congenital adrenal hyperplasia
b. Diabetes mellitus
c. Hypertension d. Peptic ulcer

173. All of the following agents act through nuclear receptors except: ***(Recent Question 2016)***
a. Thyroxine b. Rosiglitazone
c. Prednisolone d. Estrogen

174. Most potent mineralocorticoid is: ***(Recent Question 2016)***
a. Aldosterone b. DOCA
c. Fludrocortisone d. Triamcinolone

175. Systemic steroids can cause all of the following except: ***(Recent Question 2016)***
a. Hypertension b. Glaucoma
c. Cataract d. Osteoporosis

176. In Addison's disease drug to be given is: ***(Recent Question 2016)***
a. Hydrocortisone b. Betamethasone
c. Prednisolone d. DOCA

177. Corticosteroid which is given by inhalation route: ***(Recent Question 2016)***
a. Prednisolone b. Beclomethasone
c. Dexamethasone d. Hydrocortisone

178. Drug use for medical adrenalectomy: ***(Recent Question 2016)***
a. Mitotane b. Methotrexate
c. Doxorubicin d. 5-fluorouracil

179. 100 mg of hydrocortisone is equivalent to: ***(Recent Question 2016)***
a. 20 mg methylprednisolone
b. 20 mg deoxycortisone acetate
c. 10 mg dexamethasone
d. 10 mg prednisolone

180. Steroids are contraindicated in all except: ***(Recent Question 2016)***
a. Eczematous lesion b. Peptic ulcer
c. Diabetes mellitus d. Herpes simplex keratitis

181. Drug with weakest mineralocorticoid action: ***(Recent Question 2016)***
a. Deoxy corticosterone b. Cortisol
c. Triamcinolone d. Aldosterone

182. True about glucocorticoids are all except: ***(Recent Question 2016)***
a. Catabolic effects on fat and muscle
b. Acts via widely spread glucocorticoid receptors
c. Proinflammatory
d. Antiallergic

183. Antiandrogenic drugs are: ***(PGI May 2018)***
a. Abiraterone b. Anastrozole
c. Ketoconazole d. Finasteride
e. Danazol

184. Glucocorticoids do not cause: ***(Recent Question 2016)***
a. Osteoporosis b. Hypoglycemia
c. Peptic ulceration d. Cataracts

185. Which of the following antidiabetic drugs correctly match with their mechanism of action: ***(PGI Nov 2017)***
a. Acarbose – Alpha glucosidase inhibitor
b. Sitagliptin – GLP analogue
c. Exenatide – DPP-4 inhibitor
d. Canagliflozin – SGLT-2 inhibitor
e. Repaglinide – K^+ Channel inhibitor

186. Long acting insulin is/are: ***(PGI May 2017)***
a. Lispro b. Detemir
c. Glargine d. Isophane
e. Glulisine

187. All are true about bisphosphonates except: ***(PGI Nov. 2016)***
a. Prevent reabsorption of bone by osteoclast
b. Structurally similar to pyrophosphate
c. Absorption increases with food
d. Can be safely given in liver disease

188. True about effect of steroid intake in inflammatory conditions: ***(PGI Nov. 2016)***
a. Proanabolic effect on muscles
b. ↑ glucose in plasma
c. –ve feedback on corticotropin-releasing hormone (CRH) production
d. May cause osteoporosis

189. Which of the following is/are features of Triamcinolone with respect to hydrocortisone: ***(PGI June 2015)***
a. Fluorinated at carbon atom 9
b. Not used in oral form
c. Mineralocorticoid activity present
d. More potent than hydrocortisone
e. Glucocorticoid activity is 5 times of hydrocortisone

190. Which of following statement is true about canagliflozin: ***(PGI Nov 2014)***
a. SGLT-2 inhibitor
b. Blocks Na/glucose symport
c. Causes glycosuria & polyuria
d. Increases chance of vaginal infections

191. Which of following is/are true about metformin: ***(PGI Nov 2014)***
a. Cause lactic acidosis
b. PPAR γ agonist
c. Contraindicated in renal failure
d. Cause hypoglycemia
e. GI disturbances are common side effect

192. Which of the following is/are true about sulfonylurea except: ***(PGI May 2014)***
a. Increase insulin secretion
b. Cause hypoglycemia
c. Cause weight loss
d. Disulfiram-like reaction after alcohol intake
e. Safe in pregnancy

193. Use of metformin other than DM: ***(PGI Nov 2011)***
a. Impaired glucose tolerance
b. PCOS
c. Nonalcoholic fatty liver disease
d. Alcoholic fatty liver disease
e. Metabolic abnormalities associated with HIV disease

194. Features of metformin are: *(PGI Nov 2010)*
a. Notorious for causing hypoglycaemia
b. Decreases LDL
c. Increases insulin release
d. Lactic acidosis
e. Vit B deficiency

195. Long-acting insulin are: *(PGI Nov 2010)*
a. Glargine
b. Insulin lispro
c. Protamine zinc insulin
d. Insulin aspart
e. NPH

196. Which of the following is/are sulfonylureas: *(PGI Nov 2009)*
a. Glipizide
b. Glibenclamide
c. Repaglinide
d. Nateglinide
e. Exenatide

197. Aromatase inhibitors which are used in breast Ca: *(PGI June 2009)*
a. Letrozole
b. Anastrozole
c. Exemestane
d. Flutamide
e. Fluoxymesterone

198. True about drospirenone: *(PGI June 2009)*
a. Spironolactone analogue
b. Used in OCP
c. Mineralocorticoid receptor agonist
d. Third generation progesterone
e. Dose in OCP is 3 mg

199. Monomeric insulin is/are: *(PGI June 2009)*
a. Glargine
b. Detemir
c. Lispro insulin
d. Aspart insulin
e. NPH

200. Tamoxifen is: *(PGI Dec 2007)*
a. Used as adjuvant therapy in receptor positive breast cancer
b. For chemoprophylaxis against breast cancer
c. Used in renal cell carcinoma
d. Used in HCC

201. Long-acting insulin are: *(PGI Dec 2007)*
a. Glargine
b. Lispro
c. Detemir
d. Aspart
e. Glulisine

202. Table sugar is not used in treatment of hypoglycemia caused by: *(JIPMER 2017)*
a. Insulin
b. Acarbose
c. Canagliflozin
d. Pioglitazone

203. DPP inhibitor used in renal failure is: *(JIPMER 2017)*
a. Sitagliptin
b. Linagliptin
c. Saxagliptin
d. Vildagliptin

204. Regarding insulin afrezza all are true except: *(JIPMER 2017)*
a. Inhalational insulin
b. Basic insulin not needed
c. Given in multiple doses
d. Loading dose with other drug required

205. Anastrazole is a: *(JIPMER 2017)*
a. Competitive reversible aromatase inhibitor
b. Noncompetitive reversible aromatase inhibitor
c. Irreversible aromatase inhibitor
d. Suicide substrate

206. A 63-year-old male patient a known case of prostatomegaly presents to the emergency department with constipation (for almost a week), lethargy (last three days) and appears to be mildly dehydrated. Treatment with normal saline for rehydration did not improve his condition and additional laboratory tests were conducted. There is shortened QT interval on ECG. Serum calcium level is 14.7 mEq/L. After initial rehydration therapy and diuretics, which one of the following agents is indicated? *(JIPMER 2016)*
a. Gallium nitrate
b. Bisphosphonates
c. Denosumab
d. Calcitonin

207. A 57-year-old lady presents with type-II diabetes mellitus with symptoms like polyuria, excessive thirst, fatigue and blurred vision. Further investigation reveals insulin resistance. Which one of the following drug is most appropriate for initiating treatment along with diet and exercise? *(JIPMER 2016)*
a. Pioglitazone
b. Metformin
c. Glimepiride
d. Repaglinide

208. A 48-year-old woman presents with vulvale pruritus. On examination, there is erythema of external genitalia. She is a known diabetic for 10 years. Her HbA1c level reduced to 6.6% when compared to previous value of 7.8% four months ago. The medication most probably responsible for her symptoms is: *(JIPMER 2016)*
a. Sitagliptin
b. Canagliflozin
c. Acarbose
d. Exenatide

209. An experimental new drug designed for the treatment of diabetes mellitus was found to increase the levels of incretins by preventing their degradation at the endothelium. It also increases the glucose dependent insulin production. It acts most similar to: *(JIPMER 2016)*
a. Glimepiride
b. Pioglitazone
c. Canagliflozin
d. Sitagliptin

210. Drug used in both type of diabetes is: *(JIPMER 2013)*
a. Exenatide
b. Pioglitazone
c. Alpha glucosidase inhibitors
d. Pramlintide

211. Diarrhea is a side effect of: *(JIPMER 2012)*
a. Amitriptyline
b. Metformin
c. Atropine
d. Codeine

212. Intranasal calcitonin used for: *(JIPMER 2011)*
a. Postmenopausal osteoporosis
b. Page t's disease
c. Secondary hypoparathyroidism
d. Hypercalcemia

213. Which of the following antidiabetic medications does not cause weight gain? *(JIPMER 2011)*
a. Rosiglitazone
b. Glibenclamide
c. GLP-1 analogues
d. Metformin

214. All are true regarding mifepristone except: *(JIPMER 2010)*
a. It is a pure antagonist
b. Ineffective against mineralocorticoids
c. No antiestrogenic side effects
d. Antiandrogenic action

215. Which of the following best depicts the mechanism of action of thiazolidinediones? ***(JIPMER 2010)***
- a. Improving insulin sensitivity
- b. Modifying receptors of beta cells
- c. Increasing insulin secretion
- d. Increasing number of GLUT-4

216. Insulin sensitivity increases with following treatment except: ***(JIPMER 2009)***
- a. Metformin
- b. Acarbose
- c. Exercise
- d. Fasting

217. Troglitazone is the drug used in the treatment of: ***(JIPMER 2009)***
- a. Petit mal epilepsy
- b. Type 2 diabetes mellitus
- c. Hyperlipidaemia
- d. Osteoporosis

218. Bisphosphonates act by: ***(NIMHANS 2013)***
- a. Increasing the osteoid formation
- b. Increasing the mineralization of osteoid
- c. Decreasing the osteoclast mediated resorption of bone
- d. Decreasing the parathyroid hormone secretion

219. Lactic acidosis is a side effect of: ***(NIMHANS 2013)***
- a. Chlorothiazide
- b. Metformin
- c. Cyclosporine
- d. Pentamidine

220. The dosage of testosterone cypionate is ***(NIMHANS 2013)***
- a. 100 mg/2 weeks
- b. 200 mg/2 weeks
- c. 150 mg/2 weeks
- d. 300 mg/2 weeks

221. Which one of the following is long-acting steroid? ***(NIMHANS 2011)***
- a. Triamcinolone
- b. Dexamethasone
- c. Prednisolone
- d. Methylprednisolone

222. Maximum glucocorticoid potency is seen in: ***(NIMHANS 2007)***
- a. Cortisone
- b. Betamethasone
- c. Dexamethasone
- d. Methylprednisolone

Answers with Explanations to Multiple Choice Questions

1. Ans. (d) Canagliflozin

(Ref: CMDT 2017, Page 1228)

- Sitagliptin causes pancreatitis and hence cannot be given in this patient.
- Liraglutide is a parenteral drug given by SC route and as the patient does not want injectable drugs this option is out.
- Pioglitazone causes bladder cancer and as patient has family history of bladder cancer it cannot be given as well.
- Hence, we are left with canagliflozin, which is the answer here.

Note: In clinical trials an increased risk of bladder and breast cancer has been seen with dapagliflozin and not canagliflozin.

2. Ans. (a) Metformin

(Ref: CMDT 2017, Page 1224)

- Metformin is contraindicated in patients with renal failure with a serum creatinine level cut-off of 1.5 mg/dL.

3. Ans. (a) 30% amorphous + 70% crystalline

(Ref: KDT 7th edition, Page 264)

4. Ans. (a) Linagliptin

(Ref: CMDT 2017, Page 1227)

- Repaglinide can be given by oral route but only for postprandial hyperglycemia and as its excreted by kidney its dose is reduced.
- Sulfonylureas like glimepiride are contraindicated in both hepatic and renal failure.
- DPP-4 inhibitors can be given by oral route and the only drug in this class excreted by liver and can be given in renal failure in linagliptin.

5. Ans. (b) Lateral thigh

(Ref: Goodman Gilman 12th E/P 1253)

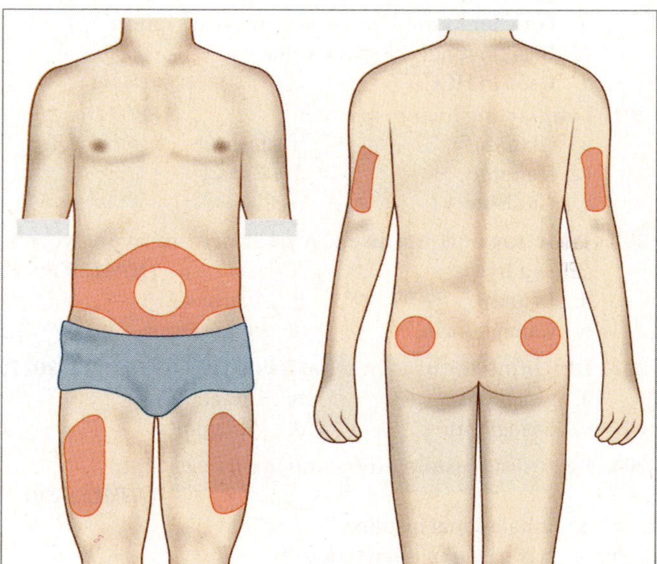

- Insulin is injected into areas with adipose tissue like abdomen > anterior thigh > buttock > dorsal arm as given in picture.
- Dorsal arm is less preferred as there can be accidental intramuscular injection due to lesser fat.
- Absorption is most rapid from the abdomen followed by dorsal arm, buttock and anterior thigh.

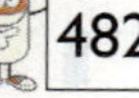

6. **Ans. (d) Smoking**

(Ref: Goodman Gilman 12th E/P 1259)

- Biguanides are excreted unchanged in urine and hence contraindicated in renal failure as the chances of lactic acidosis increases.
- Other conditions with increased lactic acid like severe respiratory disease and liver disease, CHF and chronic alcohol abuse are also contraindications.

7. **Ans. (a) Linagliptin**

(Ref: CMDT 2017/P 1227)

- All DDP-4 inhibitors are excreted by kidney and hence are contraindicated in renal failure, except linagliptin which is excreted by liver.

8. **Ans. (c) Rosiglitazone**

(Ref: Goodman Gilman 12th E/P 1259-60)

Treatment of Diabetes Mellitus

Drugs	Mechanism of action	Use
Alpha glucosidase inhibitors • Acarbose • Miglitol	Inhibit conversion of complex polysaccharides into glucose in GIT.	Postprandial hyperglycemia in type II DM.
GLP 1 agonists • Exenatide • Liraglutide	Stimulate insulin release in beta islet cells	Postprandial hyperglycemia treatment in type I DM
DPP4 inhibitors • Sitagliptin • Saxagliptin	Inhibit metabolism of GLP1 and hence end result is increase in insulin release	Treatment of type I DM along with metformin
Amylin analogue pramlintide	Inhibits gastric emptying	Postprandial hyperglycemia treatment in type I and II DM
Sulfonylureas Meglitinides	Inhibit ATP sensitive potassium channel in beta islet cell and increase insulin release	Treatment of type II DM
Metformin	Decreases insulin resistance Inhibits gastric emptying Inhibits glycogenolysis Decreases appetite (Weight loss)	Drug of choice for treatment and prophylaxis of type II DM
Thiazolidenidiones Rosiglitazone	Stimulate PPAR gamma receptors and increase GLUT4 receptors production in cells	Treatment of type II DM
Canagliflozin Dapagliflozin	SGLT2 receptor inhibitors	Treatment of type II DM
Bromocriptine	Inhibits the hyperglycemic drive of hypothalamus	Treatment of type II DM
Colesevelam	Unknown	Treatment of type II DM

9. **Ans. (c) It causes transcription of gene for carbohydrate and fat metabolism in the absence of insulin**

(Ref: Goodman Gilman 12th E/P 1260)

- Pioglitazone requires presence of insulin for its effect and hence is not used in type I DM.

10. **Ans. (b) It can be used for treatment of Type 1 diabetes mellitus**

(Ref: Goodman Gilman 12th E/P 1261)

- Exenatide is a GLP-1 analog that acts by stimulating insulin release from beta islet cells and hence would not be effective in type I DM.

11. **Ans. (c) Glucose**

(Ref: Goodman Gilman 12th E/P 1264)

- Acarbose inhibits break down of starch and disaccharides and hence glucose should be used in management of hypoglycemia.

12. **Ans. (a) Hypokalemia**

(Ref: Goodman Gilman 12th E/P 1253)

13. **Ans. (d) Ketogenesis**

(Ref: Goodman Gilman 12th E/P 1253)

- Ketogenesis is seen in the absence of insulin.

14. **Ans. (a) GLP-2 agonist**

(Ref: Goodman Gilman 13th E/P 877)

- Teduglutide is a GLP-2 agonist used for treatment of short bowel syndrome.
- Since it is a peptide, it cannot be given by oral route, rather given by subcutaneous route.

15. **Ans. (c) Glucagon like peptide 2**

(Ref: Goodman Gilman 13th E/P 939)

16. **Ans. (b) It reduces both pre- and postprandial hyperglycemia**

(Ref: Goodman Gilman 12th E/P 1264)

- Alpha glucosidase inhibitors act by inhibiting metabolism of starch and disaccharides present in food to glucose.
- Hence, they are effective in prandial and postprandial hyperglycemia but not preprandial hyperglycemia.

17. **Ans. (a) DM**

(Ref: CMDT 2017/P 1228)

18. **Ans. (a) Regular**

(Ref: CMDT 2017/P 1229)

19. **Ans. (a) Hypokalemia**

(Ref: Goodman Gilman 12th E/P 1253)

20. Ans. (c) Tolbutamide

(Ref: Goodman Gilman 12th E/P 1256)

21. Ans. (c) Neutral Protamine Hagedron

(Ref: Goodman Gilman 12th E/P 1251)

Neutral protamine hagedorn is insulin combined with zinc and protamine in a phosphate buffer is a long-acting insulin.

22. Ans. (b) Diabetes mellitus

(Ref: Goodman Gilman 12th E/P 1263)

23. Ans. (d) Once daily anytime during day

(Ref: Goodman Gilman 12th E/P 1252)

Dosing of Long-acting Insulins

NPH Detemir	Once or twice daily
Glargine	Once daily any time of day

24. Ans. (c) Pramlinitide

(Ref: Goodman Gilman 12th E/P 1265)

25. Ans. (c) Metformin

(Ref: Goodman Gilman 12th E/P 1259)

26. Ans. (b) Sulfonylureas

(Ref: Goodman Gilman 12th E/P 1261)

27. Ans. (a) Chlorpropamide

(Ref: Goodman Gilman 12th E/P 1257)

- Chlorpropamide can cause SIADH, which results in dilutional hyponatremia.

28. Ans. (d) All of the above

(Ref: Goodman Gilman 12th E/P 1261)

29. Ans. (c) Pramlintide

(Ref: Goodman Gilman 12th E/P 1265)

30. Ans. (d) Hypoglycemia is the major adverse effect

(Ref: Goodman Gilman 12th E/P 1261)

31. Ans. (a) Synthetic amylin analog

(Ref: Goodman Gilman 12th E/P 1265)

32. Ans. (a) Acts as PPAR gamma agonist

(Ref: Goodman Gilman 12th E/P 1259)

33. Ans. (a) Exenatide

(Ref: Goodman Gilman 12th E/P 1263)

- **Exenatide and liraglutide are analogs of incretin GLP-1.**

34. Ans. (c) Glargine

(Ref: Goodman Gilman 12th E/P 1251)

Ultra Short-acting	Short-acting	Long-acting	Ultra Long-acting
Glulisine Aspart Lispro	Regular insulin	NPH	Glargine Detemir

35. Ans. (a) It produces a smooth peakless effect

(Ref: Goodman Gilman 12th E/P 1252)

- Ultralong acting insulin like glargine and detemir produce a smooth peakless effect and hence cause less hypoglycemia.
- Glargine is acidic in nature whereas other insulins are neutral
- It is used for maintenance and not for postprandial hyperglycemia.

36. Ans. (a) Repaglinide

(Ref: Goodman Gilman 12th E/P 1257)

37. Ans. (d) Glargine

(Ref: Goodman Gilman 12th E/P 1252)

- **Glargine** has an acidic pH and hence **should not be mixed with other insulin as they have neutral pH.**

38. Ans. (a) Nateglinide

(Ref: Goodman Gilman 12th E/P 1257)

39. Ans. (a) Always given with insulin

(Ref: Goodman Gilman 12th E/P 1264)

- Sitagliptin, saxagliptin, alogliptin, linagliptin and vildagliptin act by inhibiting DPP-4 and increasing the endogenous GLP-1 concentration.
- Thus, they increase insulin release, but are devoid of other effects associated with GLP-1 agonists.
- These are approved for as adjuncts to other **oral hypoglycemic agents and insulin** for treatment of type II DM. Since these are chemicals with good oral absorption, they are given by oral route at OD doses.

40. Ans. (b) Acarbose

(Ref: Harrison 19th E/P2414)

- Acarbose has minimal effect on HbA1c and hence is the least preferred drug with inrceased HbA1c among the options.

41. Ans. (d) Repaglinide

(Ref: Goodman Gilman 12th E/P 1257)

42. Ans. (c) Insulin actrapid

(Ref: Goodman Gilman 12th E/P 1250)

- Actrapid is regular human insulin and not an analog.
- Other insulins in the options are ultra-short acting insulin analogs.

43. Ans. (c) Metformin

(Ref: Goodman Gilman 12th E/P 1259)

44. Ans. (a) Acarbose

(Ref: Goodman Gilman 12th E/P 1264)

- Hypoglycemia is most common with insulin and insulin releasing potent drugs like sulfonylureas and meglitinides.
- Less potent insulin releasing drugs like GLP-1 analogs and DPP-4 inhibitors can cause hypoglycemia if combined with insulin or insulin releasing drugs.

45. Ans. (c) Glargine

(Ref: Goodman Gilman 12th E/P 1250)

- Though NPH is not short rather long-acting, glargine is longest acting insulin and hence is the best possible answer in the options.
- Lispro and aspart are rapid and short acting insulins.

46. Ans. (c) Renal dysfunction is not a contraindication for their use

(Ref: Goodman Gilman 12th E/P 1264)

- Biguanides are excreted unchanged in urine and hence contraindicated in renal failure as the chances of lactic acidosis increases.
- Other conditions with increased lactic acid like severe respiratory disease and liver disease, CHF and chronic alcohol abuse are also contraindications.

47. Ans. (b) Insulin

(Ref: Goodman Gilman 12th E/P 1250)

- Insulin is administered by subcutaneous or intravenous route.

48. Ans. (b) Acetohexamide

(Ref: Goodman Gilman 12th E/P 1255)

49. Ans. (b) Phenformin

(Ref: Goodman Gilman 12th E/P 1259)

- Though both metformin and phenformin can cause lactic acidosis, it is more common with phenformin which led to its withdrawal.

50. Ans. (d) Insulin secretion

(Ref: Goodman Gilman 12th E/P 1255)

51. Ans. (c) Ultralente

(Ref: KDT 7th E/P264)

- Lente is an intermediate acting insulin invented by Hallas-Moller by combining zinc with insulin, which lead to formation of short-acting amorphous precipitate (semilente) and long-acting stable crystals (ultralente).
- Lente is made by combining 30% semilente with 70% ultralente.

52. Ans. (c) Tolbutamide

(Ref: Goodman Gilman 12th E/P 1255)

53. Ans. (b) Miglitol

(Ref: Goodman Gilman 12th E/P 1264)

54. Ans. (c) Water retention and weight gain

(Ref: Goodman Gilman 12th E/P 1261)

55. Ans. (d) Pioglitazone

(Ref: Goodman Gilman 12th E/P 1255)

- **Thiazolidenidiones like pioglitazone are metabolized and excreted by liver and hence is safe in patients with renal failure.**

56. Ans. (c) Meglitinides

(Ref: Goodman Gilman 12th E/P 1257)

57. Ans (b) It acts on transcription factor

(Ref: Goodman Gilman 13th E/P 791)

- Thyrotropin releasing hormone (TRH) acts on Gq subtype of receptors on thyrotrope cells in pituitary; this activates protein kinase C which increases synthesis of TSH.
- TSH acts on Gs subtype of receptors on thyroid cells and increases cyclic AMP, which leads to an increase in production of sodium iodide symporter, thyroid peroxidase and thiol endopeptidase. All these are crucial for synthesis and release of T_3 and T_4.
- T3 and T4 act on thyroid receptors which are nuclear receptors and hence act via modulating the transcription factors.
- Increased T_3 and T_4 levels decrease release of TSH by decreasing the transcription factors for both TSH and TRH.

58. Ans. (d) Lung fibrosis

(Ref: Goodman Gilman 12th E/P 1149)

- Thionamide group contains PTU, Carbimazole and Methimazole.
- PTU is hepatotoxic
- Carbimazole and Methimazole cause agranulocytosis and aplastic anemia.

59. Ans. (b) Contraindicated in hyperthyroidism

(Ref: Goodman Gilman 12th E/P 1152)

- Iodine in the form of Lugol's iodine or KI is used in hyperthyroidism to make the patient euthyroid before surgery.
- Side effects caused by systemic iodine is known as iodism.
- It acts by inhibiting T_3/T_4 release and hence is the fastest acting antithyroid drug.

60. Ans. (d) Methimazole

(Ref: Goodman Gilman 12th E/P 1149)

61. Ans. (c) Cleft lip/palate

(Ref: Goodman Gilman 12th E/P 1159)

Teratogenic Effects of Carbimazole/ Methimazole

- Cutis aplasia (Scalp defect)
- Choanal and esophageal atresia
- Fetal goiter

62. Ans. (a) Sodium iodide

(Ref: Goodman Gilman 12th E/P 1152)

63. Ans. (a) Propylthiouracil

(Ref: Goodman Gilman 12th E/P 1149)

- Though propylthiouracil and propranolol both inhibit peripheral conversion of T_4 to T_3, propylthiouracil is a better answer as it is a more potent inhibitor.

64. Ans. (a) Propranolol

(Ref: Goodman Gilman 12th E/P 1146)

65. Ans. (a) Iodides of Na/K

(Ref: Goodman Gilman 12th E/P 1152)

66. Ans. (a) 5% iodine and 10% KI

(Ref: KDT 7th E/P 255)

67. Ans. (b) 8 hours

(Ref: KDT 7th E/P 253)

Half-life of TP Inhibitors

PTU	1–2 hours
Carbimazole	8–10 hours
Methimazole	4–6 hours

68. Ans. (a) Inhibits peripheral conversion of T4 to T3

(Ref: Goodman Gilman 12th E/P 1149)

69. Ans. (d) Thyroid surgery

(Ref: Harrison 19th E/P 2297)

70. Ans. (c) Complete blood count

(Ref: Goodman Gilman 12th E/P 1149)

- Carbimazole and methimazole can cause agranulocytosis and hence a blood count should be done in case of sore throat.

71. Ans. (d) Agranulocytosis caused by methimazole

(Ref: Goodman Gilman 12th E/P 1149)

72. Ans. (a) Teriparatide

(Ref: Goodman Gilman 12th edition, Page 1300)

- Teriparatide increases bone formation by stimulating osteoblasts.
- Raloxifene and risedronate inhibits osteoclast mediated bone resorption.
- Strontium ranelate stimulates bone formation as well as inhibits bone resorption.

73. Ans. (d) Milnacipran

(Ref: Goodman Gilman 12th E/P 1294-98)

- Milnacipran use for long-time causes osteoporosis.
- You might be confused with PTH, but teripatatide is a PTH analog used in osteoporosis.

74. Ans. (a) Take tab before food with full glass of water

(Ref: Goodman Gilman 12th E/P 1296)

- Oral bisphosphonates have poor oral absorption and hence are given empty stomach, 30 minutes before food with a full glass of water.
- Since all drugs can cause esophagitis, the patient is asked to remain upright after drug intake.

75. Ans. (a) Strontium ranelate

(Ref: Katzung 12th E/P 777)

Drugs Used in Osteoporosis

Decrease in bone resorption	Increase in bone formation	Increase in bone formation and decrease in bone resorption
Denosumab Bisphosphonates Estrogen Raloxifene Calcitonin	Teriparatide	Strontium ranelate

76. Ans. (b) Vitamin D excess

(Ref: Goodman Gilman 12th E/P 1296)

Uses of Bisphosphonates

- Osteoporosis
- Hypercalcemia associated with malignancy
- Page t's disease
- Neoplasia – Delay development of metastases in breast cancer

Remember: The most potent bisphosphonate is zoledronic acid and is the bisphosphonate of choice.

77. **Ans. (b) Osteoporosis**

(Ref: Goodman Gilman 12th E/P 1299)

78. **Ans. (a) Increasing osteoblastic activity**

(Ref: Goodman Gilman 12th E/P 1299)

79. **Ans. (d) RANK antagonist**

(Ref: Goodman Gilman 12th E/P 1299)

80. **Ans. (c) Decreasing osteoclast mediated resorption of bone**

(Ref: Goodman Gilman 12th E/P 1295)

81. **Ans. (a) Zoledronate**

(Ref: Goodman Gilman 12th E/P 1296)

Side Effects of Bisphosphonates

Esophagitis
Osteonecrosis of jaw
Cytokine release – Flu like symptoms, myalgia, arthralgia
Hypocalcemia and Renal failure – Specifically seen with zoledronic acid

82. **Ans. (b) Increases bone resorption**

(Ref: Goodman Gilman 12th E/P 1278)

83. **Ans. (d) Postmenopausal osteoporosis**

(Ref: Goodman Gilman 12th E/P 1283)

- Salcatonin is a calcitonin analog that acts by inhibiting osteoclast mediated bone resorption.
- Subcutaneous salcatonin is used for treatment of Paget's disease, whereas intranasal salcatonin is used for prophylaxis of osteoporosis.

84. **Ans. (c) Osteoporosis**

(Ref: Goodman Gilman 12th E/P 1296)

85. **Ans. (d) Teriparatide**

(Ref: Goodman Gilman 12th E/P 1296)

86. **Ans. (a) Risedronate**

(Ref: Goodman Gilman 12th E/P 1296)

87. **Ans. (a) Acute renal failure**

(Ref: Goodman Gilman 12th E/P 1296)

88. **Ans. (d) Glioma**

(Ref: Goodman Gilman 12th E/P 113)

89. **Ans. (b) Used in secretory diarrhea**

(Ref: Goodman Gilman 12th E/P 1113)

90. **Ans. (a) Acromegaly**

(Ref: Goodman Gilman 12th E/P 1339)

91. **Ans. (c) Both a and b**

(Ref: Goodman Gilman 12th E/P 1114)

- Cabergoline is the drug of choice for treatment of both acromegaly and hyperprolactinemia.

92. **Ans. (b) Growth hormone receptor antagonist**

(Ref: Goodman Gilman 12th E/P 1109)

Drugs Related to GH

Pegvisomant	GH2 receptor antagonist
Somatrem Somatropin	GH analogues
Sermorelin	GHRH analogue
Mecasermin	IGF1 analogue
Mecasermin Rinfabate	IGF1 + IGFBP 3 analogue

93. **Ans. (c) Octreotide**

(Ref: Goodman Gilman 12th E/P 1113)

94. **Ans. (a) Octreotide**

(Ref: Goodman Gilman 12th E/P 1113)

95. **Ans. (c) Finasteride**

(Ref: Goodman Gilman 12th edition, Page 1205)

- Finasteride is used in BPH usually with large size prostate. It produces effect on long-term use by reducing prostatic epithelial cell proliferation, which reduces size of prostate improves urine flow.
- Tamsulosin just dilates prostatic urethra and hence produces fastest effect in BPH.
- Flutamide is used for treatment of metastatic prostate cancer along with GnRH agonists.

96. **Ans. (a) Hyperprolactinemia**

(Ref: Goodman Gilman 12th edition, Page 1114)

- Hyperprolactinemia can cause infertility, as prolactin inhibits secretion of GnRH, which leads to decrease secretion of LH and FSH.
- Bromocriptine can be used for treatment of hyperprolactinemia and hence is the answer here.

97. **Ans. (a) 30 mg**

(Ref: Goodman Gilman 13th E/P 820)

98. **Ans (a) Estrogen receptor**

(Ref: Goodman Gilman 13th E/P811)

99. Ans. (c) Tamoxifen dose is 20 mg for 5 years

(Ref: Goodman Gilman 13th E/P1239)

100. Ans. (b) Thromboembolism

(Ref: Goodman Gilman 13th E/P817)

101. Ans. (b) Intolerant hot flushes

(Ref: Goodman Gilman 12th edition, Page 1838)

The primary benefits of HRT in postmenopausal females is improvement of:

- Vasomotor symptoms (Hot flushes)
- Vaginal dryness
- Osteoporosis

102. Ans. (d) GnRH agonist

(Ref: Goodman Gilman 12th E/P1122)

103. Ans. (b) 600 mcg

(Ref: WHO Guidelines)

104. Ans. (d) Desogestrel

(Ref: Goodman Gilman 12th E/P1185)

Emergency Contraception

- Levonorgesterel is used within 72 hours for unprotected intercourse. Another dose is repeated after 12 hours.
- Ulipristal is a selective progesterone receptor modulator which inhibits ovulation and implantation of fertilized ovum. It is approved for emergency contraception and can be used up to 5 days.
- IUCD is more effective than levonorgesterel and can be inserted up to 5 days of unprotected intercourse.

105. Ans. (d) 600 mcg

(Ref: http://www.who.int/bulletin volumes/87/9/08-055715/en/)

"In a recent placebo-controlled trial in rural India in which babies were delivered by auxiliary nurse midwives at home or in village subcenters, a significant reduction in postpartum hemorrhage and other complications was obtained with misoprostol, **600 µg orally used alone** (i.e. without other components of the active management of the third stage of labor—umbilical cord clamping and controlled cord traction). WHO has developed guidelines supporting the use of a uterotonic when the full package of active management of the third stage of labor is not practised, which can be either oxytocin, 10 IU administered parenterally, or misoprostol, 600 µg administered orally.

Apart from its uterotonic effects, misoprostol has known pharmacologic effects on several organ systems. It inhibits platelet-activating factor and affects metabolic and physiological processes, including thermoregulation. Life-threatening hyperpyrexia has been reported following the use of misoprostol, 800 µg orally, after childbirth."

106. Ans. (b) Tamoxifen

(Ref: Goodman Gilman 12th E/P 1177-78)

- Tamoxifen is used for treatment of ER/PR positive breast cancer.
- Clomiphene is the drug of choice for ovulation induction in PCOD.
- If ovulation is not desired OCP can be used.
- Metformin is used to reverse insulin resistance associated with PCOD.

107. Ans. (d) Goserelin

(Ref: Goodman Gilman 12th E/P 1122)

108. Ans. (c) Azoospermia

(Ref: Goodman Gilman 12th E/P 1204)

109. Ans. (a) Raloxifene

(Ref: Goodman Gilman 12th E/P 1177)

110. Ans. (a) Tamoxifen

(Ref: Goodman Gilman 12th E/P 1177)

111. Ans. (a) Levonorgestrel

(Ref: Goodman Gilman 12th E/P 1185)

112. Ans. (c) Coronary heart disease

(Ref: Goodman Gilman 12th E/P 1176)

113. Ans. (b) Letrozole

(Ref: Goodman Gilman 12th E/P 1762)

114. Ans. (c) Venous thrombosis

(Ref: Goodman Gilman 12th E/P 1178)

115. Ans. (b) Levonorgestrel

(Ref: CMDT 2017/P 1198)

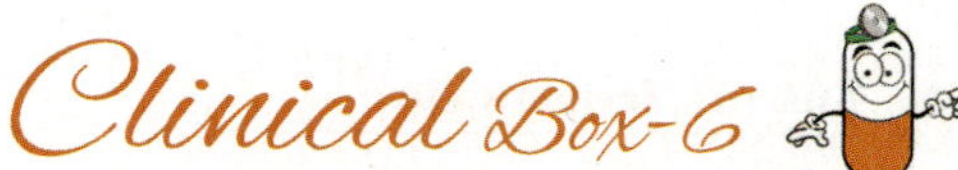

Drugs used for Treatment of Hirsutism

- Finasteride
- Flutamide
- Spironolactone
- Metformin
- Simvastatin
- Clomiphene
- GnRH agonists
- OCPs with antiandrogenic progestins (Desogesterel, Drospirenone and norgestimate)
- Topical eflornithine

116. Ans. (b) PGF$_2$ alpha

(Ref: Goodman Gilman 12th E/P 1125)

117. Ans. (a) PGF2 alpha

(Ref: Goodman Gilman 12th E/P 1125)

118. Ans. (d) Ulipristal

(Ref: Goodman Gilman 12th E/P 1185)

Emergency Contraception

- Levonorgestrel is used within 72 hours for unprotected intercourse. Another dose is repeated after 12 hours.
- Ulipristal is a selective progesterone receptor modulator which is a partial agonist at progesterone receptors and inhibits ovulation and implantation of fertilized ovum. It inhibits LH release and also inhibits LH induced follicular rupture in ovary. It is approved for emergency contraception and can be used at a dose of 30 mg up to 5 days. Side effects associated are headache and abdominal pain.
- IUCD is more effective than levonorgestrel and can be inserted up to 5 days of unprotected intercourse.
- Yuzpe regimen containing an estrogen and progesterone is less efficacious and hence not preferred.
- Mifepristone is not FDA approved but can be used for emergency contraception up to 5 days.

119. Ans. (b) Pituitary gland

(Ref: Goodman Gilman 12th E/P 1177)

120. Ans. (b) Testosterone

(Ref: Goodman Gilman 12th E/P 1200)

121. Ans. (b) 8 weeks

(Ref: Goodman Gilman 12th E/P 1185)

122. Ans. (c) Breast cancer

(Ref: Goodman Gilman 12th E/P 1178)

123. Ans. (a) Antiprogesterone

(Ref: Goodman Gilman 12th E/P 1184)

124. Ans. (b) Flutamide

(Ref: Goodman Gilman 12th E/P 1205)

- Flutamide inhibits production of DHT and hence does not cause hirsutism.

125. Ans. (a) Carcinoma colon

(Ref: Harrison 19th E/P 524)

> "Data from the Women's Health Initiative (WHI) trial showed that conjugated equine estrogens plus progestins increased the risk of breast cancer and adverse cardiovascular events but decreased the risk of bone fractures and **colorectal cancer**."

126. Ans. (b) Finasteride

(Ref: Goodman Gilman 12th E/P 1205)

127. Ans. (d) Granirelix is the most potent agent

(Ref: Goodman Gilman 12th E/P 1122)

- Granirelix is a GNRH antagonist and not agonist.

128. Ans. (b) Prostate

(Ref: Goodman Gilman 12th E/P 1205)

129. Ans. (b) SERM

(Ref: Goodman Gilman 12th E/P 1177)

130. Ans. (d) Aromatase inhibitors

(Ref: Goodman Gilman 12th E/P 1762)

131. Ans. (a) 3 months

(Ref: Goodman Gilman 12th E/P 1762)

132. Ans. (a) Estrogen

(Ref: Goodman Gilman 12th E/P 1188)

133. Ans. (d) Spironolactone

(Ref: Goodman Gilman 12th E/P 1205)

- Spironolactone is an inhibitor of androgen receptors and hence can decrease effect of testosterone.

134. Ans. (d) All of the above

(Ref: Goodman Gilman 12th E/P 1840)

- Danazol is a synthetic steroid with inhibitor effect on GNRH, which subsequently leads to decrease in LH/FSH followed by decrease in estrogen, progesterone and testosterone. It also has androgenic action.
- Uses are estrogen dependent conditions like endometriosis and gynecomastia.
- It can cause hirsutism in females due to its androgenic effect.

135. Ans. (d) Blockade of fimbrial ostia

(Ref: Goodman Gilman 12th E/P 1187)

136. Ans. (c) Finasteride

(Ref: Goodman Gilman 12th E/P 1205)

- Flutamide, spironolactone and cyproterone are all androgen receptor antagonist.
- Finasteride is an inhibitor of 5-alpha reductase and hence inhibit conversion of testosterone in DHT.

137. Ans. (b) Use in treatment of gynecomastia

(Ref: Goodman Gilman 12th E/P 1174)

- Estrogen use in males can cause gynecomastia and hence it is not used for treatment.

138. Ans. (b) Causes gynecomastia

(Ref: Goodman Gilman 12th E/P 1205)

- Cyproterone and megestrol are progesterone derivatives whereas flutamide, nilutamide and bicalutamide are synthetic inhibitors of androgen receptors.
- These are **used along with GNRH agonists or antagonists for treatment of prostate cancer** and hirsutism.
- Cyproterone and flutamide can cause hepatotoxicity. Other common side effects associated are impotence and gynecomastia.

139. Ans. (b) 5-α reductase enzyme

(Ref: Goodman Gilman 12th E/P 1205)

140. Ans. (c) Testosterone

(Ref: Goodman Gilman 12th E/P 1205)

- Testosterone is the primary cause of prostate cancer and hence not used in treatment.

141. Ans. (b) Finasteride

(Ref: Goodman Gilman 12th E/P 1205)

142. Ans. (b) Dysmenorrhea

(Ref: Goodman Gilman 12th E/P 1176)

- Dysmenorrhea is an indication for OCP.

143. Ans. (a) Dihydrotestosterone

(Ref: Goodman Gilman 12th E/P 1196)

144. Ans. (d) Mifepristone (RU 486)

(Ref: Goodman Gilman 12th E/P 1184)

145. Ans. (a) Bicalutamide

(Ref: Goodman Gilman 12th E/P 1205)

146. Ans. (a) GnRH

(Ref: Goodman Gilman 12th E/P 1121)

147. Ans. (a) Flutamide

(Ref: Goodman Gilman 12th E/P 1205)

148. Ans. (b) Antiandrogen

(Ref: Goodman Gilman 12th E/P 1205)

149. Ans. (b) 10

(Ref: Nelson 19th edition, Page 1928)

Hydrocortisone (Oral) for chronic replacement in adrenal insufficiency

- **Children:** 10 mg/m^2/day in three divided doses
- **Adults:** 15–30 mg/day in three divided doses

Fludrocortisone (Oral) for chronic replacement in adrenal insufficiency

- **Children:** 0.05–0.2 mg/day
- **Adults:** 0.05–0.3 mg/day

Hydrocortisone (IV) bolus in acute crisis of adrenal insufficiency

- **Infants:** 10 mg
- **Toddlers:** 25 mg
- **Older children:** 50 mg
- **Adults:** 100 mg

150. Ans. (a) Metyrapone

(Ref: Goodman Gilman 12th E/P 1235)

151. Ans. (a) Dexamethasone 6 mg 12 hourly 4 doses

(Ref: Nelson 20th E/P 852)

Dose of steroids for fetal lung maturation

- Dexamethasone 6mg 12 hourly 4 doses
- Betamethasone 12 mg 12 hourly 2 doses

152. Ans. (c) Kaposi sarcoma

(Ref: Goodman Gilman 12th E/P 1232)

Use of Steroids in Malignancy

- Leukemia
- Lymphoma
- Multiple myeloma
- Hypercalcemia of malignancy

Note: Steroids are associated with an increased risk of Kaposi sarcoma.

153. Ans. (b) Fever

(Ref: Goodman Gilman 12th E/P 1220)

154. Ans. (a) Dexamethasone

(Ref: Goodman Gilman 12th E/P 1230)

Pregnancy

- In pregnancy steroids are given in premature labor for fetal lung maturity; the preferred steroids are dexamethasone or betamethasone.
- In a pregnant female with baby having CAH, **dexamethasone** is preferred to inhibit fetal androgen production.

155. Ans. (d) Metabolic acidosis

(Ref: Goodman Gilman 12th E/P 1230)

156. Ans. (b) Oral steroids alone

(Ref: CMDT 2016/P 1024)

157. Ans. (c) Metyrapone

(Ref: Goodman Gilman 12th E/P 1233)

158. Ans. (a) Dexamethasone

(Ref: Goodman Gilman 12th E/P 1224)

159. Ans. (a) **Fludrocortisone**

(Ref: Goodman Gilman 12th E/P 1224)

160. Ans. (b) **Betamethasone**

(Ref: Goodman Gilman 12th E/P 1216)

Duration of Action of Steroids

- Dexamethasone and betamethasone — 36–72 hours
- Prednisolone and triamcinolone — 12–36 hours
- Hydrocortisone — 8–12 hours

161. Ans. (d) **Spironolactone**

(Ref: Goodman Gilman 12th E/P 1234)

162. Ans. (c) **3 betahydroxysteroid dehydrogenase inhibitor**

(Ref: Goodman Gilman 12th E/P 1230)

Steroid Synthesis Inhibitors

Drug	Target	Use	Side effects
Ketoconazole	17-α hydroxylase	Cushing's disease treatment	Hepatotoxicity Gynecomastia
Metyrapone	11-β hydroxylase	Cushing's disease treatment and diagnosis	Hirsutism
Etomidate	11-β hydroxylase	Emergency management of Cushing's disease	Vitamin C deficiency
Aminoglutethemide	CYP11A1	Withdrawn from market	
Trilostane	3-β dehydrogenase	Not used in humans	

163. Ans. (b) **Hydrocortisone**

(Ref: Goodman Gilman 12th E/P 1228)

- For steroid replacement in adrenal insufficiency (acute and chronic) and congenital adrenal hyperplasia the steroid of choice is hydrocortisone.
- Fludrocortisone is given for mineralocorticoid replacement.

164. Ans. (d) **Photosensitivity**

(Ref: Goodman Gilman 12th E/P 124-27)

Side Effects of Steroids

Mnemonics

- **H** : Hyperglycemia, Hypokalemia, Hypertension
- **Y** : mYopathy
- **D** : Disturbed mood (Psychosis)
- **R** : Retardation of growth
- **O** : Osteoporosis
- **C** : Cushing's syndrome, Cataract
- **O** : Osteonecrosis
- **R** : Redistribution of fat
- **T** : Topical steroid–Glaucoma, Teleangectasia
- **I** : Infections, Inflammation of follicles
- **S** : Skin atrophy

165. Ans. (a) **Hydrocortisone**

(Ref: Goodman Gilman 12th E/P 1224)

166. Ans. (d) **Prednisolone**

(Ref: Goodman Gilman 12th E/P 1225)

167. Ans. (c) **Aldosterone**

(Ref: Goodman Gilman 12th E/P 1224)

168. Ans. (c) **Hydrocortisone**

(Ref: Goodman Gilman 12th E/P 1224)

169. Ans. (c) **Loeffler's syndrome**

(Ref: Harrison 19th E/P 422)

170. Ans. (a) **Ointment**

(Ref: Goodman Gilman 12th E/P 1808)

171. Ans. (c) **Clobetasol propionate 0.5% cream**

(Ref: Goodman Gilman 12th E/P 1808)

172. Ans. (a) **Congenital adrenal hyperplasia**

(Ref: Goodman Gilman 12th E/P 1229)

173. Ans. (c) **Prednisolone**

(Ref: Goodman Gilman 12th E/P 1215)

- Glucocorticoids and mineralocorticoids act on cytoplasmic receptors.

174. Ans. (a) **Aldosterone**

(Ref: Goodman Gilman 12th E/P 1224)

175. Ans. (b) **Glaucoma**

(Ref: Goodman Gilman 12th E/P 1224-27)

- Glaucoma is seen due to topical steroids.

176. Ans. (a) **Hydrocortisone**

(Ref: Goodman Gilman 12th E/P 1228)

177. Ans. (b) **Beclomethasone**

(Ref: Goodman Gilman 12th E/P 1225)

178. Ans. (a) **Mitotane**

(Ref: Goodman Gilman 12th E/P 1234)

Mitotane is an adrenolytic drug used for treatment of inoperable adrenocortical tumors.

179. Ans. (a) **20 mg methylprednisolone**

(Ref: Goodman Gilman 12th E/P 1234)

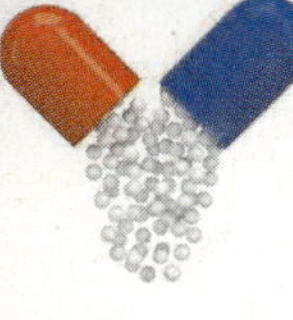

- Methylprednisolone is 5 times more potent than hydrocortisone and hence 100 mg of hydrocortisone = 20 mg methyl prednisolone.

180. Ans. (a) Eczematous lesions

(Ref: Goodman Gilman 12th E/P 1230)

181. Ans. (c) Triamcinolone

(Ref: Goodman Gilman 12th E/P 1224)

- Dexamethasone, triamcinolone and betamethasone have zero mineralocorticoid effect.

182. Ans. (c) Proinflammatory

(Ref: Goodman Gilman 12th E/P 1230)

183. Ans (a) Abiraterone, (c) Ketoconazole and (d) Finasteride

(Ref: Goodman Gilman 13th E/P 839)

Antiandrogenic drugs
- Flutamide/Bicalutamide/Apalutamide/Nilutamide/Enzalutamide
- Finasteride/Dutasteride
- Ketoconazole
- Spironolactone
- Cimetidine

184. Ans. (b) Hypoglycemia

(Ref: Goodman Gilman 12th E/P 125-27)

185. Ans. (a) Acarbose - Alpha glucosidase inhibitor, (d) Canagliflozin – SGLT-2 inhibitor, (e) Repaglinide - K+ Channel inhibitor

(Ref: Goodman Gilman 12th edition, Pages 1258-65)

Antidiabetic drugs	Mechanism of action
• Acarbose • Voglibose • Miglitol	Alpha glucosidase inhibitors
• Exenatide • Liraglutide • Albiglutide • Dulaglutide	GLP-1 Agonists
• Sitagliptin • Saxagliptin • Alogliptin • Linagliptin • Vildagliptin	DPP-4 Inhibitors
• Sulfonylureas • Meglitinides (Repaglinide)	Inhibit ATP sensitive potassium channels
Biguanides	Stimulate AMPK
Thiazolidenidiones	Stimulate PPAR gamma
• Canagliflozin • Dapagliflozin • Empagliflozin	Inhibit SGLT-2

186. Ans. (c) Glargine, (b) Detemir

(Ref: Katzung 13th edition, Page 723)

187. Ans. (c) Absorption increases with food

(Ref: Goodman Gilman 12th edition, Pages 1294-96)

- Bisphosphonates are pyrophosphate derivatives with a three-dimensional structure that increases binding to calcium in bones.
- Primary mechanism of these drugs is inhibition of osteoclast mediated bone resorption.
- Absorption of bisphosphonates is decreased by food and hence should be taken on empty stomach.
- Excretion is primarily renal and thus are safe in liver disease.

188. Ans. (b) ↑ glucose in plasma, (c) –ve feedback on corticotropin-releasing hormone (CRH) production, (d) May cause osteoporosis

(Ref: Goodman Gilman 12th edition, Page 1224)

189. Ans. (d) More potent than hydrocortisone, (e) Glucocorticoid activity is 5 times of hydrocortisone

(Ref: Goodman Gilman 12th E/P 1224)

190. Ans. (a) SGLT-2 inhibitor, (b) Blocks Na/glucose symport, (c) Causes glycosuria & polyuria, (d) Increases chance of vaginal infections

(Ref: Goodman Gilman 12th E/P 1255)

- SGLT-2 receptors present in the PCT are responsible for absorption of glucose and sodium. An upregulation of SGLT- 2 is seen particularly in type II DM.
- Canagliflozin, dapagliflozin and empagliflozin are the drugs in this class used for treatment of type II DM only.
- Glucose in urine is a medium for bacterial and fungal growth and hence UTI and vaginal infections are the most common side effect.

191. Ans. (a) Cause lactic acidosis, (c) Contraindicated in Renal failure, (e) GI disturbances are common side effect

(Ref: Goodman Gilman 12th E/P 1259)

192. Ans. (c) Cause weight loss, (e) Safe in pregnancy

(Ref: Goodman Gilman 12th E/P 1256-57)

193. Ans. (a) Impaired glucose tolerance, (b) PCOS, (c) Non-alcoholic fatty liver disease, (e) Metabolic abnormalities associated with HIV disease

(Ref: Goodman Gilman 12th E/P 1259)

194. Ans. (b) Decreases LDL, (d) Lactic acidosis, (e) Vit B deficiency

(Ref: Goodman Gilman 12th E/P 1259)

195. Ans. (a) Glargine, (c) Protamine zinc insulin, (e) NPH

(Ref: Goodman Gilman 12th E/P 1250)

196. Ans. (a) Glipizide, (b) Glibenclamide

(Ref: Goodman Gilman 12th E/P 1256)

197. Ans. (a) Letrozole, (b) Anastrozole, (c) Exemestane

(Ref: Goodman Gilman 12th E/P 1762)

198. Ans. (b) Used in OCP, (d) Third generation progesterone, (e) Dose in OCP is 3 mg

(Ref: Goodman Gilman 12th E/P 1834)

199. Ans. (c) Lispro insulin, (d) Aspart insulin

(Ref: Goodman Gilman 12th E/P 1251)

200. Ans. (a) Used as adjuvant therapy in reseptor positive breast cancer, (b) For chemoprophylaxis against breast cancer

(Ref: Goodman Gilman 12th E/P 1177)

201. Ans. (a) Glargine, (c) Detemir

(Ref: Goodman Gilman 12th E/P 1250)

202. Ans. (b) Acarbose

(Ref: Goodman Gilman 12th edition, Page 1264)

- Acarbose acts by inhibiting alpha glucosidase inhibitor in the intestine; this enzyme metabolizes starch and disaccharide (e.g. table sugar, sucrose) into glucose.
- Hence, in case of hypoglycemia caused by these drugs only glucose should be used for treatment; as disaccharide like table sugar won't be metabolized into glucose and hence will not be absorbed.

203. Ans. (b) Linagliptin

(Ref: CMDT 2018, Page 1238)

All DPP-4 inhibitors are contraindicated in renal failure as they are excreted by kidney, except linagliptin which is excreted by liver.

204. Ans. (b) Basic insulin not required

(Ref: CMDT 2017, Page 1242)

- Afrezza (technosphere) is an inhalational insulin approved for treatment of only postprandial hyperglycemia prior to meals (multiple dosing).
- For maintenance basal insulin is also given at loading dose along with afrezza.
- Absorption is rapid with peak plasma insulin level reaching within 15 minutes and then declines to baseline after 3 hours.
- Use and throw color coded cartridges of afrezza are available with 4, 8 and 12 units of insulin.
- Most common side effect is cough and few cases of lung cancer has also been seen in trials.
- It is contraindicated in smokers and patients of asthma and COPD.

205. Ans. (a) Competitive reversible aromatase inhibitor

(Ref: Goodman Gilman 12th edition, Page 1761)

206. Ans. (b) Bisphosphonates

(Ref: Goodman Gilman 12th E/P1296)

- This is a classic case of hypercalcemia associated with malignancy for which drug of choice is bisphosphonate.

207. Ans. (b) Metformin

(CMDT 2017/P 1235)

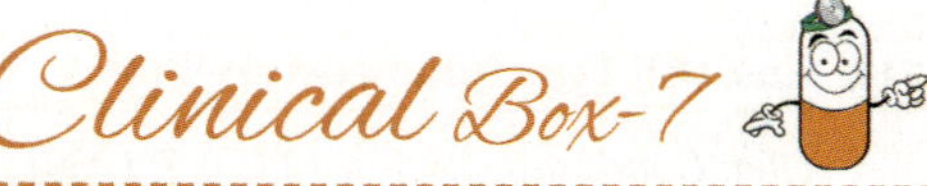
Clinical Box-7

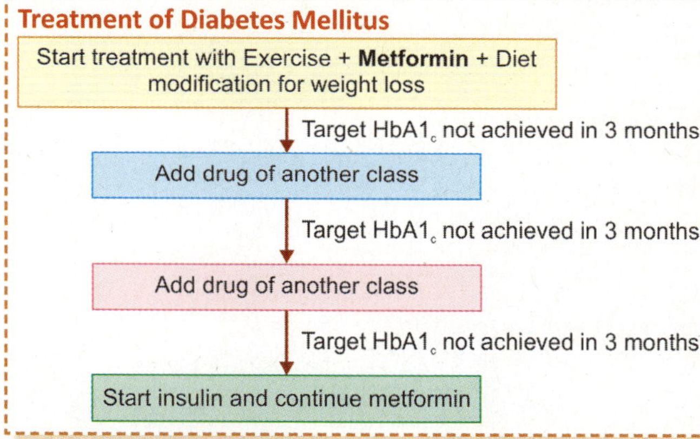
Treatment of Diabetes Mellitus
Start treatment with Exercise + Metformin + Diet modification for weight loss
Target HbA1c not achieved in 3 months
Add drug of another class
Target HbA1c not achieved in 3 months
Add drug of another class
Target HbA1c not achieved in 3 months
Start insulin and continue metformin

208. Ans. (b) Canagliflozin

(Ref: CMDT 2017/P 1228)

- SGLT-2 inhibitor like canagliflozin inhibit glucose reabsorption in renal tubules and cause glycosuria.
- Glucose in urine is a medium for bacterial and fungal growth and hence UTI and vaginal infections are the most common side effect.

209. Ans. (d) Sitagliptin

(Ref: CMDT 2017/P 1227)

210. Ans. (d) Pramlinitide

(Ref: CMDT 2017/P 1228)

211. Ans. (b) Metformin

(Ref: CMDT 2017/P 1224)

212. Ans. (a) Postmenopausal osteoporosis

(Ref: Goodman Gilman 12th E/P 1294)

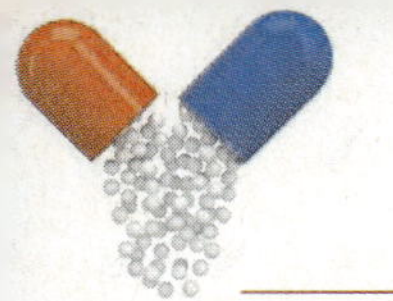

213. Ans. (d) Metformin

(Ref: Goodman Gilman 12th E/P 1259)

214. Ans. (a) It is a pure agonist

(Ref: Goodman Gilman 12th E/P1184)

- Mifepristone (RU-486) is a partial agonist at progesterone receptors and hence acts as antagonist in presence of progesterone.
- It also blocks glucocorticoid and androgen receptors.

215. Ans. (a) Improving insulin sensitivity

(Ref: Goodman Gilman 12th E/P 1260)

216. Ans. (d) Fasting

(Ref: Goodman Gilman 12th E/P 1259)

217. Ans. (b) Type 2 diabetes mellitus

(Ref: Goodman Gilman 12th E/P 1260)

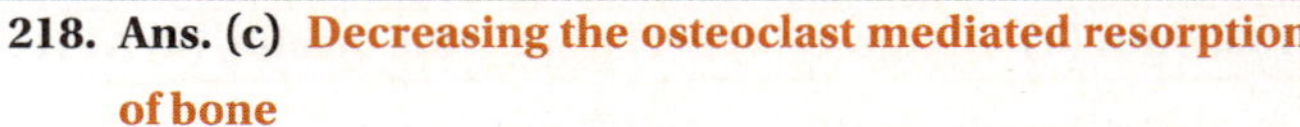

218. Ans. (c) Decreasing the osteoclast mediated resorption of bone

(Ref: Goodman Gilman 12th E/P 1294)

219. Ans. (b) Metformin

(Ref: Goodman Gilman 12th E/P 1259)

220. Ans. (b) 200 mg/2 weeks

(Ref: CMDT 2017/P 1192)

221. Ans. (b) Dexamethasone

(Ref: Goodman Gilman 12th E/P 1216)

222. Ans. (c) Dexamethasone

(Ref: Rang and Dale 6th E/P 429)

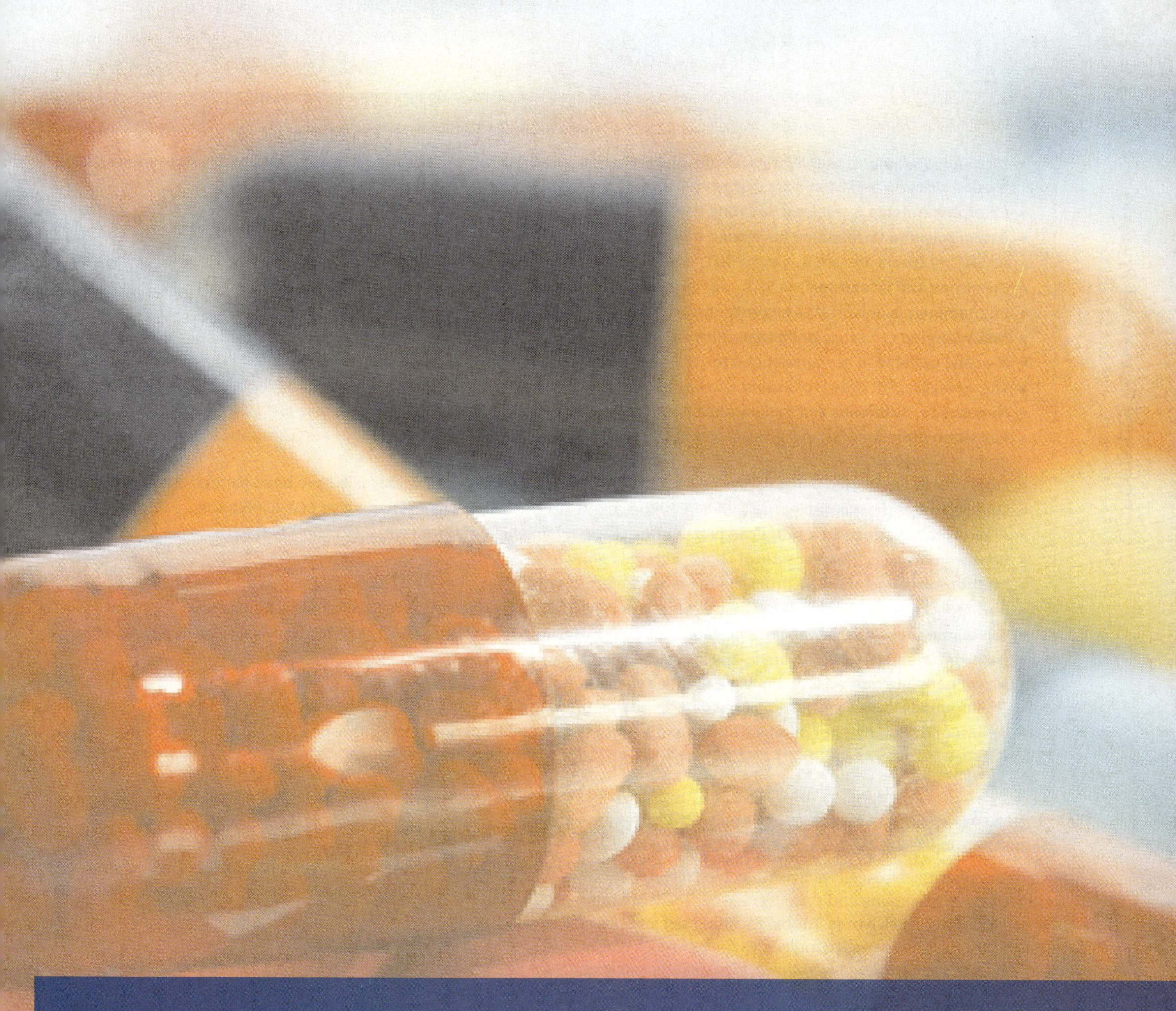

Autacoids and Immuno-modulators

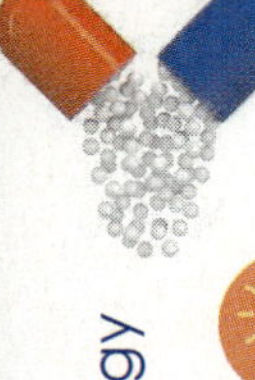

One Liners

- **Diphenhydramine, dimenhydrinate** and **promethazine** are used for the treatment of **extrapyramidal side effects (EPS), motion sickness and Meniere's disease (vertigo).**
- **Chlorpheniramine** is the **least sedating first-generation drug.**
- **Astemizole and terfenadine have been banned due to risk of QT prolongation.**
- All 5HT receptors are GPCRs except **$5HT_3$ which is a Na^+/K^+ ion channel receptors.**
- **Buspirone and ipsapirone** are $5HT_{1A}$ agonists used as **anxiolytics.**
- **Ergotamine** is a powerful **vasoconstrictor** and can cause digital gangrene.
- **Methysergide** can cause **pulmonary fibrosis.**
- **N-acetyl cysteine** in acetaminophen toxicity acts by inhibiting **NAPQI** and replenishing glutathione.
- The antiaggregant dose is of aspirin is lower, i.e. **50–320 mg/day**, whereas the anti-inflammatory dose is higher, i.e. **3–4 g/day.**
- **Nimesulide, diclofenac and meloxicam** are most **selective inhibitors of COX-II** in nonselective class which equals to celecoxib.
- **Piroxicam** is the **longest and slowest acting** nonselective COX inhibitor which undergoes enterohepatic circulation and hence given at **OD doses.**
- **Lumiracoxib** has been banned due to **hepatotoxicity** whereas r**ofecoxib and valdecoxib** have been banned due to risk of **MI**.
- **Lumiracoxib is** the most selective COX-II inhibitors whereas **celecoxib** is the least selective COX-II inhibitors.
- **Allopurinol** and **uricosuric drugs** can precipitate acute gout and hence started with colchicine or NSAIDs.
- **Benzbromarone** is the uricosuric of choice in **renal failure**.
- **Methotrexate** and **anti-TNF drugs** are the most preferred DMARDs.
- Anti-TNF drugs are absolutely contraindicated in **severe (class III/IV) heart failure and hepatitis B infection**.
- **Tacrolimus** and **cyclosporine** are calcineurin inhibitors causing common side effects line **hypertension** and **nephrotoxicity**.
- **Basiliximab** and **daclizumab** are IL-2 antagonists.
- **Mycophenolate mofetil** is an inhibitor of **IMP dehydrogenase**.
- **Thalidomide** can cause **phocomelia and peripheral neuropathy**.
- **Leflunomide**, an inhibitor of **dihydroorotate dehydrogenase** inhibits **pyrimidine synthesis.**

AUTACOIDS

Autacoids are pharmacologically active molecules secreted locally to produce effects on organs and systems nearby. The word autacoid is derived from Greek words "Autos" meaning self and "Acos" meaning relief. Thus, these active molecules for self-relief synthesized in the body are histamine, serotonin, eicosanoids, nitric oxide (NO), etc. In this section drugs action on these autacoids will be discussed.

HISTAMINE AND RELATED DRUGS

Histamine is found in most tissues and released by mast cells during and inflammatory or allergic response of the body. Histamine acts on four subtypes of receptors, i.e. **H_1, H_2, H_3 and H_4.** All of these are GPCRs and the specific effect produced by a receptor is given below in the conceptual box 1.

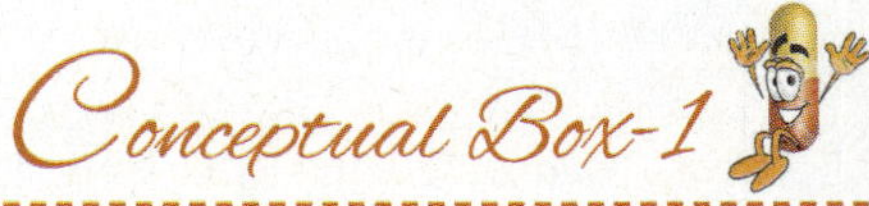

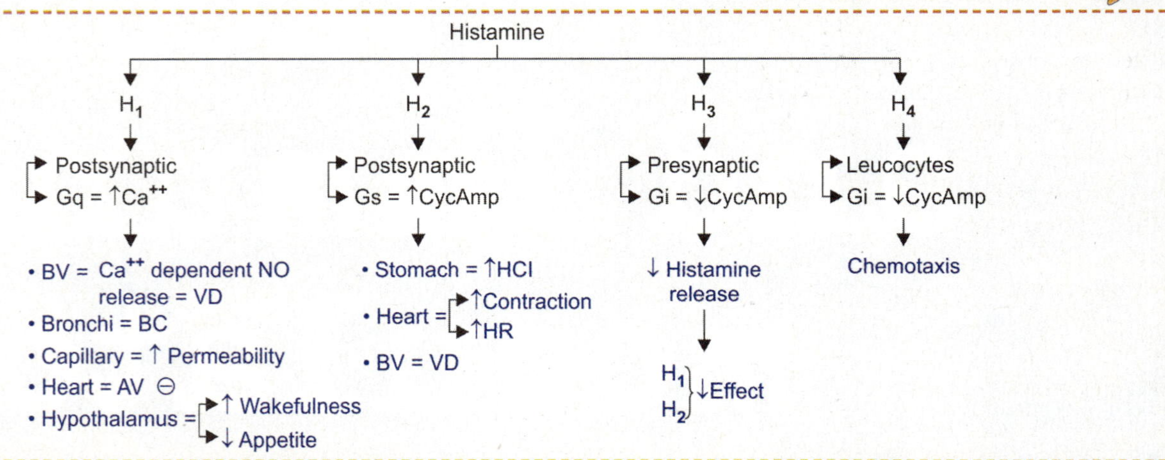

H_1 Antagonists

- The H_1 antagonists pharmacologically are inverse agonists and are broadly classified into first- and second-generation drugs.
- The first-generation drugs are highly lipid-soluble drugs, cross blood brain barrier and hence cause **sedation**. Hence, these are **contraindicated in active workers like drivers, pilots and heavy machinery workers**. These are also contraindicated in children and elderly (>65 years) due to impairment of learning and cognitive function respectively. Thus, in these age groups second-generation drugs are preferred.
- The second-generation drugs are less lipid soluble, do not cross blood brain barrier and hence are **nonsedating**. These are preferred where sedation is undesirable. The second-generation drugs are more potent and more efficacious as compared to first-generation drugs.
- Most of the first-generation drugs are short-acting except meclizine and hydroxyzine which are long-acting. The second-generation drugs are long-acting drugs.

First-generation Drugs

These are nonspecific in their mechanism of action and hence end up inhibiting other receptors like **muscarinic, serotonin and** α_1. All drugs in this class are given by oral route. Doxepin and diphenhydramine can be used by topical route as well and diphenhydramine, chlorpheniramine and hydroxyzine can be used by injectable route as well.

- **Promethazine** followed by **diphenhydramine** and **dimenhydrinate** have maximum anticholinergic effect in this class. Hence, these are preferred for the treatment of **extrapyramidal side effects (EPS), motion sickness and Meniere's disease (vertigo)** as well. Promethazine can cause α_1 block and carries risk of postural hypotension. Promethazine is also used for treatment of chemotherapy induced nausea and vomiting.
- Diphenhydramine and promethazine have local anesthetic effect as well and can be used as local anesthetics. Dimenhydrinate is used for treatment of insomnia.
- **Doxylamine** is the drug of choice for treatment of **morning sickness**. **Pyridoxine** is frequently combined with it.
- **Doxepin** is an antihistaminic later found to have inhibitory effect on monoamine reuptake and hence is used as a **TCA**. It is used for the treatment of insomnia as well.
- **Chlorpheniramine** is the **least sedating first-generation drug** and hence preferred for use in day time. It has more CNS stimulating side effects.
- **Hydroxyzine** significantly depresses CNS and produces antipruritic effect and hence is used in skin allergies. It is also used as an anxiolytic and antiemetic.
- Cyproheptadine is an antagonist at 5-HT_2 receptors and hence used for the treatment of carcinoid syndrome. It can increase appetite and cause weight gain.
- Cyclizine and meclizine can be used for motion sickness but are less effective than promethazine.

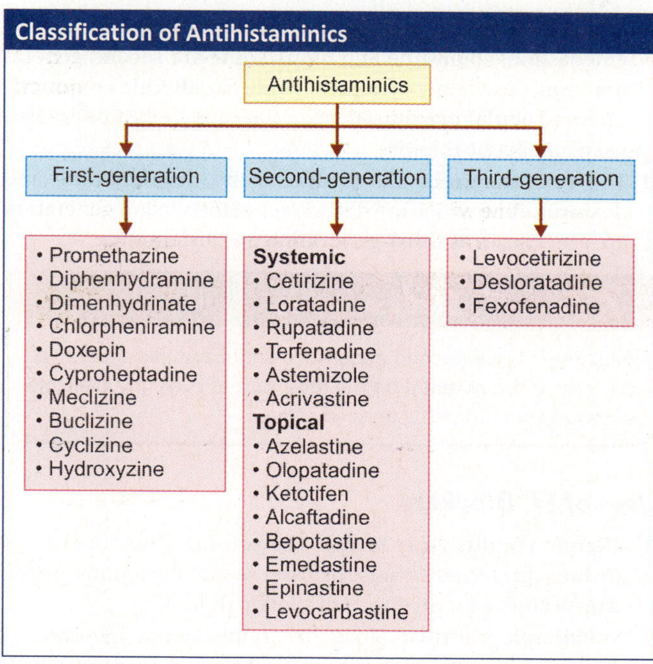

Classification of Antihistaminics
Antihistaminics
First-generation
Second-generation
Third-generation
• Promethazine
• Diphenhydramine
• Dimenhydrinate
• Chlorpheniramine
• Doxepin
• Cyproheptadine
• Meclizine
• Buclizine
• Cyclizine
• Hydroxyzine
Systemic
• Cetirizine
• Loratadine
• Rupatadine
• Terfenadine
• Astemizole
• Acrivastine
Topical
• Azelastine
• Olopatadine
• Ketotifen
• Alcaftadine
• Bepotastine
• Emedastine
• Epinastine
• Levocarbastine
• Levocetirizine
• Desloratadine
• Fexofenadine

Second-generation Drugs

- **Cetirizine** is a derivative of first-generation drug hydroxyzine and is the most sedating in this class. **Levocetirizine** is more potent than cetirizine and hence can be used at half doses of cetirizine.
- **Astemizole** is the longest acting and **terfenadine** is the fastest acting, but both have been banned due to risk of **QT prolongation** and fatal cardiac arrhythmia like torsades, especially if combined with enzyme inhibitor like ketoconazole.
- **Fexofenadine is a metabolite of terfenadine**, devoid of its side effect. It is the **least sedating** of the second generation as it is a good substrate for P-glycoprotein pump, which leads to drug efflux from CNS.

Antihistaminic and Metabolic Drugs

Antihistaminic	Metabolite drug
• Terfenadine	• Fexofenadine
• Hydroxyzine	• Cetirizine
• Loratadine	• Desloratadine

- Loratadine and its metabolite desloratadine both are marketed for use. Desloratadine is the **most potent** antihistaminic drug. Loratadine is used for prophylaxis of exercise-induced asthma.
- Cetirizine and loratadine are excreted by kidney whereas fexofenadine is excreted by liver.
- Rupatadine inhibits PAF and has significant anti-inflammatory effect as well.
- Acrivastine is used in fixed dose combination with pseudo-ephedrine for treatment of nasal congestion.

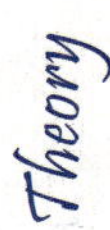

- **Azelastine**, levocabastine, ketotifen, alcaftadine, bepotastine, emedastine, epinastine and olopatadine are second generation drugs used only by **topical route for allergic conjunctivitis and ocular pruritus**. Olopatadine and azelastine are also used for allergic rhinitis.
- The antihistaminics like **levocetirizine, fexofenadine** and **desloratadine** which are derivatives of the second generation are also known as **third-generation** antihistaminics.

Recent Advances

Bilastine is a new second-generation antihistaminic under trial. It is even more potent than the most potent currently available second-generation drug desloratadine.

Uses of H_1 Blockers

- **Allergic rhinitis (Hay fever):** The second-generation drugs are more preferred because of lesser sedation. Steroids are the drug of choice for treatment of allergic rhinitis.
- **Nonallergic rhinitis:** Since histamine is not involved in nonallergic rhinitis, first-generation drugs are preferred which decrease secretions due to antimuscarinic effect.
- **Urticaria:** The second-generation antihistamines are the drug of choice for treatment of urticarial.
- Other uses for specific drugs have been discussed above.

H_2 Antagonist

This class of drug has been discussed in detail in the chapter of GIT.

H_3 Inverse Agonist

- Inverse agonism at H_3 receptors increases release of histamine which increases wakefulness and induces anorexia.
- **Tiprolisant** is an H_3 inverse agonist under trial for the treatment of narcolepsy.

Recent Advances

H_4 receptor antagonists are currently under trial for the treatment of atopic dermatitis.

BRADYKININ, KALLIDIN AND RELATED DRUGS

- Kininogens are broken down by **kallikrein** into **bradykinin** and **kallidin**. Both these products act on bradykinin receptors (B1 and B2), which are G_q subtypes of GPCRs. Once stimulated these receptors increase calcium which activates ENOS and increases NO which causes vasodilation. There is also an increase in synthesis of prostaglandins which causes pain and inflammation.

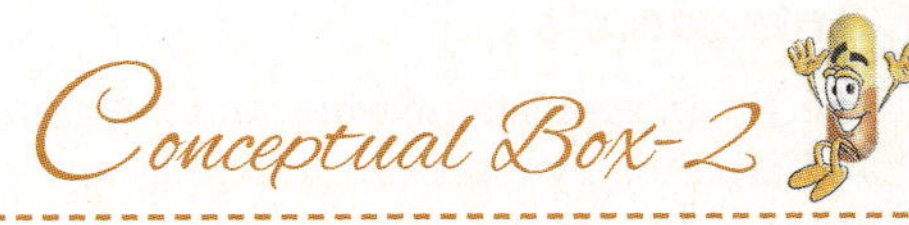

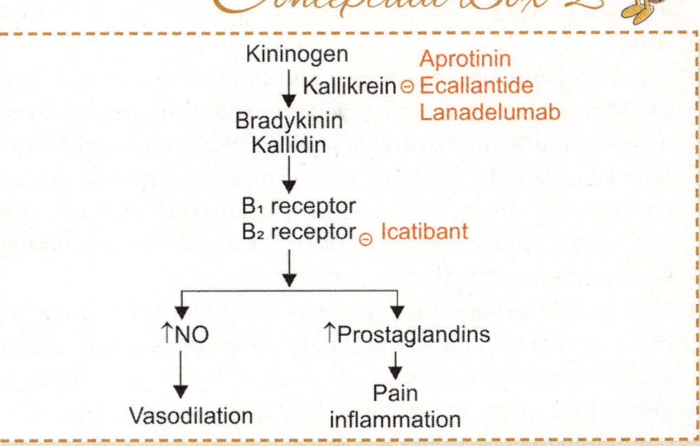

- B_2 receptor inhibitor **icatibant** and kallikrein inhibitor **ecallantide** can be used for the treatment of hereditary angioedema.
- **Lanadelumab** is a recent kallikrein inhibitor approved for prophylaxis of hereditary angioedema.
- **Aprotinin** is an inhibitor of both kallikrein and plasmin, used to decrease bleeding in patients undergoing coronary artery bypass grafting (CABG).

Clinical Box-1

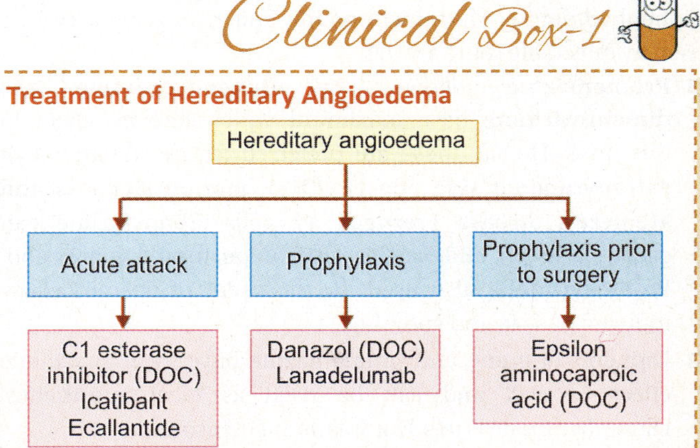

SEROTONIN AND RELATED DRUGS

- Serotonin is present throughout the body but is located maximum in the enterochromaffin cells of GIT, platelets and CNS.
- Serotonin acts on seven types of receptors $5HT_1$ to $5HT_7$; all are GPCRs except **$5HT_3$ which is a Na^+/K^+ ion channel receptors**.
- $5HT_1$ to $5HT_4$ receptors are well characterized and drugs have been developed against them. However, still little is known about the rest serotonin receptors, i.e. $5HT_5$ to $5HT_7$.
- The different functions of relevant 5HT receptors are mentioned in the conceptual box 3.

Conceptual Box-3

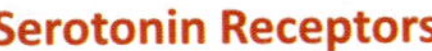

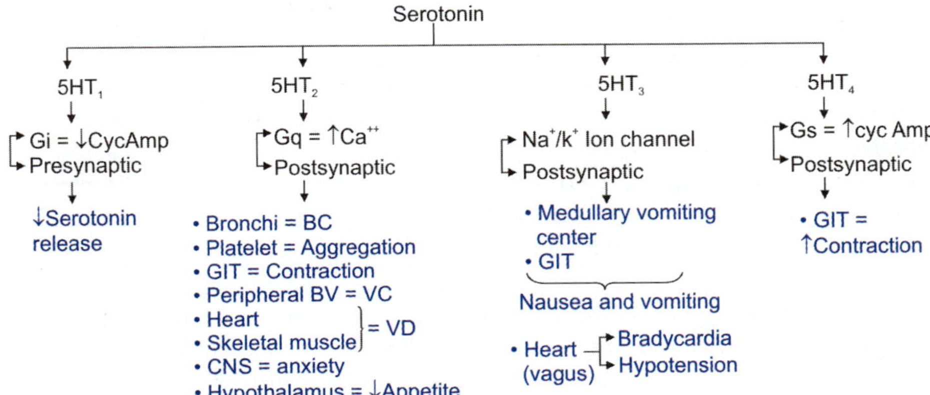

$5HT_1$ Agonists

$5HT_1$ receptors are **autoreceptors** and its agonists are of two types, i.e. $5HT_{1A}$ agonists and $5HT_{1B/1D}$ agonists.

5HT 1A Agonists

- As described in the conceptual box, these presynaptic G_I subtype of receptors decrease release of 5HT. Hence decreased activation of $5HT_2$ receptors decreases anxiety or gives anxiolytic effect.
- **Buspirone, ipsapirone** and **gepirone** are $5HT_{1A}$ partial agonists used as **anxiolytics**.

Recent Advances

Repinotan: It is a $5HT_{1A}$ agonist currently under trial for its neuroprotective effect in ischemic stroke.

$5HT_{IB/ID}$ Agonists and Migraine

Pathophysiology of Migraine

- **Migraine** is caused by spontaneous activity of trigeminal nucleus, which generates an action potential. This action potential depolarizes thalamus, which gives abnormal cutaneous (creeping movements) and visual sensations (flashing of light) known as **aura**.
- Once action potential reaches to the meningeal blood vessels, it stimulates release of calcitonin gene-related peptide (CGRP), which acts on CGRP receptors in blood vessels and causes **vasodilation**.
- Vasodilation causes meningeal edema and since meninges are highly innervated, their compression against skull causes immense pain, i.e. **headache**. Since one side of trigeminal nucleus is stimulated each time, the headache is **hemicranial and shifting**.

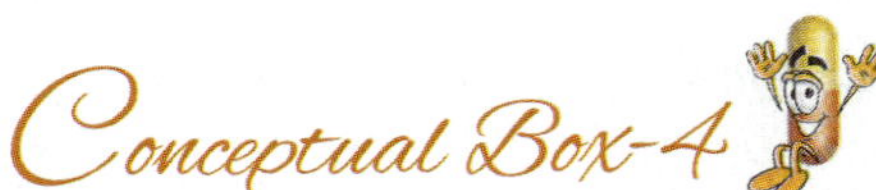

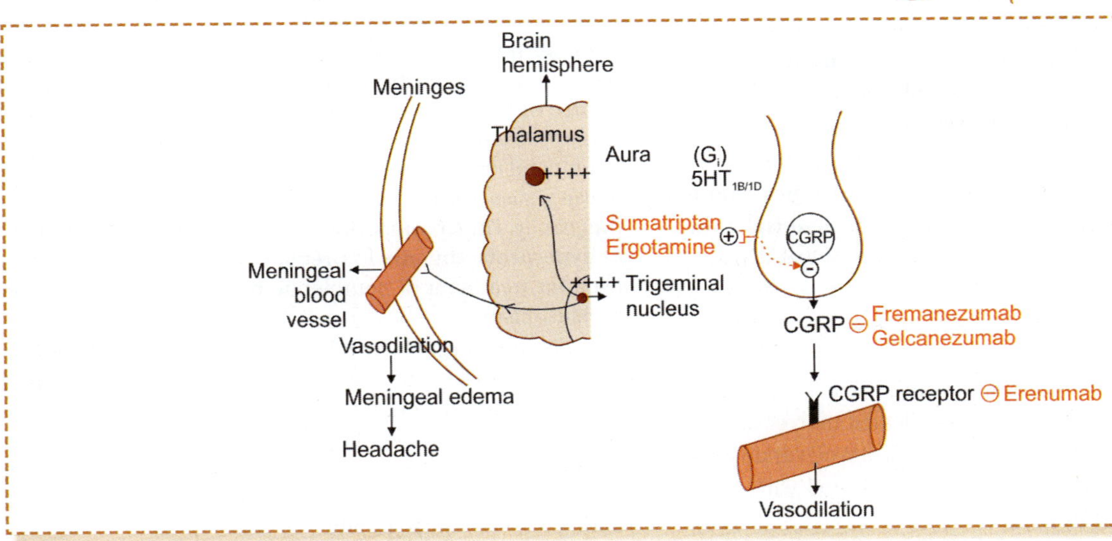

Drugs Used in Treatment of Migraine

$5HT_{1B/1D}$ partial agonists

- **$5HT_{1B/1D}$ partial agonists** are the **current drugs of choice for treatment of an acute attack** of migraine. They act by inhibiting release of CGRP, and hence if taken just after aura, it can abort an acute attack. They are also vasoconstrictors and hence can treat even if headache has begun. These are also effective in the treatment of cluster headache, but not effective in tension type headache.
- The drugs in this class are **sumatriptan, rizatriptan, frovatriptan, zolmitriptan, eletriptan, naratriptan and almotriptan.** The different aspects of pharmacokinetics and pharmacodynamics are given in the box.
- **Efficacy of these drugs is related to T_{max}** (rate of absorption). Rizatriptan > eletriptan are most efficacious due to faster onset of action.
- Frovatriptan > naratriptan have slow onset of action and hence are better tolerated.

Sumatriptan	• All parameters are least, i.e. least Bioavailability Half-life Plasma protein binding Potency Blood brain barrier penetration • Maximum toxicity • Safest in pregnancy
Naratriptan	• Maximum bioavailability and potency and hence least dose requirement • Slow onset of action
Frovatriptan	Slowest acting and hence longest acting, thus beneficial in prolonged attack or attacks precipitated by menstruation
Rizatriptan	Fastest acting and hence best in acute attack
Eletriptan	• Maximum plasma protein binding • Fast acting and hence is also good in acute attack

- All can be given by oral route; **zolmitriptan and sumatriptan** can be given by **intranasal** route as well. **Sumatriptan** can be given by **subcutaneous and rectal route** also.
- Since triptans can cause vasoconstriction, they are contraindicated in **ischemic heart disease, peripheral vascular disease, hypertension, stroke, transient ischemic attack, hemiplegic migraine and ischemic bowel disease.** Other side effects associated are arrhythmia, flushing, diaphoresis and pain in neck and jaw. Intranasal sumatriptan causes bitter taste.
- Naratriptan is contraindicated in both renal and liver failure, whereas eletriptan is contraindicated in liver failure. Zolmitriptan is contraindicated in patients of Wolf Parkinson's white syndrome. These are also contraindicated with MAO inhibitors and ergotamine.

> **Recent Advances**
>
> **CGRP receptor antagonists: Olcegepant** (IV route) and **telcagepant** (Oral route) are CGRP receptor antagonists under trial for the treatment of an acute attack of migraine. **Erenumab** is an anti CGRP receptor monoclonal antibody recently approved for prophylaxis of migraine by subcutaneous route.
>
> **CGRP ligand antagonists: Fremanezumab** and **Gaelcanezumab** are anti CGRP ligand monoclonal antibodies approved for prophylaxis of migraine by subcutaneous route.

Ergot alkaloids

Ergot alkaloids are derived from a fungus called as Claviceps purpurea, which infects crops and causes poisoning called as ergotism. All drugs in this class cause contraction of GIT and stimulate medullary vomiting center and hence end up causing nausea, vomiting and diarrhea as a common side effect. Vasoconstriction is another common side effect with these drugs (maximum with ergotamine) and hence these drugs are **contraindicated in patients of angina** and peripheral vascular disease.

- **Ergotamine** is a partial agonist/antagonist at alpha receptors and partial agonist at $5HT_2$ and $5HT_1$ receptors. It can be used in an acute attack of migraine and the primary effect is because of partial agonism at $5HT_1$ receptors like triptans. Vasoconstriction produced by alpha and $5HT_2$ receptors also play a role in its effect in migraine. Peripheral vasoconstriction of end arteries in organs like finger tips can cause **gangrene** and hence the dose should not exceed **6 mg** in an attack, and it should not be taken for more than 10 times in a month. The vasodilator of choice in such a case is **nitroprusside** or **nitroglycerine**. Ergotamine causes uterine contraction and hence should not be used in pregnancy. **Dihydroergotamine** is a derivative of ergotamine with lesser agonistic action on alpha and $5HT_2$ receptors and more antagonist action on alpha receptors. Hence, it is better tolerated than ergotamine and can also be used in acute attack of migraine. Ergotamine is given by sublingual/oral, rectal or intranasal route, whereas dihydroergotamine is given by parenteral or intranasal route. Ergotamine has poor oral absorption and hence oral tablets are formulated with caffeine, which increases its absorption as well as analgesic effect.
- **Bromocriptine, cabergoline** and **pergolide** are ergot alkaloids with primarily agonistic action on D_2 receptors. They decrease release of prolactin and hence are used for the treatment of hyperprolactinemia or prolactinoma. Cabergoline is more potent and drug of choice for **hyperprolactinemia**, however it can cause cardiac valve defects and contraindicated in pregnancy. Thus, bromocriptine is drug of choice for treatment of **hyperprolactinemia in pregnancy**. Bromocriptine is also used for treatment of neuroleptic malignant syndrome and parkinsonism.
- **Ergonovine (Ergometrine)** is primarily a $5HT_2$ agonist which produces strong uterine contraction. Hence, it is used by intramuscular route for the treatment of postpartum hemorrhage not responding to oxytocin (DOC). Its effect on alpha receptors is lesser and hence it is not a potent vasoconstrictor. It is also used for diagnosis of variant angina during coronary angiography.

- **LSD** is a D_2 and $5HT_2$ agonist in the brain and $5HT_2$ antagonist in the periphery. It is used as a peripheral $5HT_2$ antagonist in experiments. The central stimulatory effect gives hallucination and hence is commonly abused.
- **Methysergide** is primarily a $5HT_2$ partial agonist/antagonist and is effective in prophylaxis of migraine. It is not preferred due to side effects like **retroperitoneal, pulmonary and cardiac fibrosis**.
- **Dihydroergotoxine** has cholinergic effects on brain and hence can be used in Alzheimer's disease.

Dopamine Antagonists

Dopamine is increased in migraine. Hence, D_2 antagonists like chlorpromazine, prochlorperazine and metoclopramide can be given by parenteral route for an acute attack of migraine.

Opioids

Opioids like butorphanol by intranasal route or pethidine by parenteral route are also used for severe acute attack of migraine not responding to other drugs. They should not be used routinely for frequent attacks due to risk of dependence and risk of decreased response to triptans in future attacks.

NSAIDs

- NSAIDs like aspirin, acetaminophen, naproxen, and diclofenac are preferred for treatment of mild attacks of migraine. Some NSAID combinations like aspirin + acetaminophen + caffeine and aspirin + metoclopramide are also used.
- In case of no response or moderate to severe attacks triptans should be used along with NSAIDs.

Drugs Used in Prophylaxis of Migraine

Prophylactic therapy is indicated in a patient with frequent attacks (more than four in a month) or patients who respond poorly to the drugs for acute attack of migraine. Drugs are started at low doses and then gradually increased keeping adequate effect and tolerability in view. After six months of drug use, dose is gradually decreased and then as per response of patient, drug is either stopped or continued.

- Beta blockers like **propranolol** is the drug of choice for prophylaxis of migraine.
- Flunarizine is a calcium channel blocker.
- Phenelzine is a MAO inhibitor and hence should not be used along with cheese (has tyramine) due to risk of cheese reaction. It should not be used with meperidine (inhibits MAO) due to risk of serotonin syndrome.
- **Methysergide** is an ergot alkaloid effective in prophylaxis, but not preferred due to reasons described above.
- Miscellaneous drugs used in prophylaxis are butterbur, guanfacine, riboflavin and botulinum toxin.

Mnemonics

Drugs Used in Prophylaxis of Migraine

Flunarizine : Flunarizine
Can : Cyproheptadine, Clonidine, Candesartan
P : Pizotifen, Propranolol (DOC), Phenelzine
RE : Release of GABA - Gabapentin
VE : ValproatE, Venlafaxine, Verapamil
N : Nortriptyline
T : Topiramate
Migraine : Methysergide

$5HT_2$ Antagonists

- Cyproheptadine is an antagonist at **$5HT_2$, H_1 and muscarinic receptors**. It is used for the treatment of cold urticaria, carcinoid syndrome, serotonin syndrome and prophylaxis of migraine. It stimulates appetite and hence can be used in cancer patients for weight gain.
- Methysergide is used for prophylaxis of migraine and has been discussed previously.
- Ketanserin can block α_1 receptors and cause vasodilation. Hence, it can be used for the treatment of hypertension and erectile dysfunction. Ritanserin has lesser alpha blocking effect and it has not clinical use as of now.

Recent Advances

Flibanserin: Flibanserin is a latest $5HT_2$ antagonist and $5HT_{1A}$ agonist approved for hypoactive sexual desire disorder (HSDD) in females. It is contraindicated with alcohol due to risk of severe hypotension.

$5HT_2$ Agonists

- Lorcaserin is a $5HT_2$ agonist used for the treatment of obesity
- It produces anorexia by action on hypothalamus.

Clinical Box-2

Antiobesity Drugs

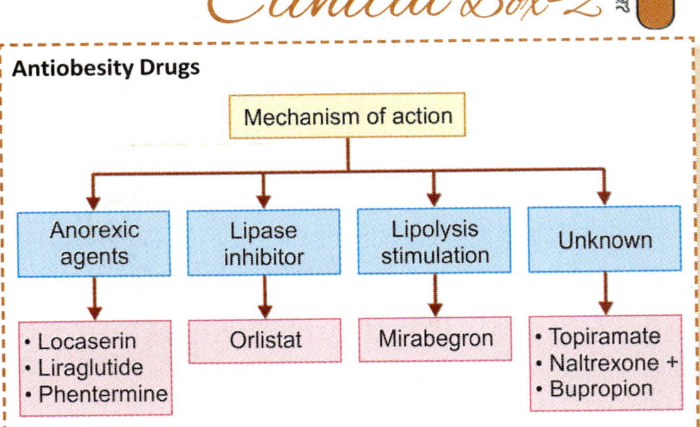

Note: Rimonabant was banned due to risk of suicidal tendency, sibutramine and phenylpropanolamine were banned due to risk of MI and stroke. Phentermine can be used alone or in combination with topiramate.

$5HT_3$ Antagonists

- **Ondansetron, palonosetron, granisetron** are $5HT_3$ antagonists used for treatment of chemotherapy induced nausea and vomiting
- **Alosetron and cilansetron** are used for treatment of diarrhea associated with irritable bowel syndrome
- These drugs have been discussed in detail in the chapter of GIT.

$5HT_4$ Agonists

- **Cisapride, tegaserod, mosapride** and **prucalopride** are $5HT_4$ agonists used as prokinetics and for treatment of constipation

- These drugs have also been discussed in detail in the chapter of GIT.

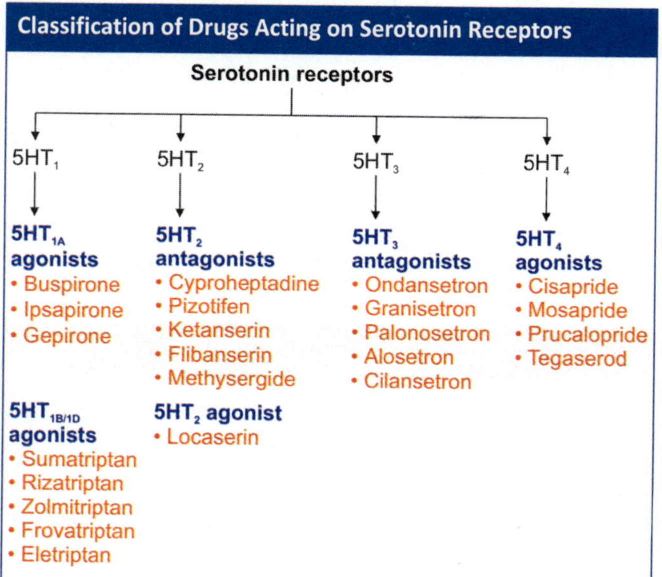

Classification of Drugs Acting on Serotonin Receptors
Serotonin receptors
5HT1
5HT2
5HT3
5HT4
5HT1A agonists
• Buspirone
• Ipsapirone
• Gepirone
5HT2 antagonists
• Cyproheptadine
• Pizotifen
• Ketanserin
• Flibanserin
• Methysergide
5HT3 antagonists
• Ondansetron
• Granisetron
• Palonosetron
• Alosetron
• Cilansetron
5HT4 agonists
• Cisapride
• Mosapride
• Prucalopride
• Tegaserod
5HT1B/1D agonists
• Sumatriptan
• Rizatriptan
• Zolmitriptan
• Frovatriptan
• Eletriptan
5HT2 agonist
• Locaserin

EICOSANOIDS AND RELATED DRUGS

Eicosanoids are autacoids like prostaglandins, thromboxane and leukotrienes derived from arachidonic acid. The drugs related to these eicosanoids are discussed in this segment.

Eicosanoid Synthesis

- Arachidonic acid is released from membrane phospholipids by phospholipase A_2 (PLA_2). Arachidonic acid is then acted upon by two enzymes cyclooxygenase (COX) I and II and 5-lipooxygenase (5-LOX).
- **COX-I** is found in most cells and it has housekeeping function like protection of gastric epithelium. **COX-II** is primarily responsible for inflammation and neoplasia. COX produces prostaglandins which are responsible for **pain, inflammation** and **pyrexia**. Selective prostaglandins have an effect as given in the conceptual box 5.
- 5-LOX pathway produces various leukotrienes, out of which leukotriene C4 and D4 are powerful bronchoconstrictors.
- AA is also precursor for synthesis of platelet-activating factor (PAF) which contributes to inflammation. Hence PAF antagonists like **apafant** have been tried in bronchial asthma, but results were not satisfactory in trials.

Conceptual Box-5

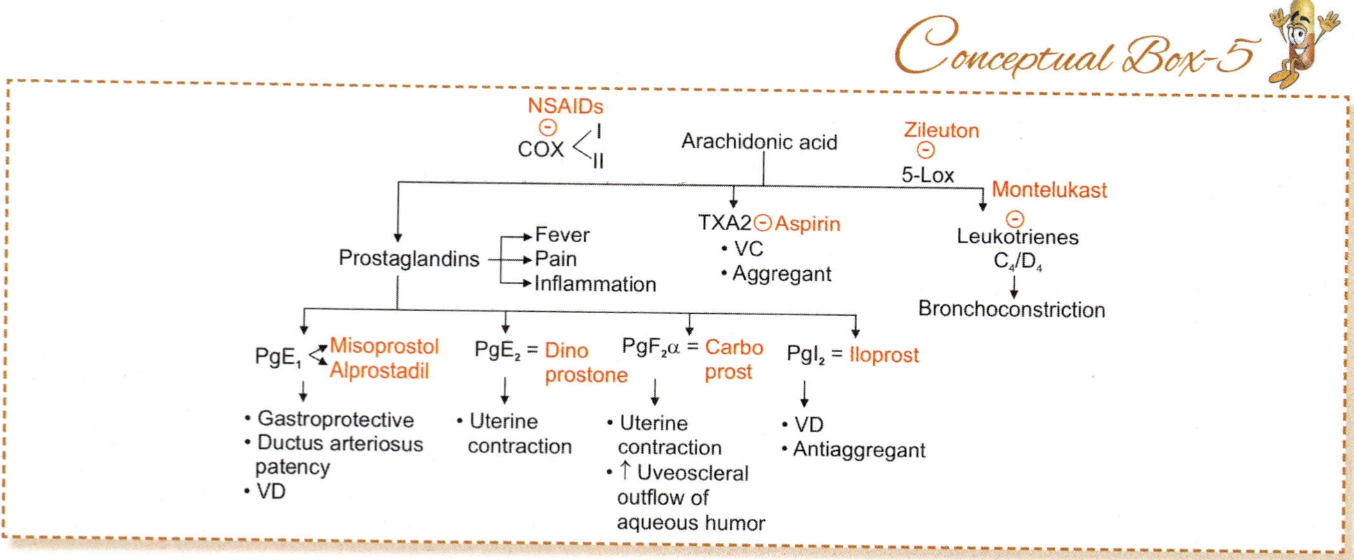

Eicosanoid Effects

Organ/symptom	Effect	Mechanism	Comments
Pain	Increased	All PG and LTB_4 increase sensitivity of nociceptive receptors	NSAIDs used as analgesics
Inflammation	Increased	PgE_2 and I_2 cause vasodilation at site of inflammation, which causes increased blood flow and leucocyte infiltration	NSAIDs used as anti-inflammatory drugs
Pyrexia	Increased	PgE_2 acts on thermosensitive neurons of hypothalamus	NSAIDs used as antipyretics

Contd...

Organ/symptom	Effect	Mechanism	Comments
Blood vessels	• Systemic vasodilation • Maintain patency of ductus arteriosus till birth	PgI_2 > PgE_2 and PgD stimulate Gs subtypes of receptors and increase cyclic AMP in smooth muscles	• Synthetic PgI_2 i.e. epoprostenol used in pulmonary hypertension • PgE_1 analogs like misoprostol and alprostadil used to maintain patency of ductus arteriosus after birth in some congenital heart disorders • PgE_1 analog like alprostadil used in erectile dysfunction • NSAIDs are used for closure of a patent ductus arteriosus
Platelet	Aggregant effect	TXA_2 acts on G_q subtype of receptors and increases calcium	Aspirin used as antiaggregant in secondary prophylaxis of MI and stroke
	Antiaggregant effect	PgI_2, PgD_2 stimulate Gs subtype receptors and increase cyclic AMP	Selective COX-II inhibitors decrease PgI_2 significantly and hence cause MI
Bronchi	Bronchoconstriction	LT C_4/D_4, $PgF_{2\alpha}$, PgD_2 stimulate G_q subtype of receptors and increase calcium	• Leukotriene inhibitors cause bronchodilation and used in asthma • NSAIDs by blocking COX, potentiate LOX pathway, increase LT synthesis and cause bronchospasm
GIT	Contraction	PgE_2, $PgF_{2\alpha}$, PgD_2 stimulate G_q subtype of receptors and cause GIT contraction	• Oral PgE_1 analog misoprostol causes abdominal cramps and diarrhea • Diarrhea in cholera is caused by prostaglandins and hence NSAIDs are effective
	Secretion	• PgE_2 and PgI_2 primarily act • Gs receptor stimulation increases mucin and bicarbonate secretion • G_i receptor stimulation decreases HCl secretion	• NSAIDs cause gastric ulcer • PgE_1 analog misoprostol is used as gastroprotective agent
Kidney	Diuresis	PgE_2 and PgI_2 cause afferent arteriole dilation in glomerulus and facilitate diuresis	• Loop diuretics produce diuresis partially by increasing prostaglandins • NSAIDs can decrease effect of loop diuretics
Uterus	Uterine contraction	PgE_2 and $PgF_{2\alpha}$ stimulate G_q subtype of receptors and increase calcium	• PgE_2 analog dinoprostone and $PgF_{2\alpha}$ analog carboprost used in abortion and induction of labor
Eye	Decreased IOP	PgE_2 and $PgF_{2\alpha}$ increases uveoscleral outflow	• $PgF_{2\alpha}$ analog latanoprost used in open angle glaucoma
Cell proliferation	Neoplasia	PgE_2 (COX-II) increases cell proliferation	• NSAIDs have been seen to have protective effect on colon cancer

Prostaglandin Analogs

- **Prostaglandin E_1 analog: Misoprostol** is used as a gastroprotective agent, to maintain patency of ductus arteriosus, for medical abortion along with mifepristone and for cervical ripening. **Alprostadil** is used to maintain patency of ductus arteriosus and for treatment of erectile dysfunction.
- **Prostaglandin E_2 analog: Dinoprostone** is used for induction of labour, abortion in second trimester of pregnancy, cervical ripening and for benign H. mole.
- **Prostaglandin $F_{2\alpha}$ analog: Carboprost** is used for induction of labour, abortion in second trimester of pregnancy and for treatment of postpartum hemorrhage. **Latanoprost** and **bimatoprost** are used for treatment of glaucoma, which act by increasing uveoscleral outflow. Latanoprost is contraindicated in patients with uveitis, as being a prostaglandin analog, it can worsen inflammation.
- **Prostaglandin I_2 (prostacyclin) related drugs: Epoprostenol** synthetic prostaglandin I_2, **iloprost** and **beraprost** are prostaglandin I_2 analogs, **treprostinil** and **selexipag** are prostaglandin I_2 receptor agonists used for treatment of pulmonary hypertension.

5-LOX Pathway Inhibitors

- **Zileuton** is a 5-LOX inhibitor and **montelukast** and **zafirlukast** are leukotriene inhibitors used in bronchial asthma.

- These drugs have been discussed in detail in the chapter of respiratory system.

NSAIDs

Nonsteroidal anti-inflammatory drugs (NSAIDs) can be broadly classified as **nonselective** and **selective COX-II inhibitors**. All of them are used as anti-inflammatory, analgesics and antipyretics.

Nonselective COX Inhibitors

Acetaminophen

- **Acetaminophen** is used as an antipyretic and analgesic but is devoid of anti-inflammatory effect. It is the **analgesic of choice in osteoarthritis.**
- Acetaminophen can cause **hepatotoxicity** due to toxic metabolite **NAPQI** that causes glutathione depletion and inactivation of liver enzymes. Glutathione depletion renders liver vulnerable to free radical damage. Histopathological finding in liver toxicity is **centrilobular necrosis with periportal sparing**. Hepatotoxicity is seen after 48–96 hours of consumption of high doses, i.e. >**10 grams or** >**150–250 mg/kg** and doses above 20 grams is fatal. The chances of hepatotoxicity are raised in conditions like fasting, malnutrition and chronic alcoholism.

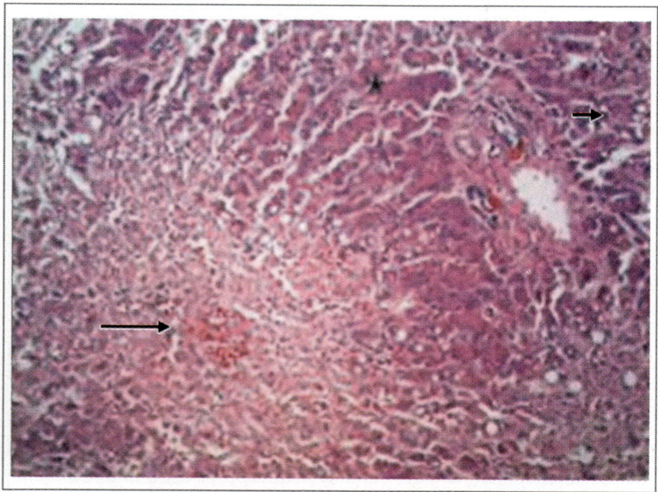

Acetaminophen-induced Centrilobular Necrosis

- The chances of hepatotoxicity can be predicted with the help of **Rumack-Mathew nomogram**, which is drawn by plotting acetaminophen plasma concentration on Y-axis and time after drug consumption on X-axis. The prognosis can be calculated only between 4 and 24 hours after drug consumption. Thus, according to nomogram, a plasma value of acetaminophen above 200 mcg/mL causes hepatotoxicity and below it is safe at 4 hours after drug consumption.
- Renal tubular necrosis and hypoglycemic coma can also be seen in case of toxicity.
- Charcoal is given to the patient if presents within 4 hours, however gastric lavage is not done. **N-acetyl cysteine** is the drug of choice which acts by **inhibiting NAPQI and replenishing glutathione in the body.** It is given at loading dose of 140 mg/kg by oral route and then a maintenance dose of 70 mg/kg every 4 hours. A total of 17 doses are given.

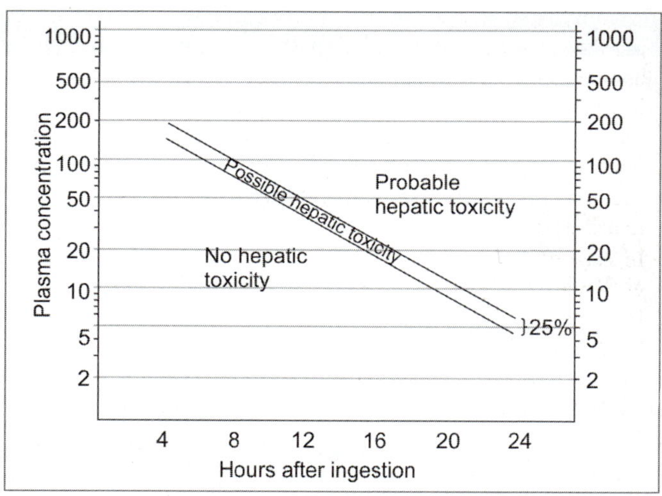

Rumack-Mathew Nomogram

Clinical Box-3

Treatment of Acetaminophen Induced Hepatotoxicity

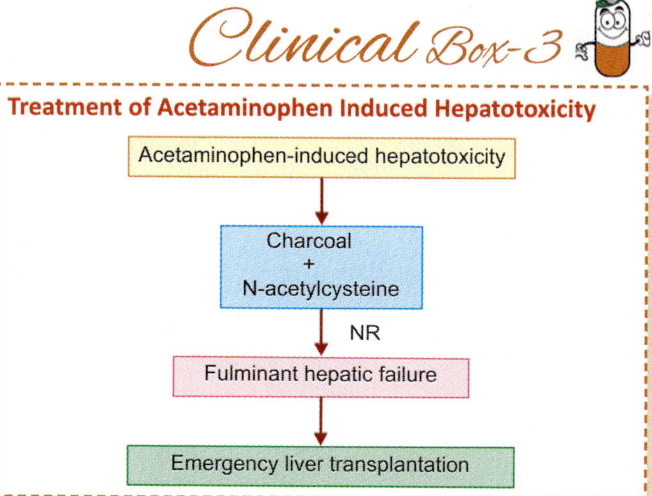

Aspirin

- **Aspirin** a **salicylate** is a noncompetitive **irreversible inhibitor of COX**. It is metabolized in liver and excreted by kidney mostly as **salicyluric acid**. Apart from anti-inflammatory, analgesic and antipyretic effects it also has **anti-aggregant effect**.
- It is the **analgesic of choice in rheumatic and rheumatoid arthritis** and is drug of choice for treatment of **niacininduced flushing**. It can also be used for treatment of systemic mastocytosis. As an antiaggregant it is used for prophylaxis of MI and stroke.
- It is usually contraindicated in children due to risk of Reye's syndrome, but the only condition where it is used in children is in **Kawasaki disease** to treat vasculitis and prevent aneurysm formation.
- Topical salicylic acid is used for treatment of dermatitis, muscle pain, warts and fungal infections.
- The antiaggregant dose is lower, i.e. **75–325 mg/day**, whereas the anti-inflammatory dose is higher, i.e. **3–4 g/day**.
- Other salicylates like mesalamine and olsalazine are used for treatment of ulcerative colitis, rheumatoid arthritis and ankylosing spondylitis.

- Diflunisal has poor antipyretic effect but is a more potent analgesic and anti-inflammatory drug than aspirin; hence it is used as analgesic in osteoarthritis and muscular pain. GIT and platelet related side effects are lesser with diflunisal than aspirin.
- Aspirintoxicity is seen at doses more than 10 grams characterized by respiratory alkalosis and compensatory metabolic acidosis, hyperthermia, ototoxicity (tinnitus, hearing loss), seizures and hyperglycemia.
- In case of aspirintoxicity forced alkaline diuresis is done to enhance excretion. It is the only NSAID that can be removed by dialysis which is indicated in case of pulmonary edema, usually seen in elderly patients.

Indomethacin

- **Indomethacin** is the **analgesic of choice in psoriatic and reactive arthritis and drug of choice for the treatment of Bartter syndrome** and **acute gout**. As it is a more potent drug but causes toxicity it is reserved for analgesia and fever in refractory cases as in Hodgkin's lymphoma.
- It also decreases intraventricular hemorrhage in LBW neonates.
- Most common side effect is headache followed by others like nephrotoxicity, pancreatitis and diarrhea.
- Sulindac is a prodrug derived from indomethacin, used as an analgesic and anti-inflammatory drug. It can also prevent colon cancer in familial adenomatous polyposis. It is less toxic as compared to indomethacin.

Diclofenac

- Diclofenac is used by oral route as an analgesic and anti-inflammatory drug, gel and transdermal patches for analgesia and as drops by ocular route for inflammation. It is used as a fixed dose combination (FDC) along with misoprostol to decrease GIT side effects.
- It is hepatotoxic but still marketed but its derivatives like lumiracoxib, bromfenac and nepafenac have been banned for the same reason. It is a highly selective COX-II inhibitor and hence GIT side effects are lesser.
- It is contraindicated in children and pregnant patients.

Ibuprofen

- **Ibuprofen** can be used by oral and intravenous route for pain, inflammation and is drug of choice for closure of PDA. Currently ibuprofen is more preferred as compared to indomethacin due to better toxicity profile for PDA closure.
- Ibuprofen interferes with the antiaggregant effect of aspirin. It is the most common cause of drug induced **aseptic meningitis**. It can cause ocular side effects like toxic amblyopia and blurring of vision and in such case, it should be discontinued. It is safe in breastfeeding though.
- **Ketoprofen** belongs to same class and has lysosomal stabilizing and bradykinin antagonizing effect. **Flurbiprofen** can be given by ocular route for intraoperative miosis.

Other NSAIDs

- **Ketorolac** is a potent analgesic providing effect equal to opioids and is rapid and short acting. Hence is used for treatment of postoperative pain but avoided for labor analgesia. **Topical ketorolac** can be used by **ocular route** for treatment of inflammation after ocular surgery and in allergic conjunctivitis.
- **Nimesulide** is contraindicated in children less than 12 years and used in adults for a maximum of 15 days due to **hepatotoxicity**.
- **Etodolac, nimesulide, diclofenac and meloxicam** are most **selective inhibitors of COX-II** in this class which equals to celecoxib. **Etodolac is the most selective** whereas ketorolac is the least selective COX-II inhibitor in this class. Etodolac is used as an analgesic in postoperative period and other inflammatory disorders.
- **Piroxicam** is the **longest and slowest acting** nonselective COX inhibitor and hence given at **OD doses** and not preferred in acute analgesia. It undergoes **enterohepatic circulation**.
- **Tolmetin** > **Indomethacin** are maximum concentrated in the synovial fluid and hence best in treatment of arthritis.
- **Mefenamic acid** used for short-term analgesia is contraindicated in pregnancy and children. It can cause autoimmune hemolytic anemia.
- **Phenylbutazone** and **antipyrine** can cause agranulocytosis and hence are not used nowadays by systemic route. **Antipyrine** is used as **drops for ear inflammation and pain**.
- **Apazone,** etodolac and aspirin have uricosuric effect.

Recent Advances

NSAIDs have been recently seen to have protective effect in colon cancer and Alzheimer's disease.

Selective COX-II Inhibitors

Selective COX-II inhibitors were synthesized to avoid the GIT side effects associated with the nonselective class. However, recent post marketing trials have shown risk of MI and stroke with these drugs and some have been banned. Thus, these drugs are not used as first line.

- **Lumiracoxib** > **etoricoxib** is the longest acting, whereas **valdecoxib** is the shortest acting selective COX-II inhibitor.
- **Lumiracoxib** > **etoricoxib** are most selective COX-II inhibitors whereas **celecoxib** is the least selective COX-II inhibitors.
- Etoricoxib and lumiracoxib have fastest absorption in this class.

Classification of NSAIDs

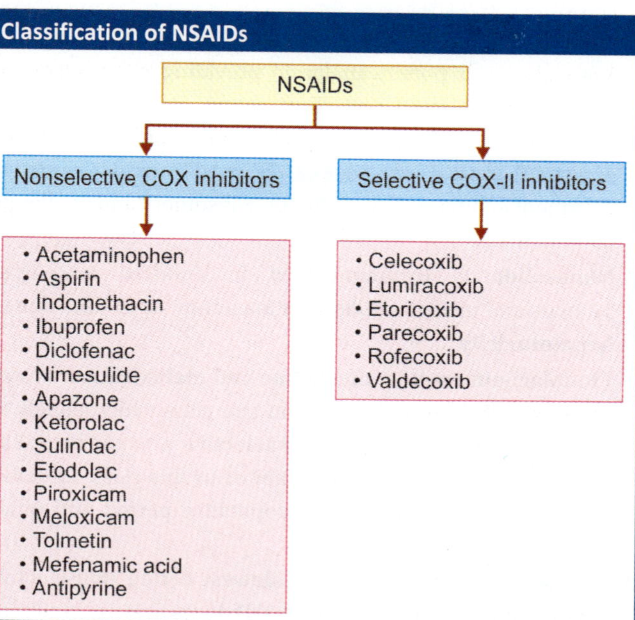

- **Lumiracoxib** is most acidic and hence is maximum concentrated at the site of inflammation. **Celecoxib** is most lipid soluble and hence easily crosses the blood brain barrier.
- **Lumiracoxib** is a derivative of **diclofenac**, has been banned due to **hepatotoxicity**. **Rofecoxib and valdecoxib** have been banned due to risk of **MI**.
- Parecoxib is a water-soluble derivative of valdecoxib used as a postoperative analgesic.
- Celecoxib, valdecoxib and parecoxib have sulfonamide group and hence can cause hypersensitivity.

Side Effects of NSAIDs

- GIT side effects like **nausea and vomiting are the most common side effects** of NSAIDs. Peptic ulcer disease can be seen, for which PPIs and misoprostol is used for treatment.
- All NSAIDs except low dose aspirin increase the risk of **adverse cardiovascular events like MI on long-term therapy**. This is due to inhibition of antiatherogenic and antithrombotic effects of prostaglandins.
- NSAIDs induce retention of salt and water and hence can cause **edema by increasing hydrostatic pressure.**
- Long-term use of NSAIDs can cause **analgesic nephropathy characterized by papillary necrosis.**

NSAID Induced Renal Papillary Necrosis

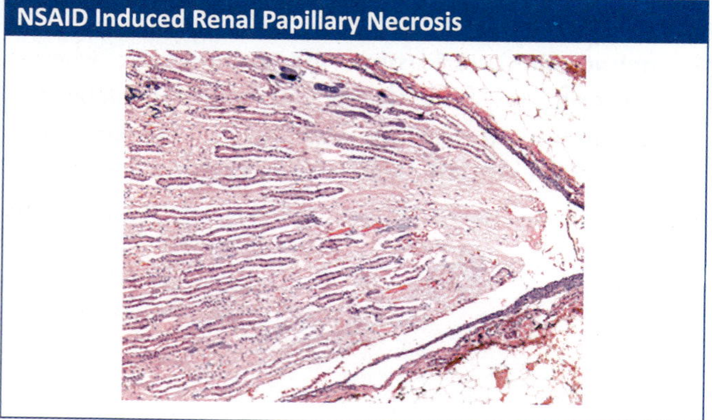

- **Reye's syndrome** characterized by encephalopathy and liver dysfunction is seen with **aspirin** if used in children with viral fever. Hence, all salicylates are contraindicated in children with viral fever.
- Hypersensitivity causing angioedema and **urticaria** is commonly seen.
- These are most common cause of drug poisoning in adults.

Drug Interactions of NSAIDs

- NSAIDs if used along with ACE inhibitors can precipitate acute renal failure, as by inhibiting prostaglandin synthesis NSAIDs prevent afferent arteriole dilation and ACE inhibitors cause efferent arteriole dilation in glomerulus; this leads to a significant decrease in GFR.
- For same reason NSAIDs can decrease the effect of diuretics.
- NSAIDs usually decrease lithium clearance and toxicity, except sulindac which decreases plasma lithium levels.
- NSAIDs also **inhibit antihypertensive effect by inhibiting prostaglandin-mediated vasodilation**.

Recent Advances

Dual LOX and XOX Inhibitors: Licofelone and tepoxalin are drugs of this class under trial as anti-inflammatory drugs. The GIT side effects of this class are minimal as compared to other NSAIDs.

GOUT

Gout is an inflammatory disorder of joints caused by deposition of urate crystals. The management of gout consists of treatment of an acute attack and prophylactic treatment to prevent further attacks.

Acute Gout

NSAIDs

NSAIDs are the drug of choice for the treatment of an acute attack of gout, the preferred agent being indomethacin. **Steroids** can also be used in acute gout in NSAID resistant cases. Aspirin at low doses inhibits uric acid excretion and hence is not used in gout (at high doses aspirin has uricosuric action).

Colchicine

- **Colchicine** is an alkaloid derived from **autumn crocus**. It inhibits adhesion of neutrophils to endothelium of blood vessels and their **migration** into joints by **inhibiting tubulin** required for their movement. Apart from that it also **inhibits phagocytosis and release of chemotactic factors** like IL-1 and leukotriene B_4 from neutrophils.
- It is FDA approved for treatment of an **acute attack of gout** and though not approved by FDA still used for **prevention of acute gout** while initiating hypouricemic drugs like allopurinol.
- Other uses are for prophylaxis of **Mediterranean fever and amyloidosis**.
- GIT-related side effects like **nausea, vomiting and diarrhea are most common**. Other side effects seen are bone marrow suppression, alopecia and rhabdomyolysis.

Chronic Gout

The aim of treatment in chronic gout is to decrease uric acid levels in the body to prevent an acute attack of gout. This can be achieved by inhibiting synthesis of uric acid by xanthine oxidase inhibitors, increasing excretion of uric acid by uricosuric drugs or by metabolism of uric acid by enzymes.

Xanthine Oxidase Inhibitors

Xanthine oxidase is the rate limiting enzyme for uric acid synthesis from hypoxanthine and xanthine. This enzyme can be inhibited by drugs like allopurinol, oxypurinol and febuxostat.

Conceptual Box-6

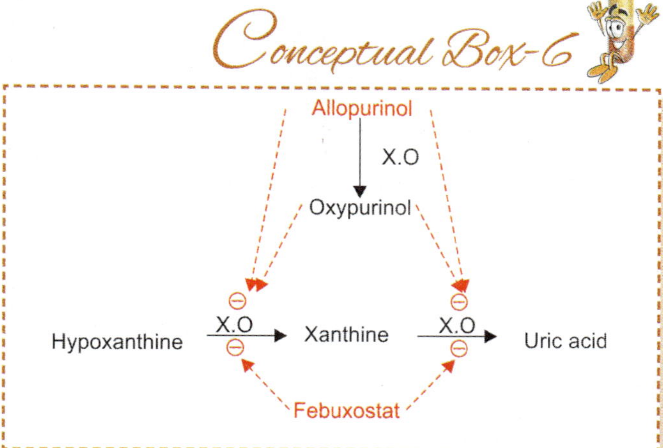

Allopurinol

- Allopurinol is metabolized by xanthine oxidase into oxypurinol (alloxanthine). Both allopurinol and oxypurinol inhibit xanthine oxidase.
- Allopurinol is the **drug of choice for the treatment of chronic gout**, however there is a **risk of an acute attack** in the beginning due to compensatory mobilization of tissue stores into plasma. Hence, colchicine or NSAIDs are given along with it at least for 6 months and then gradually stopped.
- Other uses are in hyperuricemic conditions like **tumor lysis syndrome, Lesch-Nyhan syndrome and in post-transplant patients.**

Oxypurinol

Oxypurinol is an orphan drug indicated in case of **allopurinol hypersensitivity**.

Febuxostat

Febuxostat is approved only for treatment of **chronic hyperuricemia in gout patients**.

Side Effects and Contraindication

- Most common side effect associated with allopurinol is **hypersensitivity**. It can also cause orotic aciduria by inhibiting **orotidylate decarboxylase**.
- As these drugs can increase excretion of xanthine in urine, **xanthine stones** can be seen.
- As xanthine oxidase metabolizes 6-mercaptopurine and azathioprine, the dose of these anticancer drugs is decreased by 75% along with allopurinol.
- Allopurinol increases effect of probenecid, but probenecid decreases effect of allopurinol by increasing oxypurinol excretion.

Uricosuric Drugs

- Uric acid is reabsorbed by organic anionic transporter like URAT 1 in the renal tubule. URAT 1 is competitively inhibited by other substrates of this transporter like **probenecid, benzbromarone, losartan and sulfinpyrazone.** These are used in case of intolerance or ineffectiveness of xanthine oxidase inhibitors, underexcretion of uric acid and presence of tophi.
- These drugs increase uric acid excretion and have risk of renal stones. Hence, they should not be used in patients with renal stones and overproduction of uric acid. To prevent renal stones patients should be advised to ensure adequate water intake.
- For adequate excretion of uric acid, normal kidney function is important and hence these drugs are not effective in patients of renal failure. **Benzbromarone** is the most potent uricosuric and only uricosuric drug effective in a patient of renal failure.
- Probenecid and sulfinpyrazone can cause GIT upset and aplastic anemia. Probenecid can cause nephrotic syndrome and neurotoxicity as well. Benzbromarone is a hepatotoxic drug.

Recent Advances

Lesinurad: It inhibits URAT-1 and OAT-4 transporter in kidney, which produces uricosuric effect. It is approved for treatment of gout in combination with allopurinol or febuxostat. It causes renal failure and stones especially if used as monotherapy.

Uricase Analogs

- Uricase is an enzyme that metabolizes uric acid in birds. Analogs of uricase like **rasburicase and pegloticase** have been synthesized for use in humans by genetic engineering. These drugs metabolize **uric acid into water soluble compound allantoin**, easily excreted by kidney.
- **Rasburicase** is used in pediatric hematological malignancies to prevent hyperuricemia due to **tumor lysis syndrome** following chemotherapy as an alternative to allopurinol.
- **Pegloticase** is used for treatment of chronic gout refractory to allopurinol. It can also precipitate acute gout like allopurinol.
- Side effects like hypersensitivity, hemolysis in G6PD deficiency and methemoglobinemia can be seen.

Classification of Drugs Used in Gout

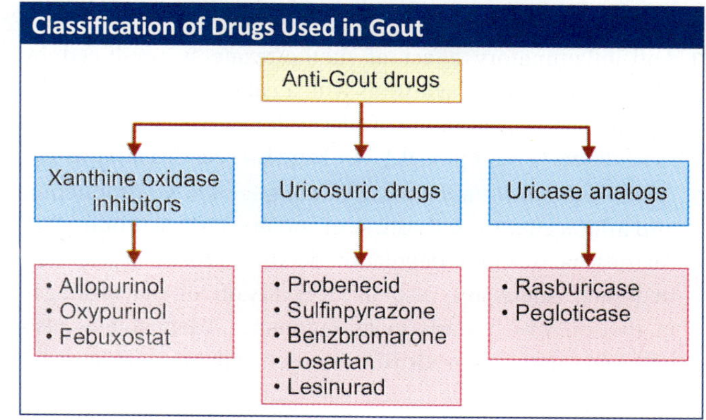

RHEUMATOID ARTHRITIS

- Rheumatoid arthritis (RA) is an autoimmune inflammation of joints where TNF and IL play a major role. There is progressive joint deformation along with signs of inflammation and pain.
- **NSAIDs** and **steroids** can be used to control acute flare of rheumatoid arthritis, whereas **disease modifying antirheumatoid drugs (DMARDs)** are the mainstay of therapy to retard the disease.
- Systemic steroids like prednisolone are used as bridge for rapid control of disease until DMARD effect kicks in. Intraarticular triamcinolone can be used for maximum of four times a year if few joints are involved.
- Drugs like gold, penicillamine and minocycline are rarely used nowadays.

DMARDs

Conventional DMARDs	Biological DMARDs	Targeted DMARDs
Methotrexate **Hydroxychloroquine** **Sulfasalazine** **Leflunomide** **Immunomodulators** • Azathioprine • Cyclosporine • Mycophenolate mofetil	**TNF alpha inhibitors** • Infliximab • Etanercept • Adalimumab • Golimumab • Certolizumab **Abatacept** **Rituximab** **Anakinra** **IL-6 inhibitors** • Tocilizumab • Sarilumab	**JAK inhibitors** • Tofacitinib • Baricitinib

Conventional DMARDs

The effect of conventional drugs is seen only after 6–12 weeks of drug use and hence steroids can be given along to bridge this period.

Methotrexate

- Methotrexate is the **drug of choice** for treatment of rheumatoid arthritis. It is also known as **anchor drug** being the most important one in the regimens as given in clinical box.
- Hepatotoxicity and liver cirrhosis are the major concern, which increases in chronic alcoholics, chronic hepatitis, CKD, obesity and diabetes mellitus. Thus, LFT should be monitored every **3 months**.
- Anti-inflammatory effect of methotrexate is produced by inhibition of purine synthesis which causes selective toxicity to lymphocytes, inhibition of effect produced by inflammatory modulators (TNF alpha, IL1, IL 6) and **increase in adenosine**.
- Adenosine causes a decrease in complement C_2 production and inhibits neutrophil adhesion and free radical production. All these factors downregulation decreases tissue destruction in joints. Adenosine also induces fusion of macrophages in tissues, which leads to granulomata. Adenosine is also believed to cause **hepatic fibrosis** seen with methotrexate.

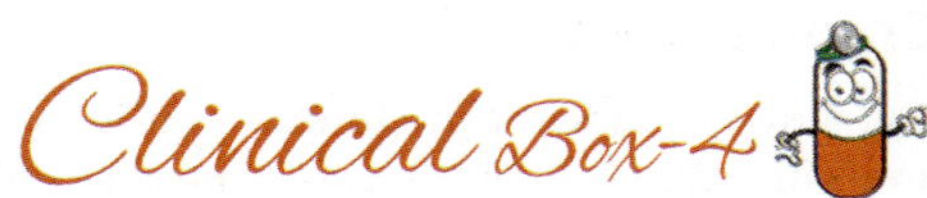
Clinical Box-4

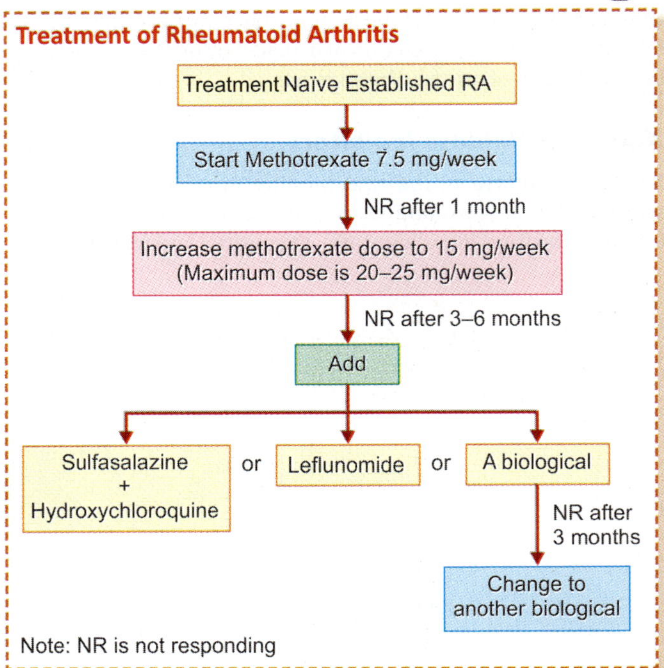
Treatment of Rheumatoid Arthritis
Treatment Naïve Established RA
Start Methotrexate 7.5 mg/week
NR after 1 month
Increase methotrexate dose to 15 mg/week (Maximum dose is 20–25 mg/week)
NR after 3–6 months
Add
Sulfasalazine + Hydroxychloroquine
or
Leflunomide
or
A biological
NR after 3 months
Change to another biological
Note: NR is not responding

Hydroxychloroquine

- Hydroxychloroquine produces anti-inflammatory effect by downregulating the effect of T lymphocytes, lysosomal stabilization and free radical scavenging effect.
- It is not a very effective drug and hence can be used as a monotherapy only in mild cases. In moderate to severe cases it is used in combination with methotrexate and sulfasalazine. It does not delay the radiological progression of disease. The standard dose is 200 to 400 mg/day.
- It is highly distributed into melanin predominant tissues like retina and hence pigmentary retinitis can be seen as a side effect. Retinitis is dose dependent and hence it should not be used at doses more than 5 mg/kg/day. Ophthalmological examination should be done once yearly to find out retinal changes.

Sulfasalazine

- Sulfasalazine is metabolized into sulfapyridine and 5 ASA.
- Sulfapyridine is absorbed into systemic circulation and then it downregulates the effect of both T and B lymphocytes, which is primarily responsible for effect in rheumatoid arthritis. It is not a very effective drug and hence can be used as a monotherapy only in mild cases. In moderate to severe cases it is used in combination with methotrexate and hydroxychloroquine. It delays the radiological progression of disease. It is started at a dose of 0.5 mg BD and then dose is gradually increased until patient responds (maximum dose is 1.5 mg BD).
- 5 ASA has anti-inflammatory effect, has poor oral absorption and hence is primarily responsible for effect in ulcerative

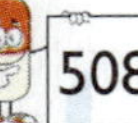

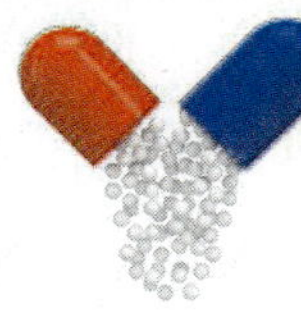

colitis. Other uses are psoriatic arthritis and ankylosing spondylitis.

- Sulfonamide related side effects like rash, bone marrow suppression, methemoglobinemia and hemolysis in G6PD deficiency can be seen.

Leflunomide

- Leflunomide inhibits pyrimidine ribonucleotide synthesis by blocking enzyme dihydroorotate dehydrogenase. This leads to arrest of lymphocyte proliferation at the G_1 phase.
- It is used along with methotrexate for cases not responding to methotrexate alone. The dose of drug is 20 mg OD.
- Side effects associated are diarrhea, bone marrow suppression, rash, alopecia, hepatotoxicity and weight loss. Since it is carcinogenic and teratogenic it is contraindicated in fertile males and females planning for conception and in pregnancy.

Immunomodulators

- Immunomodulators like azathioprine, cyclosporine and mycophenolate mofetil can be used for the treatment of rheumatoid arthritis in resistant cases.
- These drugs have been discussed in detail in the topic of immunomodulators ahead.

Biological DMARDs

Anti-TNF Drugs

- **Golimumab, certolizumab, infliximab, adalimumab** and **etanercept** are anti-TNF drugs used in rheumatoid arthritis along with methotrexate. All these drugs except infliximab have been approved to be used as monotherapy as well.
- The route of administration for all drugs is subcutaneous, whereas **infliximab and adalimumab** can also be given by **intravenous route**. Antibodies against these drugs can be produced by patient body and that can decrease efficacy. Methotrexate decreases production of these antibodies.
- Apart from rheumatoid arthritis these drugs are also used for the treatment of inflammatory bowel disease, ankylosing spondylitis, plaque, psoriasis and psoriatic arthritis.
- Side effects common to this group are **infections, SLE (rare), GIT ulceration and perforation,** and **secondary neoplasms like lymphoma and melanoma**. Since these drugs can cause reactivation of tuberculosis and hepatitis B, screening for latent TB and hepatitis B should be done before starting drug.
- These are absolutely contraindicated in **severe (class III/IV) heart failure and hepatitis B infection**.

Mnemonics

Anti-TNF Drugs

GL : GoLImumab
A : Adalimumab
C : Certolizumab
I : Infliximab
ER : EtaneRcept

Abatacept

- **Abatacept** is a novel drug produced by fusion of F_c fragment of IgG and CTLA4. It binds to CD 80/86 in T lymphocytes and prevents binding of CD28, that is required for T lymphocyte activation.
- It can be used as monotherapy or in cases resistant to methotrexate or anti-TNF drugs.
- Downregulating immune system increases risk of infection and hence it should not be combined with other biological DMARDs like anti-TNF drugs.
- Since these drugs also can cause reactivation of tuberculosis and hepatitis B, screening for latent TB and hepatitis B should be done before starting drug.
- **Belatacept** is another drug in this class used as an immunomodulator in graft rejection and hence discussed in the topic of immunomodulators.

Rituximab

- Rituximab is an anti-CD-20 monoclonal antibody which produced anti-inflammatory effect by depleting B lymphocytes.
- It is used along with methotrexate for treatment of cases resistant to TNF alpha inhibitors. It is more effective in seropositive cases.
- Side effects associated are infections, rash and progressive multifocal leukoencephalopathy. Reactivation of hepatitis B is seen but not TB.

IL-6 Inhibitors

- Tocilizumab and Sarilumab are anti-IL-6 monoclonal antibodies approved for the treatment of rheumatoid arthritis as monotherapy or with methotrexate in resistant cases. Tocilizumab is also used for the treatment of juvenile idiopathic arthritis (Still's disease).
- The route of administration is intravenous and subcutaneous.
- These drugs can cause infection, bone marrow suppression, GIT perforation and increase LDL. Both should not be combined with other biologicals like TNF alpha inhibitors.

Anakinra

- Anakinra is an IL-1 inhibitor with least efficacy among the biological DMARDS. Hence, it is not used commonly nowadays. It can cause infections and hence should not be combined with anti TNF drugs.
- It has been discussed in detail in the topic of immunomodulators.

Targeted DMARDs

Janus Kinase Inhibitors

- **Tofacitinib is an oral JAK 1 and 3 inhibitor**, currently approved for treatment of **rheumatoid arthritis** (2012), **psoriatic arthritis** (2017) and **ulcerative colitis** (2018).
- It is approved for treatment of moderate to severe rheumatoid arthritis and psoriatic arthritis in a patient not responding to or intolerant to methotrexate. It is approved for induction and maintenance of moderate to severe ulcerative colitis. It was studied for use in **Crohn's disease, but it was found ineffective**.

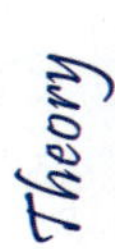

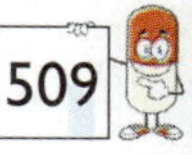

- JAK is an intracellular kinase which is activated by the cytokines acting on the cytokine receptors present on cell membrane. Activated JAK stimulates STAT which increases transcription factors required for hematopoiesis and immune cell function.
- Thus, inhibition of JAK downregulates this pathway and inhibits proliferation of lymphocytes as well as erythrocytes. This gives us anti-inflammatory and immunosuppressive effect as well as side effects for which it has **black box warning that it can cause severe infections and neoplasia (non-melanoma skin cancer)**. For same reason it is contraindicated with other immunosuppressive agents like azathioprine and cyclosporine as well as biologicals like anti-TNF drugs, abatacept, vedolizumab, anakinra, tocilizumab etc.
- Other associated side effects are anemia, hyperlipidemia (increased LDL, HDL, triglycerides), gastrointestinal perforation and paresthesia.

Recent Advances

Baricitinib: It is a JAK inhibitor recently approved for treatment of rheumatoid arthritis in patient not responding or intolerant to methotrexate.

Mnemonics

Disease Modifying Anti-Rheumatoid Drugs (DMARDS)

G : Golimumab, Gold compounds
E : Etanercept
T : Tofacitinib, Tocilizumab
S : Sulfasalazine
M : Methotrexate
A : Abatacept, Azathioprine
LL : Leflunomide
C : Cyclosporine
H : Hydroxychloroquine
A : Anakinra, Adalimumab
I : Infliximab
R : Rituximab

PSORIASIS

Retinoids

- Retinoids acts in psoriasis by stimulating retinoic acid receptor (RAR) which produces anti-inflammatory and antiproliferative effects.
- **Acitretin** is the drug of choice for the treatment of **pustular psoriasis** and it is synergistic with ultraviolet therapy and hence can be used as add on to ultraviolet therapy in mild to moderate plaque psoriasis. Other retinoids used in psoriasis are adapalene and tazarotene.
- Retinoids mentioned above can also be used for the treatment of acne and photoaging.
- Retinoids like alitretinoin and bexarotene act stimulating retinoid x receptor (RXR), which produces apoptotic effect and hence these are used topically for the treatment of Kaposi sarcoma and cutaneous T cell lymphoma respectively.
- These are teratogenic and hence should not be given in pregnancy.

Topical Steroids

- In mild cases of **plaque psoriasis** topical steroids are used along with topical vitamin D like calcipotriene and calcitriol. Tacrolimus ointment can also be used for mild cases. In a mild case less than 10%, in moderate 10–30% and in severe more than 30% body surface area is involved.
- Systemic steroids are never used for the treatment of flares of psoriasis.

Ultraviolet Therapy

- In moderate to severe cases of plaque psoriasis narrow band ultra violet B (NB-UVB) light therapy is the treatment of choice. In case patients does not respond then psoralen and ultraviolet A (PUVA) light therapy can be used.
- Ultraviolet light has immunosuppressive effect which is responsible for its clinical effect in psoriasis as well as for grave side effects like skin cancer (melanoma and nonmelanoma).
- It should not be used in patients on cyclosporine, as it is an immunosuppressant and the neoplastic effect of ultraviolet light will increase.

Other Drugs

- Systemic drugs are used in case of severe disease.
- Methotrexate is the drug of choice for the treatment of **erythrodermic psoriasis** and **psoriatic arthritis**. Methotrexate causes **keratinocyte apoptosis** and hence is beneficial in resistant psoriasis.
- Cyclosporine is used for treatment of severe and resistant cases.
- **TNF-alpha inhibitors** are used in pustular and moderate to severe chronic plaque psoriasis and are drug of choice in **methotrexate resistant psoriatic arthritis**. Infliximab is the most effective drug in this class and is used in pustular or erythrodermic flares.
- **Alefacept** prevents activation of T lymphocytes, responsible for psoriasis and hence is indicated in mild to moderate plaque psoriasis. It is discussed in detail in the topic of immunomodulators ahead.

Recent Advances

New drugs for treatment of moderate to severe plaque psoriasis

Ustekinumab	Anti-IL 12/23 monoclonal antibodies
Guselkumab **Tildrakizumab**	Anti-IL 23 monoclonal antibody
Secukinumab **Ixekizumab**	Anti-IL 17 antibodies
Brodalumab	Anti-IL-17 receptor antibody
Apremilast	PDE-4 inhibitor

Clinical Box-5

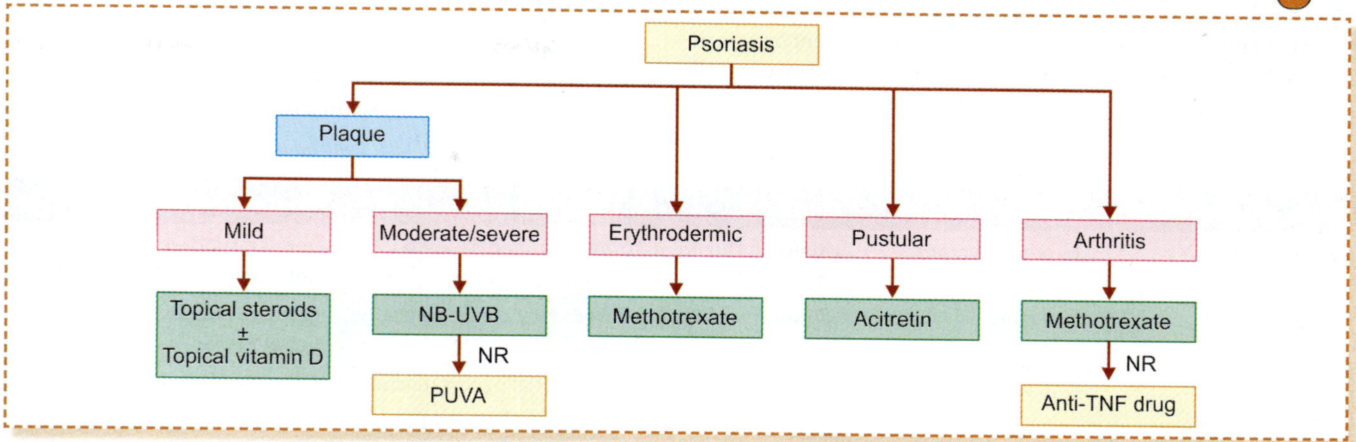

IMMUNOMODULATORS

PATHOPHYSIOLOGY OF GRAFT REJECTION

- When a solid organ is transplanted for example kidney, a foreign protein present in the organ for the recipient's body is recognized by the MHC receptors and brought out and presented to the local immune cells.
- The local immune cells produce inflammatory mediators like **IL-1, IL-6 and TNF-**α, which stimulate a phosphatase calcineurin present in the CD-4 cells of central lymphoid organs like lymph node and spleen.
- Calcineurin being a phosphatase, dephosphorylates cytoplasmic nuclear factor for activation of T lymphocytes ($NFAT_C$), which can enter into the nucleus and combines with $NFAT_N$ and increases transcription actor for synthesis of IL-2.
- IL-2 acts on the IL-2 receptors present in resting CD-8 cells and pushes it into cell cycle of proliferation; G_1-S phase being mediated by a protein called as m-tor.
- These CD-8 lymphocytes once released into systemic circulation attack the foreign protein in the kidney and cause inflammatory damage leading to graft rejection. This process can be inhibited by various drugs at various levels as given in the conceptual box 7.

Conceptual Box-7

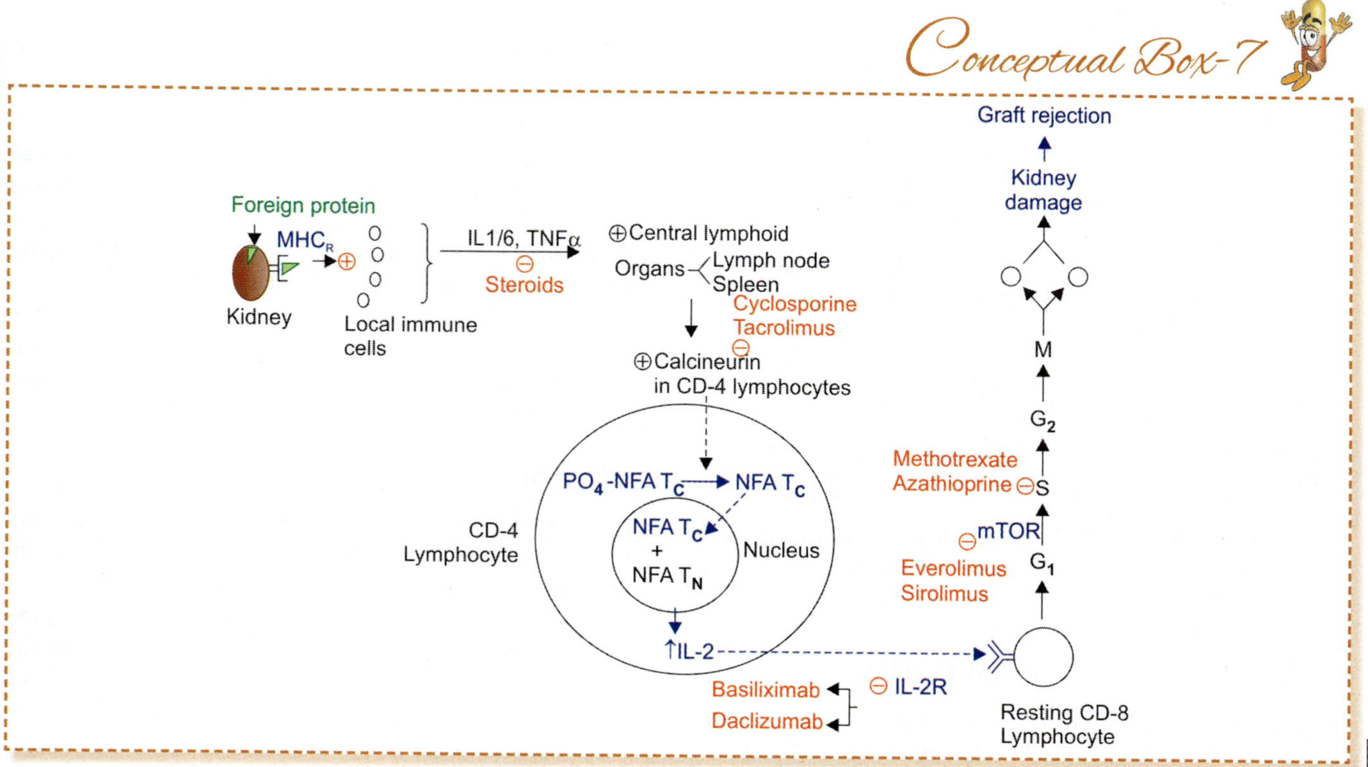

GVHD AND GRAFT REJECTION

GVHD

- Allogenic bone marrow transplantation can cause **GVHD** in which the donor T lymphocytes attack the recipient organs. It can be acute or chronic (>100 days) and responds well to all immunosuppressive drugs. All immunosuppressive drugs can be used for treatment or prophylaxis.
- Lifelong use of immunosuppressive drugs is not required, and patient may discontinue drugs after GVHD resolves.

Graft Rejection

- **Graft rejection** can be of four types as given in the table below. Immunosuppressive drugs are active against acute and chronic rejection but inactive against hyperacute and accelerated rejection.

Type of graft rejection	Time to rejection	Cause	Treatment
Hyperacute	Minutes to hours	**Humoral**: Due to preformed antibodies to donor antigens like anti blood group antibodies	Immunosuppressive drugs are not effective
Accelerated	Few days	**Humoral and cell mediated**: Previous sensitization to donor antigen	Immunosuppressive drugs are not effective
Acute	One week to months	**Cell mediated**: Development of allogenic reaction to donor antigen	All immunosuppressive drugs can be used
Chronic	Months to years	**Humoral and cell mediated**: Disturbance of host graft tolerance	All immunosuppressive drugs can be used

- In organ transplantation immunosuppressive drugs are used either for prophylaxis or treatment of graft rejection. In prophylaxis all immunosuppressive drugs can be used but in treatment only those drugs which are active against activated T cells can be used.
- **Prophylaxis** of graft rejection can be done by induction or maintenance therapy.
  - **Induction therapy** is done with biological agents like antithymocyte globulin, antilymphocyte globulin, alemtuzumab, muromonab or basiliximab. It is given to patients with high risk of rejection.
  - **Maintenance therapy** is given to all patients. All immunosuppressive drugs can be used, and multiple drugs are combined with different mechanisms of action. A regimen is made by combining drugs targeting inactive T lymphocytes with different mechanisms (Calcineurin inhibitors + yycophenolate mofetil) and a drug targeting active T lymphocytes (steroids). Lifelong use of immunosuppressive drugs is required to prevent graft rejection.
- **Treatment** of an established case of graft rejection can be done by drugs active against active T lymphocyte like steroids, muromonab, alemtuzumab and anti-lymphocyte globulins.

GLUCOCORTICOIDS

- Glucocorticoids act by downregulating the inflammatory mediators and increasing apoptosis and redistribution of lymphocytes.
- Steroids can be used for both prophylaxis and treatment of graft rejection and GVHD. They are also used to prevent first dose cytokine storm seen with muromunab.

CALCINEURIN INHIBITORS

- **Tacrolimus** binds to FKBP-12 (FK Binding Protein-12) and **cyclosporine** to cyclophilin, and then these complexes inhibit phosphatase called as calcineurin. This decreases the transcription factors for synthesis of **interleukin 2.** Both drugs can be given by oral or intravenous route.
- Both are metabolized by CYP450 enzymes and hence drug interactions are commonly seen.
- Side effects common to both these drugs are **nephrotoxicity, hyperkalemia, hypertension, hepatotoxicity, neurotoxicity (seizures), hyperglycemia, diabetes mellitus** and **neoplasia (Kaposi sarcoma and melanoma).** Cyclosporine specific side effects are **hirsutism, hyperplasia of gums, hyperlipidemia, hyperuricemia.**

Tacrolimus

- **Tacrolimus (FK-506)** is a **macrolide antibiotic** derived from bacteria Streptomyces tsukubaensis.
- It is used as a first-line drug for prophylaxis of GVHD and graft rejection. It is significantly more potent than cyclosporine and hence used as a rescue therapy for patients not responding to cyclosporine. Topical tacrolimus is used in atopic dermatitis, lichen planus, vitiligo, allergic dermatitis and rosacea.
- Since cyclosporine is also nephrotoxic, it should be avoided with tacrolimus except in rescue therapy and if patient is changed from cyclosporine to tacrolimus then a 24-hour gap is mandatory.

Cyclosporine

- Cyclosporine is also used as a first-line drug for prophylaxis of GVHD and graft rejection. It is drug of choice for the treatment of **steroid resistant nephrotic syndrome**.
- Other systemic uses are in **ulcerative colitis**, rheumatoid arthritis, myasthenia gravis, uveitis and Beçhet's syndrome. Topical cyclosporine is used in ocular GVHD, atopic dermatitis, alopecia areata, bullous pemphigoid, lichen planus, pyoderma gangrenosum and psoriasis.

IL-2 RECEPTOR (CD-25) INHIBITOR

- Monoclonal antibodies like **daclizumab** and **basiliximab** act by inhibiting IL-2 receptors in the CD-8 cells. Basiliximab is more potent but daclizumab is longer acting.
- These are approved for prevention of **acute organ rejection** and used along with cyclosporine and steroids. Daclizumab is costlier and hence used only for treatment of multiple sclerosis now a days.

M-TOR INHIBITORS

- **Everolimus, temsirolimus** and **sirolimus (rapamycin)** bind to FKBP-12 and the complex inhibits m-tor protein. This leads to inhibition of proliferation of CD-8 cells at G_1-S phase. They inhibit proliferation of B lymphocytes and immunoglobulin production also.
- M-tor inhibitors and calcineurin inhibitors are metabolized by CYP450 enzymes and hence can competitively inhibit each other's metabolism and increase side effect. Hence, if combined, the plasma levels of the drugs need monitoring.
- Side effects associated are **hypokalemia, hyperlipidemia, lymphocele, mouth ulcer, hemolytic uremic syndrome and myelosuppression (thrombocytopenia).**
- These drugs inhibit proliferation of other cells as well and hence have anticancer effect. Everolimus and temsirolimus are used as anticancer drugs. Sirolimus is the immunomodulator of choice in patients with history of neoplasia.
- Sirolimus and everolimus are used by oral route, whereas temsirolimus is used by intravenous route.

Sirolimus (Rapamycin)

Sirolimus is used along with first-line drugs, i.e. calcineurin inhibitors for prophylaxis of GVHD and graft rejection. Sirolimus is also used for **coating of cardiac stents.** It is used along with cyclosporine for treatment of **uveoretinitis.**

Temsirolimus

It is used for treatment of renal cell cancer.

Everolimus

Like sirolimus everolimus can also be used along with calcineurin inhibitors for prophylaxis of GVHD and graft rejection. It is also used for treatment of **renal angiomyolipoma, renal cell cancer, astrocytoma, pancreatic cancer and drug resistant ER positive breast cancer.**

AZATHIOPRINE

- **Azathioprine is a prodrug of anticancer drug 6-mercaptopurine**. It acts by inhibiting CD-8 cells proliferation at the "S" phase.
- It is used as add on drug to calcineurin inhibitors for prophylaxis of GVHD and graft rejection primarily in renal transplant. It is drug of choice for **steroid-dependent ulcerative colitis** and other uses are myasthenia gravis, multiple sclerosis, SLE associated glomerulonephritis, nephrotic syndrome and rheumatoid arthritis.
- **Bone marrow suppression and hepatotoxicity like grave side effects are associated with azathioprine.** Azathioprine induced hepatotoxicity is associated with **increased alkaline phosphatase**.
- **TPMT (Thiopurine Methyl Transferase)** metabolizes azathioprine and hence a decreased TPMT in patients body increases risk of toxicity.

ANTICANCER DRUGS

- Anticancer drugs can inhibit proliferation of lymphocytes and hence have immunomodulatory action.
- **Methotrexate** inhibits lymphocyte proliferation at "S" phase. It is used for prophylaxis of GVHD and also used for the treatment of inflammatory and autoimmune disorders like rheumatoid arthritis, psoriasis, multiple sclerosis.
- **Cyclophosphamide** inhibits lymphocyte proliferation in all phases. It is used for treatment of autoimmune and inflammatory disorders like nephrotic syndrome, Wegener's granulomatosis, myasthenia gravis, rheumatoid arthritis, SLE and multiple sclerosis.
- **Dactinomycin** can be used to prevent rejection in renal transplant patients.
- **Vincristine** can be used for the treatment of steroid resistant immune thrombocytopenic purpura.

ANTIBODIES

- Antibodies can be polyclonal or monoclonal. Polyclonal antibodies are produced by different clones plasma B cells and they bind to different epitopes in same antigen. Monoclonal antibodies are produced by same clone of plasma B cells and they bind to a particular epitope in an antigen.
- **Monoclonal antibodies** have been discussed in detail in the topic of anticancer drugs and hence the discussion here is limited to polyclonal antibodies.
- **Polyclonal antibodies** in clinical use are antithymocyte globulins, antilymphocyte globulins, intravenous immunoglobulins (IVIG), Rho D immune globulin and hyperimmune immunoglobulins.
- **Antithymocyte** and **antilymphocyte globulins** are produced by injection of human thymocytes and lymphocytes into animals. The antibodies generated in the animals are then collected and purified. When injected they bind to different antigens in lymphocytes and block their activation. Both can be used for prophylaxis and treatment of graft rejection.
- **Intravenous immunoglobulins (IVIG)** is prepared from serum of 1000–1500 donors. IVIG is drug of choice for treatment of Kawasaki disease, Guillain-Barre syndrome and myasthenic crisis. It can also be used in SLE and idiopathic thrombocytopenic purpura (ITP).
- **Rho D immune globulin** are antibodies against the Rho D antigen. It is given to Rh negative mother which gave birth to Rh positive baby. The Rho D antigens will be neutralized and thus prevent erythroblastosis fetalis in the next pregnancy.
- **Hyperimmune globulins** are very high titer antibodies usually produced against viruses, toxins and drugs. Some examples are digiband against digoxin, rabies hyperimmune

globulin, tetanus hyperimmune globulin and snake/scorpion antivenom.

MYCOPHENOLATE MOFETIL (MMF)

- **Mycophenolate mofetil is a prodrug, converted into mycophenolic acid**. Mycophenolic acid inhibits de novo purine synthesis by inhibiting **inosine monophosphate (IMP) dehydrogenase**. Since lymphocytes do not have salvage pathway, there is selective lymphocyte death.
- It is used by oral or intravenous route as a first-line drug for prophylaxis of graft rejection in cardiac and bone marrow transplant patients. For other cases it is used in graft rejection resistant to calcineurin inhibitors or in case there is intolerance to calcineurin inhibitors. Its other uses are in lupus nephritis, steroid resistant nephrotic syndrome, myasthenia gravis, rheumatoid arthritis and inflammatory bowel disease.
- In a regimen it can be combined with steroids, calcineurin inhibitors and sirolimus, but never with azathioprine.
- Most common side effect is **GIT upset** (nausea, vomiting, diarrhea) followed by neutropenia and hypertension.

MUROMONAB

- **Muromonab** is an **anti-CD-3 monoclonal antibody** used for treatment of acute graft rejection. Rebound rejection after drug stoppage has been seen.
- It can cause cytokine release syndrome characterized by fever, chills, nausea, myalgia, etc.

LEFLUNOMIDE

- **Leflunomide** inhibits pyrimidine ribonucleotide synthesis by blocking enzyme **dihydroorotate dehydrogenase**. This leads to arrest of lymphocyte proliferation at the G1 phase.
- It can be used for prophylaxis of GVHD as add on drug and is also used in rheumatoid arthritis.
- Side effects associated are diarrhea, **bone marrow suppression, rash**, alopecia, **hepatotoxicity** and weight loss. Since it is **carcinogenic** and **teratogenic** it is contraindicated in fertile males and females planning for conception.
- **Teriflunomide** is a metabolite of leflunomide and is used for treatment of multiple sclerosis.

INHIBITORS OF T CELL ACTIVATION

Belatacept

- CD 80/86 present in antigen presenting cells bind to CD 28 in T lymphocytes and activate their proliferation and production of inflammatory mediators. CTLA4 (Cytotoxic T Lymphocyte associated Antigen 4) in T lymphocytes bind to CD 80/86 in antigen presenting cells and prevent this activation of T lymphocytes.
- **Belatacept** is a novel drug produced by fusion of Fc fragment of IgG and CTLA4. It binds to CD 80/86 in T lymphocytes and prevents binding of CD28, that is required for T lymphocyte activation. It is used by **intravenous route** as a substitute for calcineurin inhibitors to prevent rejection in renal transplant patients. It is used in a regimen along with basiliximab, mycophenolate mofetil and steroids. In Epstein-Barr virus seronegative patients, it increases post-transplant lymphoproliferative disorders.
- **Abatacept** is another drug in this class used for the treatment of rheumatoid arthritis.
- **Ipilimumab** is anti-CTLA 4 monoclonal antibody. By inhibiting CTLA 4, it facilitates binding of CD 28 to CD 80/86 and this activates T lymphocytes, which kill the melanoma cells. Hence, ipilimumab is approved for treatment of malignant melanoma.

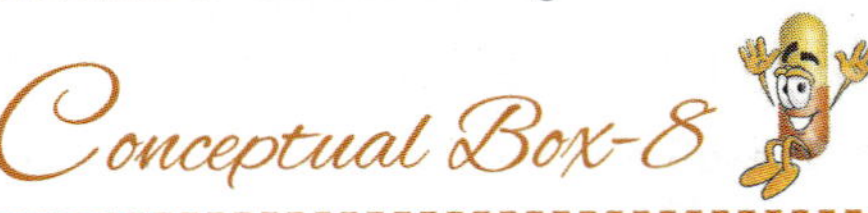

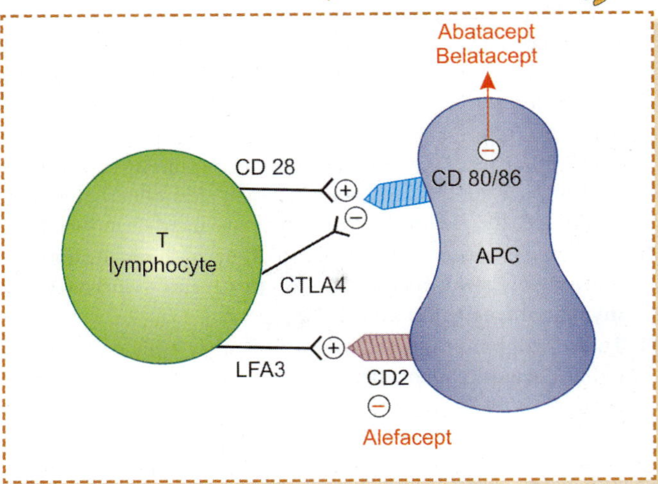

Alefacept

- Lymphocyte Function associated Antigen 3 (LFA 3) in antigen presenting cells binds to CD 2 receptors present in T lymphocytes and activate their proliferation and production of inflammatory mediators.
- Alefacept is produced by fusion of LFA 3 and Ig G1, which binds to and blocks CD 2 mediated T ell activation. It is approved for treatment of psoriasis and under trial for treatment of resistant graft rejection.

ALEMTUZUMAB

- Alemtuzumab is anti CD-52 monoclonal antibody which binds to and causes lysis of lymphocytes, macrophages and granulocytes.
- It is used for prevention of graft rejection as an induction agent and it decreases dose of steroid required. It is also reserved for treatment of resistant graft rejection. Other clinical uses are in chronic lymphocytic leukemia and multiple sclerosis.
- Prolonged neutropenia (>1 year) and autoimmune hemolytic anemia can be seen with alemtuzumab.

MISCELLANEOUS DRUGS

Thalidomide

- **Thalidomide** was first introduced as a **sedative and hypnotic** agent but later found to have antiemetic effect and was prescribed for **morning sickness**. However, due to an acute surge in the incidence of **phocomelia, i.e. limb bud formation defect**, this drug was withdrawn from the market.

Mnemonics

Uses	Side Effects
Catch : CLL, Crowe Fukase syndrome **P :** Pancreatic cancer, Pyoderma gangrenosum **R :** Renal cell cancer **O :** Oro-ocular-genital syndrome (Behçet's disease) **G :** GVHD **R :** cRohn's disease **A :** AIDS related apthous ulcer and wasting **M :** Multiple myeloma, Melanoma **M :** Myelodysplasia **E :** ENL **S :** Sarcoidosis	In **S :** Sedation **PO :** PhOcomelia, Peripheral neuropathy **R :** Rash **T :** Thrombosis **Channel :** Constipatin **Note:** Sedation and constipation are most common side effect.

- This drug has been reintroduced due to miscellaneous effects like **immunomodulatory, anti-inflammatory, antiangiogenic and antineoplastic effects.**
- **Lenalidomide** is a recent thalidomide analog that is less toxic and more preferred. It is a first-line drug currently for treatment of multiple myeloma and transfusion dependent anemia in myelodysplasia. It can cause **thrombosis** and the **risk is higher with steroids** when used in multiple myeloma.
- Pomalidomide is also a thalidomide analog approved for treatment of multip0le myeloma.

Elapegademase

- **Elapegademase** is recombinant adenosine deaminase enzyme approved for treatment of adenosine deaminase severe combined immunodeficiency syndrome (ADA-SCID). ADA-SCD is an immunodeficiency syndrome characterized by decreased adenosine deaminase.
- Elapegademase metabolizes adenosine and deoxyadenosine nucleotides which are toxic to lymphocytes and thus increases the lymphocyte count.

Cytokines

- Cytokines like interferons, TNF α, interleukins, G-CSF and GM-CSF can also have immunomodulatory effect and hence have diverse clinical uses in autoimmune, inflammatory and neoplastic disorders. These drugs have short half-lives of few minutes but become long-acting by subcutaneous route due to slow release.
- **Interferon** α is used for treatment if hepatitis (B, C and D), papilloma virus, acyclovir resistant herpes, Kaposi sarcoma, hairy cell leukemia and HIV associated thrombocytopenia, malignant melanoma and resistant CML. **Interferon** β is used for treatment if remitting type of multiple sclerosis and **interferon** γ is used for treatment of chronic granulomatous disease.

Mnemonics

Uses of Interferon α

- **C** : CML
- **H** : Hairy cell leukemia, HIV associated thrombocytopenia, Hepatitis B, C and D
- **A** : Acyclovir resistant herpes
- **M** : Malignant melanoma
- **P** : Papilloma virus
- **S** : Sarcoma (Kaposi)

- **TNF** α by intraarterial route is used for the treatment of malignant melanoma and soft tissue sarcoma of limbs.
- **IL-2 analog aldesleukin** is used for treatment of malignant melanoma and renal cell carcinoma. **G-CSF** and **GM-CSF** have been covered in detail in the topic of blood.
- Anorexia, fatigue and flu like symptoms are common side effects that can be seen with cytokines.

Interleukin 1 Antagonists

- **Anakinra,** an **IL-1 antagonist** is the drug of choice for treatment of CAPS or Cryopyrin Associated Periodic Syndrome. CAPS is a genetic disorder characterized by increased interleukin 1. There are three diseases associated with CAPS, i.e. neonatal onset multisystem inflammatory disease (NOMID), Muckle Wells syndrome and familial cold autoinflammatory syndrome. It is also used in rheumatoid arthritis, Behçet's disease, gout and Still's disease.
- **Canakinumab** is an **anti-IL-1 monoclonal antibody** used for treatment of CAPS (Cryopsin Associated Periodic Syndrome) and juvenile idiopathic arthritis. **Rilonacept** is an **IL-1 antagonist** used for treatment of and gout.
- All these drugs can increase risk of infection.

Recent Advances

Canakinumab is under trial for treatment of COPD.

Levamisole

- Levamisole is an antihelminthic drug, which is also used as an immunomodulator. It stimulated antibody production as well as activates lymphocytes.
- It is used as an immunomodulator for treatment of cancer.

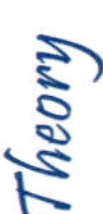

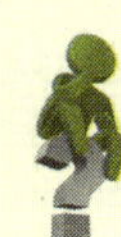

Image-based Questions

1. A patient was given an antihistaminic which caused the following changes in ECG. Which of the following drug might have caused it?

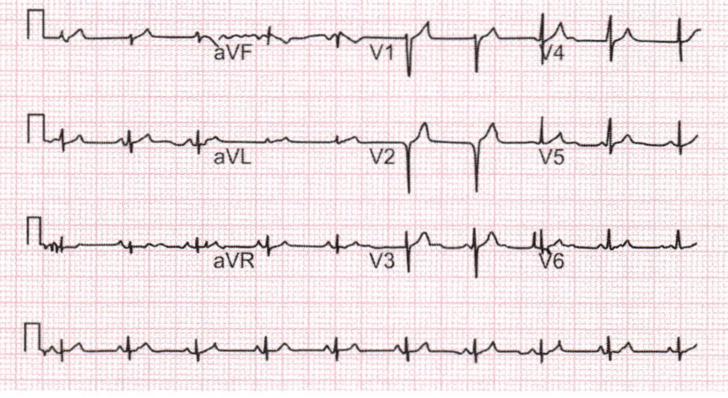

a. Astemizole
b. Fexofenadine
c. Cetirizine
d. Promethazine

2. Which of the following antimigraine drug might have caused the side effect in the picture?

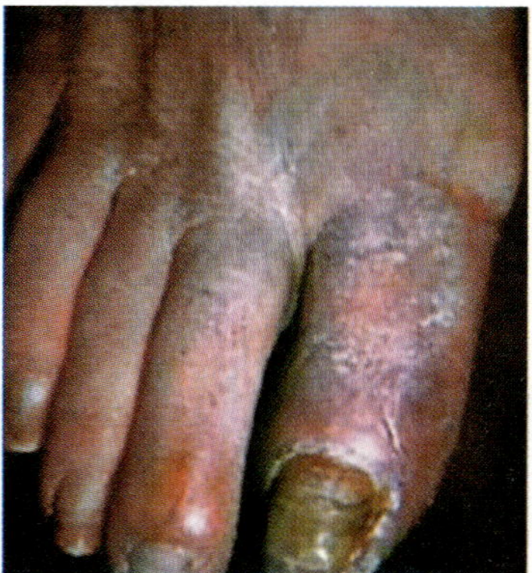

a. Sumatriptan
b. Propranolol
c. Methysergide
d. Ergotamine

3. A patient with joint pain advised for aspirate fluid analysis. The aspirate microscopy finding in given in the picture. Which is the best possible drug to prevent a further acute attack?

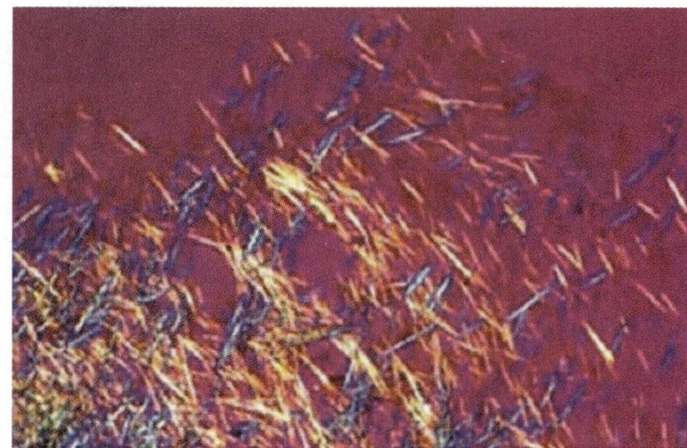

a. Rasburicase
b. Probenecid
c. Colchicine
d. Allopurinol

4. The best strategy to prevent the deformity in the picture is?

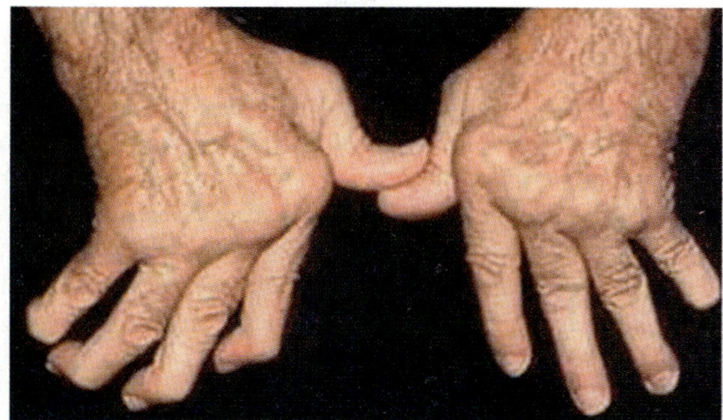

a. Methotrexate
b. Methotrexate + sulfasalazine
c. Methotrexate + penicillamine
d. Methotrexate + infliximab

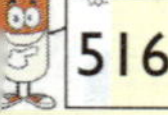

5. The teratogenic effect given in the picture is associated with?

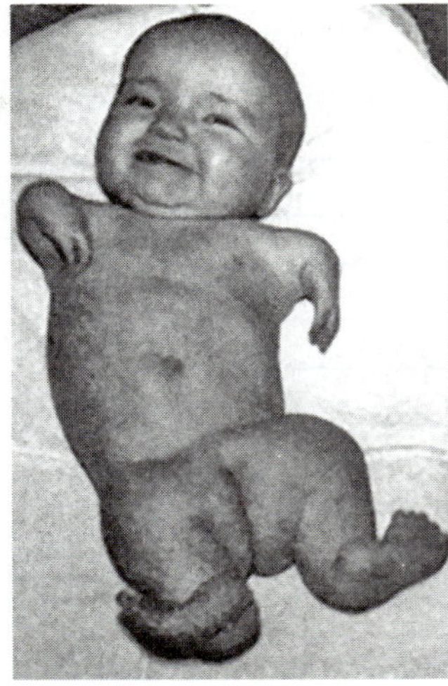

a. Lenalidomide
b. Warfarin
c. Cyclosporine
d. Thalidomide

Answers with Explanations to Image-based Questions

1. Ans. (a) Astemizole

(Ref: Katzung 12th E/P820)

- The ECG depicts QT prolongation, which can be seen with astemizole and terfenadine.

2. Ans. (d) Ergotamine

(Ref: Goodman Gilman 12th E/P347)

- Ergotamine can cause severe peripheral vasoconstriction and gangrene in organs with end arteries like fingers.

3. Ans. (d) Allopurinol

(Ref: Goodman Gilman 12th E/P996)

- The needle shaped crystals in microscopic picture is confirmatory of gout.
- The drug of choice in chronic gout to prevent an acute attack is allopurinol.

4. Ans. (d) Methotrexate + Infliximab

(Ref: Goodman Gilman 12th E/P994)

- Z deformity given in the picture is seen with rheumatoid arthritis.
- The best treatment option currently to prevent this is methotrexate plus an anti-TNF drug like infliximab.

5. Ans. (d) Thalidomide

(Ref: Goodman Gilman 12th E/P1022)

- The teratogenic defect given in the pcture is limb bud defect, i.e. phocomelia.
- It has been classically associated with thalidomide.

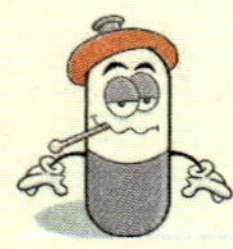

Annexures

Drugs of Choice

Acute Mountain Sickness	Acetazolamide
Acetaminophen toxicity	N-acetyl cysteine
Allergic rhinitis	Steroids
Ankylosing Spondylitis	NSAIDs
Analgesic of choice in Arthritis	• Rheumatoid Arthritis, Osteoarthritis – Acetaminophen • Rheumatic Arthritis, Arthralgia and Fever – Aspirin • Reactive Arthritis, Psoriatic arthritis– Indomethacin
Cold agglutinin disease	Rituximab
Familial Mediterranean Fever	Colchicine
Genital warts	• Males – Podophyllintoxin • Females – Imiquimod
Gout	Acute – Indomethacin Chronic – Allopurinol
Head lice	Permethrin 1% cream
Hypersensitivity reaction	Epinephrine
Pseudotumor Cerebri	Acetazolamide
Migraine	Prophylaxis – Propranolol Treatment – Sumatriptan
Morning Sickness	Doxylamine
PDA	Closure – Indomethacin Maintain patency – Misoprostol
Niacin induced flushing	Aspirin
Mild psoriasis	Oral retinoids
Psoriatic arthritis Erythrodermic psoriasis	Methotrexate
Pustular psoriasis	Acitretin
Pyrexia in children	Acetaminophen
Rheumatoid arthritis	Methotrexate
Raynaud Phenomenon	CCB (DHPs)
Tumor lysis syndrome	Allopurinol
Urticaria	2nd generation anti-histaminics

New Drugs

Tildrakizumab	Anti IL-23 monoclonal Ab	Plaque psoriasis
Erenumab	Anti CGRP-receptor monoclonal antibody	Prophylaxis of migraine
Fremanezumab and Galcanezumab	Anti CGRP ligand monoclonal antibody	Prophylaxis of migraine
Baricitinib	Oral Janus Kinase 1 and 2 inhibitor	Rheumatoid arthritis not responding to TNF alpha inhibitors
Lanadelumab	Anti-kallikrein monoclonal antibody	Prophylaxis of hereditary angioedema
Dupilumab	Anti-IL-4 receptor alpha MAb	Atopic dermatitis
Crisaborole	PDE-4 inhibitor	Atopic dermatitis

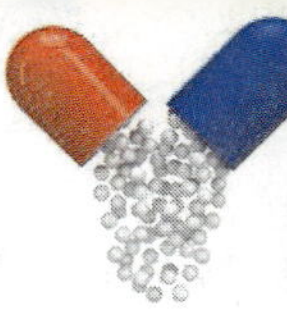

Multiple Choice Questions

HISTAMINE AND RELATED DRUGS

1. Which of the following is not a 2nd generation antihistamine? *(AIIMS Nov 2012)*
a. Cetirizine b. Cyclizine
c. Loratadine d. Fexofenadine

2. Which of the following is not a second generation antihistaminic? *(AIIMS May 2008, Nov 2006)*
a. Cyclizine b. Fexofenadine
c. Loratadine d. Acrivastine

3. Least antihistaminic property is seen with? *(Recent Question Dec 2016)*
a. Astemizole b. Dimenhydrinate
c. Desloratadine d. Cetirizine

4. Which Antihistaminic can be used in day times? *(Recent Question Dec 2016)*
a. Diphenhydramine
b. Dimenhydrinate
c. Chlorpheniramine maleate
d. Promethazine

5. True about first generation antihistaminics: *(Recent Question Dec 2016)*
a. Cause Torsades de Pointes
b. Are also used as Anti Motion sickness drugs
c. Poor lipid solubility
d. More potent

6. DOC for an acute attack of hereditary angioneurotic edema is *(Recent Question Dec 2016)*
a. Danazol b. C1 inhibitor concentrate
c. Icatibant d. Methylprednisolone

7. H_1 receptor blocker with least sedative action is *(Recent Question 2016)*
a. Terfenadine b. Promethazine
c. Astemizole d. Chlorpheniramine

8. Which of the following is not an antihistaminic drug of the ethanolamine group? *(Recent Question 2016)*
a. Clemastine b. Diphenhydramine
c. Dimenhydrinate d. Chlorpheniramine

9. This antihistaminic drug can cause cardiac arrhythmia at high dose by blocking cardiac K^+ channels. It is most likely to be *(Recent Question 2016)*
a. Levocetirizine b. Fexofenadine
c. Astemizole d. Loratadine

10. H_1 antihistaminic having best topical activity is *(Recent Question 2016)*
a. Loratadine b. Cetirizine
c. Astemizole d. Azelastine

11. Fexofenadine is metabolic product of *(Recent Question 2016)*
a. Loratadine b. Astemizole
c. Cetirizine d. Terfenadine

12. Which of the following drug causes QT prolongation? *(Recent Question 2016)*
a. Loratadine b. Levocetirizine
c. Fexofenadine d. Finasteride

SEROTONIN AND RELATED DRUGS

13. Mechanism of action of buspirone is *(Recent Question 2019)*
a. 5HT1 agonist b. Alpha agonist
c. Beta agonist d. 5HT2 antagonist

14. Which of the following is true about Triptans? *(Recent Question Dec 2016)*
a. Prophylaxis migraine
b. Indicated in heart disease
c. Variable Pharmacokinetics
d. Variable Pharmacodynamics

15. Methysergide used as drug of choice in migraine but not now because *(Recent Question Dec 2016)*
a. Peptic ulcer b. Arrhythmias
c. Pulmonary fibrosis d. MI

16. Sumatriptan acts as an agonist at this receptor– *(Recent Question Dec 2016)*
a. 5HT-1 b. 5HT-2A/2C
c. 5HT 1B/1D d. 5HT 2A/2C

17. Sumatriptan not given in *(Recent Question Dec 2016)*
a. Peptic ulcer b. Hypertension
c. IHD d. CKD

18. Which of the following is the mechanism of action of Ondansetron? *(Recent Question 2016)*
a. 5-HT2 receptor agonist
b. 5-HT3 receptor agonist
c. 5-HT2 receptor antagonist
d. 5-HT3 receptor antagonist

19. Drug used in treatment of migraine *(Recent Question 2016)*
a. 5HT1 agonist b. 5HT1 antagonist
c. D1 agonist d. DI antagonist

20. Methysergide is banned as it causes *(Recent Question 2016)*
a. Pulmonary fibrosis b. Pleural effusion
c. Syncope d. Myocarditis

21. Drug of choice for acute migraine is *(Recent Question 2016)*
a. Sumatriptan b. Ergot alkaloids
c. Ondansetron d. Ketanserin

22. Rizatriptan is a drug used for *(Recent Question 2016)*
a. Prophylaxis of migraine b. Acute migraine
c. Cluster headache d. Chronic migraine

23. Emesis receptor is: *(Recent Question 2016)*
a. 5HT 1 b. 5HT 2
c. 5HT 3 d. 5HT 4

24. Drugs used in prophylaxis of migraine are all except: ***(Recent Question 2016)***
a. Propranolol
b. Flunarizine
c. Topiramate
d. Levetiracetam

25. Which of the following is most useful for reversing severe ergot induced vasospasm? ***(Recent Question 2016)***
a. Ergotamine
b. Methysergide
c. Nitroprusside
d. Phenoxybenzamine

26. Which of the following serotonergic receptors is an auto-receptor? ***(Recent Question 2016)***
a. 5-HT1A
b. 5-HT4
c. 5-HT2A
d. 5-HT3

27. Drugs used in migraine prophylaxis are all except: ***(Recent Question 2016)***
a. Flunarizine
b. Propranolol
c. Cyproheptadine
d. Sumatriptan

28. Sumatriptan is used in ***(Recent Question 2016)***
a. Mania
b. Depression
c. Schizophrenia
d. Migraine

29. Sumatriptan is ***(Recent Question 2016)***
a. 5HT1D antagonist
b. 5HT1A agonist
c. 5HT1D agonist
d. 5HT1A antagonist

30. One of the following is not a 5-HT receptor antagonist ***(Recent Question 2016)***
a. Ketanserin
b. Lanreotide
c. Methysergide
d. Tropisetron

31. Granisetron is ***(Recent Question 2016)***
a. 5HT2 receptor antagonist
b. 5HT2 receptor agonist
c. 5HT3 receptor antagonist
d. 5HT3 receptor agonist

32. 5HT2A antagonist is ***(Recent Question 2016)***
a. Cisapride
b. Clozapine
c. Ketanserin
d. Sumatriptan

33. Granisetron is used in ***(Recent Question 2016)***
a. Motion sickness
b. Sedation in endoscopy
c. Chemotherapy induced nausea and vomiting
d. Gastro-oesophageal reflux disease

EICOSANOIDS AND RELATED DRUGS

34. Mechanism of action of colchicine in acute gout is: ***(Recent Question 2017)***
a. Mobilization of uric acid
b. Purine metabolism
c. Mobilization of leucocytes
d. Inhibition of COX

35. False about NSAIDs ***(AIIMS Nov 2014)***
a. Used in neuropathic pain
b. Decreases efficacy of antihypertensives
c. Cause renal failure
d. Can be used topically

36. Which NSAID undergoes enterohepatic circulation? ***(AIIMS Nov 2006)***
a. Phenylbutazone
b. Aspirin
c. Ibuprofen
d. Piroxicam

37. Analgesic effect of Paracetamol mediated by which receptor? ***(Recent Question 2018)***
a. NK 1
b. BK1
c. Px23
d. TRPV1

38. Which of the following is both Cox and Lox pathway inhibitor? ***(Recent Question Dec 2016)***
a. Meloxicam
b. Mefenamic acid
c. Licofelone
d. Celecoxib

39. Which of the following NSAID is used in rheumatoid arthritis? ***(Recent Question Dec 2016)***
a. Nimesulide
b. Aspirin
c. Cycloxydim
d. Diclofenac

40. Which COX II inhibitor causes hepatotoxicity? ***(Recent Question Dec 2016)***
a. Celecoxib
b. Refecoxib
c. Lumiracoxib
d. Etoricoxib

41. Drug combination avoided in Renal failure? ***(Recent Question Dec 2016)***
a. Ibuprofen + Enalapril
b. ßblocker + Enalapril
c. ßblocker + ibuprofen
d. Enalapril + Diuretics

42. Which NSAID available as eyedrops ***(Recent Question Dec 2016)***
a. Acetaminophen
b. Indomethacin
c. Aspirin
d. Ketorolac

43. Which of the following drug is Contra Indicated in Glaucoma with Acute Anterior Uveitis ***(Recent Question Dec 2016)***
a. Latanoprost
b. Timolol
c. Acetazolamide
d. Pilocarpine

44. Urgent liver transplantation done in ***(Recent Question Dec 2016)***
a. Paracetamol toxicity
b. Isoniazid toxicity
c. Rifampicintoxicity
d. Diclofenac toxicity

45. Anti-inflammatory dose of aspirin ***(Recent Question 2016)***
a. 500 mg/day
b. 1 - 2 g/day
c. 3 - 6 g/day
d. 6 - 12 g/day

46. NSAID given as a single daily dose is ***(Recent Question 2016)***
a. Naproxen
b. Ketorolac
c. Piroxicam
d. Paracetamol

47. Mechanism of action of aspirin is ***(Recent Question 2016)***
a. Inhibits COX-2 preferentially
b. Inhibits COX-1 preferentially
c. Inhibits COX 1 and COX2 reversibly
d. Inhibits COX 1 and COX2 irreversibly

48. Which of the following is the least acidic NSAID ***(Recent Question 2016)***
a. Aspirin
b. Etodolac
c. Diclofenac
d. Nabumetone

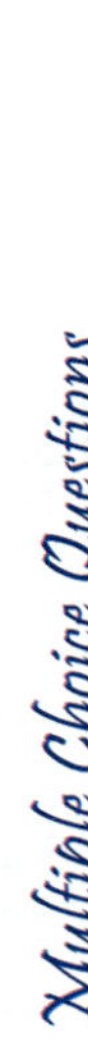

49. Which of the following drug is associated with highest cardiac mortality? *(Recent Question 2016)*
a. Rofecoxib b. Nicorandil
c. Losartan d. Metoprolol

50. Aspirin inhibits *(Recent Question 2016)*
a. Lipoprotein lipase b. Lipoxygenase
c. Cyclooxygenase d. Phospholipase

51. Misoprostol is a: *(Recent Question 2016)*
a. Prostaglandin E_1 analog
b. Prostaglandin E_2 analog
c. Prostaglandin antagonist
d. Antiprogestin

52. Which of the following drugs inhibit platelet cyclooxygenase reversibly? *(Recent Question 2016)*
a. Alprostadil b. Aspirin
c. Ibuprofen d. Prednisolone

53. Which of the following drugs inhibit an enzyme in the prostaglandin synthesis? *(Recent Question 2016)*
a. Aminocaproic acid b. Aspirin
c. Aprotinin d. Alteplase

54. Aspirin is *(Recent Question 2016)*
a. Methyl salicylate b. Para-aminobenzoic acid
c. Para-aminosalicylic acid
d. Acetyl salicylic acid

55. Ibuprofen acts on *(Recent Question 2016)*
a. Lipoxygenase pathway b. Cyclooxygenase pathway
c. Kinin system d. Serotonin system

56. Cyclooxygenase enzyme is not inhibited by *(Recent Question 2016)*
a. Aspirin b. Warfarin
c. Phenylbutazone d. Diclofenac

57. Which prostaglandin helps in cervical ripening? *(Recent Question 2016)*
a. PGI2 b. PGF2
c. PGF2 d. PGD2

58. Inhibitor of platelet aggregation includes *(Recent Question 2016)*
a. TXA2 b. PGI2
c. PGG2 d. All of the above

59. All the are reversible inhibitors of COX except: *(Recent Question 2016)*
a. Diclofenac
b. Ibuprofen
c. Aspirin
d. Indomethacin

60. Which is not a side effect of prostaglandin? *(Recent Question 2016)*
a. Vomiting b. Fever
c. Convulsion d. Diarrhea

61. Drug of choice for paracetamol poisoning: *(Recent Question 2016)*
a. Adrenaline
b. Atropine
c. Acetylcysteine
d. Insulin

62. False about NSAIDs *(Recent Question 2016)*
a. Cause addiction b. Cause gastric irritation
c. Used in acute gout d. Inhibit COX

63. Alprostadil is used in all except *(Recent Question 2016)*
a. Congenital heart disease
b. Maintain PDA
c. Erectile dysfunction
d. Closure of PDA

64. Aspirin and NSAIDs commonly causes: *(Recent Question 2016)*
a. Anaphylaxis
b. Urticaria
c. Phototoxicity
d. Photosensitivity

65. Patient presenting two hours after consumption of 40 tablets of aspirin. Immediate step in the management is: *(Recent Question 2016)*
a. Gastric lavage
b. Specific antidote
c. Forced alkaline diuresis
d. Symptomatic treatment

66. Drug causing patency of ductus *(Recent Question 2016)*
a. Alprostadil b. Apraclonidine
c. Aripiprazole d. Aspirin

67. NABPQI inhibitor used in acute acetaminophen poisoning is *(Recent Question 2016)*
a. Parabenzol b. Rotenone
c. N-acetyl cysteine d. Thermogenin

68. Renal papillary necrosis is caused by: *(Recent Question 2016)*
a. NSAIDs b. Cocaine
c. Heroin d. Morphine

GOUT

69. Drug acting by inhibition of recruitment of neutrophils is: *(Recent Question 2019)*
a. Colchicine b. Omalizumab
c. Sodium cromoglycate d. Febuxostat

70. Drug for uric acid to allantoin conversion is: *(Recent Question 2018)*
a. Sulfinpyrazone b. Rasburicase
c. Febuxostat d. Colchicine

71. Mechanism of action of colchicine is *(Recent Question 2016)*
a. Inhibits gouty inflammation
b. Inhibits the release of chemotactic factors
c. Inhibits granulocyte migration
d. All the above

72. Uricosuric drug not used in acute gout is *(Recent Question 2016)*
a. NSAIDs b. Colchicine
c. Corticosteroids d. Sulfinpyrazone

73. Febuxostat is used for *(Recent Question 2016)*
a. Hyperkalemia b. Hyperuricemia
c. Hypernatremia d. Hypercalcemia

74. Allopurinol inhibits which enzyme *(Recent Question 2016)*
a. Xanthine oxidase
b. Carbonic anhydrase
c. Pyrimidine synthase
d. Dihydro-orotate dehydrogenase

75. The most common effect of colchicines which is dose limiting is ***(Recent Question 2016)***

a. Diarrhea b. Dyspepsia
c. Retinal damage d. Loss of taste sensation

76. Treatment of tumor lysis syndrome ***(Recent Question 2016)***

a. Rasburicase b. Febuxostat
c. Probenecid d. Allopurinol

77. Acute gouty arthritis is seen early in treatment with ***(Recent Question 2016)***

a. Probenecid b. Allopurinol
c. Colchicine d. Rasburicase

78. Drug used in acute gout ***(Recent Question 2016)***

a. Allopurinol b. Febuxostat
c. Steroids d. All of the above

RHEUMATOID ARTHRITIS

79. Which of the following drugs is not used in rheumatoid arthritis? ***(AIIMS May 2018)***

a. Methotrexate b. Febuxostat
c. Etanercept d. Leflunomide

80. Which of the following anti rheumatic drug acts by increasing extracellular adenosine? ***(AIIMS May 2017)***

a. Hydroxychloroquine b. Leflunomide
c. Methotrexate d. Azathioprine

81. Which of the DMARD requires repeated hepatic function ***(AIIMS Nov 2016)***

a. Methotrexate b. Infliximab
c. Abatacept d. Cyclophosphamide

82. The treatment of choice for erythrodermic psoriasis is ***(AIIMS May 2016)***

a. Topical corticosteroid b. Corticosteroid
c. Methotrexate d. Coltar topically

83. A treatment naive 13 years old patient of rheumatoid arthritis with deformity given in picture. How will you start treatment? ***(Recent Question 2019)***

a. 3 months of NSAID
b. Single TNF alpha inhibitors
c. Start methotrexate and short course of steroids
d. Start Leflunomide

84. A patient of rheumatoid arthritis is not responding to NSAIDs and methotrexate for 6 months. What will you do next? ***(Recent Question 2019)***

a. Start single DMARD
b. Increase dose of methotrexate
c. Replace leflunomide with methotrexate
d. Add sulfasalazine and hydroxychloroquine

85. Which of the following is not a TNF alpha inhibitor? ***(Recent Question Dec 2016)***

a. Mycophenolate mofetil b. Etanercept
c. Adalimumab d. Infliximab

86. Which of the following TNF alpha inhibitor is given by IV route? ***(Recent Question Dec 2016)***

a. Etanercept b. Infliximab
c. Certolizumab d. Adalimumab

87. Not a DMARD in RA: ***(Recent Question Dec 2016)***

a. BAL b. Gold.
c. Methotrexate d. Hydroxychloroquine

88. Ustekinumab acts on: ***(Recent Question Dec 2016)***

a. IL 11 and IL 13
b. IL 12 and IL 13
c. IL 12 and 23
d. IL 11 and 23

89. Abatacept is used in: ***(AIIMS Nov 2014)***

a. Osteoarthritis
b. Rheumatoid arthritis
c. Multiple Sclerosis
d. Sarcoidosis

90. TNF-α inhibitors should not be used in: ***(AIIMS Nov 2009)***

a. Rheumatoid arthritis with HIV infection
b. Rheumatoid arthritis with hepatitis B
c. Rheumatoid arthritis with hepatitis C
d. Rheumatoid arthritis with pulmonary fibrosis

91. Anti-TNF alpha drugs are used for the treatment of all of following diseases except: ***(AIIMS Nov 2008)***

a. Systemic lupus erythematosus
b. Seronegative arthritis
c. Psoriatic arthritis

92. Sulfasalazine, which was developed as a drug for rheumatoid arthritis is now undergoing several trials for its possible role in the reversal of liver cirrhosis. The drug is a prodrug. Which among the following is an active moiety of sulfasalazine? ***(Recent Question 2016)***

a. 5-ASA b. Acrolein
c. Semustine d. Althesin

93. Which among the following is an IL-1 antagonist? ***(Recent Question 2016)***

a. Anakinra b. Adalimumab
c. Etanercept d. Inliximab

94. Which of the following is a DMARD? ***(Recent Question 2016)***

a. Desferrioxamine
b. Penicillamine
c. Succimer
d. Dimercaprol

95. First choice DMARD in RA ***(Recent Question 2016)***

a. Gold salts b. Infliximab
c. Methotrexate d. Steroids

96. Leflunomide is used in the treatment of ***(Recent Question 2016)***

a. Rheumatoid arthritis
b. Dermatomyositis
c. Bony metastasis
d. Postmenopausal osteoporosis

IMMUNOMODULATORS

97. Mechanism of action of basiliximab is: ***(Recent Question 2017)***

a. IL-2 inhibition
b. EGFR inhibition
c. VEGFR inhibition
d. Inhibition of purine synthesis

98. Which of the following is a calcineurin inhibitor? *(AIIMS Nov 2015)*
a. Cyclosporine
b. Basiliximab
c. Azathioprine
d. Sirolimus

99. Thalidomide is used in all of the following except: *(AIIMS May 2010, May 2009)*
a. HIV associated peripheral neuropathy
b. HIV associated aphthous (mouth) ulcers
c. Behçet syndrome
d. Erythema nodosum leprosum

100. A newborn baby was born with phocomelia. It results due to which drug taken by mother during pregnancy? *(AIIMS Nov 2010)*
a. Tetracycline b. Thalidomide
c. Warfarin d. Alcohol

101. Thalidomide can be used in all of the following conditions except? *(AIIMS Nov 2008)*
a. Behçet syndrome
b. HIV associated peripheral neuropathy
c. HIV associated mouth ulcers
d. Erythema nodosum leprosum

102. All of the following drugs are used as immunosuppressants except: *(AIIMS Nov 2008)*
a. Glucocorticoids b. Cyclosporine
c. Cephalosporin d. Azathioprine

103. The mechanism of action of cyclosporine is: *(Recent Question 2018)*
a. Inhibits IL2
b. Targets activated T cells
c. Decrease in transcription of IL2
d. Targets inactivated T cells

104. Thalidomide is used in *(Recent Question 2016)*
a. Mutiple myeloma b. Squamous cell carcinoma
c. Basal cell carcinoma
d. Nasopharyngeal carcinoma

105. Daclizumab acts through *(Recent Question 2016)*
a. cGMP activation b. Adenylyl cyclase inhibition
c. IL 2 receptor blocker d. IL 10 receptor blocker

106. Mechanism of action tacrolimus is *(Recent Question 2016)*
a. Inhibition of calcineurin
b. Antimetabolite
c. mTOR inhibitor
d. Inhibition of DNA synthesis

107. Which of the following statement(s) is/are true about hepatotoxic drugs except: *(PGI May 2017)*
a. Paracetamol toxicity is not dose dependent
b. Tetracycline can cause liver toxicity in high dose
c. Multiple exposure of halothane is important risk factor for halothane hepatitis
d. Rifampicin cause hepatitis
e. Chlorpropazine can cause cholestatic jaundice

108. Liver function test (LFT) monitoring is/are required in use of which of the following Disease Modifying Antirheumatic Drugs (DMARDs): *(PGI Nov. 2016)*
a. Methotrexate b. Hydroxychloroquine
c. Sulfasalazine d. Leflunomide
e. Gold

109. Which of the following is/are true about Tacrolimus: *(PGI Nov. 2016)*
a. A macrolides antibiotic
b. Structure similar to cyclosporine
c. Derived from a fungus
d. T cell inhibitor
e. Hirsutism less evident than cyclosporine

110. Disease modifying drug (s) used in treatment of rheumatoid arthritis: *(PGI June 2015)*
a. Naproxen b. Nabumetone
c. Abatacept d. Monoclonal antibodies
e. Methotrexate

111. TNF-α inhibitors are: *(PGI June 2014, Nov 2012)*
a. Bevacizumab b. Ranibizumab
c. Adalimumab d. Infliximab
e. Etanercept

112. Disease modifying agents in Rheumatoid arthritis *(PGI Nov 2009)*
a. Leflunomide b. Methotrexate
c. Abatacept d. Etanercept
e. Tacrolimus

113. True about Prostacyclin: *(PGI Nov 2007)*
a. Vasoconstriction
b. Cause aggregation of platelet
c. ↓ BP
d. Synthesis from vascular endothelium.

114. True about TXA_2: *(PGI Nov 2007)*
a. Synthesized by platelets
b. Prothrombotic
c. Formed by all cells of the body
d. Vasoconstriction
e. Permeability of vessel wall

115. Not true about Tofacitinib? *(JIPMER Nov 2018)*
a. Oral JAK inhibitor
b. Can be used in moderate to severe Crohn's disease
c. Increases triglycerides
d. Used in induction and maintenance of IBD

116. Misoprostol is analogue of: *(JIPMER Nov 2018)*
a. PGE1
b. PGE2
c. PGF2 alpha
d. PGF2 beta

117. Which is false about the following drugs used in rheumatoid arthritis? *(JIPMER May 2018)*
a. Tofacitinib inhibits JAK1 and JAK3
b. Tocilizumab used in rheumatoid arthritis
c. Tofacitinib given IV
d. Tocilizumab given IV and subcutaneous

118. Which liver enzyme is elevated in Azathioprine toxicity? *(JIPMER May 2018)*
a. GGT b. SGPT
c. ALP d. TPMT

119. Correctly matched dose of drugs used in gout is: *(JIPMER May 2018)*
a. Febuxostat 40 – 80 mg OD
b. Probenecid – 2000 mg OD
c. Sulphinpyrazone 1500 mg OD
d. Benzbromarone 15 mg OD

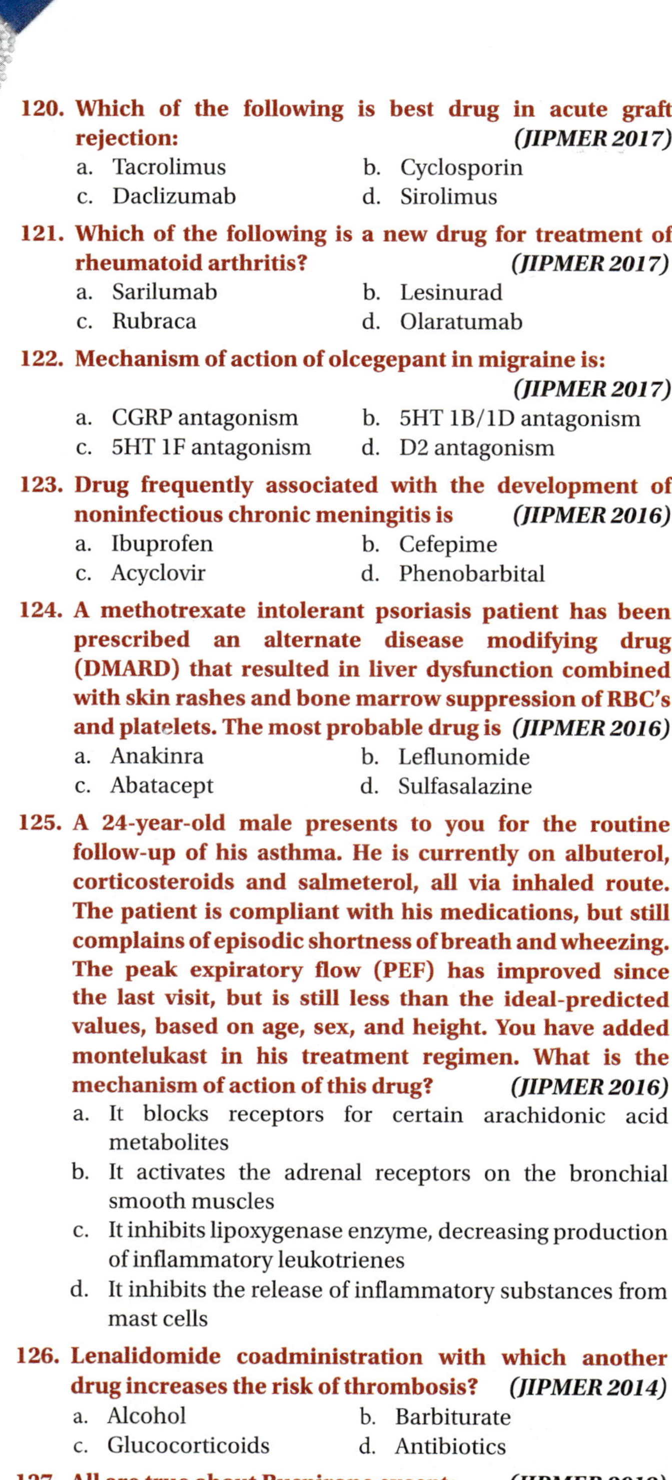

120. Which of the following is best drug in acute graft rejection: (JIPMER 2017)
a. Tacrolimus
b. Cyclosporin
c. Daclizumab
d. Sirolimus

121. Which of the following is a new drug for treatment of rheumatoid arthritis? (JIPMER 2017)
a. Sarilumab
b. Lesinurad
c. Rubraca
d. Olaratumab

122. Mechanism of action of olcegepant in migraine is: (JIPMER 2017)
a. CGRP antagonism
b. 5HT 1B/1D antagonism
c. 5HT 1F antagonism
d. D2 antagonism

123. Drug frequently associated with the development of noninfectious chronic meningitis is (JIPMER 2016)
a. Ibuprofen
b. Cefepime
c. Acyclovir
d. Phenobarbital

124. A methotrexate intolerant psoriasis patient has been prescribed an alternate disease modifying drug (DMARD) that resulted in liver dysfunction combined with skin rashes and bone marrow suppression of RBC's and platelets. The most probable drug is (JIPMER 2016)
a. Anakinra
b. Leflunomide
c. Abatacept
d. Sulfasalazine

125. A 24-year-old male presents to you for the routine follow-up of his asthma. He is currently on albuterol, corticosteroids and salmeterol, all via inhaled route. The patient is compliant with his medications, but still complains of episodic shortness of breath and wheezing. The peak expiratory flow (PEF) has improved since the last visit, but is still less than the ideal-predicted values, based on age, sex, and height. You have added montelukast in his treatment regimen. What is the mechanism of action of this drug? (JIPMER 2016)
a. It blocks receptors for certain arachidonic acid metabolites
b. It activates the adrenal receptors on the bronchial smooth muscles
c. It inhibits lipoxygenase enzyme, decreasing production of inflammatory leukotrienes
d. It inhibits the release of inflammatory substances from mast cells

126. Lenalidomide coadministration with which another drug increases the risk of thrombosis? (JIPMER 2014)
a. Alcohol
b. Barbiturate
c. Glucocorticoids
d. Antibiotics

127. All are true about Buspirone except: (JIPMER 2012)
a. Not a Benzodiazepine
b. Is a antianxiety drug
c. Used as sedative hypnotic
d. Used as antidepressant

128. Which of the following is a selective COX-2 inhibitor? (JIPMER 2010)
a. Diflunisal
b. Piroxicam
c. Sulindac
d. Parecoxib

129. Which of the following is not a uricosuric drug? (JIPMER 2010)
a. Probenecid
b. Benzbromarone
c. Sulfinpyrazone
d. Febuxostat

130. Short acting antihistamine is: (JIPMER 2009)
a. Cetirizine
b. Promethazine
c. Hydroxyzine
d. Acrivastine

131. Sumatriptan is contraindicated in: (JIPMER 2009)
a. Asthma
b. DM
c. Sepsis
d. Peripheral vascular disease

132. Which of the following has the highest affinity for 5HT3 receptors? (JIPMER 2008)
a. Dolasetron
b. Granisetron
c. Ondansetron
d. Palonosetron

133. Longest acting triptan: (JIPMER 2006)
a. Rizatriptan
b. Zolmitriptan
c. Naratriptan
d. Frovatriptan

134. Least sedative anti-histaminic is: (JIPMER 2006)
a. Cetirizine
b. Hydroxyzine
c. Chlorpheniramine
d. Carbinoxamine

135. In aspirin mechanism of action (NIMHANS 2014)
a. Lipoxygenase decreased
b. Cyclooxygenase decreased
c. Phospholipase
d. Increased Lipoxygenase

136. Aspirin acts by (NIMHANS 2011)
a. Cycloxygenase pathway
b. Lipoxygenase pathway
c. Membrane phospholipases
d. Cyclic AMP

137. NSAID Drug induced edema is due to (NIMHANS 2012)
a. Increased hydrostatic pressure
b. Protein losing enteropathy
c. Endothelial damage due to IL-2
d. Low oncotic pressure

138. Among the following TNF-alpha inhibitor is: (NIMHANS 2011)
a. Infliximab
b. Efalizumab
c. Mannose-6phosphate
d. Decorin

139. $5HT_3$ antagonist is: (NIMHANS 2008)
a. Levocetirizine
b. Metoclopramide
c. Domperidone
d. Ondansetron

140. Prophylaxis of migraine include all of the following drugs except: (NIMHANS 2008)
a. Verapamil
b. Propranolol
c. Sumatriptan
d. Topiramate

Answers with Explanations to Multiple Choice Questions

1. Ans. (b) Cyclizine

(Ref: Goodman Gilman 12th E/P921)

2. Ans. (a) Cyclizine

(Ref: Goodman Gilman 12th E/P921)

3. Ans. (b) Dipmenhydrinate

(Ref: Goodman Gilman 12th E/P920)

4. Ans. (c) Chlorpheniramine maleate

(Ref: Goodman Gilman 12th E/P923)

5. Ans. (b) Are also used as Anti Motion sickness drugs

(Ref: Goodman Gilman 12th E/P923)

- **The first generation drugs like promethazine, diphenhydramine, dimenhydrinate, meclizine and cyclizine are used in motion sickness due to anticholinergic effect.**
- **First generation drugs are less potent but more lipid soluble as compared to second generation drugs.**

6. Ans. (b) C1 inhibitor concentrate

(Ref: Harrison 19th E/P2120)

7. Ans. (a) Terfenadine

(Ref: Goodman Gilman 12th E/P921)

- Terfenadine is a second-generation drug which is less lipid soluble and hence do not cross blood brain barrier and there is not a sedative
- All other drugs in option are first generation drugs which are lipid soluble, cross blood brain barrier and cause sedation.
- Chlorpheniramine is the least sedating drug in the first generation.

8. Ans. (d) Chlorpheniramine

(Ref: Goodman Gilman 12th E/P921)

- **Chlorpheniramine is an antihistaminic of alkylamine group.**

9. Ans. (c) Astemizole

(Ref: Goodman Gilman 12th E/P924)

- Astemizole is longest acting and terfenadine is fastest acting, but both have been banned due to risk of QT prolongation and fatal cardiac arrhythmia specially if combined with enzyme inhibitor like ketoconazole.

10. Ans. (d) Azelastine

(Ref: Goodman Gilman 12th E/P922)

Mnemonics

Antihistamines given Only by Topical Route–DOKLA

D : Dibenzoxepins
O : Olopatadine
K : Ketotifen
L : Levocarbastine
A : Azelastine

11. Ans. (d) Terfenadine

(Ref: Katzung 12th E/P277)

Antihistaminic	Metabolite drug
Terfenadine	Fexofenadine
Hydroxyzine	Cetirizine
Loratadine	Desloratadine

12. Ans. (c) Fexofenadine

(Ref: Goodman Gilman 12th E/P 920)

- Terfenadine causes QT prolongation and hence it has been banned.
- Fexofenadine is a metabolite of terfenadine which causes less QT prolongation than terfenadine.

13. Ans. (a) 5HT1 agonist

(Ref: Goodman Gilman 13th E/P234)

- Buspirone and ipsapirone are nonbenzodiazepine anxiolytic, which act by stimulating 5HT1A receptors.
- 5HT1 against is a Gi subtype of presynaptic GPCR and hence its stimulation decreases release of 5HT. This decreases stimulation of postsynaptic 5HT2 receptors and causes a decrease in anxiety.

Note: SSRI increases 5HT in synapse, which leads to stimulation of postsynaptic 5HT2 and hence causes anxiety as a side effect.

14. Ans. (c) Variable pharmacokinetics

(Ref: Goodman Gilman 12th E/P346)

15. Ans. (c) Pulmonary fibrosis

(Ref: Goodman Gilman 12th E/P349)

16. Ans. (c) 5HT 1B/1D

(Ref: Goodman Gilman 12th E/P345)

17. Ans. (c) IHD

(Ref: Goodman Gilman 12th E/P346)

18. Ans. (d) 5-HT3 antagonist

(Ref: Goodman Gilman 12th E/P 1341)

19. Ans. (a) 5HT1 agonist

(Ref: Goodman Gilman 12th E/P345)

$5HT_{1A}$ Agonists used as anxiolytics	$5HT_{1B/1D}$ Agonists used in migraine
Buspirone	Sumatriptan
Ipsapirone	Zolmitriptan
	Rizatriptan

20. Ans. (a) Pulmonary fibrosis

(Ref: Goodman Gilman 12th E/P351)

21. Ans. (a) Sumatriptan

(Ref: Goodman Gilman 12th E/P351)

Drug of Choice for

- Acute migraine – Sumatriptan
- Prophylaxis of migraine – Propranolol

22. Ans. (b) Acute migraine

(Ref: Goodman Gilman 12th E/P351)

23. Ans. (c) 5HT 3

(Ref: Goodman Gilman 12th E/P340)

24. Ans. (d) Levetiracetam

(Ref: Katzung 12th E/P285)

Mnemonics

Drugs Used in Prophylaxis of Migraine

Flunarizine : Flunarizine
Can : Cyproheptadine, Clonidine
P : Pizotifen, Propranolol (DOC)
RE : Release of GABA inhibitor- Gabapentine
VE : ValproatE
N : Nortriptyline
T : Topiramate
Migraine : Methysergide

25. Ans. (c) Nitroprusside

(Ref: Goodman Gilman 12th E/P340)

- Dextran, anticoagulants and nitroprusside is used in ergot induced vasospasm to maintain circulation.

26. Ans. (a) 5HT1A

(Ref: Goodman Gilman 12th E/P339)

27. Ans. (d) Sumatriptan

(Ref: Goodman Gilman 12th E/P345)

- Sumatriptan is the drug of choice for treatment of an acute attack of migraine but is not used in prophylaxis of migraine.

28. Ans. (d) Migraine

(Ref: Goodman Gilman 12th E/P345)

29. Ans. (c) 5HT1D agonist

(Ref: Goodman Gilman 12th E/P345)

30. Ans. (b) Lanreotide

(Ref: Goodman Gilman 12th E/P350-51)

- Lanreotide is a somatostatin analog.
- Ketanserin and methysergide are 5HT2 antagonist and tropisetron is a 5HT3 antagonist.

31. Ans. (c) 5HT3 receptor antagonist

(Ref: Goodman Gilman 12th E/P350)

32. Ans. (c) Ketanserin

(Ref: Goodman Gilman 12th E/P350)

33. Ans. (c) Chemotherapy induced nausea and vomiting

(Ref: Goodman Gilman 12th E/P350)

34. Ans. (c) Mobilization of leucocytes

(Ref: Goodman Gilman 12th E/P995)

- Colchicine inhibits tubulins required for mobilization of leucocytes (neutrophils) into joints in an acute attack of gout.
- It also inhibits release of chemotactic factors form neutrophils and inhibits adhesion of neutrophils to endothelium of blood vessels.

35. Ans. (a) Used in neuropathic pain

(Ref: Goodman and Gilman 12th E/P 971)

- NSAIDs are effective for treatment of pain which arises due to sensitization of pain receptors caused by inflammation. They are effective in pain of arthritis, menstruation, migraine and many other inflammatory disorders.
- Analgesic nephropathy can be seen, which is associated with a progressive renal failure, decreased concentrating ability of tubules and sterile pyuria.
- NSAIDs can decrease efficacy of antihypertensives and diuretics. Loss of Pg induced Cl loss and vasopressin inhibition leads to retention of salt and water.
- Some NSAIDs like ketorolac are available intopical preparation of topical gel and ophthalmic solutions.

36. Ans. (d) Piroxicam

(Ref: Goodman Gilman 12th E/P987)

37. Ans (d) TRPV1

(Ref: David Golan 3rd E/P276)

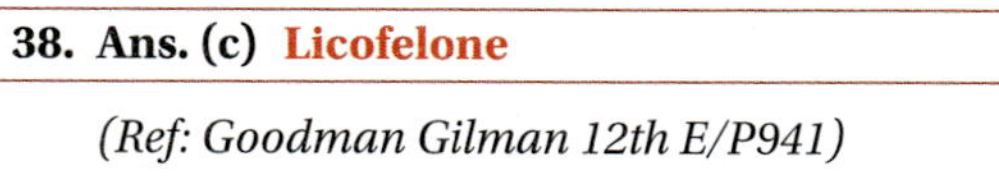

38. Ans. (c) Licofelone

(Ref: Goodman Gilman 12th E/P941)

39. Ans. (b) Aspirin

(Ref: Goodman Gilman 12th E/P979)

40. Ans. (c) Lumiracoxib

(Ref: Goodman Gilman 12th E/P965)

Hepatotoxic NSAIDs

- Acetaminophen
- Diclofenac
- Lumiracoxib

41. Ans. (a) Ibuprofen + Enalapril

(Ref: Goodman Gilman 12th E/P975)

42. Ans. (d) Ketorolac

(Ref: Goodman Gilman 12th E/P986)

43. Ans. (a) Latanoprost

(Ref: Goodman Gilman 12th E/P1787)

44. Ans. (a) Paracetamol toxicity

(Ref: Goodman Gilman 12th E/P984)

45. Ans. (c) 3-6 g/day

(Ref: Goodman Gilman 12th E/P979)

Antiaggregant dose of aspirin	Anti-inflammatory dose of aspirin
50-320 mg/day	3-4 g/day

46. Ans. (c) Piroxicam

(Ref: Goodman Gilman 12th E/P990)

- Piroxicam is the longest and slowest acting nonselective COX inhibitor and hence given at OD doses and not preferred in acute analgesia.

47. Ans. (d) Inhibits COX1 and COX2 irreversibly

(Ref: Goodman Gilman 12th E/P964)

48. Ans. (d) Nabumetone

(Ref: Goodman Gilman 12th E/P985, 986 and 977)

NSAID	Derivative of
Aspirin	Acetyl salicylic acid
Diclofenac	Phenylacetic acid
Etodolac	Acetic acid
Tolmetin Ketorolac	Heteroaryl acetic acid derivative
Ibuprofen Naproxen	Propionic acid
Piroxicam Meloxicam	Enolic acid

Contd...

49. Ans. (a) Refecoxib

(Ref: Goodman Gilman 12th E/P992)

- Refecoxib and valdecoxib were banned due to risk of MI.

50. Ans. (c) Cyclooxygenase

(Ref: Goodman Gilman 12th E/P977)

51. Ans. (a) Prostaglandin E_1 analog

(Ref: Goodman Gilman 12th E/P950)

Prostaglandin E_1 analogue	Misoprostol Alprostadil
Prostaglandin E_2 analogue	Dinoprostone
Prostaglandin $F_{2\alpha}$ analogue	Carboprost
Prostaglandin I_2 analogue	Epoprosterenol

52. Ans. (c) Ibuprofen

(Ref: Goodman Gilman 12th E/P988)

53. Ans. (b) Aspirin

(Ref: Goodman Gilman 12th E/P977)

54. Ans. (d) Acetyl salicylic acid

(Ref: Goodman Gilman 12th E/P971)

55. Ans. (b) Cyclooxygenase pathway

(Ref: Goodman Gilman 12th E/P988)

56. Ans. (b) Warfarin

(Ref: Goodman Gilman 12th E/P971, 988)

57. Ans. (c) PGF2

(Ref: Goodman Gilman 12th E/P950)

58. Ans. (b) PGI2

(Ref: Goodman Gilman 12th E/P946)

59. Ans. (c) Aspirin

(Ref: Goodman Gilman 12th E/P971)

60. Ans. (c) Convulsion

(Ref: Goodman Gilman 12th E/P946-51)

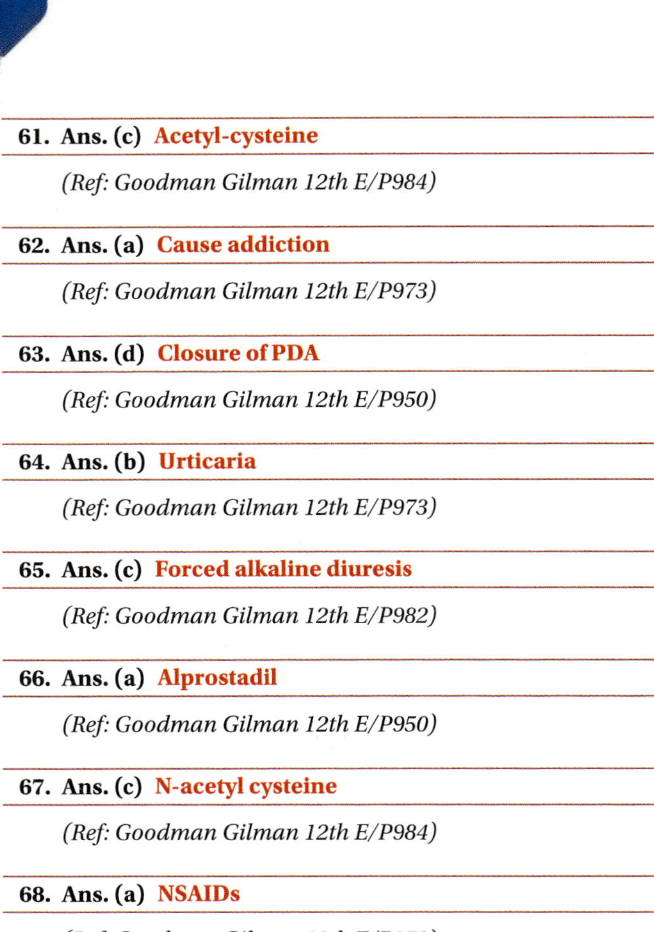

61. Ans. (c) Acetyl-cysteine

(Ref: Goodman Gilman 12th E/P984)

62. Ans. (a) Cause addiction

(Ref: Goodman Gilman 12th E/P973)

63. Ans. (d) Closure of PDA

(Ref: Goodman Gilman 12th E/P950)

64. Ans. (b) Urticaria

(Ref: Goodman Gilman 12th E/P973)

65. Ans. (c) Forced alkaline diuresis

(Ref: Goodman Gilman 12th E/P982)

66. Ans. (a) Alprostadil

(Ref: Goodman Gilman 12th E/P950)

67. Ans. (c) N-acetyl cysteine

(Ref: Goodman Gilman 12th E/P984)

68. Ans. (a) NSAIDs

(Ref: Goodman Gilman 12th E/P973)

69. Ans. (a) Colchicine

(Ref: Goodman Gilman 13th E/P702)

- Colchicine inhibits microtubules in neutrophils and hence inhibits their migration into the site of inflammation.
- Thus, it is used in an acute attack of gout.

70. Ans. (b) Rasburicase

(Ref: Goodman Gilman 13th E/P705)

71. Ans. (d) All of the above

(Ref: Goodman Gilman 12th E/P971)

72. Ans. (d) Sulfinpyrazone

(Ref: Goodman Gilman 12th E/P999)

73. Ans. (b) Hyperuricemia

(Ref: Goodman Gilman 12th E/P997)

74. Ans. (a) Xanthine oxidase

(Ref: Goodman Gilman 12th E/P996)

Xanthine oxidase inhibitors
Allopurinol
Oxypurinol
Febuxostat

75. Ans. (a) Diarrhea

(Ref: Goodman Gilman 12th E/P995)

- GIT related side effects like nausea, vomiting and diarrhea are most common. Other side effects seen are bone marrow suppression and rhabdomyolysis.

76. Ans. (d) Allopurinol

(Ref: Goodman Gilman 12th E/P996)

Tumor Lysis Syndrome

- **Allopurinol - DOC**
- **Rasburicase – Alternative in pediatric patients**

77. Ans. (b) Allopurinol

(Ref: Goodman Gilman 12th E/P996)

78. Ans. (c) Steroids

(Ref: Goodman Gilman 12th E/P1000)

79. Ans. (b) Febuxostat

(Ref: Goodman Gilman 13th E/P704)

- Febuxostat is a xanthine oxidase inhibitor used for treatment of chronic gout.

80. Ans. (c) Methotrexate

(Ref: Nijkamp's Principles of immunotherapy/P601)

Anti-inflammatory effect of methotrexate is produced by:

- Inhibition of purine synthesis which causes selective toxicity to lymphocytes.
- Inhibition of effect produced by inflammatory modulators like TNF alpha, IL1, IL 6 at the site of inflammation.
- Increase in adenosine release which leads to
  - Decrease in complement C2 production
  - Inhibition of neutrophil adhesion
  - Inhibition of free radical production
- All these factors down regulation decreases tissue destruction in joints.
- Adenosine also induces fusion of macrophages in tissues, which leads to granulomata. Adenosine is also believed to cause hepatic fibrosis seen with methotrexate.

Note: Methotrexate also causes keratinocyte apoptosis and hence is beneficial in resistant psoriasis.

81. Ans. (a) Methotrexate

(Ref: Goodman Gilman 12th E/P1820)

82. Ans. (c) Methotrexate

(Ref: Goodman Gilman 12th E/P1820)

83. Ans. (c) Start methotrexate and a short course of steroids

(Ref: Harrison 19th E/P2148)

84. Ans. (d) **Add sulfasalazine and hydroxychloroquine**

(Ref: Harrison 19th E/P2148)

85. Ans. (a) **Mycophenolate mofetil**

(Ref: Goodman Gilman 12th E/P996)

86. Ans. (b) **Infliximab**

(Ref: CMDT 2017/P838)

The route of administration for all anti-TNF drugs is subcutaneous, whereas **infliximab** can also be given by **intravenous route**.

87. Ans. (a) **BAL**

(Ref: Goodman Gilman 12th E/P994)

88. Ans. (c) **IL 12 and 23**

(Ref: CMDT 2017/P108)

Anti-IL 12 and 23 monoclonal antibodies used in psoriasis

- **Ustekinumab**
- **Guselkumab**

89. Ans. (b) **Rheumatoid arthritis**

(Ref: Goodman and Gilman 12th E/P 1825)

90. Ans. (b) **Rheumatoid arthritis with hepatitis B**

(Ref: Harrison 19th E/P2145)

Contraindications of Anti-TNF Drugs

- Severe heart failure
- RA with hepatitis B

91. Ans. (a) **Systemic lupus erythematosus**

(Ref: Harrison 19th E/P2146)

92. Ans. (a) **5-ASA**

(Ref: Goodman Gilman 12th E/P 1466)

93. Ans. (a) **Anakinra**

(Ref: Goodman Gilman 12th E/P 994)

Drugs Related to IL

IL1 antagonist	Anakinra
IL2 analogue	Aldesleukin
IL2 receptor antagonist	Basiliximab Daclizumab
IL6 antagonist	Tocilizumab
IL17 antagonist	Secukinumab

94. Ans. (b) **Penicillamine**

(Ref: Goodman Gilman 12th E/P995)

95. Ans. (c) **Methotrexate**

(Ref: Goodman Gilman 12th E/P993)

96. Ans. (a) **Rheumatoid arthritis**

(Ref: Goodman Gilman 12th E/P995)

97. Ans. (a) **IL-2 inhibition**

(Ref: Goodman Gilman 12th E/P1017)

IL-2 Receptor Inhibitors

- Basiliximab
- Daclizumab

98. Ans. (a) **Cyclosporine**

(Ref: Goodman Gilman 12th E/P1008)

Calcineurin Inhibitors
Cyclosporine Tacrolimus

99. Ans. (a) **HIV associated peripheral neuropathy**

(Ref: Goodman Gilman 12th E/P1022)

100. Ans. (b) **Thalidomide**

(Ref: Goodman Gilman 12th E/P1022)

101. Ans. (b) **HIV associated peripheral neuropathy**

(Ref: Goodman Gilman 12th E/P1022)

102. Ans. (b) **Cyclosporine**

(Ref: Goodman Gilman 12th E/P1010)

103. Ans. (c) **Decrease in transcription of IL2**

(Ref: Goodman Gilman 13th E/P640)

- Calcineurin is an enzyme which dephosphorylates NFATc (Nuclear Factor for Activation of T lymphocytes - cytoplasmic). Once dephosphorylated NFATc can enter to nucleus of T cells and combines with NFATn (Nuclear factor for activation of T lymphocytes – nuclear) and this leads to transcription of IL2, which activates T cells.
- Cyclosporine inhibits calcineurin which leads to a decrease transcription of IL-2 followed by a decreased activation of T lymphocytes.
- Calcineurin also increases TGF-beta, which inhibits IL-2 mediated T cell stimulation

104. Ans. (a) **Multiple myeloma**

(Ref: Goodman Gilman 12th E/P1022)

105. Ans. (c) **IL 2 receptor blocker**

(Ref: Goodman Gilman 12th E/P1017)

106. Ans. (a) Inhibition of calcineurin

(Ref: Goodman Gilman 12th E/P1008)

107. Ans. (a) Paracetamol toxicity is not dose dependent

(Ref: Goodman Gilman 12th E/P983)

Paracetamol Induced hepatotoxicity is dose dependent and seen at doses > 10 grams or > 150-250 mg/kg.

108. Ans. (a) Methotrexate, (d) Leflunomide, (e) Gold

(Ref: Goodman Gilman 12th E/P1694)

109. Ans. (a) A macrolide antibiotic, (d) T cell inhibitor, (e) Hirsutism less evident than cyclosporine

(Ref: Goodman Gilman 12th E/P1822)

110. Ans. (c) Abatacept, (d) Monoclonal antibodies, (e) Methotrexate

(Ref: Goodman Gilman 12th E/P995)

111. Ans. (c) Adalimumab, (d) Infliximab, (e) Etanercept

(Ref: Goodman Gilman 12th E/P995)

112. Ans. (a) Leflunomide, (b) Methotrexate

(Ref: Goodman Gilman 12th E/P995)

113. Ans. (c) ↓ BP, (d) Synthesis by vascular endothelium

(Ref: Goodman Gilman 12th E/P946)

114. Ans. (a) Synthesized by platelet, (b) Prothrombotic, (d) Vasoconstriction

(Ref: Goodman Gilman 12th E/P946)

115. Ans. (b) Can be used in moderate to severe Crohn's disease

(Ref: Goodman Gilman 13th E/P1288)

116. Ans. (a) PGE1

(Ref: Goodman Gilman 13th E/P825)

117. Ans. (c) Tofacitinib given IV

(Ref: Goodman Gilman 13th E/P1288)

118. Ans. (c) ALP

(Ref: KATZUNG 14th E/P988)

119. Ans. (a) Febuxostat 40-80 mg OD

(Ref: Goodman Gilman 13th E/P704)

120. Ans. (c) Daclizumab

(Ref: Goodman Gilman 12th E/P1017)

- Daclizumab and basiliximab are anti CD-25/IL-2 monoclonal antibodies used to prevent acute graft rejection.
- These drugs are combined with other immunomodulators used for maintenance like cyclosporine, tacrolimus and prednisolone.

121. Ans. (a) Sarilumab

(Ref: https://www.centerwatch.com/drug-information/fda-approved-drugs/drug/100205/kevzara-sarilumab)

- Sarilumab is an anti-IL-6 receptor antibody approved by FDA in 2017 for treatment of rheumatoid arthritis not responding to other existing DMARDs.
- It is given by subcutaneous route at a dose of 200 mg once every 2 weeks.
- Other anti-IL-6 receptor antibody approved for treatment of rheumatoid arthritis is tocilizumab.

122. Ans. (a) CGRP antagonism

(Ref: Journals)

- Olcegepant (IV) and telcagepant (Oral) are new drugs under trial for treatment of an acute attack of migraine.

123. Ans. (a) Ibuprofen

(Ref: Goodman Gilman 12th E/P988)

124. Ans. (b) Leflunomide

(Ref: CMDT 2017/P837)

Leflunomide

- **Leflunomide inhibits de-novo pyrimidine synthesis in lymphocytes by inhibiting dihydroorotate dehydrogenase.**
- **It can be used in GVHD as add on drug and is also used in rheumatoid arthritis.**
- **Side effects associated are bone marrow suppression, rash, alopecia, hepatotoxicity and weight loss. Since it is carcinogenic and teratogenic it is contraindicated in fertile males and females planning for conception.**

125. Ans. (a) It blocks receptors for certain arachidonic acid metabolites

(Ref: Goodman Gilman 12th E/P942)

126. Ans. (c) Glucocorticoids

(Ref: Goodman Gilman 12th E/P1022)

127. Ans. (c) Used as sedative hypnotic

(Ref: Goodman Gilman 12th E/P345)

128. Ans. (d) Parecoxib

(Ref: Goodman Gilman 12th E/P991)

129. Ans. (d) Febuxostat

(Ref: Goodman Gilman 12th E/P997)

130. Ans. (b) Promethazine

(Ref: Goodman Gilman 12th E/P921)

- Most of the first generation drugs are short acting except meclizine and hydroxyzine which are long-acting.
- The second generation drugs are long-acting drugs.

131. Ans. (d) Peripheral vascular disease

(Ref: Goodman Gilman 12th E/P346)

132. Ans. (d) Palonosetron

(Ref: Goodman Gilman 12th E/P345)

133. Ans. (d) Frovatriptan

(Ref: Goodman Gilman 12th E/P346)

134. Ans. (a) Cetirizine

(Ref: Goodman Gilman 12th E/P921)

- First generation drugs are less sedating as compared to second generation drugs. Hence, cetirizine the only second generation drug in the options is the answer.
- However cetirizine is most sedating among the second generation drugs.

135. Ans. (b) Cyclooxygenase decreased

(Ref: Goodman Gilman 12th E/P977)

136. Ans. (a) Cyclooxygenase pathway

(Ref: Goodman Gilman 12th E/P977)

137. Ans. (a) Increased hydrostatic pressure

(Ref: Goodman Gilman 12th E/P973)

138. Ans. (a) Infliximab

(Ref: Goodman Gilman 12th E/P994)

139. Ans. (d) Ondansetron

(Ref: Goodman Gilman 12th E/P346)

140. Ans. (c) Sumatriptan

(Ref: Goodman Gilman 12th E/P347)

NOTES

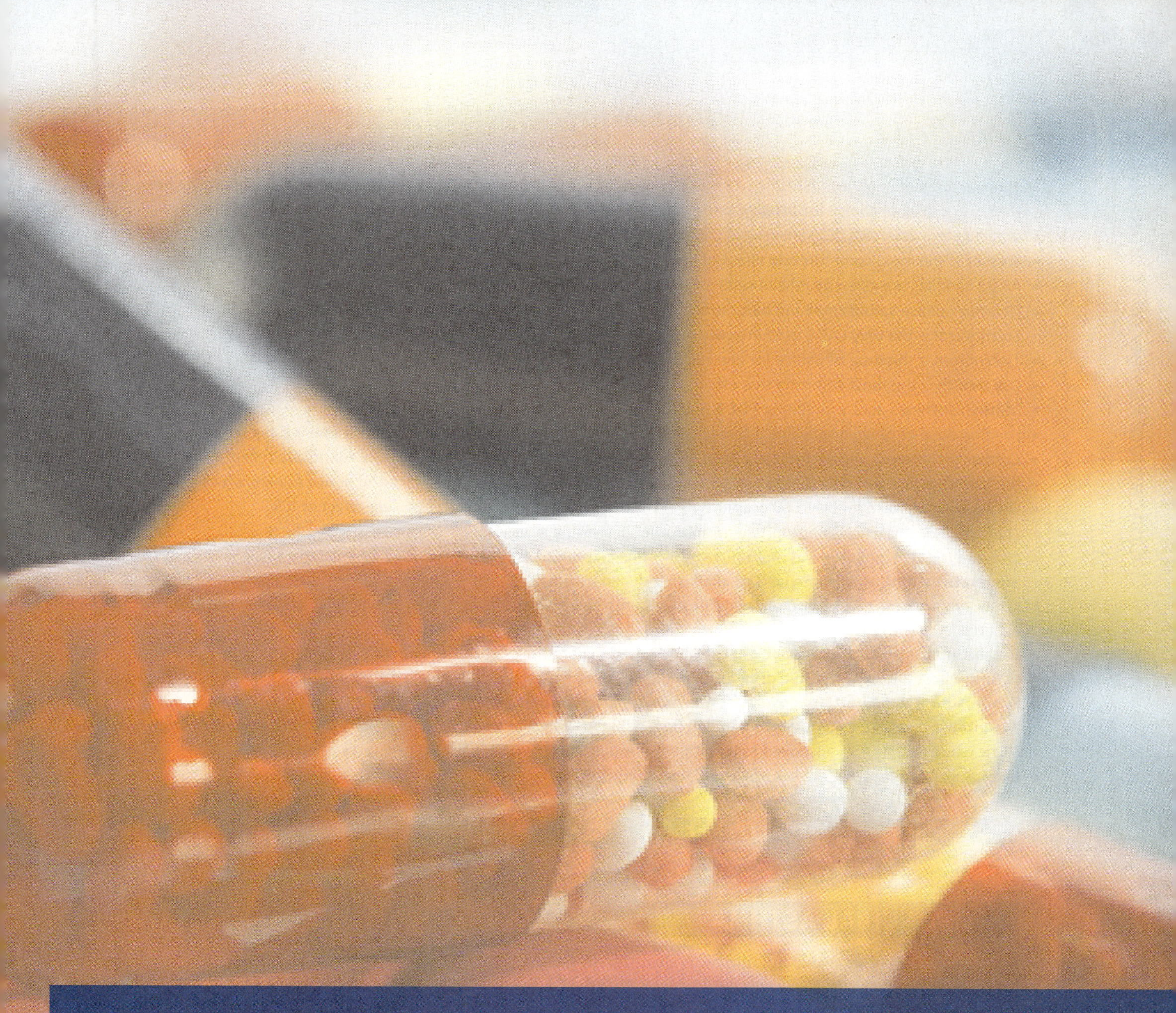

Respiratory System

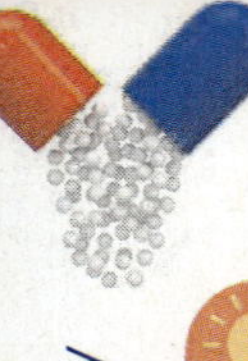

One Liners

- Short-acting beta-agonists (SABA) are drug of choice for **acute attack** of bronchial asthma, whereas long-acting beta-agonists (LABA) are drug of choice for **prophylaxis** of bronchial asthma.
- Inhaled corticosteroids (ICS) are drug of choice for **persistent** bronchial asthma and for prophylaxis of **exercise induced asthma**.
- **Tremor** is the most common side effect of β_2 agonists.
- All β2 agonists are given by inhalational route except **terbutaline which is given by subcutaneous route**.
- Delayed release **salbutamol** and **bambuterol** are given by **oral route** for prophylaxis of nocturnal asthma.
- **Formoterol** is the only LABA used in **acute attack of asthma** due to its faster onset of action.
- **Tiotropium** is the drug of choice for chronic obstructive pulmonary disease (COPD).
- **Dry mouth** is the most common side effect of inhalational anticholinergics due to local effect.
- **Methylxanthines** act by inhibiting **PDE 3 and 4**.
- Loading dose of IV aminophylline is **6 mg/kg** and oral dose of theophylline and aminophylline is **8 mg/kg BD**.
- **Cardiac arrhythmia** and **seizures** are seen at toxic doses of **methylxanthines** due to A1 adenosine receptor antagonism.
- **Beclomethasone** and **ciclesonide** are ICS activated by esterases in respiratory tract and hence are known as **soft steroids**.
- **Hoarseness of voice** followed by **oropharyngeal candidiasis** is the most common side effect of ICS.
- The size of drug particles appropriate for inhalational therapy is **2–5 μm**.
- **Zileuton** is a **LOX** inhibitor and **montelukast/zafirlukast/pranlukast** are **competitive leukotriene antagonists** used for **mild** to **moderate asthma** and **prophylaxis of exercise induced asthma**.
- **Cromolyn sodium** and **nedocromil sodium** are mast cell stabilizers used in prophylaxis of allergen and exercise induced asthma.
- **Omalizumab** is an **anti IgE monoclonal antibody** used in persistent bronchial asthma.
- **CCBs** are **best antihypertensive drug** for pulmonary artery hypertension.
- **Epoprostenol** is the **best drug overall** for pulmonary artery hypertension.
- **Bosentan** is drug of choice for **class II and III (low risk) PAH** whereas **epoprostenol** is drug of choice in **class IV (high risk) PAH**.
- **Nitric oxide (NO)** is FDA approved for treatment of **pulmonary hypertension in neonates**.
- **Doxapram** and **almitrine** are specific ventilatory stimulants.

BRONCHIAL ASTHMA

- Bronchial asthma (BA) is a chronic inflammatory disorder of the lower respiratory tract with predominant involvement of the bronchi. On repeated exposure to an allergen T_{helper}-2 cells are activated, which release IL-4.
- IL-4 induces mast cells to produce IgE, which binds to mast cells and causes its degranulation.
- The mast cells release inflammatory mediators which cause chronic inflammation of the airway.
- Histamine and leukotrienes produced are powerful bronchoconstrictors and hence all these factors together lead to the symptoms of bronchial asthma.
- For treatment of an acute attack bronchodilators are used whereas for long-term control the inflammatory process can be inhibited by various drugs as given in conceptual Box-1.

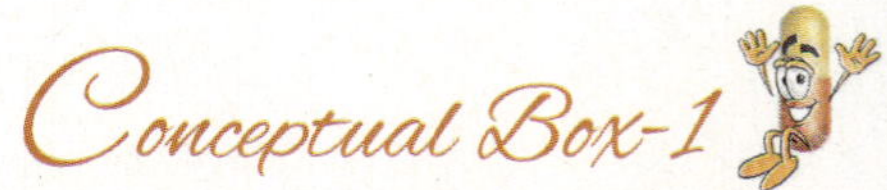

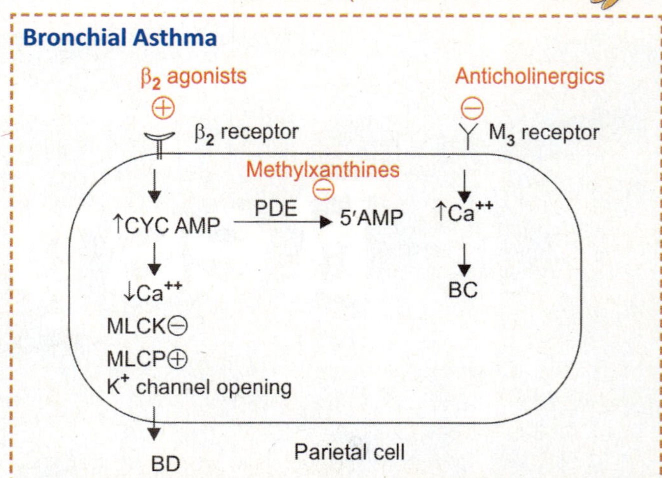

BRONCHODILATORS

Bronchodilators used to relieve an acute attack of bronchial asthma are β_2 agonists, anticholinergics and methylxanthines.

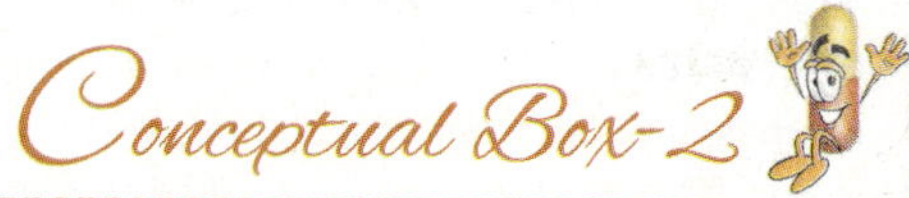

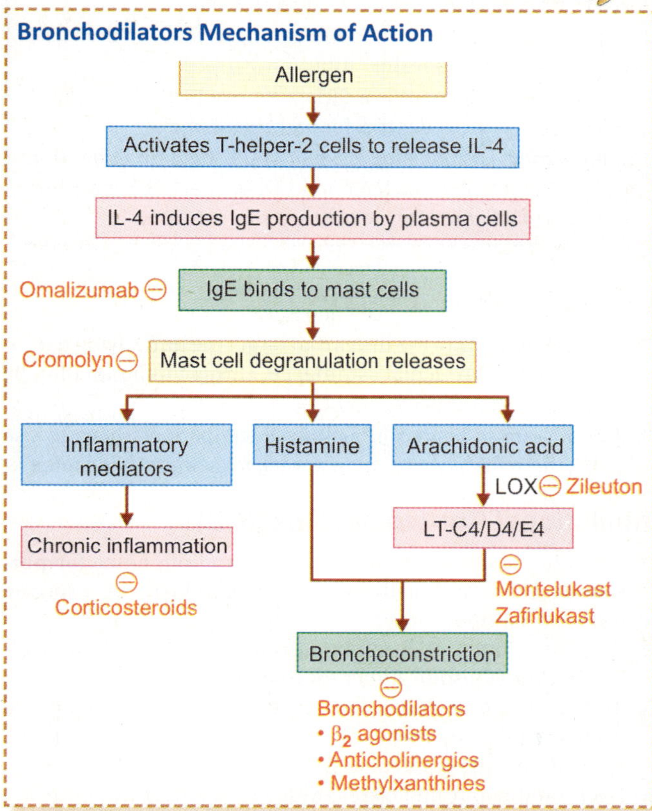

β_2 Agonists

- β_2 agonists are the functional/physiological antagonists of the bronchoconstrictors (histamine and LT) and hence are best bronchodilators in bronchial asthma.
- As depicted in the conceptual Box-2, β_2 agonists cause bronchial smooth muscle relaxation by decreasing calcium, opening potassium channels, inhibiting myosin light chain kinase (MLCK) and stimulating myosin light chain phosphorylase (MLCP).

Short-acting β_2 Agonists (SABA)

- SABA are short- and fast-acting (within 5 minutes) and hence used at SOS doses, as the drugs of choice for an **acute attack of bronchial asthma**.
- Salbutamol (albuterol), levalbuterol, metaproterenol and pirbuterol are given by inhalational route, whereas **terbutaline by subcutaneous** route for an acute attack of BA.
- Inhalational SABA are used for prophylaxis of exercise induced asthma as well.
- Delayed release oral formulation of salbutamol and bambuterol is used for nocturnal asthma, as inhalational SABA is not effective due to shorter duration of action (4–6 hours).
- Levalbuterol, the S-enantiomer of albuterol is more β_2 selective and **most potent SABA**.

Long-acting β_2 Agonists (LABA)

- Salmeterol is a partial agonist whereas formoterol is a full agonist at β_2 receptors.
- LABA have a duration of action near to 12 hours and hence at BD doses by inhalational route are used for prophylaxis of asthma, exercise induced asthma and nocturnal asthma.
- LABA use along with ICS decreases asthma exacerbation as well as required dose for ICS in persistent asthma. LABA should never be used as monotherapy in asthma, as they have no effect on the disease pathophysiology; thus by improving symptoms they will mask the severity.
- **Salmeterol** is slow acting and used **only in prophylaxis**, but **formoterol** being fast-acting can be used for an **acute attack** as well.
- Arformoterol, the R enantiomer of formoterol is approved only for COPD. Salmeterol and formoterol can also be used for treatment of COPD.
- These drugs are available as fixed dose combinations with inhalational corticosteroids in inhalers.

Very Long-acting β_2 Agonists (VLABA)

- VLABA has a duration of action near to 24 hours and hence used at OD doses for treatment of COPD.
- Indacaterol, vilanterol and olodaterol are approved by FDA for COPD. These drugs are not used for treatment of bronchial asthma.

Side Effects of β_2 Agonists

- **Tremors** are the most common side effect seen due to β_2 receptor stimulation in skeletal muscles.
- Other side effects associated are palpitation, hypokalemia, hyperglycemia, ventilation perfusion mismatch and QT prolongation.

Recent Advances

- **Abediterol:** Abediterol is VLABA under trial for COPD.

Classification of Bronchodilators

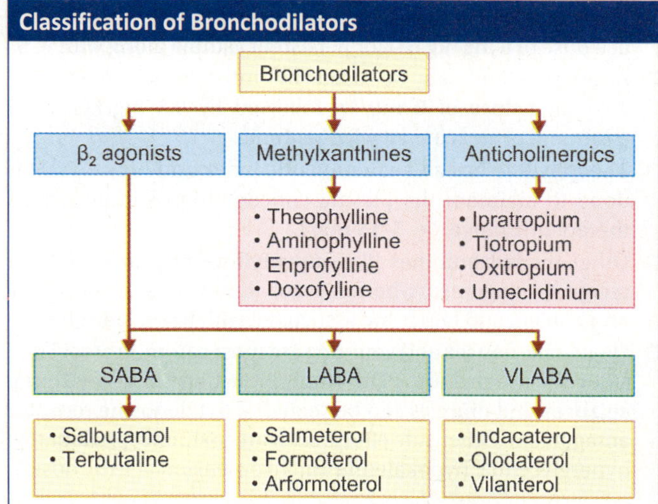

Anticholinergics

- Anticholinergics act by inhibiting M3 receptor induced bronchoconstriction. Since atropine is a lipid soluble tertiary amine that can cause systemic side effects even by inhalational route, lipid insoluble quaternary amines like ipratropium, oxitropium and tiotropium were derived from it.
- **Anticholinergics** are the **bronchodilator of choice in COPD** as the only reversible component of bronchoconstriction in COPD is cholinergic effect. In bronchial asthma these drugs are not approved by FDA but used off label in case patient is not responding to or is intolerant to β_2 agonists.
- **Tiotropium** and **umeclidinium** are longest acting anticholinergic in this class and hence are **drug of choice for treatment of COPD** as they can be used by OD dosing.
- **Ipratropium** (QID dosing) and **aclidinium** (BD dosing) are other drugs in this class used for treatment of COPD.
- **Oxitropium** is intermediate acting and can be used in nocturnal asthma.
- Most common side effect seen with this class is **dry mouth** due to anticholinergic effect. Other side effects associated are glaucoma and urine retention.

Recent Advances

Revefenacin: It is a long acting anticholinergic (M3 antagonist) approved for treatment of COPD.

Roflumilast: Roflumilast is a selective PDE-4 inhibitor recently approved by FDA for the treatment of COPD.

Methylxanthines

- Methylxanthines act by inhibiting **PDE 3 and 4**, which increases cyclic AMP and cause bronchodilation by mechanisms like β_2 agonists. **Adenosine receptor antagonism** also contributes to bronchodilation. Stimulation of histone **deacetylase, release of interleukin 10, apoptosis of neutrophils/eosinophils** and inhibition of PDE-4 in lymphocytes give additional anti-inflammatory effect.
- These drugs are rarely used nowadays in bronchial asthma and COPD; reserved for patients not responsive to previous bronchodilators.
- **Theophylline** and **aminophylline** can be used by oral route at a dose of **8 mg/kg BD** for persistent asthma along with ICS.
- Aminophylline can be used by intravenous route with a loading dose of **6 mg/kg** followed by 0.5 mg/kg/hr for treatment of an acute attack of asthma.
- Theophylline has a low therapeutic index and hence TDM is done to maintain the plasma concentration within normal therapeutic range, i.e. **5–15 mg/L.**
- Other methylxanthines like **enprofylline** has no adenosine receptor antagonism whereas doxofylline has lesser adenosine antagonism and hence are associated with lesser side effects.
- Headache, nausea and vomiting are most common associated side effects seen due to PDE-4 inhibition. **Cardiac arrhythmia, seizures** and diuresis can be seen due to adenosine receptor antagonism. Other side effects seen are toxic encephalopathy, hyperglycemia, hypokalemia and hypotension at toxic doses.

Recent Advances

Magnesium: Magnesium can cause bronchodilation by inhibiting calcium transport into smooth muscle cells. It is under trial for treatment of an acute attack of bronchial asthma.

Cromakalim: Cromakalim is a potassium channel opener under trial as a bronchodilator for bronchial asthma.

Aviptadil: Aviptadil is a VIP analog under trial for bronchial asthma as a bronchodilator.

Fevipiprant: Fevipiprant is a CRTH2 (Chemotactic Factor for T Helper2) inhibitor under trial for bronchial asthma.

Losmapimod: Losmapimod is a p38 MAPK inhibitor under trial for the treatment of asthma and COPD. It acts by inhibiting synthesis of inflammatory mediators.

CORTICOSTEROIDS

- Corticosteroids are the drugs that target the underlying pathophysiology of bronchial asthma, i.e. chronic inflammation by their anti-inflammatory effect.
- Steroids are indicated in asthma if the patients have to use SABA more than two times in a week for symptomatic relief.

Inhalational Corticosteroids (ICS)

- Inhalational corticosteroids are the drug of choice for **persistent bronchial asthma** and **prophylaxis of exercise induced asthma**.
- The drugs in this class are budesonide, ciclesonide, flunisolide, beclomethasone, fluticasone and mometasone.
- All ICS except beclomethasone and triamcinolone undergo extensive first pass metabolism after absorption into systemic circulation and hence cause lesser systemic side effects.
- **Beclomethasone** and **ciclesonide** are prodrugs which are activation by esterase in lungs and are known as **"soft steroids"** due to lesser associated side effects.
- Fluticasone is the most potent whereas flunisolide is the least potent ICS.
- **Hoarseness of voice** due to deposition of steroids on vocal cords is the most common side effect followed by **oropharyngeal candidiasis**. Systemic side effects can also be seen, when used at high doses.

Systemic Corticosteroids

- Systemic steroids are reserved for patients not responding to ICS.
- Intravenous hydrocortisone and methylprednisolone or oral prednisolone can be used in acute attack of asthma if patients do not respond to β_2 agonists. Hydrocortisone is the IV steroid of choice as it is the fastest acting systemic steroid.
- In acute attack steroids act by decreasing mucous secretion and inflammatory cell response. In addition to this steroids increase transcription of β_2 receptor genes and hence increase responsiveness to β_2 agonists.
- On the other hand the β_2 agonists increase effect of steroid by enhancing action of glucocorticoid receptors. Theophylline also increases effect of steroids by stimulating enzyme histone deacetylase, which is a target for steroids as well.

- Oral prednisolone and intramuscular depot formulation triamcinolone can be used for persistent asthma.

Recent Advances

Mapracorat: Mapracorat is a selective glucocorticoid receptor agonist that targets receptors for inflammation only and is devoid of systemic side effects.

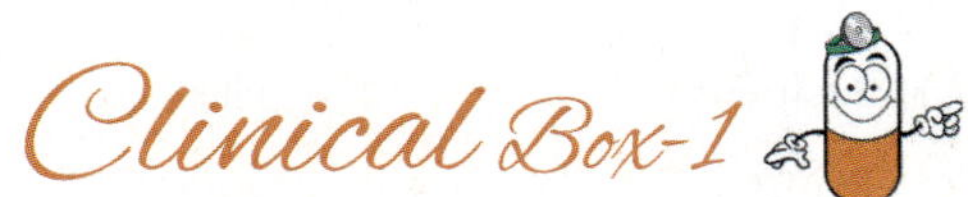

Inhalational Devices

Inhalational route produces immediate effect and causes lesser systemic side effects. The size of drug particle appropriate for inhalational route is **2–5 µm**.

- **Metered dose inhalers (MDI):** MDI when pressed, the drug is propelled by hydrofluoroalkane (HFA) and is then inhaled. MDI pressing, and inhalation must coincide for effect and hence is difficult by children to maneuver.
- **Dry powder inhalers (DPI):** The act of inspiration creates a negative pressure in the DPI, which sucks the powder. No coordination is required and hence is easier for children.
- **Nebulizers:** Passing of a compressed gas through the liquid drug makes a mist that is inhaled by patient. It is the preferred device in neonates and acute attack of bronchial asthma and COPD.

LEUKOTRIENE PATHWAY INHIBITORS

- Leukotriene (LT) pathway produces **LT C4/D4** which causes bronchoconstriction, mucus secretion and mucosal edema, and LT B4 which causes chemotaxis. This can be prevented by inhibiting LOX and LT receptors. **Zileuton** is a **LOX inhibitor,** whereas **montelukast, zafirlukast** and **pranlukast** are **LT D4 receptor inhibitors**.
- These are most preferred for the treatment of aspirin induced asthma, which is caused by COX inhibition which potentiates the LOX pathway. Monteleukast is the preferred drug in this condition.
- Leukotriene pathway inhibitors are given by oral route for **mild to moderate bronchial asthma progressive on ICS** and for prophylaxis of **exercise induced asthma**. In allergic rhinitis leukotriene inhibitors are as good as antihistaminics. These are easier to administer in children (oral route) than inhalational corticosteroids.
- **Zileuton** is associated with hepatotoxicity and hence routine liver function test is mandatory. **Montelukast, zafirlukast** and **pranlukast are competitive LT D4 receptor inhibitors**, also associated with hepatotoxicity. Montelukast and zafirlukast can cause Churg-Strauss syndrome also.

CROMOLYNS

- **Cromolyns** were invented by Roger Altounyan, who synthesized two compounds, i.e. **cromolyn sodium** and **nedocromil sodium**.
- Their primary mechanism of action as depicted in conceptual Box-1, is by inhibition of **mast cell degranulation** and hence are also known as **mast cell stabilizer**.
- Hence, by preventing release of bronchoconstrictors they are beneficial in **prophylaxis of allergen induced asthma (QID dosing)** and **exercise induced asthma** (just before exercise) by inhalational route.
- These drugs are more effective in children as compared to other age groups.
- Side effects are negligible, and these are the **safest antiasthmatic drugs**.

KETOTIFEN

- Ketotifen acts by **inhibiting mast cell degranulation** and **H_1 receptors and stimulating NO synthesis**.
- Like cromolyns it is also used for prophylaxis of asthma but by oral route.

MONOCLONAL ANTIBODIES

Anti IgE Monoclonal Antibody

- **Omalizumab** is an **anti IgE monoclonal antibody** used for treatment of severe asthma, allergic rhinitis, chronic urticaria and peanut allergy.
- It is administered by subcutaneous route every 2–4 weeks. The dose is calculated based on both weight of patient and plasma IgE titer.
- Omalizumab is called as a steroid sparing drug as the dose required to control asthma is decreased.
- In coexisting atopic dermatitis omalizumab is ineffective due to high titer of IgE.

Anti-interleukin 4 and 5 Monoclonal Antibodies

- Interleukin 4 is responsible for proliferation of T-helper 2 cells which produce interleukin 5. Interleukin 5 acts on interleukin 5 receptors on eosinophils and promote their maturation, activation and survival. Interleukin 4 and 13 also promote IgE production from the B cells.
- Thus, inhibitors of interleukin 4 and 5 have been developed for treatment of severe eosinophilic asthma not responding to inhalational corticosteroids.
- **Reslizumab** and **mepolizumab** are anti-interleukin 5 monoclonal antibodies and **benralizumab** is anti-interleukin 5 receptor monoclonal antibody. These drugs can cause hypersensitivity however anaphylaxis is seen only with reslizumab.
- **Dupilumab** is an anti-interleukin 4Rα monoclonal antibody which downregulates effects of both interleukin 4 and 13. It is approved for both asthma and atopic dermatitis. It can also cause hypersensitivity and anaphylaxis.

Clinical Box-2

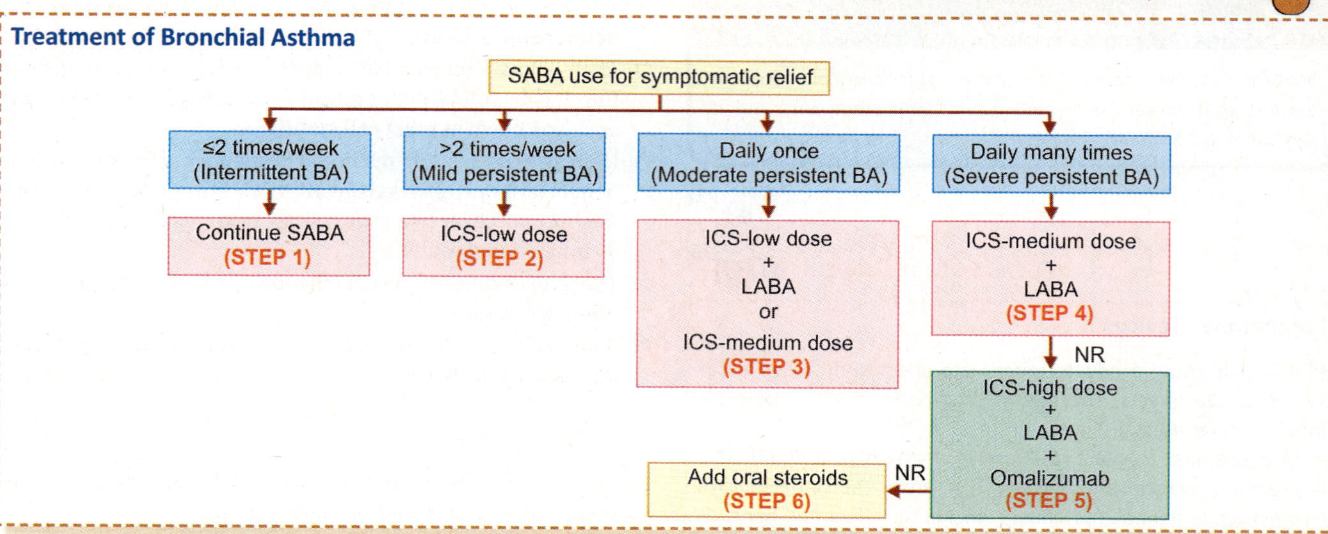

Note: Omalizumab is added only in step 5 and 6 if patient has allergic symptoms as well.

PULMONARY ARTERY HYPERTENSION

- Pulmonary hypertension is a pulmonary artery pressure of more than 25 mm Hg, which is caused by vascular smooth muscle hypertrophy.
- The cause can be idiopathic or secondary due to scleroderma, COPD, interstitial lung disease etc.
- On long-standing pulmonary hypertension, left ventricular hypertrophy occurs which can cause heart failure.
- The main aim is to relieve this pulmonary artery resistance by vasodilators like endothelin antagonists, prostaglandin I2 analogs, PDE-5 inhibitors, guanylate cyclase stimulators and calcium channel blockers.
- Class I PAH does not require drug therapy, whereas class II and III (low-risk groups) and IV (high-risk groups) require drug therapy to target morbidity and mortality.
- Warfarin as well is given to all patients of pulmonary hypertension.

Clinical Box-3

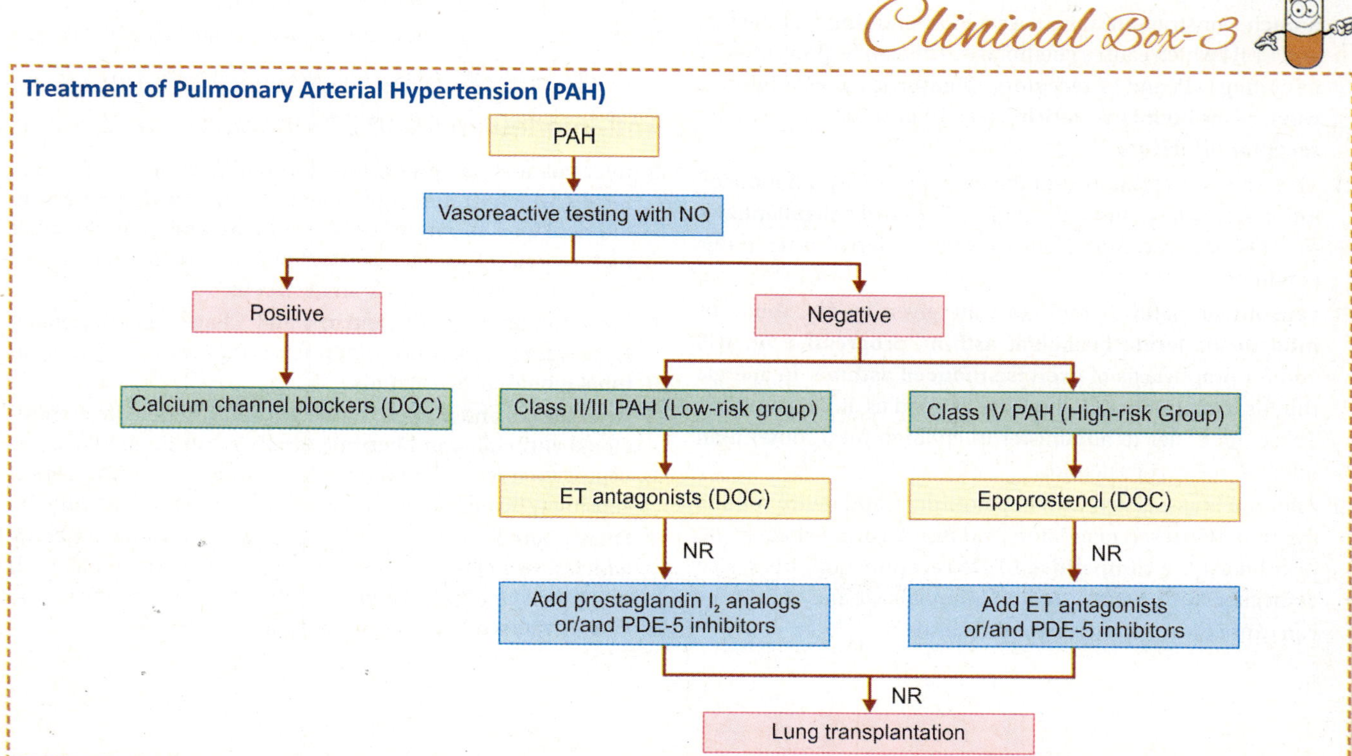

CALCIUM CHANNEL BLOCKERS

- Only some patients of pulmonary hypertension respond to CCBs and hence a vasoreactive testing is done first with nitric oxide.
- On positive and sustained response CCB like nifedipine is the first line drugs.
- **CCBs** are the **best antihypertensives** for treatment of PAH, whereas **prostaglandin I_2 analogs** are the **best drugs** overall for treatment of PAH.

ENDOTHELIN ANTAGONISTS

Endothelin produced in PAH causes powerful vasoconstriction by acting on ET_A receptor, whereas ET_B mediates release of NO and prostaglandin I_2.

- ET antagonists are the drug of choice for treatment of **class II and III (low risk) PAH**.
- **Bosentan** and **macitentan** are nonselective ET antagonists. Bosentan is associated with side effects like hepatotoxicity and anemia.
- **Ambrisentan** and **sitaxsentan** are selective ET_A antagonists.

PROSTAGLANDIN I_2 ANALOGS

- **Prostaglandin I_2 (prostacyclin)** causes vasodilation by cyclic AMP pathway and apart from that it has antiaggregant and antiproliferative effect. These are overall most effective and best drugs for treatment of pulmonary hypertension.
- Epoprostenol is synthetic prostaglandin I_2 which is very short acting and hence long acting prostaglandin I_2 analogs like iloprost and beraprost were synthesized. The latest drugs are prostaglandin I_2 receptor agonists like treprostinil and selexipag.
- **Epoprostenol** is shortest acting (6 minutes) and needs to be given by continuous intravenous infusion. Epoprostenol is the drug of choice for **class IV (high risk) PAH**. Side effects associated are headache and flushing due to vasodilation.
- **Iloprost** by inhalation route or **beraprost** by oral route may be used for class III (low risk) PAH.
- **Treprostinil** is longer acting (4 hours) and can be given by continuous subcutaneous infusion and inhalational route. It is indicated in class III (low risk) PAH.

PDE-5 INHIBITORS

- PDE-5 metabolizes cyclic GMP in smooth muscles of blood vessels. Thus, its inhibition increases cyclic GMP which causes vasodilation.
- This class is used along with ET antagonists or prostaglandin I_2 analogs for treatment of class II, III and IV PAH.
- **Sildenafil** is short-acting and requires TDS dosing, whereas **tadalafil** is longer acting that can be given at OD doses.
- Erectile dysfunction is a secondary use of these drugs, as this came into picture after PDE-5 inhibitors were approved for PAH. Sildenafil is the drug of choice for the treatment of erectile dysfunction.

Recent Advances

Riociguat: Riociguat is a guanylate cyclase stimulator and causes vasodilatation by increasing cyclic GMP. It has been recently approved for the treatment of PAH.

ANTITUSSIVES

- Cough is a protective reflex of the respiratory tract to remove exogenous substances and secretions.
- It can be associated with drugs (ACEIs), respiratory tract infection, bronchial cancer, asthma, GERD etc.
- Cough can be suppressed by various drugs which act on the cough center in medulla (centrally acting) or on the stretch receptors respiratory tract (peripherally acting).

CENTRALLY ACTING

Opioids

- Opioids act by inhibiting μ receptors in the cough center.
- **Codeine** and **pholcodine** are used for treatment of mild to moderate cough. Codeine is overall the antitussive of choice.
- **Morphine** and **methadone** are indicated in sever persistent cough associated with bronchial cancer.
- Most common opioid related side effect is **constipation**.

Dextromethorphan

- Dextromethorphan is D isomer of opioid levomethorphan but is devoid of opioid agonistic effect.
- Rather it acts by **inhibiting NMDA receptors** in CNS.
- It is not only associated with lesser side effects but also is less effective than opioids and is an over the counter medication for mild cough. It can be combined with opioids if required.
- Hallucinations and addiction are associated drawbacks.

Diphenhydramine

- Diphenhydramine is an antihistaminic that produces antitussive effect by central mechanisms.
- Sedation and anticholinergic side effects are associated.

Caramiphen

Caramiphen is a central anticholinergic used as antitussive in combination with decongestant drug phenylpropanolamine.

Recent Advances

Aprepitant: Aprepitant is a NK1 antagonist under trial for treatment of cough associated with bronchial cancer.

Gabapentin and pregabalin: These can be used for the treatment of chronic idiopathic cough.

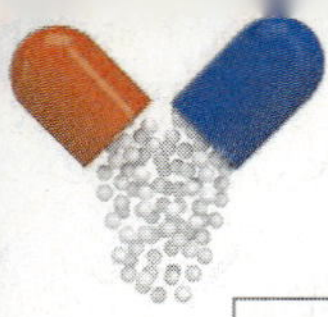

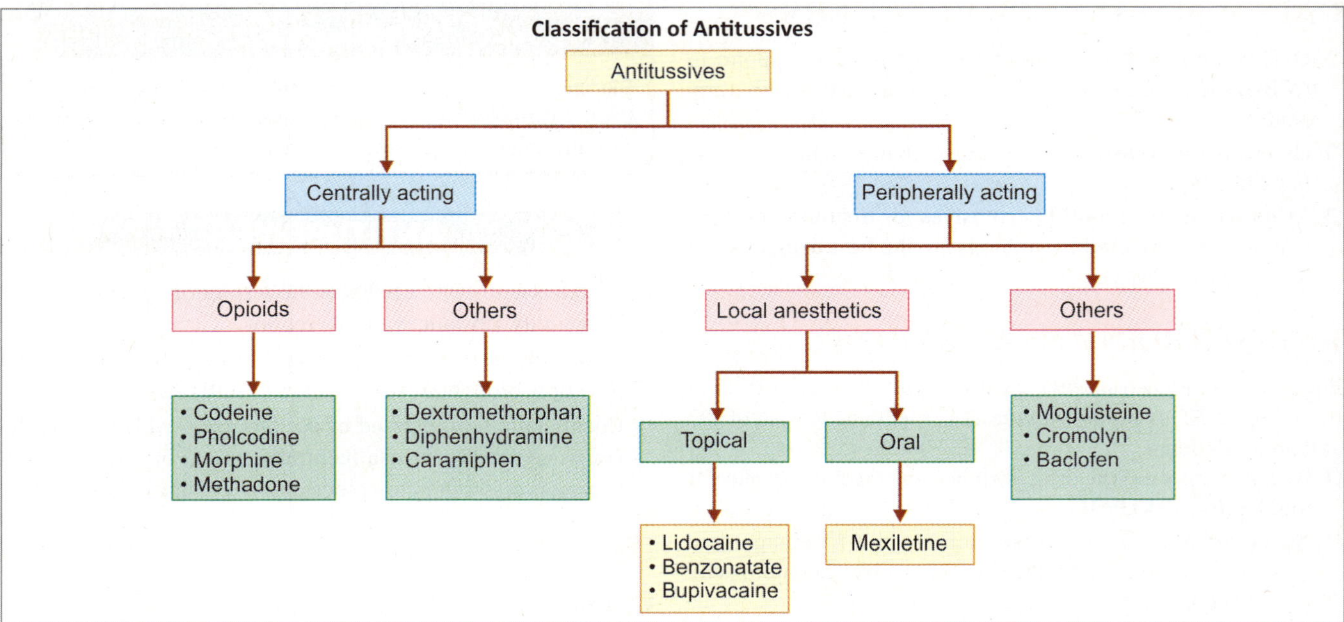

PERIPHERALLY ACTING

Local Anesthetics

- Local anesthetics inhibit peripheral stretch receptors in the sensory nerves of respiratory tract and blunts cough reflex.
- These can be used in case the central drugs are ineffective.
- **Benzonatate, lidocaine** and **bupivacaine** can be used topically, whereas **mexiletine** by oral route.
- The antitussive effect of benzonatate is not reliable and more over it is commonly associated with side effects like drowsiness and dysphagia.

Moguistine

Moguistine produces antitussive effect by opening K channels and hyperpolarizing the peripheral sensory nerves of respiratory tract.

Cromolyn

Cromolyn acts by persistently depolarizing the peripheral sensory nerves in respiratory tract and increases threshold for action potential. It is effective in ACEIs induced cough.

Recent Advances

Baclofen: Baclofen is a $GABA_B$ agonist which has inhibitory effect if used peripherally on the sensory nerves of respiratory tract and produces antitussive effect.

MUCOLYTICS AND EXPECTORANTS

Mucolytics and expectorants are commonly combined with antitussive drugs for removal of secretions in case of productive cough.

EXPECTORANTS

- Expectorants are drugs that increase removal of secretions from respiratory tract due to reflex stimulation caused by gastric irritation.
- The only FDA approved drug in this class is **guaifenesin**. It is also used as cough suppressant in patients with upper respiratory tract infection.
- The other off label used expectorants are ammonium chloride, hypertonic saline and iodides.
- Expectorants are not effective in COPD and associated with side effects like nausea and vomiting.

MUCOLYTICS

- Mucolytics are drugs that liquefy the mucus in respiratory tract and facilitate removal.
- Mucolytics with free **sulfhydryl group like N-acetyl cysteine, ethyl cysteine and methyl cysteine** are cysteine analogs that act by **breaking the disulfide bonds** in mucus to decrease viscosity.
- Mucolytics with blocked sulfhydryl group like **carbocisteine, erdosteine, letosteine** and **stepronine** cannot break the disulfide bond. These drugs act by stimulating secretion of sialomucins. These are given by oral route as tablets or combined with antitussives in cough syrups.
- **Bromhexine** and its **metabolite** ambroxol act by depolymerization of mucopolysaccharides in mucus.
- **DNase** is an enzyme that liquefies mucus and is used in cystic fibrosis.
- Mucolytics as well are not effective in COPD.

SURFACTANTS

- Surfactant analogs like **beractant** and **poractant alpha** are used for prophylaxis and treatment of RDS in premature babies.
- They are delivered directly into the lower respiratory tract, after which they decrease surface tension in alveoli and prevent its collapse.

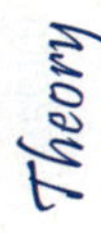

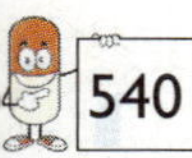

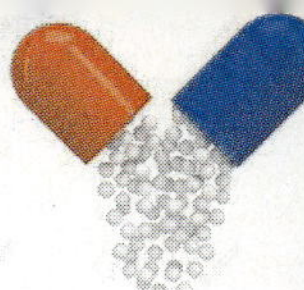

Image-based Questions

1. Which of the following is incorrect regarding the device in the picture?

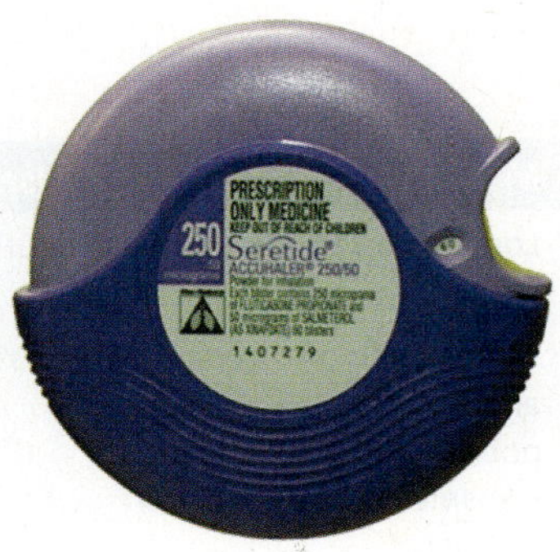

a. Requires coordination with inspiration
b. Easier to maneuver
c. Known as dry powder inhaler
d. Insulin can be used

2. The device connected to the metered-dose inhaler (MDI) in the picture is known as:

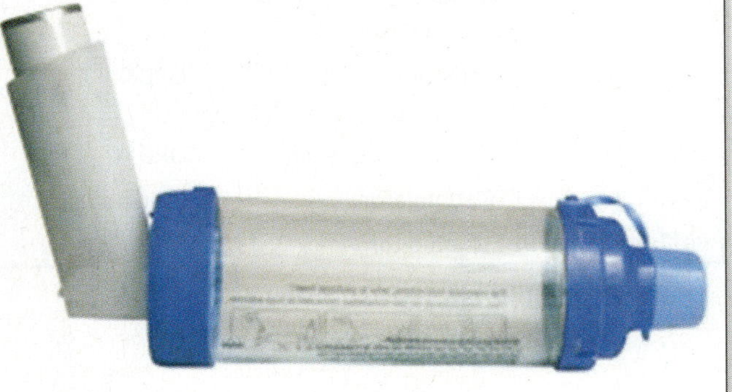

a. Connector
b. Facilitator
c. Spacer
d. Inhaler

3. Which of the following drug is preferred in WHO stage IV for the condition given in the picture?

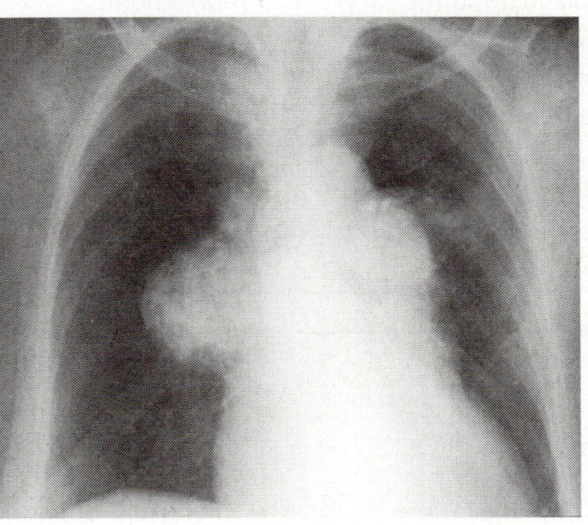

a. Bosentan
b. Sildenafil
c. Epoprostenol
d. Nifedipine

Answers with Explanations to Image-based Questions

1. Ans. (a) Requires coordination with inspiration

(Ref: Goodman Gilman 12th E/P 1035)

- The device in the picture is a dry powder inhaler, which does not require coordination with inspiration. Rather the inspiratory drive pulls drug out of the device.
- MDIs require coordination with inspiration.

2. Ans. (c) Spacer

(Ref: Goodman Gilman 12th E/P 1035)

- Spacer is a device that connects to the MDI and patient inhales drug from the spacer.
- This causes lesser deposition of steroid in oropharyngeal cavity and hence lesser oropharyngeal candidiasis and systemic side effects are seen.
- This device makes it easier to use MDI in children.

3. Ans. (c) Epoprostenol

(Ref: CMDT 2016/P 428)

- The prominent pulmonary arteries in the X-ray are consistent with the diagnosis of PAH.
- For stage IV PAH, the drug of choice is IV epoprostenol.

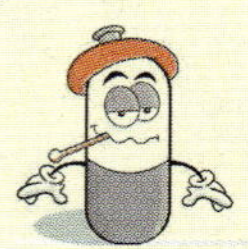

Annexures

Drugs of Choice

Condition	Drug of choice
Allergic bronchopulmonary aspergillosis Proliferative bronchiolitis Cryptogenic organizing pneumonia Eosinophilic pneumonia Pulmonary vasculitis Sarcoidosis	Prednisolone
Bronchial asthma	• **Acute attack:** Short-acting β_2 agonist • **Prophylaxis:** Long-acting β_2 agonist • **Exercise induced:** Inhalational corticosteroids • **Persistent:** Inhalational corticosteroids • **Brittle:** Epinephrine
Chylothorax	Octreotide via chest tube
COPD	Anticholinergics (Tiotropium)
Cough	• **Nonspecific:** Codeine • **Bronchial cancer:** Morphine
Pleurodesis Pericardiodesis	Doxycycline
Pulmonary hypertension	• **Class II and III (Low risk):** Bosentan • **Class IV (High risk):** Epoprostenol
Pulmonary edema (Diuretic of choice)	Loop diuretics

New Drugs

Drugs	Mechanism of action	Uses
Revefenacin	Long-acting anticholinergic (M3 antagonist)	COPD
Tezacaftor + ivacaftor	Tezacaftor is a corrector and ivacaftor is a potentiator of cystic fibrosis transmembrane regulator	Cystic fibrosis
Reslizumab	Anti-IL-5 monoclonal antibody	Severe bronchial asthma
Pirfenidone	Oral antifibrotic p38 MAP kinase inhibitor that reduces growth factor signaling	Idiopathic pulmonary fibrosis
Nintedanib	Inhibits multiple receptor tyrosine kinases (RTKs) like PDGFR, FGFR, VEGFR and nonreceptor tyrosine kinases (nRTKs)	Idiopathic pulmonary fibrosis
Umeclidinium	Antimuscarinic (Long-acting)	COPD
Olodaterol	Long-acting β_2 agonist	COPD
Ivacaftor	CFTR stimulator	Cystic fibrosis
Roflumilast	PDE-4 inhibitor	COPD

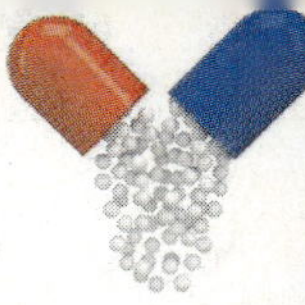

Multiple Choice Questions

1. In a case of acute exacerbation of asthma, salbutamol was given and no improvement noticed. Intravenous corticosteroids and aminophylline was given and condition improved. What is the mechanism of corticosteroids? *(AIIMS Nov 2017)*
   a. Corticosteroids increase bronchial responsiveness to salbutamol
   b. Corticosteroids cause direct bronchodilation when used with xanthines
   c. Corticosteroids indirectly increase the effect of xanthines on adenosine receptor
   d. Corticosteroids increase mucociliary clearance

2. Which of the following is best hypertensive drug for treatment of pulmonary hypertension *(AIIMS May 2015)*
   a. Bosentan b. Amlodipine
   c. Furosemide d. Digoxin

3. Which of the following is not used in the treatment of pulmonary hypertension? *(AIIMS May 2010)*
   a. Calcium-channel blockers
   b. Alpha blockers
   c. Prostacyclins
   d. Endothelin receptor antagonists

4. All are used for treatment of pulmonary hypertension except: *(AIIMS May 2008)*
   a. Endothelin receptor antagonists
   b. Phosphodiesterase inhibitors
   c. Calcium-channel blockers
   d. Beta blockers

5. Which of the following drugs can be administered by subcutaneous route? *(AIIMS May 2013)*
   a. Albuterol b. Terbutaline
   c. Metaproterenol d. Pirbuterol

6. The loading dose of aminophylline is: *(AIIMS May 2006)*
   a. 50–75 mg/kg b. 0.5–1 mg/kg
   c. 2–3.5 mg/kg d. 5–6 mg/kg

7. Which of the following does not have sulfhydryl group? *(Recent Question Dec 2016)*
   a. Bromhexine b. N-acetyl cysteine
   c. Carboxycysteine d. Methyl cysteine

8. Which of the following is not true about aminophylline? *(Recent Question Dec 2016)*
   a. Anti-inflammatory effect
   b. Bronchodilator
   c. Low therapeutic index therefore used
   d. Histone deacetylase stimulator

9. All of the following are inhaled corticosteroid except: *(Recent Question Dec 2016)*
   a. Budesonide b. Triamcinolone
   c. Sodium cromoglicate d. Fluticasone

10. Which drug is not used for acute bronchial asthma? *(Recent Question 2016)*
   a. Salmeterol b. Formoterol
   c. Salbutamol d. Corticosteroids

11. Omalizumab is: *(Recent Question 2016)*
   a. Anti-IgM antibody b. Anti-IgG antibody
   c. Anti-IgE antibody d. Anti-IgD antibody

12. Montelukast is: *(Recent Question 2016)*
   a. Leukotriene antagonist b. Potassium channel opener
   c. Smooth muscle relaxant d. Anti-inflammatory

13. LT antagonists are used in asthma for: *(Recent Question 2016)*
   a. Along with beta agonists to reduce steroids
   b. In place of beta blockers as sole therapy
   c. Prophylactic therapy for mild to moderate asthma
   d. Definitive therapy in acute attack of asthma

14. Mechanism of action of theophylline in bronchial asthma is: *(Recent Question 2016)*
   a. Inhibition of phosphodiesterase-IV
   b. Beta 2 agonism
   c. Anticholinergic action
   d. Inhibition of mucociliary clearance

15. To prevent exercise induced bronchial asthma drug used is: *(Recent Question 2016)*
   a. Sodium cromoglycate b. Ipratropium bromide
   c. Terbutaline d. Epinephrine

16. Which of the following drugs has been found to be useful in acute severe asthma? *(Recent Question 2016)*
   a. Magnesium sulfate b. Anti leukotrienes
   c. Cromolyn sodium d. Cyclosporine

17. Enzyme inhibited by aminophylline: *(Recent Question 2016)*
   a. Monoamine oxidase b. Alcohol dehydrogenase
   c. Phosphodiesterase d. Cytochrome P 450

18. Inhibition of 5-lipoxygenase is useful in: *(Recent Question 2016)*
   a. Cardiac failure b. Bronchial asthma
   c. Hepatic failure d. Arthritis

19. The drug not used in acute asthma is: *(Recent Question 2016)*
   a. Salbutomol b. Ipratropium
   c. Montelukast d. Hydrocortisone

20. Which of the following antiasthma drugs is not a bronchodilator? *(Recent Question 2016)*
   a. Ipratropium bromide b. Theophylline
   c. Formoterol d. Sodium cromoglycate

21. Relatively higher dose of theophylline is required to attain therapeutic plasma concentration in: *(Recent Question 2016)*
   a. Smokers
   b. Congestive heart failure patients
   c. Those receiving erythromycin
   d. Those receiving cimetidine

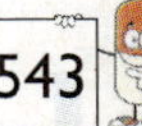

22. Most common side effect of inhaled corticosteroids: *(Recent Question 2016)*
a. Pneumonia
b. Oropharyngeal candidiasis
c. Atrophic rhinitis
d. Pituitary adrenal suppression

23. Which of the following drugs is effective in the treatment of acute asthmatic attack? *(Recent Question 2016)*
a. Zafirlukast b. Nedocromil
c. Prednisolone d. Albuterol

24. The following drug is not useful during acute attack of bronchial asthma: *(Recent Question 2016)*
a. Salbutamol b. Hydrocortisone
c. Cromolyn sodium d. Theophylline

25. All of the following drugs useful in bronchial asthma are bronchodilators except: *(Recent Question 2016)*
a. Theophylline b. Salmeterol
c. Beclomethasone d. Ipratropium

26. Which of the following is a bronchodilator? *(Recent Question 2016)*
a. Corticosteroids b. Salmeterol
c. Ketotifen d. Sodium cromoglycate

27. All of the following drugs can precipitate acute attack of asthma except: *(Recent Question 2016)*
a. Phenylbutazone b. Naproxen
c. Glucocorticoids d. Aspirin

28. Dextromethorphan is an: *(Recent Question 2016)*
a. Antihistaminic b. Antitussive
c. Expectorant d. Antiallergic

29. Which is a 'soft steroid' used in bronchial asthma? *(Recent Question 2016)*
a. Budesonide b. Dexamethasone
c. Ciclesonide d. Flunisolide

30. Directly acting cough suppressant is: *(Recent Question 2016)*
a. Dextromethorphan b. Bromhexine
c. Acetylcysteine d. Carbapentate

31. Complications of aerosol steroids used include: *(Recent Question 2016)*
a. Oral candidiasis b. Cushing's syndrome
c. Decreased ACTH d. Systemic complications

32. Release of histamine and leukotrienes from mast cells is prevented by: *(Recent Question 2016)*
a. Zileuton b. Nedocromil sodium
c. Zafirlukast d. Fexofenadine

33. Theophylline overdose causes: *(Recent Question 2016)*
a. Bradycardia b. Seizures
c. Drowsiness d. Bronchospasm

34. In theophylline metabolism, drug interactions occurs with all except: *(Recent Question 2016)*
a. Cimetidine b. Phenobarbitone
c. Rifampin d. Tetracyclines

35. Which of the following is not a bronchodilator? *(Recent Question 2016)*
a. Ipratropium bromide b. Methylxanthines
c. Steroids d. Anticholinergic

36. Mechanism of action of zileuton is: *(Recent Question 2016)*
a. Inhibits production of IgE
b. Inhibits lipoxygenase
c. Inhibits cyclooxygenase
d. Inhibits activity of mast cells

37. Montelukast mechanism of action is: *(Recent Question 2016)*
a. Competitive inhibitor of leukotriene synthesis
b. Inhibits alpha receptor
c. Beta receptor agonist
d. Noncompetitive inhibitor of leukotriene synthesis

38. An opioid which has an antitussive action is: *(Recent Question 2016)*
a. Dextromethorphan b. Oxeladin
c. Codeine d. Narcotine

39. Drug not used in the treatment of acute asthma is: *(Recent Question 2016)*
a. Oral prednisolone b. Inhalational salbutamol
c. Inhalational salmeterol d. IV corticosteroid

40. Theophylline levels in blood are increased by: *(Recent Question 2016)*
a. Barbiturates b. Methotrexate
c. Cimetidine d. All of the above

41. Epinephrine in asthma acts on: *(Recent Question 2016)*
a. β_1 receptors b. β_2 receptors
c. α_1 receptors d. α_2 receptors

42. Leukotriene receptor inhibitor is: *(Recent Question 2016)*
a. Ipratropium b. Salbutamol
c. Steroids d. Zafirleukast

43. Theophylline metabolism is increased by: *(Recent Question 2016)*
a. Barbiturates b. Carbamazepine
c. Phenytoin d. Smoking

44. All are inhalational steroids except: *(Recent Question 2016)*
a. Sodium cromoglycate b. Triamcinolone
c. Beclmethasone d. Budesonide

45. Drug inhibits histamine release: *(Recent Question 2016)*
a. d-penicillamine b. Tubocurarine
c. Atracurium d. Nedocromil sodium

46. Size of particle for aerosol therapy is: *(Recent Question 2016)*
a. 2–5 μm b. 1–2 μm
c. 5–10 μm d. 10–15 μm

47. The only FDA approved application of nitric oxide is: *(Recent Question 2016)*
a. Primary pulmonary hypertension
b. Newborn with pulmonary hypertension
c. Congestive cardiac failure
d. HAPE

48. True-IgE antibodies used in asthma is? *(Recent Question 2016)*
a. Active against
b. Fragilis
c. Superior to ceftriaxone for treatment of meningitis
d. Poor CSF penetration
e. Excreted rapidly by kidney

49. Mechanism of action of ketotifen is? *(Recent Question 2016)*

a. Stabilising mast cell
b. H1-receptor antagonism
c. Leukotriene receptor antagonist
d. All of the above

50. Corticosteroid has which action in asthma: *(Recent Question 2016)*

a. Inhibition of antigen antibody reaction
b. Antagonist at LT receptor
c. Inhibition of leukotriene synthesis
d. None of the above

51. Corticosteroid which is given by inhalation route is: *(Recent Question 2016)*

a. Prednisolone b. Beclomethasone
c. Dexamethasone d. Hydrocortisone

52. Which drug used in bronchial asthma needs monitoring? *(Recent Question 2016)*

a. Theophylline b. Cromoglycate
c. Salmeterol d. Terbutaline

53. Which of the following drug(s) is/are used for acute asthma? *(PGI May 2018)*

a. Terbutaline b. Budesonide
c. Salbutamol d. Formoterol
e. Ipratropium

54. Drug which can be given by inhalation route: *(PGI Nov. 2016)*

a. Zileuton b. Steroid
c. Salbutamol d. Tobramycin

55. All adverse effects of theophylline are mediated by A1 receptor except: *(JIPMER May 2018)*

a. Cardiac arrhythmias b. Diuresis
c. Seizures d. GI Discomfort

56. A 24-year-old male presents to you for the routine follow-up of his asthma. He is currently on albuterol, corticosteroids and salmeterol, all via inhaled route. The patient is compliant with his medications, but still complains of episodic shortness of breath and wheezing. The peak expiratory flow (PEF) has improved since the last visit, but is still less than the ideal-predicted values, based on age, sex, and height. You have added montelukast in his treatment regimen. What is the mechanism of action of this drug? *(JIPMER 2016)*

a. It blocks receptors for certain arachidonic acid metabolites
b. It activates the adrenal receptors on the bronchial smooth muscles
c. It inhibits lipoxygenase enzyme, decreasing production of inflammatory leukotrienes
d. It inhibits the release of inflammatory substances from mast cells

Practice Questions & Answers from 57 to 62 are given at the end of the chapter.

Answers with Explanations to Multiple Choice Questions

1. Ans. (a) Corticosteroids increase bronchial responsiveness to salbutamol

(Ref: Goodman Gilman 12th edition, Page 1049)

- Mechanism of steroids in acute asthma attack
  - Increased responsiveness to β_2 agonists
  - Decreased mucous secretion
- Decreased inflammatory cell response
  - Steroids increase transcription of β_2 receptor genes and hence increase responsiveness to β_2 agonists.
  - β_2 agonists on the other hand increase effect of steroids by enhancing action of glucocorticoid receptors.
  - Theophylline increase effect of steroids by activating enzyme histone deacetylase which is a target for steroids as well.

2. Ans. (b) Amlodipine

(Ref: CMDT 2016/P 428)

- The only hypertensive class of drugs used in pulmonary hypertension are calcium channel blockers and hence amlodipine is the answer.
- CCBs are the best hypertensive drugs for treatment of pulmonary hypertension.
- Prostaglandin I_2 analogs are the best drugs for treatment of pulmonary hypertension and hence are reserved for class IV patients (high risk).

3. Ans. (b) Alpha blockers

(Ref: CMDT 2016/P 428)

Drugs used in Pulmonary Hypertension

- CCBs
- Prostaglandin I_2 or prostacyclin analogs
- ET receptor antagonists
- PDE-5 Inhibitors
- Guanylate cyclase stimulator (Riociguat)

4. Ans. (d) Beta blockers

(Ref: CMDT 2016/P 428)

5. Ans. (b) Terbutaline

(Ref: Goodman Gilman 12th E/P 1038)

6. Ans. (d) 5–6 mg/kg

(Ref: Goodman Gilman 12th E/P 1042)

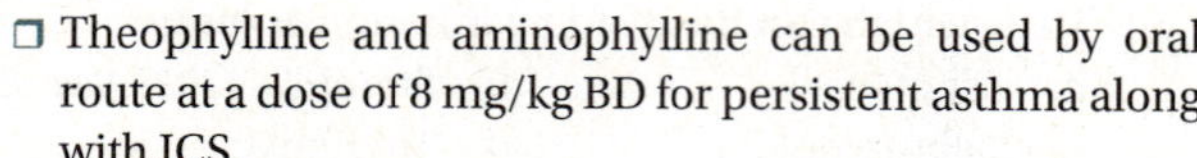

- Theophylline and aminophylline can be used by oral route at a dose of 8 mg/kg BD for persistent asthma along with ICS.
- Aminophylline can be used by intravenous route with a loading dose of 6 mg/kg followed by 0.5 mg/kg/hr for treatment of an acute attack of asthma.

7. Ans. (a) Bromhexine

(Ref: Goodman Gilman 12th E/P 1057)

8. Ans. (c) Low therapeutic index therefore used

(Ref: Goodman Gilman 12th E/P 1042)

9. Ans. (c) Sodium cromoglicate

(Ref: Goodman Gilman 12th E/P 1051)

10. Ans. (a) Salmeterol

(Ref: Goodman Gilman 12th E/P 1038)

- Salmeterol has a slower onset of action and hence not useful in acuteasthma attack.
- Formoterol and salbutamol are faster acting and hence used in acute attack as bronchodilators.
- Corticosteroids either IV or oral can be used for an acute attack.

11. Ans. (c) Anti-IgE antibody

(Ref: Goodman Gilman 12th E/P 1054)

12. Ans. (a) Leukotriene antagonist

(Ref: Goodman Gilman 12th E/P 1052)

13. Ans. (c) Prophylactic therapy for mild to moderate asthma

(Ref: Goodman Gilman 12th E/P 1052)

14. Ans. (a) Inhibition of phosphodiesterase-IV

(Ref: Goodman Gilman 12th E/P 1041)

15. Ans. (a) Sodium cromoglycate

(Ref: Goodman Gilman 12th E/P 1054)

- Leukotriene pathway inhibitors are given by oral route in bronchial asthma progressive on ICS and for prophylaxis of **exercise induced asthma**.

16. Ans. (a) Magnesium sulfate

(Ref: Goodman Gilman 12th E/P 1046)

- Magnesium can cause bronchodilation by inhibiting calcium transport into smooth muscle cells. It is under trial for treatment of an acute attack of bronchial asthma.

17. Ans. (c) Phosphodiesterase

(Ref: Goodman Gilman 12th E/P 1041)

18. Ans. (b) Bronchial asthma

(Ref: Goodman Gilman 12th E/P 1052)

19. Ans. (c) Monteleukast

(Ref: Goodman Gilman 12th E/P 1052)

- Monteleukast is a LT inhibitor given by oral route in bronchial asthma progressive on ICS and for prophylaxis of **exercise-induced asthma**.

20. Ans. (d) Sodium cromoglycate

(Ref: Goodman Gilman 12th E/P 1052)

- **Cromolyn sodium and nedocromil sodium are mast cell stabilizers, which prevent mast cell degranulation and is used for prophylaxis of bronchial asthma.**

21. Ans. (a) Smokers

(Ref: Goodman Gilman 12th E/P 1043)

- Smoke of cigarette is an enzyme inducer and hence higher dose of theophylline is required in smokers.

22. Ans. (b) Oropharyngeal candidiasis

(Ref: Goodman Gilman 12th E/P 1050)

- Hoarseness of voice is the most common side effect of inhalational steroids followed by oropharyngeal candidiasis.
- Hence oropharyngeal candidiasis is best answer.

23. Ans. (d) Albuterol

(Ref: Goodman Gilman 12th E/P 1038)

24. Ans. (c) Cromolyn sodium

(Ref: Goodman Gilman 12th E/P 1052)

25. Ans. (c) Beclomethasone

(Ref: Goodman Gilman 12th E/P 1050)

26. Ans. (b) Salmeterol

(Ref: Goodman Gilman 12th E/P 1038)

27. Ans. (c) Glucocorticoids

(Ref: Goodman Gilman 12th E/P 1038)

- Glucocorticoids are drugs of choice for persistent asthma and for prophylaxis of exercise induced asthma.
- All other drugs in the options are NSAIDs and can precipitate asthma by potentiating the LOX pathway.

28. Ans. (b) Antitussive

(Ref: Goodman Gilman 12th E/P 1057)

29. Ans. (c) Ciclesonide

(Ref: Goodman Gilman 12th E/P 1050)

- Ciclesonide and beclomethasone are activated in the respiratory tract by esterases and are known as soft steroids due to lesser side effects associated.
- Butoxocort and tipredene are other soft steroids that have been developed but not approved due to poor clinical effect.

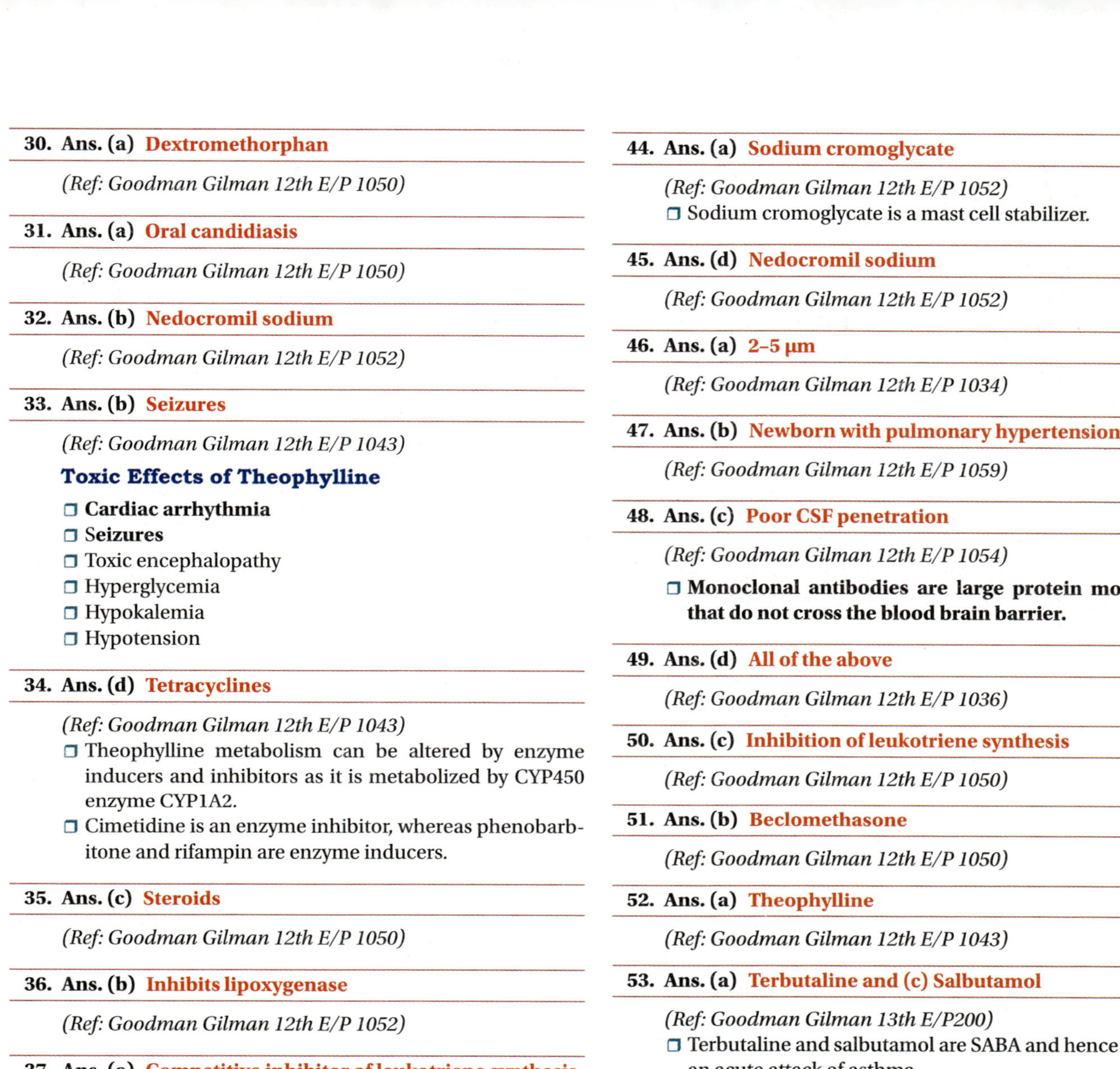

30. Ans. (a) Dextromethorphan

(Ref: Goodman Gilman 12th E/P 1050)

31. Ans. (a) Oral candidiasis

(Ref: Goodman Gilman 12th E/P 1050)

32. Ans. (b) Nedocromil sodium

(Ref: Goodman Gilman 12th E/P 1052)

33. Ans. (b) Seizures

(Ref: Goodman Gilman 12th E/P 1043)

Toxic Effects of Theophylline

- **Cardiac arrhythmia**
- **Seizures**
- Toxic encephalopathy
- Hyperglycemia
- Hypokalemia
- Hypotension

34. Ans. (d) Tetracyclines

(Ref: Goodman Gilman 12th E/P 1043)

- Theophylline metabolism can be altered by enzyme inducers and inhibitors as it is metabolized by CYP450 enzyme CYP1A2.
- Cimetidine is an enzyme inhibitor, whereas phenobarbitone and rifampin are enzyme inducers.

35. Ans. (c) Steroids

(Ref: Goodman Gilman 12th E/P 1050)

36. Ans. (b) Inhibits lipoxygenase

(Ref: Goodman Gilman 12th E/P 1052)

37. Ans. (a) Competitive inhibitor of leukotriene synthesis

(Ref: Goodman Gilman 12th E/P 1052)

38. Ans. (c) Codeine

(Ref: Goodman Gilman 12th E/P 1058)

39. Ans. (c) Inhalational salmeterol

(Ref: Goodman Gilman 12th E/P 1038)

40. Ans. (c) Cimetidine

(Ref: Goodman Gilman 12th E/P 1043)

41. Ans. (b) β_2 receptors

(Ref: Goodman Gilman 12th E/P 1050)

42. Ans. (d) Zafirleukast

(Ref: Goodman Gilman 12th E/P 1052)

43. Ans. (d) Smoking

(Ref: Goodman Gilman 12th E/P 1043)

44. Ans. (a) Sodium cromoglycate

(Ref: Goodman Gilman 12th E/P 1052)

- Sodium cromoglycate is a mast cell stabilizer.

45. Ans. (d) Nedocromil sodium

(Ref: Goodman Gilman 12th E/P 1052)

46. Ans. (a) 2–5 µm

(Ref: Goodman Gilman 12th E/P 1034)

47. Ans. (b) Newborn with pulmonary hypertension

(Ref: Goodman Gilman 12th E/P 1059)

48. Ans. (c) Poor CSF penetration

(Ref: Goodman Gilman 12th E/P 1054)

- **Monoclonal antibodies are large protein molecules that do not cross the blood brain barrier.**

49. Ans. (d) All of the above

(Ref: Goodman Gilman 12th E/P 1036)

50. Ans. (c) Inhibition of leukotriene synthesis

(Ref: Goodman Gilman 12th E/P 1050)

51. Ans. (b) Beclomethasone

(Ref: Goodman Gilman 12th E/P 1050)

52. Ans. (a) Theophylline

(Ref: Goodman Gilman 12th E/P 1043)

53. Ans. (a) Terbutaline and (c) Salbutamol

(Ref: Goodman Gilman 13th E/P200)

- Terbutaline and salbutamol are SABA and hence used in an acute attack of asthma.
- Budesonide is an ICS used in persistent asthma.
- Formoterol is a LABA used along with ICS in persistent bronchial asthma and are also first line drugs in nocturnal asthma.
- Ipratropium can be used along with LABA in persistent bronchial asthma.

54. Ans. (b) Steroid; (c) Salbutamol; (d) Tobramycin

(Ref: Katzung 13th edition, Page 346)

- Steroids are used by inhalational route in bronchial asthma
- Salbutamol is an inhalational β_2 agonist used in bronchial asthma
- Tobramycin is an aminoglycoside given by inhalational route for treatment of pseudomonas infection in patients of cystic fibrosis.

55. Ans (d) GI discomfort

(Ref: Goodman Gilman 13th E/P 735)

56. Ans. (a) It blocks receptors for certain arachidonic acid metabolites

(Ref: Goodman Gilman 12th E/P 1052)

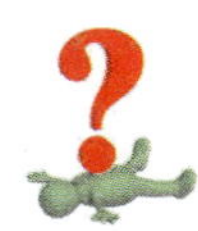

Practice Questions

57. Which of the following is the drug of choice for treatment of brittle asthma?

a. Salbutamol b. ICS
c. Ipratropium d. Epinephrine

Ans. (d) Epinephrine

(Ref: Harrison 19th E/P 1680)

- Brittle asthma is characterized by fluctuation in the symptoms being on adequate clinical treatment.
- For such patients the cause is thought to be anaphylactoid reaction of bronchi and hence epinephrine is best drug.
- In type 1 brittle asthma there is a stable pattern of fluctuation, whereas in type 2 there is a rapid fluctuation that might even cause death.

58. Which of the following is the safest antiasthmatic drug?

a. Salbutamol b. Ipratropium
c. Zileuton d. Cromolyn

Ans. (d) Cromolyn

(Ref: Goodman Gilman 12th E/P 1052)

59. The preferred drug for low-risk group patients of PAH is

a. Sildenafil b. Bosentan
c. Epoprosterenol d. Riociguat

Ans. (b) Bosentan

(Ref: CMDT 2016/P 428)

60. Omalizumab is contraindicated in bronchial asthma associated with:

a. Allergic rhinitis b. COPD
c. PAH d. Atopic dermatitis

Ans. (d) Atopic dermatitis

(Ref: Goodman Gilman 12th E/P 1054)

- Omalizumab is contraindicated in bronchial asthma associated with atopic dermatitis, due to high levels of IgE.

61. ALT/AST monitoring is required with the use of following drug for asthma:

a. Theophylline b. Salbutamol
c. ICS d. Zileuton

Ans. (d) Zileuton

(Ref: Goodman Gilman 12th E/P 1052)

62. Which of the following is drug of choice for prophylaxis of exercise induced asthma?

a. Salbutamol b. Salmeterol
c. ICS d. Cromolyn

Ans. (c) ICS

(Ref: Goodman Gilman 12th E/P 1050)

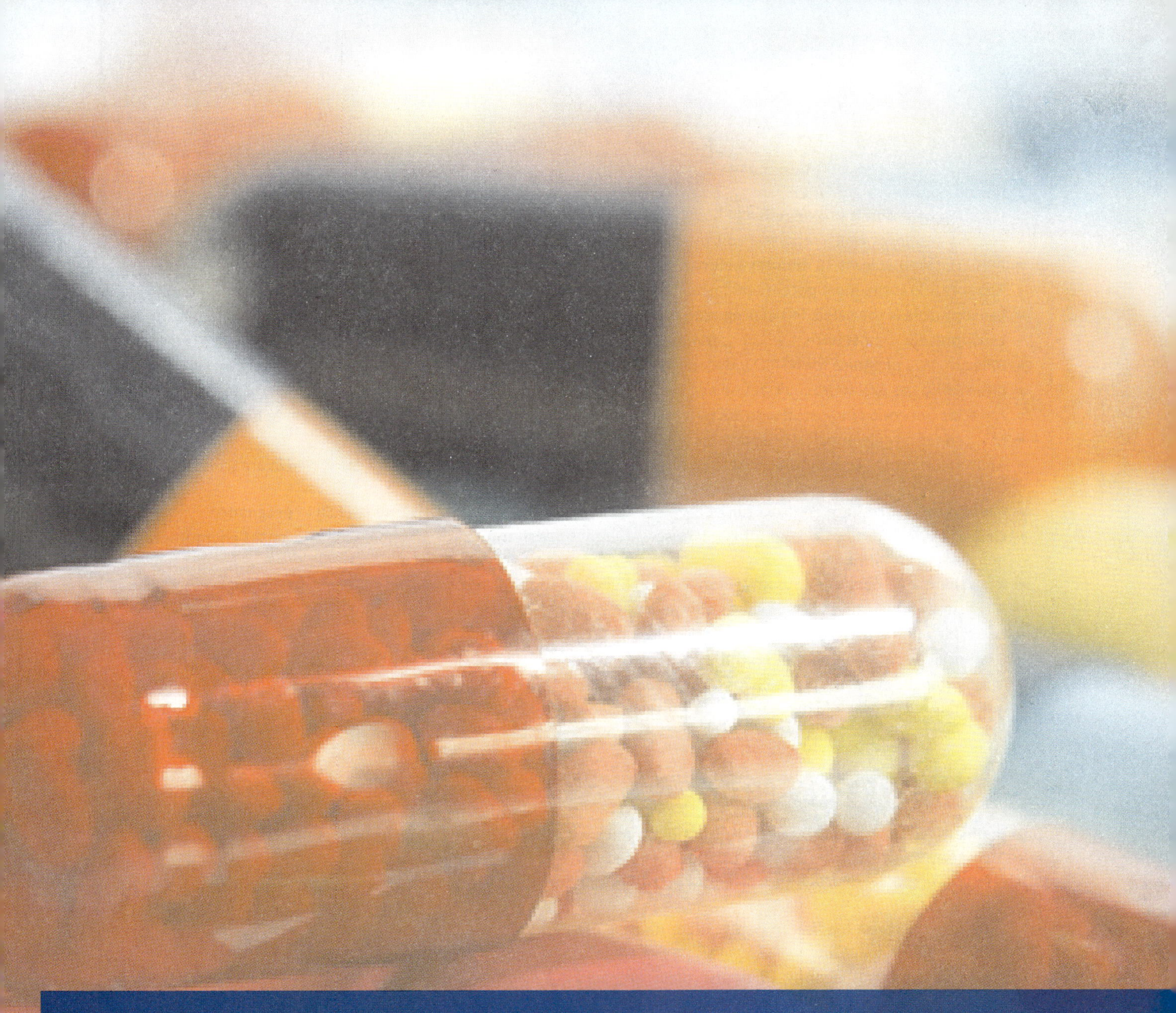

Gastro-intestinal Tract

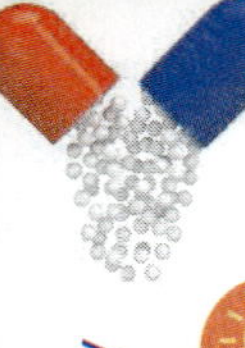

One Liners

- Proton pump inhibitors (PPIS) are called as hit and run drugs because they have a **short half-life** of 30–120 minutes, but their **duration of action is prolonged** (>24 hours) due to irreversible binding.
- PPIs are prodrugs which require **acidic medium** for their activation.
- PPIs are taken at least **30 minutes before meal** for adequate clinical effect.
- **Rabeprazole** is the most potent and fastest acting PPI.
- **Lansoprazole** is the safest PPI in **pregnancy**.
- **Lansoprazole** is most potent whereas **pantoprazole** is least potent enzyme inhibitor.
- **PPIs** are drug of choice for NSAID induced gastric ulcer, but **misoprostol** is the most specific drug for same.
- **Cimetidine** has antiandrogenic action and hence it causes **gynecomastia** and impotence in males.
- **Antacids** are **contraindicated** with **sucralfate**, as the former can prevent crosslinking of sucralfate by increasing gastric pH.
- Most common side effect of **misoprostol** and **cisapride** is **diarrhea**.
- **Aluminium** causes **constipation** whereas **magnesium** causes **diarrhea**, thus both are combined in antacids to neutralize each-others effect.
- **Antacids** and **sucralfate** are the drug of choice for **gastroesophageal reflux disease (GERD) in pregnancy**.
- **Ondansetron** is drug of choice for **early onset** whereas **aprepitant** is drug of choice for **late onset chemotherapy induced nausea and vomiting**.
- **Dronabinol** and **nabilone** cause hypotension and hence **BP monitoring** should be done.
- **Metoclopramide causes EPS** whereas domperidone is devoid of same.
- **Cisapride** and **tegaserod** were banned due to risk of **QT prolongation**.
- **Octreotide** is drug of choice in **secretory diarrhea** as in case of **HIV**.
- **Mesalamine** is the drug of choice for **ulcerative colitis**.
- **Infliximab** is the drug of choice for **Chron's disease**.

PEPTIC ULCER DISEASE

- A peptic ulcer is a breach in the gastric or duodenal mucosa due to depletion of protective factors. The damage is added upon by action of gastric hydrochloric acid and pepsin on the exposed area.
- The most common cause leading to peptic ulcer disease are NSAIDs and *H. pylori* infection.
- The treatments aimed at healing of peptic ulcer are acid antisecretory agents, gastroprotective agents, antacids and anti-*H. pylori* agents.
- The antisecretory agents are first line drugs whereas others are second line.

ACID ANTISECRETORY AGENTS

- Hydrochloric acid is secreted by parietal cells and regulated by other cells like G and D cells.
- The receptors present in a parietal cell are M3, H2 and CCK2, for which the ligands are acetylcholine, histamine and gastrin respectively.
- The action of ligands on the receptors activate **proton pumps (H^+ K^+ ATPase)**, which secrete H+ into the lumen in exchange for K^+.
- G cells release gastrin, which stimulates the enterochromaffin like cells (ECL) to release histamine, which stimulates parietal cells.
- D cells secrete somatostatin which has antagonistic action on G cells and decrease gastrin release.
- The antisecretory agents can target the mentioned receptors and proton pumps. Thus we have drugs like **proton pump inhibitors, anticholinergic drugs, H2 antagonist and CCK2 antagonist.**

Conceptual Box-1

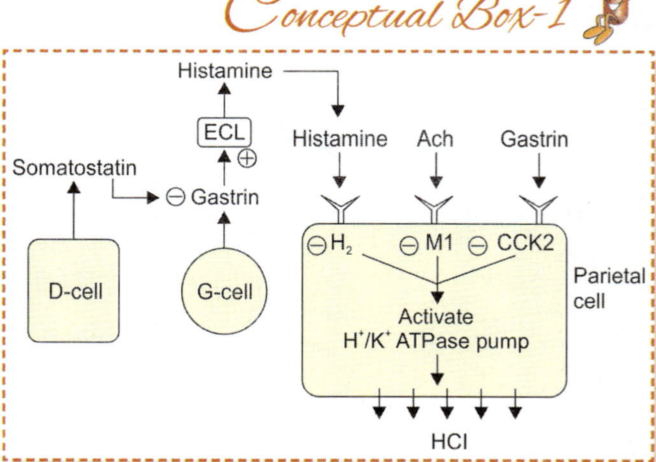

Proton Pump Inhibitors

Mechanism of Action of PPIs

- Proton pump inhibitors (PPIs) are the most effective anti-acid secretory agents as they block the terminal step in hydrochloric acid secretion, i.e. **proton pumps (H^+ K^+ ATPase)**. Omeprazole, esomeprazole, lansoprazole, rabeprazole, pantoprazole etc. are the drugs in this class.

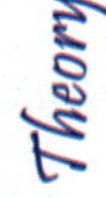
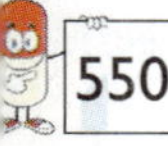

- After PPIs are ingested, they are absorbed into systemic circulation and secreted into the canaliculi of parietal cells.
- During food intake there is release of hydrochloric acid into these canaliculi, and the **acidic medium activates the PPIs**, which are prodrugs. The activated PPIs block the proton pumps.
- This is the reason for which PPIs are given **at least 30 minutes before food** intake **(usually before breakfast)**, so that they are present in the canaliculi at the time of hydrochloric acid secretion.
- Maximum inhibition of acid secretion is seen after **2 hours** and after stopping it takes **2–5 days** to normalize.

Pharmacokinetics and Pharmacodynamics of PPIs

- Though PPIs have a **short half-life** of 30–120 minutes, their **duration of action is prolonged** (>24 hours) due to irreversible binding the reason why they are called as **hit and run drugs**.
- Since PPI are acid labile they are given as enteric coated capsules. The order of acid stability of PPI is **pantoprazole > omeprazole > lansoprazole > rabeprazole**. Thus pantoprazole is most acid stable and rabeprazole is most acid labile PPI. Rabeprazole has the highest pKa of 5.
- Omeprazole is a racemic mixture of R and S enantiomer; since S enantiomer is slowly eliminated due to insensitivity to CYP2C19, **esomeprazole** has been synthesized, which is **longer acting than omeprazole**.
- **Rabeprazole is the most potent, longest and fastest acting PPI**.
- Esomeprazole and lansoprazole are excreted by liver and hence dose reduction is required in liver failure.

Uses of PPIs

- PPIs are the drug of choice for treatment of **peptic ulcer disease, NSAID induced ulcer, stress ulcer, Zollinger-Ellison syndrome, GERD and empirical treatment of dyspepsia.**
- In NSAID induced gastric ulcers, PPIs are drugs of choice, whereas **misoprostol** is the **most specific drug**.
- Intravenous PPIs are also drugs of choice in an **acutely bleeding gastric ulcer** as an increase in gastric pH promotes coagulation and prevents clot dissolution.
- PPIs are usually avoided in pregnancy and **lansoprazole is the PPI of choice in pregnancy**.

Side Effects of PPIs

- Most common side effects related to indigestion of food are nausea, flatulence, constipation, diarrhea etc. PPIs can also cause interstitial nephritis.
- An increase in gastric pH decreases the antimicrobial barrier of gastrointestinal tract (GIT) and hence **pneumonia** and **pseudomembranous enterocolitis** can be seen.
- A decrease in gastric acid secretion also causes a compensatory increase in gastrin release and causes **hypergastrinemia**.
- Long-term therapy decreases absorption of **calcium (osteoporosis, hip fracture), iron, vitamin B12** and **magnesium (hypomagnesemia)**

Drug Interactions of PPIs

- All PPI are metabolized by CYP2C19 and CYP2C19 activates clopidogrel. Hence PPIs can decrease activation clopidogrel and its antiaggregant effect. The PPI with least effect on clopidogrel is pantoprazole.
- The order of enzyme inhibition is **omeprazole > lansoprazole > rabeprazole > pantoprazole.** Thus pantoprazole being the least potent enzyme inhibitor has least drug interactions.
- **Omeprazole** is both **enzyme inducer** (CYP1A2) and **inhibitor** (CYP2C19) whereas **lansoprazole** is an enzyme inhibitor.
- **PPIs** can also competitively decrease elimination of methotrexate and precipitate its toxicity.

Recent Advances

Tenatoprazole: It is a reversible PPI, which is longer acting than others and thus can inhibit nocturnal acid secretion beneficial in GERD. Tenatoprazole is the only PPI not metabolized by CP450 enzymes and has longest half-life of 9 hours. It is more acid stable than pantoprazole.

Vonoprazan and **Revaprazan:** These are potassium competitive acid blockers (P-CAB), which compete with potassium to bind to proton (H^+K^+ ATPase) pump and inhibit it. They are irreversible inhibitors and cause faster acid suppression.

H_2 Blockers

- Histamine is primarily responsible for nocturnal acid secretion, which is inhibited by H_2 blockers.
- The first H_2 blocker cimetidine was invented by **James Black**, which followed others like ranitidine, famotidine and nizatidine.
- Cimetidine is least potent and shortest acting whereas famotidine is the longest acting and most potent H_2 blocker.
- Food increases and antacids decrease absorption of H_2 blockers.
- H_2 blockers are used but less preferred for peptic ulcer disease, Zollinger-Ellison syndrome, stress ulcer and GERD treatment.
- H_2 blockers are the drugs of choice for **prophylaxis of aspiration pneumonia in patients undergoing surgery**. Maximum ulcer healing effect is seen at least after **8 weeks** of therapy.
- **Cimetidine** causes **antiandrogenic** action along with **inhibition of estradiol metabolism** and **increase in prolactin levels**. This causes gynecomastia and impotence in males and galactorrhea in females.
- Cimetidine is also an enzyme inhibitor and causes drug interactions. Ranitidine is a less potent enzyme inhibitor as compared to cimetidine.
- CNS (confusion, delirium etc.) and GIT (nausea, **constipation** etc.) side effects can be seen with this class. Pancytopenia and **elevated ALT/AST** can be rarely associated.
- **Tolerance** is another drawback that can be seen within 3 days of treatment in patients.

Anticholinergics

- Pirenzepine and telenzepine decrease acid secretion by inhibiting M_1 receptors of the intramural ganglia, though M_3 receptors are present in parietal cells, which can be blocked by other anticholinergics.
- These drugs are less preferred now because of availability of better classes of drugs.

Recent Advances

Netazepide is a CCK2 or B/gastrin receptor antagonist, which is under trial for treatment of gastric neuroendocrine tumors like carcinoid tumor.

Classification of Drugs used in Peptic Ulcer Disease

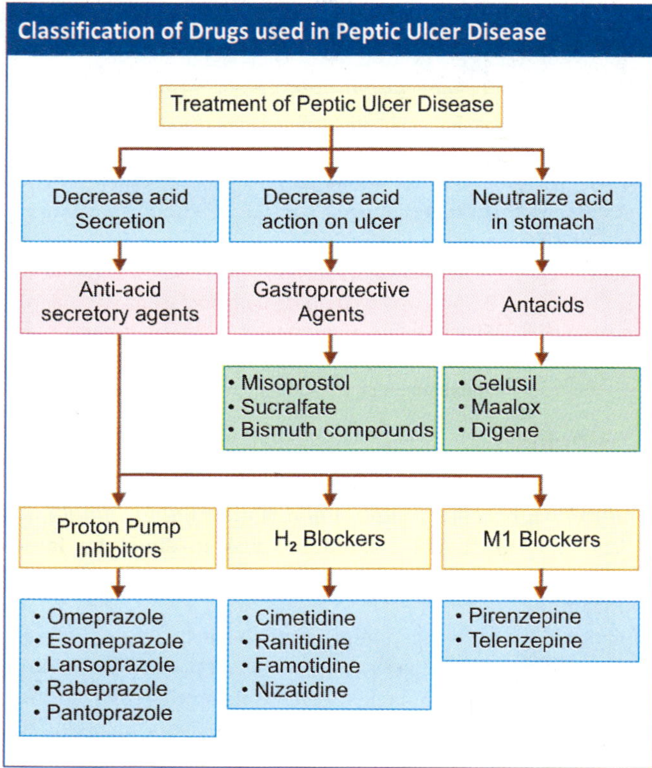

GASTROPROTECTIVE AGENTS

- Prostaglandins are the physiological gastroprotectors. They stimulate Gs subtype prostaglandin receptors like EP_2 and EP_4, thus increasing cyclic AMP which **stimulates mucin and bicarbonate production**.
- Stimulation of Gi subtype prostaglandin receptor, i.e. EP_3 decreases cyclic AMP resulting in **decreased hydrochloric acid secretion**.
- Prostaglandins also act by **inhibiting gastrin release** and increasing mucosal blood flow.

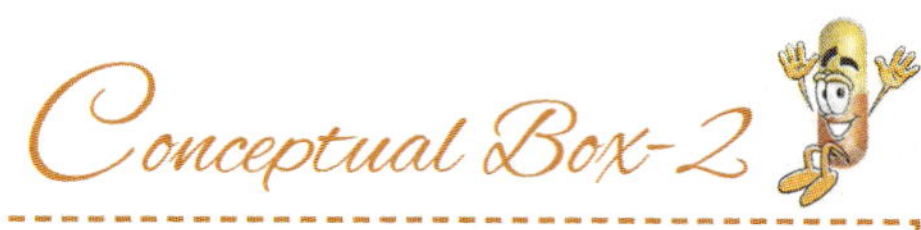

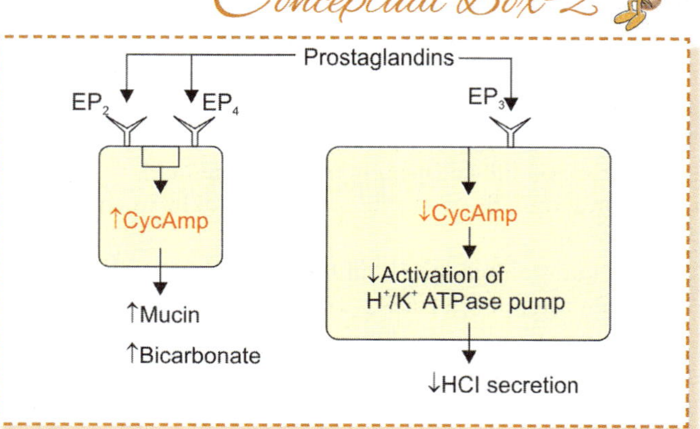

Misoprostol

- **Misoprostol** is a **prostaglandin E_1 analog**, which acts by the mechanism mentioned above. It is a prodrug that is activated into misoprostol acid.
- Misoprostol is the **most specific drug** for treatment of NSAID induced gastric ulcer (200 micrograms QID) and hence is available in fixed dose combination with diclofenac.
- It is also used to **maintain patency of ductus arteriosus** and for **medical abortion** along with mifepristone.
- It has both dose dependent effects as well as side effects. Most common side effect is **diarrhea** with abdominal cramps that begins after 2 weeks of therapy but is self-limiting.
- It is contraindicated in **inflammatory bowel disease** as it can be worsened.

Sucralfate

- Sucralfate is made up of sucrose and aluminum hydroxide.
- It is given on empty stomach before meal (1 g QID) as **acid stimulates crosslinking that produces a viscous polymer** that sticks to ulcer base and protects it.
- Apart from this, it also stimulates prostaglandin and epithelial growth factor(EGF) synthesis and binds to bile acid.
- Because of its protective effect it is used for prophylaxis of stress ulcer, peptic ulcer, as rectal enema in radiation proctitis and solitary rectal ulcers.
- Since it binds to bile acid, biliary gastritis and esophagitis are also its indications.
- **Constipation** is the most common side effect, whereas hypophosphatemia and gastric bezoars can be rarely seen.
- Renal failure can cause aluminum toxicity and hence is **contraindicated in renal failure**. Since acid activates sucralfate, antacids are contraindicated within 30 minutes of intake. Though PPIs and H_2 blockers can be used with sucralfate, as these drugs take time to decrease secretion of hydrochloric acid.

Bismuth Compounds

- **Colloidal bismuth subcitrate (CBS)** and **bismuth subsalicylate** are the drugs in this class, which act by physically **binding to ulcers and promoting mucin** and **bicarbonate production**.
- The anti-*H. pylori* action has led to emergence of this class in treatment of *H. pylori* **associated ulcer**.
- Bismuth subsalicylate is also used for prophylaxis and treatment of **traveller's diarrhea** due to its antisecretory effect.
- Side effects associated with this class are **constipation** and **black discoloration** of **stool** and **tongue**.
- Bismuth subsalicylate can precipitate **Reye's syndrome** whereas colloidal bismuth subcitrate is associated with **neurotoxicity**.

Miscellaneous Gastroprotective Agents

Carbenoxolone	Carbenoxolone is a gastroprotective agent derived from **licorice root**. It increases mucin production and its viscosity. Mineralocorticoid receptor activation causes **hypertension** and **hypokalemia**.
Rebamipide	Rebamipide stimulates prostaglandin synthesis and has antioxidant effect.
Ecabet	Ecabet stimulates prostaglandin synthesis.

ANTACIDS

- Antacids use began with sodium bicarbonate and calcium carbonate but are less preferred due to side effects like **milk alkali syndrome** (alkalosis, hypercalcemia and renal failure), when administered with milk.
- The currently preferred antacids are mixtures of aluminum and magnesium salts; **Al** relaxes smooth muscles and causes **constipation** and **Mg** contracts smooth muscles and causes **diarrhea**. Hence both neutralize each-others side effect related to smooth muscle activity.
- The preferred antacids are maalox, gelusil, digene etc. The dosing for uncomplicated ulcer is 1 and 3 hours after meals whereas every 30-60 minutes for complicated ulcers.
- Their use is primarily for **ulcer healing** as well as acute relief from symptoms of dyspepsia.
- **Antacids** and **sucralfate** are the drugs of choice for **GERD in pregnancy**.
- Antacids are also drug of choice for **GERD in children**; PPI are used in severe cases of GERD due to safety concerns.
- Aluminum is associated with osteoporosis, encephalopathy and myopathy. Antacids are contraindicated in **renal failure** due to risk of aluminum toxicity.
- **Simethicone** is a surfactant added to decrease surface tension of gas bubbles in stomach that bursts bubbles and **expels gas thereby relieving flatulence**. There is also a decreased foaming and associated GERD.
- **Alginate** is also combined with antacids which form a viscous layer that floats over gastric contents and prevents GERD.

ANTI-*H. PYLORI* AGENTS

Anti-*H. pylori* agents are used for treatment of associated gastric ulcer by combination of multiple antimicrobials with PPIs or H_2 blockers along with bismuth in resistant cases. Combination of three drugs (triple therapy) started and in case of poor response four drugs combination is preferred (quadruple therapy) for **14 days**.

Drugs for Triple Therapy and Quadruple Therapy

Triple Therapy	Quadruple Therapy
PPI BD Clarithromycin Metronidazole or amoxicillin	PPI BD Metronidazole Tetracycline Bismuth subsalicylate
PPI BD Levofloxacin Amoxicillin	PPI BD Tinidazole Clarithromycin Amoxicillin

ANTIEMETICS

$5HT_3$ ANTAGONISTS

- $5HT_3$ receptors are present in CTZ area that cause nausea and vomiting when stimulated by 5HT released from enterochromaffin like cells in response to anticancer drugs.
- Thus, inhibitors of 5HT3 are effective in **chemotherapy induced nausea and vomiting**.
- **Ondansetron** is shortest acting and is **drug of choice in early onset chemotherapy induced nausea and vomiting**.
- Palonosetron is most potent and longest acting and hence preferred in late onset chemotherapy induced nausea and vomiting.
- Other uses are nausea and vomiting post **abdominal irradiation**, in **pregnancy** and **postoperative patients**.
- The route of administration is IV, oral, IM (ondansetron) and transdermal (granisetron).
- $5HT_3$ antagonists are not used for **apomorphine** induced emesis due to risk of severe hypotension. These drugs are not effective in **motion sickness**.

NEUROKININ-1 (NK-1) ANTAGONIST

- Substance P acts on NK-1 receptors and cause nausea and vomiting. Hence NK-1 antagonist like **aprepitant** ($T_{1/2}$ = 13 hours) is **drug of choice for late onset chemotherapy induced nausea and vomiting**.
- Aprepitant is given by oral route whereas fosaprepitant is given by IV route.
- Rolapitant ($T_{1/2}$ = 180 hours) and netupitant (T1/2 = 90 hours) are ultra-long acting NK-1 antagonists.

CANNABINOID RECEPTOR AGONIST

- Cannabinoids are released after depolarization of postsynaptic neurons into the synapse. These cannabinoids act on presynaptic CB1 receptor and inhibit release of neurotransmitters in the vomiting centre.
- **Dronabinol** and **nabilone** are CB1 receptor agonist which have antiemetic effect and are used for chemotherapy induced nausea and vomiting resistant to previous class drugs.

- They can also stimulate appetite and are used in **anorexia**.
- Central sympathomimetic effect can decrease NE release, which causes hypotension, tachycardia and conjunctival injections, i.e. **blood shot eyes**. Thus, **blood pressure** of patients on these drugs should be monitored regularly.
- It can cause symptoms of marijuana and hence has potential for abuse.

MISCELLANEOUS DRUGS

Scopolamine	Motion sickness (DOC) Migraine and vertigo associated nausea and vomiting
Doxylamine + vitamin B6	Morning sickness (DOC)
Antihistaminics (Promethazine/ Diphenhydramine)	• Motion sickness • Migraine and vertigo associated nausea and vomiting
Antipsychotics (Phenothiazines)	• Motion sickness • Hiccups (DOC-Chlorpromazine)
Dexamethasone	Chemotherapy induced nausea and vomiting

PROKINETICS

- The normal contraction of GIT is in the craniocaudal direction. Prokinetics are drugs that stimulate this contraction and increase emptying of GIT.
- The primary neurotransmitter responsible for GIT contraction is acetylcholine.
- Dopaminergic and serotonergic neurons form synapse on axons of cholinergic neurons where D_2 and $5HT_4$ receptors are located on the postsynaptic membrane.
- D_2 is an inhibitory receptor ($G\alpha_i$) and 5HT4 is a stimulatory receptor ($G\alpha_s$); hence dopamine decreases GIT contraction by decreasing acetylcholine release and 5HT increases GIT contraction by increasing acetylcholine release.
- Cholecystokinin (CCK) and motilin are other stimulators that act on CCK_1 and motilin receptors in GIT respectively and increase contraction.
- Thus prokinetic effect can be achieved by inhibiting D_2 receptors and stimulating $5HT_4$, CCK_1 and motilin receptors.

Conceptual Box-3

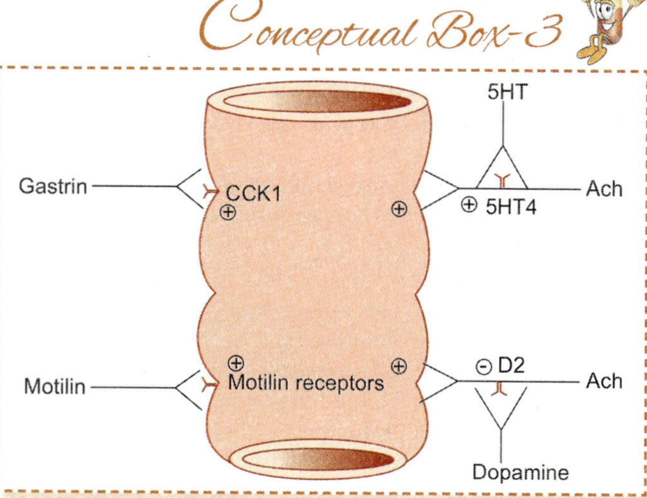

D_2 ANTAGONISTS

The drugs in this class are metoclopramide, domperidone and levosulpiride. Apart from prokinetic effect, inhibition of D_2 receptors in the CTZ area gives **antiemetic effect** as well. D_2 antagonists **increase lower esophageal sphincter, gastric antral and small intestinal contraction, however they do not have any effect on large intestine**.

Metoclopramide

- Metoclopramide is not only a D_2 antagonist but also antagonist at $5HT_3$ receptors and agonist at $5HT_4$ receptors.
- **Inhibition of D_2 and $5HT_3$ receptors in CTZ area** gives adequate antiemetic effect and hence is commonly used for same seen with GIT motility disorders and chemotherapy.
- Metoclopramide has more affinity for D_2 receptors than 5HT and hence at normal doses antiemetic effect is because of D_2 block. $5HT_3$ block is seen only at high doses.
- Antagonism at D_2 and agonism at $5HT_4$ gives strong prokinetic effect which makes it useful in treatment of **gastroparesis, GERD, postoperative ileus** and **hiccups**.
- Since it is a lipid soluble drug, it can easily cross blood brain barrier and due to central D_2 block, causes **extrapyramidal side effects** and **hyperprolactinemia**.
- **Methemoglobinemia** can be seen in neonates.

Domperidone

- Domperidone is a specific D_2 antagonist with limited use for treatment of GERD and dyspepsia.
- It is lipid insoluble and hence does not cause extrapyramidal side effects (EPS).

Levosulpiride

Levosulpiride is levo isomer of antipsychotic sulpiride, which can be used as prokinetic due to D_2 antagonism in GERD, irritable bowel syndrome and dyspepsia.

$5HT_4$ AGONISTS

- $5HT_4$ agonists like **cisapride** and **tegaserod** have been banned due to risk of prolonged **QT interval**.
- Available drugs like **prucalopride, itopride** and **mosapride** are used for treatment of GERD, chronic constipation and gastroparesis.
- Due to increased contraction of GIT **diarrhea (most common)** and abdominal pain can be seen.
- **Central nervous system (CNS)** side effects like headache and insomnia can also be associated.

MOTILIN RECEPTOR AGONISTS

- Erythromycin is a motilin receptor agonist which can be used for gastroparesis, bezoar removal and paralytic ileus.
- The limitation of erythromycin is rapid development of tolerance, i.e. tachyphylaxis.

Recent Advances

Mitemcinal and camicinal: Mitemcinal and camicinal are motilin receptor agonists under trial for treatment of gastroparesis.

Dexloxiglumide: These are **CCK 1 or A** receptor antagonist under trial for gastroparesis and IBS associated constipation treatment.

Relamorelin: Relamorelin is a ghrelin receptor agonist under trial as a prokinetic for treatment of gastroparesis and chronic idiopathic constipation.

Velusetrag and **naronapride:** These are under trial as prokinetics for treatment of gastroparesis and chronic idiopathic constipation.

Sincalide: It is CCK analogue used for stimulating movement of barium through organs of GIT for diagnostic tests.

LAXATIVES

Laxatives are drugs that facilitate movement of formed fecal material out of the rectum. These are the primary drugs used for treatment of constipation. Chronic laxative abuse causes renal **ammonium urate stone** formation.

PROBIOTICS, PREBIOTICS AND SYMBIOTICS

- These drugs increase the bulk of stool and attract water into the intestine. Thus, they are beneficial both in constipation and diarrhea.
- In constipation by attracting water stool gets soften. In diarrhea by increasing stool bulk the stool consistency is improved. Probiotics are also used in antibiotic associated diarrhea.
- **Probiotics** are live organisms that provide benefits to health when taken in adequate amounts. For example, Bifidobacterium, saccharomyces, lactobacillus, *Bacillus clausii*, etc.
- **Prebiotics** are food ingredients that are composed of oligosaccharides, not digestible by humans, but have a beneficial effect on the growth of intestinal microorganisms. For example, psyllium husk, bran, methyl cellulose, etc.
- **Symbiotics** are synergistic combination of probiotics and prebiotics.

STIMULANTS

- **Bisacodyl, cascara** and **senna** irritate colon by inducing inflammation that removes fecal material by promoting water and solute accumulation.
- **Castor oil** is hydrolyzed by lipase into ricinoleic acid, which stimulates intestine and increases solute and water.
- Bisacodyl is **activated by esterase in bowel**; hence the effect is seen after at least 5–6 hours. However, by rectal route effect can be seen after 30 minutes.
- These are indicated for short term use in constipation as prolonged use can cause atonic colon.
- Bisacodyl overdose can cause electrolyte deficiency like **hypokalemia**.
- Senna and cascara use can cause **melanosis coli**. They are **absolutely contraindicated** in case of **intestinal obstruction**.

OSMOTIC AGENTS

Nondigestible Sugars

- **Lactulose, sorbitol** and **mannitol** are nondigestible sugars metabolized into short chain fatty acids (SFA) which are osmotic and draw water into intestinal lumen.
- They are used for treatment of constipation.
- Lactulose when metabolized into SFA, makes intestinal pH acidic which converts ammonia into polar ammonium ion and facilitates its excretion. Hence, it is used in **hepatic encephalopathy**.

Polyethylene Glycol

- Polyethylene glycol is osmotic in nature and draws water into the intestine due to its high molecular weight.
- It is commonly used for irritable bowel syndrome (IBS) associated with constipation and bowel cleaning prior to various procedures in colon.

Saline Laxatives

- Saline laxatives are various salts containing magnesium and phosphate like magnesium sulfate, sodium phosphate, etc. These are used for treatment of IBS associated with constipation.
- These are **fast acting laxatives** as effect is seen within 6 hours.
- **Magnesium citrate** is a purgative laxative used in acute constipation.
- Since these salts are excreted by kidney, toxicity can be seen in renal failure and hence should be avoided.
- **Magnesium hydroxide** can **decrease absorption of fat soluble vitamins** and hence should be avoided in elderly.

STOOL SOFTENERS

- **Docusate sodium and calcium** are anionic surfactants that induce stool softening by decreasing surface tension.
- **Mineral oils** can penetrate and then soften the stool. They can cause **pneumonitis** due to aspiration.

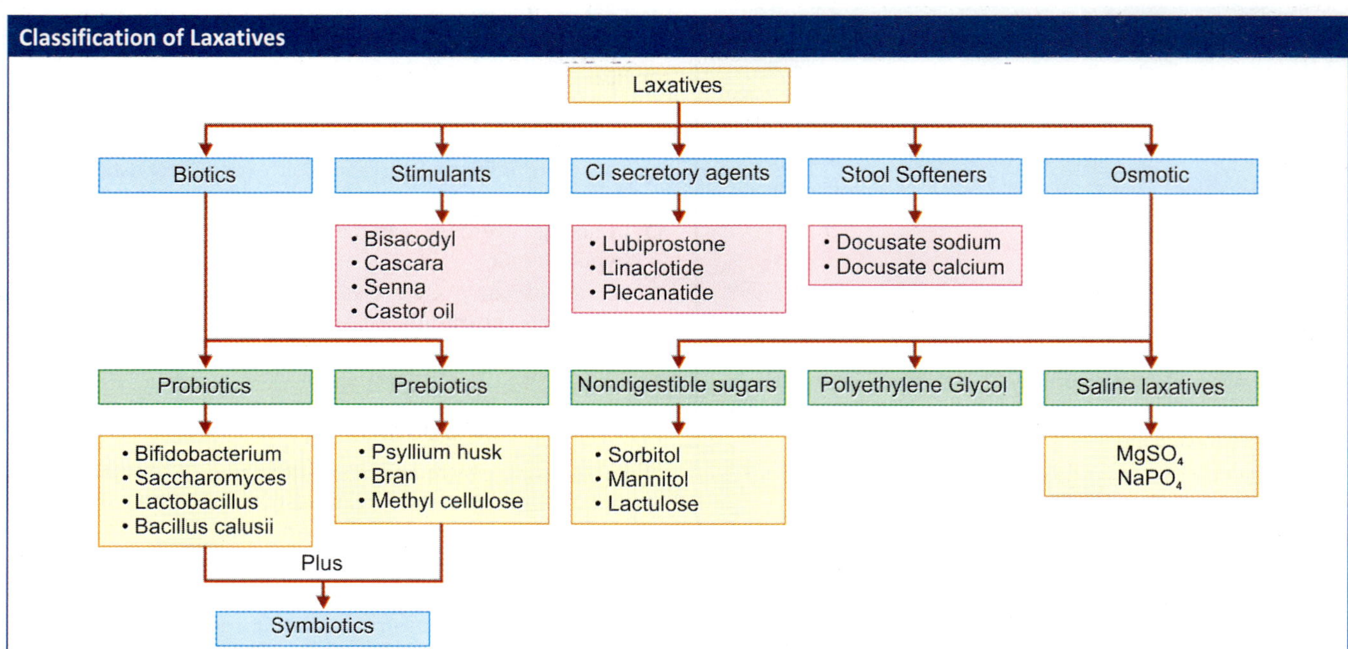

CHLORIDE SECRETORY DRUGS

Drugs in these classes like lubiprostone and linaclotide are costlier and hence reserved for cases refractory to other agents.

Lubiprostone

- Lubiprostone is a bicyclic fatty acid derivative of prostaglandin E1.
- It stimulates **type 2 chloride ion channels (ClC2)** on apical membrane of intestinal epithelial cells, which leads to secretion of chloride ions into intestinal lumen followed by sodium secretion by paracellular pathways to maintain isoelectric neutrality.
- This leads to secretion of water into the lumen to maintain isotonic equilibrium.
- It is approved for treatment of chronic constipation, IBS associated with constipation and opioid induced constipation.
- Nausea can be seen as a side effect due to a delay in gastric emptying.
- It is avoided in pregnancy (category C).

Linaclotide

- **Linaclotide and plecanatide** stimulate **guanylate cyclase** and increases cyclic GMP, which stimulates cystic fibrosis transmembrane regulator (CFTR) resulting in increased chloride and water secretion into lumen.
- These are also approved for chronic constipation and IBS associated with constipation.
- These are avoided in pregnancy (category C) and contraindicated in children.
- Side effect associated is diarrhea.

Recent Advances

Fedotozine: Fedotozine is a kappa opioid receptor antagonist that can be used for IBS associated with constipation.

Plecanatide: Plecanatide is a drug with similar mechanism to linaclotide uses and has been recently approved by FDA.

Clinical Box-1

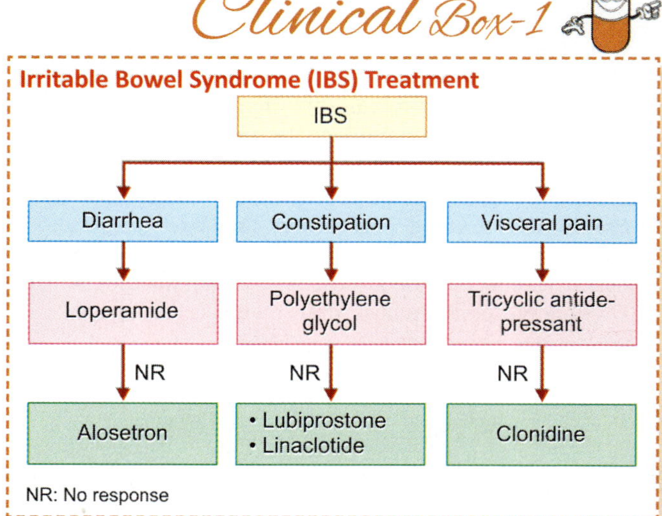

ANTIDIARRHEAL DRUGS

OPIOIDS

- **Loperamide** is a potent μ receptor agonist which acts by decreasing intestinal motility and secretion and increasing anal sphincter tone.

- It is the **drug of choice for treatment of nonsecretory diarrhea, i.e. IBS and irinotecan associated diarrhea** and also used for traveller's diarrhea.
- In **children less than 2 years it is absolutely contraindicated** and in **inflammatory bowel disease,** relatively contraindicated due to risk of toxic megacolon.
- **Diphenoxylate** is an opioid that is metabolized into difenoxin. Both parent compound and metabolite can be used for treatment of diarrhea. Atropine is given along with these drugs to prevent abuse.

SOMATOSTATIN ANALOGS

- **Octreotide** inhibits secretion of various hormones in GIT like serotonin, gastrin, VIP, etc. which leads to decrease GIT secretion and contraction.
- Hence it is drug of choice in **secretory diarrhea** of **pancreatic and gut tumors, chemotherapy, HIV associated** and in **diabetes**.
- Decreased contraction of GIT makes it useful in dumping syndrome seen after gastric surgery.
- Octreotide can also be used for prophylaxis and treatment of acute pancreatitis as it decreases pancreatic enzyme secretion as well.

BILE ACID BINDING RESINS

- Cholestyramine, colesevelam and colestipol can be used for treatment of biliary diarrhea, gastritis and esophagitis.
- Apart from this it can be used for treatment of pseudomembranous enterocolitis and pruritus seen in biliary obstruction.

Recent Advances

Racecadotril: Racecadotril is an enkephalinase inhibitor, which increases endogenous opioid, i.e. encephalin that produces antidiarrheal effect. It is used for treatment of acute diarrhea in children.

Alosetron: Alosetron is a $5HT_3$ antagonist which decreases GIT contraction and increases fluid absorption. It is approved for IBS associated with diarrhea in females who are not responding to other therapies. It carries a risk of ischemic colitis.

Crofelemer: It acts by cystic fibrosis transmembrane conductance regulator (CFTR) chloride channels in intestine and inhibits chloride secretion into intestine. It is approved for treatment of diarrhea associated with AIDS treatment.

Eluxadoline: It is an agonist at mu and kappa receptor and antagonist at delta receptor. It is approved for treatment of diarrhea associated with IBS.

INFLAMMATORY BOWEL DISEASE

- Inflammatory bowel disease encompasses two disorders namely ulcerative colitis (UC) and Crohn's disease (CD).
- Ulcerative colitis is generalized involvement of the intestinal mucosal layer which is continuous whereas CD is transmural involvement which is not continuous and associated with fistulas.
- The treatment is aimed at an acute attack and maintaining remission.
- For acute attack anti-inflammatory drugs are used (Sulfasalazine and steroids) whereas to maintain remission, the immune system is toned down for longer period of time by immunomodulators (azathioprine, cyclosporine).
- Biological agents like anti-TNF drugs and anti-integrin drugs are used in both induction as well as maintenance.

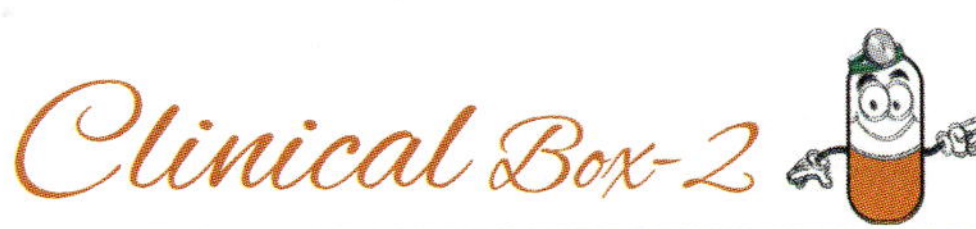

Treatment of Ulcerative Colitis

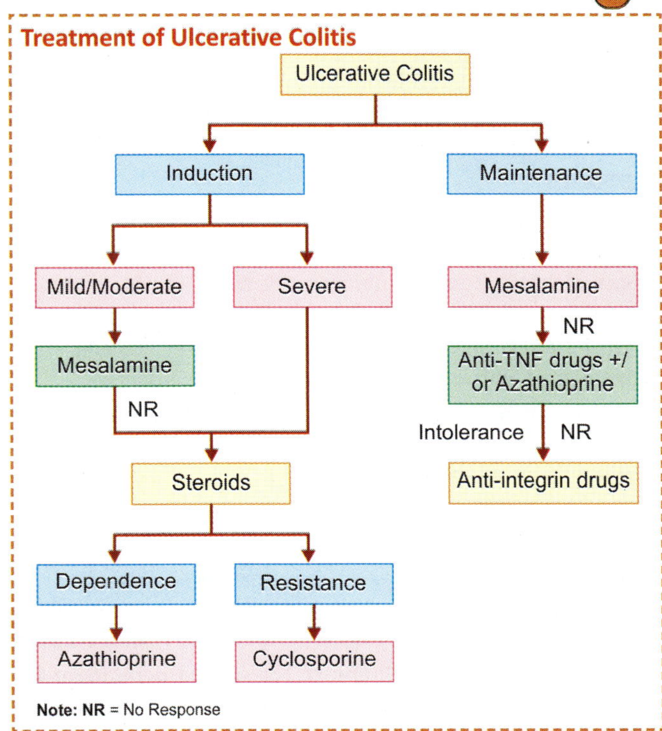

Note: NR = No Response

5-ASA Compounds

5-ASA compounds (Mesalamine) are drug of choice for treatment of an acute attack in mild to moderate UC and for maintenance of remission. They are not effective in CD and hence not recommended according to current guidelines.

Sulfasalazine

- **Sulfasalazine** is made up of anti-inflammatory molecules **5-ASA and antibiotic sulfapyridine** (1 g of sulfasalazine = 400 mg 5-ASA + 600 mg sulfapyridine) attached by an azo bond which prevents absorption in stomach and small intestine.
- This bond is broken down by colonic bacteria and releases the active compound 5-ASA in the colon. The anti-inflammatory effect of 5-ASA is not by COX inhibition, rather by decreasing production of inflammatory mediators and free radicals.
- The sulfapyridine molecule causes sulfonamides related hypersensitivity reactions, oligospermia and folic acid deficiency. Thus, sulfasalazine is less preferred.

Mesalamine

- **Mesalamine** is only 5-ASA and hence devoid of sulfonamide related side effects. Thus, it is **more preferred 5-ASA drug currently**.
- It is given by oral and topical route. For oral administration mesalamine is coated in acid resistant polymers and time release capsules (pentasa).

Olsalazine and Balsalazide

- **Olsalazine** is made up of two 5-ASA molecules attached by azo bond and **balsalazide** is made up of 5-ASA and an inert molecule 4-ABA by azo bond.
- Hence these are also activated in the colon and act like sulfasalazine but devoid of sulphonamide related side effects.
- Though these are associated with secretory diarrhea.

Steroids

- **Steroids** are used **only for treatment of an acute attack of UC (DOC in moderate/severe cases)** and **CD (DOC in mild cases)** but not for maintenance of remission as long-term therapy is associated with deleterious side effects.
- **Oral budesonide** is the initial steroid of choice as it is associated with lesser side effects.
- Patients with no response to budesonide can be given intravenous (methyl prednisolone or dexamethasone) or oral (prednisolone) steroids.

Immunomodulators

- Immunomodulators like azathioprine, 6-MP, cyclosporine and tacrolimus are used along with anti-TNF drugs for added benefit and in case of **steroid dependent and resistant cases.**
- **Azathioprine is drug of choice for steroid dependent UC whereas cyclosporine is drug of choice for steroid resistant UC.**
- Azathioprine can be used alone or along with anti-TNF drugs to maintain remission in UC and CD.
- **Methotrexate** is reserved for patients intolerant to azathioprine.

Anti-TNF Drugs

- Anti-TNF monoclonal antibodies like **infliximab, golimumab, certolizumab** and **adalimumab** are used not only for induction in acute attack but also for maintenance of remission.
- These are **drug of choice for an acute attack of moderate to severe CD and maintenance in CD (along with azathioprine).**
- These are effective for **fistulas** and **extra intestinal manifestations of CD** as well.
- In UC, they are preferred for maintenance in patients not responding to mesalamine.

Anti-integrin Drugs

- Anti-integrin antibodies like **natalizumab** and **vedolizumab** inhibit adhesion and migration of lymphocytes to the site of inflammation.
- These are used for treatment of UC and CD in case of anti-TNF drug toxicity or ineffectiveness.
- Natalizumab is not preferred due to risk of progressive multifocal leucoencephalopathy.

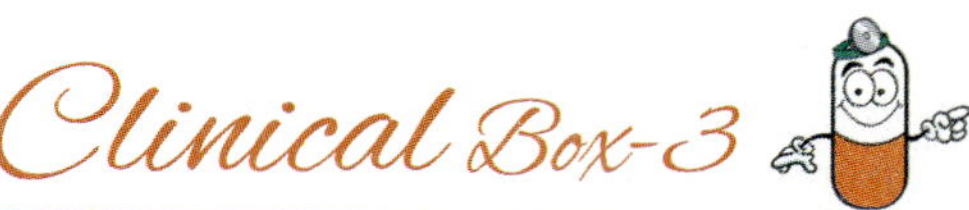

Treatment of Crohn's Disease

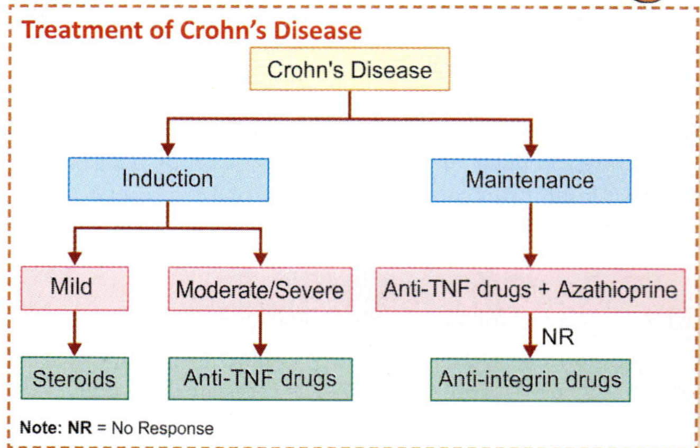

Note: NR = No Response

Recent Advances

Ustekinumab: Ustekinumab is an anti-IL-12 and IL-23 monoclonal antibody under trial for treatment of CD.

Tofacitinib: Tofacitinib is an anti-Janus kinase 1 and 3 monoclonal antibody under trial for treatment of UC.

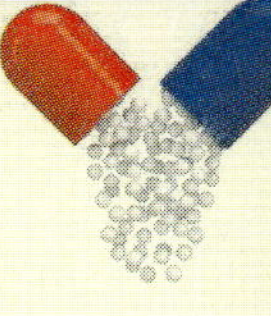

Image-based Questions

1. **A patient with dyspepsia and pain in epigastric region for last one year undergoes endoscopy, for which the findings are given in the picture. History confirmed nonsteroidal anti-inflammatory drug (NSAID) abuse for last 2 years for fibromyalgia. Which of the following drugs is best for the patient?**

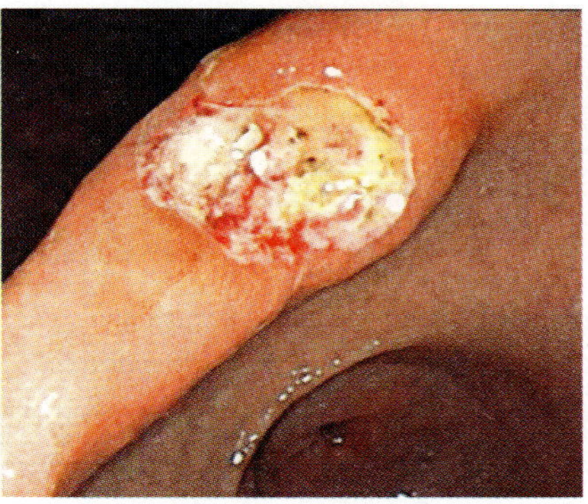

a. TCA　　b. Omeprazole
c. Sucralfate　　d. Misoprostol

2. **Which of the following drugs might have caused the side effect given in the picture?**

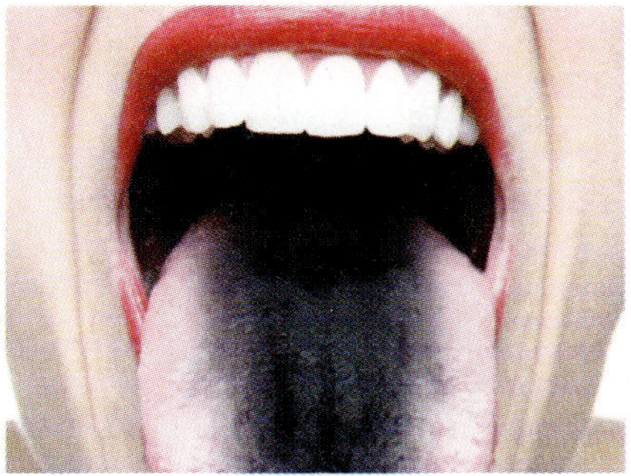

a. Antacids　　b. Bismuth
c. Cisapride　　d. Sucralfate

3. **The drug whose structure is given in the picture is effective against**

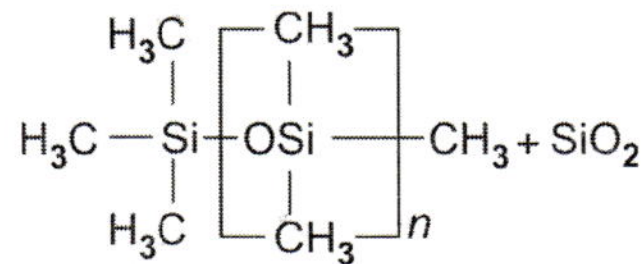

a. Ulcer　　b. Gastric bleeding
c. *H.pylori*　　d. Reflux

4. **A positive result in the kit given in the picture for a patient having dyspepsia for last 3 months, warrants administration of all except:**

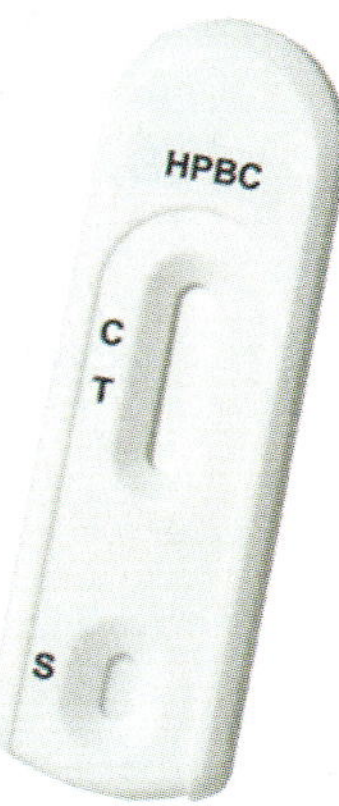

a. Metronidazole　　b. Ampicillin
c. Clarithromycin　　d. Carbapenems

5. **Which of the following drugs has effect against the microorganism in the picture?**

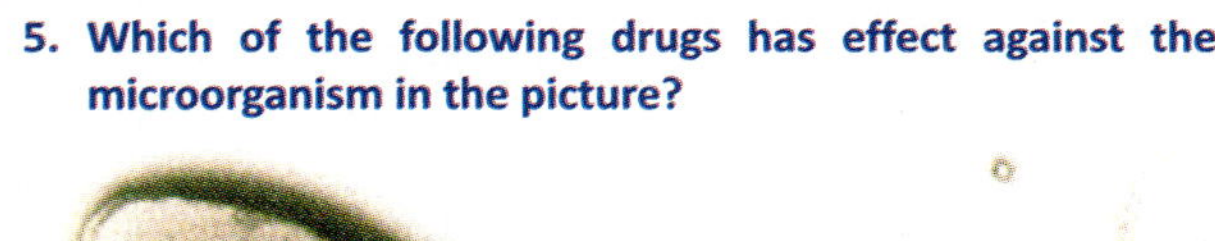

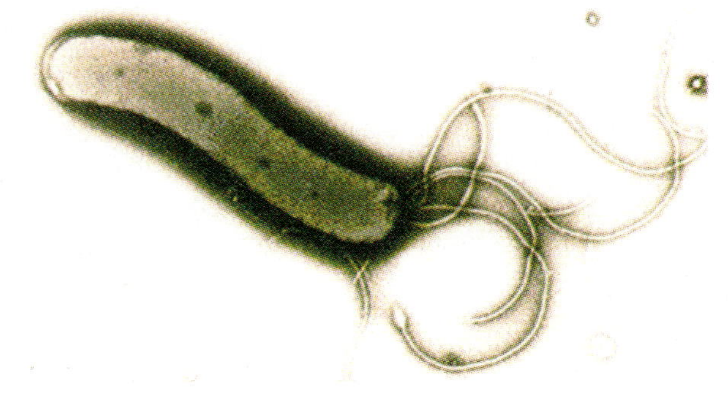

a. Sucralfate　　b. Alginate
c. Simethicone　　d. Bismuth

6. Which of the following antiemetic can cause the side effect given in the picture?

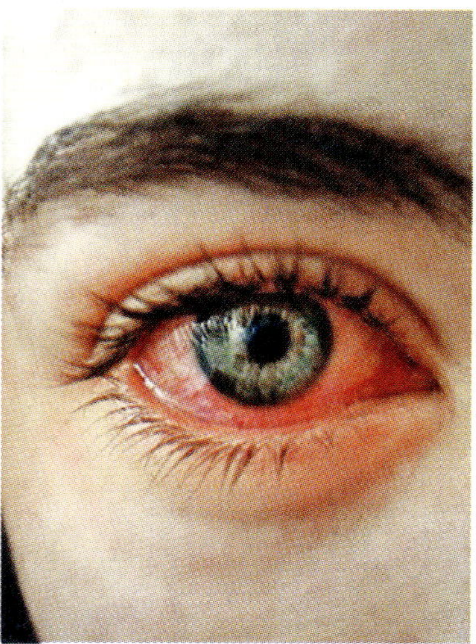

a. Domperidone
b. Nabilone
c. Ondansetron
d. Aprepitant

7. The 5-ASA compound given in the picture is:

NaO_2C CO_2Na
HO— —N=N— —OH

a. Sulfasalazine
b. Mesalamine
c. Olsalazine
d. Balsalazide

8. A patient on steroids for the condition in the X-ray, responded but relapsed on discontinuation. Which of the following is the drug used for this condition?

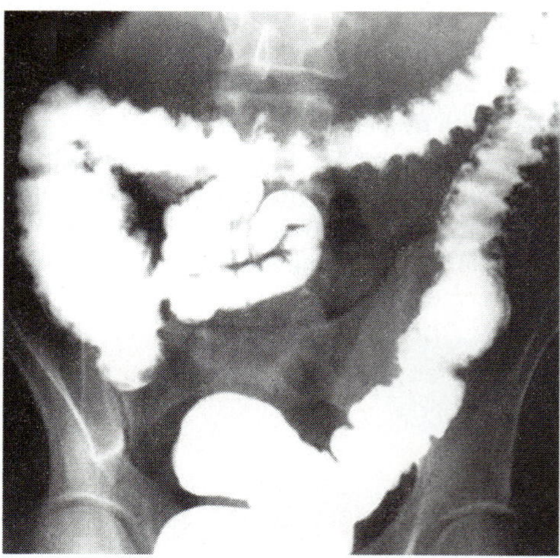

a. Sulfasalazine
b. Infliximab
c. Azathioprine
d. Cyclosporine

9. Which of the following is the drug of choice for the condition given in the X-ray?

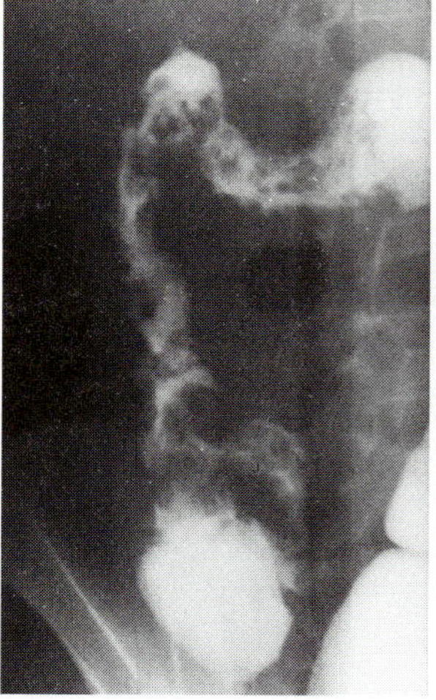

a. Steroids
b. Sulfasalazine
c. Infliximab
d. Azathioprine

Answers with Explanations to Image-based Questions

1. Ans. (b) Omeprazole

(Ref: Goodman Gilman 12th edition, page 1312)

- History of NSAID abuse and endoscopic findings are consistent with the diagnosis of NSAID induced gastric ulcer.
- The best drugs for ulcer healing are PPIs.
- Misoprostol though is the most specific drug.

2. Ans. (b) Bismuth

(Ref: Goodman Gilman 12th edition, page 1317)

- Bismuth can cause black discoloration of stool and tongue.

3. Ans. (d) Reflux

- The compound containing silicon dioxide and siloxane polymers is simethicone.
- Simethicone decreases foaming in GIT and prevents reflux as well as flatulence.

4. Ans. (d) Carbepenams

(Ref: Goodman Gilman 12th edition, page 1320)

- The kit given in the picture for rapid diagnosis of *H. pylori* infection in blood sample.
- The antibiotics used in *H. pylori* are ampicillin, clarithromycin, metronidazole and tetracycline.

5. Ans. (d) Bismuth

(Ref: Goodman Gilman 12thedition, page 1320)

- The microorganism in the picture is *H.pylori*.
- Antibiotics effective against this organism are metronidazole, tetracycline, clarithromycin and ampicillin.
- Only gastroprotective agent affective against *H.pylori* is bismuth.

6. Ans. (b) Nabilone

(Ref: Goodman Gilman 12th edition, page 1343)

- Cannabinoid receptor agonists like dronabinol and nabilone can cause conjunctival congestion known as blood shot eyes.

7. Ans. (c) Olsalazine

(Ref: Goodman Gilman 12th edition, page 1354)

- The given compound contains only two 5-ASA molecules and hence it is olsalazine.

8. Ans. (c) Azathioprine

(Ref: Goodman Gilman 12th edition, page 1357)

- Pancolitis with pseudopolyps in X-ray are confirmatory of ulcerative colitis.
- Since patient responded to steroids but relapsed on discontinuation, it is a case of steroid dependent ulcerative colitis.
- The drug of choice for same is azathioprine.

9. Ans. (c) Infliximab

(Ref: Goodman Gilman 12th edition, page 1359)

- The string sign present in the given X-ray is confirmatory of Crohn's disease.
- The drug of choice for same in anti-TNF drugs like infliximab.

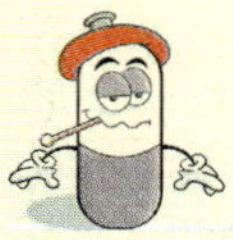

Annexures

Drugs of Choice

Acute Bleeding gastric ulcer	I/V Proton Pump Inhibitor

Acute Colonic Pseudo-Obstruction (Ogilive Syndrome)	Neostigmine

Aspiration pneumonia prophylaxis in surgical patients	H_2 blockers

Chemotherapy induced nausea and vomiting	
Early onset Late onset	Ondansetron Aprepitant

Dyspepsia Gastrinoma Gastroesophageal reflux disease (GERD) NSAID Induced Ulcer Peptic Ulcer Disease Zollinger-Ellison Syndrome Stress Ulcer	Proton Pump Inhibitors

GERD in Pregnancy	Antacids or Sucralfate

Hemochromatosis	Deferoxamine

Hiccups	Chlorpromazine

HIV associated secretory diarrhea	Octreotide

Inflammatory bowel disease

Ulcerative colitis
- For maintenance and induction – Mesalamine
- Mesalamine nonrespondents in induction – Steroids
- Steroid dependence in induction – Azathioprine
- Steroid resistance in induction – Cyclosporine

Crohn's disease (For maintenance and induction): Anti-TNF drugs (Infliximab)
(Exclusion: Only for induction of mild cases steroids are first preferred)

Note: Steroids are used only for induction in ulcerative colitis and Crohn's disease.

Irritable Bowel Syndrome	• Diarrhea – Loperamide • Constipation – Polyethelene glycol

Morning Sickness	• Pyridoxine Plus • Doxylamine

Motion Sickness	Scopalamine

Sclerosing Cholangitis	Glucocorticoids

Whipple's Disease	Cotrimoxazole (Double strength for 1 year)

Wilson's Disease	
Without hepatic decompensation or neuropsychiatric features With hepatic decompensation With neuropsychiatric features	Zinc Zinc + Trientene Tetrathiomolybdate

Xerostomia	Cevimeline > Pilocarpine

New Drugs

Drugs	Mechanism of Action	Uses
Eluxadoline	mu-opioid receptor agonist and delta-opioid receptor antagonist	Irritable bowel syndrome associated with diarrhea
Rifaximin	Rifamycin derivative	Irritable bowel syndrome associated with diarrhea
Golimumab	Anti-TNF Ab	Ulcerative colitis
Crofelemer	Latex of the *Croton lechleri* tree, which reduces excess chloride ion secretion via the cystic fibrosis transmembrane conductance regulator (CFTR) channel.	Diarrhea in HIV patients
Teduglutide	GLP-2 analogue, which decreases HCl production and increases intestinal and portal blood flow.	Short bowel syndrome
Linaclotide plecanatide	Stimulate guanylate cyclase-c, followed by increase in cyc-GMP which increases Cl and bicarbonate secretion	Irritable bowel syndrome associated with constipation
Lubiprostone	Increases Cl ion secretion by stimulation of EP-4 receptors	Irritable bowel syndrome associated with constipation

Multiple Choice Questions

PEPTIC ULCER DISEASE

1. A patient with 5 episodes of loose stools after eating in a hotel. He is afebrile, has tachycardia and mild dehydration. What is treatment? *(AIIMS Nov. 2017)*
  a. Ciprofloxacin and tinidazole
  b. Because it may not be giardia give only ciprofloxacin
  c. Ciprofloxacin, tinidazole and ORS
  d. Only ORS

2. Which stone is common in chronic laxative use? *(Recent Question 2017)*
  a. Xanthine b. Cysteine
  c. Ammonia urate d. Struvite

3. Which drug causes melanosis coli? *(Recent Question 2017)*
  a. Senna b. Bisacodyl
  c. Magnesium hydroxide d. Bismuth

4. The drug that produces least inhibition of CYP_{450} is *(AIIMS May 2016)*
  a. Omeprazole b. Rabeprazole
  c. Lansoprazole d. Pantoprazole

5. The anti-emetic activity of metoclopramide is mainly because of *(AIIMS May 2016)*
  a. D2 antagonism b. 5-HT4 antagonism
  c. 5-HT4 agonism d. 5-HT3 antagonism

6. Which of the following is not a long-term side effect of PPI? *(AIIMS Nov 2014)*
  α. Hypothyroidism
  β. Pelvic fracture
  χ. Increased risk of Pneumonia
  δ. Increased risk of C.difficile infection

7. Drug not used in *H. pylori* is: *(AIIMS May 2008, Nov 2006)*
  a. Metronidazole b. Omeprazole
  c. Mosapride d. Amoxicillin

8. Shortest acting purgative is? *(Recent Question Dec 2016)*
  a. Senna b. Docusate
  c. Sodium phosphate d. Methyl cellulose

9. Which is CCK- A receptor antagonist? *(Recent Question Dec 2016)*
  a. Dexloxiglumide b. Natezpide
  c. Ondansetron d. Pirenzepine

10. Most potent H2 blocker is? *(Recent Question Dec 2016)*
  a. Cimetidine b. Ranitidine
  c. Famotidine d. Loratidine

11. Longest acting PPI? *(Recent Question Dec 2016)*
  a. Rabeprazole b. Pantoprazole
  c. Lansoprazole d. Esomeprazole

12. DOC for nonsecretory diarrhea? *(Recent Question Dec 2016)*
  a. Loperamide
  b. Alosteron
  c. Octreotide d. Colesevelam

13. Which of the following drug is used for treatment of irritable bowel syndrome associated diarrhea? *(Recent Question Dec 2016)*
  a. Senna b. Alosetron
  c. Lubiprostone d. Linaclotide

14. Enterocutaneous Fistula closure is seen due which drug *(Recent Question Dec 2016)*
  a. Corticosteroid b. Infliximab.
  c. 5ASA d. Sulfasalazine

15. Drug of choices in children for GERD. *(Recent Question Dec 2016)*
  a. Antacids B. PPI
  c. H2 blockers d. Sucralfate

16. Which of the following drugs has both 5HT4 agonist and D2 antagonist property :- *(Recent Question Dec 2016)*
  a. Ondansetron b. Metoclopramide
  c. Benzhexol d. Ibutilide

17. Drugs causing peptic ulcer are all except *(Recent Question 2016)*
  a. Clopidogrel b. NSAID
  c. Mycophenolate mofetil d. Propylthiouracil

18. Which of the following proton pump inhibitor has enzyme inhibitory activity? *(Recent Question 2016)*
  a. Rabeprazole b. Lansoprazole
  c. Pantaprazole d. Omeprazole

19. Drug is not used for *H. pylori* treatment: *(Recent Question 2016)*
  a. Oxytetracycline
  b. Bismuth compounds
  c. Amoxicillin
  d. Omeprazole

20. Which of the following agents is beneficial in NSAID induced gastric ulcer? *(Recent Question 2016)*
  a. PGE_1 agonist b. PGE_2 agonist
  c. PGD_2 agonist d. PGF_{2a} agonist

21. Proton pump inhibitors are most effective when they are given *(Recent Question 2016)*
  a. After meals
  b. Shortly before meals
  c. Along with H_2 blockers
  d. During prolonged fasting periods

22. The drugs employed for anti-*H. pylori* therapy include all of the following except *(Recent Question 2016)*
  a. Ciprofloxacin b. Clarithromycin
  c. Tinidazole d. Amoxicillin

23. Drug of choice for the treatment of peptic ulcer caused due to chronic use of NSAIDs is *(Recent Question 2016)*
  a. Pirenzepine
  b. Loxatidine
  c. Misoprostol
  d. Esomeprazole

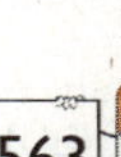

24. Most specific drug for the treatment of peptic ulcer disease due to chronic use of aspirin is: ***(Recent Question 2016)***

a. Omeprazole b. Misoprostol
c. Pirenzipine d. Ranitidine

25. M_1 blocker used in peptic ulcer disease is: ***(Recent Question 2016)***

a. Pirenzepine b. Pyridostigmine
c. Atropine d. Oxybutynin

26. Drug used in the treatment gastric ulcer due to *H. pylori* is ***(Recent Question 2016)***

a. Anticholinegics b. Carbenoxolone sodium
c. Bismuth subcitrate d. Corticosteroid

27. Esomeprazole acts by inhibiting ***(Recent Question 2016)***

a. $H^+ K^+$ ATPase pump b. $H^+ Na^+$ ATPase pump
c. H^+ pump d. Any of the above

28. Diarrhea is side effect of ***(Recent Question 2016)***

a. Omeprazole b. Sucralfate
c. Metoclopramide d. Misprostol

29. Antacid drug that typically causes diarrhea is ***(Recent Question 2016)***

a. Sodium bicarbonate b. Magnesium hydroxide
c. Calcium bicarbonate d. Aluminium hydroxide

30. All are H_2 blockers except ***(Recent Question 2016)***

a. Omeprazole b. Cimetidone
c. Famatodine d. Ranitidine

31. Primary role of antacids in peptic ulcer is ***(Recent Question 2016)***

a. Pain relief b. Ulcer healing
c. H pylori eradication d. All

32. Drug not used in the treatment of *H. pylori* is ***(Recent Question 2016)***

a. Clarithromycin b. Metronidazole
c. Cisapride d. Omeprazole

33. Which drug has maximum relief of symptoms and cure rate of reflux oesophagitis? ***(Recent Question 2016)***

a. Omeprazole b. Ranitidine
c. Mosapride d. Cimetidine

34. Mechanism of action of prostaglandins ***(Recent Question 2016)***

a. Decreases acid secretion
b. Increases bicarbonate secretion
c. Form a protective mucus covering over the stomach
d. All of the above

35. H_2 blocker therapy in a case of peptic ulcer should be given for ***(Recent Question 2016)***

a. 4 weeks b. 6 weeks
c. 8 weeks d. 12 weeks

36. Antacids should not be given along with ***(Recent Question 2016)***

a. Sucralfate b. H_2 blockers
c. Proton pump inhibitors d. Prostaglandins

37. Which of the following is PPI? ***(Recent Question 2016)***

a. Ranitidine
b. Lansoprazole
c. Misoprostol
d. Amoxycillin

38. Ranitidine differs from cimetidine because of ***(Recent Question 2016)***

a. Ranitidine does not have anti androgenic side effect
b. Shorter half life
c. More side effects
d. Less potent

39. Drug used in *H. pylori* are all except ***(Recent Question 2016)***

a. Chloramphenicol b. Tetracycline
c. Amoxicillin d. Omeprazole

40. A patient of peptic ulcer disease was prescribed ranitidine and sucralfare in the morning hours. Why is this combination incorrect? ***(Recent Question 2016)***

a. Ranitidine combines with sucralfate and prevents its action
b. Combination of these two drugs produce serious side effects like agranulocytosis.
c. Ranitidine increases gastric pH so that sucralfate is unable to act
d. Sucralfate inhibits the absorption of ranitidine

41. All are H_2 blockers except: ***(Recent Question 2016)***

a. Omeprazole b. Cimetidine
c. Famotidine d. Ranitidine

42. Gynaecomastia and infertility is caused by? ***(Recent Question 2016)***

a. Flutamide b. Cimetidine
c. Ranitidine d. Methotrexate

43. Irrational combination among the following ***(Recent Question 2016)***

a. Sucralfate + bismuth b. Sucralfate + ranitidine
c. Sucralate + simethicone d. Sucralate + omeprazole

ANTIEMETICS

44. Which of the following drugs is not an antiemetic? ***(AIIMS May, 2007)***

a. Ondansetron b. Domperidone
c. Metoclopramide d. Cinnarizine

45. Most specific drug for treatment of chemotherapy induced nausea and vomiting is ***(Recent Question 2019)***

a. Granisetron b. Metoclopramide
c. Haloperidol d. Dexamethasone

46. All are antiemetic except ***(Recent Question 2016)***

a. Ondansetran b. Metoclopramide
c. Chlorpromazine d. Bismuth

47. Regarding aprepitant all are true except ***(Recent Question 2016)***

a. Agonist at NK_1 receptors
b. Crossed blood brain barrier
c. Ameliorate nausea and vomiting induced by chemotherapy
d. Metabolized by CYP_{450} enzymes

48. The most effective antiemetic for controlling cisplatin induced vomiting is ***(Recent Question 2016)***

a. Prochlorperazine b. Ondansetron
c. Metoclopramide d. Aprepitant

49. Ondansetron acts by inhibiting which of the following receptors? *(Recent Question 2016)*
a. 5-HT_1 b. 5-HT
c. 5-HT_3 d. 5-HT_4

50. Drug that should not be given with apomorphine is *(Recent Question 2016)*
a. Dopamine agonist b. Spironolactone
c. Ondansetron d. Aspirin

51. Not an anti-emetic *(Recent Question 2016)*
a. Nabilone b. Ondansetron
c. Pentazocine d. Dronabinol

PROKINETICS, LAXATIVES, ANTI-DIARRHEA DRUGS AND IBS

52. Medical student with protracted vomiting was given anti emetic and he develops abnormal posturing. Which drug was given? *(AIIMS May 2018)*
a. Ondansetron b. Metoclopramide
c. Domperidone d. Dexamethasone

53. Commonest side effect of cisapride *(Recent Question 2016)*
a. Abdominal cramps b. Headache
c. Diarrhea d. Convulsions

54. Drug used in irritable bowel syndrome with constipation is *(Recent Question 2016)*
a. Lubiprostone
b. Loperamide
c. Alosetron
d. Clonidine

55. True about octreotide is *(Recent Question 2016)*
a. Stimulates growth hormone
b. Used in secretory diarrhea
c. Used orally
d. Contraindicated in acromegaly

56. Drug implicated in prolonging QT interval is *(Recent Question 2016)*
a. Domperidone b. Metoclopramide
c. Cisapride d. Omeprazole

57. Metoclopramide *(Recent Question 2016)*
a. Increase lower esophageal sphincter tone
b. Prokinetic action is blocked by atropine
c. Increase gastric peristalsis
d. Increase large intestinal peristalsis

58. Which of the following prokinetic drugs produces extrapyramidal side effects? *(Recent Question 2016)*
a. Metoclopramide
b. Cisapride
c. Domperidone
d. All of the above

59. Stimulant purgatives are contraindicated in *(Recent Question 2016)*
a. Bed ridden patients
b. Before abdominal radiography
c. Subacute intestinal obstruction
d. All of these

60. Which of the following prokinetic drugs has been implicated in causing serious ventricular arrhythmias, particularly in patients concurrently receiving erythromycin or ketoconazole? *(Recent Question 2016)*
a. Domperidone b. Cisapride
c. Mosapride d. Metoclopramide

61. Bisacodyl is *(Recent Question 2016)*
a. Bulk forming b. Stool softner
c. Stimulant purgative d. Osmotic purgative

62. Drug useful in hepatic encephalopathy is *(Recent Question 2016)*
a. Magnesium sulphate b. Lactulose
c. Bisacodyl d. Bisphosphonates

63. Drug of choice for diarrhea in HIV is: *(Recent Question 2016)*
a. Loperamide
b. Somatostatin
c. Octreotide
d. Codeine

64. Laxative acting by opening of chloride channels *(Recent Question 2016)*
a. Docusate b. Anthraquinone
c. Lubiprostone d. Bisacodyl

65. Aloe, senna, and cascara are *(Recent Question 2016)*
a. Laxatives b. Emetics
c. Anti-diarrheals d. Anti-emetics

66. Mosapride is a *(Recent Question 2016)*
a. $5HT_4$ Agonist b. $5HT_3$ Agonists
c. $5HT_3$ Antagonists d. $5HT_4$ Antagonists

67. Cisapride is a *(Recent Question 2016)*
a. $5HT_4$ Agonist b. $5HT_3$ Agonists
c. $5HT_3$ Antagonists d. $5HT_4$ Antagonists

68. True regarding metoclopramide are all except *(Recent Question 2016)*
a. Acts through the blockade of D2 receptors
b. Increases gastric peristalsis
c. Stimulates CTZ
d. Associated with extrapyramidal effects

69. Antiobesity drug withdrawn from Indian market due to cardiac side effects is? *(Recent Question 2016)*
a. Orlistat b. Sibutramine
c. Rimonabant d. Clofibrate

70. Enzyme papain is used? *(Recent Question 2016)*
a. To decreases intestinal gas produced during digestive process
b. As Anti helminthic
c. To treat Herpes zoster
d. To treat infected wounds in nucleus pulposus

71. Which of the following don't have prokinetic activity? *(Recent Question 2016)*
a. Erythro
b. Amoxicillin
c. Metacloprmide
d. Domepridone

72. Hyperprolactinemia is a side effect of? *(Recent Question 2016)*
a. Bromocriptine
b. Levodopa
c. Amantadine
d. Metoclopramide

INFLAMMATORY BOWEL DISEASE

73. Sulfa drug used in inflammatory bowel disease includes
a. Sulfasalazine b. Sulfamethoxazole
c. Sulfinpyrazone d. Sulphadoxine

74. Which one of the drugs is useful in treating crohn's disease
a. Infliximab b. Azathioprine
c. Tacrolimus d. Cyclosporine

75. Initial management of ulcerative colitis is with
a. Sulfasalazine b. Mesalazine
c. Prednisolone d. Suphamethoxazole

76. Drug of choice for crohn's disease
a. Infliximab b. Azathioprine
c. Tacrolimus d. Steroids

77. Which of the following statement about proton pump inhibitors is/are true except: ***(PGI Nov 2014)***
a. Hit & run drug
b. Acidic medium is essential for activity
c. Act on H+/K+ ATPase
d. Forms an integral component of anti-H.pylori regimens
e. Act best in alkaline medium

78. Adverse effect of Cimetidine includes: ***(PGI Nov 2010)***
a. Constipation b. Impotence
c. ↑ In plasma Aminotranferase
d. ↓ In prolactin level e. Gynecomastia

79. Alginates and simethicone are given with antacids in peptic ulcer disease because of: ***(PGI Nov 2010)***
a. Alginates decrease proton secretion from stomach
b. Alginates prevent GERD
c. Simethicone relieve flatulence
d. Simethicone forms protective layer over ulcer
e. Simethicone prevent GERD

80. Drug used to control post-operative vomiting: ***(PGI Nov 2008)***
a. Diazepam b. Phenobarbitone
c. Apretitant d. Droperidol
e. Ondansetron

81. Which drug acts via stimulating chloride channel? ***(JIPMER 2017)***
a. Lubiprostone b. Lincosamide
c. Linaclotide d. Linezolid

82. Which of the following drug acts via stimulating guanylate cyclase? ***(JIPMER 2017)***
a. Linaclotide b. Lubiprostone
c. Lincosamide d. Linezolid

83. Which of the following is a new drug approved for treatment of constipation? ***(JIPMER 2017)***
a. Plecanatide b. Lixisenatide
c. Venetoclax d. Alosetron

84. A 45 years old male patient a known case of Crohn's disease presents with recent flare-ups suggestive of fistulas. He was admitted and treated with immune-suppressive. Unfortunately, he got reactivation of his tuberculosis as a result of the side effects of the treatment. Which of the following immunosuppressive medication is the most likely cause of his TB reactivation?
a. Methotrexate b. Infliximab ***(JIPMER 2016)***
c. Azathioprine d. Mizorbine

85. A 40 year old woman with Crohn's Disease reports multiple bowel movements with frequent stools. She was previously treated with a mesalamine derivative "Pentasa" and in the latest episode of the disease flare up she didn't tolerate the oral steroid therapy with budesonide. What is the next appropriate step in her treatment? ***(JIPMER 2016)***
a. Hydrocortisone (I.V) b. Prednisolone (oral)
c. Azathioprine d. Sulfasalazine

86. Mesalamine is used in: ***(JIPMER 2012)***
a. Ulcerative colitis b. Diabetes
c. Erectile dysfunction d. Tinea corporis

87. Proton pump inhibitors for peptic ulcer disease should be taken: ***(JIPMER 2011)***
a. Before Breakfast b. After Breakfast
c. Before Dinner d. After Dinner

88. Sucralfate does not interfere with the absorption of:
a. Phenoxy methyl penicillin ***(JIPMER 2010)***
b. Ciprofloxacin
c. Phenytoin
d. Digoxin

89. Anti Helicobacter pylori drugs include all of the following except: ***(JIPMER 2008)***
a. Amoxicillin b. Clarithromycin
c. Metronidazole d. Sucralfate

90. Which of the following proton pump inhibitors is known to inhibit CYP2C19? ***(JIPMER 2008)***
a. Pantoprazole b. Omeprazole
c. Rabeprazole d. Dexlansoprazole

91. Ondansetron is not useful for: ***(JIPMER 2006)***
a. Chemotherapy-induced nausea and vomiting
b. Postoperative and postradiation emesis
c. Reduce carving in alcoholism
d. Chemotherapy induced hypercuriemia

92. A patient is taking regular laxative and develop hypokalemia. The probable causative drug is ***(NIMHANS 2012)***
a. Isopsyllium b. Bisacodyl
c. Liquid paraffin d. Phenolphthalein

93. Which of the following is a true match among antiemetics?
a. Domperidone-5H2 antagonist ***(NIMHANS 2011)***
b. Ondansetron selective-5HT3 antagonist
c. Metoclopramide-5HT1 antagonist
d. Meclizine-5HT4 antagonist

94. Antiemetic causing extra pyramidal symptoms includes ***(NIMHANS 2010)***
a. Prochlorpromazine b. Ondansetron
c. Domperidone d. Option D

95. Mechanism of action of antiemtic-incorrect match
a. Ondansetron-5HT3 agonist ***(NIMHANS 2010)***
b. Meclizine-5HT4 agonist
c. Metoclopramide-D2-5HT3 antagonist
d. Domperidone-D2-agonist

Answers with Explanations to Multiple Choice Questions

1. Ans. (d) Only ORS

(Ref: CMDT 2017, Page 1305)

- It is a case of acute diarrhea which can be managed by just ORS in stable patients.
- If patient is afebrile antibiotics are not given.
- Patients with mild to moderate symptoms of dehydration are treated with ORS. In case of severe dehydration IV fluids are given.
- In a febrile patient antibiotics are used empirically; in Asian countries ciprofloxacin is used. In countries like Russia, giardia is common and hence metronidazole or tinidazole is also recommended. However, if giardia infection is suspected in India, the same may be added.
- Since patient is afebrile in this case, we can use only ORS.

2. Ans. (c) Ammonia urate

(Ref: Campbell's Urology, Page 210)

Chronic laxative use leads to decreased sodium in the urine, as most sodium is excreted by GIT. Hence, urate binds more with ammonia and this leads to ammonia urate stones.

3. Ans. (a) Senna

(Ref: Goodman Gilman 12th edition, Page 1334)

Senna and cascara can cause melanotic pigmentation of colonic mucosa known as melanosis coli.

4. Ans. (d) Pantoprazole

(Ref: Goodman Gilman 12th E/P1312)

The order of enzyme inhibitory effect of PPI is Omeprazole > Lansoprazole > Rabeprazole > Pantoprazole.

5. Ans. (a) D2 antagonism

(Ref: Goodman Gilman 12th E/P1343)

- **Metoclopromide has more affinity for D2 as compared to 5HT3 receptors.**
- **Hence at normal doses the antiemetic effect is due to D2 receptors.**
- **However at high doses 5HT3, antagonism also plays a role.**

6. Ans. (a) Hypothyroidism

(Ref: Goodman and Gilman 12th E/P 1312)

Side effects of PPI

- **Increased risk of hospital acquired pneumonia**
- **Increased risk of bone fractures**
- **Increased risk of *C. difficile* infection**
- Gastrinoma
- Vitamin B12, iron, calcium and magnesium deficiency
- GIT upset (Nausea, flatulence, constipation, diarrhea) - M.C side effect

7. Ans. (c) Mosapride

(Ref: Goodman Gilman 12th E/P1320)

Anti-H. pylori Regimen

Triple therapy	Quadruple therapy
PPI OD Clarithromycin Metronidazole or Amoxicillin or Tetracycline	PPI BD Metronidazole Tetracycline Bismuth subsalicylate

8. Ans. (c) Sodium phosphate

(Ref: Goodman Gilman 12th E/P1332)

9. Ans. (a) Dexloxiglumide

(Ref: Goodman Gilman 12th E/P1328)

CCK-A agonist - Loxiglumide and Dexoxiglumide
CCK-B antagonist – Natezepide

10. Ans. (c) Famotidine

(Ref: Goodman Gilman 12th E/P1313)

11. Ans. (a) Rabeprazole

(Ref: Goodman Gilman 12th E/P1312)

12. Ans. (a) Loperamide

(Ref: Goodman Gilman 12th E/P1337)

13. Ans. (b) Alosetron

(Ref: Goodman Gilman 12th E/P1340)

14. Ans. (b) Infliximab

(Ref: Goodman Gilman 12th E/P1359)

15. Ans. (a) Antacids

(Ref: Nelson 19th E/P1268)

16. Ans. (b) Metoclopramide

(Ref: Goodman Gilman 12th E/P1343)

17. Ans. (d) Propylthiouracil

(Ref: Harrison 19th E/P1918)

Drugs Causing Peptic Ulcer

- Anticancer drugs
- Mycophenolate mofetil
- NSAID
- Clopidogrel
- Bisphosphonates

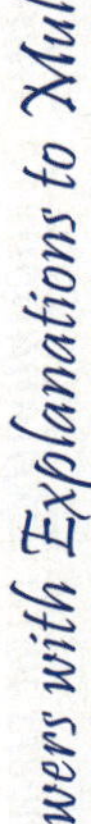

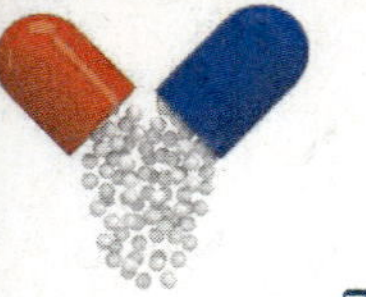

- KCl
- Glucocorticoids

18. Ans. (d) Omeprazole

(Ref: Goodman Gilman 12th E/P1312)

- **Omeprazole** is both **enzyme inducer** (CYP1A2) and **inhibitor** (CYP2C19).

19. Ans. (a) Oxytetracycline

(Ref: Goodman Gilman 12th E/P1320)

Anti-*H. pylori* drugs

Triple therapy	Quadruple therapy
PPI OD Clarithromycin Metronidazole or Amoxicillin or Tetracycline	PPI BD Metronidazole Tetracycline Bismuth subsalicylate

20. Ans. (a) PGE_1 agonist

(Ref: Goodman Gilman 12th E/P1314)

- **PGE_1 analog misoprostol is beneficial for treatment of NSAID induced gastric ulcer.**
- **Though it is rarely used because of qid dosing and diarrhea.**

21. Ans. (b) Shortly before meals

(Ref: Goodman Gilman 12th E/P1312)

- After PPIs are ingested, they are absorbed into systemic circulation and secreted into the canaliculi of parietal cells. During food intake there is release of HCl into these canaliculi, and the acidic medium activates the PPIs, which are prodrugs. The activated PPIs block the proton pumps.
- This is the reason for which PPIs are given **at least 30 minutes before food** intake, so that they are present in the canaliculi at the time of HCl secretion.

22. Ans. (a) Ciprofloxacin

(Ref: Goodman Gilman 12th E/P1320)

- Tinidazole can be used in place of metronidazole for *H. pylori*.

Triple therapy	Quadruple therapy
PPI OD Clarithromycin Metronidazole or Amoxicillin or Tetracycline	PPI BD Metronidazole Tetracycline Bismuth subsalicylate

23. Ans. (d) Esomeprazole

(Ref: Goodman Gilman 12th E/P1312)

- **PPIs are the drug of choice for NSAID induced ulcer whereas misoprostol is the most specific drug.**

24. Ans. (b) Misoprostol

(Ref: Goodman Gilman 12th E/P1314)

- PPIs are drug of choice but misoprostol is the most specific drug for treatment of NSAID induced gastric ulcer.

25. Ans. (a) Pirenzepine

(Ref: Goodman Gilman 12th E/P1310)

- Pirenzepine and telezepine are M1 blockers used in peptic ulcer disease.

26. Ans. (c) Bismuth subcitrate

(Ref: Goodman Gilman 12th E/P1320)

27. Ans. (a) $H^+ K^+$ ATPase pump

(Ref: Goodman Gilman 12th E/P1311)

28. Ans. (d) Misoprostol

(Ref: Goodman Gilman 12th E/P1314)

- Most common side effect of misoprostol is **diarrhea** with abdominal cramps that begins after 2 weeks of therapy but is self-limiting.

29. Ans. (b) Magnesium hydroxide

(Ref: Goodman Gilman 12th E/P1315)

- Magnesium contracts smooth muscles and causes diarrhea.
- Aluminum relaxes smooth muscles and causes constipation.
- Hence both are combined as antacids to neutralize each others effect.

30. Ans. (a) Omeprazole

(Ref: Goodman Gilman 12th E/P1311)

31. Ans. (b) Ulcer healing

(Ref: Goodman Gilman 12th E/P1315)

32. Ans. (c) Cisapride

(Ref: Goodman Gilman 12th E/P1320)

33. Ans. (a) Omeprazole

(Ref: Goodman Gilman 12th E/P1311)

- PPIs are the drug of choice for GERD. Maximum acid secretion inhibition gives maximum clinical benefit by PPIs.

34. Ans. (d) All of the above

(Ref: Goodman Gilman 12th E/P1314)

- Prostaglandins are the physiological gastroprotectors.
- They stimulate Gs subtype Pg receptors like EP_2 and EP_4, thus increasing cyc AMP which **stimulates mucin and bicarbonate production**.

- Stimulation of G_i subtype Pg receptor, i.e. EP_3 decreases cyc AMP resulting in **decreased HCl secretion**.

35. Ans. (c) 8 Weeks

(Ref: KDT 7th E/P651)

36. Ans. (a) Sucralfate

(Ref: Goodman Gilman 12th E/P1315)

- Gastric acid is required for polymerization of sucralfate and hence antacids will inhibit the same.

37. Ans. (b) Lansoprazole

(Ref: Goodman Gilman 12th E/P1312)

38. Ans. (a) Ranitidine does not have anti androgenic effect

(Ref: Goodman Gilman 12th E/P1314)

39. Ans. (a) Chloramphenicol

(Ref: Goodman Gilman 12th E/P1320)

40. Ans. (c) Ranitidine increases gastric pH so that sucralfate is unable to act

(Ref: Goodman Gilman 12th E/P 1315)

41. Ans. (a) Omeprazole

(Ref: Goodman Gilman 12th E/P 1313)

42. Ans. (b) Cimetidine

(Ref: Goodman Gilman 12th E/P 1314)

43. Ans. (c) Sucralfate + simethicone

(Ref: Goodman Gilman 12th E/P 1315)

- Simethicone is combined with antacids to prevent foaming and associated GERD.

44. Ans. (d) Cinnarizine

(Ref: Goodman Gilman 12th E/P1343)

Antiemetics	
5HT3 antagonists	Ondansetron
D2 antagonists	Metoclopromide, Domperidone
H1 antagonists	Promethazine, Diphenhydrinate, Doxylamine
Anticholinergics	Scopalamine
Antipsychotics	Haloperidol, Chlorpromazine
Steroids	Dexamethasone
NK1 antagonist	Aprepitant
Cannabinoid agonist	Dronabinol, Nabilone

45. Ans. (a) Granisetron

(Ref: Goodman Gilman 13th E/P935)

- Anticancer drugs stimulate enterochromaffin cells to release serotonin, which stimulates 5HT3 receptors. This is responsible for chemotherapy induced nausea and vomiting.
- Thus, the most specific drugs for treatment of chemotherapy induced nausea and vomiting are 5HT3 antagonists like granisetron and ondansetron.
- 5HT-3 antagonists are effective only against early onset nausea and vomiting i.e. seen within 24 hours and hence are drug of choice for early onset nausea and vomiting.
- For late onset nausea and vomiting seen beyond 24 hours, NK1 antagonist aprepitant is the drug of choice.

Note: With all drugs nausea and vomiting is early onset and with only few drugs it is late onset. Hence if it is asked drug of choice for chemotherapy induced nausea and vomiting with both ondansetron and aprepitant in options, ondansetron is a better answer.

46. Ans. (d) Bismuth

(Ref: Goodman Gilman 12th E/P1343)

47. Ans. (a) Agonist at NK_1 receptors

(Ref: Goodman Gilman 12th E/P1343)

- Aprepitant is an antagonist at the NK1 receptors and not agonist.
- It is the drug of choice for late onset chemotherapy induced nausea and vomiting.

48. Ans. (b) Ondansetron

(Ref: Goodman Gilman 12th E/P1344)

- Cisplatin causes early onset (within 24 hours) and late onset (after 48 hours) nausea and vomiting. All patients experience early onset, whereas only some have late onset nausea and vomiting.
- For early onset 5HT3 antagonists like ondansetron is drug of choice but are ineffective in late onset.
- Aprepitant is drug of choice for late onset nausea and vomiting associated with cisplatin.
- Since early onset is seen in all patients ondansetron is best possible answer.

49. Ans. (c) 5-HT_3

(Ref: Goodman Gilman 12th E/P1344)

50. Ans. (c) Ondansetron

(Ref: Goodman Gilman 12th E/P1344)

- For apomorphine induced emesis 5HT3 antagonists and antipsychotics are not used.
- 5HT3 antagonist increase risk of severe hypotension whereas antipsychotics being D2 antagonists, decrease the D2 agonistic effects of apomorphine.

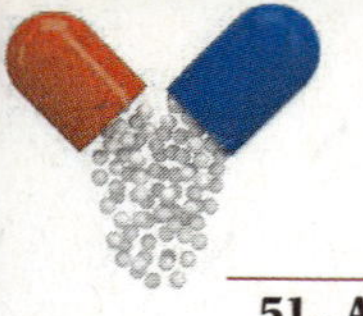

51. Ans. (c) Pentazocine

(Ref: Goodman Gilman 12th E/P1344)

52. Ans. (b) Metoclopramide

(Ref: Goodman Gilman 13th E/P923)

- Metoclopramide a D2 antagonist is a lipid soluble drug and hence can cross blood brain barrier and cause EPS.
- In the given question, the student is having acute dystonia, the EPS that can be seen earliest.

53. Ans. (c) Diarrhea

(Ref: KDT 7th E/P667)

54. Ans. (a) Lubiprostone

(Ref: Goodman Gilman 12th E/P 1334)

55. Ans. (b) Used in secretory diarrhea

(Ref: Goodman Gilman 12th E/P 1328)

56. Ans. (c) Cisapride

(Ref: Goodman Gilman 12th E/P1326)

- $5HT_4$ agonists like cisapride and tegaserod can cause QT prolongation and hence were banned.

57. Ans. (a) Increase lower esophageal sphincter tone

(Ref: Goodman Gilman 12th E/P 1325)

- D_2 antagonists increase lower esophageal sphincter, gastric antral and small intestinal contraction, however they don't have any effect on large intestine.
- Thus best possible answer is option (a), as option (c) which states increased gastric peristalsis is partially correct, as the effect in stomach is confined only to antrum.

58. Ans. (a) Metoclopromide

(Ref: Goodman Gilman 12th E/P 1325)

- Metoclopromide being lipid soluble can easily cross blood brain barrier and hence associated with EPS.
- Domperidone does not cross blood brain barrier and is devoid of EPS.

59. Ans. (c) Subacute intestinal obstruction

(Ref: Goodman Gilman 12th E/P 1333)

- Stimulants are absolutely contraindicated in patients of intestinal obstruction.

60. Ans. (b) Cispride

(Ref: Goodman Gilman 12th E/P1326)

61. Ans. (c) Stimulant purgative

(Ref: Goodman Gilman 12th E/P 1333)

62. Ans. (b) Lactulose

(Ref: Goodman Gilman 12th E/P 1332)

- Lactulose when metabolized into SFA, makes intestinal pH acidic which converts ammonia into polar ammonium ion and facilitates its excretion. Hence it is used in **hepatic encephalopathy**.

63. Ans. (c) Octreotide

(Ref: Goodman Gilman 12th E/P 1338)

64. Ans. (c) Lubiprostone

(Ref: Goodman Gilman 12th E/P 1334)

- Lubiprostone increases chloride ion secretion along with water into intestinal lumen by stimulating prostanoid receptor (EP_4).

65. Ans. (a) Laxatives

(Ref: Goodman Gilman 12th E/P 1333)

66. Ans. (a) $5HT_4$ agonist

(Ref: Goodman Gilman 12th E/P 1314)

67. Ans. (a) $5HT_4$ Agonist

(Ref: Goodman Gilman 12th E/P 1314)

68. Ans. (c) Stimulates CTZ

(Ref: Goodman Gilman 12th E/P 1325)

69. Ans. (b) Sibutramine

(Ref: CMDT 2015/P 1248)

Drugs used for obesity	Drugs under trial for obesity	Drugs banned for treatment of obesity
• Orlistat – Inhibits intestinal lipase • Locaserin – Selective serotonin receptor agonist • Phenteramine and topiramate combination	• Beta 3 receptor agonist • H3 antagonist – Tiprolisant • Bupropion and naltrexone combination – Increased CVS risk seen in trial • Cetilistat – Pancreatic lipase inhibitor • Exenatide	• Sibutramine – Cardiovascular side effects • Rimonabant – Suicidal tendencies

70. Ans. (a) To decrease intestinal gas produced during digestive process

(Ref: Gary Walsh Pharmaceutical biotechnology/P 365)

- Enzyme papain digests dietary proteins and is helpful as an anti-flatulence agent.

71. Ans. (b) Amoxicilline

(Ref: Goodman Gilman 12th E/P 1326-28)

72. Ans. (d) Metoclopromide

(Ref: Goodman Gilman 12th E/P 1325)

73. Ans. (a) Sulfasalazine

(Ref: Goodman Gilman 12th E/P 1355)

74. Ans. (a) Infliximab

(Ref: Goodman Gilman 12th E/P 1359)

75. Ans. (b) Mesalazine

(Ref: Goodman Gilman 12th E/P 1355)

- Mesalazine is the preferred 5-ASA compound due to better side effect profile.

76. Ans. (a) Infliximab

(Ref: Goodman Gilman 12th E/P 1359)

77. Ans. (e) Acts best in alkaline medium

(Ref: Goodman Gilman 12th E/P1311)

- **PPIs are prodrugs which are activated by the acid in canaliculi, following which they inhibit proton pumps.**
- Though PPIs have a **short half-life** of 30-120 minutes, their **duration of action is prolonged** (>24 hours) due to irreversible binding; the reason why they are called as **hit and run drugs**.

78. Ans. (a) Constipation, (b) Impotence, (c) ↑ In plasma Aminotranferase, (e) Gynecomastia

(Ref: Goodman Gilman 12th E/P1314)

- **Cimetidine** causes **antiandrogenic** action along with **inhibition of estradiol metabolism** and **increase in prolactin levels**. This causes **gynecomastia** and **impotence in males** and galactorrhea in females.
- Cimetidine is also an enzyme inhibitor and causes drug interactions. Ranitidine is a less potent enzyme inhibitor as compared to cimetidine.
- CNS (confusion, delirium etc.) and GIT (nausea, **constipation** etc.) side effects can be seen with this class.
- Tolerance is another drawback that can be seen within 3 days of treatment in patients. Pancytopenia and **elevated ALT/AST** can be rarely associated.

79. Ans. (b) Alginates prevent GERD, (c) Simethicone relieve flatulence, (e) Simethicone prevent GERD

(Ref: Goodman Gilman 12th E/P1315)

- **Simethicone** is a surfactant added to decrease surface tension of gas bubbles in stomach that bursts bubbles and **expels gas thereby relieving flatulance**. There is also a decreased foaming and associated **GERD**.
- **Alginate** is also combined with antacids which forms a viscous layer that floats over gastric contents and **prevents GERD**.

80. Ans. (a) Diazepam, (d) Droperidol, (e) Ondansetron

(Ref: Goodman Gilman 12th E/P1344)

81. Ans. (a) Lubiprostone

(Ref: Katzung 13th edition, Page 1064)

- Lubiprostone stimulates type 2 chloride ion channels (ClC_2) on apical membrane of intestinal epithelial cells, which leads to secretion of chloride ions into intestinal lumen followed by sodium secretion by paracellular pathways to maintain isoelectric neutrality.
- This leads to secretion of water into the lumen to maintain isotonic equilibrium.

82. Ans. (a) Linaclotide

(Ref: Katzung 13th edited, Page 1064)

Linaclotide stimulates **guanylate cyclase** and increases cyclic guanosine monophosphate (cGMP), which stimulates cystic fibrosis transmembrane regulator (CFTR) resulting in increased chloride and water secretion into lumen.

83. Ans. (a) Plecanatide

(Ref: https://www.centerwatch.com/drug-information/fda-approved-drugs/drug/100183/trulance-plecanatide)

- Plecanatide is a new drug approved by FDA in 2017 for treatment of chronic idiopathic constipation.
- It stimulates guanylate cyclase and increases cyclic AMP, which stimulates cystic fibrosis transmembrane regulator (CFTR) in intestinal epithelial cells. This leads to secretion of chloride ions and water into the lumen.
- The dose is 3 mg by oral route once daily.

84. Ans. (b) Infliximb

(Ref: Goodman Gilman 12th E/P1359)

85. Ans. (c) Azathioprine

(Ref: Godman Gilman 12th E/P1357)

86. Ans. (a) Ulcerative colitis

(Ref: Goodman Gilman 12th E/P1354)

87. Ans. (a) Before breakfast

(Ref: Goodman Gilman 12th E/P1312)

88. Ans. (a) Phenoxy methyl penicillin

(Ref: Goodman Gilman 12th E/P1315)

Sucralfate Decreases Absorption of

- Phenytoin
- Digoxin
- Cimetidine
- Ketoconazole
- Fluoroquinolones

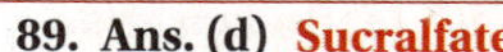

89. Ans. (d) Sucralfate

(Ref: Goodman Gilman 12th E/P11320)

90. Ans. (b) Omeprazole

(Ref: Goodman Gilman 12th E/P1312)

91. Ans. (d) Chemotherapy induced hyperuricemia

(Ref: Goodman Gilman 12th E/P1343)

92. Ans. (b) Bisacodyl

(Ref: Goodman Gilman 12th E/P1333)

93. Ans. (b) Ondansetron selective-5HT3 antagonist

(Ref: Goodman Gilman 12th E/P1343)

94. Ans. (a) Prochlorpromazine

(Ref: Goodman Gilman 12th E/P1343)

95. Ans. (b) Meclizine-5HT4 agonist

(Ref: Goodman Gilman 12th E/P1343)

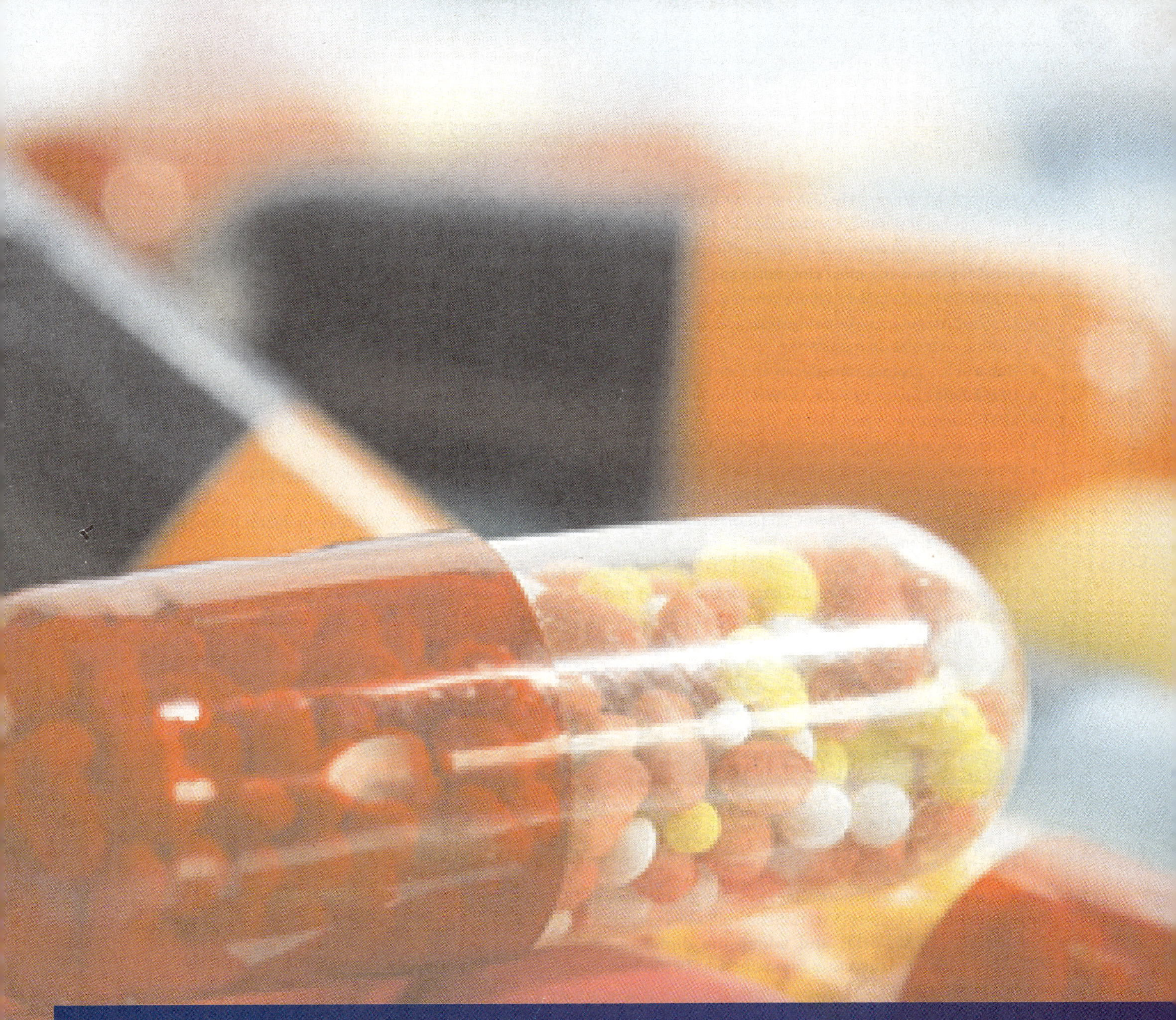

Blood

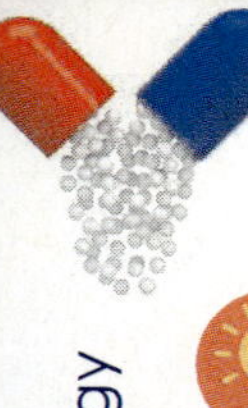

One Liners

- Aspirin is an **irreversible COX inhibitor and decreases TXA2 synthesis.**
- Antiaggregant potency can be rated as **glycoprotein IIb/IIIa inhibitors > ADP inhibitors > Aspirin.**
- **Epsilon aminocaproic acid is the antifibrinolytic of choice** for hemorrhagic states in **fibrinolytic overdose**.
- **Tenecteplase is the most clot/fibrin specific drug.**
- **Lepirudin** is safe in liver failure whereas argatroban is safe in renal failure.
- Oral anticoagulants like **dabigatran** and **apixaban** and parenteral anticoagulants like **LMWH** and **fondaparinux** don't require routine coagulation monitoring.
- **Heparin** is a **glycosaminoglycan** and strongest acid found in mast cells.
- **UFH** inhibits factor Xa = IIa, **LMWH** inhibits factor Xa > IIa and **fondaparinux** inhibits only factor Xa.
- aPTT monitoring is required for heparin whereas PT monitoring is required for warfarin.
- **Protamine sulphate** is the antidote of choice for heparin toxicity.
- **Vitamin K** is the antidote of choice in symptomatic whereas **FFP** is the treatment of choice in symptomatic warfarin toxicity.
- The incidence of HIT is **UFH > LMWH > Fondaparinux**.
- The first to decrease is **factor VII (shortest acting)** followed by protein C and last to decrease in factor II (longest acting) after warfarin therapy.
- **Skin necrosis** is seen with warfarin due to a rapid decrease in **anticoagulant protein C**.
- Desferrioxamine is the iron chelator of choice and deferiprone is preferred in case of desferrioxamine intolerance.
- **Filgrastim** and lenograstim are granulocyte colony stimulating factor (G-CSF) analogs whereas sargramostim is granulocyte macrophage colony stimulating factor (GM-CSF) analog.
- **Trisodium citrate** is the anticoagulant of choice for practical studies.
- **Dextran 40** is a plasma expander used in shock, also has antithrombotic effect due to inhibition of platelet aggregation.

ANTI-AGGREGANTS

PLATELET AGGREGATION PATHOPHYSIOLOGY

- Whenever there is an injury to blood vessels, then collagen and von Willebrand's factors (Vwf) activate platelets to secrete aggregants like **TXA2, 5HT, and adenosine diphosphate (ADP)**. The aggregates then undergo adhesion to the Vwf in subendothelial membrane.
- Activation of **glycoprotein IIb/IIIa** in the platelets further promotes aggregation and binding of aggregates to fibrinogen.
- Exposed phospholipid from platelet surface promotes thrombin formation in the coagulation pathway, which converts fibrinogen to fibrin and stabilizes the clot. Thrombin acts on protease activated receptor 1 (PAR1) in platelets and further promotes aggregation.
- To prevent excessive clot formation, the fibrinolytic pathway may be stimulated. **Plasminogen is activated into plasmin by tissue plasminogen activator (tPA)**. Plasmin breaks fibrin and reshapes the thrombus. Thus, a balance must be stroked in between thrombus formation and dissolution as both can be fatal, if present in excess.

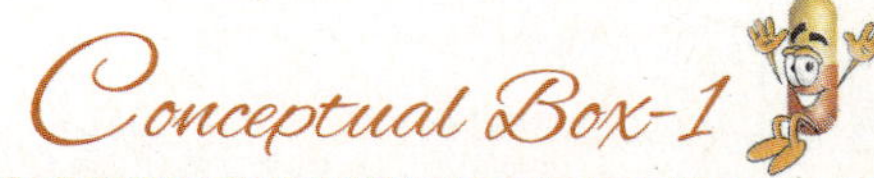

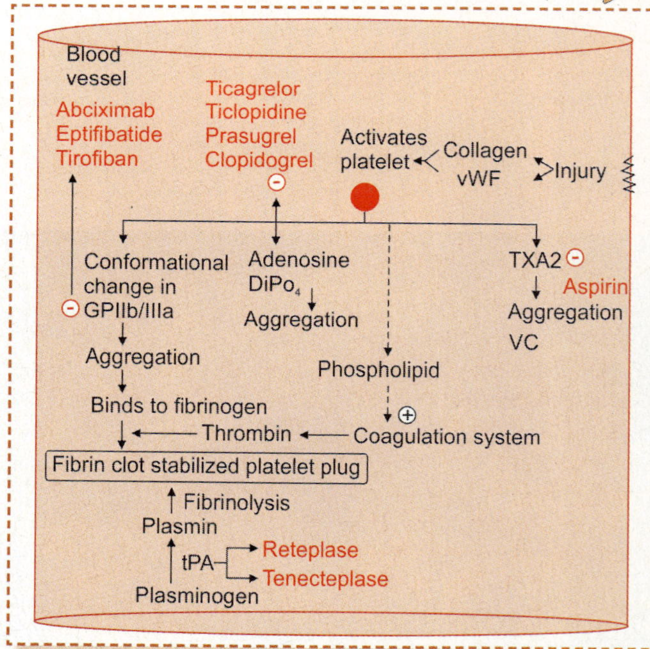

ASPIRIN

- Aspirin is an **irreversible COX inhibitor and decreases TXA2 synthesis**. Since platelets do not have nucleus and cannot synthesize new COX, the effect is seen until platelet lives i.e. **7 to 10 days**.
- Antiaggregant effect seen at **lower doses is primarily due to inhibition of COX 1**. The antiaggregant dose is in between 75–325 mg/day.
- Aspirin is the first line drug for secondary prophylaxis of MI and stroke i.e. a patient who already had an attack of MI or stroke. Because of its side effects it is not used for primary prophylaxis. Aspirin along with clopidogrel is also used for treatment of unstable angina.
- Being an NSAID it retains the side effect of GIT like ulcers and there is always risk of bleeding. According to recent guidelines aspirin need not be stopped before surgery. But the **ADP inhibitors being more potent drug, should be stopped 1 week before surgery.**

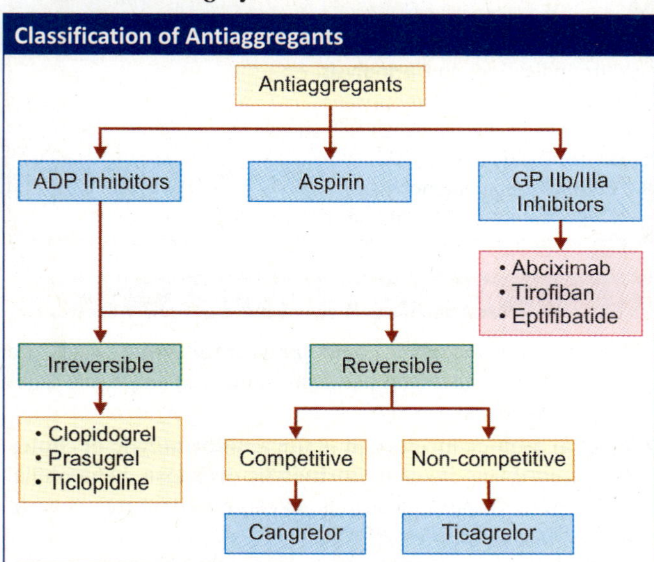

ADENOSINE DIPHOSPHATE RECEPTOR (P_2Y_{12}) INHIBITORS

- Older drugs in this class like clopidogrel, ticlopidine, prasugrel are **prodrugs and irreversible inhibitors** of P_2Y_{12} receptor.
- Recent drugs like **ticagrelor and cangrelor are not prodrugs and reversible** inhibitors of P2Y12 receptor.
- Aspirin, clopidogrel, ticlopidine and prasugrel, though have short half-life, their effect is prolonged due to irreversible inhibition. Thus, these are known as **hit and run** drugs.

Ticlopidine

- Ticlopidine is a prodrug activated by CYP_{450} enzymes.
- It is associated with side effects like agranulocytosis, thrombocytopenia, TTP-HUS and GIT side effects (most common) like nausea and vomiting.
- Hence it is not commonly used nowadays and has been replaced by clopidogrel which is more potent and less toxic than ticlopidine.

Clopidogrel

- **Clopidogrel** is a **prodrug** activated by **CYP2C19** and hence genetic polymorphism with decreased CYP2C19 activity can compromise its activity.
- A black box warning has been issued against it that patients with genetic polymorphism might be at an increased risk of MI and stroke. **PPIs** are metabolized by CYP2C19 and hence can **decrease activation of clopidogrel**.
- Only 15% of clopidogrel is activated, whereas the rest 85% is inactivated by esterases.
- It is approved for prophylaxis of stroke, MI, peripheral vascular disease and acute coronary syndrome. The recommended dose is 75 mg OD for prophylaxis.
- It is synergistic with aspirin and hence frequently combined. **Clopidogrel along with aspirin** is the standard antiaggregant of choice in patients with PCI followed by stenting.
- As it is more potent, it has a higher risk of bleeding than aspirin.

Prasugrel

- **Prasugrel** is also a prodrug that is completely absorbed and activated by CYP_{450} enzymes. It is the fastest acting and most efficacious drug in this class.
- However, because of more efficacy the chances of bleeding are also higher and hence is contraindicated in patients with **cerebrovascular disorders like stroke**.
- Thus, it is used as an antiaggregant only in patients undergoing percutaneous coronary intervention.

Cangrelor

- **Cangrelor** is an adenosine analog and hence the inhibition of P_2Y_{12} receptor is competitive and reversible.
- Being adenosine analog, it cannot be given by oral route and is immediately metabolized with a half-life of 3-6 minutes.
- It is given by intravenous route to patients undergoing percutaneous coronary intervention.

Ticagrelor

- **Ticagrelor** is a non-competitive reversible inhibitor of P2Y12 receptor. Since it is not a prodrug, it is fast acting and even is more potent antiaggregant than clopidogrel.
- It is an oral drug that is used along with aspirin in patients with acute coronary syndrome (MI or unstable angina).
- Bleeding, dyspnea and asymptomatic ventricular pauses can be seen as side effects.

DIPYRIDAMOLE

- Dipyridamole increases cyclic AMP in platelets by inhibiting phosphodiesterase and adenosine uptake proteins. Cyclic AMP decreases intraplatelet calcium and gives antiaggregant effect.
- Dipyridamole along with aspirin can be used for prophylaxis of stroke.
- By increasing cyclic AMP in blood vessel smooth muscles, it can cause vasodilation. This can result in **coronary steal phenomenon** and hence not used in MI.

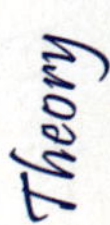

- Vasodilation can result in side effects like flushing, hypotension and headache.

GLYCOPROTEIN IIB/IIIA INHIBITORS

- Abciximab, tirofiban and eptifibatide inhibit $\alpha_{IIb}\beta_3$ receptors in glycoprotein IIb/IIIa of platelets. These drugs are used in patients of MI undergoing PCI along with anticoagulants, unstable angina and NSTEMI. These are the **most potent anti-aggregants**. Antiaggregant potency can be rated as **glycoprotein IIb/IIIa inhibitors > ADP inhibitors > Aspirin**.
- **Abciximab** is not specific for glycoprotein IIb/IIIa as it also inhibits vitronectin and hence is more effective as compared to eptifibatide and tirofiban. It has the shortest half-life in this class but is longest acting due to high affinity binding to $\alpha_{IIb}\beta_3$.
- **Eptifibatide** is a peptide and **tirofiban** is a nonpeptide inhibitor of only $\alpha_{IIb}\beta_3$ receptors. Eptifibatide has longest half-life but is shortest acting due to least affinity for $\alpha_{IIb}\beta_3$ receptors. Both these drugs are excreted by **kidney**.
- Side effects like **bleeding and thrombocytopenia** are more commonly seen with **abciximab**.

Recent Advances

Vorapaxar: Vorapaxar inhibits thrombin and thrombin receptor agonist peptide (TRAP) induced aggregation by inhibiting protease activated-1 (PAR-1) receptors in platelets. It is approved by FDA recently for prophylaxis of MI and peripheral artery disease along with aspirin or clopidogrel. It has a high risk of intracranial bleeding and hence should not be used in a patient with history of stroke, transient ischemic attack or intracranial bleeding.

FIBRINOLYTICS

Streptokinase

- **Streptokinase** is a protein synthesized from streptococci.
- It binds to plasminogen and together the streptokinase-plasminogen complex activates **plasminogen to plasmin**, which breaks down fibrin present in thrombi as well as plasma. Hence it is clot/fibrin nonspecific drug.
- It is used for thrombolysis in MI at a dose of 1.5 million units over 30–60 minutes by continuous infusion.
- Its use is limited by neutralizing antibodies produced against it due to its **antigenic nature**. As it is an exogenous reaction, hypersensitivity can be seen characterized by rash, fever and anaphylaxis. It can cause transient hypotension due to bradykinin release by plasmin.
- Other clot/fibrin nonspecific drugs are urokinase and anistreplase. Anistreplase is streptokinase combined with lys-plasminogen. It is similar to streptokinase in all aspects, except that it is long acting and hence once bolus dosing is possible. It is much costlier than streptokinase and hence not widely used.
- Urokinase is a serine protease that activates plasminogen to plasmin. It can be used for thrombolysis in arteries and veins via catheter. It is not commonly used now days due to unavailability.

Tissue Plasminogen Activator (tPA) Analogs

- Recombinant tPA produced by genetic engineering like **alteplase and recombinant tPA derivatives like tenecteplase** and duteplase have more affinity for **plasminogen bound to fibrin** than plasminogen in plasma. Hence these are known as **clot/fibrin specific drugs**.
- Alteplase has a half-life of **5 minutes**. It is given as a bolus dose of 15 mg followed by **0.75 mg/kg continuous infusion**. Tenecteplase is longest acting and hence given as single IV bolus dose and reteplase is given as two IV doses 30 minutes apart.
- **Tenecteplase is the most clot/fibrin specific drug.**
- These are given by intravenous route for thrombolysis in MI, ischemic stroke and massive pulmonary embolism. In case of arterial and proximal venous thrombosis they can be administered directly in to the thrombus via catheter.
- Most common side effect of fibrinolysis therapy is **bleeding**.

Mnemonics

Contraindications to Fibrinolysis

B : Brain tumor and aneurysms
R : Recent ischemic stroke or trauma
A : Aortic dissection
I : Intracranial haemorrhage
N : Noncompressible vascular punctures

ANTI-FIBRINOLYTICS

- **Epsilon aminocaproic acid** and **tranexamic acid** are lysine analogs that competitively bind and inactivate both plasminogen and plasmin.
- **Epsilon aminocaproic acid is the antifibrinolytic of choice** for hemorrhagic states in **fibrinolytic overdose**, hemophilia, surgery etc. Tranexamic acid is also approved for treatment of metrorrhagia.

ANTICOAGULANTS

PHYSIOLOGY OF COAGULATION SYSTEM

- In the extrinsic coagulation pathway, tissue injury releases tissue factor, which along with factor VIIa and calcium converts factor X to Xa.
- Factor Xa along with Va and calcium converts prothrombin (II) to thrombin (IIa).
- Thrombin converts fibrinogen to fibrin which forms the permanent clot.
- Antithrombin III is a protease that breaks down factors IIa, IXa, Xa, XIa and XIIa.
- Thus, one way of achieving anticoagulant effect is by inhibiting coagulation pathway at the level of thrombin by giving direct thrombin inhibitors like lepirudin.
- Another way is to stimulate anticoagulation pathway by activating antithrombin III by giving indirect thrombin inhibitors like heparin.

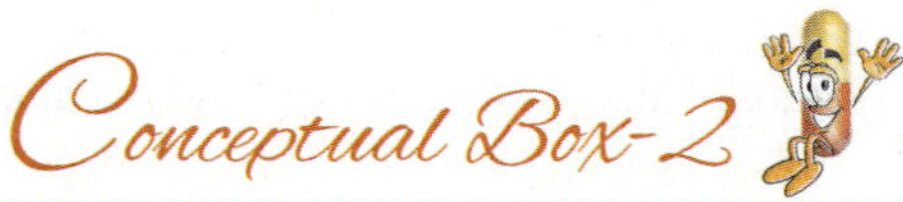

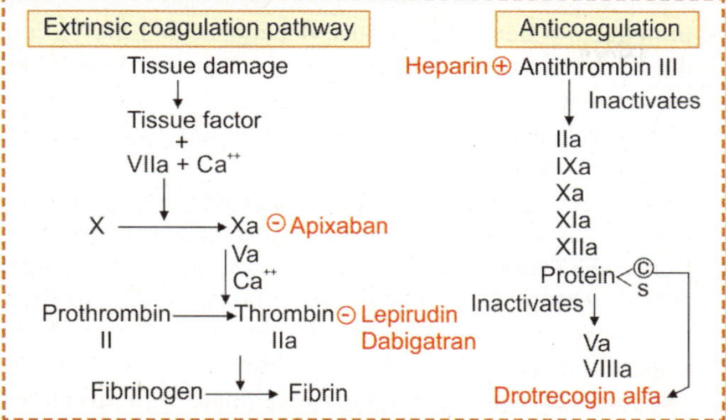

DIRECT THROMBIN INHIBITORS (DTI)

Parenteral DTI

All parenteral DTI are bivalent compounds and inhibit catalytic site as well as substrate recognition site in thrombin. The only exception is **argatroban which is univalent** and inhibits only catalytic site.

- **Hirudin** was the first DTI derived from leech saliva. This followed development of recombinant drugs from hirudin like desirudin and lepirudin. The recent ones like bivalirudin and argatroban are purely synthetic.
- **Hirudin and lepirudin** are clinically not used. Argatroban is the drug of choice for treatment of **heparin induced thrombocytopenia**; desirudin and bivalirudin can also be used.
- **Desirudin** is approved for DVT prophylaxis in lower limb surgeries and **bivalirudin** can be used in patients of MI undergoing PCI.
- **All drugs are** excreted by kidney except argatroban and hence dose adjustment is required in renal failure. **Argatroban** is excreted by liver and hence dose adjustment is required in liver failure and is the **preferred anticoagulant in renal failure**.
- **aPTT monitoring is required for all drugs in this class, whereas argatroban also requires PT monitoring.**

Oral DTI

- **Ximelagatran** was the first oral DTI, but was withdrawn due to **hepatotoxicity**.
- **Dabigatran** is the recent one approved for DVT prophylaxis in lower limb surgeries and also for treatment of acute venous thromboembolism.
- The major side effect is bleeding and to reverse it an anti dabigatran monoclonal antibody called as **idarucizumab** has been recently approved**.**
- These drugs **don't require aPTT monitoring** like the parenteral drugs.
- Dabigatran a is substrate for p-glycoprotein and hence can interact with inducers and inhibitors of p-glycoprotein. Since majority of the drugs administered are excreted by kidneys, dose reduction is required in renal failure.

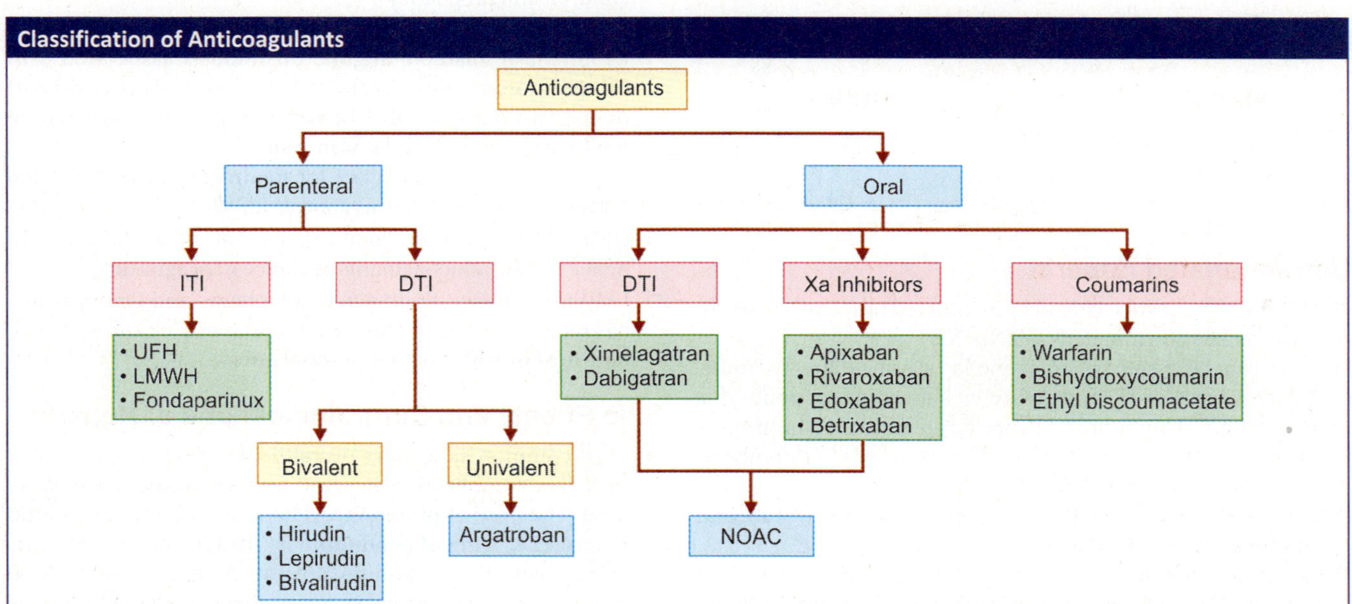

Note: NOAC is Novel Oral Anti-Coagulants.

INDIRECT THROMBIN INHIBITORS (ITI)

- As mentioned in the conceptual box ITI acts indirectly by binding to antithrombin III (AT-III) and activating it. Activated AT-III is active against most of the factors like IIa, IXa, Xa, Xa, XIa and XIIa, except **factor VIIa**.
- **Unfractionated heparin (UFH)** is a **glycosaminoglycan** derived from mast cells of porcine intestinal mucosa. It is made up of an active pentasaccharide that binds to AT-III and a long chain **heteropolysaccharide** attached to this pentasaccharide.
- **Low molecular weight heparin (LMWH)** is a semisynthetic derivative of heparin with pentasaccharide and a shorter chain.
- **Fondaparinux** is a synthetic drug containing only active pentasaccharide.
- Activation of AT-III by pentasaccharide of **UFH, LMWH and fondaparinux** increases affinity of AT-III only for factor **Xa**. However, because of a long chain of **UFH** it can also facilitate binding of **IIa** to thrombin. **LMWH** has a shorter chain and hence it has **lesser effect on IIa** and **fondaparinux** does not have any chain and hence is **not active at all against IIa**.
- Because of long chain UFH binds to endothelium and plasma proteins, whereas LMWH has lesser binding and fondaparinux does not bind at all.

Conceptual Box-3

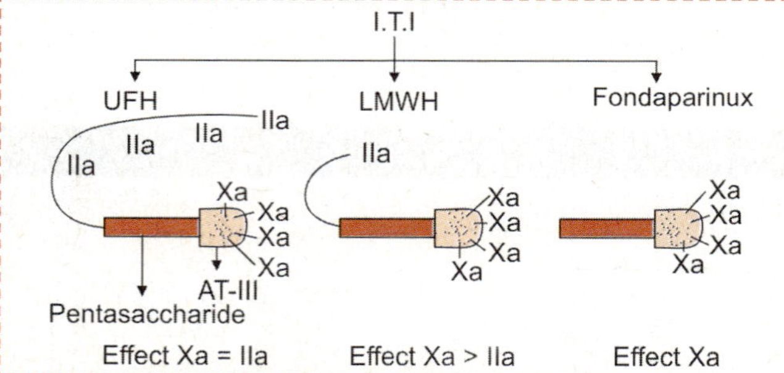

Unfractionated Heparin

- UFH inhibits **in vitro** coagulation initiated by factor XII and **in vivo** coagulation initiated by factor XI.
- UFH can be given by intravenous or subcutaneous route. Heparin has low bioavailability by subcutaneous route due to endothelial binding and hence for treatment of thrombosis intravenous route is preferred. For prophylaxis of thrombosis subcutaneous route can be used.
- Since it is short acting **QID dosing is required by IV route and BD dosing is required by subcutaneous route.**
- The only place where UFH is preferred more than LMWH and fondaparinux is for **prevention of catheter induced thrombosis** caused by factor XII in cardiopulmonary bypass and in patients with high risk of bleeding. In patients of DVT or pulmonary embolism with concurrent thrombolysis (increased risk of bleeding) unfractionated heparin is preferred because it has a short half-life and protamine is more effective against unfractionated heparin than LMWH.
- Heparin is cleared primarily by the **reticuloendothelial system (macrophages) and only a minor part by kidney**. Hence it can be safely used in renal failure. It binds to macrophages, endothelium of blood vessels and plasma proteins and hence has a dose dependent half-life. At low doses it has short, whereas at high doses it has longer half-life.
- Since heparin also binds to a protein called as "platelet factor 4" released by activated platelets, it is less active against platelet rich thrombi.
- Due to inter individual variability in heparin binding proteins, the anticoagulant effect is variable and unpredictable as well. Hence **aPTT monitoring** is absolutely required with heparin. For this reason, LMWH and fondaparinux are more preferred nowadays.
- Heparin at high doses has antiaggregant effect and it also induces release of lipoprotein lipase and decreases plasma triglyceride, VLDL and chylomicrons. Hence on discontinuation, hyperlipidemia can be seen.

LMWH and Fondaparinux

- LMWH (Enoxaparin, tinzaparin) and fondaparinux are given by **subcutaneous route. They have longer half-life and hence LMWH can be given by once or twice daily dosing and fondaparinux by twice daily dosing.**
- Unlike UFH, LMWH has lesser binding to endothelium and plasma proteins and fondaparinux does not bind at all and hence both have a more bioavailability and longer duration of action **(fondaparinux > LMWH > Heparin)**. Thus, routine **aPTT monitoring is not required**.
- To monitor the effect of LMWH **anti-factor Xa assay** is done in selective cases like patients with renal failure, obesity, in children and pregnancy.
- These are the preferred parenteral anticoagulants of choice for treatment of **unstable angina, thrombosis associated with MI, pulmonary embolism, DVT**. However, fondaparinux is not preferred in **post MI PCI and stenting** because it cannot inhibit catheter induced thrombosis.
- LMWH is the drug of choice for treatment of cancer related thrombosis; edoxaban is as good as LMWH.
- UFH, LMWH and fondaparinux cannot cross placenta and hence are the anticoagulants of choice in **pregnancy**.
- LMWH has lesser binding to macrophages and fondaparinux has nil and hence both are cleared primarily by kidney. Thus, both are **contraindicated in renal failure**.

Side Effects and Contraindications of Heparin

- Most common side effect overall is bleeding. To prevent or treat this complication intravenous **protamine sulphate** is used. The dose of protamine to heparin in body is in a ratio of **1:100 i.e. 1 mg of protamine is used for every 100 units of heparin**. The maximum dose of protamine used is 50 mg. Protamine sulphate is more effective against UFH as compared to LMWH, but is not active against fondaparinux.
- Autoantibodies against heparin bound to platelets can cause platelet aggregation, thrombosis and **heparin induced thrombocytopenia (HIT)**.
- Other side effects associated are hyperkalemia, alopecia and osteoporosis.

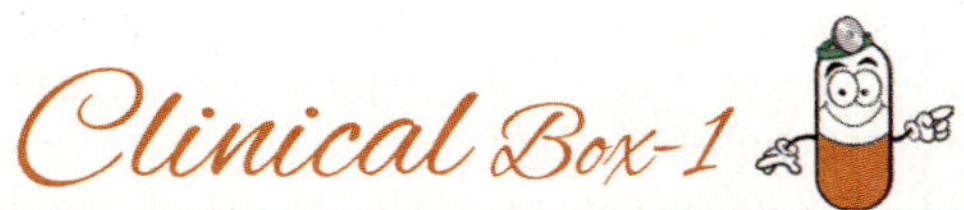

Heparin Induced Thrombocytopenia

- Heparin induced thrombocytopenia (HIT) is caused due to antibodies developed against antigens on PF4 (Platelet Factor 4) which are exposed due to heparin's heteropolysaccharide and PF4 binding. These antibodies activate platelets through Fc receptors which lead to platelet aggregation and thrombosis. In this due process platelets are consumed which leads to thrombocytopenia, which is not severe.
- Since LMWH has a shorter heteropolysaccharide chain, the risk of HIT is lesser and fondaparinux does not cause HIT due to absence of heteropolysaccharide chain.
- HIT develops after 1–2 weeks of exposure to heparin for the first time. In case of repeated exposure HIT develops usually in initial days if patient was exposed within 100 days.
- It is more common in **females** and in surgical and cancer patients. Thrombosis is usually **venous more than arterial** and incidence is **UFH > LMWH**.
- After diagnosis of HIT heparin is stopped. The drug of choice for HIT is **argatroban**. Fondaparinux, bivalirudin, danaparoid and rivaroxaban are also used in treatment. Once a platelet count of 100,00/mcl is achieved, warfarin is started and continued for at least 30 months. Argatroban is stopped once the INR with warfarin comes to 2 to 3.
- However warfarin should not be used in the beginning for treatment as in HIT protein C level is decreased. Thus heparin can cause skin necrosis by further decreasing protein C.

Mnemonics

Side effects of Heparin

A : Alopecia
H : Hyperkalemia, Haemorrhage
O : Osteoporosis
T : Thrombocytopenia

Contraindications of Heparin

T : Thrombocytopenia
E : Endocarditis
A : Alcoholics
C : Cirrhosis of liver
H : Hypertension
E : pEptic ulcer
R : Renal failure

COUMARINS

Bishydroxycoumarin is the longest acting whereas ethyl biscoumacetate and phenindione are shortest acting coumarins. Warfarin is intermediate acting and more preferred in this group.

- Vitamin K is activated by **vitamin K epoxide reductase-1 (VKORC-1)** enzyme. Activated vitamin K activates **gamma carboxylase** that activates coagulation factors **II, VII, IX and X;** anticoagulant **protein C and S**; and synthesizes bone matrix protein **osteocalcin** as well. Hence warfarin inhibits coagulation only in vivo stimulated by tissue factor and **factor VIIa**.
- There is a gradual decrease in these factors and hence the anticoagulant effect of warfarin is delayed. Hence in setting of acute thrombosis, parenteral anticoagulant (UFH/LMWH/Fondaparinux) is given for 5 days, known as heparin bridging.
- Warfarin produces anticoagulant effect by inhibiting VKORC-1 enzyme. It has good oral absorption, high albumin binding, metabolized by liver and has a half-life of around **40 hours**.
- The first to decrease is **factor VII (shortest acting)** followed by protein C and last to decrease in factor II (longest acting) after warfarin therapy.
- Interindividual variability in the effect of warfarin can be seen due to polymorphisms in CYP2C9 and VKORC1 gene as discussed in the topic of clinical pharmacology.

Conceptual Box-4

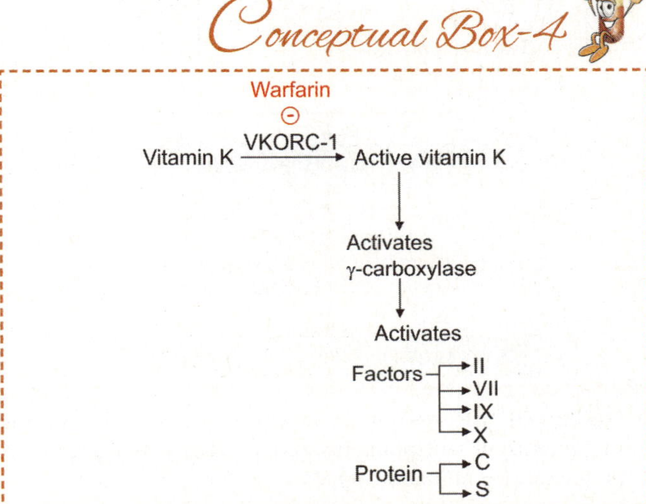

Uses of Warfarin

Warfarin by oral route is the drug of choice for **prophylaxis of venous thrombosis e.g. DVT and pulmonary thrombosis** and in patients of valvular atrial fibrillation.

Clinical Box-2

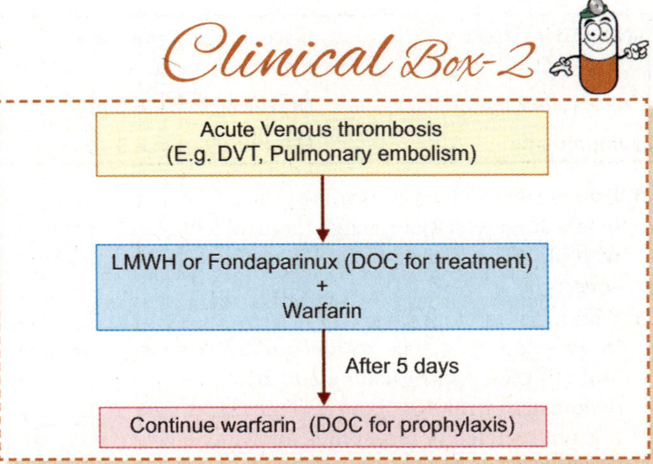

Note: Anticoagulation therapy is given for at least 3 months.

- Warfarin is also used to prevent thrombosis in pregnant females with prosthetic valve. However it crosses placenta and increases risk of fetal intraventricular hemorrhage and hence **should be stopped after 36 weeks and LMWH is started on the 37th week**.

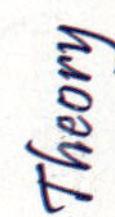

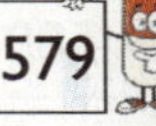

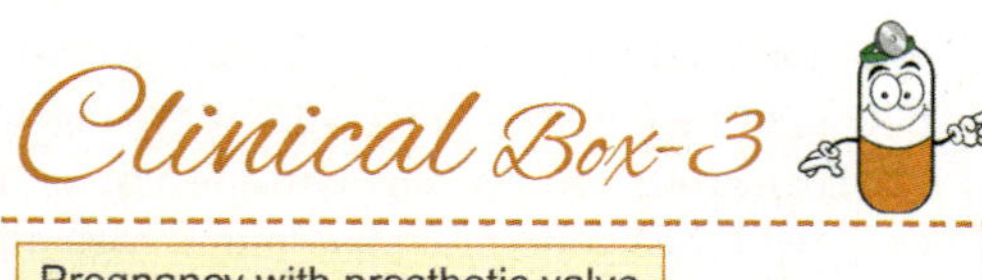
Clinical Box-3

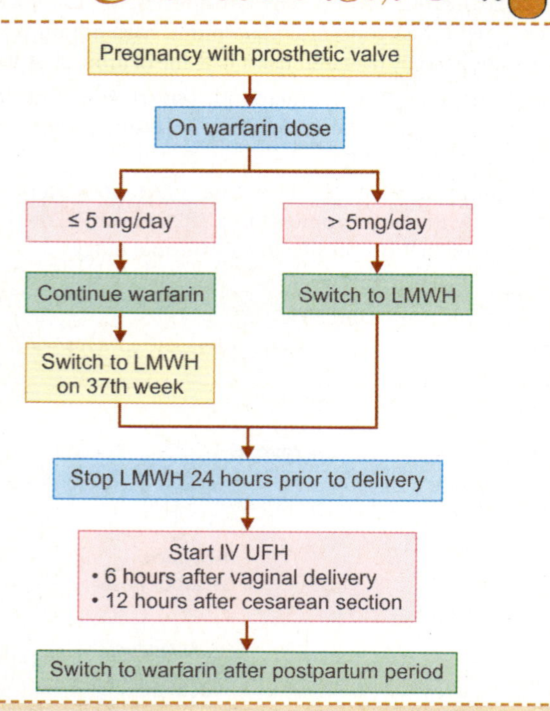
Pregnancy with prosthetic valve
On warfarin dose
≤ 5 mg/day
> 5mg/day
Continue warfarin
Switch to LMWH
Switch to LMWH on 37th week
Stop LMWH 24 hours prior to delivery
Start IV UFH
• 6 hours after vaginal delivery
• 12 hours after cesarean section
Switch to warfarin after postpartum period

- Warfarin is preferred anticoagulant to prevent thrombosis in patients of **antiphospholipid antibody syndrome**. In pregnancy, combination of LMWH and aspirin is used.

Side Effects and Contraindications

- **Bleeding** is the most common side effect and hence PT monitoring is done to maintain INR in a range of **2–3** (Normal INR = **0.9–1.3**). Bleeding is usually seen with INR > 4. Management of warfarin toxicity based on INR or symptoms is given below.

INR < 10 (Asymptomatic)	Discontinue warfarin and resume once INR is normal
INR ≥ 10 (Asymptomatic)	**Oral Vitamin K 2.5-5 mg**
Symptomatic	**FFP + IV Vitamin K 5-10 mg**

- Due to risk of bleeding warfarin should be stopped 4-5 days before surgery. If there is high risk of bleeding it is substituted with LMWH and then LMWH is stopped 12-24 hours before surgery.
- Warfarin is teratogenic and hence absolutely contraindicated in pregnancy. It can cause **midfacial/nasal hypoplasia and stippled epiphyseal calcifications** due to a decreased **osteocalcin** synthesis. It can also cause **CNS defects**. However, it is not secreted in breast milk and can be given to lactating females.
- **Skin necrosis** is a common complication seen after 2-5 days of treatment and the most common site is **breast in females**. The cause is a rapid decline in anticoagulant protein C or S.
- Other side effects seen are alopecia, blue discoloration of feet and worsening of HIT.
- Warfarin a mixture of R and S enantiomers, is metabolized by CYP2C9, hence enzyme inducers and inhibitors can affect its metabolism and effect.
- Antibiotics can decrease vitamin K production in gut by bacteria and hence increase effect of warfarin.

NOVEL ORAL ANTICOAGULANTS (NOAC)/DIRECT ACTING ORAL ANTICOAGULANTS (DOAC)

- This class contains the oral DTI like **dabigatran** and **oral factor Xa inhibitors** like **rivaroxaban, edoxaban and apixaban**.
- These drugs are used for **prophylaxis of thrombosis in a patient of nonvalvular atrial fibrillation** and are used for treatment and secondary prophylaxis of DVT or pulmonary embolism and prevention of DVT in patients of hip surgery.
- In treatment of DVT or pulmonary embolism apixaban and rivaroxaban can be used as monotherapy, whereas dabigatran and edoxaban are used only after initial 5 days of parenteral anticoagulation with heparin or fondaparinux.
- There is a faster onset of action with these drugs and hence heparin bridging is not required. Warfarin takes longer to produce adequate effect and hence heparin bridging is required.
- The best benefit of these drugs is that they **don't require routine coagulation monitoring**.
- The major side effect of these drugs is also bleeding which can be reversed by a factor Xa analog called as **andexanet alfa**.
- Excretion of these drugs is renal and hence dose should be decreased in patients with renal failure. Edoxaban is contraindicated even in case of high creatinine clearance (>95 ml/min) as it can decrease efficacy due to rapid excretion of drug.
- These drugs are contraindicated in patients with mechanical heart valves, thrombosis caused by antiphospholipid antibody syndrome and in splanchnic vein thrombosis.

Recent Advances

Betrixaban: Betrixaban is a recent oral factor Xa inhibitor approved for prophylaxis of venous thromboembolism in high risk patients.

Ciparantag: Ciparantag is an inhibitor of dabigatran, factor Xa inhibitors, heparin and LMWH under trial to reverse their effects.

DRUGS USED IN ANEMIA

IRON

- Iron is an important element in human metabolism and plays central role in erythropoiesis. Dietary iron in small quantity is present in meat and meat products in haem iron which has good absorption, whereas iron in vegetables is non-haem iron which is not absorbed. Thus, in case of deficiency therapeutic iron must be given from outside.
- Iron can be given by oral or parenteral route. As the rise in haemoglobin level is similar by both routes, **oral route is**

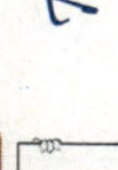
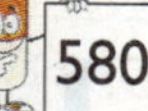

preferred, with parenteral being used in case of intolerance to oral route.

Iron Deficiency Anemia

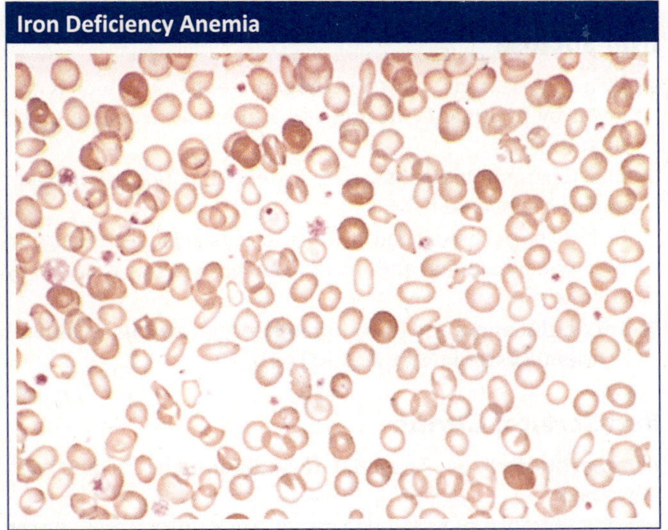

Oral Iron Therapy

- Iron is absorbed from upper small intestine and the proportion absorbed decreases with increasing dose. The absorption for example is 40% at 35 mg dose i.e. 14 mg is absorbed, whereas absorption is only **12% at 325 mg dose** i.e. 39 mg is absorbed.
- The oral iron preparations available are ferrous salts, iron-polysaccharide complex and carbonyl iron.
- Though side effects are lesser with food, absorption is decreased and hence **iron should be given on empty stomach**. Iron is absorbed at acidic pH hence antacids, PPI and H2 blockers should not be combined.
- Vitamin C (ascorbic acid) and succinic acid can increase iron absorption, however vitamin C can cause iron toxicity, which is not seen with succinic acid. Hence ferrous succinate has better oral absorption than other preparations but is many times costlier.
- The best marker of response to therapy is an increase in **reticulocyte count**, which begins at least after **1 week** of starting therapy. However, the increase in **hemoglobin level** is seen at least after **1 month** as daily increase is 2 g/L and if it does not increase more than 20 g/L, the diagnosis of iron deficiency should be questioned.
- Replenishment of iron stores requires 3 - 6 months and hence iron therapy should be continued for same duration after treating the cause of iron deficiency.
- Response failure is usually due to incompliance, but other reasons could be possible like achlorhydric stomach (add vitamin C), anaemia of chronic disease, thalassemia, celiac disease and chronic blood loss.
- Side effects for oral route are related to GIT like **nausea, vomiting** which are dose dependent. **Diarrhea and constipation** are dose independent and seen due to effects on intestinal microbes.
- In case of intolerance, patient should be started at low doses and then gradually increased, or patient can be asked to take drug just after food.

Ferrous Salts

- These are the **cheapest available iron preparation** and hence more preferred.
- The oral formulation of choice is **ferrous sulphate** and available agents are ferrous succinate, ferrous gluconate and ferrous fumarate.
- Ferrous sulphate **325 mg OD in adults** and **5 mg/kg in children** is the drug of choice for treatment of iron deficiency anaemia and should be continued for at least **3–6 months** after restoration of normal hemoglobin level and iron store.
- In pregnancy the prophylactic dose in 15–30 mg OD.

Ferrous Salts	Elemental Iron
Ferrous fumarate	**33% (Maximum)**
Ferrous sulphate (Dried)	32%
Ferrous sulphate (Hydrated)	20%
Ferrous gluconate	**12% (Minimum)**

Iron Polysaccharide Complex

- It is as effective as ferrous sulphate but associated with lesser incidence of side effects.
- The drawback is, it is much costlier.

Carbonyl Iron

- It is metallic iron powder with particle size less than 5 mm available as tablets.
- It also has lesser side effects but is much costlier.

Classification of Iron

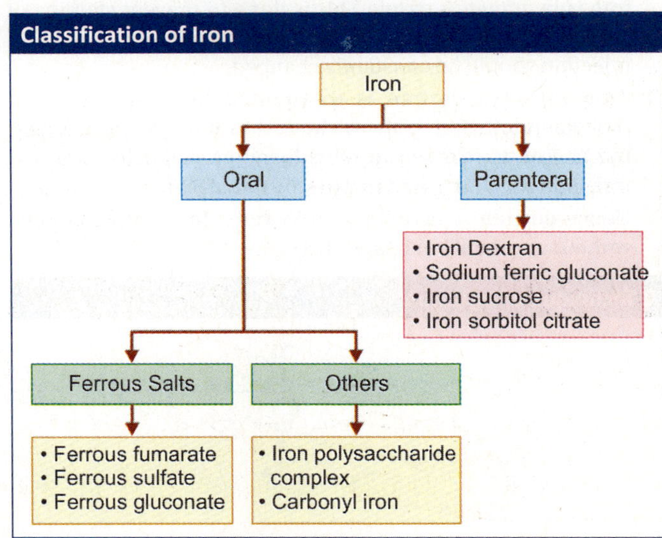

Parenteral Iron Therapy

- The parenteral formulations like **iron dextran**, iron sorbitol citrate, sodium ferric gluconate and iron sucrose are used.
- These are preferred in case oral route is not preferable as in case of poor compliance, intolerance to oral iron, rapid blood loss, GIT disorders (peptic ulcer disease, inflammatory bowel disease), sprue, short bowel syndrome, hemodialysis (inability to maintain iron homeostasis), pregnant woman with severe iron deficiency anemia presenting late in pregnancy and patient donating huge amount of blood for self-transfusion.

- The most severe side effect of parenteral iron is **anaphylaxis** which is **dose independent** and is seen within first few minutes after drug administration.
- Since risk of anaphylaxis is higher with dextran it is given by slow IV infusion, whereas sodium ferric gluconate and iron sucrose have lesser risk and can be given by rapid IV infusion.
- Other side effects are arthralgia-myalgia syndrome, urticaria, lymphadenopathy and skin pigmentation at site of injection (permanent).
- Dose of parenteral iron to be administered can be calculated by the formula given below.

Dose of Parenteral Iron
Iron Dose in mg = 15 – Patient Hb in g/dL × Body weight in kg × 3

Iron Dextran

- Iron dextran is a colloid of ferric hydroxide and dextran.
- It can be administered by **IV or IM** route but IV is more preferred due to local tissue irritation and malignancy risk by IM route.
- It is the only iron that is given as single total dose infusion. Each ml contains 50 mg of iron. Since dextran can cause anaphylaxis a **test dose** must be given prior to initiation of therapy.
- IM iron can be given daily, on alternate days or once/week at dose of 1.5 to 2 ml. The IM injection is given on the upper outer quadrant of buttock by **Z technique**, in which the injection site on skin is away from the entry point of needle into subcutaneous tissue. This is done to prevent staining of skin which can be permanent. For same reason the site of injection should be constantly changed.
- After injection dextran is transported by lymphatics into reticuloendothelial cells **without binding to transferrin**, but as iron is released in reticuloendothelial cells then it is transported to erythroid marrow by transferrin.
- Hence dextran is **metabolized in reticuloendothelial cells** without any renal or hepatic clearance

Z Technique of Injection

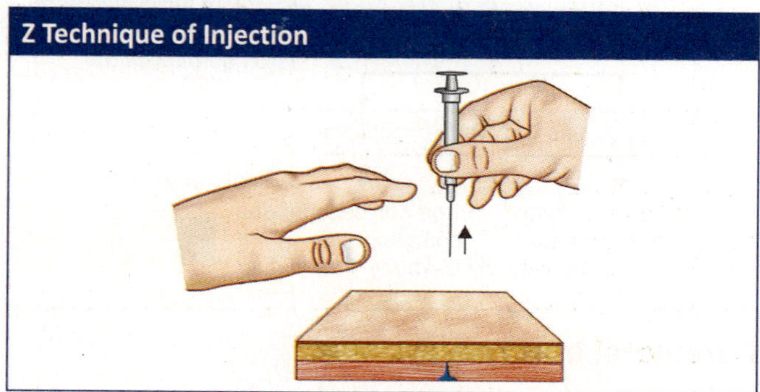

Sodium Ferric Gluconate

- Ferric gluconate is safer than dextran and iron sorbitol citrate and hence **test dose is not required**.
- It is given as multiple IV injections as single dose infusion causes rapid saturation of transferrin due to rapid release of iron from this drug, as it doesn't require reticuloendothelial cells for iron release.
- Currently it is the parenteral iron of choice and dextran is reserved for incompliant patients.

Iron Sucrose

- Iron sucrose is the safest form of parenteral iron, which is also given by multiple IV dosing and it **does not require a test dose**.
- Like dextran it is also taken up by reticuloendothelial system and iron is released.
- It has been associated with osteomalacia secondary to hypophosphatemia and renal tubular damage caused by sucrose.
- **Ferric gluconate** and **iron sucrose** are approved for treatment of **anemia associated with CKD** only.

Iron Sorbitol Citrate

Iron sorbitol citrate is an IM formulation that is not used nowadays.

Parenteral iron	Route	Test dose requirement
Iron dextran	IV > IM (Slow)	Yes
Iron sorbitol citrate	IM (Slow)	Yes
Sodium ferric gluconate Iron sucrose	IV (Rapid)	No

Recent Advances

Ferric pyrophosphate citrate has been recently approved for treatment of anemia associated with CKD. It is added to dialysate at dose of 5–7 mg.

Treatment of Iron Toxicity

Acute Toxicity

- Acute iron toxicity is usually seen in small children who accidentally consume iron tablets.
- This can cause GIT symptoms as mentioned earlier and death can be due to hemorrhagic gastritis and shock.
- Treatment is directed at removing the iron tablets by lavage with sodium bicarbonate solution and at end of lavage 5-10 mg of Desferrioxamine and 60 mL of sodium bicarbonate is left in the stomach.
- Patient is also given iron chelator parenteral **desferrioxamine 0.5-1 g by IM route**. It is a parenteral chelator but given by oral route also to chelate iron in GIT as described earlier.
- Long term effect of iron toxicity can present as gastric and intestinal fibrosis and stenosis.

Chronic Toxicity

- Chronic iron toxicity is seen in conditions like thalassemia.
- **Desferrioxamine** is the preferred agent in these patients.
- In case of intolerance, oral chelator **deferiprone** can also be used.

PYRIDOXINE

- Pyridoxine is used for treatment of acquired sideroblastic anemia caused by drugs like isoniazid, pyrazinamide, OCP, penicillamine and cycloserine. However, it is not effective in sideroblastic anemia caused by chloramphenicol and lead. The dose of pyridoxine given is 50 mg OD in case of drug induced sideroblastic anemia.
- Pyridoxine is also used for treatment of pyridoxine sensitive anemia. In these cases, higher dose up to 600 mg/day is required.
- In case of pyridoxine resistance parenteral pyridoxal phosphate can be given.
- Pyridoxine toxicity can present as sensory neuropathy.

Drug Induced Sideroblastic Anemia

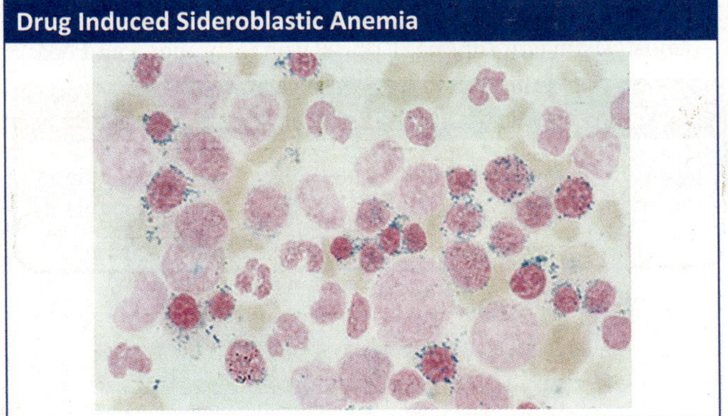

FOLIC ACID

- Folic acid in our body is metabolized in to THF, which donates methyl group for DNA synthesis. Hence deficiency of folic acid can also cause megaloblastic anemia.
- The source of folic is fruits and vegetables. The daily requirement is 50–100 mcg and the body has a store of 5 mg.
- Deficiency of folic acid is mostly due to inadequate consumptions of fruit and vegetables, however certain drugs like phenytoin and sulphonamides can also cause deficiency.
- Folic acid is used for treatment of megaloblastic anemia at a dose of 1 mg oral daily. For prophylaxis of NTD in pregnant females the dose is **400 mcg daily**, however in case of a history of NTD **4000 mcg daily** is given. Folic acid prophylactically is also given in homocystinemia and conditions with rapid cell turnover like haemolytic anemia at dose of 1000 mcg daily.
- Folic acid deficiency might coexist with vitamin B12 deficiency as deficiency of the later can cause intestinal mucosal atrophy and decrease folic acid absorption. However folic acid should never be given alone in case both are deficient as the hematological picture improves neurological damage progresses.
- Synthetic form of active folic acid i.e. **folinic acid or leucovorin** is used for prevention of toxicity to antifolate drugs like **methotrexate** and increase effect of anticancer drug like **5-FU**. Folic acid in large doses can compromise antiepileptic effects of **phenobarbital, phenytoin and primidone**.

VITAMIN B_{12}

- Vitamin B12 as methylcobalamin is an important cofactor for various enzymes required for synthesis of DNA in the erythroid precursor cells. Hence its deficiency can be associated with megaloblastic anemia.
- The source of vitamin B_{12} is from animal source food like meat and eggs. The daily requirement of vitamin B_{12} is **3–5 mcg** and the body has a store of **2–5 mg** in the liver.
- Deficiency of vitamin B_{12} is seen in case of pernicious anaemia, gastrectomy, H. pylori infection, blind loop syndrome, fish tape worm infection and Crohn's disease.
- Vitamin B_{12} is used for treatment in the cases of deficiencies in above mentioned cases. The preferred route of administration is IM or SC 100 mcg daily for one week followed by once weekly for a month and then continue once a month lifelong. Oral or sublingual route is less preferred as absorption is unreliable.
- It can also be used in **Schilling test** and given with **pemetrexed** to prevent severe bone marrow suppression.
- Side effect associated with vitamin B_{12} therapy is transient hypokalemia.

Megaloblastic Anemia

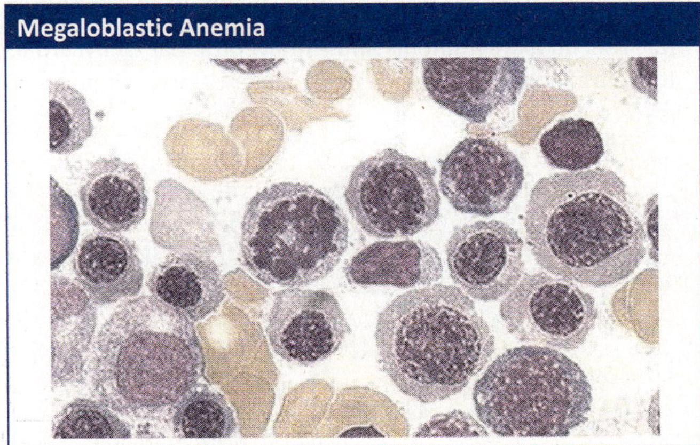

HEMATOPOIETIC GROWTH FACTORS

Erythropoietin Analogs

- **Epoetin alpha, epoetin beta and darbepoetin** are erythropoietin analogs, the latter being the longest acting.
- These are used for treatment of **anemia associated with chemotherapy, chronic renal failure, premature infants, dialysis and zidovudine.**
- Side effects associated are flu like symptoms, iron deficiency, hypertension, thrombosis and pure red cell aplasia.

Recent Advances

Peginesatide: Peginesatide is a recent erythropoietin receptor agonist approved for treatment of anemia associated with chronic renal failure.

Colony Stimulating Factor Analogs

- **Filgrastim** and **lenogsatrim** are granulocyte colony stimulating factor (G-CSF) analogs whereas **sargamostim** is granulocyte macrophage colony stimulating factor (GM-CSF) analog. Both can be given by IV or SC route.
- These are used for treatment of **neutropenia** associated with autologous bone marrow transplantation, chemotherapy,

HIV, aplastic anemia and myelodysplasia. They are also given before leukapharesis to harvest leucocytes.

- These drugs are used to mobilize the peripheral blood stem cells from the marrow for collection and transplantation in patients on high dose of chemotherapy. Patients of multiple myeloma and Non-Hodgkin's lymphoma have poor response to these drugs alone. Hence a new drug **plerixafor** can be combined, which blocks CXCR4 receptors on stem cells in marrow and facilitates mobilization to periphery.
- Filgrastim has a short half-life (3.5 hours) and needs to be injected daily for many days in a chemotherapy cycle. Hence **long acting formulation like pegfilgrastim** and **lipegfilgrastim** were synthesized, which can be used only once in a chemotherapy cycle.
- **Sargamostim** is a GM-CSF analog produced in yeast by genetic engineering. In low doses it increases only neutrophils but at high doses it increases eosinophils and monocytes also. Side effects associated are capillary leak syndrome, bone pain malaise, flu like symptoms and supraventricular tachycardia. It is less effective and more toxic than filgrastim and hence less preferred.
- Filgrastim is G-CSF analog produced in E. coli by genetic engineering. Side effects associated are bone pain, cutaneous necrotizing vasculitis, splenomegaly and splenic rupture.

Thrombopoiesis Stimulator

- **Oprelevkin** is an IL-11 analog used for treatment of chemotherapy induced thrombocytopenia. Most common side effect is fluid retention and related cardiac side effects.
- Thrombopoietin analogs like **recombinant human megakaryocyte growth and development factor** and **recombinant human thrombopoietin** used for treatment of chemotherapy induced thrombocytopenia.
- **Romiplostim** and **eltrombopag** are thrombopoietin agonists used for treatment of ITP. These drugs can cause hepatotoxicity (mostly with eltrombopag), portal vein thrombosis and AML.

Recent Advances

Lusutrombopag and **Avatrombopag:** These are thrombopoietin receptor agonists recently approved for thrombocytopenia in patients with chronic liver disease prior to any procedure.

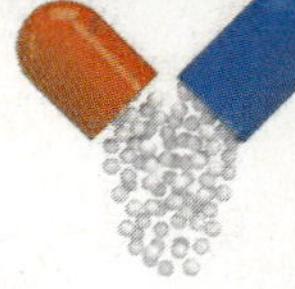

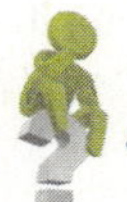

Image-based Questions

1. Which of the following is started after the procedure given in the picture?

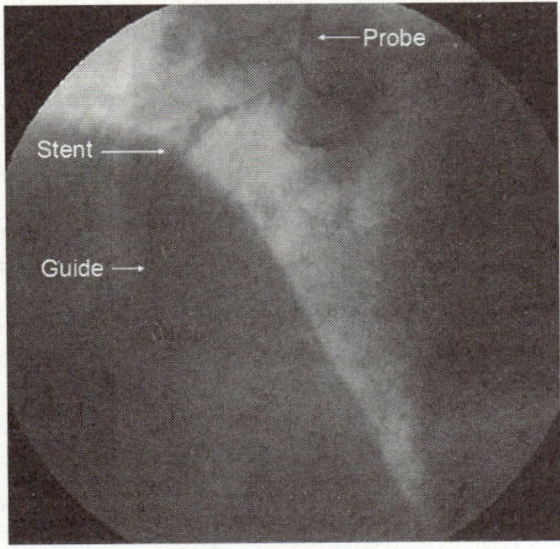

a. Aspirin
b. Clopidogrel
c. Aspirin + clopidogrel
d. None

2. A patient on unfractionated heparin developed the following digital changes. Which of the following drug cannot be used in this patient?

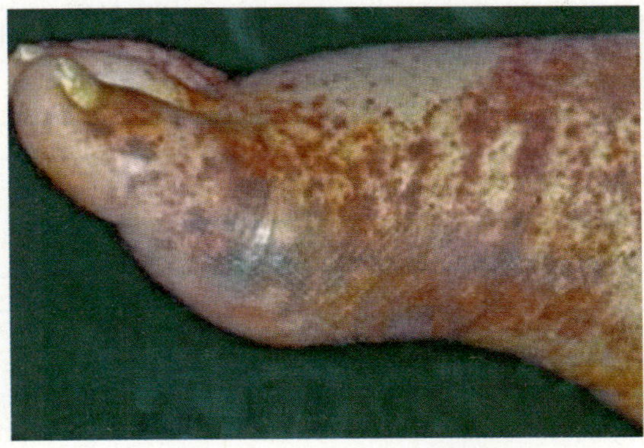

a. LMWH
b. Fondaparinux
c. Argatroban
d. L epirudin

3. Which of the following anticoagulant might have caused the features seen in USG?

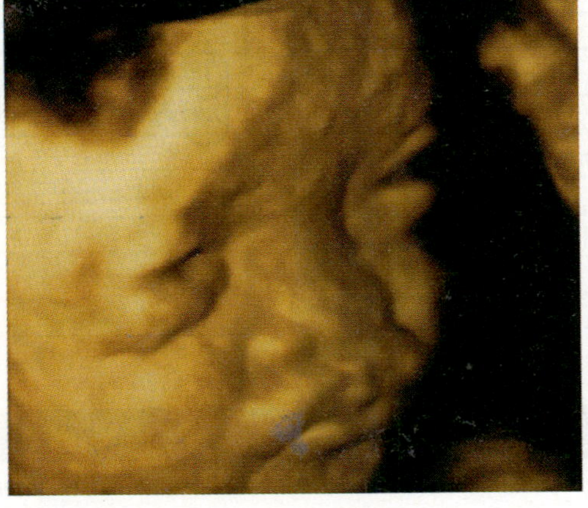

a. Heparin
b. Fondaparinux
c. Warfarin
d. Dabigatran

Answers with Explanations to Image-based Questions

1. Ans. (c) Aspirin + Clopidogrel

(Ref: Goodman Gilman 12th E/P871)

- In the picture a stent placement has been demonstrated.
- In case of PCI without stent only aspirin can be used as an antiaggregant.
- In case of PCI with stent placement dual antiaggregant therapy with aspirin and clopidogrel is indicated.

2. Ans. (a) LMWH

(Ref: Goodman Gilman 12th E/P859)

- UFH can cross react with LMWH and hence in case of HIT none of these should be used.
- However as fondaparinux does not cross react it can be used.
- Lepirudin is the drug of choice and argatroban is an alternative for treatment of HIT.

3. Ans. (c) Warfarin

(Ref: Goodman Gilman 12th E/P864)

Nasal hypoplasia seen in the USG is a classical teratogenic feature of warfarin.

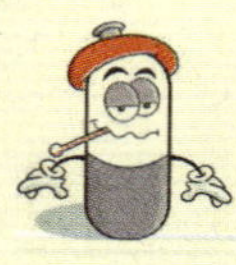

Annexures

Condition	Drug
Anemia associated with CKD or Inflammation	Erythropoetin analogue (Darbopoetin alfa)
Antiaggregant of choice	PCI without stenting – Aspirin PCI with stenting – Aspirin + Clopidogrel
Atrial fibrillation associated thrombosis prophylaxis	Dabigatran Or Apixaban
(Autoimmune hemolytic anemia)	• Prednisolone Plus • Rituximab
Deep Vein Thrombosis	Treatment – LMWH Prophylaxis – Warfarin
Essential thrombocythemia	• Hydroxyurea Plus • Aspirin
Fibrinolysis	Epsilon aminocaproic acid
Heparin toxicity	Protamine sulphate
Heparin induced thrombocytopenia	Lepirudin
Immune thrombocytopenic purpura	Prednisolone
(Iron deficiency anemia)	Symptomatic – RBC transfusion Asymptomatic – Oral iron
Myelodysplasia	Azacitidine
Neutropenia	Filgrastim
Paroxysmal nocturnal hemoglobinuria	Eculizumab
Polycythemia vera	Anagrelide > Hydroxyurea
Pure red cell aplasia	Glucocorticoids
Sickle cell anemia Myelofibrosis	Hydroxyurea
Thrombocytopenia	Oprelvekin
Transfusional hemosiderosis	Desferrioxamine
Von Willebrand disease	Desmopressin
Warfarin toxicity	Asymptomatic – Vitamin K Symptomatic – FFP

New Drugs

Drug	Mechanism of action	Uses
Avatrombopag and Lusutrombopag	Oral thrombopoietin receptor agonist	Thrombocytopenia in patients with chronic liver disease, prior to any procedure
Andexanet alfa	Modified form of factor Xa	Reverse anticoagulant effect of factor Xa inhibitors
Ravulizumab Eculizumab	Anti-compliment C5 monoclonal antibody	PNH
Fostamatinib	Spleen tyrosine kinase inhibitor	Immune thrombocytopenic purpura

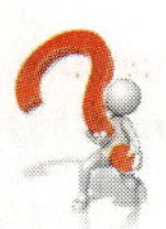

Multiple Choice Questions

1. In a rheumatic heart disease pregnant female with prosthetic valve, when should we switch to heparin *(AIIMS Nov 2018)*

a. 32 weeks b. 36 weeks
c. 37 weeks d. 40 weeks

2. Anticoagulant used for treatment of cancer related thrombi is *(AIIMS May 2018)*

a. LMWH
b. Vitamin K inhibitor
c. Direct thrombin inhibitor
d. Xa inhibitors

3. Heparin acts via which of the following adjuvants *(AIIMS May 2018)*

a. Antithrombin 3 b. Protein C
c. Protein S d. Thrombomodulin

4. Antidote of fibrinolytic drug is *(AIIMS May 2017)*

a. Heparin b. Epsilon aminocaproic acid
c. Protamine d. Alteplase

5. Which of the following is true regarding iron replacement therapy in iron deficiency anaemia *(AIIMS Nov 2016)*

a. Parenteral iron to be given till the haematocrit normalizes and should be discontinued afterwards because of gastric side effects
b. Before giving parenteral iron dilute the dose and give to check for anaphylaxis
c. 50% of the iron given is absorbed in 325 mg of ferrous sulphate tablets
d. Because of side effects of oral iron always give parenteral iron for treatment

6. You are attending your practical examination and you are given a patient. The lab findings of the patient shows prolonged bleeding time. You take a detailed history and ask the patient for any intake of NSAIDs as it is known to prolong the bleeding time. The patient categorically refuses intake of any form of NSAIDs. No other drug history was obtained. All the group of drugs can prolong bleeding time except? *(AIIMS Nov 2016)*

a. Vitamin K b. Cephalosporins
c. Antidepressants d. Theophylline

7. All of the following are GpIIb/IIIa receptor inhibitor except *(AIIMS May 2016)*

a. Abciximab b. Prasugrel
c. Eptofibatide d. Tirofiban

8. Antidote for overdose of fibrinolytic therapy *(AIIMS Nov 2015)*

a. Heparin b. Epsilon aminocaproic acid
c. Protamine d. Warfarin

9. Which of the following is a factor Xa inhibitor? *(Recent Question 2019, 2018)*

a. Rivaroxaban b. Dabigatran
c. Argatroban d. Fondaparinux

10. Which of the following is an oral DTI *(Recent Question 2019)*

a. Edoxaban b. Enoxaparin
c. Lepirudin d. Dabigatran

11. Which of the following statements is true regarding pegfilgrastim? *(Recent Question 2019)*

a. Used in neutropenia b. Oral drug
c. Short acting d. GM-CSF analog

12. Which of the following is used in antiphospholipid antibody syndrome? *(Recent Question 2019)*

a. Heparin b. Warfarin
c. Aspirin d. Dabigatran

13. All of the following are false regarding prasugrel except: *(Recent Question 2017)*

a. Not much metabolism in body
b. Slow onset of action than clopidogrel
c. Reversible inhibitor of ADP
d. Contraindicated in cerebrovascular accident

14. Mechanism of action of apixaban is: *(Recent Question 2017)*

a. Inhibition of factor Xa
b. Inhibition of thrombin
c. Stimulation of antithrombin
d. Vitamin K antagonism

15. Coagulation testing is needed for: *(Recent Question 2017)*

a. Lepirudin b. Enoxaparin
c. Fondaparinux d. Dabigatran

16. What is the single best agent to be given in homocysteinemia? *(Recent Question Dec 2016)*

a. Pyridoxine b. B12
c. Folic acid d. Iron

17. Which of the following does not act on ADP? *(Recent Question Dec 2016)*

a. Prasugrel b. Ticlopidine
c. Clopidogrel d. Aspirin

18. Teratogenic effect of Warfarin is? *(Recent Question Dec 2016)*

a. Absent nasal bone b. Midfacial hypoplasia
c. Neural tube defects d. Cardiac anomalies

19. Anticoagulant with both invitro and invivo activity is *(Recent Question Dec 2016)*

a. Heparin b. Warfarin
c. Apixaban d. Dabigatran

20. aPTT indicates *(Recent Question Dec 2016)*

a. Extrinsic pathway b. Intrinsic pathway
c. Both d. None

21. Anticoagulant effect was compromised after vitamin K was started. Which of the following anticoagulant the patient was on? *(Recent Question Dec 2016)*

a. Heparin b. Warfarin
c. Dabigartan d. Apixaban

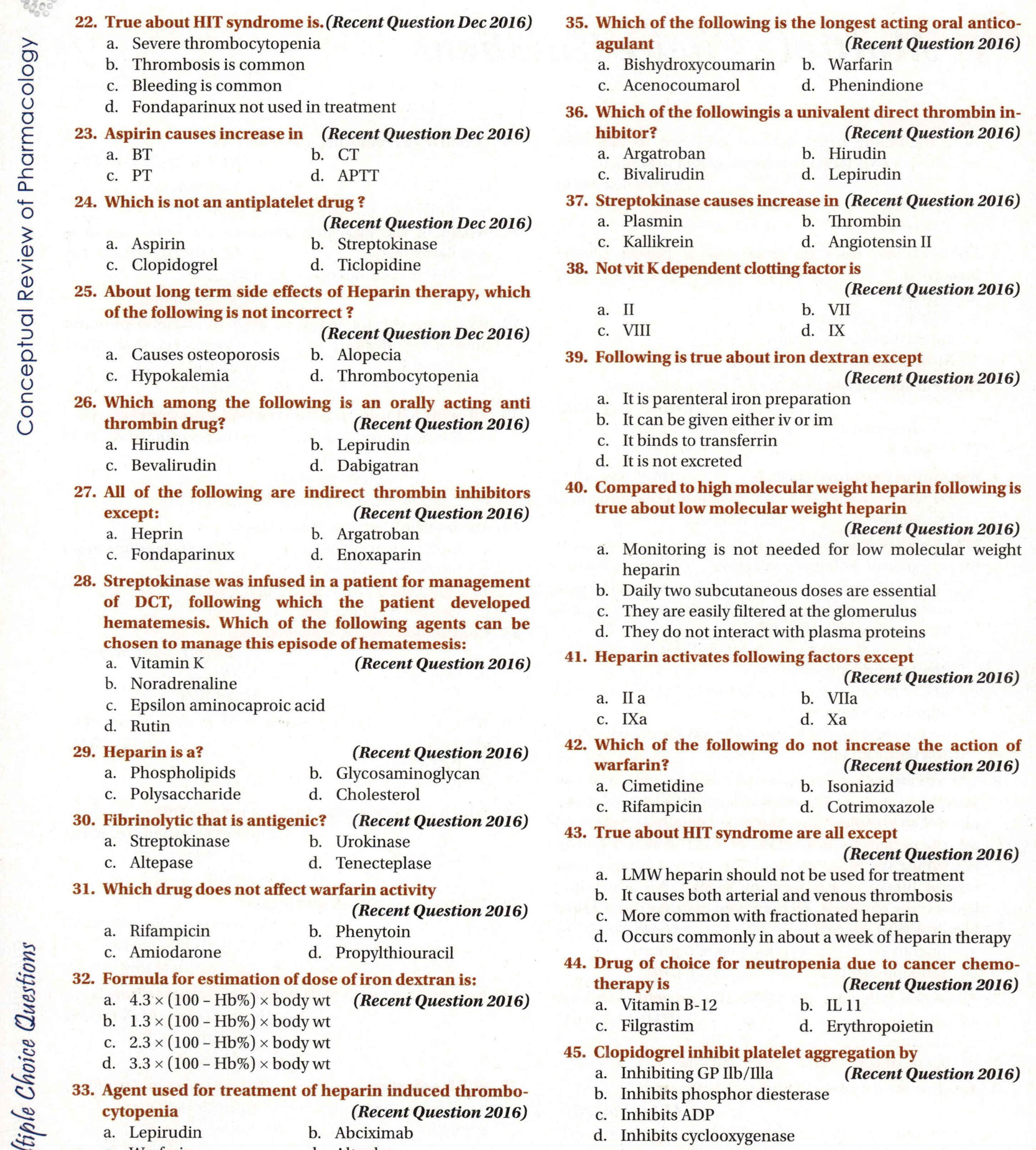

22. True about HIT syndrome is. *(Recent Question Dec 2016)*
a. Severe thrombocytopenia
b. Thrombosis is common
c. Bleeding is common
d. Fondaparinux not used in treatment

23. Aspirin causes increase in *(Recent Question Dec 2016)*
a. BT b. CT
c. PT d. APTT

24. Which is not an antiplatelet drug ? *(Recent Question Dec 2016)*
a. Aspirin b. Streptokinase
c. Clopidogrel d. Ticlopidine

25. About long term side effects of Heparin therapy, which of the following is not incorrect ? *(Recent Question Dec 2016)*
a. Causes osteoporosis b. Alopecia
c. Hypokalemia d. Thrombocytopenia

26. Which among the following is an orally acting anti thrombin drug? *(Recent Question 2016)*
a. Hirudin b. Lepirudin
c. Bevalirudin d. Dabigatran

27. All of the following are indirect thrombin inhibitors except: *(Recent Question 2016)*
a. Heprin b. Argatroban
c. Fondaparinux d. Enoxaparin

28. Streptokinase was infused in a patient for management of DCT, following which the patient developed hematemesis. Which of the following agents can be chosen to manage this episode of hematemesis: *(Recent Question 2016)*
a. Vitamin K
b. Noradrenaline
c. Epsilon aminocaproic acid
d. Rutin

29. Heparin is a? *(Recent Question 2016)*
a. Phospholipids b. Glycosaminoglycan
c. Polysaccharide d. Cholesterol

30. Fibrinolytic that is antigenic? *(Recent Question 2016)*
a. Streptokinase b. Urokinase
c. Altepase d. Tenecteplase

31. Which drug does not affect warfarin activity *(Recent Question 2016)*
a. Rifampicin b. Phenytoin
c. Amiodarone d. Propylthiouracil

32. Formula for estimation of dose of iron dextran is: *(Recent Question 2016)*
a. 4.3 × (100 – Hb%) × body wt
b. 1.3 × (100 – Hb%) × body wt
c. 2.3 × (100 – Hb%) × body wt
d. 3.3 × (100 – Hb%) × body wt

33. Agent used for treatment of heparin induced thrombocytopenia *(Recent Question 2016)*
a. Lepirudin b. Abciximab
c. Warfarin d. Alteplase

34. Drug not acting on P2y12 receptor is *(Recent Question 2016)*
a. Ticlopidine b. Clopidrogel
c. Dipyridamole d. Prasugrel

35. Which of the following is the longest acting oral anticoagulant *(Recent Question 2016)*
a. Bishydroxycoumarin b. Warfarin
c. Acenocoumarol d. Phenindione

36. Which of the followingis a univalent direct thrombin inhibitor? *(Recent Question 2016)*
a. Argatroban b. Hirudin
c. Bivalirudin d. Lepirudin

37. Streptokinase causes increase in *(Recent Question 2016)*
a. Plasmin b. Thrombin
c. Kallikrein d. Angiotensin II

38. Not vit K dependent clotting factor is *(Recent Question 2016)*
a. II b. VII
c. VIII d. IX

39. Following is true about iron dextran except *(Recent Question 2016)*
a. It is parenteral iron preparation
b. It can be given either iv or im
c. It binds to transferrin
d. It is not excreted

40. Compared to high molecular weight heparin following is true about low molecular weight heparin *(Recent Question 2016)*
a. Monitoring is not needed for low molecular weight heparin
b. Daily two subcutaneous doses are essential
c. They are easily filtered at the glomerulus
d. They do not interact with plasma proteins

41. Heparin activates following factors except *(Recent Question 2016)*
a. II a b. VIIa
c. IXa d. Xa

42. Which of the following do not increase the action of warfarin? *(Recent Question 2016)*
a. Cimetidine b. Isoniazid
c. Rifampicin d. Cotrimoxazole

43. True about HIT syndrome are all except *(Recent Question 2016)*
a. LMW heparin should not be used for treatment
b. It causes both arterial and venous thrombosis
c. More common with fractionated heparin
d. Occurs commonly in about a week of heparin therapy

44. Drug of choice for neutropenia due to cancer chemotherapy is *(Recent Question 2016)*
a. Vitamin B-12 b. IL 11
c. Filgrastim d. Erythropoietin

45. Clopidogrel inhibit platelet aggregation by *(Recent Question 2016)*
a. Inhibiting GP IIb/IIIa
b. Inhibits phosphor diesterase
c. Inhibits ADP
d. Inhibits cyclooxygenase

46. All about warfarin are true except *(Recent Question 2016)*
a. Half-life is 36 hours
b. Crosses placenta
c. Contraindicated in hepatic failure
d. Inhibits all Vit-K dependent clotting factors

47. Which of the following drugs is ADP receptor inhibitor? ***(Recent Question 2016)***

a. Aspirin b. Clopidogrel
c. Abciximab d. Tirofiban

48. Apixaban is a new drug that acts by ***(Recent Question 2016)***

a. Inhibiting TNF alpha
b. Inhibiting factor Xa
c. Inhibiting platelet aggregation
d. Activating plasminogen

49. Which of the following is given to treat thrombocytopenia secondary to anti-cancer therapy and is known to stimulate progeniotor megakaryocytes? ***(Recent Question 2016)***

a. Filgrastim b. Oprelvrkin
c. Erythropoletin d. Iron dextran

50. Which of the following is vitamin K-dependent clotting factor? ***(Recent Question 2016)***

a. Factor VII b. Factor I
c. Factor XI d. Factor XII

51. Anti-coagulant of choice for heparin induced thrombocytopenia is ***(Recent Question 2016)***

a. Lepirudin b. Aprotinin
c. Abciximab d. Plasminogen

52. Vitamin K dependent clotting factors are ***(Recent Question 2016)***

a. Factor IX and X b. Factor IV
c. Factor XII d. Factor I

53. Drug used in heparin overdose is ***(Recent Question 2016)***

a. Protamin sulphate b. Phylloquinone
c. Ticlopidine d. Clopidogrel

54. Filgrastim is used for the treatment of ***(Recent Question 2016)***

a. Neutropenia b. Anemia
c. Polycythemia d. Neutrophilia

55. Hemorrhage secondary to heparin administration can be corrected by the administration of ***(Recent Question 2016)***

a. Vitamin K b. Whole blood
c. Protamine d. Ascorbic acid

56. In low does aspirin acts on ***(Recent Question 2016)***

a. Cyclooxygenase b. Thromboxane A2
c. PGI2 d. Lipoxygenase

57. Vitamin K is a cofactor in ***(Recent Question 2016)***

a. Carboxylation b. Hydroxylation
c. Deamination d. Hydrolysis

58. A patient of thrombosis of veins has been receiving coumarin therapy for three years. Recently she developed bleeding tendency. How will you reverse the effect of coumarin therapy? ***(Recent Question 2016)***

a. Protamin injection b. Vit K injection
c. Infusion of fibrinogen d. Whole blood transfusion

59. Urgent reversal of warfarin induced bleeding can be done by the administration of ***(Recent Question 2016)***

a. Cryoprecipitate b. Platelet concentrates
c. Fresh frozen plasma d. Packed red blood cells

60. Which of the following is most likely to be used in a young child with chronic renal insufficiency? ***(Recent Question 2016)***

a. Cyanocobalamin b. Desferrioxamine
c. Erythropoietin d. Filgrastim (G-CSF)

61. The difference between iron sorbitol-citric acid and iron dextran is that the former ***(Recent Question 2016)***

a. Cannot be injected
b. Is not bound to transferring in plasma
c. Is not excreted in urine
d. Produces fewer side effect

62. The anticoagulant of choice for performing coagulation studies is ***(Recent Question 2016)***

a. EDTA b. Heparin
c. Trisodium citrate d. Double oxalate

63. Alteplase differs from streptokinase as it ***(Recent Question 2016)***

a. Is longer acting
b. Is derived from human kidney
c. Is cheap
d. Activates plasminogen bound to fibrin

64. Which of the following has proved antithrombotic property ***(Recent Question 2016)***

a. Gelatin b. Dextran 40
c. Dextran 100 d. Hexastarch

65. Heparin acts via activation of ***(Recent Question 2016)***

a. Antithrombin III b. Factor VIII
c. Factor II and X d. Factor V

66. Glycoprotein IIb/IIIa receptor antagonist is ***(Recent Question 2016)***

a. Clopidogrel b. Abciximab
c. Tranexamic acid d. Ticlopidine

67. All are antiplatelet drugs except ***(Recent Question 2016)***

a. Aspirin b. Clopidogrel
c. Dipyridamole d. Warfarin

68. All of the following are anticoagulants except ***(Recent Question 2016)***

a. Phytonadione b. Warfarin
c. LMW heparin d. Lepirudin

69. Abciximab is ***(Recent Question 2016)***

a. Antibody against IIb/IIIa receptors
b. Antibody against Ib/IX receptors
c. Topoisomerase inhibitor
d. Adenosine inhibitor

70. Erythropoietin is mainly produced in ***(Recent Question 2016)***

a. Liver b. Kidney
c. Intestine d. Bone

71. Tirofiban is a ***(Recent Question 2016)***

a. Monoclonal antibody
b. Antiplatelet drug
c. Anti-Inflammatory drug
d. Antianginal drug

72. Methotrexate should be given with which of the following to decrease its side effects? ***(Recent Question 2016)***

a. Folic acid b. Cyanocoblamin
c. Thiamine d. Folinic acid

73. Orally acting direct thrombin inhibitor is ***(Recent Question 2016)***
a. Bivalirudin b. Ximelgatran
c. Melagatran d. Argatroban

74. Heparin does not cause ***(Recent Question 2016)***
a. Osteoporosis b. Factor V inhibition
c. Thrombocytopenia d. Prolongation of aPTT

75. All are seen with heparin therapy except ***(Recent Question 2016)***
a. Skin necrosis
b. Thrombosis and thrombocytopenia
c. Osteoporosis
d. Alopecia

76. A useful thrombolytic agent that leads to plasmin activation is ***(Recent Question 2016)***
a. Vitamin K b. Heparin
c. Streptokinase d. Aspirin

77. Oral anticoagulants are monitored by ***(Recent Question 2016)***
a. Bleeding time (BT)
b. Coagulation time (CT)
c. Prothrombin time (PT)
d. partial thromboplastin time (PTT)

78. Structurally, heparin is ***(Recent Question 2016)***
a. Homopolysaccharide b. Heteropolysaccharide
c. Glycoprotein d. Mucoprotein

79. Relative contraindication to thrombolytic therapy includes all the following except ***(Recent Question 2016)***
a. Hypotension b. Recent surgery
c. Active peptic ulcer d. Pregnancy

80. Epsilon amino caproic acid is used to reduce bleeding due to ***(Recent Question 2016)***
a. Heparin b. Warfarin
c. Thrombocytopenia d. Hyperplasminemia

81. Which is the most potent anticoagulant? ***(Recent Question 2016)***
a. Tirofiban b. Aspirin
c. Clopidogrel d. Cilostazole

82. Anticoagulant given in renal insufficiency ***(Recent Question 2016)***
a. Heparin b. Argatroban
c. Ximelagatran d. Warfarin

83. Which does not increase the anticoagulant action of warfarin ***(Recent Question 2016)***
a. Cimetidine b. Griseofulvin
c. Aspirin d. Probenecid

84. Half-life of alteplase ***(Recent Question 2016)***
a. 4-8 minutes b. 4-8 hours
c. 4-8 days d. 40-80 minutes

85. Dose of altepase ***(Recent Question 2016)***
a. 7.5 mg/kg b. 75 mg/kg
c. 0.75 mg/kg d. 0.075 mg/kg

86. Fondaparinux acts by inhibiting ***(Recent Question 2016)***
a. Blocks plasminogen activity
b. Stimulates fibrinolysis
c. Anticoagulant
d. Thrombolytic

87. Which of the following anti-platelet drug acts through adenosine receptor antagonism: ***(PGI May 2018)***
a. Aspirin b. Prasugrel
c. Cloipidogrel d. Abciximab
e. Ticagrelor

88. All are true about oral iron therapy in anemia except: ***(PGI Nov. 2016)***
a. May worsen inflammatory bowel disease
b. It takes minimum 2 weeks for reticulocyte count to increase
c. Generally 3-6 month therapy is required to replenish iron stores
d. Gastrointestinal side effects limits its dose
e. Hb level is generally attained in 1-3 month

89. True about Low molecular weight heparin (LMWH): ***(PGI Nov. 2016)***
a. Anti-factor Xa assay monitoring required in every patient
b. It increases aPTT more than UFH
c. Can be safely given in renal failure
d. Toxicity is totally reversed by protamine sulphate
e. Inactivate factor Xa selectively

90. Which of the following drug interact with Warfarin: ***(PGI Nov 2014)***
a. ACE inhibitor b. Azithromycin
c. Fluconazole d. Aspirin
e. Benzodiazepine

91. Oral iron chelating agent (s) is/are: ***(PGI June 2009)***
a. Desferrioxamine b. Deferiprone
c. Desferiroxamine d. BAL
e. Succimer

92. Heparin is the most widely used antithrombotic agent. It act by activating: ***(PGI June 2009)***
a. Plasmin b. Antithrombin III
c. Fibrinolysin d. Factor X
e. Thrombin

93. In a warfarin treated patient, skin necrosis found in: ***(PGI June 2006)***
a. Protein C deficiency
b. Protein S deficiency
c. AT III deficiency

94. Eltrombopag is a ***(JIPMER Nov 2018)***
a. Thrombopoietin agonist
b. Thrombopoietin antagonist
c. Erythropoietin agonist
d. Erythropoietin antagonist

95. Warfarin embryopathy is due to action of: ***(JIPMER May 2018)***
a. Osteophysin b. Osteotensin
c. Osteocalcin d. Osteogenin

96. Regarding neuraxial anesthesia, which of the following statement is true? ***(JIPMER May 2018)***
a. Aspirin should be stopped 7 days before surgery
b. Unfractionated heparin should be stopped 7 days before surgery
c. Fondaparinux should be stopped 7 days before surgery
d. Clopidogrel should be stopped 7 days before surgery

97. Limitations with direct thrombin inhibitor is: ***(JIPMER 2017)***

a. Needs regular monitoring of aPTT and INR
b. Lacks antidote
c. Causes more thrombocytopenia than heparin
d. Parenteral route of administration

98. Which of the following drug causes capillary leak syndrome? ***(JIPMER 2014)***

a. GM CSF b. GCSF
c. Filgristin d. Peg filgrastim

99. Heparin injection releases which of the following: ***(JIPMER 2014)***

a. Lipoprotein lipase b. Nitric oxide
c. cGMP d. hormone sensitive lipase

100. Heparin induced thrombocytopenia is reversed by: ***(JIPMER 2006)***

a. Warfarin b. Enoxaparin
c. Danaparoid d. Ardeparin

101. Proton pump inhibitor used along which of the following antiplatelet drug can decrease its anti-platelet activity? ***(JIPMER 2013)***

a. Clopidogrel b. Aspirin
c. Ticlodipine d. Thrombospondin

102. Which of the following is prothrombotic? ***(JIPMER 2009)***

a. Thrombomodulin b. PGI2
c. Heparin d. ADP

103. Heparin treatment is monitored by: ***(JIPMER 2008)***

a. aPTT b. PT
c. CT d. BT

104. Which one of the following is FALSE about Ticlopidine? ***(NIMHANS 2013)***

a. Inhibits platelet function by inducing a thrombasthenia like state
b. Stimulates platelet aggregation and clot retraction
c. Prolongs the bleeding time
d. Directly interacts with platelet membrane glycoprotein IIb/IIIa receptors

Answers with Explanations to Multiple Choice Questions

1. Ans. (c) 37 weeks

(Ref: ACC/AHA guidelines 2018)

"Anticoagulation should be held prior to delivery because therapeutic anticoagulation increases the risk for hemorrhagic complications with regional anesthesia, and warfarin (which crosses the placenta) increases the risk for fetal intraventricular hemorrhage. Warfarin should be held after **36 weeks gestation** and replaced with LMWH or unfractionated heparin."

- Pregnancy itself is a hypercoagulable state and the risk of thrombosis further increases in case the female has prosthetic valves. The risk of thrombosis continues postpartum as well and is maximum in the first 6 weeks postpartum
- The use of anticoagulants during pregnancy is complicated by the fact that warfarin is most effective to prevent thrombosis, but is associated with teratogenicity, which is maximum in 6-12 weeks of gestation. Teratogenicity is dose dependent and the risk is higher at doses > 5 mg/day and is less or like LMWH at doses ≤ 5 mg/day.
- Thus, if female is on warfarin ≤ 5 mg/day, it is continued in all three trimesters.
- However, if the female is on warfarin > 5mg/day, then LMWH is used in all three trimesters and factor Xa level is monitored after 4-6 hours of every dose.
- Low dose aspirin is also used in the second and third trimester.
- Warfarin crosses placenta and increases risk of fetal intraventricular hemorrhage and hence should be stopped after 36 weeks and LMWH is started on the 37th week.
- Anticoagulants are stopped 24 hours prior to delivery and then intravenous UFH can be started 6 hours after vaginal delivery and 12 hours after cesarean section.
- Warfarin is started after postpartum period and continued as it is safe during breast feeding.

2. Ans. (a) LMWH

(Ref: Goodman Gilman 13th E/P 589)

3. Ans. (a) Antithrombin 3

(Ref: Goodman Gilman 13th E/P 589)

4. Ans. (b) Epsilon aminocaproic acid

(Ref: Goodman Gilman 12th edition, Page 867)

Antidotes for fibrinolysis:

- Epsilon amino capreoic acid
- Tranexamic acid

5. Ans. (b) Before giving parenteral iron dilute the dose and give to check for anaphylaxis

(Ref: Goodman Gilman 12th E/P 1084)

- Gastric side effects are seen with oral and not parenteral iron.
- As parenteral iron like dextran can cause anaphylaxis, a test dose should be given prior to infusion.
- Only 12% of a 325mg dose of oral iron is absorbed.
- Because of risk of anaphylaxis with parenteral iron, oral iron is always preferred.

6. Ans. (a) Vitamin K

(Ref: Goodman Gilman 12th E/P 861)

- SSRI have antiaggregant effect.
- Theophylline also have antiaggregant effect due to PDE inhibition.
- Some cephalosporins produce antiaggregant effect

7. Ans. (b) Prasugrel

(Ref: Goodman Gilman 12th E/P 870)

8. Ans. (b) Epsilon aminocaproic acid

(Ref: Goodman Gilman 12th E/P 867)

- **Epsilon aminocaproic acid** and **tranexamic acid** are lysine analogs that competitively bind and inactivate both plasminogen and plasmin.
- **Epsilon aminocaproic acid is the antifibrinolytic of choice** for hemorrhagic states in fibrinolytic overdose, haemophilia, surgery etc. Tranexamic acid is also approved for treatment of metrorrhagia.

9. Ans. (a) Rivaroxaban

(Ref: Goodman Gilman 13th E/P 594)

10. Ans. (d) Dabigatran

(Ref: Goodman Gilman 13th E/P 594)

11. Ans. (a) Used in neutropenia

(Ref: Goodman Gilman 13th E/P 756)

- Filgrastim is a G-CSF analog used for treatment of neutropenia caused by chemotherapy, HIV, bone marrow transplantation and aplastic anemia. It has a short half-life (3.5 hours) and needs to be injected daily for many days in a chemotherapy cycle.
- Hence long acting formulation like pegfilgrastim and lipegfilgrastim were synthesized, which can be used only once in a chemotherapy cycle.
- It is given by subcutaneous or intravenous route.

12. Ans. (b) Warfarin

(Ref: CMDT 2019/P 857)

- Life long warfarin is the anticoagulant of choice for prevention of thrombosis in antiphospholipid antibody syndrome.
- However, as it is teratogenic, in pregnancy a combination of LMWH and aspirin is used.
- In catastrophic cases, intravenous heparin + corticosteroids + IVIG or plasmapheresis is done.

13. Ans. (d) Contraindicated in cerebrovascular accident

(Ref: Goodman Gilman 12th edition, Page 870)

- Prasugrel is most efficacious ADP inhibitor and the chances of bleeding is higher. Hence it is contraindicated in patients with history of cardiovascular accident like stroke.
- Most of the absorbed prasugrel undergoes activation, whereas its clopidogrel which undergoes only partial activation (15%).
- Prasugrel is the fastest acting ADP inhibitor.
- Prasugrel, clopidogrel and ticlopidine are irreversible inhibitors of ADP.

14. Ans. (a) Inhibition of factor Xa

(Ref: Goodman Gilman 12th edition, Page 866)

Oral factor Xa Inhibitors

- Apixaban
- Rivaroxaban
- Edoxaban

15. Ans. (a) Lepirudin

(Ref: Goodman Gilman 12th E/P 859)

Coagulation Testing

Drugs	Test
Heparin (Unfractionated) Lepirudin Bivalirudin Argatroban	aPTT
Warfarin Argatroban	PT
LMWH: Enoxaparin, Tinzaparin Apixaban Rivaroxaban Ximelagatran Dabigatran Fondaparinux	Not required

16. Ans. (c) Folic acid

(Ref: Goodman Gilman 12th E/P 1095)

17. Ans. (d) Aspirin

(Ref: Goodman Gilman 12th E/P 871)

18. Ans. (b) Midfacial hypoplasia

(Ref: Goodman Gilman 12th E/P 864)

Teratogenic effects of warfarin

- Nasal/Midfacial hypoplasia
- Stippled epiphyseal calcifications
- CNS defects

19. Ans. (a) Heparin

(Ref: Goodman Gilman 12th E/P 852)

20. Ans. (a) Extrinsic pathway

(Ref: Goodman Gilman 12th E/P 857)

21. Ans. (b) Warfarin

(Ref: Goodman Gilman 12th /P 861)

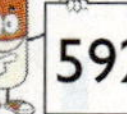

22. Ans. (b) **Thrombosis is common**

(Ref: Harrison 19th E/P 728)

23. Ans. (a) **BT**

(Ref: Goodman Gilman 12th E/P 868)

24. Ans. (b) **Streptokinase**

(Ref: Goodman Gilman 12th E/P 868)

25. Ans. (c) **Hypokalemia**

(Ref: Goodman Gilman 12th E/P 859)

26. Ans. (d) **Dabigatran**

(Ref: Goodman Gilman 12th E/P 865)

Direct Thrombin Inhibitors

Oral	Parenteral
Dabigatran Ximelagatran	Hirudin Lepirudin Bivalirudin Argatroban

27. Ans. (b) **Argatroban**

(Ref: Goodman Gilman 12th E/P 858)

Indirect Thrombin Inhibitors

Heparin	LMWH	Fondaparinux
	• Enoxaparin • Tinzaparin • Ardeparin • Reviparin • Nadoparin	

28. Ans. (c) **Epsilon aminocaproic acid**

(Ref: Goodman Gilman 12th E/P 867)

Inhibitors of Fibrinolysis

- Aminocaproic acid
- Tranexemic acid

29. Ans. (b) **Glycosaminoglycan**

(Ref: Goodman Gilman 12th E/P 866)

30. Ans. (a) **Streptokinase**

(Ref: Goodman Gilman 12th E/P 867)

31. Ans. (d) **Propylthiouracil**

(Ref: Goodman Gilman 12th E/P 867)

- **Rifampicin and phenytoin are enzyme inducers and amiodarone is an enzyme inhibitor and hence they can affect warfarin metabolism.**

32. Ans. (a) **4.3 × (100 – Hb%) × body wt**

(Ref: KDT 7th E/P604)

33. Ans. (a) **Lepirudin**

(Ref: Goodman Gilman 12th E/P 859)

Drugs Used for Treatment of HIT
Lepirudin – Drug of choice Argatroban Fondaparinux

34. Ans. (c) **Dipyridamole**

(Ref: Goodman Gilman 12th E/P 871)

ADP Receptor P_2Y_{12} Inhibitors
Clopidogrel Prasugrel Ticlopidine Ticagrelor Cangrelor

35. Ans. (a) **Bishydroxycoumarin**

(Ref: KDT 7th E/P 621)

- Bishydroxycoumarin is longest acting whereas ethylbiscoumacetate and phenindione are shortest acting coumarins.

36. Ans. (a) **Argatroban**

(Ref: Goodman Gilman 12th E/P 866)

- All parenteral DTI are bivalent compounds and inhibit catalytic site as well as substrate recognition site in thrombin.
- The only exception is **argatroban which is univalent** and inhibits only catalytic site.

37. Ans. (a) **Plasmin**

(Ref: Goodman Gilman 12th E/P 866)

- **Streptokinase** is a protein synthesized from streptococci. It binds to plasminogen and together the streptokinase-plasminogen complex activates plasminogen to **plasmin**, which causes fibrinolysis.
- Its use is limited by neutralizing antibodies produced against it due to its **antigenic nature**.

38. Ans. (c) **VIII**

(Ref: Goodman Gilman 12th E/P 866)

Vitamin K dependent coagulation factors	Vitamin K dependent anticoagulation factors
II VII IX X	Protein C Protein S

39. Ans. (c) It binds to transferrin

(Ref: KDT 7th E/P 604)

- Dextran is transported to reticuloendothelial cells without binding to transferrin, but as iron is released in reticuloendothelial cells then iron is transported to erythroid marrow by transferrin.
- Hence dextran is metabolized in reticuloendothelial cells without any renal or hepatic clearance.

40. Ans. (a) Monitoring is not needed for low molecular weight heparin

(Ref: Goodman Gilman 12th E/P 858)

- The anticoagulant effect of LMWH is predictable as compared to UFH and hence coagulation monitoring is not required.
- The smaller fragments of heparin, LMWH and fondaparinux are all filtered easily by kidney.
- UFH by subcutaneous route is given at BD doses, whereas LMWH is given at OD doses.

41. Ans. (b) VIIa

(Ref: Goodman Gilman 12th E/P 854)

42. Ans. (c) Rifampicin

(Ref: Goodman Gilman 12th E/P 864)

- Rifampicin being an enzyme inducer decreases the effect of warfarin.

43. Ans. (c) More common with fractionated heparin

(Ref: Goodman Gilman 12th E/P 859)

Heparin Induced Thrombocytopenia

- Autoantibodies against heparin bound to platelets can cause platelet aggregation, thrombosis and heparin induced thrombocytopenia (HIT).
- It is more common in females and thrombosis is usually venous more than arterial.
- The incidence is UFH > LMWH > Fondaparinux.
- The drug of choice for HIT is lepirudin; argatroban can also be used. For HIT associated with UFH, a LMWH cannot be used but fondaparinux can be used.

44. Ans. (c) Filgrastim

(Ref: Goodman Gilman 12th E/P 1074)

45. Ans. (c) Inhibits ADP

(Ref: Goodman Gilman 12th E/P 871)

46. Ans. (c) Contraindicated in hepatic failure

(Ref: Goodman Gilman 12th E/P 864)

47. Ans. (b) Clopidogrel

(Ref: Goodman Gilman 12th E/P 871)

48. Ans. (b) Inhibiting factor Xa

(Ref: Goodman Gilman 12th E/P 866)

Oral Factor Xa Inhibitors
Apixaban
Rivaroxaban

49. Ans. (b) Oprelevkin

(Ref: Goodman Gilman 12th E/P 1075)

- Oprelevkin is an IL-11 analog used for treatment of chemotherapy induced thrombocytopenia. Most common side effect is fluid retention.

50. Ans. (a) Factor VII

(Ref: Goodman Gilman 12th E/P 861)

51. Ans. (a) Lepirudin

(Ref: Goodman Gilman 12th E/P 859)

52. Ans. (a) Factor IX and X

(Ref: Goodman Gilman 12th E/P 861)

53. Ans. (a) Protamine sulphate

(Ref: Goodman Gilman 12th E/P 858)

54. Ans. (a) Neutropenia

(Ref: Goodman Gilman 12th E/P 1074)

55. Ans. (c) Protamine

(Ref: Goodman Gilman 12th E/P 858)

56. Ans. (a) Cyclooxygenase

(Ref: Goodman Gilman 12th E/P 868)

57. Ans. (a) Carboxylation

(Ref: Goodman Gilman 12th E/P 861)

- Vitamin K is a cofactor in gamma carboxylation of coagulation factors.

58. Ans. (b) Vit K injection

(Ref: Goodman Gilman 12th E/P 864)

Management of Warfarintoxicity

INR < 5 (Asymptomatic)	Discontinue warfarin and resume once INR is normal
INR ≥ 5 (Asymptomatic)	**Vitamin K**
INR > 20 or Symptomatic	**FFP**

59. Ans. (c) Fresh frozen plasma

(Ref: Goodman Gilman 12th E/P 864)

60. Ans. (c) Erythropoetin

(Ref: Goodman Gilman 12th E/P1071)

- Erythropoetin is produced by kidney and in renal failure its deficiency causes anemia.
- Hence erytropoetin analogs are used for treatment of anemia associated with CRF.

61. Ans. (a) Cannot be injected IV

(Ref: KDT 7th E/P604)

62. Ans. (c) Trisodium citrate

(Ref: G.K.Pal's Practical Physiology 2nd E/P8)

- Trisodium Citrate is the anticoagulant of choice in practical studies.
- It produces anticoagulation by chealating calcium ions.

63. Ans. (d) Activates plasminogen bound to fibrin

(Ref: Goodman Gilman 12th E/P866)

64. Ans. (b) Dextran 40

(Ref: Joyce fluid and electrolytes 3rd E/P158)

65. Ans. (a) Antithrombin III

(Ref: Goodman Gilman 12th E/P854)

66. Ans. (b) Abciximab

(Ref: Goodman Gilman 12th E/P871)

Glycoprotein IIb/IIIa Inhibitors
Abciximab
Tirofiban
Eptifibatide

67. Ans. (d) Warfarin

(Ref: Goodman Gilman 12th E/P871)

68. Ans. (a) Phytonadione

(Ref: Goodman Gilman 12th E/P865)

69. Ans. (a) Antibody against IIb/IIIa receptors

(Ref: Goodman Gilman 12th E/P1071)

70. Ans. (b) Kidney

(Ref: Goodman Gilman 12th E/P1069)

71. Ans. (b) Antiplatelet drug

(Ref: Goodman Gilman 12th E/P871)

72. Ans. (d) Folinic acid

(Ref: Goodman Gilman 12th E/P1095)

73. Ans. (b) Ximelagatran

(Ref: Goodman Gilman 12th E/P865)

74. Ans. (b) Factor V inhibition

(Ref: Goodman Gilman 12th E/P858)

75. Ans. (a) Skin necrosis

(Ref: Goodman Gilman 12th E/P 858)

- Skin necrosis is a side effect of warfarin and not heparin.

76. Ans. (c) Streptokinase

(Ref: Goodman Gilman 12th E/P866)

77. Ans. (c) Prothrombin time (PT)

(Ref: Goodman Gilman 12th E/P862)

- Oral anticoagulants of coumarin class like warfarin require PT monitoring whereas the lastest ones like dabigatran and apixaban don't require monitoring.

78. Ans. (b) Heteropolysaccharide

(Ref: Goodman Gilman 12th E/P1071)

- Heparin is a glycosaminoglycan made up of different saccharides, i.e. it's a heteroplolysaccharide.

79. Ans. (a) Hypotension

(Ref: KDT 7th E/P619)

- Hypertension is a contraindication to anticoagulant therapy.

80. Ans. (d) Hyperplasminemia

(Ref: Goodman Gilman 12th E/P867)

81. Ans. (a) Tirofiban

(Ref: Goodman Gilman 12th E/P870)

82. Ans. (b) Argatroban

(Ref: Goodman Gilman 12th E/P860)

- Argatroban is excreted by liver and hence preferred in renal failure.

83. Ans. (b) Griseofulvin

(Ref: Goodman Gilman 12th E/P864)

- Griseofulvin is an enzyme inducer and hence decreases the anticoagulant effect of warfarin.

84. Ans. (a) 4–8 minutes

(Ref: Goodman Gilman 12th E/P866)

85. Ans. (c) 0.75 mg/kg

(Ref: Goodman Gilman 12th E/P866)

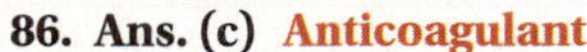

86. Ans. (c) Anticoagulant

(Ref: Goodman Gilman 12th E/P857)

87. Ans. (b) Prasugrel, (c) Clopidogrel and (e) Ticagrelor

(Ref: Goodman Gilman 13th E/P597)

88. Ans. (b) It takes minimum 2 weeks for reticulocyte count to increase

(Ref: Goodman Gilman 12th edition, Page 1082)

- Inflammatory bowel disease is associated with iron deficiency anemia and hence iron therapy is used. Oral iron therapy however can worsen inflammatory bowel disease.
- An increase in reticulocyte count is the earliest response to iron therapy and it takes at least 1 week.
- The rise in hemoglobin levels begin only after 1 month and attained within 3 months.
- Nausea, vomiting, constipation and diarrhea are the dose limiting side effect.
- Iron stores are replenished after 3-6 months of therapy and hence iron should be given for this duration after treatment of the cause of iron deficiency.

89. Ans. (e) Inactivates factor Xa selectively

(Ref: Goodman Gilman 12th edition, Page 858)

90. Ans. (d) Aspirin

(Ref: Goodman Gilman 12th E/P863)

- Aspirin being an antiaggregant can increase bleeding with anticoagulants like warfarin.

91. Ans. (b) Deferiprone, (c) Desferioxamine

(Ref: Goodman Gilman 12th E/P1083)

- Desferioxamine can be given by both oral and parenteral route
- Deferiprone is given only by oral route.

92. Ans. (b) Antithrombin III

(Ref: Goodman Gilman 12th E/P854)

93. Ans. (a) Protein C deficiency

(Ref: Goodman Gilman 12th E/P864)

94. Ans. (a) Thrombopoietin agonist

(Ref: Goodman Gilman 13th E/P756)

95. Ans. (c) Osteocalcin

(Ref: Meyler's side effects/P708)

- Vitamin K is required for activation of gamma carboxylase which not only activates coagulation factor, but also synthesizes noncollagenous bone matrix i.e. osteocalcin.
- Hence warfarin by inhibiting activation of vitamin K decreases osteocalcin synthesis, which leads to defective bone formation leading to nasal hypoplasia and stippled epiphyseal calcification.

96. Ans. (d) Clopidogrel should be stopped 7 days before surgery

(Ref: Goodman Gilman 13th E/P597)

97. Ans. (b) Lacks antidote

(Ref: Katzung 13th edition, Page 593)

- Oral direct thrombin inhibitors usually don't require monitoring as they have a predictable effect; however parenteral drugs do require aPTT monitoring.
- Most of the direct thrombin inhibitors don't have antidotes, though recently idarucizumab an anti-dabigatran monoclonal antibody has been approved for reversal of dabigatran effect. Hence it is the best answer in this MCQ.

98. Ans. (a) GM CSF

(Ref: Goodman Gilman 12th E/P1074)

99. Ans. (a) Lipoprotein lipase

(Ref: Goodman Gilman 12th E/P855)

100. Ans. (c) Danaparoid

(Ref: Harrison 19th E/P728)

101. Ans. (a) Clopidogrel

(Ref: Goodman Gilman 12th E/P870)

102. Ans. (d) ADP

(Ref: Goodman Gilman 12th E/P869)

103. Ans. (a) aPTT

(Ref: Goodman Gilman 12th E/P857)

104. Ans. (b) Stimulates platelet aggregation and clot retraction

(Ref: Goodman Gilman 12th E/P869)

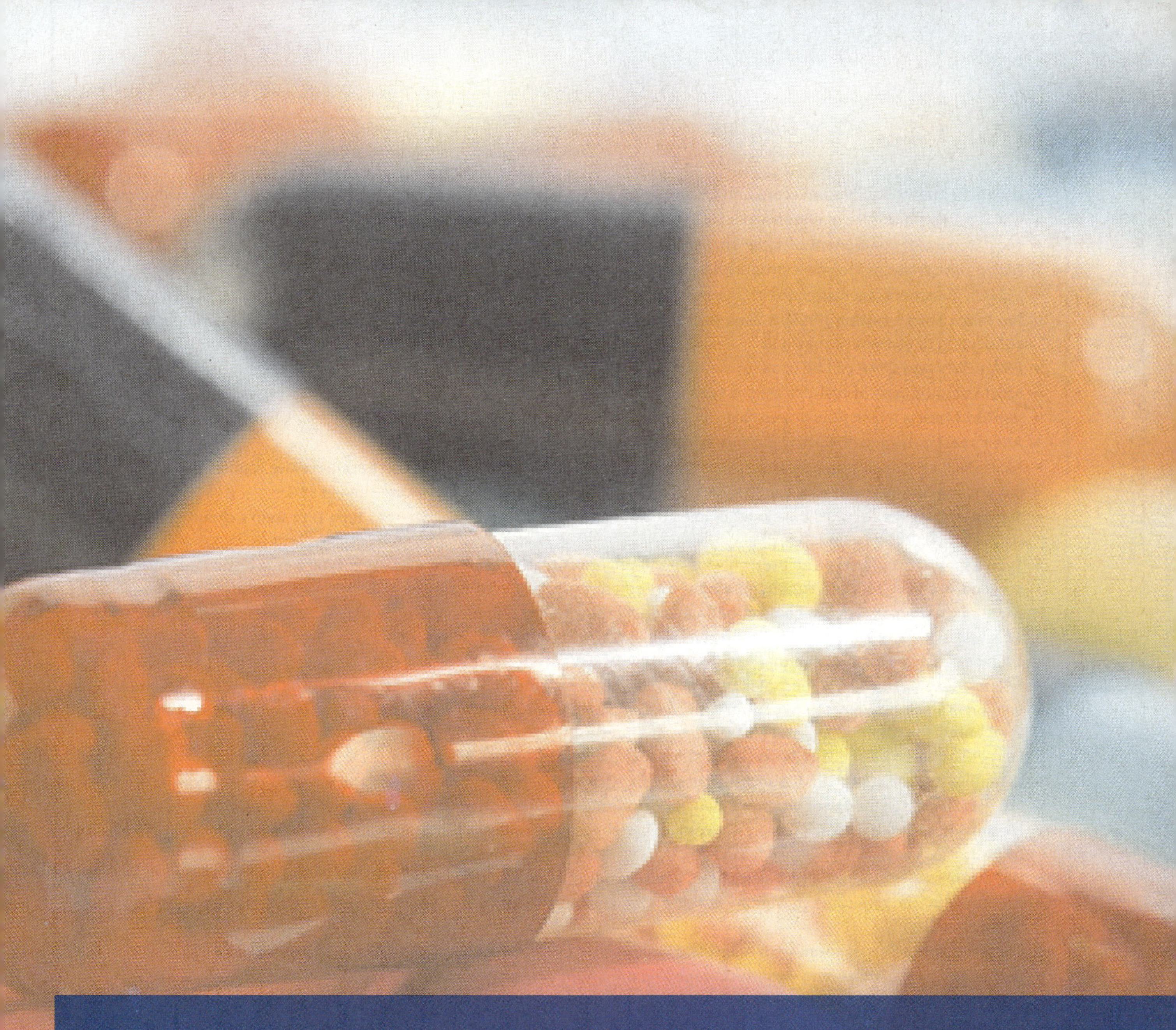

Anesthesia

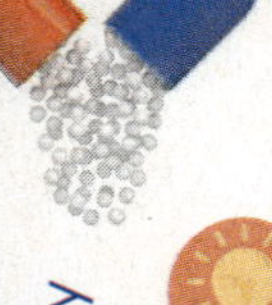

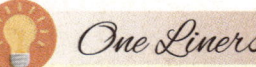

One Liners

- A class **III and IV Mallampati score and thyromental distance of less than 6.5 cm** is associated with difficult intubation.
- The most common size of endotracheal tube used in an **adult male is 8–8.5 mm** and in **adult female is 7–8 mm.**
- Most important component of soda lime in carbon dioxide absorbing canister is **calcium hydroxide.**
- Maximum carbon monoxide is produced by **desflurane** and minimum with **halothane** and **sevoflurane.**
- Volatile anesthetic agents require different vaporizers due to their different **vapor pressure.**
- **Pin Index Safety system (PISS)** is used for cylinders and **DISS Diameter index safety system (DISS)** for pipelines for correct connection to anesthetic machine.
- **PSV, ACMV and CPAP** can be used for weaning of patients from ventilators.
- Most common type of cylinder used is **type E.**
- **Venturi Mask** is a high flow device that can deliver a maximum of **60% oxygen.**
- **Allen's test** is used to check the **patency of ulnar artery** before invasive BP monitoring.
- Most ideal site for core temperature measurement is **distal esophagus** whereas most accurate site is **pulmonary artery.**
- In **light anesthesia** β waves are seen whereas in **deep anesthesia θ and σ waves** are seen in EEG.
- **Type A or Magill's circuit** is the circuit of choice for spontaneous ventilation, whereas **type D or Bain's circuit** is the circuit of choice for controlled ventilation.
- **Type E or Ayre's T piece** can be used only for spontaneous ventilation in children, whereas **type F or Jackson Rees modification** is circuit of choice for both spontaneous and controlled ventilation in children.
- For confirmation of endotracheal intubation, **capnography** is most commonly used, whereas **fiberoptic bronchoscopy** is best.
- All anesthetic agents act by stimulating **glycine** and **GABA** receptors, whereas, only ketamine, cyclopropane, N_2O and xenon act by opening **potassium channel** and by inhibiting **NMDA** receptors.
- IV anesthetic agent with highest plasma protein binding is **propofol** followed by **barbiturates** and lowest with **ketamine**.
- Pain on intravenous injection is caused by maximum with **propofol** followed by other drugs like barbiturates (methohexital > thiopental) and etomidate.
- Pain on intraarterial injection is caused by **thiopental sodium**.
- Ketamine is associated with **dissociative anesthesia, strong analgesia, hallucinations and emergence reaction.**
- Etomidate is associated with **vitamin C deficiency, adrenal suppression** and **maximum nausea and vomiting**.
- **Methoxyflurane > Halothane** undergo maximum metabolism, whereas **isoflurane > desflurane** undergo minimum metabolism by liver.
- **Hepatotoxicity** is maximum with halothane, whereas it is minimum with **sevoflurane**.
- **Methoxyflurane** generates maximum fluoride ions and **desflurane < isoflurane** generates least fluoride ions that cause nephrotoxicity.
- Ozone depletion is **maximum with halothane**, whereas no effect is seen with **sevoflurane and desflurane**.
- **Global warming** is **maximum with desflurane** and **minimum with halothane**.
- **MAC** is the measure of **potency** of inhalational agents; MAC 1/α potency.
- **Blood gas partition** coefficient is a measure of **speed of onset and offset of effect** of inhalational agents; Blood gas partition coefficient 1/α (inversely proportional to) Speed of onset and offset of action.
- **Methoxyflurane** has least MAC and hence is most potent, whereas **nitrous oxide** has maximum MAC and is least potent.
- **Methoxyflurane** has highest whereas **xenon < desflurane** has lowest blood gas partition coefficient.
- **Sevoflurane** can react with lime to produce **compound A** which is nephrotoxic.
- **Trielene** can react with lime to produce **phosgene gas** which causes ARDS and **dichloroacetylene** which causes neurotoxicity.
- **Enflurane** causes epilepsy at normal doses, whereas **sevoflurane** causes **epilepsy** at high doses.
- **Halothane** causes a maximum increase in ICP, whereas **sevoflurane** and **nitrous oxide** cause a minimum increase in ICP.
- **Nitrous oxide** has a low blood gas partition coefficient, which produces effects like **concentration effect, second gas effect and diffusion hypoxia**.
- NDMRs safe in renal failure are **rocuronium, vecuronium, atracurium** and **cis-atracurium**.
- **Doxacurium** is most potent and longest acting NDMR; **rapacuronium** is shortest acting and **rocuronium** is fastest acting NDMR.
- The central muscles like **diaphragm**, larynx and muscles of **head and neck** have **fastest onset and offset of action**. The peripheral muscles like that of hands like **adductor pollicis** have **slowest onset and offset of action**.
- The **peripheral muscles are more sensitive to NDMR as compared to central muscles like diaphragm**.
- **Fade intoF stimulation** is seen with **NDMRs** and **phase II block** of depolarizing muscle relaxants.

Contd...

- **Ester local anesthetics** are metabolized by plasma esterases and hence are **shorter acting**, whereas **amides** are metabolized in liver by amidase and hence are **long acting**.
- The orders of sensitivity of block fibre by local anesthetics in tissue is type **A > B (preganglionic sympathetic) > C (Temperature)**. In fibre type A the order is **gamma (muscle tone) > delta (Pin prick) > beta (touch) and alpha (motor)**. Thus, the sequence of block is **muscle tone > pin prick > touch > motor > preganglionic sympathetic > temperature**.
- **Potency** of local anesthetics is directly proportional to their **lipid solubility**, whereas **duration of action** is directly proportional to **plasma protein binding**.
- The onset of action of **local anesthetics** is directly proportional to the **pK_a**.
- In spinal anesthesia the sequence is **B (preganglionic sympathetic) > C (Temperature) > A**. The sequence of block in **A fibres is A delta (Pin prick) > A beta (touch) > A alpha (motor)**. The sequence of block is **temperature > pin prick > touch > motor**. The order of reversal of block is opposite, i.e. **motor > touch > pin prick > temperature**.
- **Epinephrine** increases duration of action and decreases toxicity of local anesthetics, whereas **bicarbonate** decreases pain on injection.
- Systemic absorption of local anesthetics is maximum by **intercostal route** and minimum by **subcutaneous route**.
- Bupivacaine is most cardiotoxic local anesthetic.
- **Dibucaine** is most potent and the longest acting local anesthetic, whereas **chlorprocaine < procaine** is the shortest acting and least potent local anesthetic.
- For application on intact skin **eutectic mixture of local anesthetic (EMLA)**, i.e. **lidocaine (2.5%) and prilocaine (2.5%) is preferred**.
- In spinal anesthesia drugs commonly used are **lidocaine, bupivacaine and tetracaine**; **procaine** is used for diagnostic block due to its shorter duration of action.
- Post-spinal headache is seen after **12–24 hours** of procedure, within **48 hours** in most cases and resolves spontaneously within **7 days**.

HISTORY

Milestones in the History of Anesthesia

Achievements	Persons associated
Term anesthesia was first used by	Dioscorides
Term anesthesia coined by	Oliver Wendell Homes
Term balanced anesthesia coined by	John Lundy and Ralph Waters
Father of anesthesia	WTG Morton
Father of modern anesthesia	Crawford Long
Spinal anesthesia first demonstrated by	August Bier
Epidural anesthesia first demonstrated by	Cathelin and Sicard
Ether's effect first demonstrated by	WTG. Morton
Ether anesthesia was first used by	Crawford Long
Nitrous oxide effect first demonstrated by	Horace Wells
First IV agent thiopentone used by	John Lundy
First muscle relaxant curare used by	Harold Griffith
First endotracheal intubation was done by	Ivan Magill
First local anesthetic cocaine was isolated from cocoa shrubs and introduced by	Albert Niemann
First local anesthetic cocaine used by	Carl Koller
Chloroform was introduced by	James Simpson
Capnography introduced by	Bethune and Brethren
Laryngeal mask airway invented by	Archie Bain
Ketamine was synthesized by	Stevens
Ketamine was first used clinically by	Corssen and Domino

Contd...

Overall anesthesia can be broadly classified into **general** and **local** anesthesia.

GENERAL ANESTHESIA

- The term anesthesia was coined by **Oliver Wendell Homes.** For an uneventful surgery a balanced anesthesia is required, and the term "balanced anesthesia" was coined by Lundy.
- Balanced anesthesia includes four components mentioned below,
  - Amnesia
  - **Analgesia**
  - **Muscle relaxation**
  - **Abolition of reflexes with maintenance of homeostasis**
- The process of general anesthesia begins with premedication which includes drugs like sedative hypnotics, opioids, glycopyrrolate and anti-emetics.
- This is followed by preoxygenation for three minutes to increase the oxygen reserve of the body.
- Induction of anesthesia is done usually with intravenous agents and then muscle relaxants are given for facilitation of intubation.
- After intubation anesthesia is maintained with either inhalational or intravenous agents.

- After the planned surgery is over, reversal follows and then patient is extubated.

Clinical Box-1

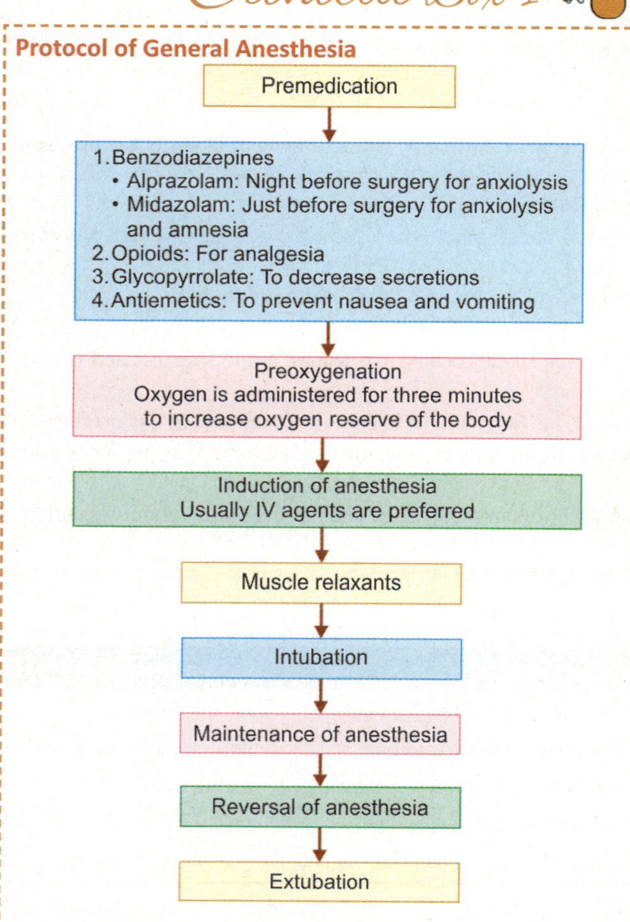

Protocol of General Anesthesia
Premedication
1. Benzodiazepines
• Alprazolam: Night before surgery for anxiolysis
• Midazolam: Just before surgery for anxiolysis and amnesia
2. Opioids: For analgesia
3. Glycopyrrolate: To decrease secretions
4. Antiemetics: To prevent nausea and vomiting
Preoxygenation
Oxygen is administered for three minutes to increase oxygen reserve of the body
Induction of anesthesia
Usually IV agents are preferred
Muscle relaxants
Intubation
Maintenance of anesthesia
Reversal of anesthesia
Extubation

ANESTHETIC ASSESSMENT

- The anesthetic assessment before surgery is important for the preanesthetic clearance (PAC).
- In this process, history of patient is taken for disorders of cardiovascular system (CVS), central nervous system (CNS), respiratory system and other important systemic disorders that can alter the outcome of anesthesia.
- This is followed by family history with anesthetic agents, history of drug allergies, smoking and alcohol consumption.
- After this, examination is done focusing more on the disorders mentioned in history.
- After systemic examination patient's airway is assessed for any problems that can be encountered later during intubation.

AIRWAY ASSESSMENT

Airway can be assessed commonly by Mallampati score and thyromental distance.

- **Mallampati score:** Patient sitting upright is asked to open mouth and protrude tongue. Based on the visible structures the patient is assigned a class from I to IV as given in the Table. A class **III and IV Mallampati score is associated with difficult intubation.**

Mallampati Score

Classes	Structures Visible
Class I	S: Soft Palate U: Uvula F: Faucial Pillars
Class II	S: Soft Palate U: Uvula
Class III	S: Soft Palate
Class IV	Only hard palate visible

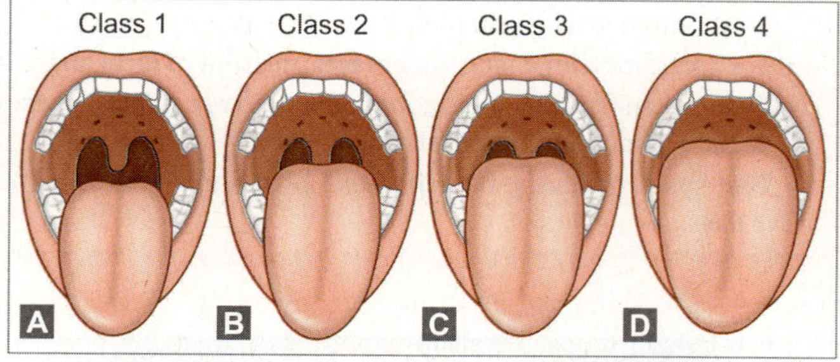

Mallampati classes; A. Class 1; B. Class 2; C. Class 3; D. Class 4

- **Thyromental distance:** The distance between thyroid cartilage and chin is measured with an extended head. A distance of **more than 6.5 cm** predicts normal intubation.

Thyromental Distance and its Outcome

Thyromental Distance	Outcome
> 6.5 cm	Normal intubation
6.0 – 6.5 cm	Difficult intubation
< 6 cm	Impossible intubation

Mnemonics

Indicator of difficult laryngoscopy/intubation

SMALL PALATE

- **S :** Short thyromental distance, short neck
- **M :** Mallampati class III and IV, Mouth opening small
- **A :** Arched, high palate
- **L :** Long upper incisors
- **L :** Limited cervical mobility
- **Palate :** Prominent overbite

RISK ASSESSMENT

There are various risks associated with anesthesia and based upon physical status of the patient, ASA classification is commonly used to calculate risk. The most common cause of death after surgery is myocardial infarction.

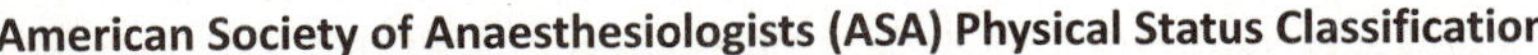

American Society of Anaesthesiologists (ASA) Physical Status Classification

Class	Physical status	Mortality risk
I	**Normal healthy patient:** No organic, physiologic or psychiatric disturbance; excludes very young and very old; healthy with good exercise tolerance	0–0.3%
II	**Patients with mild systemic disease:** No functional limitations; has a well-controlled disease of one body system; controlled hypertension or diabetes without systemic effects, cigarette smoking without chronic obstructive pulmonary disease (COPD); mild obesity, pregnancy	0.3–1.4%
III	**Patients with severe systemic disease:** Some functional limitation; has a controlled disease of more than one body system or one major system; no immediate danger of death; controlled congestive heart failure (CHF), stable angina, old heart attack, poorly controlled hypertension, morbid obesity, chronic renal failure; bronchospastic disease with intermittent symptoms	1.5–5.4%
IV	**Patients with severe systemic disease that is a constant threat to life:** Has at least one severe disease that is poorly controlled or is at an end stage; possible risk of death; unstable angina, symptomatic COPD, symptomatic CHF, hepatorenal failure	7.8–25.9 %
V	**Moribund patients who are not expected to survive without the operation:** Not expected to survive > 24 hours without surgery; imminent risk of death; multiorgan failure, sepsis syndrome with hemodynamic instability, hypothermia, poorly controlled coagulopathy	9.4–57.8%
VI	A declared brain-dead patient whose organs are being removed for donor purposes	

EQUIPMENT IN ANESTHESIA

LARYNGOSCOPE

Laryngoscopes can be of two types, i.e. **direct and indirect**.

Direct Laryngoscope

The direct laryngoscopes are the conventional ones which facilitate direct visualization of larynx for tracheal tube insertion. It is made up of a handle and a blade is attached to it.

- **Macintosh blade** is a curved one, which is the most common blade used.
- **McCoy blade** has a movable tip that helps to elevate epiglottis for visualization of larynx.
- **Miller blade** is a straight one with curved tip, that is less commonly used.

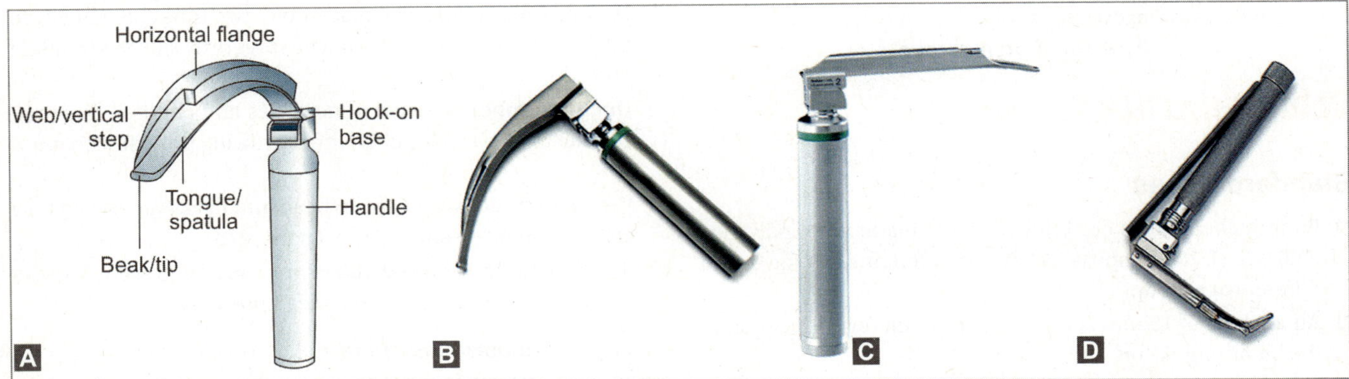

Direct Laryngoscopes: A. Parts of laryngoscope; B. Macintosh laryngoscope; C. Miller laryngoscope; D. McCoy laryngoscope

Indirect Laryngoscope

Indirect laryngoscopes are recent advancements where the larynx is visualized indirectly through various devices.

- **McGrath laryngoscope** is a laryngoscope with a small camera at the tip which projects the image of larynx on a screen. It is also known as video laryngoscope.
- **Fiberoptic laryngoscope** is a flexible laryngoscope that transmits the image of larynx through glass piece or to a monitor. It is used in difficult intubation.
- **Airtraq** is a laryngoscope that uses a prism for visualization of larynx.
- Optical stylets are like fiberoptic laryngoscope but are rigid and can be used only in patients on general anesthesia.

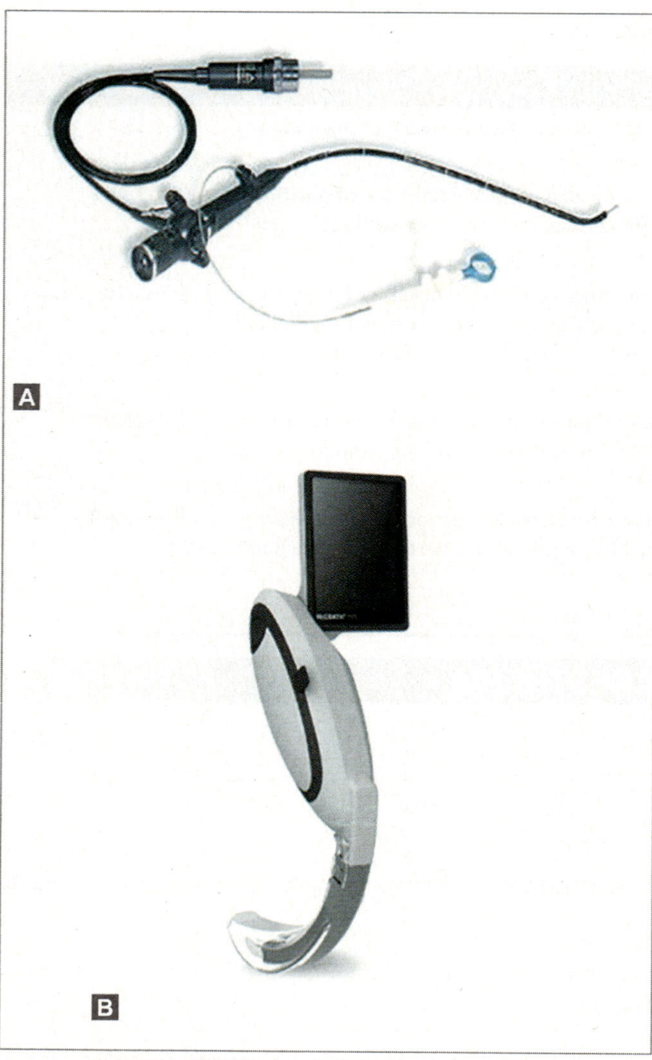

Indirect Laryngoscope: A. Fiberoptic laryngoscope; B. McGrath laryngoscope

ENDOTRACHEAL TUBE

Standard Tubes

- Endotracheal tubes currently used are made up of polyvinyl chloride (PVC) (disposable) are of different sizes for use in different age groups.
- An adaptor of 15 mm is attached to the tip for connection to the breathing circuit.
- A high volume low pressure cuff is provided that is inflated with air with a pressure less than 25 cm of H_2O to prevent leakage of gas and aspiration.
- Saline is used for inflation in case of laser surgeries and when hyperbaric oxygen is used.
- Another distal opening on the side wall of tube called as **Murphy eye** is there for ventilation as an additional port.
- The tip of the tube should lie at least **4–5 cm above the carina**.
- The most common size used in an **adult male is 8–8.5 mm** and in **adult female is 7–8 mm.**

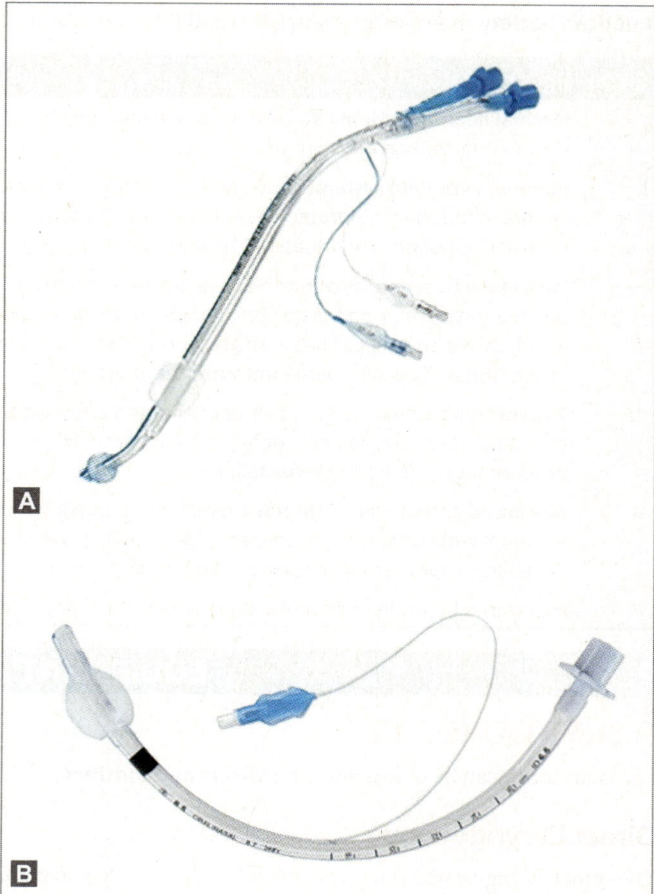

Endotracheal Tubes: A. Double lumen ET tube; B. Standard ET tube

Other Types of Tubes

- **Double lumen tubes** are made up of two tubes attached side by side. These are used in thoracic surgery to selectively inflate one lung.
- **Uncuffed tubes** are used in neonates and children less than 10 years of age as the subglottic narrowing provides a natural cuff.
- **Preformed tubes** are used in head and neck surgery to allow connection diversions away from the area.
- **Reinforced or armored tubes** are used to prevent kinking that can be seen at a particular head position.

Diameter of Endotracheal Tube

Age group	Diameter (mm)
Premature neonate	2.5
0-6 months	3–3.5
≥ 6 months – 1 year	3.5–4
≥ 1 year – 6 years	Age (in years)/3 + 3.5
≥ 6 years	Age (in years)/4 + 4.5

Note: The maximum size of tube is 10.5 mm.

Length of Endotracheal Tube

Age Group	Length (cm)
Children	Age/2 + 12
Adult male	23
Adult female	21

Note: The tube should lie 4–5 cm above the carina.

ANESTHETIC MACHINE

The primary function of an anesthetic machine is to **reduce the pressure of gas** supplied from source cylinder and to control the flow of gas to deliver a required amount to the breathing system. The machine contains various parts to achieve this which are mentioned below. Various other equipment loaded in the machine are: Carbon dioxide absorbing canister, cylinders of gases, vaporizers for volatile agents, rebreathing bag, display unit and bellows assembly.

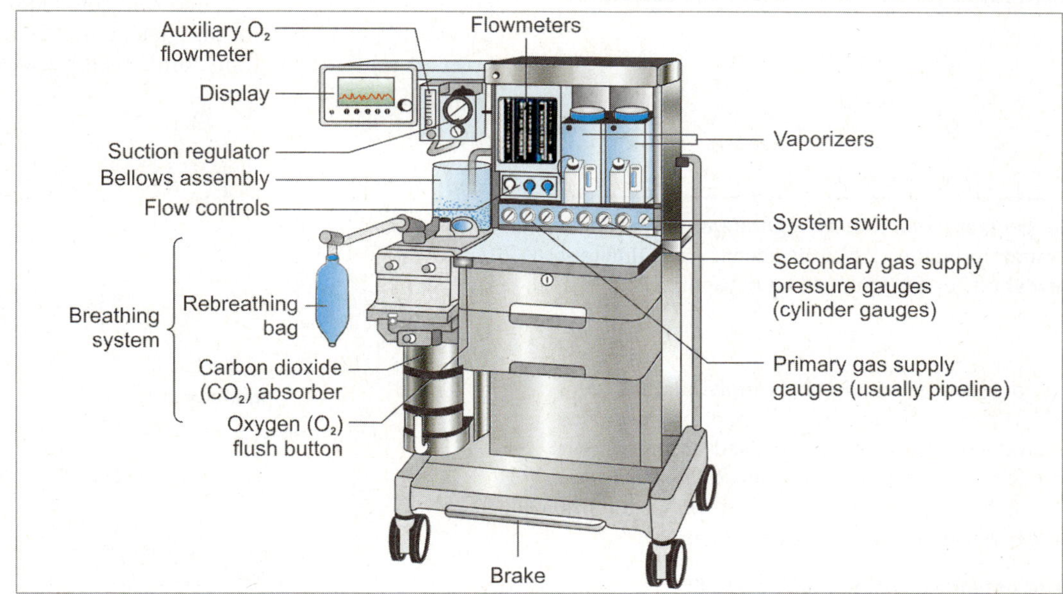

Anesthetic machine

- **Reducing valves:** These valves decrease the pressure of gases from the cylinders to 400 kPa.
- **Flowmeters or Rotameters:** There are different flowmeters for different gases like oxygen, nitrous oxide, air, etc. with oxygen being on extreme left.

Carbon Dioxide Absorbing Canister

- The function of these canisters is to absorb excessive carbon dioxide from the circulation. Currently **calcium hydroxide (soda lime)** and **lithium hydroxide based absorbers** are used; barium hydroxide (bary lime) based absorber is not preferred now.
- Soda lime is made up of calcium hydroxide, sodium hydroxide, potassium hydroxide, silica and an indicator. Calcium hydroxide poorly reacts with CO_2, hence CO_2 first reacts with water to form bicarbonate, which further reacts with NaOH and KOH to form Na_2CO_3 and K_2CO_3. Finally the later compounds react with $Ca(OH)_2$ to form $CaCO_3$ and this is the **rate limiting step**.
- There are various factors that can affect CO_2 absorption; these are
    - **Surface area of granules:** Smaller is the size of granules more is the area exposed to gas and more is CO_2 absorption.
    - **Airway resistance:** Smaller is the size of granules more is airway resistance and lesser is CO_2 absorption. Hence to maintain a higher surface area exposure with lesser resistance a medium size of 4–8 mesh is preferred for granules.
    - **Channeling:** Passage of gas through the gaps in between the granules is called channeling, which can decrease CO_2 absorption.
- The bases NaOH and KOH can react with some agents to produce toxic compounds. **Trielene** can react with these bases to produce dichloroacetylene which is neurotoxic and phosgene gas which can cause ARDS. **Sevoflurane** can react with bases to produce compound A which is nephrotoxic. Sevoflurane can also react with bases (mainly bary lime) to create an exothermic reaction that can cause airway burn.
- Volatile agents can react with bases in dry soda lime to produce carbon monoxide, which is **maximum with desflurane** and **minimum with halothane and sevoflurane**.
- Lithium hydroxide base absorbers can directly react with CO_2 and has no bases, hence does not cause above reactions.

Soda Lime
Calcium Hydroxide: 94% (Most Important)
Sodium hydroxide: 5%
Potassium hydroxide: 1%
+
Silica: For consolidation
+
Indicators: Phenolphthalein, Ethyl violet, Momosaz, Durasorb

Vaporizers

- Vaporizers are used to heat the volatile liquid anesthetic agents that form vapors and then can be delivered to the patient. The concentration of anesthetic agent delivered can be controlled by the gas passing through vaporizer.
- A color coding is used for different vaporizers as given in Table.

Color coding for different vaporizers

Volatile anesthetic agent	Vaporizer color
Desflurane	Blue
Halothane	Red
Isoflurane	Purple
Sevoflurane	Yellow
Enflurane	Orange

- When volatile agents are heated, they evaporate and form vapors to generate vapor pressure. Different agents have different **vapor pressures** and hence require different vaporizers.

Cylinders

- The cylinders for gases are made up of molybdenum, steel or aluminum. Different colors for cylinders are used for identification and a **pin index** system is used for prevention of errors in connection of cylinder to the anesthetic machine.
- Cylinders come in different sizes from A to H, however the size **E cylinders** are most commonly used in anesthesia.

Cylinder color and pin index (Mnemonic: At ONCE)

Gas	Pin index	Forms of physical content	Cylinder color
At: Air	1, 5	Gas	Gray body with black and white shoulders
O: Oxygen	2, 5	Gas or Liquid	Black with white shoulders
N: Nitrous oxide	3, 5	Liquid	Blue
C: $CO_2 \geq 7.5\%$	1, 6	Liquid	Grey
$CO_2 < 7.5\%$	2, 6	Liquid	Orange
Cyclopropane	3, 6		
Entonox	7	Liquid	Blue body with blue and white shoulder

Note: The color of helium cylinder is brown

SAFETY SYSTEMS FOR GAS CONNECTIONS

- The medical gases can be delivered to the patient from either a cylinder or a gas pipeline.
- The cylinders have gases at a very high pressure, e.g. 2000 psig for oxygen and air, whereas the hospital pipeline has gases at a pressure of 50–55 psig. Hence gases from cylinders must pass through a high pressure regulator to decrease pressure.
- To prevent mistake in attachment of cylinders two systems are used namely **pin index safety system (PISS)** for cylinders and **diameter index safety system (DISS)** for pipelines.

Pin Index Safety System

- The anesthetic machines have a yoke assembly which have pins numbering 1 to 7 for safe attachment of cylinders and a Bodok seal to prevent gas leak.
- There are two holes for these pins on the cylinder at specific positions, which gives a pin index, e.g. pin index for oxygen is 2,5 which means the pins for attachment of oxygen cylinder holes are present at position 2 and 5 on the yoke assembly.

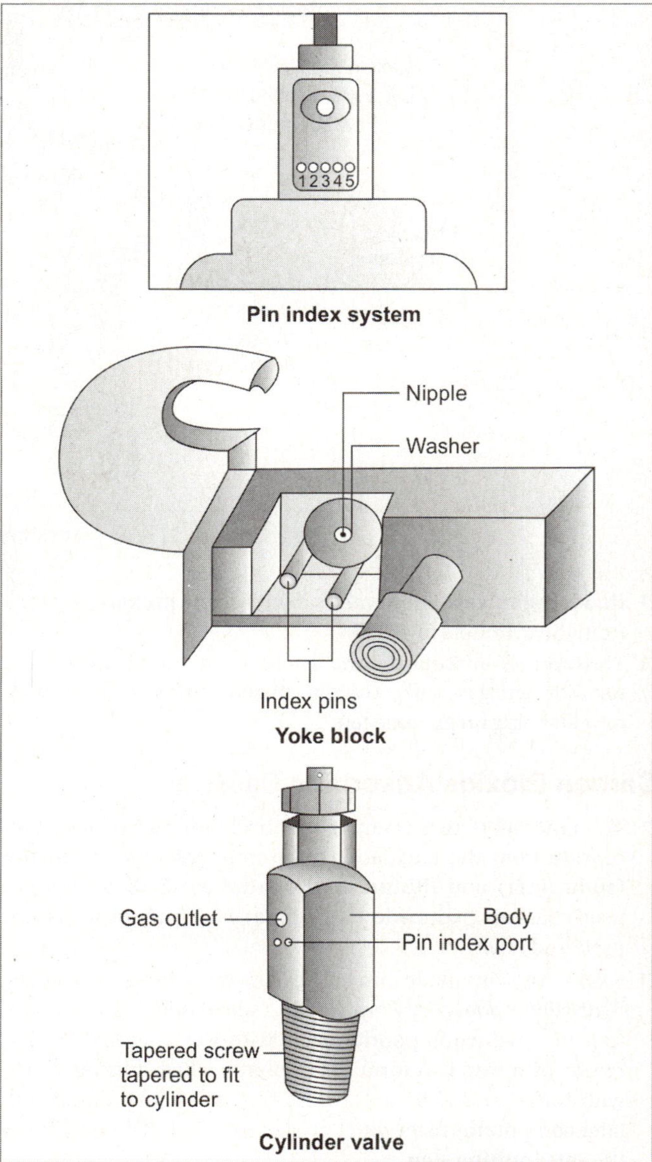

Pin Index Safety System

Diameter Index Safety System (DISS)

- On the other hand, for connection of gas pipeline in hospital, different diameter pipes with different colors are used for different gases to prevent wrong attachment.

- The oxygen connector is different from other gases in that it has a threaded texture.

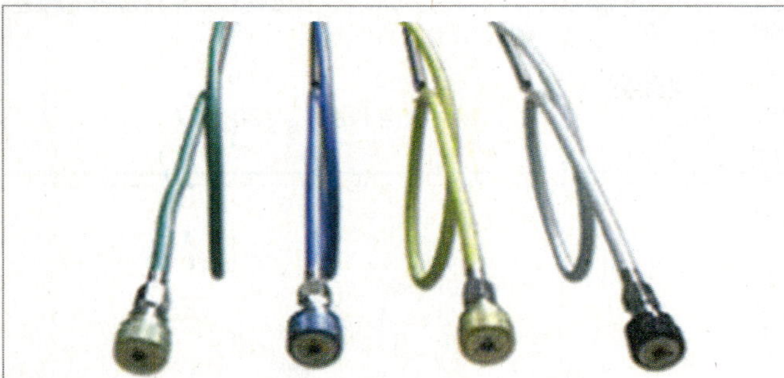

Diameter Index Safety System

VENTILATOR

- Ventilation can be facilitated via endotracheal tube known as invasive ventilation, whereas if it is facilitated via mask on the face and nose it is called as noninvasive ventilation.
- Invasive ventilation is associated with infection of respiratory tract known as ventilator-associated pneumonia (VAP) and **ventilator-associated tracheobronchitis (VAT)**.
- Noninvasive ventilation is associated with lesser incidence of ventilator associated pneumonia and sepsis and lesser sedation required. It is indicated in COPD exacerbation, postoperative respiratory failure and acute cardiogenic pulmonary edema.
- Ventilators are primarily of three types, i.e. time cycled, pressure cycled and volume cycled.

Types of Ventilators

Time cycled	Expiration begins after a definite time set. It is preferred in **neonates**.
Pressure cycled	Expiration begins after a definite pressure is reached.
Volume cycled	Expiration begins after a definite volume is delivered; the gas flow rate is 30–50 L/minute. It is preferred in **ICU**.

- The different ventilation modes are mentioned in detail below.

MODES OF VENTILATION

Controlled Mechanical Ventilation

- In controlled mechanical ventilation (CMV) there is no patient effort and the tidal volume is delivered by ventilator.
- Thus, it is preferred in patients without effort in cases like paralysis and head injury. It **cannot be used for weaning**.

Assisted-Controlled Mechanical Ventilation

- In assisted-controlled mechanical ventilation (ACMV) inspiration is initiated by patient and continued by ventilator, if required. It is the most commonly used mode of **initiation of mechanical ventilation**.
- ACMV requires heavy sedation and muscle relaxants. If patient is tachypneic then ventilator can continue that can cause **respiratory alkalosis**.
- Similarly, it can cause over inflation, known as **auto PEEP** which can **decrease cardiac output** and cause **barotrauma** as well.
- It is not suitable for weaning as patient is supported in each breath.

Synchronized Intermittent Mandatory Ventilation

- In synchronized intermittent mandatory ventilation (SIMV) only a definite number of breaths are assisted by ventilator.
- Since patient can exercise respiratory muscles to full capacity in between assisted breaks, **SIMV can be used for weaning**. It is hemodynamically more stable and requires lesser sedation and muscle relaxants.
- However, if patient is tachypneic then an inspiration of patient and machine can coincide and in the case, the machine assisted breath is abolished; this is known as **patient-ventilatory asynchrony**. This can also be seen in case of **ACMV**.

Positive End-Expiratory Pressure

- In positive end-expiratory pressure (PEEP) a positive pressure is applied by the machine at end of expiration that prevents alveolar collapse and **increases fractional residual capacity (FRC).**
- PEEP is used in case of **pulmonary edema, emergency thoracic surgery, ARDS, refractory hypoxemia (PaO_2 < 60 mm Hg for 1 hour while getting FiO_2 of 1.0) and to prevent atelectasis**.
- The drawbacks are the pressure can cause a **decrease in cardiac output and hypotension, pulmonary hypertension and barotrauma**.

Mnemonics

Uses of PEEP

P : Pulmonary edema
E : Emergency thoracic surgery
E : Emergency in ARDS
P : Prevent atelectasis, PaO_2 < 60 mmHg

Pressure Support Ventilation

- Pressure support ventilation (PSV) is preferred in patients with spontaneous respiration having normal rate with inadequate tidal volume. In this case the machine supports with a definite pressure.
- PSV helps in the process of **weaning**.

Pressure-Controlled Ventilation

- Pressure-controlled ventilation (PCV) differs from PSV in that PSV is ventilator triggered and machine supports ventilation with a definite pressure and time to regulates peak airway pressure.
- PCV is used in patients with **barotrauma** and **postoperative thoracic surgery patients**.

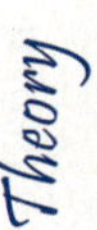

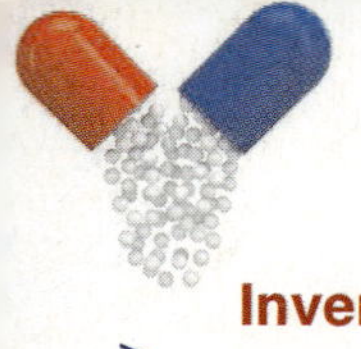

Inverse Ratio Ventilation

- In this case the ratio of inspiration to expiration is 2:1, which behaves like a PEEP. Normally the ratio is 1:2.
- It is used in patients with severe hypoxemic respiratory failure.

Continuous Positive Airway Pressure

- Continuous positive airway pressure (CPAP) is **noninvasive positive pressure ventilation** in which the ventilator does not control breathing, rather just infuses fresh gas with a definite pressure.
- **CPAP is used to assess the weaning capacity** of the patients. It is also used for treatment of **COPD** and is treatment of choice for **obstructive sleep apnea (OSA)** and used for **ventilation in preterm neonates less than 1 kg or less than 28 weeks**.

Nonconventional Ventilation

- **Extracorporeal membrane oxygenation (ECMO):** It is nonconventional in which it **does not use a ventilator**. A large cannula is inserted into inferior IVC and venous blood drawn is allowed to pass through an artificial lung for oxygenation and then the oxygenated blood is passed through small cannula into peripheral vein. It is reserved for treatment of hypoxia resistant to conventional therapy.
- **High frequency oscillatory ventilation (HFOV):** It is nonconventional in that it maintains a tidal volume lesser than dead space volume. HFOV maintains a relatively high pressure as compared to low tidal volume and hence is protective for lungs. Thus, it is preferred in ARDS to prevent alveolar collapse.

OXYGEN DELIVERY DEVICES

Oxygen delivery devices can be broadly classified into high-flow and low-flow devices.

High-Flow Devices

- High-flow devices deliver a fixed amount of oxygen irrespective of other variables of patients like respiratory rate.
- These are best for treatment of severe hypoxemia.
- Venturi mask is most commonly used device in this section, which can deliver **60% oxygen**.

Low-Flow Devices

- Low flow devices ability to deliver oxygen depends on patient variables.
- These are devices like oxygen mask, nasal cannula, rebreathing mask and non-rebreathing mask.

Percentage of Oxygen Delivered from the Oxygen Delivery Devices

Oxygen delivery devices	Percentage of oxygen delivered
Venturi mask	60%
Oxygen mask	60%
Rebreathing mask	100%
Nonrebreathing mask	80%
Non-rebreathing mask with reservoir	95%
Nasal cannula	44%
Face mask with reservoir connected to Ambu bag	100%

Contd...

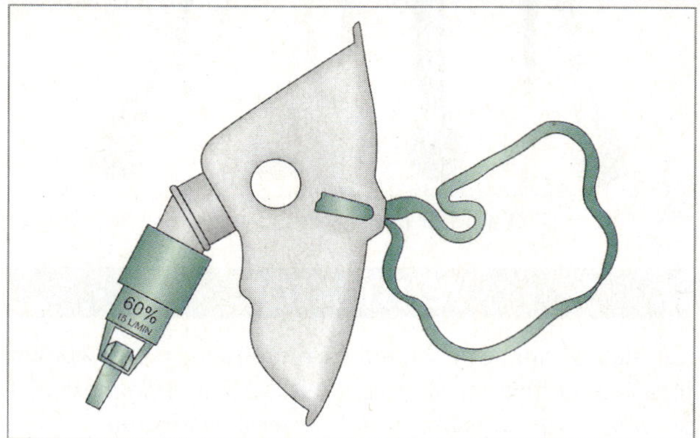

Venturi Mask

MONITORING IN ANESTHESIA

ELECTROCARDIOGRAM

- ECG is used to detect the rate, rhythm and development of cardiac pathologies.
- Cardiac arrhythmia is best detected in second lead, whereas ischemia is best detected in lead V_5.

TRANSESOPHAGEAL ECHOCARDIOGRAPHY

It is best for detection of ischemia and air embolism.

BLOOD PRESSURE

- Blood pressure is usually measured by noninvasive method.
- Invasive blood pressure monitoring can be done by catheterization of radial artery.
- However, before it the patency of ulnar artery is confirmed by **Allen's test**.

Steps in Allen's Test

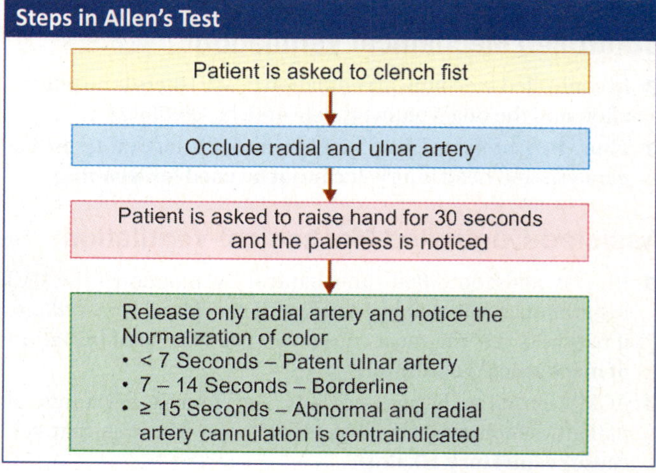

Patient is asked to clench fist
Occlude radial and ulnar artery
Patient is asked to raise hand for 30 seconds and the paleness is noticed
Release only radial artery and notice the Normalization of color
• < 7 Seconds – Patent ulnar artery
• 7 – 14 Seconds – Borderline
• ≥ 15 Seconds – Abnormal and radial artery cannulation is contraindicated

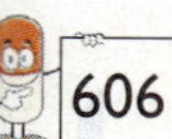

CENTRAL VENOUS PRESSURE

- Central venous pressure is measured in the left jugular vein.
- A normal value in adults is 3–10 cm of H_2O and in children is 3–6 cm of H_2O.

CARDIAC OUTPUT

Pulse Contour Continuous Cardiac Output Monitoring (PiCCO)

- In this system, a central venous catheter and a femoral artery catheter is placed.
- A definite amount of cold saline is injected into the central venous catheter and then a drop in temperature is estimated via femoral artery is used to calculate cardiac output.

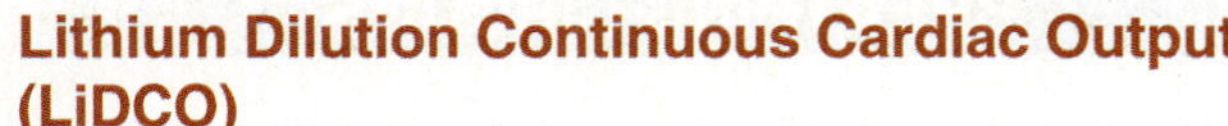

Lithium Dilution Continuous Cardiac Output (LiDCO)

- Catheters are established as previous case.
- But in this case lithium chloride is injected into central venous catheter and change of lithium chloride concentration in femoral artery sample is used to calculate cardiac output.

Flotrac

This system is connected to an arterial catheter which is further connected to a transducer and monitor, which detects changes in arterial waveform to calculate cardiac output.

PULSE OXIMETER

- Pulse oximeter probe contains a light emitting diode and a photodetector which is applied to the nail bed, ear lobule or nose tip.
- Based on the amount of light absorbed by tissues, oxyhemoglobin and deoxyhemoglobin and rest detected by photodetector, the oxygen saturation of **hemoglobin** is measured.
- The normal value of oxygen saturation is 97–98%.

CAPNOGRAPHY

- Capnography was introduced in the year 1965 by **Bethune and Brethren**.
- It works on the principle that **carbon dioxide absorbs infrared** corresponding to its concentration. A capnograph plots CO_2 pressure on Y axis and time on Y axis.
- It is useful in measuring the end tidal carbon dioxide, for which the normal value is **32–42 mm Hg**.
- A normal capnograph has four phases, i.e. 0, 1, 2 and 3. **Phase 0** corresponds to inspiration whereas others correspond to expiration. **Phase 1** measures exhaled gas of dead space, **phase 2** measures dead space gas along with CO_2 from the alveoli and phase 3 measures CO_2 exhaled from alveoli. The maximum height reached by the graph is called as the **ET_{CO2} (End-Tidal CO_2)**.
- The α **angle** tells about degree of airway obstruction whereas the β **angle** tells about the rebreathing of exhaled CO_2 rich gas. The slope of graph provides information about ventilation perfusion ratio.

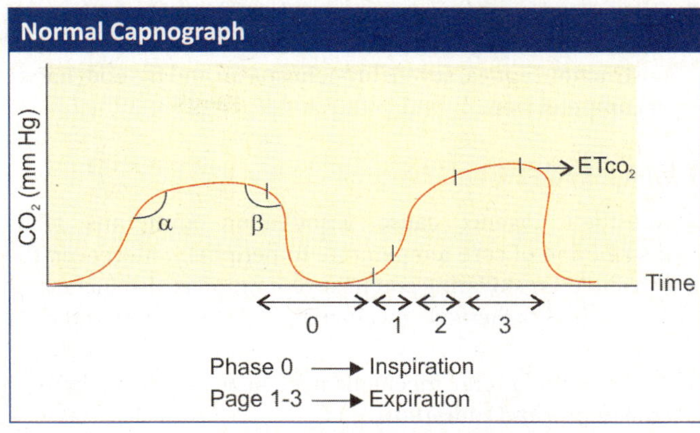

Normal Capnograph

- The uses of capnography are mentioned in the Box below.

Uses of Capnography

- Confirmation of intubation
- Disconnection indicator
- Alveolar ventilation indicator
- Cardiac output indicator
- Indicator of pulmonary embolism: Fall in capnogram
- Diagnosis of malignant hyperthermia: End-tidal CO_2 is highly raised and can be > 100 mm Hg
- Indicator of ET tube displacement/obstruction or ventilator failure: Flat capnogram

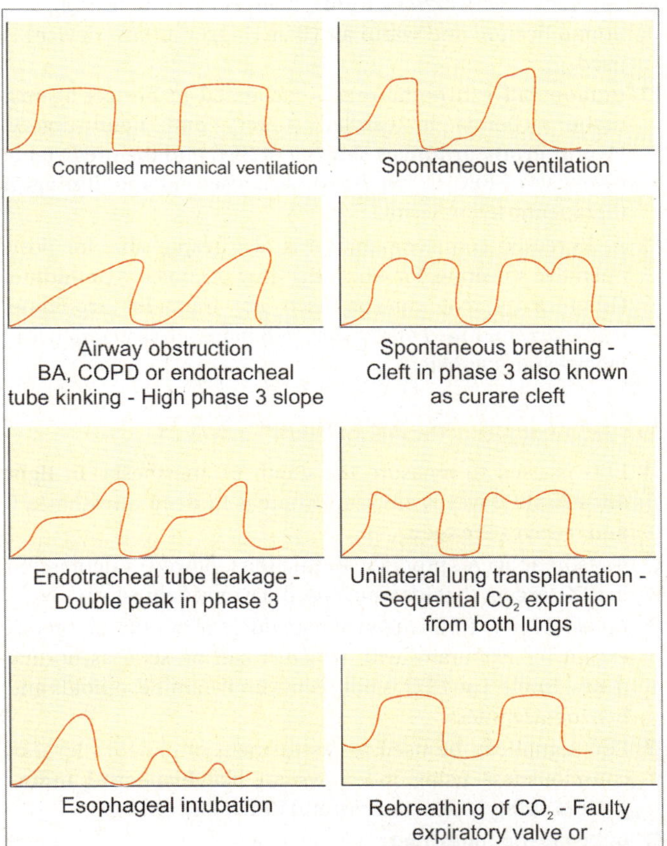

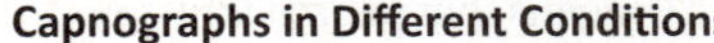
Capnographs in Different Conditions

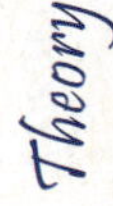

- Capnography might not detect endotracheal intubation and show a flat capnogram in patients with **cardiac arrest**, airway obstruction, apnea, severe bronchospasm and hemodynamic decompensation.

TEMPERATURE

- Anesthetic agents cause vasodilation and thus allow distribution of core temperature to periphery. Moreover, the threshold for shivering and heat generation is also increased. The most preserved mechanism of heat regulation **is sweating**.
- The most common mechanism of heat loss in patients is **convection and radiation**.
- Hypothermia is seen if the temperature goes below 35°C.
- During anesthesia core temperature monitoring is preferred in distal esophagus, pulmonary artery, nasopharynx and tympanic membrane.

Preferred sites for measuring body temperature

Temperature measurement sites	
Distal esophagus	Most ideal site
Pulmonary artery	Most accurate site for core body temperature
Tympanic membrane	Most accurate site for brain temperature

- To prevent hypothermia the ideal OT temperature maintained in children is 28°C and in adults is 21°C. If hypothermia develops then **warm IV fluids**, blankets, airway heating and humidification and warm air (Bair Hugger airflow device) is used.
- Intraoperative hypothermia is facilitated to protect against tissue ischemia in cardiac surgery and neurosurgery. **Hypothermia produces slowing of EEG** and the predictable response of EEG to hypothermia is used for monitoring of therapeutic hypothermia
- A decreased core temperature is also responsible for post-operative shivering, for which the drug of choice is **pethidine**. Other drugs that can be used are tramadol, clonidine, dexmedetomidine, Ketanserine, nefopam, physostigmine and magnesium sulphate.

ELECTROENCEPHALOGRAM

- EEG is used to measure the depth of anesthesia. In **light anesthesia** β waves are seen whereas in **deep anesthesia** θ **and σ waves are seen**.
- Anesthetic agents produce stimulation followed by depression in EEG, except opioids which produce only depression.
- An **isoelectric EEG** is seen at high doses of anesthetic agents, except for isoflurane with which it can be seen as normal doses. Isoelectric EEG is not seen with ketamine, opioids and benzodiazepines.
- EEG signal can be used for assessment of patient's level of consciousness using index system like **bispectral index, patient safety index, narcotrend index and entropy**.
- In bispectral index there is a scale of 0 to 100; a score of 100 means the patient is fully awake, 40–60 means anesthesia is adequate and 0 means that patient is in coma.
- In patient safety index also, there is a scale of 0 to 100 and a value of 25–50 signifies adequate anesthesia.

EEG in Different Stages of Anesthesia

Clinical stage	EEG
Awake	Alpha waves
Excitation	Beta waves
Early anesthesia	Alpha-Theta waves
Surgical tolerance	Delta
Deep surgical tolerance	Delta
High dose/Toxicity	Isoelectric EEG

BREATHING CIRCUITS

The breathing circuits have kept on evolving from time to time.

OPEN SYSTEM

- In an open system a **Schimmelbusch mask** is placed and anesthetic agent is poured on the mask. Since the anesthetic agent can escape into the environment it is called as open system.
- A modification of this is **semi open** system in which a towel is placed on mask and then anesthetic agent is poured on the towel. This prevents an early escape of the agent into the environment.
- These systems lead to wastage of anesthetic agents as well as environmental pollution and hence are not preferred.

SEMI-CLOSED CIRCUITS

- Semi-closed circuits are partially connected with the environment and hence there is lesser wastage and pollution.
- These circuits are known as **Mapleson** circuit.

Type A

- Type A circuit is also known as **Magill's circuit** which has an inlet for fresh gas flow, a breathing bag and an expiratory valve.
- There is no separation of the inhaled gas and exhaled gas and hence rebreathing of exhaled gas takes place.
- If patient goes into hypoxia then compensatory mechanisms can kick in like an increase in respiratory rate and hence it is the semi closed circuit of choice for **spontaneous ventilation**.

Type B

Type B circuit is a modification of type A with change in position of fresh gas inlet and breathing bag, that does not give any extra benefit and hence is not used.

Type C

Type C circuit is also known as **Water's circuit,** which is just a smaller version of type A without any extra benefit and hence is also not used.

Type D

- Type D circuit is also known as **Bain's circuit**.
- As compared to type A, this one is a coaxial circuit in which there are separate tubes for the inhaled and exhaled gases and hence there is no mixing.
- Since the chance of hypoxia are lesser, it is the semi closed circuit of choice for **controlled ventilation**.
- Though it can also be used for spontaneous ventilation.

Type E

Type E circuit is also known as **Ayre's T piece**, used in children for **spontaneous ventilation**.

Type F

- Type F circuit is **Jackson's Rees modification** of the Ayre's T piece.
- It is used in children for both **spontaneous** and **controlled** ventilation.

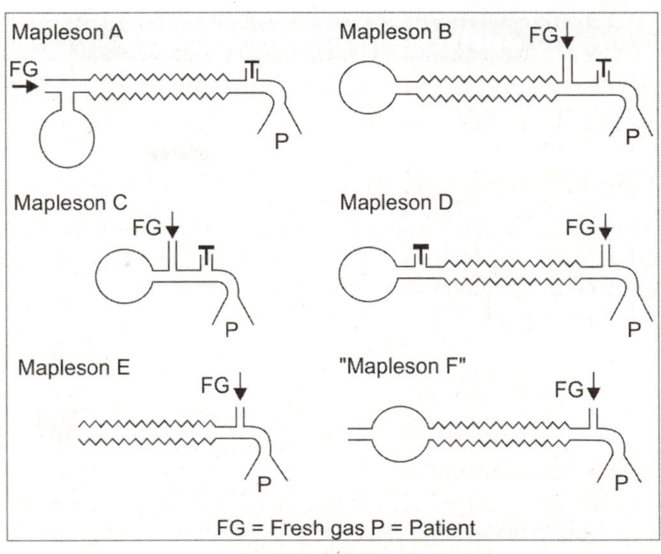
Mapleson A
FG
P
Mapleson B
FG
P
Mapleson C
FG
P
Mapleson D
FG
P
Mapleson E
FG
P
"Mapleson F"
FG
P
FG = Fresh gas P = Patient

Semi Closed Circuits

CLOSED CIRCUIT

- Intoday's anesthetic world closed circuits are used.
- In closed circuit as given in the picture there is an inlet for fresh gas flow from the anesthetic machine to the patients through a one way valve.
- Then the exhaled gas passes through the one way valve and the excess gas is let out of the system by an API valve.
- Remaining gas is then passed through the CO_2 absorbing canister and it is again passed to the patient.

Excess gas is vented out through the pop-off (APL) valve to the scavenging
6 ... through the expiratory limb one-way valve..
5 ... from the patient through the expiratory breathing tube..
7 ... in & out of the reservoir bag ...
4 ... through the Y-piece to the patient ...
8 ... through the absorbent canister where CO_2 is removed ...
9 ... and then back towards the patient.
3 ... then flows through the inspiratory breathing tube...
Fresh gas enters the circle from the common gas outlet of the anesthetic machine...
2 ... flows through the inspiratory limb one-way valve...

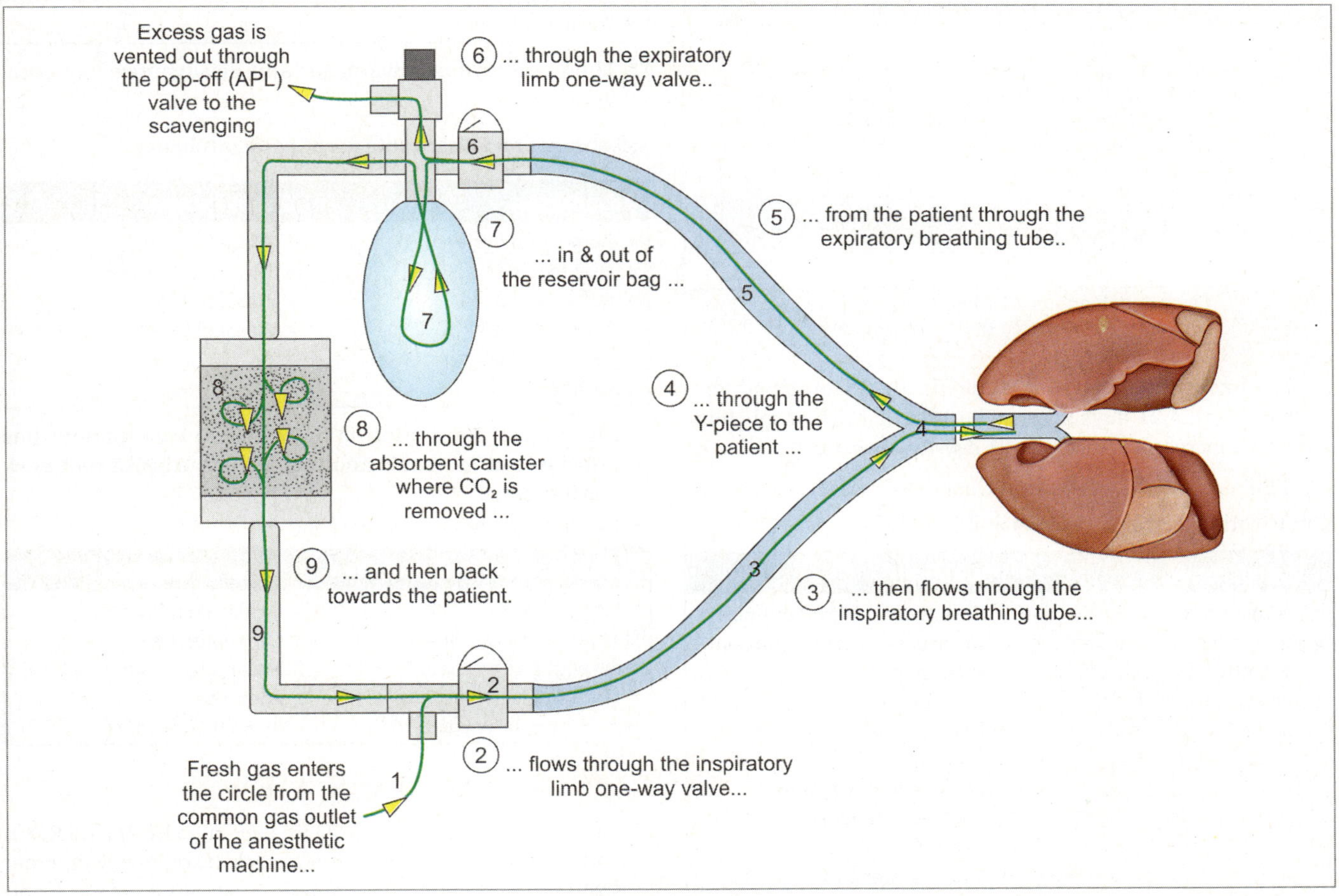

Closed Circuit

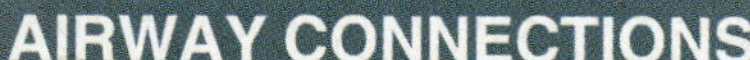

AIRWAY CONNECTIONS

The airway can be connected to the anesthetic machine by endotracheal intubation, nasal intubation or a laryngeal mask airway.

ENDOTRACHEAL INTUBATION

As described in the section of anesthetic equipment, laryngoscope and endotracheal tube are required for endotracheal intubation. It is done after induction of anesthesia with an IV agent and administration of muscle relaxant.

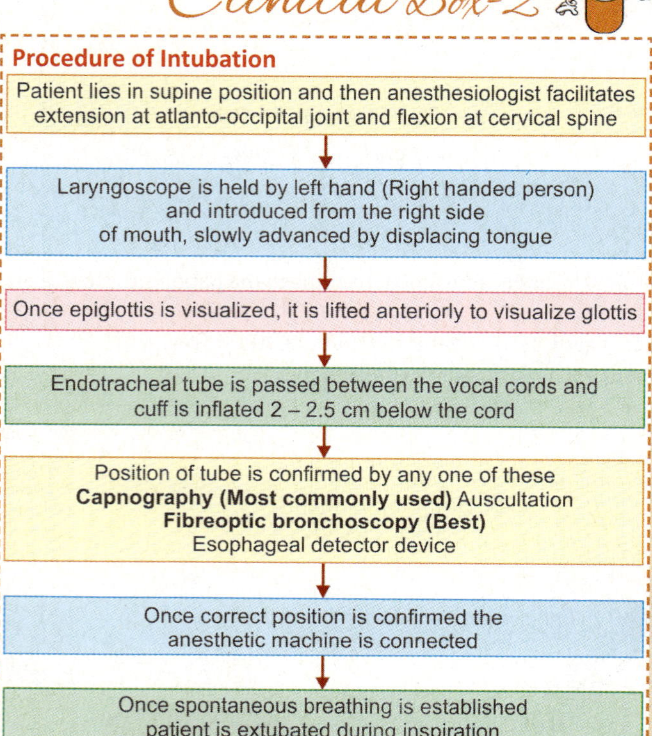

Clinical Box-2
Procedure of Intubation
Patient lies in supine position and then anesthesiologist facilitates extension at atlanto-occipital joint and flexion at cervical spine
Laryngoscope is held by left hand (Right handed person) and introduced from the right side of mouth, slowly advanced by displacing tongue
Once epiglottis is visualized, it is lifted anteriorly to visualize glottis
Endotracheal tube is passed between the vocal cords and cuff is inflated 2 – 2.5 cm below the cord
Position of tube is confirmed by any one of these
Capnography (Most commonly used) Auscultation
Fibreoptic bronchoscopy (Best)
Esophageal detector device
Once correct position is confirmed the anesthetic machine is connected
Once spontaneous breathing is established patient is extubated during inspiration

- Endotracheal intubation if required can be continued for a maximum of **21 days** because beyond that risk of subglottic edema increases. Thus after 21 days tracheostomy should be done.

Complications of Laryngoscopy and Intubation

Laryngoscopy	Intubation
• Upper incisor damage • Cervical spinal cord damage • Hemodynamic alterations • Soft tissue and nerve damage	• **Sore throat: Most common postoperative complication** • Pneumonia • Laryngeal edema • Emphysema • Atelectasis • Laryngeal nerve injury (anterior branch) – Vocal cord paralysis • Tracheal stenosis • Vocal cord granuloma

RAPID SEQUENCE INTUBATION

- Rapid sequence intubation is used in conditions associated with increased risk of regurgitation and aspiration like patient with full stomach, GERD, morbid obesity, gastroparesis, pregnancy after 20 weeks gestation, cardiac arrest.
- Patient is administered an IV agent followed by IV Succinylcholine after preoxygenation with 100% oxygen for 3 minutes.
- Then **cricoid pressure is applied (Sellick maneuver)** to occlude esophagus and intubation is done.
- Cricoid pressure is applied until endotracheal tube is placed and cuff inflations are confirmed.
- The chin of the patient is elevated without **cervical spine displacement** and then **cricoid cartilage is pushed posteriorly** toward the esophagus.
- It impairs laryngoscopic view and hence is contraindicated in patients of cardiac arrest.

NASAL INTUBATION

Nasal intubation is preferred in many cases as described below.

Indications to Nasal Intubation
• Long-term intubation • Obstructing mass in oral cavity • Mandibular fracture • Temporomandibular joint dysfunction • Oral surgery • Awake intubation

- There are various advantages and disadvantages of nasal intubation.

Advantages and disadvantages of nasal intubation

Advantages	Disadvantages
• Better oral hygiene • Oral feeding possible • Better tolerated • No tube biting • Less chance of accidental extubation	• More bleeding • More bacteremia • Nasal trauma • Nasal deformity

- Blind nasal intubation is indicated in case patient has **ankyloses of temporomandibular joint, trismus and neck contractures.**
- Contraindications of intubation.

Both nasal and oral intubation	Nasal intubation
Intact gag reflex Unstable cervical spine Transaction of trachea High risk of laryngospasm (epiglottitis, laryngitis)	Basilar skull fracture CSF rhinorrhea Nasal polyps, abscess, adenoids Bleeding disorders

LARYNGEAL MASK AIRWAY

- Laryngeal mask airway (LMA) was invented by **Archie Brain** and hence is also known as Brain mask. It comes in 8 different sizes; the most common size used in an adult male is 5 and female is 4.

Laryngeal Mask Airway Sizes

Age group	Size
Neonate	1
Infant 5–10 kg	1.5
Children 10–20 kg	2
Children 20–30 kg	2.5
Children or Adult 30–50 kg	3
Adult 50–70 kg	4
Adult > 70–100 kg	5
Adult > 100 kg	6

- LMA consists of a mask that sits over **the hypopharynx**. The LMA is inserted blindly into the oropharyngeal cavity and then cuff is inflated with a pressure 40–60 cm of H_2O that seals around the **periglottic tissue**. Then the LMA is connected to anesthetic machine.
- LMA is preferred in case of **difficult and emergency intubation** and in **minor surgeries**.
- The drawbacks are: It **does not prevent aspiration** and there is an increased incidence of laryngospasm. Complications like sore throat and injuries to oral cavity, larynx and pharynx can be seen.
- LMAs are contraindicated in patients with high risk for aspiration (**pregnancy**, hiatus hernia), full stomach and oropharyngeal mass.
- LMA proseal and LMA supreme are second generation LMAs which have better cuffs that can be used with lesser pressure and hence lesser incidence of sore throat. These also have a drain tube to remove gastric secretions, with the end of tube sitting **above esophageal opening**.

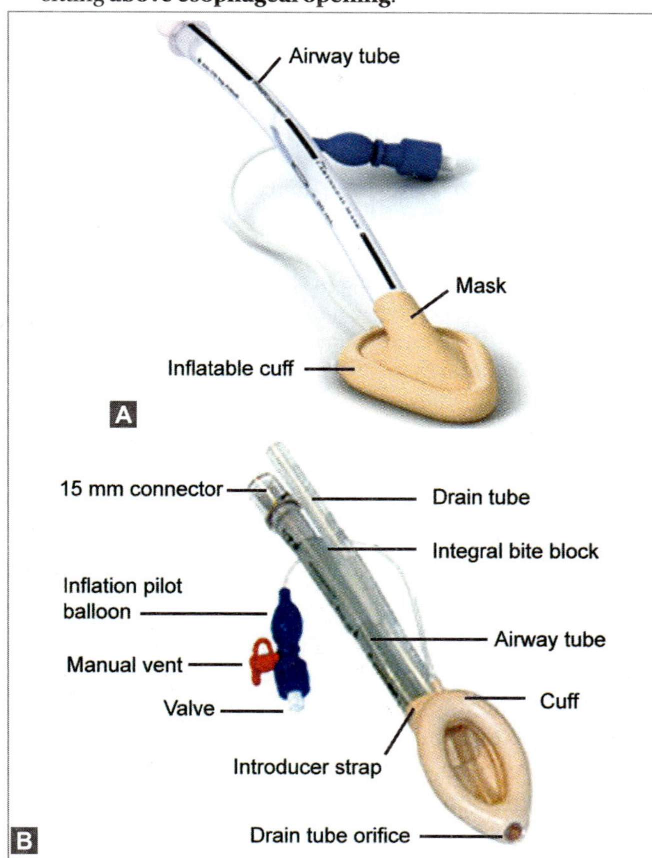

Laryngeal Mask Airway: A. LMA classical; B. LMA proseal

GENERAL ANESTHETIC AGENTS

The general anesthetic agents have ability to produce loss of consciousness, anterograde amnesia, loss of response to noxious stimuli and these effects are reversible. These effects are seen both at the level of spinal cord, brain, thalamus and limbic system.

- The effects described above are possible in two ways; stimulation of inhibitory neurotransmitter pathway (glycine and GABA) and inhibition of stimulatory neurotransmitters (glutamate).
- All anesthetic agents act by stimulating **glycine** and **GABA** receptors. The site of action for GABA is in the α subunit, whereas for benzodiazepines is between α and γ subunits and for all general anesthetics it is located on the β subunit.
- Only ketamine, cyclopropane, N_2O and xenon act by opening **potassium channel** and by inhibiting **NMDA** receptors.
- The potency of the general anesthetic agents is related to lipid solubility because of the lipophilicity of the protein binding sites.
- The general anesthetic agents can be broadly classified into intravenous and inhalational anesthetic agents.

Conceptual Box-1

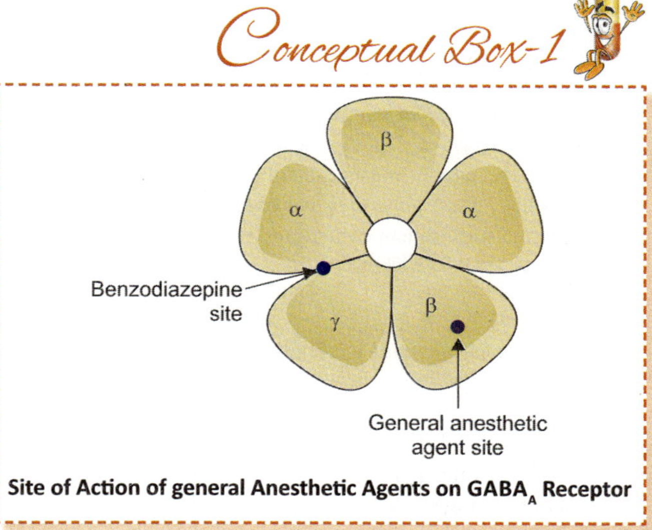

Site of Action of general Anesthetic Agents on $GABA_A$ Receptor

INTRAVENOUS ANESTHETIC AGENTS

- Intravenous anesthetic agents are drugs that produce loss of consciousness in one arm brain circulation time. The only intravenous agent that does not produce anesthesia in one arm brain circulation is **ketamine**.
- Intravenous agents are primarily used for **induction** as many inhalational agents are pungent.
- The potency of intravenous agents is measured by the free plasma concentration that produces loss of response to surgical incision in 50% of patients.
- This class contains drugs like barbiturates, propofol, etomidate and ketamine.
- The steroidal compounds like **althesin** are not used nowadays because of poor lipid solubility and **anaphylaxis** due to use of **cremophor** as dissolving agent.

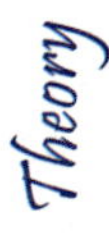

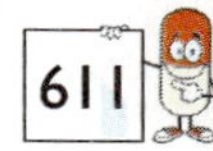

Barbiturates

- Barbiturates are GABA facilitatory agents and increase duration of chloride ion channel opening, but at high doses they produce GABA mimetic effect which is responsible for anesthetic effect. They also inhibit effect of excitatory neurotransmitters like glutamate and acetylcholine.
- The first barbiturate used clinically was **thiopental**, which was introduced by **Waters and Lundy**. Other barbiturates used now are methohexital and thiamylal.
- These drugs are highly lipid soluble, have high plasma protein binding and are metabolized by liver.
- The primary use of barbiturates in anesthesia is for induction, maintenance and premedication. The amnestic effect is lesser with barbiturates than with benzodiazepines.
- Thiopental causes analgesia but is missing with methohexital.
- After reconstitution thiopental can be used after storing in refrigerator for 1 week, whereas methohexital can be used for 6 weeks. When stored in refrigerator.

Thiopental Sodium

- Thiopental sodium is synthesized by combining pentobarbital with sulfur and sodium carbonate, which forms a **pale yellow powder**.
- Sulfur increases lipid solubility which is important to cross the blood brain barrier, whereas sodium carbonate increases water solubility required for parenteral use.
- Sodium carbonate reacts with water to form sodium bicarbonate, which makes the solution highly alkaline with a pH of 10.5. This alkaline pH gives **bacteriostatic effect**.
- Thiopental sodium is reconstituted with distil water or normal saline and used as **2.5% solution**.

Pharmacokinetics

- Though thiopental has a long half-life it is short acting because of redistribution into adipose tissue because of its high lipid solubility.
- It has a pK_a of 7.6 and hence is 60% unionized in plasma.
- Thiopental sodium and methohexital have a **high plasma protein binding of 85%**.

Uses

- Induction is fast because of high lipid solubility and hence it is the most common IV anesthetic agent used for induction.
- It decreases cerebral oxygen consumption, cerebral metabolic rate and ICT; hence it is the agent of choice for **cerebral protection**.
- Being a parenteral barbiturate, it is also used for treatment of and as anesthetic agent of choice for **status epilepticus**.
- Owing to its anti-thyroid effect it is the agent of choice in **hyperthyroidism**.

Side Effects

- Side effects that can be associated are **hypokalemia, hypotension (vasodilation and decreased cardiac output), garlic/onion taste and transient apnea (known as double apnea).**
- Being a barbiturate, it is an enzyme inducer and hence can precipitate **acute intermittent porphyria**.
- Alkalinity can cause **thrombophlebitis** and for the same reason if it is injected by intramuscular and intradermal route can cause muscle and dermal necrosis respectively.

Contraindications

- Thiopental sodium is contraindicated with acidic solutions like **ringer lactate** as it precipitates.
- It is also contraindicated by **intra-arterial route** as it crystalizes in the acidic pH of blood and can cause vasoconstriction and thrombosis leading to severe pain and gangrene. If it is accidentally injected into arteries the **first thing done is that the needle is left *in situ*** and normal saline is injected into same needle to dilute thiopental. This is followed by injection of drugs like heparin, vasodilators, lignocaine and urokinase into the needle. Stellate ganglion block can also be done.
- Thiopental sodium is also contraindicated in patients with respiratory obstruction, shock and status asthmaticus.
- ECG changes like QT prolongation and T wave flattening can be seen and hence it is avoided in patients with ventricular arrhythmia.

Methohexital

- Methohexital is three times more potent than thiopental and hence used as 1% solution.
- Addition of methyl group makes it faster acting but causes excitatory side effects like seizures. Hence it is the anesthetic agent of choice in **electroconvulsive therapy**.
- Methohexital is given by rectal route in children as premedication. Since methohexital is cleared faster than thiopental, it is preferred for maintenance.
- **Methohexital** > **Thiopental** can also cause pain on intravenous injection but lesser than **propofol**.

Propofol

- Propofol has **GABA facilitatory effect** by stimulating the beta subunit of receptor. At high doses it has GABA mimetic effect as well. It inhibits excitatory neurotransmitter receptors of glutamate like **NMDA**.
- Propofol is an **alkylphenol**, which are highly lipid soluble compounds and hence **1% propofol** is combined with **10% soybean oil, 2.25% glycerol to adjust tonicity and 1.2% egg phospholipid for emulsification**. This combination gives a **milky white color**.
- Because this medium is suitable for bacterial growth, EDTA or metabisulphite is used as preservative in some countries. In India as preservative is not used, once reconstituted the solution **should be used within six hours**.

Pharmacokinetics

- Propofol has a pK_a of 11 and hence is completely unionized in plasma (pH of 7.4).
- It has a very short duration of action due to rapid clearance and redistribution.
- It is metabolized primarily in liver along with some extrahepatic metabolism in lungs and kidney.
- It is an enzyme inhibitor and hence can increase concentration of other anesthetic agents like midazolam and alfentanil, thus the doses of these drugs should be decreased.

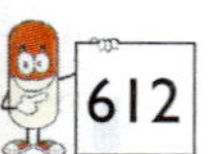

- Propofol is the IV anesthetic agent with **highest plasma protein binding, i.e. 98%.**

Uses

- Currently propofol is the **most commonly used intravenous anesthetic agent** for induction and maintenance.
- It is the intravenous anesthetic agent of choice for **day care surgery (recovery faster than thiopental), total intravenous anesthesia (TIVA), sedation in ICU and surgery and in patients susceptible to malignant hyperthermia.**
- Propofol has antiemetic effect by decreasing serotonin in area postrema; it can be used for prevention of **postoperative and chemotherapy-induced nausea and vomiting.**
- It has antipruritic effect as well and hence used to relieve **cholestatic and opioid induced pruritus.**
- It can decrease ICP and IOP and has a **neuroprotective effect**.
- Bronchodilation can be seen and hence is safe in bronchospastic disorders.
- There is a decrease in cardiac out output along with vasodilation and hence it has **cardioprotective** effect as well, for which it is used for maintenance in cardiac surgery.

Side Effects

- Due to its oil content it can cause **pain on intravenous injection**, which can be decreased by using lidocaine and injecting into large veins.
- The egg phospholipid accounts for **hypersensitivity** and **pancreatitis**.
- Other side effects seen are myoclonus, **choreiform movements/opisthotonus**, hallucinations, sexual fantasies, apnea (more common than thiopental).
- It has both epileptic and antiepileptic effect; because it can precipitate seizure it is used for cortical mapping of epileptogenic foci.
- It can cause a green discoloration of urine and hair.
- The most severe side effect is known as **propofol infusion syndrome (PRIS)**, characterized by refractory bradycardia (asystole) with metabolic acidosis, hyperlipidemia, rhabdomyolysis or hepatomegaly (fatty liver).
- Propofol increases dopamine in nucleus accumbens which gives pleasurable effect and hence addiction and abuse has been seen in medical professionals.

Fospropofol

- Fospropofol is water-soluble propofol, which does not require the oily medium for injection and hence there is no pain on injection.
- It is metabolized by alkaline phosphatase in liver into propofol, formaldehyde and phosphate metabolite.
- The phosphate metabolite causes perineal paresthesia and pruritus.
- Fospropofol has slower induction and is associated with lesser side effects than propofol.

Ketamine

- Ketamine was synthesized by **Stevens** but first used clinically by **Corssen and Domino**.
- Ketamine primarily acts by inhibiting **NMDA subtype of glutamate receptors** in the association area of cortex and thalamus which produces **dissociative anesthesia and strong analgesia respectively**. In this dissociative or cataleptic state, patient appears awake with preserved reflexes (corneal, laryngeal and pharyngeal) but is detached from the surrounding with eyes open.
- On the other hand, it stimulates limbic system, which causes **hallucinations and emergence reaction**. Emergence reaction seen during awakening from ketamine anesthesia is characterized by vivid dreams, sensation of floating out of body, illusions, confusion and euphoria. The **drug of choice** for treatment of same is **benzodiazepines**.
- It produces amnesia but is lesser as compared to other drugs.
- Apart from this it also has stimulatory effect on sympathetic and opioid receptors and inhibitory effect on muscarinic receptors. Sympathetic receptor stimulation **stimulates heart (tachycardia)** and causes vasoconstriction (increase in blood pressure) and bronchodilation.
- Other effects are: An **increase in intracranial pressure, cerebral blood flow and cerebral oxygen consumption and increase in intraocular pressure.**

Pharmacokinetics

- It is a **phencyclidine** with high lipid solubility and poor plasma protein binding; hence It has a very high volume of distribution.
- It is a racemic mixture of R and S enantiomer with the S one being 3 times more potent than R.
- Phencyclidine also known as **"angel dust"** has been discontinued due to psychiatric side effects.

Uses

- Ketamine is the intravenous anesthetic agent of choice in various conditions as described ahead. As it causes **bronchodilation**. It is preferred IV anesthetic agent in **reactive airway disease like, bronchial asthma and status asthmaticus**.
- Since it has cardio-stimulatory effect and increases blood pressure. It is IV anesthetic agent of choice in **shock (hypovolemic, hemorrhagic, septic), DIC** and preferred in cardiac tamponade, restrictive pericarditis and **cyanotic congenital heart diseases with right to left shunt** also.
- Since it preserves pharyngeal and laryngeal reflexes, it is IV anesthetic agent of choice in patients with **full stomach**.
- Due to profound analgesic effect it can be used in low doses for pain in post-operative period, cancer, neuropathy, fibromyalgia, migraine and phantom limb.
- It is preferred for sedation in children for procedures not done in operation theatre.

Contraindications

- Ketamine is contraindicated in **schizophrenia** as it stimulates limbic system.
- As it increases intraocular pressure it is contraindicated in **glaucoma and ocular injury**.

- Because of cardiostimulatory effect it is contraindicated as single agent in **ischemic heart disease and vascular aneurysms**.
- Due to increase in intracranial pressure it is contraindicated in **epilepsy**.
- Ketamine increases muscle tone and hence should be avoided in patients with malignant hyperthermia.
- At high doses it can cause cystitis.

Etomidate

- Etomidate is an imidazole derivative which primarily acts only by $GABA_A$ facilitatory and mimetic effects on the β_2 and β_3 subunits of $GABA_A$ receptor.
- It is used only for induction of anesthesia due to rapid onset and offset of action. It is the **most hemodynamic stable** IV anesthetic agent as it does not affect sympathetic nervous system and baroreceptors; hence is preferred for induction in **old patients, cardiovascular disorders (aneurysm, cardiomyopathy, CHF, CAD, aortic stenosis)** and in **altered hemodynamic states (splenic rupture, hemorrhagic shock)**.
- Side effects associated are **pain on injection**, thrombophlebitis and **vitamin C deficiency**. It inhibits 11-β-hydroxylase and inhibits cortisol synthesis and hence causes **adrenocortical suppression**; for same reason it can be used for treatment of hypercortisolemia. It is the IV anesthetic agent causing **maximum nausea and vomiting**.

Intravenous Anesthetic Agents Properties

Features	Thiopental	Propofol	Ketamine	Etomidate
Half-life	6-15 hours	5-12 hours	2 hours	1-4 hours
Volume of distribution	2.5 L/Kg	4 L/Kg	3 L/Kg	3 L/Kg
Plasma protein binding	80%	**98%**	25%	75%
Nausea and vomiting	**Absent**	**Antiemetic**	Present	**Maximum**
Pain on IV injection	**Present**	**Present (Maximum)**	Absent	**Present**
Blood Pressure	Decreased	**Maximum decreased**	**Increased**	No effect
Cardiac output	Decreased	**Maximum decreased**	**Increased**	No effect
Intracranial pressure	Decreased	Decreased	**Increased**	No effect
Intraocular Pressure	Decreased	Decreased	**Increased**	No effect
Respiratory Rate	Decreased	Decreased	Increased	Decreased

Benzodiazepines

- Benzodiazepines are GABA facilitatory agents and increase frequency of chloride ion channel opening.
- The benzodiazepines which are used in anesthesia are midazolam, lorazepam, diazepam and temazepam. These are highly lipid soluble drugs and hence have rapid onset of action (midazolam > diazepam > lorazepam).
- Potency of these drugs at GABA receptor is maximum with lorazepam > midazolam > diazepam.
- Flumazenil, a benzodiazepine antagonist is used for reversal of effects of benzodiazepines in anesthesia. It is more effective in reversing sedation, hypnosis and respiratory depression than anterograde amnesia.
- The uses of these drugs in anesthesia is diverse and are discussed below.

Premedication

- Benzodiazepines are the most commonly drugs used for premedication in anesthesia and the most commonly used benzodiazepine is midazolam because of its faster onset of action and recovery.
- However, if prolonged effect is required as in case of cardiac surgery, then lorazepam is preferred.
- The aim in premedication is to achieve sedation, anterograde amnesia, vagolytic, sympatholytic and antiemetic effect.

Induction and Maintenance of Anesthesia

The benzodiazepine of choice for induction and maintenance of anesthesia is midazolam, however lorazepam and diazepam can also be used.

Sedation

Benzodiazepines can be used for sedation in ICU and minor procedures (diagnostic and therapeutic).

Antiemetics

- Benzodiazepines can be used for prevention of postoperative nausea and vomiting.
- The preferred benzodiazepine is midazolam.

Recent Advances

Remimazolam: It is a new benzodiazepine which has an ester moiety and hence is metabolized by esterases, which makes it very short acting. It has faster onset of action and recovery and greater depth of sedation than midazolam. It is currently under trial for
- Premedication for sedation in general anesthesia
- Sedation in ICU
- Procedural sedation

Dexmedetomidine

- Dexmedetomidine is an α_2 receptor agonist which produces sedation, hypnosis, analgesia and sympatholytics. It is more selective for α_2 receptors as compared to other drugs in this class like, clonidine.
- The uses of clonidine are described below.
  - **Sedative:** It is FDA approved only for short-term sedation in ICU for weaning off patients from ventilators. It can

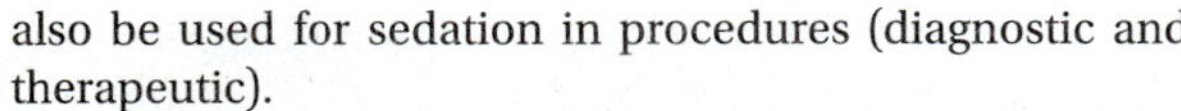

also be used for sedation in procedures (diagnostic and therapeutic).

- **Hypnotic:** It is used for hypnosis in awake craniotomy, deep brain stimulation and awake endarterectomy.
- **Analgesic:** It is used as an adjuvant to local anesthetic agents to decrease their doses for local and regional blocks.
- **Premedicant:** It is used as a premedication in anesthesia.
- **Intubation:** Since it decreases salivation and does not cause respiratory depression, it can be used for awake fiberoptic intubation.
- **Addiction treatment:** It can be used for treatment of addiction to opioid, cocaine withdrawal and benzodiazepine and opioid tolerance.

- It can be used for induction of anesthesia, but requires to be used at 10 times higher doses which increases risk of severe hypotension; hence it is **not used for induction**.
- **Atipamezole** is an α_2 receptor antagonist used to reverse effects of dexmedetomidine in animals; yet to be approved in humans.
- **Hypotension (most common side effect)** and bradycardia can be seen due to central sympatholytic effect. However, during beginning of infusion it can cause transient hypertension due to stimulation of postsynaptic α_2 receptors which cause vasoconstriction.

Droperidol

- Droperidol is a butyrophenone neuroleptic derived from haloperidol.
- It can be used along with fentanyl for neurolept anesthesia, however it is less preferred nowadays.
- Currently it is more commonly used as sedative, antiemetic and antipruritic (opioid induced) in anesthesia.

INHALATIONAL ANESTHETIC AGENTS

- Inhalational anesthetic agents are either gases like **nitrous oxide, cyclopropane** and **xenon** or volatile liquids like **halothane, isoflurane, sevoflurane, desflurane, enflurane** and **methoxyflurane**.
- All volatile inhalational agents are primarily **excreted unchanged with minor metabolism by liver**.
- The most common enzyme responsible for metabolism is **CYP2E1**. The agent which undergoes maximum metabolism is **methoxyflurane followed by halothane**, followed by others (methoxyflurane > halothane > enflurane > isoflurane > desflurane). This metabolism directly correlates well with **hepatotoxicity** as well.
- **Nitrous oxide** does not undergo any metabolism and excreted as such by lungs.
- The order of lipid solubility is also same and hence methoxyflurane and halothane are sequestered in adipose tissues for longer period. **Hepatotoxicity** is maximum with halothane, whereas it is minimum with **sevoflurane**.
- Metabolism of anesthetic agents generate fluoride ions, hence **methoxyflurane** generates maximum fluoride ions and **desflurane < isoflurane** generate least fluoride ions that cause nephrotoxicity.
- Reaction of some volatile agents containing -CHF_2 group, produces **carbon monoxide** with lime which is maximum with desflurane followed by enflurane and isoflurane **(desflurane > enflurane > isoflurane)**.
- Inhaled agents can **deplete ozone**; the effect is **maximum with halothane**, whereas **no effect is seen with sevoflurane and desflurane**.
- Inhalational agents can also cause **global warming**, which is **maximum with desflurane** and **minimum with halothane**.
- All volatile agents are bronchodilators (maximum with halothane) except desflurane.
- All agents decrease myocardial contractility except ether which increases contractility due to release of catecholamines. Trielene does not have any effect on myocardial contractility. All of them are coronary vasodilators with maximum effect by isoflurane and hence can cause coronary steal phenomenon.
- All inhalational agents have uterine relaxant effect **except nitrous oxide**.
- **Tachypnea** can be seen with **trielene** > **ether**.

Properties of Inhalational Agents

- **Minimum alveolar concentration (MAC)**
  - 1 MAC is the minimum alveolar concentration that prevents movement in response to surgical stimulation in 50% of patients. It is described in percentage of agent required in alveolar air to produce the above effect. Sevoflurane has a MAC of 2%; this means out of 100% space in alveoli 2% should be occupied by sevoflurane to produce effect in 50% patients. Thus to produce effect in 100% patients 2 MAC is required, i.e. 4% of sevoflurane in the alveolar space.
  - Comparing MAC to pharmacodynamics, it is like the minimum dose required for a particular effect, hence **MAC is a measure of potency of inhalational agents.**
  - An ideal anesthetic agent should have a MAC as less as possible for lesser drug requirement. **Methoxyflurane has least MAC and hence is most potent**, whereas **nitrous oxide has maximum MAC and is least potent.**
  - Nitrous oxide has a MAC of 104%; 104% of nitrous oxide in 100% of alveolar space is practically not possible and hence 1 MAC is never achievable. Thus, it is always combined with other agents.

Mnemonics

Factors Decreasing MAC–HEAT

H: Hypoxia
Hypercarbia
Hypotension
Hypothermia
Hypothyroidism
E: Electrolyte imbalance
Hyponatremia
Hypercalcemia
Hypermagnesemia
A: Age
Anemia
Anesthetic agents (IV, Local, Opioids, Sedatives)
Acute alcohol intake
T: Trimester of pregnancy

Note: MAC is increased by factors opposite to described above like hypernatremia etc.

- **Blood gas partition coefficient**
  - **Blood gas partition coefficient** is the ratio of solubility of inhalational anesthetic agent, in blood to gas.
  - When an inhalational anesthetic agent is started it diffuses out of alveoli into pulmonary capillaries and depending on its solubility, it takes time to saturate in blood. An agent with high solubility in blood will take more time and vice versa.
  - After the blood is saturated, the inhalational agent starts to exert a partial pressure and this is responsible for anesthetic effect by acting on CNS. Thus, a drug with high solubility in blood takes more time to exert a partial pressure and hence effect is delayed.
  - Similarly, on discontinuation of drug, effect is terminated after the free agent plus the one soluble in blood is exhaled or metabolized. Thus, for agents with high solubility in blood, recovery is also slower.
  - Thus, agents with **high blood gas partition coefficient have slower induction and recovery** and agents with **low blood as partition coefficient have faster induction and recovery**.
  - Methoxyflurane has highest whereas xenon < desflurane has lowest blood gas partition coefficient.

Conceptual Box-2

Effect of Inhalational Agents

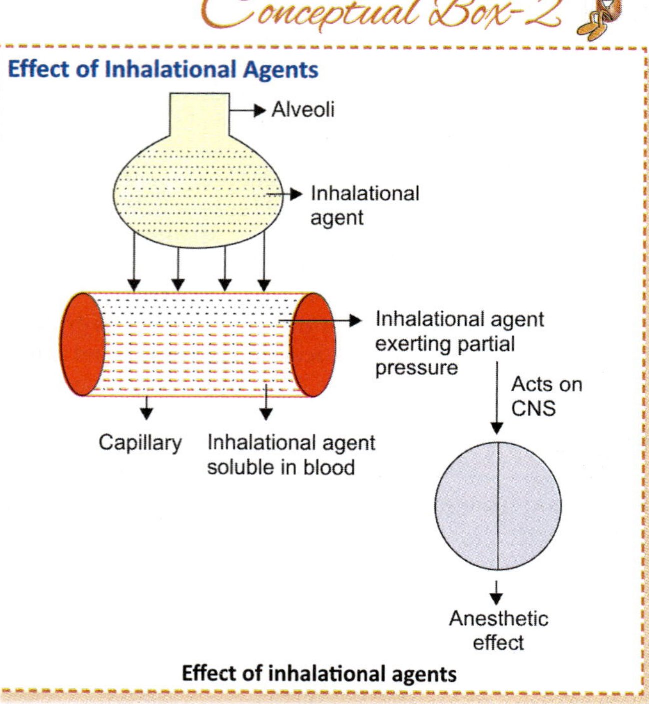

Effect of inhalational agents

Inhalational Anesthetic Agent Properties

Inhalational agent	MAC	Blood gas partition coefficient	Odor
Nitrous oxide	**104**	**0.47**	Nil
Halothane	0.75	2.5	**Sweet**
Enflurane	1.58	1.9	Nil
Isoflurane	1.28	1.4	**Irritant**
Desflurane	6.0	**0.45**	**Pungent**
Sevoflurane	2.05	0.65	Nil
Methoxyflurane	**0.2**	**12**	Nil
Xenon	**71**	**0.14**	Nil

Contd...

Halothane

- Halothane is a volatile, photosensitive liquid and hence stored in **amber colored bottles**.
- **Thymol** is added as a preservative to prevent liberation of free bromine. A **red color vaporizer** is used for this liquid and in the circuit it **diffuses into the rubber tubes**. It is a potent anesthetic without **analgesic effect**.

Uses

- High blood-gas partition coefficient is responsible for slower induction and hence it is used in **maintenance** in adults.
- Though it is used for **induction in children** because of it is non-pungent. High lipid-blood partition coefficient leads to accumulation for longer period and hence recovery is slow.
- As it is the **most potent bronchodilator**, it is the inhalational agent of choice in **asthma**.
- It **relaxes uterus** and has a **tocolytic effect** and hence is used in internal version, manual removal of placenta.

Side Effects

- An inhibitory effect on heart produces hypotension with bradycardia or a normal heart rate.
- It causes a decrease in cerebral metabolism.
- Stimulation of ryanodine receptors can cause **malignant hyperthermia**.
- A metabolite of halothane called as trifluoroacetyldehyde can behave as a heptane, acetylate liver proteins and generate antibodies against hepatocytes which causes **hepatic necrosis**. Hepatic necrosis can be seen with **enflurane** also, though incidence is lesser than halothane. The factors predisposing to hepatotoxicity are **repeated exposure (avoided within 3 months of use), female sex, obesity and middle age**.
- Postoperative chills and shivering can be seen with halothane due to a decrease in the core temperature of the body.
- It causes muscle relaxation and hence potentiates action of NDMRs.

Contraindications

- There is an increase in ICP and hence is **contraindicated in CNS surgery**.
- Halothane sensitizes myocardium to epinephrine and hence is contraindicated in patients of pheochromocytoma.

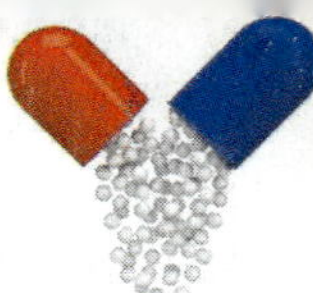

Mnemonics

HALOTHANE

H: High blood gas and lipid blood partition coefficient
A: Amber colored bottle for storage
L: Lowers blood pressure
O: Obstetric use as tocolytic in internal version and manual removal of placenta
T: Thymol used as preservative
H: Hyperthermia (malignant) and Hepatotoxic
A: Asthma safe for use
N: No analgesia
E: Epinephrine's effect is increased in heart

Isoflurane

- Isoflurane an isomer of enflurane, causes cough and laryngospasm and hence it is not used in induction; rather it is **preferred for maintenance**.
- It is the anesthetic agent of choice for various conditions as mentioned in Table.

Anesthetic agent of choice for various conditions

Isoflurane is anesthetic agent of choice in:	Cause
Cardiac surgery	Maintains cardiac output
Controlled hypotension	Vasodilation

- Though it causes bronchodilation, cough and laryngospasm are the limitations in hyperreactive disorders of airway. It potentiates action of NDMR more than halothane.
- It can cause coronary vasodilation and hence precipitate **coronary steal phenomenon** in patients with angina

Sevoflurane

- Sevoflurane has a low blood gas partition coefficient and hence causes a faster induction and recovery; thus, preferred in **day care surgery**.
- As it is non-pungent it does not cause cough and laryngospasm and is the inhalational **induction agent of choice in infants and children**.
- It maintains a normal heart rate and does not increases oxygen demand; hence preferred in **myocardial ischemia**.
- It causes **least increase in intracranial pressure** and hence preferred in **neurosurgery**.
- Reaction with lime produces **compound A** which is nephrotoxic and causes proximal tubular necrosis. To prevent nephrotoxicity fresh gas flow should be at least 2 liters/minute.
- It can undergo exothermic reaction with dry lime and produce ignition and airway burn.
- Sevoflurane can also increase ICP like halothane and isoflurane. At high doses it can cause nephrotoxicity and epilepsy.

Inhalational agents	Increase in ICP	Seizure activity
Halothane	+++++++++ (Maximum)	+
Sevoflurane	+ **(Minimum)**	+/–
Nitrous oxide	+	+
Isoflurane	++	+
Desflurane	++	+

Enflurane

- Enflurane has a high blood gas partition coefficient, which causes a slow induction and recovery. Hence it is used only in maintenance of anesthesia.
- Enflurane is **epileptogenic** and hence contraindicated in patients with epilepsy. Other effects seen are an increase in ICP, hypotension and uterine relaxation.

Desflurane

- Desflurane chemically is a **fluorinated methyl ethyl ester**.
- Desflurane has least blood gas partition coefficient and hence causes fastest induction and recovery, but is not used for induction as it is associated with cough and laryngospasm.
- Because of faster recovery it is used for maintenance in day care surgery.
- It has a high vapor pressure and **boiling point less than 23 °C**.
- It produces maximum carbon monoxide among all agents by reacting with lime.
- It causes vasodilation and reflex tachycardia.
- It has mild **muscle relaxant effect** as well.

Methoxyflurane

- Methoxyflurane has highest blood gas partition coefficient and hence causes slowest induction and recovery. Clinically it is not preferred because of side effects.
- It has least MAC and thus is the most potent inhalational agent used.
- It has a boiling point more than water i.e. 104 °C.
- Since it is highly inflammable fluoride ions are added (maximum among all agents) to reduce the same. These fluoride ions can **cause high output renal failure**; a plasma concentration above 50 μM produces **nephrotoxicity**.
- Like halothane it is also a hepatotoxic agent and absorbed into the tubes of circuit.

Mnemonics

METHI

M: Maximum potency, Maximum metabolized
E: Easily catches fire and hence combined with fluoride
T: Tubes soluble
H: Hepatotoxic, Highest blood gas partition coefficient

Ether

- Ether was the first anesthetic agent used by Crawford Long, however the first public demonstration was done by W.T.G. Morton, an American dentist.
- It is a **highly inflammable and explosive liquid and hence is contraindicated with cautery**. Fluorine is added to decrease inflammability and the compound is called fluroxene.
- Since it has a high blood gas partition coefficient, induction and recovery is slow and hence Guedel studied the stages of anesthesia with ether.
- Because of slower induction it is relatively safer in inexperienced hands.

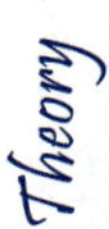

- It stimulates sympathetic nervous system and hence causes hyperglycemia and bronchodilation (safe in asthma).
- It is the only anesthetic agent that preserves ciliary reflex.
- There is a pungent odor which causes cough and laryngospasm on induction. It causes maximum nausea and vomiting among all inhalational agents.
- Ether is also a good analgesic and muscle relaxant.

Mnemonics

HIGH Partition Coefficient In MAN

- **H :** High blood gas partition coefficient
- **I :** Inflammatory and explosive
- **G :** Guedel studied stages of anesthesia
- **H :** Hyperglycemia
- **Partition :** Pungent odor
- **Coefficient :** Ciliary activity is preserved
- **In :** Inexeprienced hands its safe
- **M :** Muscle relaxation
- **A :** Analgesia
- **N :** Nausea and vomiting

Cyclopropane

- Cyclopropane has a low blood gas partition coefficient and hence has a faster induction and recovery.
- It is also a highly inflammable agent.
- It stimulates sympathetic nervous system and raises blood pressure; was used in shock.
- However now it stands discontinued due to cyclopropane shock caused by its withdrawal.

Trielene (Trichloroethylene)

- Trielene is the second most potent inhalational agent after methoxyflurane.
- It is the most potent analgesic among all inhalational agents.
- It is not routinely used nowadays as it **reacts with soda lime** in closed circuit to produce toxic compounds; dichloroacetylene causes **neurotoxicity** involving fifth cranial nerve most commonly and phosgene causes **ARDS**.

Chloroform

- Chloroform is not used routinely nowadays due to side effects like cardiotoxicity, hepatotoxicity and hyperglycemia.

Nitrous Oxide

- Nitrous oxide also known as **laughing gas** is synthesized by heating of ammonium nitrate at 250°C.
- It produces anesthesia by antagonizing **NMDA receptors** and analgesia by stimulating **opioid receptors**.
- It has a boiling point of -89°C critical temperature of 36.5°C.
- It has **maximum MAC (lest potent)** i.e. 104%, which is practically not possible and hence it is used at a concentration of 66% with 33% oxygen as a carrier to other inhalational agents. The benefit is a **decreased MAC or dose requirement for other agents and a faster induction**.
- A low blood gas partition coefficient produces effects like **concentration effect, second gas effect and diffusion hypoxia**.
- It diffuses immediately out of alveoli into capillaries and creates a negative pressure in the alveoli which draws more nitrous oxide from the cylinder; this is known as **concentration effect**.
- This negative pressure can pull oxygen or other volatile agents also into the alveoli; this is known as **second gas effect**.
- After nitrous oxide is discontinued, the alveoli are flooded back with nitrous oxide from the capillaries; this is called as **diffusion hypoxia**. Diffusion hypoxia is prevented by administering **100% oxygen to the patient for five minutes** before discontinuation of nitrous oxide. These effects are seen only with nitrous oxide, as it is the only agent used at high concentration.
- Nitrous oxide **inactivates vitamin B_{12}** and its deficiency results in **peripheral neuropathy, megaloblastic anemia** and **subacute combined degeneration of spinal cord**. It can diffuse into cavities and accumulate and hence contraindicated in patients with **pneumothorax, pneumoperitoneum, volvulus, laparoscopic procedures ocular surgery and middle ear surgery**. It can increase homocysteine, which increases vascular inflammation and thrombosis. Other side effects associated are methemoglobinemia, pulmonary edema and laryngospasm (due to impurities). It can also cause **pulmonary vasoconstriction** and hence is avoided in patients with pulmonary hypertension.
- Entonox is 50% nitrous oxide used along with 50% oxygen. Both dissolve with each other by losing individual properties and this phenomenon is called as "Poynting effect".

Xenon

- Xenon is a noble and inert gas with **viscosity and density more than air**.
- Antagonism of **NMDA receptors** produces anesthesia whereas **potassium channel** opening causes analgesia.
- It has **least blood gas partition coefficient** and hence causes fastest induction and recovery.
- Though it has **low potency** with a **high MAC of 71** only second to that of nitrous oxide.
- It is **not metabolized** and excreted unchanged by lungs.
- It is the most ideal gas as it has **limited effect on CVS, CNS and respiratory system**. It can also be used in place of nitrous oxide as **oxygen carrier**.
- However, it is not widely used, as it cannot be synthesized and needs to be extracted from air. This considerably increases costing.
- Since it has **more density than air**, it increases resistance to flow and can cause difficult breathing in airway disorders.

Mnemonics

XENON

- **X :** Xtremely safe agent
- **E :** Elevated MAC (71), i.e. low potency
- **N :** NMDA antagonist
- **O :** Onset of anesthesia is fastest, Oxygen carrier
- **N :** Nausea and vomiting

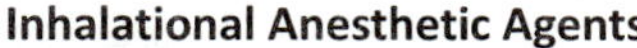

Inhalational Anesthetic Agents

Properties	Halothane	Isoflurane	Sevoflurane	Desflurane	Enflurane
Cardiac output	**Maximum decrease**	Decreases	Decreases	**Minimum decrease**	Decreases
Heart rate	**Maximum decrease**	**Maximum increase**	**No effect**	Increases	Increases
Blood Pressure	Decreases	Decreases	**Minimal decrease**	Decreases	Decreases
Respiratory rate	**Minimum increase**	Increases	Increases	Increases	Increases
Intracranial pressure	**Maximum increase**	**Minimum increase**	Increases	Increases	Increases
Splanchnic blood flow	**Decreases**	Normal	Normal	Normal	**Decreases**
Sensitization to catecholamines	**Maximum**	Absent	Absent	Absent	Minimum
Effect on uterus	**Maximum relaxation**	Relaxation	Relaxation	Relaxation	Relaxation
Analgesia	**Absent**	Present	Present	Present	Present
Bronchodilation	**Maximum in asthmatics**	Present	Maximum in nonasthmatics	Present	Present

NONANESTHETIC GASES

HELIUM

- Helium is an **inert gas** stored in brown colored cylinders. **Heliox is 79% helium plus 21% oxygen**, stored in **brown cylinders** with white shoulders.
- As helium is **lighter than air**, has **viscosity higher than air** and has a **low density,** heliox is used in case of airway obstruction to decrease turbulence.
- Low solubility is the reason for its use in diving; nitrogen is also used but it causes narcosis.
- High thermal conductivity makes it ideal for use in laser surgery.

OXYGEN

- Oxygen is stored in **black cylinders with white shoulders**.
- The primary use is to prevent or treat hypoxia and is also combined with nitrous oxide.
- Side effects can be seen at high partial pressure, like neurological, lung collapse due to lipid peroxidation of alveoli and retrolental fibroplasia in neonates.

CARBON DIOXIDE

- Carbon dioxide is a pungent gas stored in grey colored cylinders.
- The use of carbon dioxide is as a respiratory stimulant, in cryotherapy and in laparoscopy to insufflate.

MUSCLE RELAXANTS

- Muscle relaxants are used to facilitate intubation and ventilation followed by surgical procedure.
- Muscle relaxants used in anesthesia can be broadly classified into **depolarizing and nondepolarizing ones**.
- The general side effects seen with these agents are prolonged apnea, cardiovascular collapse and **anaphylaxis**.

Classification of Muscle Relaxants

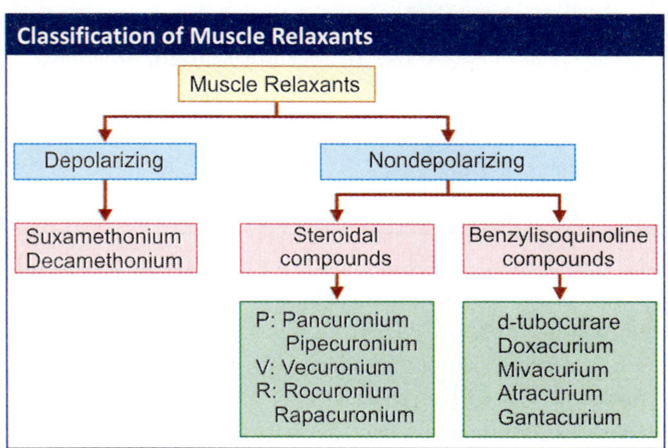

DEPOLARIZING MUSCLE RELAXANTS

Suxamethonium

- Suxamethonium or succinylcholine (Sch) is made up of two molecules of acetylcholine joined by their acetyl groups. It should be stored at **2–8°C** and has a shelf life of **2 years**.
- Succinylcholine is metabolized by **butyryl cholinesterase**, also known as **plasma cholinesterase** and **pseudocholinesterase**.
- As this enzyme is not present in the synapse, Sch is metabolized only after it diffuses out to plasma. Thus, Sch induced persistent stimulation of N_M receptors causes persistent depolarization of postsynaptic membrane and inactivation of sodium channel, which causes muscle relaxation. This is called **as phase I block**, which is worsened by AchE inhibitors.
- At further higher doses there can be receptor desensitization mimicking tachyphylaxis called as **phase II block**, which can be reversed by increasing Ach in synapse by AchE inhibitors.
- **Sch is the shortest and fastest acting muscle relaxant** and hence it is commonly used for intubation.
- Persistent depolarization of postsynaptic membranes can cause **hyperkalemia** and contraction of muscles leading to side effects mentioned in Table.

Side effects Due to Persistent Depolarization of Postsynaptic Membranes

Increased muscle contraction	Fasciculations **Masseter spasm** Myalgia Muscle damage – Raised myoglobin and CPK
Increased abdominal muscle contraction	Increased intragastric pressure
Increased oxygen consumption and carbon dioxide production due to muscle contraction cause cerebral vasodilation	Increased ICP
Increased tonic myofibrils contraction and dilation of choroidal blood vessels	Increased IOP
Increased catecholamine release	Increased blood pressure Ventricular tachyarrhythmia
Depolarization of muscles	Hyperkalemia
Cardiac muscarinic receptor stimulation	**Sinus bradycardia** Junctional rhythms
Stimulation of ryanodine receptor	**Malignant hyperthermia**

- Myalgia is seen usually in females, after minor surgeries and ambulatory patients. Prostaglandin inhibitors can decrease the incidence of myalgia.
- Fasciculations can be prevented by **precurarization**, i.e. premedication with an NDMR.
- **Hyperkalemia** is a side effect that can cause refractory asystole and hence other conditions with increased potassium levels are absolute contraindication. These are conditions like burn patients, myopathy, neuropathy, spinal cord damage, etc.
- **Succinylcholine** is the most common cause of anaphylaxis during anesthesia.
- Patients with atypical pseudocholinesterase due to genetic variability are unable to metabolize Sch and hence there is prolonged apnea. **Dibucaine number** is used to find out the amount of normal enzyme; dibucaine a local anesthetic inhibits 80% of normal enzyme but only 20% of abnormal enzyme. If it is said that the dibucaine number in a patient is 80, it means dibucaine inhibits 80% of normal enzyme.

Dibucaine number	Pseudocholinesterase type	Response to Sch
70–80	Homozygous typical	Normal
50–60	Heterozygous atypical	Abnormal
20–30	Homozygous atypical	Abnormal

- AchE inhibitors like neostigmine can also inhibit pseudocholinesterase and hence prolong the effect of Sch.

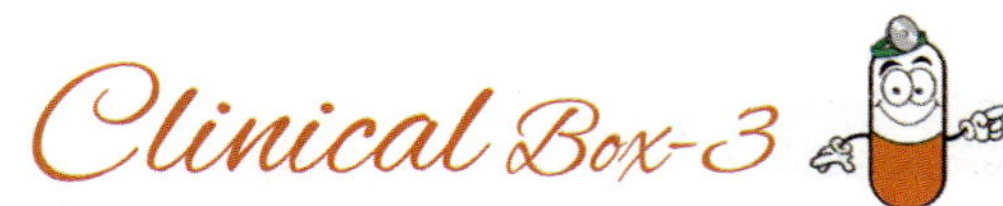

Malignant Hyperthermia
- Increased activity of genes increase ryanodine receptors, which are present is sarcoplasmic reticulum and release calcium. Anesthetic agents act on this receptor increases excessive release of calcium (passive), which is then taken up by sarcoplasmic reticulum (active). This depletes a huge number of ATP, generating heat energy and leads to malignant hyperthermia.
- Most common cause is succinylcholine, whereas most common inhalational agent causing malignant hyperthermia is **halothane** and most common local anesthetic is **lidocaine**. Other agents causing malignant hyperthermia are volatile agents, cyclopropane and ether.
- Apart from hyperthermia other presenting features are **metabolic acidosis, raised CPK, arrhythmia, hypertension, hyperkalemia, decreased oxygen saturation and increased end tidal carbon dioxide**.
- In management part, the first thing to be done is to stop all drugs. Then the drug of choice for malignant hyperthermia **dantrolene** is administered. **100% oxygen**, **bicarbonate** for acidosis and other supportive measures like **cooling** are also important.

NONDEPOLARIZING MUSCLE RELAXANTS

- Nondepolarizing muscle relaxants (NDMR) are competitive inhibitors of the N_M receptors, which prevent Ach-mediated depolarization of muscles and that results in muscle relaxation.
- The NDMRs can be broadly classified into **benzylisoquinolinium** and **aminosteroidal** compounds.
- NDMRs are quaternary amines, i.e. ionized and are lipid insoluble and hence have low volume of distribution.
- The **speed of onset of muscle relaxation is inversely proportional to the potency of NDMRs**, except for atracurium.
- All NDMRs are excreted primarily by kidney (maximum with **pancuronium**) except with rocuronium which are excreted by liver. Vecuronium is excreted almost equally by liver and kidney. Atracurium and cis-atracurium undergo spontaneous degradation, i.e. **Hoffman's elimination**.
- The effect of muscle relaxants is prolonged by volatile anesthetics (maximum with **desflurane**), antibiotics (aminoglycosides, colistin, polymyxin B, clindamycin and lincomycin), local anesthetics, lithium, calcium channel blockers, hypothermia, acidosis and hypomagnesemia.
- **Myasthenia gravis decreases effect of muscle relaxants** as there are anti N_M antibodies.

Benzylisoquinolinium Compounds

- This group has drugs like **d-tubocurare, doxacurium, mivacurium, atracurium and gantacurium**.
- This class is notorious for causing **histamine release** and **autonomic ganglionic block**, which is maximum with d-tubocurare and hence is not used.

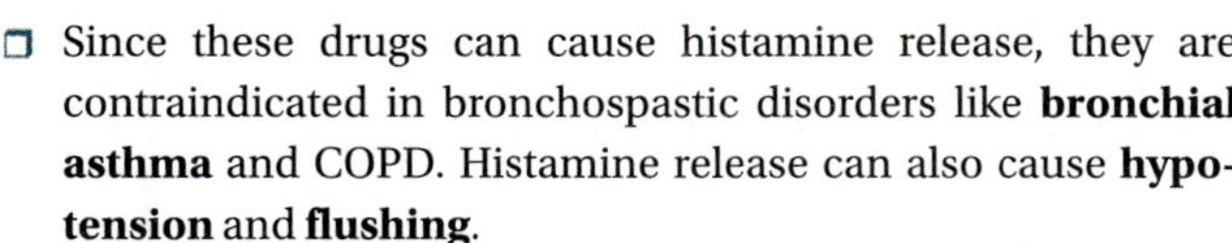

- Since these drugs can cause histamine release, they are contraindicated in bronchospastic disorders like **bronchial asthma** and COPD. Histamine release can also cause **hypotension** and **flushing**.
- **Doxacurium** is the **longest acting** and **most potent** NDMR.
- **Mivacurium** is metabolized by pseudocholinesterase in plasma and hence is a **short-acting NDMR**. It is the NDMR of choice for **day care surgery**.
- Atracurium undergoes ester hydrolysis and spontaneous degradation known as **Hofmann elimination**, in which it is converted into a tertiary amine. Hence, it is the muscle relaxant of choice in **hepatic failure, renal failure, myasthenia gravis, old age and newborn**. High pH and temperature stimulate Hofmann elimination. At high dose it produces a compound called as **laudanosine** which is glycine antagonist and can cause seizures. It can also cause critical illness myopathy.
- There is correlation between **total body weight** and duration of action of atracurium. The duration of action is prolonged when atracurium is given based on ideal body weight.
- **Cis-atracurium** an isomer of atracurium is four time more potent than atracurium and hence has a **slower onset of action**. It **does not cause histamine release** and the amount of **laudanosine** produced at high doses is also **five times lesser**. Unlike atracurium it does not undergo ester hydrolysis and is primarily metabolized by **Hofmann elimination**.
- Gantacurium is a ultrashort acting NDMR, currently under trial. It is overall the shortest acting NDMR. Its shorter duration of action is due to unique inactivation by addiction of cysteine which makes a compound that cannot bind to N_M receptors.

Steroidal Compounds

- **Pancuronium** the **second longest acting NDMR**. It causes vagolysis and increases NE by inhibiting its reuptake and hence is associated with hypertension and tachycardia. Since it causes vasoconstriction is the muscle relaxant of choice in **congenital heart diseases with right to left shunt**. It increases arrhythmogenic effect of halothane. It is an inhibitor of pseudocholinesterase as well. The shelf-life of pancuronium is 6 months.
- Pipecuronium is a derivative of pancuronium with no vagolytic effect and hence is cardiostable.
- **Vecuronium** is the most cardiovascular stable NDMR and hence is the muscle relaxant of choice in **cardiac surgeries**. It can cause polyneuropathy, critical illness myopathy and its use is contraindicated in **biliary obstruction** as it is excreted by bile.
- **Rocuronium** is the **fastest acting** NDMR due to its low potency and hence is the NDMR of choice for **intubation** and precurarization in case of Sch. It can cause **pain on injection**. Its effect can be reversed by both AchE inhibitors and sugammadex. The shelf life at room temperature is 60 days.
- **Rapacuronium** is the **shortest acting** NDMR, but not used commonly nowadays.

Histamine release	Benzylisoquinolinium compounds Max – d-tubocurare Not seen – cis-atracurium
Autonomic ganglion block	d-tubocurare
Autonomic ganglion stimulation	Succinylcholine
Vagolytic effect	Max – Pancuronium None – Vecuronium
Vagomimetic effect	Succinylcholine
Fastest acting	Rocuronium
Shortest acting	Rapacuronium
Metabolism and elimination	• Pseudocholinesterase Succinylcholine Mivacurium • Hofmann elimination Atracurium > cis-atracurium • Renal – Pancuronium • Liver – Rocuronium • Equally by liver and kidney - Vecuronium

Reversal Agents

- AchE inhibitors like **edrophonium** and **neostigmine** are routinely used for reversal of muscle relaxants. The details of this class are discussed in the chapter on autonomic nervous system.
- **Sugammadex** is a gamma cyclodextrin which encapsulates the muscle relaxants and removes them from plasma and neuromuscular junction. It is used for emergency reversal of **rocuronium** and **vecuronium**. It can cause hypersensitivity and bradycardia.

MONITORING OF MUSCLE RELAXANTS

- There are two distinct points one needs to understand about muscle relaxation; one is-speed of onset and recovery of muscle relaxation and second is-sensitivity of the muscles to muscle relaxants.
- The central muscles with abundant blood supply like **diaphragm**, larynx and muscles of **head and neck** have **fastest onset and offset of action**. The peripheral muscles like that of hands like **adductor pollicis** have **slowest onset and offset of action**. The **peripheral muscles are more sensitive to NDMR as compared to central muscles like diaphragm**.
- Thus, while induction and maintenance of anesthesia **orbicularis oculi muscle is most ideal**, as if it is relaxed then other central muscles must have relaxed and intubation can be done. However, for induction and reversal **adductor pollicis (ulnar nerve)** is **most commonly used** as if it has recovered, the central muscles must have recovered and the patient can be taken off ventilator.

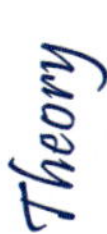

- The degree of neuromuscular block is assessed by applying a supramaximal stimulus (current of 25% above maximal stimulus) to a peripheral nerve and then measuring the muscular response.
- The different patterns of nerve stimulation used are train of four (TOF) stimulation, tetanic stimulation, post-tetanic facilitation, double burst stimulation and post-tetanic count.
- The muscular response can be recorded by **kinemography (KMG)**, electromyography (EMG) and acceleromyography (AMG). KMG measures the electrical response in a piezoelectric film attached to the muscle. EMG measures the evoked electrical response of muscle. AMG measures the acceleration of muscle response.

Train of Four (TOF) Stimulation

- IntoF the ulnar nerve is stimulated four times with a frequency of 2 Hz for 2 seconds and each stimulation separated by 0.5 seconds. The TOF then can be repeated after **10 seconds**.
- The four stimulations are called as T_1, T_2, T_3 and T_4. The ratio between T_1 and T_4 is known as TOF ratio which in a normal muscle is 1.
- In case of NDMR there is a gradual decrease in height of stimulations followed by their disappearance; T_4 disappears at 75% depression of T_1, T_3 disappears at 80% depression of T_1 and T_2 disappears at 90% depression of T_1. The gradual decrease in twitch height is known as fade of TOF. For safe extubation a TOF ratio must be 0.9 or more.
- TOF is less useful for depolarizing muscle relaxant like succinylcholine as the decrease in height is same in all four twitches. Hence the TOF ratio is 1. However, in excessive doses if there is **phase II block**, a **fade intoF** can be seen as in case of NDMRs.

Tetanic Stimulation

- For tetanic stimulation a high frequency stimulus of 50Hz for 5 seconds is delivered.
- In absence of NDMR, the contraction is sustained and there is no fade. In the presence of NDMR there is a gradual fade in contraction. It is useful in postoperative recovery room for extubation.
- The drawback is it is highly painful due to the high frequency stimulation.

Post-tetanic count

- A 50 Hz frequency stimulation is given for 5 seconds and then after 3 seconds a 1Hz stimulus is given to see response. Response might be seen to 1 Hz stimulus due to Ach release by the 50 Hz stimulus. This is called as post-tetanic facilitation or potentiation.
- The number of responses seen after 50 Hz stimulus is called as post-tetanic count, which is inversely proportional to the time of recovery from neuromuscular block.
- During deep neuromuscular blockade when TOF is not effective, post-tetanic count can be used.

Double Burst Stimulation

- In double burst stimulation two stimulation of 50 Hz frequency are given–750 milliseconds apart.
- In muscle without NDMR effect, the two contractions are of equal height whereas in case of NDMR the second contraction is reduced.
- It can be used to detect even small degree of residual block.

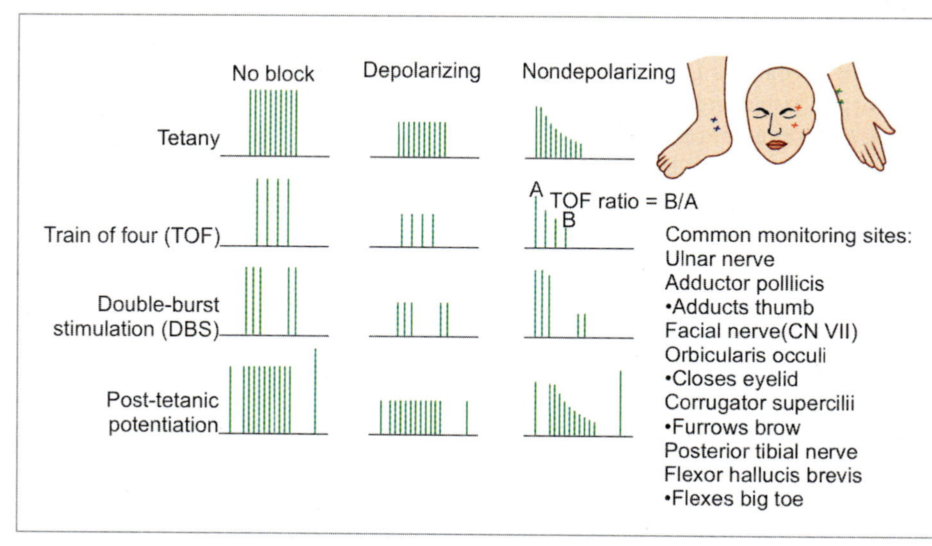

Muscle Relaxation Monitoring

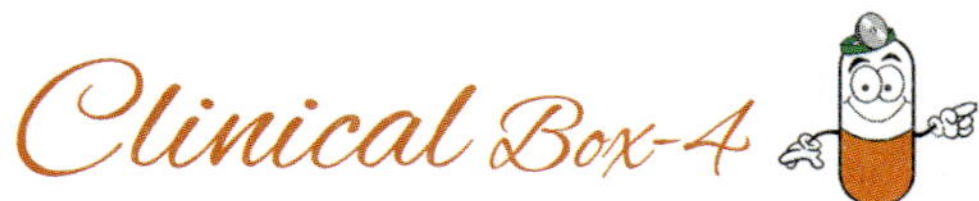

Anaphylaxis in Anesthesia

- Anaphylaxis during anesthesia is most commonly caused by **muscle relaxants > latex > antibiotics**. The other causes are intravenous anesthetic agents (thiopental and Propofol), NSAIDs, colloids and benzodiazepines.
- Most common muscle relaxant responsible for anaphylaxis is **Succinylcholine**. Since muscle relaxants are given before intubation, anaphylaxis is seen in the beginning of surgery.
- Latex induced anaphylaxis can be seen in health workers and patients of neural tube defects, spinal cord trauma, urogenital malformations who have chronic exposure to latex gloves because of procedures. As time is required for allergen to be absorbed to systemic circulation, anaphylaxis with latex is seen toward the end of surgery.
- **NSAIDs usually cause anaphylaxis toward the end of surgery** when given as an analgesic.
- Most common antibiotic responsible for anaphylaxis is **penicillin**. Since antibiotics are administered before surgery, anaphylaxis is seen before or in the beginning of surgery.
- Colloids like dextran and hydroxyethyl starch can cause anaphylaxis after 20 minutes of beginning of infusion.
- Intravenous anesthetic agents like thiopental and Propofol can also cause anaphylaxis. Women are at greater risk of anaphylaxis than men in case of thiopental
- The most common benzodiazepine associated with anaphylaxis is diazepam and the safest one is midazolam.
- Opioids though can cause anaphylaxis are rarely associated.
- To prevent anaphylaxis patients can be preloaded with antihistaminics and steroids (1 gram of methylprednisolone).

OPIOIDS

Opioids have a diverse use in anesthesia ranging from analgesia to induction of anesthesia.

- **Fentanyl** is 100 times more potent than morphine. It is used as an analgesic and used along with IV agents in induction. It is used along with neuroleptic droperidol in neurolept analgesia and neurolept anesthesia (along with nitrous oxide). It causes **maximum muscle rigidity known as wooden chest syndrome**. Pentazocine followed by fentanyl is used as sequential analgesic anesthesia.
- **Alfentanil** is 20 times more potent than morphine. It is used along with propofol for **total intravenous anesthesia (TIVA)** in day care surgery patients.
- **Sufentanil** is 1,000 times more potent than morphine; it is the **most potent opioid and opioid with maximum plasma protein binding**. It is used to inhibit stress response to laryngoscopy and intubation.
- **Remifentanil** is the opioid with **fastest onset of action and recovery**. Hence it is the opioid of choice in **day care surgery**. It is metabolized by esterase and hence is ultrashort acting. Since it contains glycine that can cause neurotoxicity it is not used by epidural route.
- **Pethidine** is the drug of choice for treatment of **postoperative chills**; tramadol is an alternative.

LOCAL ANESTHESIA

- Local anesthetics are drugs which act by blocking the **sodium channels in closed state at inner vestibule**.
- Broadly local anesthetics can be classified into esters and amides based on their chemical structure.
- **Esters** are metabolized by plasma esterases and hence are **shorter acting**, whereas **amides** are metabolized in liver by amidase and hence are **longer acting**.

Classification of Local Anesthetics

Amides	Esters
• Lidocaine	• Procaine
• Articaine	• Cocaine
• Mepivacaine	• Chlorprocaine
• Bupivacaine	• Benzocaine
• Prilocaine	• Tetracaine
• Etidocaine	
• Ropivacaine	

FACTORS AFFECTING LOCAL ANESTHETIC EFFECT

- **Type of fibre**: The orders of sensitivity of fibres is type **A > B (preganglionic sympathetic) > C (Temperature)**. In fibre type A the order is **gamma (muscle tone) > delta (Pin prick) > beta (touch) and alpha (motor)**. Thus the sequence of block is **muscle tone > pin prick > touch > motor > preganglionic sympathetic > temperature**.
- **pH:** Local anesthetics are weak bases and hence added with bicarbonate, which makes them unionized or lipid soluble. In this form they can traverse through the lipid barrier, but in the neurons, they turn into ionized form and inhibit sodium channels. The addiction of bicarbonate makes onset of block faster, quality of block better and **injection less painful**. In ischemic and infected tissues as the medium is acidic, local anesthetics are less effective. **Bupivacaine precipitates with bicarbonate** and hence these should not be combined.
- **Addition of vasoconstrictors:** Epinephrine (5 µg/mL or **1:200,000**) as a vasoconstrictor **increases duration of action** and **decreases toxicity** of local anesthetics. Local anesthetics with epinephrine are contraindicated in some conditions mentioned below.
- Onset and duration of action depends on the site of injection. **Fastest onset and shortest duration of action is seen with subarachnoid and subcutaneous injection**, whereas **slowest onset and longest duration of action is seen in brachial plexus block**.

Mnemonics

Contraindications to use of LA with Epinephrine–BHIM

B : Block of areas with end arteries, e.g. Digital block
H : Hypertension, Hyperthyroidism, with Halothane
I : Intravenous regional anesthesia
M : Myocardial ischemia

- Local anesthetic induced systemic toxicity is increased in case of **hypercapnia, hypoxia, acidosis, old age and pregnancy**.

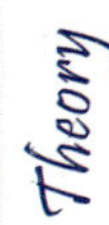

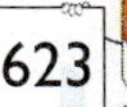

PROPERTIES OF LOCAL ANESTHETICS

- **Potency** of local anesthetics is directly proportional to their **lipid solubility**.
- Local anesthetics have intrinsic vasodilatory activity at low concentration (Maximum - Prilocaine, Minimum - Ropivacaine) and vasoconstriction at high concentration. The only exception is **cocaine** which causes only **vasoconstriction**.
- **Duration of action** of local anesthetics is directly proportional to the **plasma protein binding**. Amides have more plasma protein binding as compared to esters. Local anesthetics bind maximum with albumin, but bind with higher affinity with α_1-acid glycoprotein.
- The **onset of action is directly proportional to the pK_a**. Local anesthetics with higher pK_a have more ionized form and have slower onset of action, whereas those with lower pK_a have more unionized form and have faster onset of action.
- The systemic absorption of local anesthetic depends on the site of application or injection. The order of absorption is **intercostal** > caudal > epidural > brachial plexus > **subcutaneous**.

AMIDES

Lidocaine

- Lidocaine is the most commonly used local anesthetic. Clinically it is used for different indications like postherpetic neuralgia, dental procedures, dermal procedures and in neuraxial anesthesia. The different uses and concentration used is given in Table.

Different Uses and Concentration of Lidocaine

Lidocaine Uses	Concentration (%)
Topical	Ointment: 2.5 – 5 Solution: 2 – 4 Jelly: 2 Suppositories: 10 Aerosol: 10
Spinal	1.5 5
Epidural	1–2
Major nerve block	1–2
Minor nerve block	1

- Lidocaine is the most preferred agent for **intravenous reginal anesthesia (IVRA) i.e. Bier's block**.
- Lidocaine also belongs to class I_a antiarrhythmic and is drug of choice for treatment of **digoxin and MI induced ventricular tachycardia and fibrillation**.
- Side effects are mostly neurological like-drowsiness, tinnitus, dizziness, twitching, **seizures** and coma. In genetically susceptible patients it can also cause malignant hyperthermia. Treatment of neurological side effects is supportive and for seizures **benzodiazepines is the drug of choice**.

Prilocaine

- Prilocaine has a high volume of distribution and causes lesser neurological side effects.
- It is metabolized to o-toluidine which causes **methemoglobinemia** and hence its use is mostly limited to dental procedures. Since neonates are more sensitive to toxic effect of methemoglobinemia, prilocaine is not used.
- Prilocaine is preferred next to lidocaine for intravenous regional anesthesia.

Bupivacaine

- Bupivacaine is a long acting local anesthetic because of its slow dissociation from sodium channels.
- It is used in labor and postoperative analgesia.
- As it is the **most cardiotoxic** local anesthetic it is contraindicated in IVRA or Bier's block. The most common ECG finding in patients with bupivacaine cardiotoxicity is **slow idioventricular rhythm** with broad QRS complexes. Currently antiarrhythmic drugs like bretylium, amiodarone and lidocaine are not advised for treatment of bupivacaine toxicity. Rather the ACLS advised drugs like **atropine** and **epinephrine** are used along with cardioversion for ventricular fibrillation. **Lipid emulsion** is also advised for treatment of cardiotoxicity.
- Ropivacaine, a derivative of bupivacaine is lesser cardiotoxic.
- **Bupivacaine** and **ropivacaine** are preferred local anesthetics of choice for **epidural analgesia in labor** as they have a higher sensory to motor block ratio as compared to other drugs like lidocaine.

Dibucaine

- Dibucaine is the **longest acting** and **most potent** local anesthetic.
- It is used for spinal and topical anesthesia.

Mepivacaine

- Mepivacaine causes increased toxicity in neonates due to ion trapping and hence is contraindicated in labor.
- It is not effective by topical route.

Articaine

- Articaine is the only amide metabolized by esterases and hence is short acting.
- It is primarily used in dental procedures.

Esters

The common side effects of ester local anesthetics is hypersensitivity.

Cocaine

- Cocaine was the first local anesthetic used. It is derived from leaves of cocoa shrubs.
- As it inhibits NE reuptake and **causes vasoconstriction**, it is contraindicated with vasoconstrictors like epinephrine.

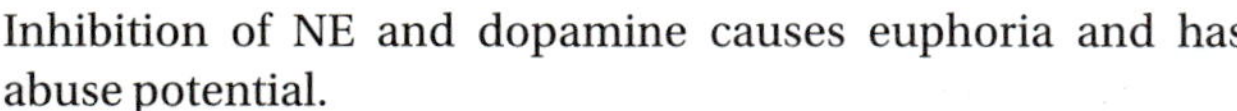

Inhibition of NE and dopamine causes euphoria and has abuse potential.

- It is used only as topical solution of 4% in ENT.

Procaine

- Procaine was the first synthetic local anesthetic used. As it is less potent, short acting (second shortest acting after chlorprocaine) with slow onset of action, it is used only for infiltrative anesthesia and diagnostic nerve block.
- It is the local anesthetic of choice in patients susceptible to malignant hyperthermia.
- As it is metabolized into PABA, it decreases effect of antifolate drugs like sulfonamides and PAS.

Chlorprocaine

- Chlorprocaine is **least potent** and **shortest acting** local anesthetic.
- It has preservatives like sodium metabisulphite which is neurotoxic and hence **contraindicated for spinal anesthesia**.
- Ca EDTA preservative chlorprocaine can be used for epidural anesthesia and is associated with backpain due to paraspinal muscle contraction.

Tetracaine

- Tetracaine is long acting and hence preferred for spinal anesthesia for procedures requiring longer duration.
- Since it has a slow onset of action it is not preferred in peripheral nerve blocks.

Benzocaine

- Benzocaine has a low water solubility and hence is slowly absorbed; thus, it can be directly applied on cut surfaces.
- It can also cause methemoglobinemia like prilocaine.

Safe dose of Local Anesthetics

Safe dose of local anesthetics	
Lidocaine	Without adrenaline: 3 mg/kg or 200 mg With adrenaline: 7 mg/kg or 500 mg
Bupivacaine	2 mg/kg
Chlorprocaine Procaine	12 mg/kg or 1000 mg
Tetracaine	3 mg/kg
Prilocaine	8 mg/kg
Mepivacaine	4.5 mg/kg
Etidocaine	4 mg/kg
Dibucaine	1 mg/kg

TYPES OF LOCAL ANESTHESIA

Topical Anesthesia

- Local anesthetics preferred for topical anesthesia commonly are **lidocaine, dibucaine, tetracaine, cyclonine, hexylcaine and benzocaine**. These drugs are used for anesthesia of mucous membranes or denuded skin.
- Spray of lidocaine and tetracaine are used in intubation, bronchoscopy and esophagoscopy.
- For application on intact skin **eutectic mixture of local anesthetic (EMLA)** i.e. **lidocaine (2.5%) and prilocaine (2.5%) is preferred**.
- An eutectic mixture has a melting point lesser than individual drugs and hence the mixture is in oil form at room temperature.
- The cream is applied 45–60 minutes before the procedure with an occlusive dressing.
- It is preferred for **circumcision in children**, venipuncture, cannulation and skin grafting.

Tumescent Anesthesia

- A huge volume of diluted local anesthetic like lidocaine along with epinephrine is injected into subcutaneous space for liposuction by plastic surgeons.
- It carries risk of systemic toxicity.

Infiltration Anesthesia

- Infiltration anesthesia is performed by injecting the local anesthetics **directly into the tissue** of interest.
- The local anesthetics preferred are lidocaine, procaine and bupivacaine.
- It is used for minor procedures like CLW suturing and hydrocele operation.

Intravenous Regional Anesthesia or Bier's Block

- Intravenous regional anesthesia (IVRA) is used for the surgery of legs and the arm. A proximal tourniquet is applied with a pressure of **100–150 mm Hg** more than systolic blood pressure. Then a local anesthetic is applied into the cannula and analgesia is seen within 5–10 minutes.
- The drug of choice for **IVRA is lidocaine**; prilocaine is less commonly used nowadays.
- **Bupivacaine is contraindicated for IVRA** due to risk of cardiotoxicity. IVRA is contraindicated in patients of sickle cell anemia.

Spinal Anesthesia

- In spinal anesthesia local anesthetic is injected into the subarachnoid space (between pia and arachnoid mater) after a lumbar puncture.
- In adults the level of lumbar puncture is L_{3-4} and in children it is L_{4-5}. After the site for spinal anesthesia is selected on back, local anesthetic is applied and then needle is inserted at 10–15 degrees of a cephalad angle through skin, subcutaneous tissue, **supraspinous ligament** and **interspinous ligament** until a **resistance is felt while piercing through ligamentum flavum and dura mater.**
- Then after passing through **dura there is a click or pop sensation** and when needle is removed CSF appears.
- The sequence of block of nerves in spinal anesthesia is different from local anesthesia in tissues (A>B>C). In spinal

anesthesia the sequence is **B (preganglionic sympathetic)** > **C (Temperature)** > **A**. The sequence of block in A fibers is **A delta (Pin prick)** > **A beta (touch)** > **A alpha (motor)**. The sequence of block is **temperature** > **pin prick** > **touch** > **motor**. The order of reversal of block is opposite, i.e. **motor** > **touch** > **pin prick** > **temperature**.

- For lumbar puncture two types of needles can be used.
  - **Traumatic (dura cutting) needles** like **Quinke-Babcock** leave space for CSF leak and hence are associated with more post spinal headache.
  - **Atraumatic (dura separating) needles** like **Whitacre** and **Sprotte** do not leave space for CSF leak and hence are associated with lesser incidence of post spinal headache.

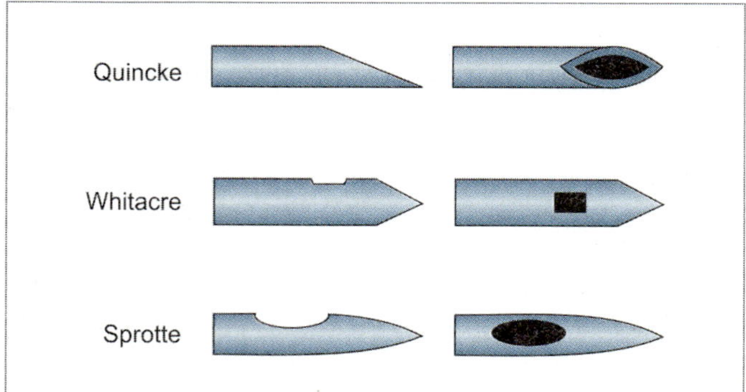

Spinal Needles

- The drugs commonly used are **lidocaine, bupivacaine and tetracaine**; procaine is used for diagnostic block due to its shorter duration of action.

Duration of procedure	La of choice	Safe dose in mg
Short	Lidocaine 0.5% or 5%	50–100
Intermediate to long	**Bupivacaine 0.5%** or 0.75%	4–5
Long	Tetracaine 0.25% or 1%	5–15
Diagnostic block	Procaine 10%	50–200

- Opioids like **morphine, fentanyl** and **sufentanil** are used by spinal route for analgesia.
- Spinal anesthesia is preferred for surgery in the lower limbs (orthopedic surgeries), obstetric and gynecological surgeries (caesarean section), surgeries of lower abdomen, pelvis and perineum.
- **Saddle block** is a type of spinal anesthesia given to the patient in sitting position to block the sacral segment for perianal surgeries like hemorrhoids, fissure and perineal procedures like **forceps delivery**.
- The level of block depends on dose of drug injected, its baricity, age, pregnancy, CSF volume, position of patient and epidural injection post spinal. Old age, pregnancy, high dose, high level injection and hypobaricity is associated with a higher level block. Higher level block can affect sympathetic nervous system and cause asystole.

Mnemonics

Factors Affecting Height of Block in Spinal Anesthesia
SPREAD
- **S :** Solution baricity
- **P :** Position of patient, Pregnancy
- **R :** Relative CSF volume
- **E :** Epidural injection post spinal
- **A :** Age
- **D :** Dose of drug

Note: Level of injection, volume/concentration/temperature of solution, needle type are less important factors.

- Most common intraoperative side effect is **hypotension** due to venodilation; the drug of choice for same is **ephedrine**, though phenylephrine can also be used. To prevent hypotension patient is placed in head down position, also known as **Trendelenburg's position**.
- Risk of hypotension is more in hypertensives and hence spinal anesthesia is avoided in patients of preeclampsia.
- Most common postoperative side effect is occipital > frontal headache seen after **12 to 24 hours** of procedure, within **48 hours** in most cases and resolves spontaneously within **7 days**. The patient can be given analgesics, intravenous caffeine, sumatriptan, supine positioning, and hydration, however autologous blood patch is definitive management which is applied only after 24 hours of lumbar puncture and development of headache. The incidence of headache can be decreased by using a **small bore** and **atraumatic needle** (dura separating), **removing the stylet prior to needle** and by placing the needle bevel in long axis of neuraxis. Incidence of headache is more in young patients, females sex and pregnant females.
- Bradycardia can be seen in spinal anesthesia due to three reasons.
  - A high level block at the level of T1 to T4 can block **cardiac accelerator fibers.**
  - **Reverse Bainbridge reflex:** In Bainbridge reflex an increase in blood volume in heart causes atrial stretch and the atrial stretch receptors inhibit parasympathetic activity in the heart causing tachycardia. In reverse Bainbridge reflex a decrease in blood volume in heart conversely can cause bradycardia. This can be seen by a decrease in preload due to venodilation caused by spinal and epidural anesthesia.
  - **Bezold-Jarisch reflex:** When noxious stimuli in the ventricles stimulate chemoreceptors and mechanoreceptors a triad of hypotension, bradycardia and coronary artery dilation are seen. It is usually seen with associated hypovolemia when a small systolic volume stimulates mechanoreceptors.
- Other side effects related to the procedure are infection, hematoma, neurological deficits and cranial nerve palsies. All cranial nerves can be affected except 1, 9 and 10, however the **6th cranial nerve** is most commonly affected.
- **Cauda equine syndrome** is a side effect of local anesthetics administered by spinal route. It is usually seen with high doses of local anesthetic like 5% lidocaine.

Level of Block Required for Surgical Procedures

Surgical procedure	Level of block
Upper abdominal surgery Cesarean delivery	T4
Transurethral resection of prostate (TURP) Hip surgery	T10
Foot and ankle surgery	L2

- Local anesthetic requirement is considerably decreased in pregnancy and old age due to reasons mentioned below. This causes high level block and is most common cause of maternal mortality.

Pregnancy	• There is an increased abdominal pressure causes epidural veins engorgement and a decreased subarachnoid space and CSF volume. • There is increased local anesthetic diffusion across the membranes due to decrease in serum bicarbonate and elevated CSF pH. • There is increased sensitivity of the nerves to local anesthetics due to elevated progesterone levels.
Old age	• There is decreased leakage of local anesthetic from intervertebral foramina. • There is decreased compliance of subarachnoid space. • There is increased sensitivity to local anesthetics in elderly.

Epidural Anesthesia

- The local anesthetic is injected by **Tuohy's needle** into the epidural space bounded by **ligamentum flavum posteriorly and dura mater anteriorly**. It can be performed at cervical, thoracic, lumbar and caudal regions.
- Epidural anesthesia requires more expertise as there is no confirmatory CSF through lumbar puncture needle in case of spinal anesthesia.
- It is preferred for treatment of postoperative pain, chronic cancer pain, labor analgesia etc. Lidocaine and bupivacaine are most commonly used local anesthetics.
- It is the anesthesia of choice in **preeclampsia patients planned for cesarean section.**
- **Caudal block** is a type of epidural anesthesia used in **children** for perineal, anal, rectal, genital and urethral surgeries. Child is positioned in left lateral decubitus position and after sacral hiatus is identified a Tuohy's needle is inserted at an angle of 45 degrees to sacrum till it enters the caudal space.
- The important factors deciding the level of epidural block are: Volume and dose of drug, age, pregnancy and level of injection.

Mnemonics

Factors Affecting Height of Block in Epidural Anesthesia–EPID

E : Elderly age
P : Pregnancy
I : Injection level
D : Dose and volume of drug

Note: Patient's position, weight and height are less important factors.

- The risk of **systemic toxicity is higher** with epidural anesthesia due to presence of rich venous plexus; for same reason the risk of **accidental intravascular injection is also high**.

Mnemonics

Contraindication of Spinal and Epidural Anesthesia–SHARP Injection

S : Stenotic valvular heart disease
H : Hypovolemia
A : Antiaggregant therapy
R : Raised ICP
P : Platelet count < 80,000
Injection: Infection at local site

Difference between Spinal and Epidural Anesthesia:

Spinal anesthesia	Epidural anesthesia
• Simple and cheap procedure	• Complex and costly procedure
• Rapid onset of action	• Delayed onset of action
• Reliable	• Less reliable
• Side effects like hypotension, headache etc.	• No hypotension and headache
• Limited duration of action	• Can be used for longer duration
• Higher concentration of LA used	• Lower concentration of LA used
• Lesser amount of LA required	• Large amount of LA required
• Good quality block	• Patchy block
• Lesser chances of intravascular injection and total spinal block	• High chances of intravascular injection and total spinal block
• Low failure chances	• High failure chances

Nerve Block Anesthesia

- To perform a nerve block anesthesia, the drug is injected around a nerve or nerve plexuses, but never into the nerve itself as it can cause severe pain and nerve damage.
- Most common nerve block anesthesia used clinically is **brachial plexus block** for surgical procedures on upper extremity and shoulders. The most common associated complication is **pneumothorax**.
- **Intercostal nerve block** is done for relaxation and anesthesia of abdominal wall and is used for post-operative analgesia and rib fractures. It is associated with maximum systemic absorption. The drug is injected in the **mid or posterior axillary line** at inferior border of rib. **Pneumothorax** is a complication that can be associated.
- **Cervical plexus block** is done for surgery in head and neck area.
- Sciatic and femoral nerve blocks are done for surgeries distal to knee.
- **Pudendal nerve block** can be used for procedures around perineum. For **vaginal delivery with forceps** and for episiotomy it is preferred; a trans vaginal approach is preferred taking **ischial spine** as anatomical land mark and then needle is passed through vaginal mucosa towards ischial spine and after passing through sacrospinous ligament drug is injected.
- Celiac plexus block is done **bilaterally** for treatment of abdominal pain associated with malignancy. The most common side effects associated are **hypotension** and **diarrhea**.

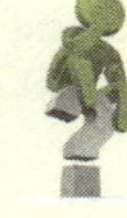

Image-based Questions

1. The distance shown in the picture is for assessment of:

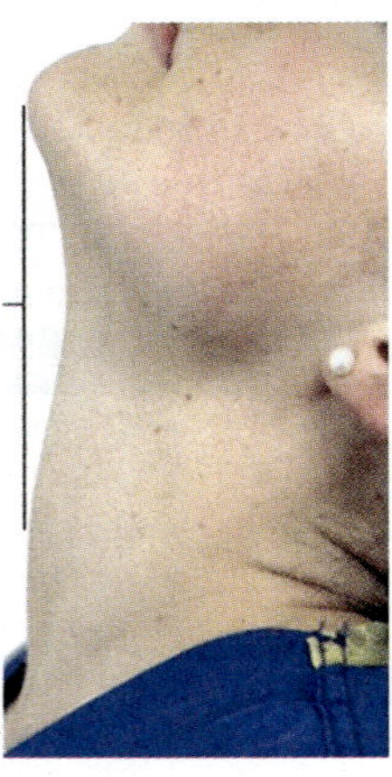

a. Intubation
b. Extubation
c. Bronchoscopy
d. LMA placement

2. The most important component of the anesthetic machine component given in the picture is?

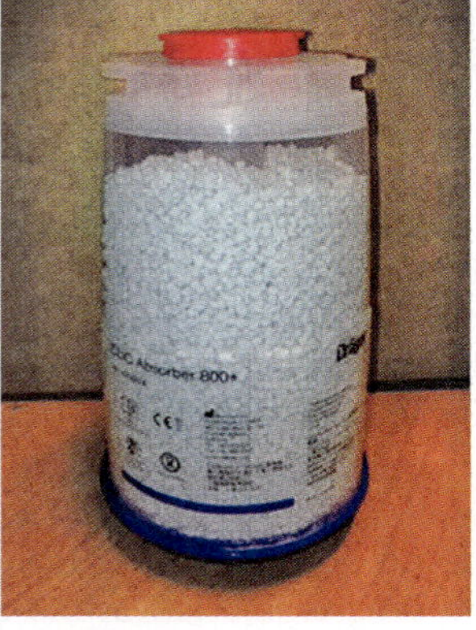

a. Calcium hydroxide
b. Potassium hydroxide
c. Sodium hydroxide
d. Water

3. The cylinder given in the picture is used to store:

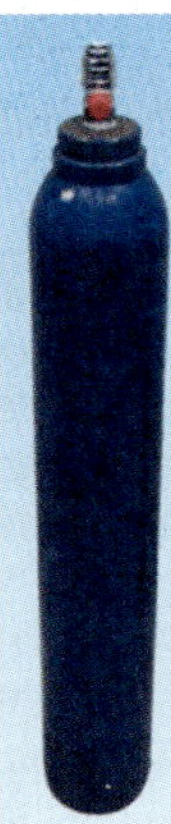

a. Air
b. Oxygen
c. Entonox
d. Nitrous oxide

4. The test done in the picture is to test the patency of:

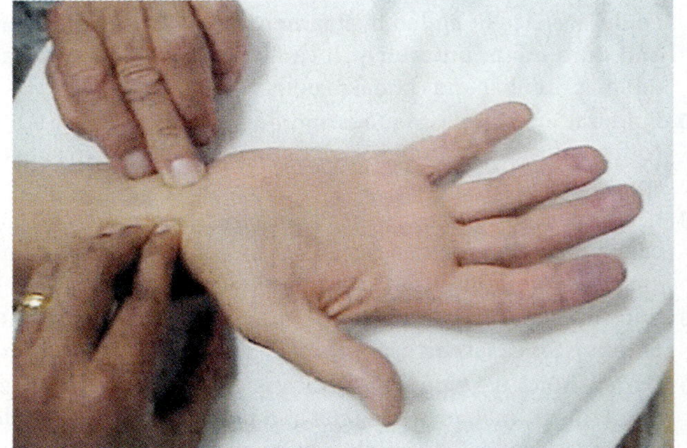

a. Ulnar artery
b. Radial artery
c. Ulnar vein
d. Radial vein

5. The bottle given in the picture is used to store:

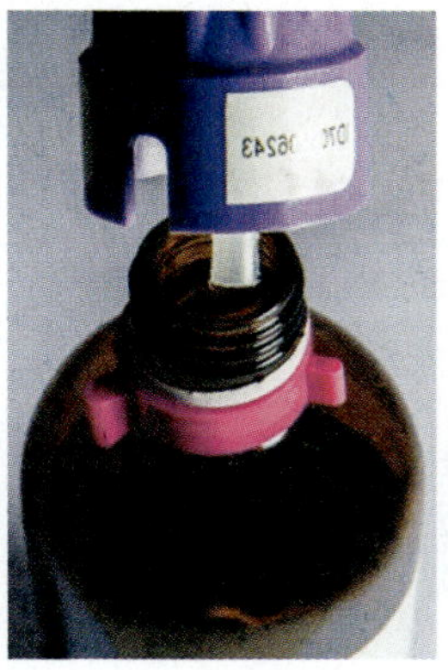

a. Isoflurane b. Enflurane
c. Halothane d. Desflurane

6. Which of the following drug is not used for the procedure given in the picture?

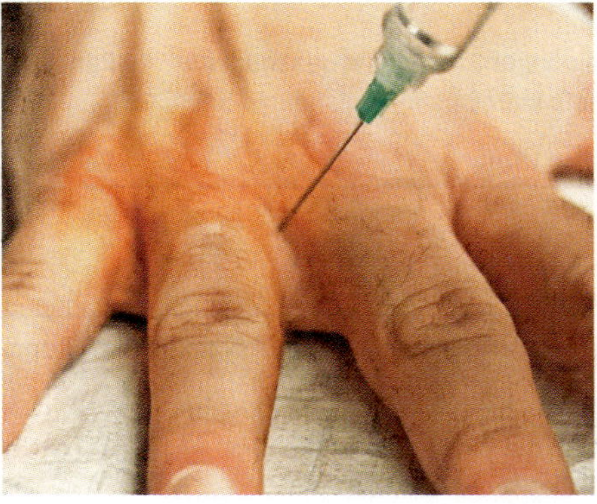

a. Lidocaine b. Tetracaine
c. Benzocaine d. Cocaine

7. The apparatus given in the picture is used for monitoring:

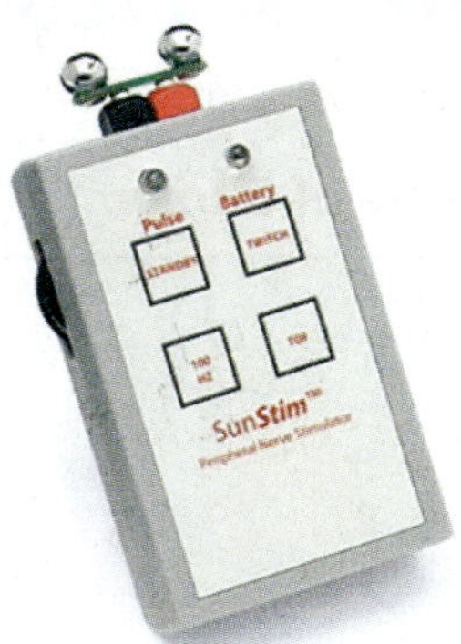

a. Pain b. Muscle relaxation
c. Nerve conduction d. Blood vessel patency

Answers with Explanations to Image-based Questions

1. Ans. (a) Intubation

❒ The distance given in the picture known as thyromental distance is for assessment of difficulty in intubation. A distance of less than 6.5 cm indicates difficult intubation.

2. Ans. (a) Calcium hydroxide

❒ The anesthetic equipment given in the picture is carbon dioxide absorbing canister, which has sodalime. The most important component of sodalime is calcium hydroxide.

3. Ans. (d) Nitrous oxide

❒ Blue colour cylinders are used to store nitrous oxide.

4. Ans. (a) Ulnar artery

❒ The test shown in the picture is called as Allen's test which is done to check patency of ulnar artery.

5. Ans. (c) Halothane

❒ Amber coloured bottles are used to store halothane.

6. Ans. (d) Cocaine

❒ Cocaine being a vasoconstrictor is contraindicated for block of organs with end arteries like fingers.

7. Ans. (b) Muscle relaxation

❒ The apparatus given in the picture is a peripheral nerve stimulator to monitor muscle relaxation.

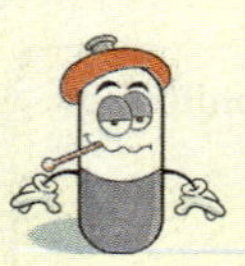

Annexures

Anesthetic Agents of Choice

• Cerebral protection • Raised ICT • Status epilepticus • Epilepsy • Hyperthyroidism • LSCS induction	Thiopental Sodium
• Electroconvulsive therapy	Methohexital
• Day care surgery • Total intravenous anesthesia (TIVA) • Sedation in ICU • Patients susceptible to malignant hyperthermia	Propofol
• Bronchial asthma induction agent • Status asthmaticus • Shock (hypovolemic, hemorrhagic, septic) • DIC • Cyanotic congenital heart diseases with right to left shunt • Hypothyroidism	Ketamine
• Old patients • Cardiovascular disorders (aneurysm, cardiomyopathy, CHF, CAD, aortic stenosis) • Altered hemodynamic states (splenic rupture, hemorrhagic shock)	Etomidate

Inhalational Agents of Choice

• Bronchial asthma maintenance agent • Tocolysis	Halothane
• Cardiac surgery • Controlled hypotension • LSCS Maintenance	Isoflurane
• Induction in infants, children and day care surgery • Myocardial ischemia • Neurosurgery	Sevoflurane
• Day care surgery maintenence • Renal failure • Obese	Desflurane

Muscle Relaxants of Choice

Muscle relaxant of choice for: • Intubation • Day care surgery	Succinylcholine
• NDMR of choice for intubation	Rocuronium
• NDMR of choice for day care surgery	Mivacurium
• Hepatic failure • Renal failure • Myasthenia gravis • Old age • New born • Obese	Atracurium
• Precurarization	Rocuronium
• Cardiac surgery	Vecuronium
• Cyanotic congenital heart diseases with right to left shunt	Pancuronium
• Bronchial asthma	Vecuronium

LA of Choice

• Epidural analgesia in labor	Bupivacaine and Ropivacaine
• IVRA or Bier's Block • Digoxin and MI induced VT and V.fibrillation	Lidocaine
• LA induced neurotoxicity	Benzodiazepines
• LA induced cardiotoxicity	Lipid emulsion
• Skin	2.5% lignocaine + 2.5% prilocaine (EMLA)
• Mucous membranes	Lidocaine Tetracaine Benzocaine
• Gastritis	Oxethazine
• History of malignant hyperthermia	Procaine

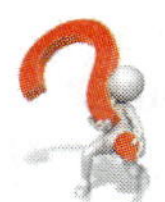

Multiple Choice Questions

HISTORY OF ANESTHESIA

1. General anesthetic effects of ether was demonstrated by *(Recent Question Dec 2016)*

a. Priestly
b. Morton
c. Liston
d. Simpson

2. Endotracheal intubation was first performed by: *(Recent Question Dec 2016)*

a. Joseph Dwyer
b. Friedrich
c. Ivan Magill
d. Trendlenberg

3. Cocaine was introduced as a local anesthetic by: *(Recent Question Dec 2016)*

a. Niemanm
b. Morton
c. Joseph Priestley
d. Griffith

4. The term anesthesia was first used by: *(Recent Question Dec 2016)*

a. Niemann
b. Morton
c. Joseph priestley
d. Dioscorides

5. Father of anesthesia *(Recent Question Dec 2016)*

a. Morton
b. Wallace
c. Augustus Bier
d. Holmes

6. Cocaine was first used as local anaesthetic by: *(Recent Question Dec 2016)*

a. Carl kollar
b. Horace wells
c. Morton
d. None

ANESTHETIC ASSESSMENT

7. What is the time for pre-oxygenation before ET tube insertion: *(AIIMS Nov 2017)*

a. 2 mins
b. 3 mins
c. 4 mins
d. 5 mins

8. Modified Mallampati grading is used in assessment of *(Recent Question 2018)*

a. Inspection of oral cavity
b. Assessing Airway
c. Tracheostomy
d. Intubation

9. Malampatti score is for: *(Recent Question 2017)*

a. Difficulty in intubation
b. Assessment of physical status
c. Risk assessment
d. Morbidity assessment

10. ASA grade in hypertensive patient which is under control by medications? *(AIIMS Nov 2012)*

a. ASA 1
b. ASA 2
c. ASA 3
d. ASA 4

11. For anesthesiology mild systemic disease included in ASA grade

a. 1
b. 2
c. 3
d. 4

12. ASA classification is done for

a. Status of the patient
b. Risk
c. Pain
d. Lung capacity

EQUIPMENTS IN ANESTHESIA

13. A patient is undergoing MRND for laryngeal malignancy; While dissecting the venous tributaries the surgeon elevated the internal jugular vein for ligation. Suddenly the patients EtCO2 dropped from 38 mmHg to 12 mmHg and the patient developed hypotension along with cardiac arrhythmia. Which of the following is most likely cause? *(AIIMS May 2018)*

a. Sympathetic over activity
b. Vagal stimulation
c. Venous air embolism
d. Carotid body stimulation

14. Murphy's eye is seen in *(Recent Question 2018)*

a. Macintosh laryngoscope
b. Endotracheal tube
c. LMA
d. Flexible laryngoscope

15. Anasthetic equipment that can provide 100 percent oxygen is: *(AIIMS Nov 2017)*

a. Venturi mask
b. Oxygen mask
c. Nasal canula
d. Face mask with reservoir

16. A patient on ventilator gets agitated and pulls out his ET tube. The patent's attendant rushes to you. What will be your next step. *(AIIMS Nov 2017)*

a. Sit the patient up and to chest physiotherapy
b. Give bag and mask ventilation and reassess spontaneous breathing
c. Face mask and 100% oxygen
d. Reintubate the patient under sedation

17. A sevofluorane vapourizer will deliver the accurate concenteration of an unknown anesthetic if the it has the same ____ as sevofluorane *(AIIMS May 2016)*

a. Blood gas partition co-efficient
b. Vapour pressure
c. Oil gas partition co-efficient
d. Molecular weight

18. A patient was in surgery when following Capnography picture was noticed. What is the next most appropriate step? *(AIIMS Nov 2015)*

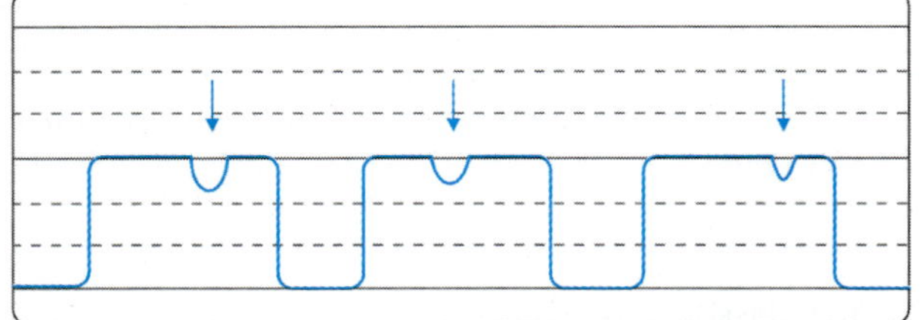

a. Administer skeletal muscle relaxant
b. Check for anaesthetic machine connections
c. Check endotracheal tube position
d. Change soda lime container

19. What is true about medical Oxygen cylinder? *(AIIMS Nov 2015)*
a. Black body white shoulder
b. Black body grey shoulder
c. Grey body white shoulder
d. Grey body black and white shoulder

20. Identify the instrument shown below (ANES PLATE 6 A):

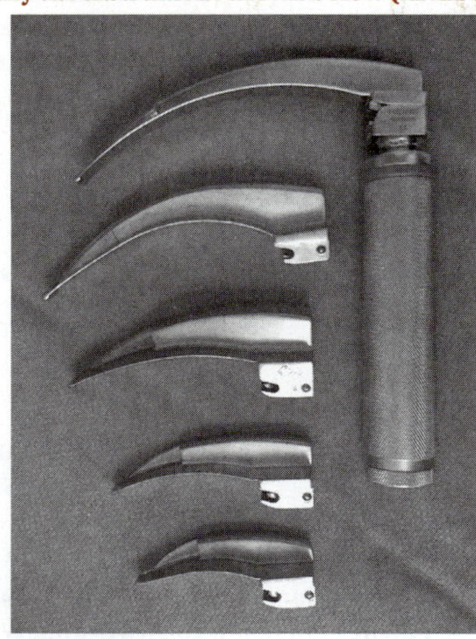

a. Straight blade high pressure laryngoscope
b. Curved blade laryngoscope
c. Macintosh laryngoscope
d. LMA

21. The names Bethune and Brethren are associated with which of the following monitoring devices? *(AIIMS Nov 2014)*
a. Plethysmography
b. End tidal capnography
c. Transesophageal echo
d. Precordial Doppler

22. All of the following are methods for improving oxygenation using a ventilator, EXCEPT: *(AIIMS Nov 2014)*
a. Extracorporeal membrane oxygenation (ECMO)
b. Low tidal volume high peep
c. Prone ventilation
d. High frequency ventilation

23. A patient of head injury is intubated and ventilated. Which would be the ideal mode of ventilation in him? *(AIIMS May 2014)*
a. CMV
b. CPAP
c. AMV
d. SIMV

24. A child is intubated for craniotomy. During surgery after 2 min, bellows of the anaesthetic machine collapse. What would be the next step? *(AIIMS Nov 2012)*
a. Ventilate Manually
b. Continue the operation
c. Use Bigger Size Tube
d. Increase Flow rate

25. An infant present with respiratory distress, was intubated. Which is the fastest and accurate method to confirm intubation? *(AIIMS Nov 2012)*
a. Capnography
b. Clinically by auscultation
c. Chest radiography
d. Airway pressure measurement

26. Which is the most important constituent in soda lime for reabsorption of CO_2 in a closed circuit? *(AIIMS May 2012)*
a. Sodium hydroxide
b. Barium hydroxide
c. Calcium hydroxide
d. Potassium hydroxide

27. In which of the following condition, flat capnogram is NOT seen? *(Recent Question 2018)*
a. Apnea
b. Complete laryngospasm
c. Foreign body obstructing the upper airway
d. None of the above

28. Peep (Positive end expiratory pressure) has the following effect *(Recent Question Dec 2016)*
a. Increased airway resistance
b. Increased FRC
c. Increase cardiac output
d. Increased renal blood flow

29. Composition of soda lime includes all except *(Recent Question Dec 2016)*
a. NaOH
b. KOH
c. $Ca(OH)_2$
d. $Mg(OH)_2$

30. Standard method to differentiate between endotracheal and esophageal intubation is *(Recent Question Dec 2016)*
a. End tidal CO_2
b. Chest X-rays
c. Auscultation
d. Partial pressure of O_2

31. VAT in mechanical ventilation stands for *(Recent Question Dec 2016)*
a. Ventilator associated trauma
b. Ventilator associated treatment
c. Ventilator associated tracheobronchitis
d. None of the above

32. DISS is used for *(Recent Question Dec 2016)*
a. Correct application of cylinder to anaesthesia machine
b. To provide analgesia
c. To monitor BP
d. To monitor CVP

33. In venturi mask oxygen concentration attained is *(Recent Question Dec 2016)*
a. 90%
b. 100%
c. 60%
d. 80%

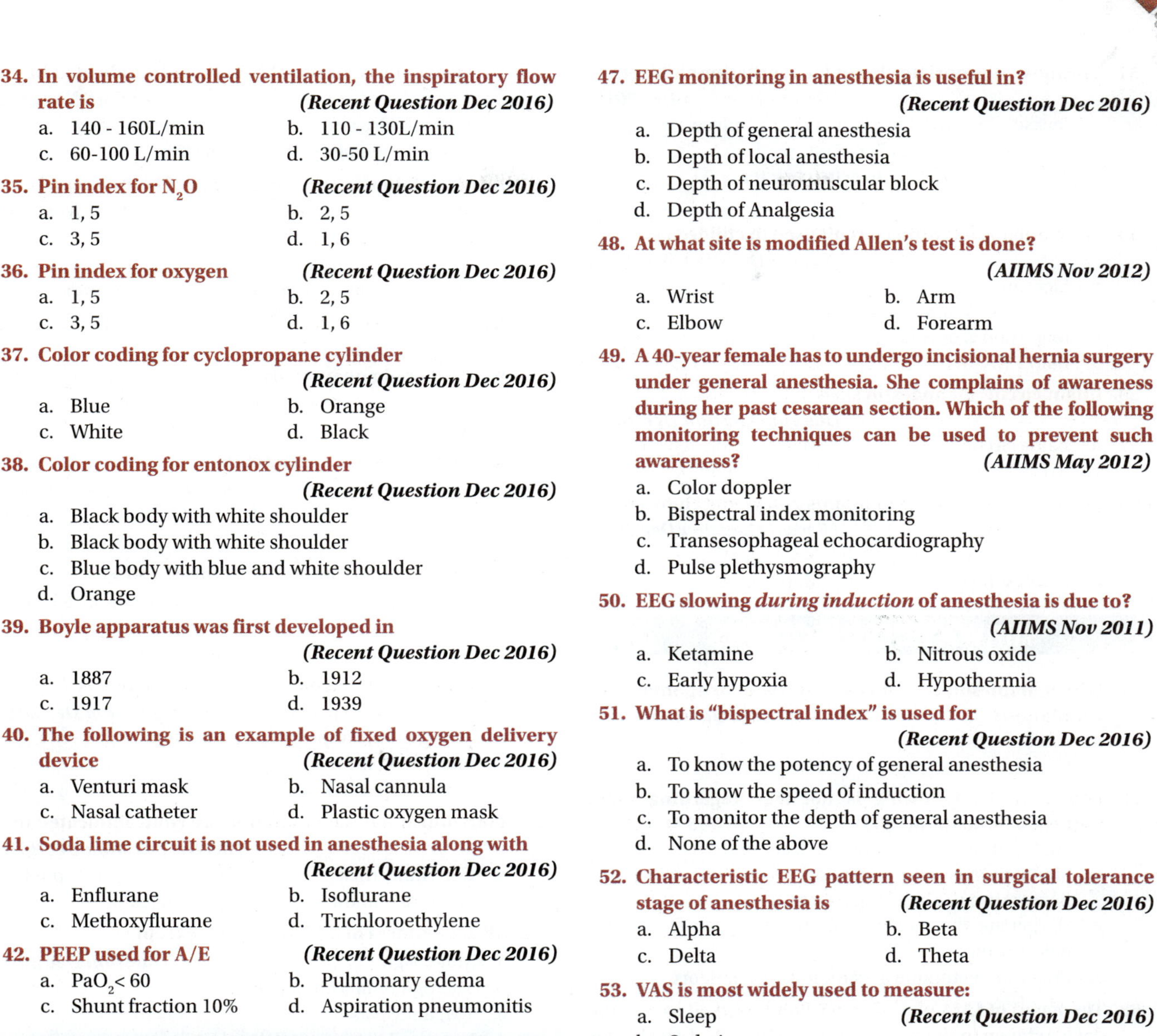

34. In volume controlled ventilation, the inspiratory flow rate is *(Recent Question Dec 2016)*
a. 140 - 160L/min b. 110 - 130L/min
c. 60-100 L/min d. 30-50 L/min

35. Pin index for N_2O *(Recent Question Dec 2016)*
a. 1, 5 b. 2, 5
c. 3, 5 d. 1, 6

36. Pin index for oxygen *(Recent Question Dec 2016)*
a. 1, 5 b. 2, 5
c. 3, 5 d. 1, 6

37. Color coding for cyclopropane cylinder *(Recent Question Dec 2016)*
a. Blue b. Orange
c. White d. Black

38. Color coding for entonox cylinder *(Recent Question Dec 2016)*
a. Black body with white shoulder
b. Black body with white shoulder
c. Blue body with blue and white shoulder
d. Orange

39. Boyle apparatus was first developed in *(Recent Question Dec 2016)*
a. 1887 b. 1912
c. 1917 d. 1939

40. The following is an example of fixed oxygen delivery device *(Recent Question Dec 2016)*
a. Venturi mask b. Nasal cannula
c. Nasal catheter d. Plastic oxygen mask

41. Soda lime circuit is not used in anesthesia along with *(Recent Question Dec 2016)*
a. Enflurane b. Isoflurane
c. Methoxyflurane d. Trichloroethylene

42. PEEP used for A/E *(Recent Question Dec 2016)*
a. $PaO_2 < 60$ b. Pulmonary edema
c. Shunt fraction 10% d. Aspiration pneumonitis

MONITORING IN ANESTHESIA

43. Which nerve is tested for adequacy of anesthesia *(Recent Question 2018)*
a. Median Nerve b. Ulnar Nerve
c. Radial nerve d. Mandibular nerve

44. Ideal site for measuring temperature during anesthesia? *(Recent Question Dec 2016)*
a. Rectum b. Tympanic membrane
c. Pulmonary artery d. Lower end of oesophagus

45. At supra MAC concentrations, anesthetics lead to shift of EEG wave from? *(Recent Question Dec 2016)*
a. Alpha to theta waves b. Theta to delta waves
c. Delta to theta waves d. Theta to delta waves

46. All of the following is true about hypothermia in anaesthesia? *(Recent Question Dec 2016)*
a. Occurs in all patients irrespective of the type of anesthesia
b. Can be prevented by administration of warm fluids
c. Is beneficial to the patient
d. The most common mechanism of heat loss is conduction

47. EEG monitoring in anesthesia is useful in? *(Recent Question Dec 2016)*
a. Depth of general anesthesia
b. Depth of local anesthesia
c. Depth of neuromuscular block
d. Depth of Analgesia

48. At what site is modified Allen's test is done? *(AIIMS Nov 2012)*
a. Wrist b. Arm
c. Elbow d. Forearm

49. A 40-year female has to undergo incisional hernia surgery under general anesthesia. She complains of awareness during her past cesarean section. Which of the following monitoring techniques can be used to prevent such awareness? *(AIIMS May 2012)*
a. Color doppler
b. Bispectral index monitoring
c. Transesophageal echocardiography
d. Pulse plethysmography

50. EEG slowing *during induction* of anesthesia is due to? *(AIIMS Nov 2011)*
a. Ketamine b. Nitrous oxide
c. Early hypoxia d. Hypothermia

51. What is "bispectral index" is used for *(Recent Question Dec 2016)*
a. To know the potency of general anesthesia
b. To know the speed of induction
c. To monitor the depth of general anesthesia
d. None of the above

52. Characteristic EEG pattern seen in surgical tolerance stage of anesthesia is *(Recent Question Dec 2016)*
a. Alpha b. Beta
c. Delta d. Theta

53. VAS is most widely used to measure: *(Recent Question Dec 2016)*
a. Sleep
b. Sedation
c. Pain intensity
d. Depth of anesthesia

54. Pulse oximetry monitors *(Recent Question Dec 2016)*
a. Oxygen saturation of hemoglobin
b. Oxygen content of blood
c. Pulse pressure
d. Oxygen partial pressure

BREATHING CIRCUITS

55. Which of the following is the circuit of choice for spontaneous ventilations? *(AIIMS Nov 2014)*
a. Mapleson B b. Mapleson C
c. Mapleson D d. Mapleson A

56. Most effective circuit in spontaneous anesthesia is *(Recent Question 2018)*
a. Mapleson A
b. Mapleson B
c. Mapleson C
d. Mapleson D

57. The most appropriate circuit for ventilating children *(Recent Question Dec 2016)*
a. Jackson Rees modification of ayre's T piece
b. Mapleson A or Magill's circuit
c. Mapleson C or water to & fro canister
d. Brain's circuit

58. Spontaneous breathing circuit used in children is *(Recent Question Dec 2016)*
a. Jackson Rees modification of Ayre's T piece
b. Mapleson A or Magill's circuit
c. Mapleson C or water's to & fro canister
d. Bain's circuit

59. Infant circuit for anaesthesia is *(Recent Question Dec 2016)*
a. Bains circuit b. Magill circuit
c. Ayers T piece d. Waters circuit

60. Mapleson circuit used in infants and young children: *(Recent Question Dec 2016)*
a. Mapleson A b. Mapleson C
c. Mapleson D d. Mapleson E

AIRWAY CONNECTIONS

61. Which Mapleson circuit is appropriate for spontaneous ventilation? *(Recent Question 2017)*
a. A b. B
c. C d. D

62. Which of the following is not true regarding rapid sequence intubation(RSI) *(AIIMS May 2016)*
a. High volume low pressure cuffs are preferred
b. Simultaneous administration of an induction and neuromuscular blocking agents
c. Oxygenate the patient with 100% oxygen for 3 mins before intubation
d. Preferred technique in cardiac arrest patients

63. Tip of cuff of LMA placed over? Point marked as a in the device shown in the picture is placed over? *(AIIMS Nov 2015)*

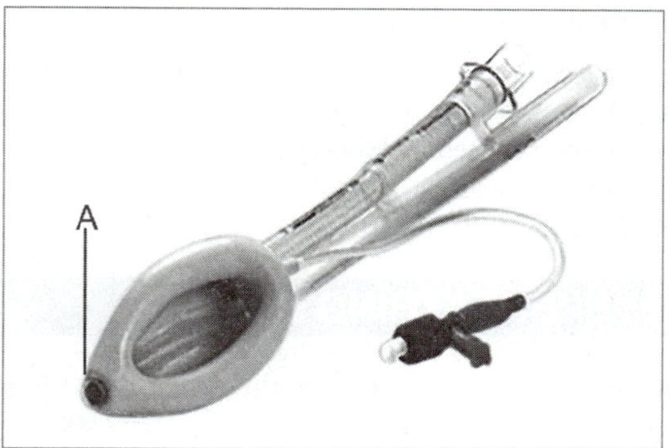

a. Above oesophagus b. Above epiglottis
c. Above vocal cords d. Above thyroid cartilage

64. A What is the appropriate size of LMA for an average adult patient weighing 50 kg is? *(AIIMS May 2014)*
a. 2.5 b. 3.0
c. 4.0 d. 5.0

65. Laryngeal mask airway (LMA) is contraindicated in *(AIIMS Nov 2012)*
a. Difficult airways b. Ocular surgeries
c. Pregnant female d. In CPR

66. All of the following are advantages of LMA except
a. More reliable than face mask *(AIIMS Nov 2012)*
b. Prevent aspiration
c. Alternative to Endotracheal intubation
d. Does not require laryngoscope & visualization

67. Laryngeal mask airway is used for *(AIIMS Nov 2012)*
a. Airway maintenance
b. Cardiopulmonary resuscitation
c. Positive pressure ventilation
d. All of the above

68. Size of LMA used for 25 kg child is *(Recent Question Dec 2016)*
a. 1 b. 1.5
c. 2.5 d. 4

69. Contraindication for laryngeal mask airway is *(Recent Question Dec 2016)*
a. Empty stomach b. Hiatus hernia
c. Minor surgery d. Young age

70. Indication for blind nasotracheal intubation is
a. Uncooperative patient *(Recent Question Dec 2016)*
b. Ankylosis of temperomandibular joint
c. Fracture mandible
d. Cervical spondylosis

71. Both oral and nasal intubation are contraindicated in: *(Recent Question Dec 2016)*
a. CSF rhinorrhea b. Fracture cervical spine
c. Fracture mandible d. Short neck

72. All are features of difficult airway except
a. Miller sign *(Recent Question Dec 2016)*
b. Micrognathia with macroglossia
c. TMJ ankylosis
d. Increased thyromental distance

73. Blind nasal intubation is not indicated in *(Recent Question Dec 2016)*
a. Temporo mandibular joint ankylosis
b. Locked jaw
c. Neck contractures
d. Base of skull fracture

74. Most common indication for intubation *(Recent Question Dec 2016)*
a. To maintain airway patency during GA
b. Pneumothorax
c. To remove foreign bodies
d. Airway Aspiration

INTRAVENOUS ANESTHETIC AGENTS

75. Which of the following is given in induction of anaesthesia: *(AIIMS Nov 2017)*
a. Lorazepam b. Bupivacaine
c. Neostigmine d. Dexmeditomidine

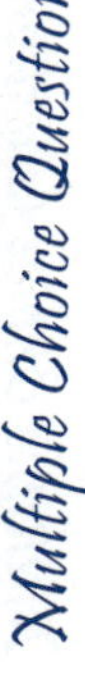

76. In a pediatric patient while surgery is being done, heart rate drops from 120 to 40 beats per minute. What is the immediate step: *(Recent Question 2017)*
a. Give atropine
b. Stop surgery
c. Lighten plane of anesthesia
d. Trans cutaneous Cardiac Pacing

77. A pregnant female presents with placenta previa, bleeding and systolic BP of 85 mm Hg, induction and maintenance of anesthesia for Cesarean section is done by? *(AIIMS Nov 2015)*
a. Ketamine followed by Intubation and GA
b. Propofol followed by intubation and GA
c. Thiopentone followed by muscle relaxant

78. Which anesthetic agent can cause pain on IV administration? *(AIIMS May 2015)*
a. Thiopentone b. Propofol
c. Ketamine d. Midazolam

79. Which of the following combinations can be used for day care surgery? *(AIIMS May 2015)*
a. Remifentanyl, midazolam, propofol
b. Fentanyl, midazolam, thiopentone sodium
c. Morphine, midazolam, propofol
d. Morphine, ketamine, diazepam

80. Which of the following agent is used in day care surgery? *(AIIMS Nov 2014)*
a. Propofol b. Ketamine
c. Diazepam d. Thiaopentone

81. Which of the following intravenous anesthetic agents is contraindicated in epileptic patients posted for general anesthesia? *(AIIMS May 2014, Nov 2013, May 2013)*
a. Ketamine b. Thiopentone
c. Propofol d. Midazolam

82. A patient presented with blunt trauma to the abdomen to the emergency department. His heart rate is 150/min and his BP is 80/50 mm Hg. He is scheduled to undergo an emergency laparotomy. Which of the following is the anaesthetic agent of choice? *(AIIMS May 2012)*
a. Thiopentone b. Midazolam
c. Ketamine d. Propofol

83. A 32-year old male with no past medical history is brought to the emergency department after being injured in a bomb blast. On examination he is suspected to have a splenic injury and is supposed to undergo an emergency laparotomy. Which of the following is the ideal anaesthetic agent of choice? *(AIIMS May 2012)*
a. Remifentanil b. Morphine
c. Etomidate d. Halothane

84. IV anesthetic agent that doesn't cause pain on intravenous injection is *(Recent Question 2019)*
a. Propofol b. Etomidate
c. Ketamine d. Thiopentone

85. IV anesthetic agent with cardiostimulant effect *(Recent Question 2019)*
a. Propofol b. Ketamine
c. Etomidate d. Thiopentone

86. Which of the following determines the speed of recovery from IV anesthetic? *(Recent Question 2018)*
a. Liver metabolism of drug
b. Protein binding of drug
c. Redistribution of the drug from sites in the CNS
d. Plasma clearance of the drug

87. Adverse effects of Etomidate: *(Recent Question 2018)*
a. Myoclonus & adrenal suppression
b. Adrenal suppression & Seizures
c. Seizures & Vomiting
d. Seizures & myoclonus

88. A patient with subdural hematoma has to undergo elbow surgery, best anesthetic agent among following is *(Recent Question Dec 2016)*
a. Ketamine b. Sevolurane
c. Thiopentone d. Succinylcholine

89. Ketamine is useful as an anesthetic agent in *(Recent Question Dec 2016)*
a. Ischemic heart disease
b. Intracranial hemorrhage
c. Hyperactive airways d. Glaucoma

90. Which of the following intravenous induction agent is the most suitable for day care surgery *(Recent Question Dec 2016)*
a. Morphine b. Ketamine
c. Propofol d. Diazepam

91. Which of the following anesthetic agent is a potent bronchodilator *(Recent Question Dec 2016)*
a. Propofol b. Ketamine
c. Thiopentone d. Methoxytone

92. Which of the following drugs produces dissociative anesthesia *(Recent Question Dec 2016)*
a. Ketamine b. Propofol
c. Thiopentone d. Enflurane

93. Thiopentone is contraindicated in *(Recent Question Dec 2016)*
a. Acute intermittent porphyria
b. Electro convulsive therapy
c. Sarcoidosis
d. Diabetic patients

94. Induction agent that may cause adrenal cortex suppression is *(Recent Question Dec 2016)*
a. Ketamine b. Etomidate
c. Propofol d. Thiopentione

95. Inducing agent of choice in shock *(Recent Question Dec 2016)*
a. Isoflurane b. Desflurane
c. Ketamine d. Thiopentone

96. Anaphylaxis is caused by *(Recent Question Dec 2016)*
a. N_2O b. Althesin
c. Halothane d. Propofol

97. Anesthesia with involuntary movements as a side effect is *(Recent Question Dec 2016)*
a. Ketamine b. Propofol
c. Halothane d. Isoflurane

98. Pain during injection occurs with all except *(Recent Question Dec 2016)*

a. Propofol b. Thiopentone
c. Ketamine d. Etomidate

99. Which of the following is safe in heart failure *(Recent Question Dec 2016)*

a. Etomidate b. Propofol
c. Thiopentone d. Ketamine

100. Benefit of ketamine is *(Recent Question Dec 2016)*

a. Causes decrease in BP b. Good analgesic action
c. Decrease ICT d. Decrease IOP

101. Induction agent of choice in asthma is *(Recent Question Dec 2016)*

a. Thiopentone b. Methoxyexitone
c. Ketamine d. Propofol

102. Induction agent of choice in DIC is *(Recent Question Dec 2016)*

a. Thiopentane b. Ketamine
c. Methohexitone d. Propofol

103. Intraoperative wheezing can be managed by *(Recent Question Dec 2016)*

a. Thiopental b. Propofol
c. Ketamine d. All of the above

104. Percentage of thiopentone used for induction is *(Recent Question Dec 2016)*

a. 0.5% b. 1.5%
c. 2.5% d. 4.5%

105. Anaesthetic agent used for maintenance in ICU is *(Recent Question Dec 2016)*

a. Thiopentane b. Propofol
c. Ketamine d. None of the above

106. The following drug is not safe in malignant hyperthermia *(Recent Question Dec 2016)*

a. Nitrous oxide
b. Pancuronium
c. Diazepam
d. Ketamine

107. Highly protein bound intravenous anesthetic agent *(Recent Question Dec 2016)*

a. Propofol b. Etomidate
c. Barbiturates d. Ketamine

108. Which of the following is true about thiopentone? *(Recent Question Dec 2016)*

a. Decreases cerebral metabolism and increases intracranial tension
b. Decreases cerebral metabolism and decreases intracranial tension
c. Increases cerebral metabolism and increases cerebral blood flow
d. Increases cerebral metabolism and decreases perfusion pressure

109. Hallucinations are seen with *(Recent Question Dec 2016)*

a. Propofol b. Sevoflurane
c. Ketamine d. Isoflurane

110. Bradycardia is caused by all except *(Recent Question Dec 2016)*

a. Halothane b. Isoflurane
c. Thiopentone d. Ketamine

111. Anesthetic of choice for status asthmaticus *(Recent Question Dec 2016)*

a. Ketamine b. Thiopentone
c. Ether d. Propofol

112. Anesthesia of choice in a child with cyanotic heart disease *(Recent Question Dec 2016)*

a. Propofol
b. Ketamine
c. Thiopentone
d. Sevoflurane

113. Intraocular pressure is increased by *(Recent Question Dec 2016)*

a. Thiopentone b. Halothane
c. Hexamethonium d. Ketamine

114. Intracranial pressure is increased by *(Recent Question Dec 2016)*

a. Barbiturate b. Ketamine
c. Etomidate d. Propofol

115. Which of the following intravenous induction cells agent suppresses steroid synthesis *(Recent Question Dec 2016)*

a. Thiopentone b. Propofol
c. Ketamine d. Etomidate

116. Pain on intravenous administration is caused by *(Recent Question Dec 2016)*

a. Propofol b. Etomidate
c. Methohexitone d. All the above

117. Ketamine is the preferred anaesthetic in the following cases except *(Recent Question Dec 2016)*

a. Hypertension
b. Trauma cases that have bled significantly
c. Burn dressing
d. Short operations on asthmatics

118. Structural analogue of phencyclidine? *(Recent Question Dec 2016)*

a. Propofol b. Etomidate
c. Ketamine d. Thiopentone

INHALATIONAL ANESTHETIC AGENTS

119. The correct relation of age and MAC requirements are represented correctly in which of the following *(AIIMS May 2016)*

a. Neonates> adults > infants
b. Infants >neonates > adults
c. Infants >adults>neonates
d. Adults>infants>neonates

120. Which of the following drugs does not affect absorption and secretion of cerebrospinal fluid? *(AIIMS May 2014)*

a. Halothane
b. Nitrous oxide
c. Ketamine
d. Thiopentone sodium

121. Induction of inhalational agent is faster with which of the following? ***(AIIMS Nov 2013)***
a. Agent with high blood gas solubility
b. Combined with nitrous oxide
c. Person with increased residual volume
d. Right to left shunt

122. A patient posted for surgery has raised intracranial tension. Which of the following anesthetics would be preferred in him? ***(AIIMS May 2013)***
a. Halothane b. Isoflurane
c. Sevoflurane d. Desflurane

123. Most potent analgesic agent among following? ***(AIIMS Nov 2012)***
a. Nitrous oxide b. Nitric oxide
c. CO_2 d. Oxygen

124. Which of the following is not true about xenon anaesthesia? ***(AIIMS Nov 2011)***
a. Non explosive
b. Minimal cardiovascular side effects
c. Slow induction and slow recovery
d. Low blood gas solubility

125. Most respiratory irritant anesthetic drug ***(Recent Question 2019)***
a. Desflurane b. Sevoflurane
c. Halothane d. Enflurane

126. Anesthesia of choice for induction in children among the following is: ***(Recent Question 2018)***
a. Desflurane b. Halothane
c. Sevoflurane d. Isoflurane

127. Which of the following inhalational agent is the best uterine relaxant? ***(Recent Question Dec 2016)***
a. Halothane b. Isoflurane
c. Sevoflurane d. Desflurane

128. Most potent bronchodilator among inhalational anesthetic agents is ***(Recent Question Dec 2016)***
a. Isoflurane b. Sevoflurane
c. Halothane d. Desflurane

129. Potency of inhalational anesthetic agent is measured by ***(Recent Question Dec 2016)***
a. Minimum alveolar concentration
b. Diffusion coefficient
c. Dead space concentration
d. Alveolar blood concentration

130. Which anesthetic gas was used by WTG Morton in his experiment ***(Recent Question Dec 2016)***
a. Nitrous oxide b. Ammonia
c. Diethyl ether d. Trichloroethylene

131. Blood: Gas (B:G) partition coefficient is a measure of ***(Recent Question Dec 2016)***
a. Potency of anaesthetic agent
b. Speed of induction and recovery
c. Lipid solubility of agent
d. None

132. Hepatotoxic agent is: ***(Recent Question Dec 2016)***
a. Halothane b. Ketamine
c. N_2O d. Ether

133. All inhalational anesthetics cause uterine relaxation except for ***(Recent Question Dec 2016)***
a. Halothane b. Sevofluorane
c. Desfluorane d. Nitrous oxide

134. Following is the most severe adverse effect of halothane ***(Recent Question Dec 2016)***
a. Asthma b. Hepatitis
c. Tachycardia d. Hypertension

135. 5 minutes before recovery from anesthesia, nitrous oxide is removed and 100% oxygen is administered to the patient to prevent ***(Recent Question Dec 2016)***
a. Diffusion hypoxia b. Second gas effect
c. Hyperoxia d. Bronchospasm

136. Second gas effect is seen with ***(Recent Question Dec 2016)***
a. Ether b. Nitrous oxide
c. Desflurane d. Sevoflurane

137. Gas cylinder with single pin index ***(Recent Question Dec 2016)***
a. Oxygen b. Air
c. Nitrogen d. Entonox

138. Which of the following is nephrotoxic ***(Recent Question Dec 2016)***
a. Halothane b. Methoxyflurane
c. Ether d. Cyclopropane

139. Malignant hyperthermia is caused by ***(Recent Question Dec 2016)***
a. Succinycholine + halothane
b. Propranolol
c. Lidocaine
d. Bupivacaine

140. Inhalation agent of choice in children ***(Recent Question Dec 2016)***
a. Methoxyfulrane b. Sevoflurane
c. Desflurane d. Isoflurane

141. Guedels stages of anaesthesia is seen classically with ***(Recent Question Dec 2016)***
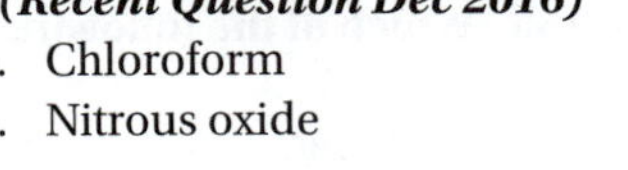
a. Ether b. Chloroform
c. Morphine d. Nitrous oxide

142. Coronary steal syndrome is associated with ***(Recent Question Dec 2016)***
a. Desflurane b. Sevoflurane
c. Isoflurane d. Halothane

143. Which of the following inhalational agent is contraindicated in renal disease ***(Recent Question Dec 2016)***
a. Desflurane b. Isoflurane
c. Methoxyflurane d. Halothane

144. MAC of desflurane is ***(Recent Question Dec 2016)***
a. 1.15 b. 2
c. 4 d. 6

145. Diffusion hypoxia seen during ***(Recent Question Dec 2016)***
a. Induction of anesthesia b. Reversal of anesthesia
c. Post operative period d. None of the above

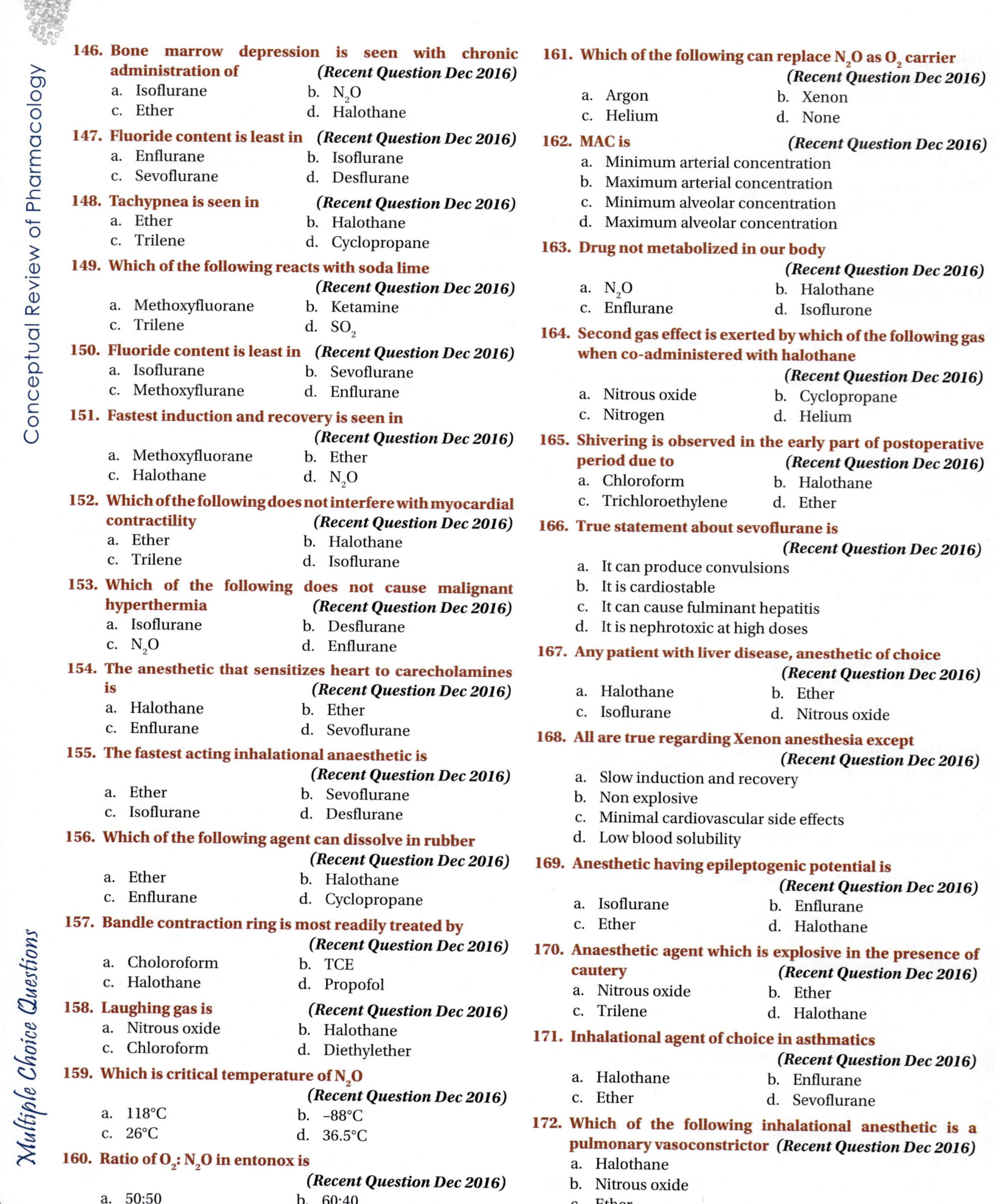

146. Bone marrow depression is seen with chronic administration of *(Recent Question Dec 2016)*
a. Isoflurane b. N_2O
c. Ether d. Halothane

147. Fluoride content is least in *(Recent Question Dec 2016)*
a. Enflurane b. Isoflurane
c. Sevoflurane d. Desflurane

148. Tachypnea is seen in *(Recent Question Dec 2016)*
a. Ether b. Halothane
c. Trilene d. Cyclopropane

149. Which of the following reacts with soda lime *(Recent Question Dec 2016)*
a. Methoxyfluorane b. Ketamine
c. Trilene d. SO_2

150. Fluoride content is least in *(Recent Question Dec 2016)*
a. Isoflurane b. Sevoflurane
c. Methoxyflurane d. Enflurane

151. Fastest induction and recovery is seen in *(Recent Question Dec 2016)*
a. Methoxyfluorane b. Ether
c. Halothane d. N_2O

152. Which of the following does not interfere with myocardial contractility *(Recent Question Dec 2016)*
a. Ether b. Halothane
c. Trilene d. Isoflurane

153. Which of the following does not cause malignant hyperthermia *(Recent Question Dec 2016)*
a. Isoflurane b. Desflurane
c. N_2O d. Enflurane

154. The anesthetic that sensitizes heart to carecholamines is *(Recent Question Dec 2016)*
a. Halothane b. Ether
c. Enflurane d. Sevoflurane

155. The fastest acting inhalational anaesthetic is *(Recent Question Dec 2016)*
a. Ether b. Sevoflurane
c. Isoflurane d. Desflurane

156. Which of the following agent can dissolve in rubber *(Recent Question Dec 2016)*
a. Ether b. Halothane
c. Enflurane d. Cyclopropane

157. Bandle contraction ring is most readily treated by *(Recent Question Dec 2016)*
a. Choloroform b. TCE
c. Halothane d. Propofol

158. Laughing gas is *(Recent Question Dec 2016)*
a. Nitrous oxide b. Halothane
c. Chloroform d. Diethylether

159. Which is critical temperature of N_2O *(Recent Question Dec 2016)*
a. 118°C b. –88°C
c. 26°C d. 36.5°C

160. Ratio of O_2: N_2O in entonox is *(Recent Question Dec 2016)*
a. 50:50 b. 60:40
c. 40:60 d. 25:75

161. Which of the following can replace N_2O as O_2 carrier *(Recent Question Dec 2016)*
a. Argon b. Xenon
c. Helium d. None

162. MAC is *(Recent Question Dec 2016)*
a. Minimum arterial concentration
b. Maximum arterial concentration
c. Minimum alveolar concentration
d. Maximum alveolar concentration

163. Drug not metabolized in our body *(Recent Question Dec 2016)*
a. N_2O b. Halothane
c. Enflurane d. Isoflurone

164. Second gas effect is exerted by which of the following gas when co-administered with halothane *(Recent Question Dec 2016)*
a. Nitrous oxide b. Cyclopropane
c. Nitrogen d. Helium

165. Shivering is observed in the early part of postoperative period due to *(Recent Question Dec 2016)*
a. Chloroform b. Halothane
c. Trichloroethylene d. Ether

166. True statement about sevoflurane is *(Recent Question Dec 2016)*
a. It can produce convulsions
b. It is cardiostable
c. It can cause fulminant hepatitis
d. It is nephrotoxic at high doses

167. Any patient with liver disease, anesthetic of choice *(Recent Question Dec 2016)*
a. Halothane b. Ether
c. Isoflurane d. Nitrous oxide

168. All are true regarding Xenon anesthesia except *(Recent Question Dec 2016)*
a. Slow induction and recovery
b. Non explosive
c. Minimal cardiovascular side effects
d. Low blood solubility

169. Anesthetic having epileptogenic potential is *(Recent Question Dec 2016)*
a. Isoflurane b. Enflurane
c. Ether d. Halothane

170. Anaesthetic agent which is explosive in the presence of cautery *(Recent Question Dec 2016)*
a. Nitrous oxide b. Ether
c. Trilene d. Halothane

171. Inhalational agent of choice in asthmatics *(Recent Question Dec 2016)*
a. Halothane b. Enflurane
c. Ether d. Sevoflurane

172. Which of the following inhalational anesthetic is a pulmonary vasoconstrictor *(Recent Question Dec 2016)*
a. Halothane
b. Nitrous oxide
c. Ether
d. Sevoflurane

173. **Inhalational agent associated with maximum nephrotoxicity** ***(Recent Question Dec 2016)***
a. Halothane b. Enflurane
c. Methoxyflurane d. Isoflurane

174. **The following inhalation anaesthetic should be avoided in middle ear surgery** ***(Recent Question Dec 2016)***
a. Halothane b. Nitrous oxide
c. Ether d. Isoflurane

175. **High output renal failure is caused by** ***(Recent Question Dec 2016)***
a. Methoxyflurane b. Ether
c. Ketamine d. Halothane

176. **MAC is least with** ***(Recent Question Dec 2016)***
a. Isoflurane b. Halothane
c. Sevoflurane d. Desflurane

177. **All are true about Halothane except:** ***(Recent Question Dec 2016)***
a. Excellent anaesthetic, poor analgesic
b. Preferred in hypotensive surgeries
c. Lowers ICT, hence preferred in CNS surgeries
d. Causes centrilobular necrosis of liver

178. **Which among the following inhalational anesthetic agent is least hepatotoxic?** ***(Recent Question Dec 2016)***
a. Enflurane b. Halothane
c. Isoflurane d. Ether

MUSCLE RELAXANTS

179. **Adavantage of cisatracurium over atracurium is** ***(Recent Question 2019)***
a. Short duration b. Doesn't release histamine
c. Less potent d. Faster onset of action

180. **Mechanism of action of tubocurare is** ***(Recent Question 2019, 2018)***
a. Blocks Ach synthesis
b. Blocks Ach release
c. Blocks Ach receptors
d. Depolarizes postsynaptic membrane

181. **Which will help in rapid recovery from rocuronium-** ***(Recent Question 2018)***
a. Neostigmine b. Sugammadex
c. Edrophonium d. Atropine

182. **What is the mechanism of action of d-tubocurare:** ***(Recent Question 2017)***
a. Depolarization
b. Decreased release of acetylcholine
c. Inhibition of acetylcholine receptors
d. Inhibition of ACHE

183. **Which nerve is most commonly used to assess the effect of muscle relaxants in anesthesia:** ***(Recent Question 2017)***
a. Ulnar b. Radial
c. Median d. Axillary

184. **All of the following act on neuromuscular junction except** ***(AIIMS May 2016)***
a. Pipercurium b. Dantrolene sodium
c. Succinylcholine d. Mivacurium

185. **Allergic reactions occurring during the immediate peri-operative period is due to administration of** ***(AIIMS May 2016)***
a. Local anaesthetics b. Neuromuscular blockers
c. Opiods d. Induction agents

186. **A drug that undergoes Hoffmann elimination is** ***(AIIMS May 2016)***
a. Atracurium b. Vecuronium
c. Pancuronium d. Mivacurium

187. **Which of the following muscle relaxant can be used in a patient with high bilirubin of 6 mg/ dL and serum Creatinine of 4.5mg/dL?** ***(AIIMS May 2015)***
a. Vecuronium b. Atracurium
c. Pancuronium d. Mivacurium

188. **An eye surgery was performed using propofol as the intravenous anaesthetic agent and succinylcholine as the muscle relaxant. Recovery from anaesthesia was uneventful. However the patient complains of pain in the muscles. Which of the following is the likely reason for this?** ***(AIIMS Nov 2014)***
a. Propofol b. Succinylcholine
c. Muscle infarction d. None of the above

189. **Which muscle is first affected by Tubocurare ?** ***(AIIMS Nov 2013)***
a. Head and neck b. Limbs
c. Respiratory muscles d. Abdominal muscles

190. **Which of the following drug causes malignant hyperthermia?** ***(AIIMS Nov 2013)***
a. Cisatracurium b. Suxamethonium
c. Propofol d. Thiopentone

191. **Suxamethonium is available as a clear, colourless liquid. What is the shelf life of suxamethonium?** ***(AIIMS May 2013)***
a. 6 months b. 1 year
c. 2 year d. 6 year

192. **Dose of which neuromuscular blocking agent in an obese female requires calculation of total body weight instead of ideal body weight?** ***(AIIMS Nov 2012)***
a. Atracurium b. Vecuronium
c. Pancuronium d. Rocuronium

193. **Kinemyography is used for?** ***(AIIMS Nov 2012)***
a. Monitoring neuromuscular function
b. Monitoring muscle spindle activity
c. Monitoring exercise capacity
d. Monitoring depth of anesthesia

194. **All of the following is true in scoline apnea, EXCEPT:** ***(AIIMS May 2012)***
a. It is due to succinylcholine
b. It can be inherited
c. Patients usually do not die of scoline apnea if they are properly managed
d. It occurs due to deficiency of cholinesterase

195. **Cis-atracurium is preferred over atracurium due to advantage of?** ***(AIIMS Nov 2011)***
a. Rapid onset b. Short duration of action
c. No histamine release d. Less cardiodepressant

196. **Laudanosine is metabolite of?** ***(AIIMS Nov 2011)***
a. Cisatracurium b. Atracurium
c. Pancuronium d. Gallamine

197. Suxamethonium acts through which channels *(Recent Question Dec 2016)*
a. Sodium channels b. Potassium channels
c. Calcium channels d. Chloride channels

198. Which drug can be eliminated by nonenzymatic degradation *(Recent Question Dec 2016)*
a. Atracurim b. Pancuronium
c. Mivacurium d. Dexacurium

199. Only available depolarizing muscle relaxant is *(Recent Question Dec 2016)*
a. Decamethonium b. Suxamethonium
c. Mivacurium d. None

200. Which of the following regarding succinylcholine is true *(Recent Question Dec 2016)*
a. Produces bradycardia
b. Long acting
c. Safe to use in head injury
d. Non-depolarizing muscle relaxant

201. In bronchial asthma patient, muscle relaxant safe to use is: *(Recent Question Dec 2016)*
a. Mivacurium b. Atracurium
c. Suxamethonium d. Pancuronium

202. Non depolarizing blocking agent among the following is *(Recent Question Dec 2016)*
a. Suxamethonium b. Decamethonium
c. Pancuronium d. Beclofen

203. Which of the following is directly acting skeletal muscle relaxant *(Recent Question Dec 2016)*
a. Dantrolene b. Suxamethonium
c. Pancuronium d. Atracurium

204. Shortest acting muscle relaxant *(Recent Question Dec 2016)*
a. Pancuronium b. Atracurium
c. Mivacurium d. Vecuronium

205. Post-operative muscle ache is caused by *(Recent Question Dec 2016)*
a. d-TC b. suxamethonium
c. Gallamine d. Pancuronium

206. Regarding mivacurium false is *(Recent Question Dec 2016)*
a. Hypertension
b. Increasing dose produces rapid onset of action
c. Bronchospasm
d. Flushing

207. Long acting non depolarizing competitive blocker is *(Recent Question Dec 2016)*
a. Doxacurium b. Rocuronium
c. Mivacurium d. Atracurium

208. Which neuromuscular blocker releases histamine *(Recent Question Dec 2016)*
a. Pancuronium b. Rocuronium
c. Vecuronium d. Atracurium

209. Which of the following is neither metabolized by liver nor by kidney *(Recent Question Dec 2016)*
a. Atracurium b. Pancuronium
c. Vecuronium d. Rocuronium

210. Muscle relaxant with ganglion blocker action is *(Recent Question Dec 2016)*
a. Pancuronium b. Trimethapan
c. Curare d. Halothane

211. Drug used for d-TC reveral is *(Recent Question Dec 2016)*
a. Atropine b. Atracurium
c. Diazepam d. Neostigmine

212. Receptor responsible for malignant hyperthermia *(Recent Question Dec 2016)*
a. Nicotinic receptor b. Muscarinic receptor
c. Ryanodine receptor d. NMDA receptor

213. Non depolarizing muscle relaxant, with chemical structure like a steroid *(Recent Question Dec 2016)*
a. Atracurium b. Mivacurium
c. Doxacurium d. Pancuronium

214. Skeletal muscle relaxant whose structure is not steroidal *(Recent Question Dec 2016)*
a. Rocuronium b. Pancuronium
c. Doxacurium d. Pipecuronium

215. Dantrolene acts by *(Recent Question Dec 2016)*
a. Inhibiting calcium release from smooth muscle cells
b. Inhibiting sodium release from smooth muscle cells
c. Inhibiting potassium release from smooth muscle cells
d. Increase calcium release from smooth muscle cells

216. Longest acting muscle relaxant *(Recent Question Dec 2016)*
a. Rocuranium b. Pipecuranium
c. Pancuranium d. Mivacurium

217. Muscle relaxant with fastest onset and intermittent duration of action *(Recent Question Dec 2016)*
a. Rocuronium b. d-tubocuranium
c. Gantacurium d. Pancuronium

218. Muscle relaxant excreted through kidney *(Recent Question Dec 2016)*
a. Rocuranium b. Pancuronium
c. Cis-atracurium d. Vecuronium

219. Baclofen is a *(Recent Question Dec 2016)*
a. Peripherally acting muscle relaxant
b. Both centrally and peripherally acting muscle relaxant
c. Directly acting muscle relaxant
d. Centrally acting muscle relaxant

220. Shortest acting neuromuscular blocker is *(Recent Question Dec 2016)*
a. Gallamine b. Mivacurium
c. Succinylcholine d. d- TC

221. Which one of the following drugs is not a long acting neuromuscular blocking agent? *(Recent Question Dec 2016)*
a. Doxacurium b. Mivacurium
c. Pancuronium d. Pipecuronium

222. Feature of depolarizing blockade *(Recent Question Dec 2016)*
a. Tetanic fade
b. Post tetanic potentiation
c. Progression to dual blockade
d. Antagonism by anticholinesterases

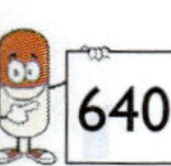

223. Laudanosine is a metabolite of *(Recent Question Dec 2016)*

a. Atracurium b. Cis-atracurium
c. Pancuronium d. Vecuronium

224. Which of the following drugs is hydrolyzed by a plasma esterase that is abnormally low in activity in about 1 in every 2500 humans?

a. Ethanol b. Rifampicin
c. Cimetidine d. Succinylcholine

225. Muscle relaxant safe in renal disease *(Recent Question Dec 2016)*

a. Doxacurium b. Pancuronium
c. Vecuronium d. Pipecuronium

226. Dibucaine number refers to *(Recent Question Dec 2016)*

a. Ach cholinesterase activity derangement
b. Potency of muscle relaxants
c. Potency of general anaesthetics
d. None

227. Dibucaine number of pseudocholinesterase *(Recent Question Dec 2016)*

a. 40 b. 60
c. 80 d. 100

228. Pseudocholinesterase eliminates *(Recent Question Dec 2016)*

a. Mivacurium b. Gallamine
c. Pancuronium d. Atracuronium

229. Most common muscle which is monitored during neuro-muscular blockade *(Recent Question Dec 2016)*

a. Levator palpebrae superioris
b. Masseter
c. Adductor pollicis
d. Brachioradialis

230. Sign which is helpful in making a pre-hyperthermic diagnosis of malignant hypertherrnia *(Recent Question Dec 2016)*

a. Metabolic acidosis b. Sinus tachycardia
c. Central cyanosis d. Masseter spasm

231. Which of the following is a skeletal muscle relaxant that acts as a central a_2 adrenergic agonist *(Recent Question Dec 2016)*

a. Tizanidine b. Brimoniodine
c. Chlorrnezanone d. Quinine

232. Which of the following skeletal muscle relaxants causes pain on injection? *(Recent Question Dec 2016)*

a. Succinylcholine b. Vecuronium
c. Rocuronium d. Pancuronium

PREMEDICATION

233. Which Anti-cholinergic drug is most commonly used pre anesthetic medication? *(AIIMS Nov 2015)*

a. Glycopyrrolate
b. Neostigmine
c. Propantheline
d. Atropine

234. Midazolam causes all EXCEPT: *(AIIMS May 2014)*

a. Anterograde amnesia
b. Retrograde amnesia
c. Causes tachyphylaxis during high dose infusions
d. Decreased cardiovascular effects as compared to propofo

235. Which of the following drugs is to treat postoperative shivering? *(Recent Question Dec 2016)*

a. Ondanestron b. Diclofenac sodium
c. Pethidine d. Paracetamol

236. Pre-anaesthetic medication is given to *(Recent Question Dec 2016)*

a. Reduce anxiety and fear
b. Reduction of secretion of saliva
c. To produce amnesia
d. All of the above

237. Which of the following agent causes muscle rigidity *(Recent Question Dec 2016)*

a. Fentanyl b. Halothane
c. Ketamine d. Droperidol

238. Which of the following cannot be given by epidural anaesthesia *(Recent Question Dec 2016)*

a. Morphine b. Remifentanil
c. Alfentanil d. Fentanyl

239. Least sedative narcotic is *(Recent Question Dec 2016)*

a. Morphine b. Codeine
c. Papaverine d. Noscapine

LOCAL ANESTHETICS

240. Which nerve fibre is least susceptible to local anesthetic: *(AIIMS Nov 2017)*

a. A-alpha type b. B type
c. C type d. A-delta type

241. All of the following are true regarding the procedure performed with the instrument shown below EXCEPT: *(AIIMS May 2017)*

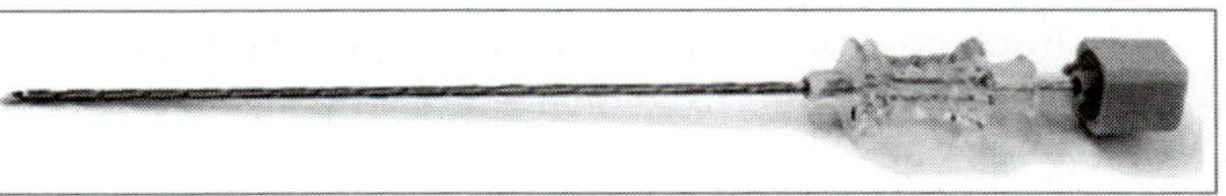

a. Absolutely contraindicated in coagulation disorder
b. Done in lateral recumbent position
c. Bevel of needle faces upwards
d. Breath holding not required

242. A patient is having preeclampsia is planned for cesarean section. Which is preferred anesthesia: *(Recent Question 2017)*

a. Spinal b. Epidural
c. Both spinal and epidural d. General

243. A 46-year-old male was given a subarachnoid block using 12 mg of bupivacaine (heavy). After 10 minutes of administration the BP dropped to 72/44 mm Hg and heart rate was 52/min. The level of sensory loss was T6. What is the reason for bradycardia in this patient *(AIIMS May 2016)*

a. Bezold-jarish reflex
b. Bainbridge reflex
c. Reverse Bainbridge reflex
d. Blockade of cardiac accelerator nerve fibres

244. The instrument shown below (MED PLATE 2 B) is used for which procedure? *(AIIMS Nov 2015)*

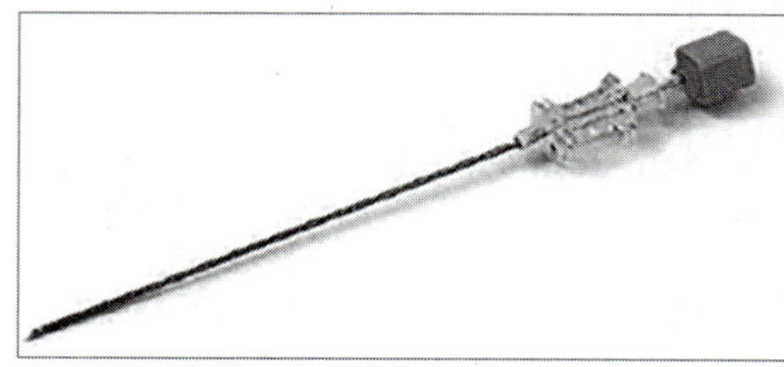

a. Bone marrow aspiration b. Lumbar puncture
c. Pleural biopsy d. Suction

245. Which structure, when pierced, causes First snap/ Resistance during epidural anesthesia?
a. Supra spinous ligament *(AIIMS Nov 2015)*
b. Inter-spinous ligament
c. Ligamentum flavum
d. Posterior longitudinal ligament

246. Sensory block for lower segment caesarian section is achieved at which level? *(AIIMS Nov 2013)*
a. T4 b. T6
c. T8 d. T10

247. All of the following are not a contraindication for neuraxial block EXCEPT: *(AIIMS Nov 2013)*
a. Platelet count < 50,000
b. Patient on clopidogrel
c. Local infection
d. Patient on antihypertensive medication

248. All of the following are effective strategies to decrease the risk of post dural puncture headache EXCEPT:
a. Use of small bore needle *(AIIMS Nov 2013)*
b. Use of atraumatic needle
c. Supplementation of fluids
d. Replacement of stylet prior to removal of needle

249. Lidocaine all are true EXCEPT: *(AIIMS Nov 2012)*
a. It acts on sodium channels in both active and inactive state
b. It is most cardiotoxic local anesthetic
c. It is given iv in cardiac arrhythmias
d. Extensive first pass metabolism

250. In a pregnant female, there is decreased requirement of the spinal anaesthetic agent because of all of the following EXCEPT: *(AIIMS May 2012)*
a. Exaggerated lumbar lordosis
b. Decreased volume of sub arachnoid space
c. Engorgement of epidural veins
d. Increased sensitivity of the nerves to anesthetic agent

251. What is the maximum dose of lignocaine with adrenaline for local blocks in ophthalmic surgeries?
a. 3mg/kg b. 5mg/kg *(AIIMS May 2012)*
c. 7mg/kg d. 10mg/kg

252. A 26 year old primigravida with severe rheumatic heart disease (MS with MR) is in early labour. For trial of normal labour, ideal intervention for labour analgesia is? *(AIIMS May 2012)*
a. Parenteral analgesia b. Neuraxial analgesia
c. Inhalational analgesia d. Spinal analgesia

253. Most cardiotoxic LA is *(Recent Question Dec 2016)*
a. Bupivacaine b. Ropivacaine
c. Prilocaine d. Etidocaine

254. In a patient with severe aortic stenosis which of the following anesthetic techniques is least preferred:
a. Propofol induction *(Recent Question 2018)*
b. Etomidate induction
c. Spinal anesthetic with 15 mg bupivacaine
d. Epidural anesthesia with 2%lidocaine

255. Anesthesia of choice for cesarean section in severe pre-eclampsia: *(Recent Question 2018)*
a. Spinal b. GA
c. Epidural d. Spinal + epidural

256. In majority of cases post spinal headache is initiated during *(Recent Question Dec 2016)*
a. One hour b. 48 hours
c. Seven days d. One month

257. Mucosal anesthesia is possible with all of the following local anesthetics, except *(Recent Question Dec 2016)*
a. Prilocaine
b. Lidocaine
c. Dyclonine (0.5% to 1.0%)
d. Hexylcaine

258. Intravenous regional anesthesia is used in *(Recent Question Dec 2016)*
a. PPS surgeries b. Upper limb surgeries
c. Lower limb surgeries d. Neurosurgeries

259. Longest acting local anesthetic agent is *(Recent Question Dec 2016)*
a. Procaine b. Lidocaine
c. Prilocaine d. Dibucaine

260. Local anesthetic act by *(Recent Question Dec 2016)*
a. Na^+ channel inhibition b. Ca^{++} channel inhibition
c. Mg^{++} channel inhibition d. K^+ channel inhibition

261. Contraindication to neuraxial block is *(Recent Question Dec 2016)*
a. Hypertension b. Renal disease
c. Clotting disorders d. Diabetes

262. Not included in neuraxial block *(Recent Question Dec 2016)*
a. Spinal block b. Epidural block
c. Bier's block d. Caudal block

263. Post dural puncture headache usually present with in *(Recent Question Dec 2016)*
a. 0-6 Hrs b. 6-12 Hrs
c. 12-72 Hrs d. 72-96 Hrs

264. Landmark for pudendal nerve block is *(Recent Question Dec 2016)*
a. Ischial tuberosity b. Iliac spine
c. Sacroiliac joint d. None of the above

265. Shortest acting local anaesthetics *(Recent Question Dec 2016)*
a. Lignocaine b. Bupivacaine
c. Etidocaine d. Chlorprocaine

266. Most common cause of maternal mortality in spinal anesthesia is ***(Recent Question Dec 2016)***

a. Allergy to local anesthesia
b. Nerve injury
c. High block
d. Hypotension

267. The afferent nerve fibres which are most sensitive to local anaesthetic belong to group ***(Recent Question Dec 2016)***

a. A
b. B
c. C
d. D

268. Shortest acting local anesthetic anesthetic agent is ***(Recent Question Dec 2016)***

a. Procaine
b. Lidocaine
c. Tetracaine
d. Bupivacaine

269. Cauda equine syndrome is associated with ***(Recent Question Dec 2016)***

a. Lidocaine
b. Halothane
c. N_2O
d. Ether

270. Local anaesthetic injected directly into the tissue ***(Recent Question Dec 2016)***

a. Infiltration anaesthesia
b. Nerve block
c. Field block
d. Bier's block

271. All are methods of regional anaesthesia except ***(Recent Question Dec 2016)***

a. Topical anaesthesia
b. Bier's block
c. Nerve block
d. Total intravenous anesthesia

272. Drug of choice in lignocaine toxicity ***(Recent Question Dec 2016)***

a. Bretylium
b. Amiodarone
c. Isoprenaline
d. Diazepam

273. Which of the following is NOT an amide ***(Recent Question Dec 2016)***

a. Lignocaine
b. Procaine
c. Mepivacaine
d. Dibucaine

274. All are surface anesthetics except ***(Recent Question Dec 2016)***

a. Lignocaine
b. Bupivacaine
c. Priloocaine
d. Cinchocaine

275. Best anesthesia for low forceps delivery ***(Recent Question Dec 2016)***

a. General anesthesia
b. Epidural block
c. Saddle block
d. Caudal block

276. Drug contraindicated for Bier's block ***(Recent Question Dec 2016)***

a. Lidocaine
b. Prilocaine
c. Dibucaine
d. Bupivacaine

277. In epidural anaesthesia drug injected ***(Recent Question Dec 2016)***

a. Outside the dura
b. Inside the duramater
c. Inside arachnoidmater
d. Inside piamater

278. Pudendal block is indicated in ***(Recent Question Dec 2016)***

a. Manual removal of placenta
b. Forceps delivery
c. IUCD insertion
d. Internal podalic version

279. Anatomical landmark for pudendal block is ***(Recent Question Dec 2016)***

a. Iliac crest
b. Iliac spine
c. Ischial spine
d. Iliac tubercle

280. Which of the following is used in coronary angiography technique ***(Recent Question Dec 2016)***

a. Local anesthesia
b. High thoracic epidural block
c. Caudal anesthesia
d. General anaesthesia

281. Commonest cranial nerve affected in spinal anaesthesia is ***(Recent Question Dec 2016)***

a. 2
b. 3
c. 4
d. 6

282. Concentration of bupivacine used in spinal anaesthesia is ***(Recent Question Dec 2016)***

a. 0.5%
b. 2%
c. 4%
d. 5%

283. Percentage of xylocaine used in spinal anaesthesia ***(Recent Question Dec 2016)***

a. 1%
b. 2%
c. 4%
d. 5%

284. Xylocaine in subarachnoid space has concentration ***(Recent Question Dec 2016)***

a. 1%
b. 2%
c. 3%
d. 5%

285. The best anesthetic agent for acute paronychia is ***(Recent Question Dec 2016)***

a. 1% xylocaine
b. 2% xylocaine
c. Ketamine
d. Xylocaine + adrenaline

286. Post spinal headache can last for ***(Recent Question Dec 2016)***

a. Upto 10 min
b. Upto 10 hours
c. 7 - 10 days
d. Upto 10 months

287. Epidural narcotic is preferred over epidural LA because ***(Recent Question Dec 2016)***

a. Less respiratory depression
b. Less dose is required
c. No motor paralysis
d. No retention of urine

288. Local anaesthetic causing methemoglobinemia ***(Recent Question Dec 2016)***

a. Procaine
b. Prilocaine
c. Etidocaine
d. Ropivacaine

289. LA with vasoconstrictor is contraindicated in ***(Recent Question Dec 2016)***

a. Digital block
b. Spinal block
c. Epidural block
d. Regional anaesthesia

290. Which of the following nerve fiber is most susceptible to local anesthetic ***(Recent Question Dec 2016)***

a. Aa
b. Ab
c. Aγ
d. C

291. Agent added to local anesthetics to speed the onset of action is ***(Recent Question Dec 2016)***

a. Methylparaben
b. Bicarbonate
c. EDTA
d. Adrenaline

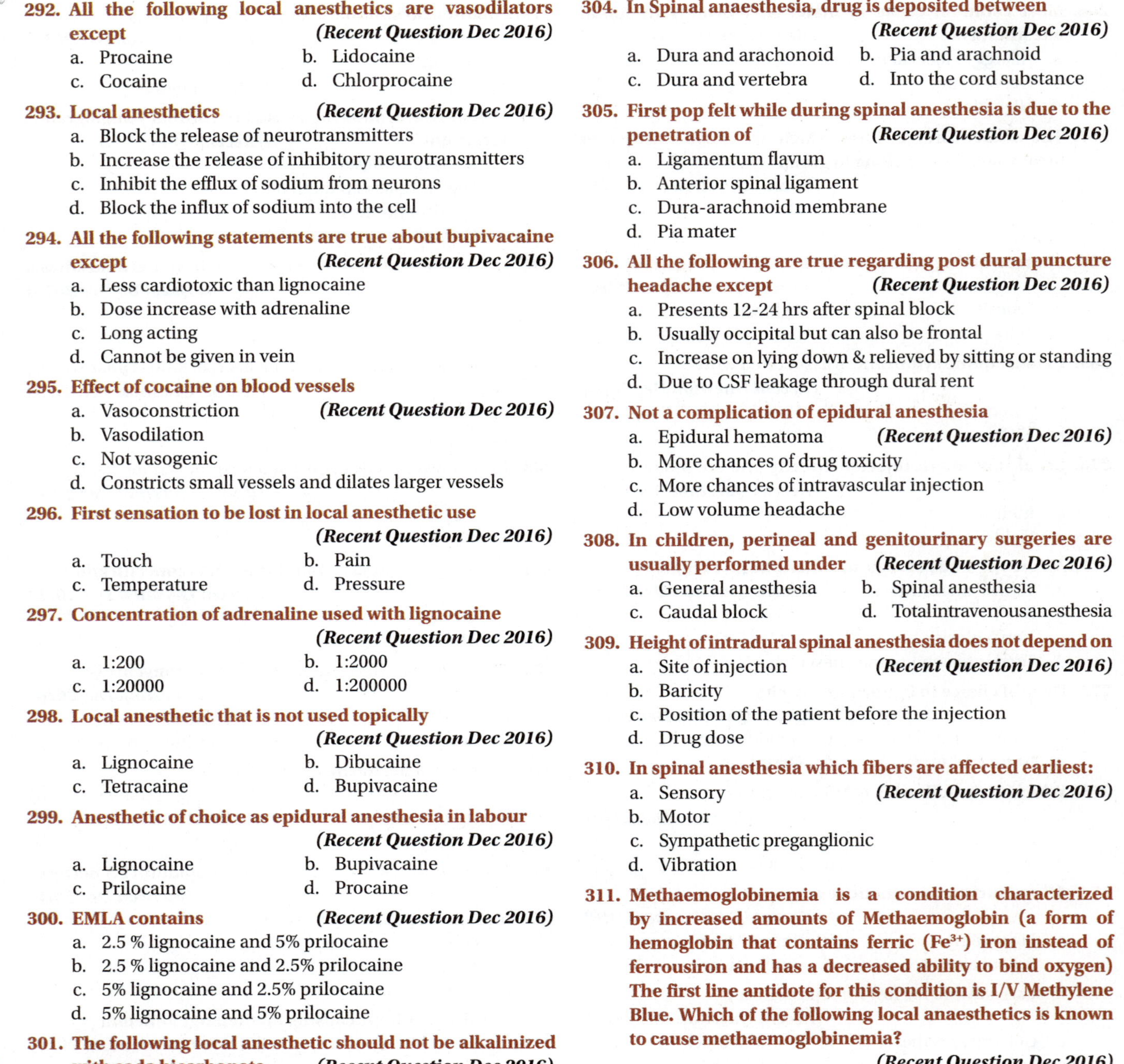

292. All the following local anesthetics are vasodilators except ***(Recent Question Dec 2016)***

a. Procaine b. Lidocaine
c. Cocaine d. Chlorprocaine

293. Local anesthetics ***(Recent Question Dec 2016)***

a. Block the release of neurotransmitters
b. Increase the release of inhibitory neurotransmitters
c. Inhibit the efflux of sodium from neurons
d. Block the influx of sodium into the cell

294. All the following statements are true about bupivacaine except ***(Recent Question Dec 2016)***

a. Less cardiotoxic than lignocaine
b. Dose increase with adrenaline
c. Long acting
d. Cannot be given in vein

295. Effect of cocaine on blood vessels ***(Recent Question Dec 2016)***

a. Vasoconstriction
b. Vasodilation
c. Not vasogenic
d. Constricts small vessels and dilates larger vessels

296. First sensation to be lost in local anesthetic use ***(Recent Question Dec 2016)***

a. Touch b. Pain
c. Temperature d. Pressure

297. Concentration of adrenaline used with lignocaine ***(Recent Question Dec 2016)***

a. 1:200 b. 1:2000
c. 1:20000 d. 1:200000

298. Local anesthetic that is not used topically ***(Recent Question Dec 2016)***

a. Lignocaine b. Dibucaine
c. Tetracaine d. Bupivacaine

299. Anesthetic of choice as epidural anesthesia in labour ***(Recent Question Dec 2016)***

a. Lignocaine b. Bupivacaine
c. Prilocaine d. Procaine

300. EMLA contains ***(Recent Question Dec 2016)***

a. 2.5 % lignocaine and 5% prilocaine
b. 2.5 % lignocaine and 2.5% prilocaine
c. 5% lignocaine and 2.5% prilocaine
d. 5% lignocaine and 5% prilocaine

301. The following local anesthetic should not be alkalinized with soda bicarbonate ***(Recent Question Dec 2016)***

a. Bupivacaine b. Lignocaine
c. Procaine d. Benzocaine

302. The following is not true about the effect of adding a vasoconstrictor to a local anesthetic ***(Recent Question Dec 2016)***

a. Prolongs duration of action
b. Reduces systemic toxicity
c. Makes the injection less painful
d. Increases the chances of subsequent local tissue edema

303. The most common ECG finding with bupivacaine intoxication ***(Recent Question Dec 2016)***

a. Narrow QRS complex b. Slow idioventricular rhythm
c. 2nd degree AV block d. Absence of P waves

304. In Spinal anaesthesia, drug is deposited between ***(Recent Question Dec 2016)***

a. Dura and arachonoid b. Pia and arachnoid
c. Dura and vertebra d. Into the cord substance

305. First pop felt while during spinal anesthesia is due to the penetration of ***(Recent Question Dec 2016)***

a. Ligamentum flavum
b. Anterior spinal ligament
c. Dura-arachnoid membrane
d. Pia mater

306. All the following are true regarding post dural puncture headache except ***(Recent Question Dec 2016)***

a. Presents 12-24 hrs after spinal block
b. Usually occipital but can also be frontal
c. Increase on lying down & relieved by sitting or standing
d. Due to CSF leakage through dural rent

307. Not a complication of epidural anesthesia ***(Recent Question Dec 2016)***

a. Epidural hematoma
b. More chances of drug toxicity
c. More chances of intravascular injection
d. Low volume headache

308. In children, perineal and genitourinary surgeries are usually performed under ***(Recent Question Dec 2016)***

a. General anesthesia b. Spinal anesthesia
c. Caudal block d. Totalintravenousanesthesia

309. Height of intradural spinal anesthesia does not depend on ***(Recent Question Dec 2016)***

a. Site of injection
b. Baricity
c. Position of the patient before the injection
d. Drug dose

310. In spinal anesthesia which fibers are affected earliest: ***(Recent Question Dec 2016)***

a. Sensory
b. Motor
c. Sympathetic preganglionic
d. Vibration

311. Methaemoglobinemia is a condition characterized by increased amounts of Methaemoglobin (a form of hemoglobin that contains ferric (Fe^{3+}) iron instead of ferrousiron and has a decreased ability to bind oxygen) The first line antidote for this condition is I/V Methylene Blue. Which of the following local anaesthetics is known to cause methaemoglobinemia? ***(Recent Question Dec 2016)***

a. Lignocaine b. Dibucaine
c. Bupivacaine d. Prilocaine

312. Maximum safe dose of lignocaine for spinal anesthesia is ***(Recent Question Dec 2016)***

a. 5-15 mg b. 25-100 mg
c. 100-200 mg d. 150-300 mg

313. In Caesarean section operation, after 8 min of spinal anesthesia, female develop hypotension. Which of the following drug(s) is/are used for management of hypotension: ***(PGI May 2018)***

a. Ephedrine b. Adrenaline
c. Dopamine d. Phenylephrine
e. Mephentermine

314. In renal disease, which of the following agents should not be used: ***(PGI May 2018)***
a. Succinylcholine b. Methoxyflurane
c. Pancuronium d. Atracurium
e. Desflurane

315. True statement(s) about local anesthetics: ***(PGI May 2018)***
a. Lidocaine is used for awake intubation
b. Bupivacaine more cardiotoxic and longer acting than lidociane
c. Intralipid is used for cardiotoxicity of bupivacaine
d. Ropivacaine- used in peripheral nerve block
e. Cocaine can produce hypotension

316. True about muscle relaxants: ***(PGI May 2018)***
a. Succinylcholine is short acting muscle relaxant
b. Succinylcholine is used for rapid-sequence induction in full stomach patients
c. Recuronium is muscle relaxant of choice in paediatric patients
d. Rocuronium can be used for rapid-sequence induction
e. Pancuronium is used in day care surgery

317. Which of the following is/are false regarding gases used in anesthesia: ***(PGI May 2018)***
a. Sevoflurane is the agent of choice for children & asthma patients
b. In day care surgery, halothane is most commonly used inhalational agent
c. Sevoflurane can be safely used in liver disease
d. Desflurane should not be used for induction in children
e. Sevoflurane fresh gas flow rates should be at least 2 L/min for exposures greater than 1 hour

318. Post-dural headache is controlled by: ***(PGI Nov 2017)***
a. Caffeine b. Blood patch
c. Steroids d. Hydration
e. Sumatriptan

319. Sugammadex developed for? ***(PGI Nov 2017)***
a. Induction of anesthesia
b. Intubation
c. Reversal of muscle relaxants
d. Opioid detoxification

320. Drugs known to trigger malignant hyperthermia: ***(PGI May 2017)***
a. Halothane b. Succinylcholine
c. Pancuronium d. Fentanyl
e. Propofol

321. When will you suspect malignant hyperthermia in post appendectomy patient shifted to ICU with high fever and: ***(PGI May 2017)***
a. Hypotonia b. Seizure
c. Masseter spasm d. Metabolic acidosis
e. Hypokalemia

322. Anaesthesia used for induction is/are: ***(PGI May 2017)***
a. Propofol
b. Thiopentone
c. Ketamine
d. Diazepam
e. Midazolam

323. Which of the following is/are used in Bupivacaine toxicity: ***(PGI May 2017)***
a. $CaCl_2$ b. Bretylium
c. Intralipids d. Esmolol
e. Epinephrine

324. Which of the following criteria is/are used for setting mechanical ventilator for adult in ICU: ***(PGI May 2017)***
a. Age b. Gender
c. Weight d. Height
e. Underlying condition of patient

325. True about endotracheal tube: ***(PGI May 2017)***
a. Non cuffed tube is used in pediatric age group
b. Made of PVC and disposable
c. Can be put either oral or nasal according to different situations
d. Cuffed PVC tubes- low pressure, low volume
e. More tendency to go to right bronchus thereby decreasing left lung ventilation

326. True about endotracheal intubation: ***(PGI May 2017)***
a. Head trauma patient presenting with a GCS score 8 or less should be intubated
b. Done in patients with increased risk of aspiration
c. Can be used in patient with full stomach
d. In cervical injury, patient neck is stabilized before intubation
e. Done in patients who need anaesthesia

327. Which of the following is/are feature(s) of epidural anaesthesia than spinal anaesthesia: ***(PGI May 2017)***
a. Smaller size of needle is used
b. Drug used is less in concentration
c. Less chance of spinal headache
d. Onset of action is delayed
e. Density of anesthetic agent is less in epidural than spinal

328. Anesthetic agents(s) having epileptogenic potential: ***(PGI Nov. 2016)***
a. Atracurium b. Etomidate
c. Enflurane d. Pethidine
e. Propofol

329. True about xenon is are: ***(PGI Nov. 2016)***
a. Environment friendly b. Cheap
c. Low blood solubility d. Inert
e. Stable

330. In gas tubing, flow rate of turbulent flow depends upon: ***(PGI Nov. 2016)***
a. Viscosity of gas b. Pressure gradient
c. Length of tube d. Radius of tube
e. Density of gas

331. Gas stored in liquid state in cylinders: ***(PGI Nov. 2016)***
a. Nitrogen b. Helium
c. CO_2 d. Cyclopropane
e. Nitrous oxide

332. True about desflurane: ***(PGI June 2016)***
a. Boiling point is <23 °C
b. Chemically it is Flourinated methyl ethyl ether
c. It increases the effect of muscle relaxant
d. Can be given safely to patient susceptible to malignant hyperthermia
e. More potent than isoflurane

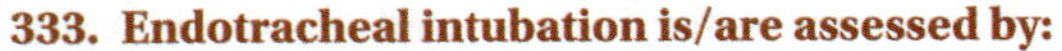

333. Endotracheal intubation is/are assessed by: ***(PGI June 2016)***

a. Mallampati grading
b. ASA physical status grading
c. Thyromental distance
d. Teeth arrangement

334. Which of the following statement(s) is/are correct regarding management of malignant hyperthermia except: ***(PGI Nov 2015)***

a. Discontinue all anaesthetics immediately
b. Dantrolene is mainstay of therapy for MH
c. Hyperventilation with 100% oxygen is helpful
d. Sodium bicarbonate is given to correct alkalosis
e. Correct hyperkalemia by giving dextrose & insulin

335. Which of the following is/are true about pre-anaesthetic checkup (PAC): ***(PGI Nov 2015)***

a. Not necessary in children
b. Used to assess patient condition to tolerate anaesthesia & surgery
c. Can be performed by surgical faculty
d. Relieves anxiety of patient
e. Help in planning anaesthesia technique

336. Which of the following is/are true regarding anaesthetic gas: ***(PGI May 2015)***

a. N_2O-increases efficacy of other inhalational agents
b. Halothane-agent of choice in children
c. Sevoflurane is agent of choice in children
d. Isoflurane-smooth induction

337. All are true about malignant hyperthermia except: ***(PGI May 2015)***

a. Occurs due to defect in ryanodine receptor
b. Caffeine–halothane test on muscle fiber is used for diagnosis
c. Halothane precipitates
d. Thiopentone triggers
e. Usually AD in inheritance

338. True about Endotracheal tube: ***(PGI May 2015)***

a. Most common used size for adult male is 8-8.5
b. Most common used size for adult female is 7-7.5
c. PVC tube is reusable by cleaning
d. In children cuffed tube is not used
e. Cuff is for aspiration of secretions

339. True about subarachnoid block (spinal anesthesia):

a. Cannot be used in infant and children ***(PGI May 2015)***
b. Can be given by unskilled doctor
c. May be used when I. V access is not possible for intravenous drugs
d. Hypotension is most common side effect

340. A Patient has hypersensitivity to neostigmine. He has to undergo upper abdominal surgery. Muscle relaxant of choice is: ***(PGI Nov 2014)***

a. Pancuronium
b. Ropacuronium
c. Vecuronium
d. Atracurium
e. Piperacurium

341. Which of the following condition (s) can cause exaggerated hyperkalemia in patients with use of succinylcholine: ***(PGI Nov 2014)***

a. Burn
b. Spinal cord injury
c. Muscular dystrophy
d. Tetanus
e. Abdominal organ injury

342. Which of the following does not increase intracranial pressure: ***(PGI Nov 2014)***

a. Sodium thiopentone
b. Desflurane
c. Mannitol
d. Sevoflurane
e. Propofol

343. Mechanism of action of general anesthesia is/are: ***(PGI Nov 2014)***

a. GABA-A receptor
b. GABA-B receptor
c. NMDA receptor
d. Na+ channel blockage

344. Which of the following statement is correct regarding mechanism of action of local anaesthesia: ***(PGI Nov 2014)***

a. Blockage of resting sodium channel more is than activated sodium channel
b. Faster conducting fibers blocked easily
c. Block Na-K ATPase channel
d. Fine touch goes before pain
e. In regional block i.v injection is used

345. All are true regarding Laryngeal Mask Airway except: ***(PGI May2014)***

a. Big oral tumor is contraindication for its use
b. May be used when intubation with ETT is not possible
c. Can be used in child 's eye surgery
d. May be used in CPR

346. Which of the following circuit is preferred in child for spontaneous respiration: ***(PGI May2014)***

a. Mapleson A
b. Jackson and Rees circuit
c. Mapleson C
d. Mapleson E
e. Mapleson F

347. Weaning is generally done by: ***(PGI May2014)***

a. SIMV
b. Controlled mode ventilation(CMV)
c. CPAP
d. Pressure controlled Ventilation
e. Assisted controlled Ventilation

348. A child on immediate postoperative, is complaining of nausea & vomiting after squint surgery. Which of the following drugs may be not used during operation in controlling this symptom: ***(PGI May2014)***

a. Propofol
b. Ketamine
c. Dexamethasone
d. Ondansetron
e. Palonosetron

349. True about intercostal analgesia: ***(PGI Nov 2013)***

a. Performed for postoperative analgesia
b. Usually performed in anterior axillary line
c. Drug usually given at superior border of rib
d. Pneumothorax may occur as a complication

350. Characteristics of isoflurane is/are: *(PGI Nov 2013)*
a. Very smooth induction
b. It is the inhalational agent of choice for controlled hypotension
c. Good analgesia
d. Cardiac stable agent

351. Not true about procedure of cricoid pressure: *(PGI Nov 2013)*
a. Neck is extended
b. Direction of pressure should be backward & upward
c. Preoxygenation with 100% oxygenation for 3-4 minute is mandatory
d. In case of emergency 4 deep breaths with 100% oxygen can be used as an alternative to preoxygenation
e. Cricoid pressure is released only once cuff is inflated & the position of ETT is confirmed

352. Acronym AMBU stands for : *(PGI May 2013)*
a. Automated Manual Breathing Unit
b. Artificial Manual Breathing Unit
c. Artificial Mechanical Breathing Unit
d. Automated Mechanical Breathing Unit
e. Artificial Mechanical Baloon Unit

353. Which of the following local anesthetic is/are not used for surface analgesia: *(PGI May 2013)*
a. Benzocaine
b. Prilocaine
c. Mepivacaine
d. Legnocaine
e. Bupivacaine

354. Which of the increases chance of malignant hyperthermia: *(PGI May 2013)*
a. Diazepam
b. Halothane
c. Suxamethonium
d. Nitrous oxide
e. Ketamine

355. True about Xenon: *(PGI Nov 2012)*
a. Blood:gas partition coefficient is 0.14
b. Minimum alveolar concentration is high
c. Minimal hemodynamic effect
d. Heavier than air
e. High blood solubility

356. Which of the following 1anesthetics does not depress ciliary function: *(PGI Nov 2012)*
a. Ketamine
b. Enflurane
c. Ether
d. Sevoflurane
e. Desflurane

357. Anesthetics agents associated with epilepsy: *(PGI Nov 2012)*
a. Enflurane
b. Desflurane
c. Propofol
d. Sevoflurane
e. Thiopentone

358. Most commonly used cylinder in anaesthesia machine is: *(PGI May 2012)*
a. A
b. B
c. D
d. E
e. F

359. Which of the following statement is/are not true about Dibucaine : *(PGI May 2012)*
a. Shorter acting than tetracaine
b. Longer acting than tetracaine
c. More potent than tetracaine
d. More potent than bupivacaine
e. Dibucaine no. < 30 indicates more quantity of atypical pseudocholinesterase

360. Feature of malignant hyperthermia includes: *(PGI May 2012)*
a. Tachycardia
b. Hypotension
c. Excessive sweating
d. ↓ed $ETCO_2$
e. ↓ed O_2 saturation

361. All are true statement about capnography except: *(PGI May 2012)*
a. ↓ $ETCO_2$ in pulmonary embolism
b. Elevated baseline represent exhausted absorbent in the circle system
c. To check cofirmation of ETT
d. Curare cleft or notch represent start of spontaneous ventilation
e. In malignant hyperthermia $ETCO_2$ decreases

362. Local anesthetic system toxicity(LAST) is/are increased by: *(PGI May 2012)*
a. Hypoxia
b. Metabolic acidosis
c. Extreme age
d. Renal failure

363. True about xenon anaesthesia: *(PGI Nov 2010)*
a. Rapid induction and recovery
b. Low potency
c. High blood solubility
d. Non-explosive
e. Heavier than air

364. True about Heliox: *(PGI Nov 2010)*
a. Helium is an inert gas
b. Less viscous than air
c. Higher density than air
d. Reduces work of breathing
e. Mixture of He & O_2

365. Which of following is/are false: *(PGI Nov 2010)*
a. Enflurane interacts with sodalime
b. Sevoflurane causes seizures
c. Rapid recovery from propofol
d. Ketamine acts through GABA-A receptors
e. MAC indicates potency of inhalational agents

366. Treatment of bupivacaine toxicity includes: *(PGI Nov 2010)*
a. Isoprenaline
b. Epinephrine
c. Bretylium
d. Metoprolol
e. Lignocaine

367. True about propofol: *(PGI May 2010)*
a. Indicated in egg allergy
b. Can be used in porphyria
c. It is of barbiturate group
d. Used in day care surgery

368. True about Bain circuit: *(PGI May 2010, June 2009)*
a. Mapleson type B
b. Mapleson type D
c. Can be used for spontaneous respiration
d. Can be used for controlled ventilation
e. Coaxial

369. True about Laryngeal mask airway: *(PGI May 2010, June 2009)*
a. More reliable than face mask
b. Prevent aspiration
c. Alternative to Endotracheal tube (E.T.T)
d. Does not require laryngoscope & visualisation
e. Indicated in full stomach to prevent aspiration

370. True statement regarding pin index: *(PGI May 2010)*
a. Pin is present on cylinder
b. Pin is present on machine
c. Not effective if wrong gas is filled in cylinder

371. True about Epidural anesthesia: *(PGI May 2010)*
a. Effects start immediately
b. C/I in coagulopathies
c. Given in subarachnoid space
d. Venous return decreases

372. Pungent volatile anesthetic agents are : *(PGI Nov 2009)*
a. Halothane b. Isoflurane
c. Sevoflurane d. Desflurane
e. Nitrous oxide

373. Sellick manouever is used to prevent: *(PGI Nov 2009)*
a. Alveolar collapse
b. Hypertension
c. Aspiration of Gastric content
d. Bradycardia
e. Glaucoma

374. Which of the following is/are *not* local anesthesia : *(PGI Nov 2009)*
a. Bupivacine b. Mepivacine
c. Mivacurium d. Butorphenol
e. Buprenorphine

375. Anesthetic agent contraindicated in porphyria: *(PGI Nov 2009, Dec 2007)*
a. Thiopentone b. Propofol
c. Ketamine d. Etomidate
e. Methadone

376. Which ones are Non-Depolaring Muscle Relaxants: *(PGI Nov 2009)*
a. Mivacurium b. Halothane
c. Desflurane d. Isoflurane
e. Ether

377. Anesthetic agent(s) safe to use in ↑ICP : *(PGI Nov 2009)*
a. Halothane b. Thiopentone
c. Ketamine d. Ether

378. Which of the following are used to protect airways: *(PGI Nov 2009)*
a. LMA b. Endotracheal tube
c. Ryles tube d. Combitube
e. Sengsten Blackmore tube

379. Structure (s) pierce in Lumbar spinal puncture is/are: *(PGI June 2009)*
a. Ligamentum flavum
b. Duramater
c. Supraspinous ligament
d. Anterior longitudinal ligament
e. Posterior longitudinal ligament

380. All of the following cause myocardial depression *except:* *(PGI June 2009)*
a. Halothane b. Etomidate
c. Thiopentone d. Ketamine
e. Propofol

381. Placement of a double lumen tube (DLT) is best confirmed by: *(PGI Dec 2008)*
a. Clinically by Auscultation
b. Fibreoptic bronchoscopy
c. Capnography
d. Chest radiography
e. Chest inflation on positive pressure

382. Treatment of malignant Hyperthermia includes: *(PGI Dec 2008)*
a. Dantrolene
b. Cooling
c. Deepening plane of inhalational anaesthesia
d. Discontinue inhalational anesthesia
e. Give O_2 therapy with 100% O_2.

383. True about malignant hyperthermia: *(PGI June 2008)*
a. Succinylcholine & halothane predisposes
b. Dantrolene usefull in all cases
c. Ketanserine can be used as an alternative to Dantrolene
d. Propofol is safe
e. Muscle biopsy is diagnostic

384. Anaesthesia of choice in renal disease: *(PGI June 2008)*
a. Atracurium b. Cisatracurium
c. Vecuronium d. Rocuronium
e. Mivacurium

385. Inhalational agent of choice in children: *(PGI June 2008)*
a. Sevoflurane b. Isofurane
c. Desflurane d. Halothane
e. N_2O

386. True about anaesthesia breathing circuit: *(PGI June 2008)*
a. Cylinder is a part of high pressure system
b. O_2 flush delivers < 35lts
c. O_2 flush delivers > 35lts
d. Pipelines is a part low pressure system

387. True about LMA (Laryngeal Mask Airway): *(PGI June 2008)*
a. Available in 8 sizes
b. Intubation can be done
c. Size 1 for neonates
d. Size 3 for adults
e. Full protection from aspiration

388. True about N_2O: *(PGI June 2008)*
a. Pin index 3,5 b. Blue in colour
c. Stored as liquid d. MAC 105

389. Which of the following have analgesic property *(PGI June 2008)*
a. N_2O b. Ketamine
c. Thiopentone d. Etomidate

390. Bupivacaine toxicity treated with: *(PGI Dec 2007)*
a. Esmolol b. Sotalol
c. Lignocaine d. 5 percent Dextrose
e. Benzodiazepines

391. **Gas is filled as liquid in cylinder in:** ***(PGI Dec 2007)***
a. O_2 b. CO_2
c. N_2O d. Cyclopropane
e. Halothane

392. **Concentration of Lignocaine used:** ***(PGI Dec 2007)***
a. 2% b. 4%
c. 5% d. 10%
e. 1%

393. **Characteristics of Remifentanyl:** ***(PGI Dec 2007)***
a. Metabolised by plasma esterase
b. Short half life
c. More potent than Alfentanyl
d. Dose reduced in hepatic and renal diseases
e. Duration of action more than Alfentanyl

394. **All ↓ CO_2 absorption in circuit except:** ***(PGI Dec 2007)***
a. Resistance in circuit b. High flow
c. Small granules size d. Medium granules size
e. Channeling

395. **Which of the following skeletal muscle relaxants undergo Hoffman elimination:** ***(PGI June 2007)***
a. Atracurium b. Cis-atracurium
c. Mivacurium d. Vecuronium

396. **True about Halothane:** ***(PGI Dec 2006)***
a. Non - irritant b. Antiarrhythmic
c. It antagonises bronchospasm
d. Vasodilator

397. **Skeletal muscle relaxant having no CVS side effects:** ***(PGI Dec 2006)***
a. Vecuronium b. Doxacurium
c. Pancuronium d. Rocuronium
e. Mivacurium

398. **True about EMLA:** ***(PGI Dec 2006)***
a. Can be used for intubation
b. Mixture of local anesthesia
c. Faster acting
d. Used in children

399. **Anesthetic agent known to cause pain on intravenous injection:** ***(JIPMER 2018)***
a. Ketamine b. Etomidate
c. Thiopentone d. Propofol

400. **Anesthetic agent with least minimum alveolar concentration (MAC):** ***(JIPMER 2018)***
a. Nitrous oxide b. Isoflurane
c. Desflurane d. Xenon

401. **Inhalational agent with lowest blood gas coefficient is:** ***(JIPMER 2018)***
a. Isoflurane b. N2O
c. Xenon d. Enflurane

402. **A resident at the emergency department is preparing for a lumbar puncture in a 26 years old female with suspected bleeding. Although she presented with altered sensorium, CT brain was found to be normal. During LP, which structure is pierced after the spinal needle crosses interspinous ligament?** ***(JIPMER 2018)***
a. Ligamentum flavum b. Arachnoid membrane
c. Areolar tissue d. Subarachnoid space

403. **Local anesthetic acts by:** ***(JIPMER 2018)***
a. Blocking sodium gated channel
b. Blocking calcium gated channel
c. Blocking potassium gated channel
d. Blocking chloride gated channel

404. **Anaphalylaxis at end of general anaesthesia is due to:** ***(JIPMER 2017)***
a. Opiods
b. Antibiotics
c. NSAIDs d. Benzodiazepines

405. **Structure pierced during spinal anesthesia after interspinous ligament?** ***(JIPMER 2015)***
a. Ligamentum flavum b. Aeriolar space
c. Arachnoid space d. Supraspinous ligament

406. **Not a complication of LSCS with regional anesthesia?** ***(JIPMER 2015)***
a. Delayed respiratory depression
b. Venous air embolism
c. Hypotension
d. Ischemia of lower limbs

407. **What is done to reduce pain after administration of local anesthetic?** ***(JIPMER 2015)***
a. Alkalinize the LA
b. Add adrenaline
c. Cool the LA
d. All of the above

408. **Which is the correct statement regarding esophageal intubation?** ***(JIPMER 2015)***
a. Cannot be detected by stethoscope
b. It does't occur for an inexperienced person
c. Capnography may not detect esophageal intubation during cardiac arrest
d. None of the above

409. **Bradycardia is most common in** ***(JIPMER 2014)***
a. Midazolam
b. Succinylcholine
c. Isoprenaline
d. Dopamine

410. **The most potent anti-emetic agent in pre-operative period is** ***(JIPMER 2014)***
a. Ondansetron b. Metoclopramide
c. Perchlorperazine d. Chlorpromazine

411. **Delivery of high concentration of oxygen (more than 90%) is delivered via** ***(JIPMER 2014, 2013)***
a. Partial rebreathing mask
b. Nasal cannula with oxygen flow at 5L/min
c. Simple face mask
d. Non rebreathing face mask with oxygen reservoir

412. **A patient on epidural anesthesia with 15 ml of 1.5% lignocaine with adrenaline for hernia surgery develops hypotension and respiratory depression in three min. Most common cause for this clinical condition is** ***(JIPMER 2014)***
a. Systemic toxicity of anesthetic agents
b. Drug allergy
c. Vaso vagal shock
d. Drug entering into sub arachnoid space

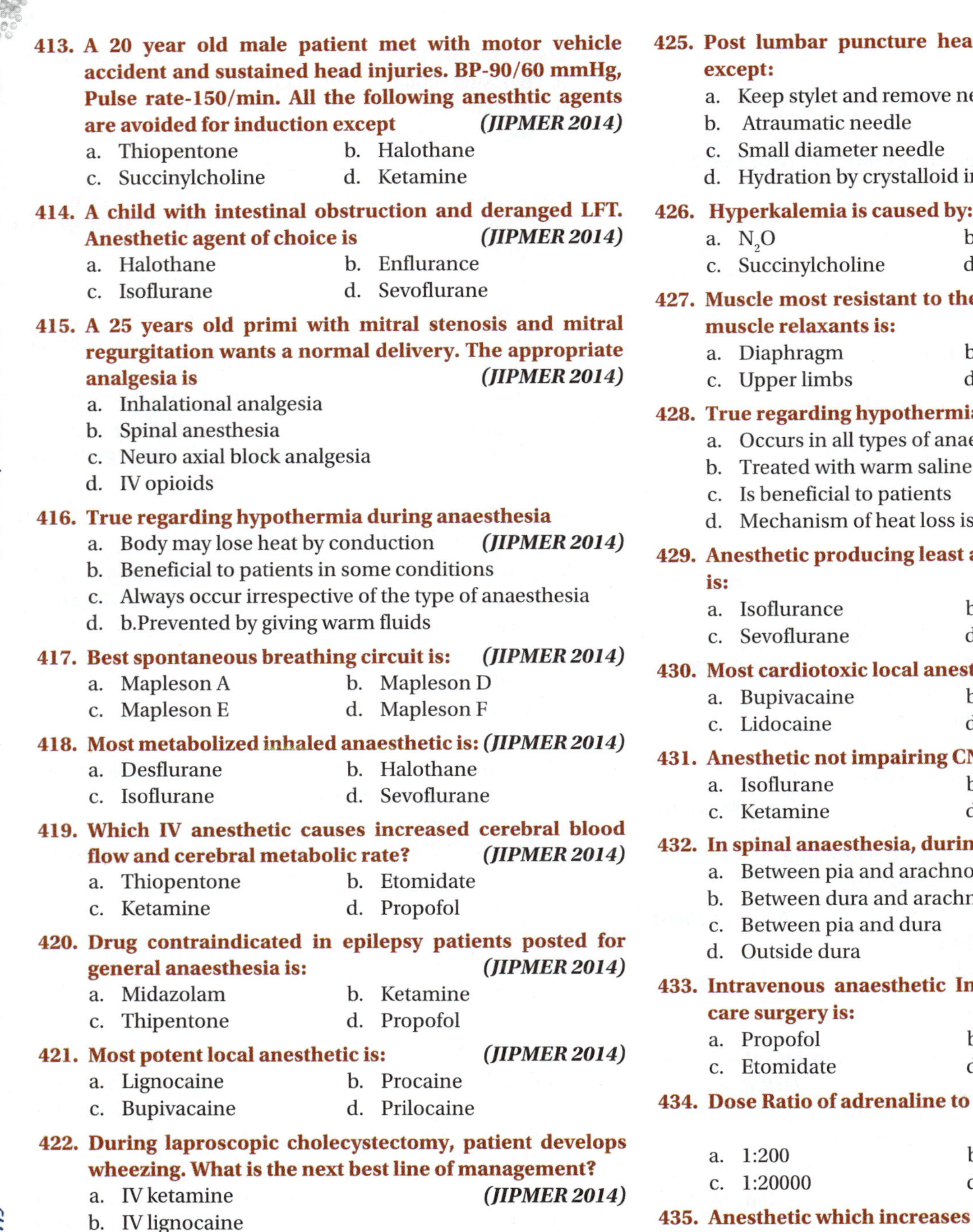

413. **A 20 year old male patient met with motor vehicle accident and sustained head injuries. BP-90/60 mmHg, Pulse rate-150/min. All the following anesthtic agents are avoided for induction except** ***(JIPMER 2014)***
a. Thiopentone b. Halothane
c. Succinylcholine d. Ketamine

414. **A child with intestinal obstruction and deranged LFT. Anesthetic agent of choice is** ***(JIPMER 2014)***
a. Halothane b. Enflurance
c. Isoflurane d. Sevoflurane

415. **A 25 years old primi with mitral stenosis and mitral regurgitation wants a normal delivery. The appropriate analgesia is** ***(JIPMER 2014)***
a. Inhalational analgesia
b. Spinal anesthesia
c. Neuro axial block analgesia
d. IV opioids

416. **True regarding hypothermia during anaesthesia**
a. Body may lose heat by conduction ***(JIPMER 2014)***
b. Beneficial to patients in some conditions
c. Always occur irrespective of the type of anaesthesia
d. b.Prevented by giving warm fluids

417. **Best spontaneous breathing circuit is:** ***(JIPMER 2014)***
a. Mapleson A b. Mapleson D
c. Mapleson E d. Mapleson F

418. **Most metabolized inhaled anaesthetic is:** ***(JIPMER 2014)***
a. Desflurane b. Halothane
c. Isoflurane d. Sevoflurane

419. **Which IV anesthetic causes increased cerebral blood flow and cerebral metabolic rate?** ***(JIPMER 2014)***
a. Thiopentone b. Etomidate
c. Ketamine d. Propofol

420. **Drug contraindicated in epilepsy patients posted for general anaesthesia is:** ***(JIPMER 2014)***
a. Midazolam b. Ketamine
c. Thipentone d. Propofol

421. **Most potent local anesthetic is:** ***(JIPMER 2014)***
a. Lignocaine b. Procaine
c. Bupivacaine d. Prilocaine

422. **During laproscopic cholecystectomy, patient develops wheezing. What is the next best line of management?**
a. IV ketamine ***(JIPMER 2014)***
b. IV lignocaine
c. Bronchodialators beta 2 agonist and oxygenation
d. Deepen plane of anaestheisa

423. **Not a contraindication for combined spinal and epidural anaestheisa:** ***(JIPMER 2014)***
a. Platelet count <50,000
b. Patient on clopidogrel
c. Local infection
d. Patient on antihypertensive medication

424. **Regarding celiac plexus block true is:** ***(JIPMER 2014)***
a. Bilaterally done
b. Diarrhea and hypotension are common side effects
c. Done in painful conditions of lower abdomen
d. Done around L3

425. **Post lumbar puncture headache is minimized by all except:**
a. Keep stylet and remove needle ***(JIPMER 2014)***
b. Atraumatic needle
c. Small diameter needle
d. Hydration by crystalloid infusion

426. **Hyperkalemia is caused by:** ***(JIPMER 2014)***
a. N_2O b. Atracurium
c. Succinylcholine d. Pancuronium

427. **Muscle most resistant to the action of non depolarizing muscle relaxants is:** ***(JIPMER 2013)***
a. Diaphragm b. Head and neck muscles
c. Upper limbs d. Abdomen

428. **True regarding hypothermia during anaesthesia is:**
a. Occurs in all types of anaesthesia ***(JIPMER 2013)***
b. Treated with warm saline
c. Is beneficial to patients
d. Mechanism of heat loss is conduction

429. **Anesthetic producing least amount of carbon monoxide is:** ***(JIPMER 2013)***
a. Isoflurance b. Desflurane
c. Sevoflurane d. Enflurane

430. **Most cardiotoxic local anesthetic is:** ***(JIPMER 2013)***
a. Bupivacaine b. Lignocaine
c. Lidocaine d. Ropivacaine

431. **Anesthetic not impairing CNS activity is:** ***(JIPMER 2013)***
a. Isoflurane b. Enflurane
c. Ketamine d. Desflurane

432. **In spinal anaesthesia, during is deposited between:**
a. Between pia and arachnoid ***(JIPMER 2013)***
b. Between dura and arachnoid
c. Between pia and dura
d. Outside dura

433. **Intravenous anaesthetic Induction agent used in Day care surgery is:** ***(JIPMER 2013)***
a. Propofol b. Ketamine
c. Etomidate d. Thiopentone

434. **Dose Ratio of adrenaline to be used with lidocaine is:** ***(JIPMER 2013)***
a. 1:200 b. 1:2000
c. 1:20000 d. 1:200000

435. **Anesthetic which increases intracranial tension** ***(JIPMER 2013, 2009)***
a. Ketamine b. Propofol
c. Etomidate d. Ether

436. **Intravenous anaesthetic causing suppression of steroid synthesis:** ***(JIPMER 2013)***
a. Etomidate
b. Thiopentone
c. Ketamine
d. Propofol

437. **Anesthetic which is least metabolized in the body is:** ***(JIPMER 2013)***
a. Xenon b. Ether
c. Halothane d. Methoxyflurane

438. Intravenous anaesthetic drug that doesn't induce cerebral metabolism: ***(JIPMER 2013)***
a. Thiopentone b. Ketamine
c. Propofol d. Methohexitone

439. Stage 2 block (Phase II block) is seen with: ***(JIPMER 2013)***
a. Suxamethonium b. Isoflurane
c. Sevoflurane d. Enflurane

440. Malignant hyperthermia is caused by: ***(JIPMER 2013)***
a. Succinylcholine b. N_2O
c. Atropine d. Dantolene

441. Mechanism of action of Local anesthetics: ***(JIPMER 2013)***
a. Inhibition of Na+ channels
b. Inhibition of Na+K+ATPase
c. Inhibition of K+channels
d. Inhibition of Ca2+channels

442. Which of the following Drug has least t1/2? ***(JIPMER 2012)***
a. Thiopentone b. Propofol
c. Midazolam d. Ketamine

443. Which of the following is an ultrashort acting anesthetic? ***(JIPMER 2012)***
a. Propofol b. Thiopentone
c. Succinylcholine d. Midazolam

444. Which of the following disease show resistance to Succinylcholine? ***(JIPMER 2012)***
a. Myasthenia gravis
b. Polymyositis
c. Eaton lambert myasthenia syndrome
d. Muscular dystrophy

445. Minimum alveolar concentration of an inhaled anesthetic is a marker of: ***(JIPMER 2012)***
a. Potency b. Efficacy
c. Elimination d. Distribution

446. In anesthesia, fitting of wrong gas cylinder to the anesthesia machine can be prevented by: ***(JIPMER 2012, 2009)***
a. Pin index system b. Yolk assembly
c. Bodock seal d. Gas analyser

447. Which of the following is a short acting muscle relaxant? ***(JIPMER 2012)***
a. Suxamethonium b. Pancuronium
c. Vecuronium d. Atracurium

448. A patient in ICU is weaned from ventilator. The mode least used for this purpose is: ***(JIPMER 2012)***
a. ASV b. CPAP
c. SIMV d. CMV

449. Fixed performance device: ***(JIPMER 2011, 2007)***
a. Venturi mask b. Nasal cannula
c. Simple mask d. Non rebreathing mask

450. Which gas accumulates in cavities post general anaesthesia? ***(JIPMER 2011)***
a. Nitrous oxide b. Halothane
c. Ether d. Sevoflurane

451. Malignant hyperthermia is common with: ***(JIPMER 2011)***
a. Local anesthetics b. Succinylcholine
c. Propofol d. Barbiturates

452. Hypotension is caused by all except: ***(JIPMER 2011)***
a. Halothane b. Propofol
c. Ketamine d. Thiopentone

453. Plasma potassium concentration is increased with: ***(JIPMER 2010)***
a. Succinylcholine b. Atracurium
c. Pancuronium d. Propofol

454. Drug used to prevent nausea and vomiting: ***(JIPMER 2010)***
a. Propofol b. Fentanyl
c. Nitrous oxide d. Sevoflurane

455. Drug producing haematological side effect is: ***(JIPMER 2010)***
a. Nitrous oxide b. Halothane
c. Ketamine d. Sevoflurane

456. Best treatment for relieving pain during intra-partum period is: ***(JIPMER 2010)***
a. Neuraxial block b. Epidural anesthesia
c. IV ketamine d. General Anesthesia

457. Centrineuraxial anaesthesia is not contra-indicated in: ***(JIPMER 2009)***
a. Platelets <80,000
b. Patients on aspirin
c. Patient on anticoagulants
d. Raised intracranial pressure

458. All are true about ether except: ***(JIPMER 2009)***
a. It has additional sympathomimetic effect
b. Can undergo spontaneous decomposition when exposed to light
c. It has additional bronchodilator and analgesic effects
d. It inhibits salivation

459. Dead space is increased by all except: ***(JIPMER 2009)***
a. Anticholinergic drugs b. Standing
c. Hyperextention of neck d. Endotracheal intubation

460. Which is non-invasive positive pressure ventilation? ***(JIPMER 2008)***
a. CPAP b. SIMV
c. CMV d. IMV

461. Anesthetic drug of choice in asthmatic: ***(JIPMER 2008)***
a. Ketamine b. Propofol
c. Etomidate d. Propofol

462. Neuromuscular blocker of choice in real failure: ***(JIPMER 2008)***
a. Atracurium b. Pancuronium
c. Rocuronium d. Tubocurare

463. Hoffman's elimination is seen with: ***(JIPMER 2008)***
a. Atracurium b. Pancuronium
c. Suxamethonium d. Rocuronium

464. Anaesthetic agent which can cause massive hepatic necrosis? ***(JIPMER 2008)***
a. Halothane
b. Isoflurane
c. Methoxyflurane
d. N_2O

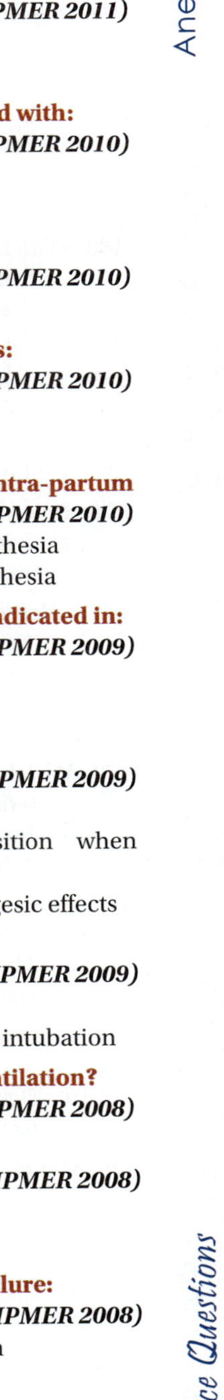

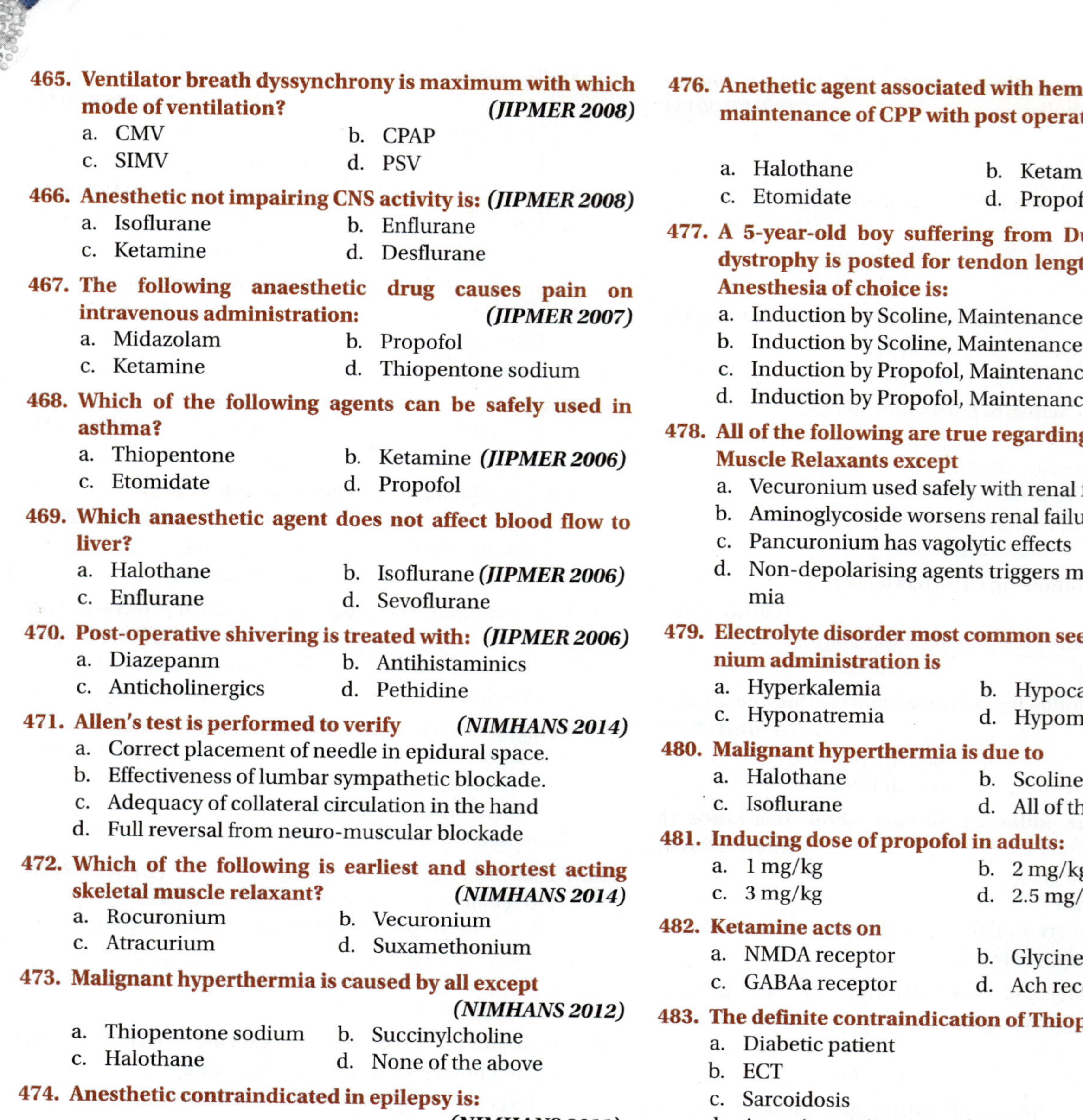

465. Ventilator breath dyssynchrony is maximum with which mode of ventilation? *(JIPMER 2008)*
a. CMV
b. CPAP
c. SIMV
d. PSV

466. Anesthetic not impairing CNS activity is: *(JIPMER 2008)*
a. Isoflurane
b. Enflurane
c. Ketamine
d. Desflurane

467. The following anaesthetic drug causes pain on intravenous administration: *(JIPMER 2007)*
a. Midazolam
b. Propofol
c. Ketamine
d. Thiopentone sodium

468. Which of the following agents can be safely used in asthma? *(JIPMER 2006)*
a. Thiopentone
b. Ketamine
c. Etomidate
d. Propofol

469. Which anaesthetic agent does not affect blood flow to liver? *(JIPMER 2006)*
a. Halothane
b. Isoflurane
c. Enflurane
d. Sevoflurane

470. Post-operative shivering is treated with: *(JIPMER 2006)*
a. Diazepanm
b. Antihistaminics
c. Anticholinergics
d. Pethidine

471. Allen's test is performed to verify *(NIMHANS 2014)*
a. Correct placement of needle in epidural space.
b. Effectiveness of lumbar sympathetic blockade.
c. Adequacy of collateral circulation in the hand
d. Full reversal from neuro-muscular blockade

472. Which of the following is earliest and shortest acting skeletal muscle relaxant? *(NIMHANS 2014)*
a. Rocuronium
b. Vecuronium
c. Atracurium
d. Suxamethonium

473. Malignant hyperthermia is caused by all except *(NIMHANS 2012)*
a. Thiopentone sodium
b. Succinylcholine
c. Halothane
d. None of the above

474. Anesthetic contraindicated in epilepsy is: *(NIMHANS 2011)*
a. Desflurane
b. Sevoflurane
c. Isoflurane
d. Enflurane

475. Delirium and hallucination is seen with: *(NIMHANS 2011)*
a. Halothane
b. Ketamine
c. Etomidate
d. Propofol

476. Anethetic agent associated with hemodynamic stability, maintenance of CPP with post operative myoclonus is: *(NIMHANS 2011)*
a. Halothane
b. Ketamine
c. Etomidate
d. Propofol

477. A 5-year-old boy suffering from Duchenne muscular dystrophy is posted for tendon lengthening procedure. Anesthesia of choice is: *(NIMHANS 2011)*
a. Induction by Scoline, Maintenance by Halothane
b. Induction by Scoline, Maintenance by N_2O and O_2
c. Induction by Propofol, Maintenance by N_2O and O_2
d. Induction by Propofol, Maintenance by Halothane

478. All of the following are true regarding Non Depolarising Muscle Relaxants except *(NIMHANS 2010)*
a. Vecuronium used safely with renal failure
b. Aminoglycoside worsens renal failure
c. Pancuronium has vagolytic effects
d. Non-depolarising agents triggers malignant hyperthermia

479. Electrolyte disorder most common seen with suxamethonium administration is *(NIMHANS 2009)*
a. Hyperkalemia
b. Hypocalcemia
c. Hyponatremia
d. Hypomagnesemia

480. Malignant hyperthermia is due to *(NIMHANS 2009)*
a. Halothane
b. Scoline
c. Isoflurane
d. All of the above

481. Inducing dose of propofol in adults: *(NIMHANS 2008)*
a. 1 mg/kg
b. 2 mg/kg
c. 3 mg/kg
d. 2.5 mg/kg

482. Ketamine acts on *(NIMHANS 2008)*
a. NMDA receptor
b. Glycine receptor
c. GABAa receptor
d. Ach receptor

483. The definite contraindication of Thiopentone *(NIMHANS 2008)*
a. Diabetic patient
b. ECT
c. Sarcoidosis
d. Acute intermittent porphyria

484. All of the following are true regarding post spinal headache, except *(NIMHANS 2007)*
a. Occurs within 48 hrs
b. Increased by sitting
c. Due to CSF Leak
d. Associated with photophobia

Answers with Explanations to Multiple Choice Questions

1. Ans. (b) Morton

(Ref: Goodman Gilman 12th E/P527)

General anesthetic effect of ether was first demonstrated by Morton, but it was first clinically used by Crawford Long.

2. Ans. (c) Ivan Magill

(Ref: Ajay Yadav 4th E/P21)

3. Ans. (a) Niemann

(Ref: Goodman Gilman 12th E/P565)

- Cocaine was first isolated from leaves of cocoa shrubs and introduced to the world by Albert Niemann.
- Cocaine was first used for local anesthesia by Carl Koller.

4. Ans. (d) Dioscoriodes

(Ref: Ajay Yadav 4th E/P20)

5. Ans. (a) Morton

(Ref: Goodman Gilman 12th E/P527)

6. Ans. (a) Carl Kollar

(Ref: Goodman Gilman 12th E/P565)

Cocaine was

- First studied by Sigmund Freud
- First used by **Carl Kollar**

7. Ans. (b) 3 mins

(Ref: Ajay Yadav 5th E/P67)

8. Ans. (b) Assessing Airway

(Ref: Miller's Anesthesia 8th E/P1093)

9. Ans. (a) Difficulty intubation

(Ref: Ajay Yadav 5th E/P124)

- Mallampati score is used for airway assessment to predict difficult intubation.
- A class III and IV Mallampati score is associated with difficult intubation.

10. Ans. (b) ASA 2

(Ref: Miller's Anesthesia 8th E/P3257)

ASA physical status classification

Class	Physical status	Mortality risk
I	**Normal healthy patient:** No organic, physiologic, or psychiatric disturbance; excludes the very young and very old; healthy with good exercise tolerance	0–0.3%
II	**Patients with mild systemic disease:** No functional limitations; has a well-controlled disease of one body system; controlled hypertension or diabetes without systemic effects, cigarette smoking without chronic obstructive pulmonary disease (COPD); mild obesity, pregnancy	0.3–1.4%
III	**Patients with severe systemic disease:** Some functional limitation; has a controlled disease of more than one body system or one major system; no immediate danger of death; controlled congestive heart failure (CHF), stable angina, old heart attack, poorly controlled hypertension, morbid obesity, chronic renal failure; bronchospastic disease with intermittent symptoms	1.5–5.4%
IV	**Patients with severe systemic disease that is a constant threat to life:** Has at least one severe disease that is poorly controlled or at end stage; possible risk of death; unstable angina, symptomatic COPD, symptomatic CHF, hepatorenal failure	7.8–25.9 %
V	**Moribund patients who are not expected to survive without the operation:** Not expected to survive > 24 hours without surgery; imminent risk of death; multiorgan failure, sepsis syndrome with hemodynamic instability, hypothermia, poorly controlled coagulopathy	9.4–57.8%
VI	A declared brain-dead patient whose organs are being removed for donor purposes	

11. Ans. (b) 2

(Ref: Miller's Anesthesia 8th E/P3257)

12. Ans. (b) Risk

(Ref: Miller's Anesthesia 8th E/P3257)

13. Ans. (c) Venous air embolism

(Ref: Millers anesthesia 8th E/P2170)

14. Ans. (b) Endotracheal Tube

(Ref: Miller's Anesthesia 8th E/P1665)

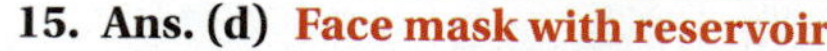

15. Ans. (d) Face mask with reservoir

(Ref: Ajay Yadav 5th E/P51, Fleisher's Pediatric Emergency Medicine)

- A face mask with oxygen reservoir bag attached to ambu bag can supply up to 100% oxygen.
- Venturi and oxygen mask supply 60% oxygen.
- A nasal cannula supplies 44% oxygen.

16. Ans. (b) Give bag and mask ventilation and reassess spontaneous breathing

(Ref: Ajay Yadav 5th E/P234)

17. Ans. (b) Vapor pressure

(Ref: Miller's Anesthesia 8th E/P767)

- When volatile agents are heated, they evaporate and form vapors to generate vapor pressure. Different agents have different **vapor pressures** and hence require different vaporizers.
- Thus to deliver accurate concentration the unknown agent must have a similar vapor pressure to sevoflurane.

18. Ans. (a) Administer skeletal muscle relaxant

(Ref: Miller's Anesthesia 8th E/P1554)

- **A notch in the phase 3 of inspiration is present in the capnogram given in the picture.**
- **This signifies rebreathing which can be seen due to wearing off effect of muscle relaxants and hence is also known as curare notch.**
- **Hence the patient is administered a dose of muscle relaxant.**

19. Ans. (a) Black body and white shoulder

(Ref: Ajay Yadav 4th E/P24)

Cylinder Color and Pin Index (Mnemonic: At ONCE)

Gas	Pin Index	Cylinder Color
At: Air	1,5	Grey body with black and white shoulders
O: Oxygen	2,5	**Black body with white shoulders**
N: Nitrous oxide	3,5	Blue
C: $CO_2 \geq 7.5\%$ $CO_2 < 7.5\%$ Cyclopropane	1,6 2,6 3,6	Grey Orange
Entonox	7	Blue body with blue and white shoulder

20. Ans. (c) Macintosh laryngoscope

(Ref: Ajay Yadav 4th E/P35)

21. Ans. (b) End tidal capnography

(Ref: David's The Neuroanesthesia Handbook/P221)

Procedure	Introduced by
End Tidal Capnography	Bethune and Brethren in 1965
Precordial Doppler	Maroon in 1968
Plethismography	Christopoulous and Nicolades in 1980
Transesophageal ECHO	Gosling and Side

22. Ans. (a) Extracorporeal membrane oxygenation (ECMO)

(Ref: Miller's Anesthesia 8th E/P3080)

- **Extracorporeal Membrane Oxygenation (ECMO):** It is nonconventional in that it **does not use a ventilator**. A large cannula is inserted into IVC and venous blood drawn is allowed to passed through an artificial lung for oxygenation and then the oxygenated blood is passed through small cannula into peripheral vein. It is reserved for treatment of hypoxia resistant to conventional therapy.

23. Ans. (a) CMV

(Ref: Miller's Anesthesia 8th E/P3064)

Controlled Mechanical Ventilation (CMV)

- In CMV there is no patient effort and the tidal volume is delivered by ventilator.
- Thus it is preferred in patients without effort in cases like paralysis and head injury.

24. Ans. (a) Ventilate Manually

(Ref: Miller's Anesthesia 8th E/P3064)

- Bellows of anesthetic machine collapse can be caused by a leak in the bellow assembly.
- To maintain perfusion manual ventilation should be continued.

25. Ans. (a) Capnography

(Ref: Miller's Anesthesia 8th E/P1670)

- Capnography is fastest as well as accurate method to confirm intubation; normal capnogram in at least 3 breaths.
- If capnography is equivocal, then fibreoptic bronchoscopy can be done.

26. Ans. (c) Calcium hydroxide

(Ref: Miller's Anesthesia 8th E/P787)

- Soda lime is made up of calcium hydroxide, sodium hydroxide, potassium hydroxide, silica and an indicator.
- Calcium hydroxide poorly reacts with CO_2, hence CO_2 first reacts with water to form bicarbonate, which further reacts with NaOH and KOH to form Na_2CO_3 and K_2CO_3.
- Finally the later compounds react with $Ca(OH)_2$ to form $CaCO_3$ and this is the **rate limiting step**.

27. Ans. (d) None of the above

(Ref: Morgan's 5th E/P127)

28. Ans. (b) Increased FRC

(Ref: Miller's Anesthesia 8th E/P3068)

Positive End Expiratory Pressure (PEEP)

- In PEEP a positive pressure is applied by the machine at end of expiration that prevents alveolar collapse and increases fractional residual capacity (FRC).
- PEEP is used in case of pulmonary edema, emergency thoracic surgery, ARDS and to prevent atelectasis.
- The drawbacks are the pressure can cause a decrease in cardiac output and hypotension, pulmonary hypertension and barotrauma.

29. Ans. (d) Mg $(OH)_2$

(Ref: Miller's Anesthesia 8th E/P788)

Soda lime
Calcium hydroxide: 94% Sodium hydroxide: 5% Potassium hydroxide: 1% + Silica: For consolidation + Indicators: Phenopthalein, Ethyl violet, Momosaz, Durasorb

30. Ans. (a) End tidal CO_2

(Ref: Miller's Anesthesia 8th E/P1670)

31. Ans. (c) Ventilator associated tracheobronchitis

(Ref: Miller's Anesthesia 8th E/P3049, https://www.ncbi.nlm.nih.gov/pmc/articles/PMC4188458/)

- Ventilator associated tracheobronchitis is considered to happen after colonization and before development of ventilator associated pneumonia (VAP).
- The diagnostic criteria for VAT are
  - Fever >38° C with no other cause
  - Purulent tracheal secretions
  - Positive tracheal aspirate (≥105cfu/mL)
  - Absence of new infiltrate on chest X-ray
- The causative organisms are mostly gram negative like pseudomonas followed by others like staphylococcus and acinetobacter.
- VAP is defined as pneumonia that develops after 48 hours of intubation.

32. Ans. (a) Correct application of cylinder to anaesthesia machine

(Ref: Miller's Anesthesia 8th E/P759)

- **DISS (Diameter Index Safety System):** For connection of gas pipeline in hospital, different diameter pipes with different colours are used for different gases to prevent wrong attachment. The oxygen connector is different from other gases in that it has a threaded texture.

33. Ans. (c) 60%

(Ref: Ajay Yadav 4th E/P43)

Oxygen delivery devices	Percentage of oxygen Delivered
Venturi Mask	**60%**
Oxygen Mask	60%
Rebreathing Mask	100%
Nonrebreathing Mask	80%
Nasal Cannula	44%

34. Ans. (d) 30 – 50 L/min

(Ref: Clinical Application of Mechanical Ventilation, 4th ed, David W. Chang, p-224-26)

35. Ans. (c) 3, 5

(Ref: Ajay Yadav 4th E/P24)

36. Ans. (b) 2, 5

(Ref: Ajay Yadav 4th E/P24)

37. Ans. (b) Orange

(Ref: Ajay Yadav 4th E/P24)

38. Ans. (c) Blue body with blue and white shoulder

(Ref: Ajay Yadav 4th E/P24)

39. Ans. (c) 1917

40. Ans. (a) Venturi mask

(Ref: Ajay Yadav 4th E/P42)

Fixed oxygen delivery device	Variable oxygen delivery device
Venturi Mask	Oxygen Mask Nasal cannula Breathing Mask Rebreathing Mask

41. Ans. (d) Tricholoethylene

(Ref: Miller's Anesthesia 8th E/P789)

- The bases NaOH and KOH can react with some agents to produce toxic compounds.
- Trielene can react with these bases to produce dichloracetylene which is neurotoxic and phosgene gas which can cause ARDS.
- Sevoflurane can react with bases to produce compound A which is nephrotoxic. Sevoflurane can also react with bases (mainly barylime) to create an exothermic reaction that can cause airway burn.

42. Ans. (d) Aspiration pneumonitis

(Ref: Miller's Anesthesia 8th E/P3079)

Mnemonics

Uses of PEEP
- **P** : Pulmonary edema
- **E** : Emergency thoracic surgery
- **E** : Emergency in ARDS
- **P** : Prevent atelectasis, PaO2 < 60 mmHg

- **Shunt fraction of 10% means a PaO_2 of > 350 mmHg at FiO_2 of 1.0 and hence it also requires PEEP.**

43. Ans. (b) Ulnar nerve

(Ref: Miller's Anesthesia 8th E/P1610)

Sites of Nerve Stimulation and Different Muscle Responses
- In principle, any superficially located peripheral motor nerve can be stimulated.
- In clinical anesthesia, the ulnar nerve is the most popular site; the median, posterior tibial, common peroneal, and facial nerves are also sometimes used.
- For stimulation of the ulnar nerve, the electrodes are best applied to the volar side of the wrist.

44. Ans. (d) Lower end of esophagus

(Ref: Ajay Yadav 4th E/P52)

For Temperature Measurement During Anesthesia

- Most ideal site: Lower end of esophagus
- Most accurate site for core body temperature: Pulmonary artery
- Most accurate site for measuring brain temperature: Tympanic membrane

45. Ans. (d) Theta to delta waves

(Ref: Ajay Yadav 4th E/P54)

EEG in different stages of anesthesia

Clinical stage	EEG
Awake	Alpha waves
Excitation	Beta waves
Early anesthesia	Alpha-Theta waves
Surgical tolerance	Delta
Deep surgical tolerance	Delta
High dose/Toxicity	Isoelectric EEG

46. Ans. (b) Can be prevented by administration of warm fluids

(Ref: Miller's Anesthesia 8th E/P1638)

- **Hypothermia is usually seen with volatile anesthetic agents.**
- **It can be prevented by warm IV fluids.**
- **Hypothermia is beneficial only in cases to prevent ischemia in cardiac surgery and neurosurgery.**
- **The most common mechanism of heat loss is convection and radiation.**

47. Ans. (a) Depth of general anesthesia

(Ajay Yadav 4th E/P54)

48. Ans. (a) Wrist

(Ref: Miller's Anesthesia 8th E/P1349)

- Invasive blood pressure monitoring can be done by catheterization of radial artery. However before it the patency of ulnar artery is confirmed by Allen's test.

Allen's Test

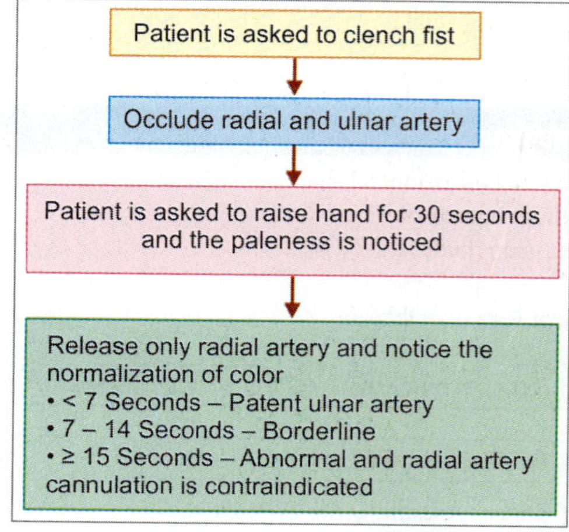

Patient is asked to clench fist
Occlude radial and ulnar artery
Patient is asked to raise hand for 30 seconds and the paleness is noticed
Release only radial artery and notice the normalization of color
• < 7 Seconds – Patent ulnar artery
• 7 – 14 Seconds – Borderline
• ≥ 15 Seconds – Abnormal and radial artery cannulation is contraindicated

49. Ans. (b) Bispectral index monitoring

(Ref: Miller's Anesthesia 8th E/P1527)

- EEG signal can be used for assessment of patient's level of consciousness using index system like bispectral index, patient safety index, narcotrend index and entropy.
- In bispectral index there is a scale of 0 to 100; a score of 100 the patient is fully awake, at 40-60 anesthesia is adequate and at 0 patient is in coma.
- In patient safety index also there is a scale of 0 to 100 and a value of 25 - 50 signifies adequate anesthesia.
- Bispectral index and patient safety index are less accurate in determining conscious level in children and with drugs like ketamine, dexmedetomidine and nitrous oxide.

50. Ans. (d) Hypothermia

(Ref: David's Monitoring in Anesthesia and Perioperative care/ P204)

- Hypothermia produces slowing of EEG and the predictable response of EEG to hypothermia is used for monitoring of therapeutic hypothermia.

51. Ans. (c) To monitor the depth of general anesthesia

(Ref: Miller's Anesthesia 8th E/P1527)

52. Ans. (c) Delta

(Ref: Ernst's Electroencephalography)

EEG in different stages of anesthesia	
Clinical Stage	EEG
Awake	Alpha waves
Excitation	Beta waves
Early anesthesia	Alpha-Theta waves
Surgical tolerance	Delta
Deep surgical tolerance	Delta
High dose/Toxicity	Isoelectric EEG

53. Ans. (c) Pain intensity

(Ref: Miller's Anesthesia 7th E/P1631)

Visual Analog Scale (VAS) is commonly used for assessment of pain.

54. Ans. (a) Oxygen saturation of hemoglobin

(Ref: Miller's Anaesthesia 8th E/P1546-47)

55. Ans. (d) Mapelson A

(Ref: Miller's Anesthesia 8th E/P791)

56. Ans. (a) Jackson Rees modification of ayre's T piece

(Ref: Miller's Anesthesia 8th E/P791)

57. Ans. (a) Mapleson A

(Ref: Miller's Anesthesia 8th E/P791)

58. Ans. (a) Jackson Rees modification of Ayre's T piece

(Ref: Miller's Anesthesia 8th E/P791)

59. Ans. (c) Ayers T piece

(Ref: Miller's Anesthesia 8th E/P791)

60. Ans. (d) Mapleson E

(Ref: Miller's Anesthesia 8th E/P791)

61. Ans. (a) A

(Ref: Ajay Yadav 5th E/P34)

62. Ans. (b) Simultaneous administration of an induction and neuromuscular blocking agents

(Ref: Miller's Anesthesia 8th E/P1655)

Rapid Sequence Intubation

- Rapid sequence intubation is used in conditions associated with increased risk of regurgitation and aspiration like patient with full stomach, GERD, morbid obesity, gastroparesis, pregnancy after 20 weeks gestation, cardiac arrest.
- Patient is administered an IV agent followed by IV Succinylcholine after preoxygenation with 100% oxygen for 3 minutes. Then cricoid pressure is applied (Sellick maneuver) to occlude esophagus and intubation is done.
- The cuffs commonly used nowadays are high volume low pressure cuffs as the older low volume high pressure coughs are associated with musical injury.

63. Ans. (a) Above oesophagus

(Ref: Miller's Anesthesia 8th E/P1664)

- The equipment in the picture is a second generation laryngeal mask airway like proseal or supreme.
- Unlike classical ones it has a drain attached and the tip designated as A in the picture is placed above esophagus.

64. Ans. (c) 4.0

(Ref: Miller's Anesthesia 8th E/P1663)

65. Ans. (c) Pregnant female

(Ref: Ajay Yadav 4th E/P40)

Contraindication of LMA

- High risk for aspiration patients (**pregnancy**, hiatus hernia)
- Patients with full stomach
- Patients with oropharyngeal mass.

66. Ans. (b) Prevent aspiration

(Ref: Ajay Yadav 4th E/P40)

67. Ans. (d) All of the above

(Ref: Ajay Yadav 4th E/P40)

68. Ans. (c) 2.5

(Ref: Ajay Yadav 4th E/P40)

LMA sizes	
Age Group	Size
Neonate	1
Infant 5–10 kg	1.5
Children 10–20 kg	2
Children 20–30 kg	**2.5**
Children or Adult 30–50 kg	3
Adult 50–70 kg	4
Adult > 70–100 kg	5
Adult > 100 kg	6

69. Ans. (c) Minor surgery

(Ref: Ajay Yadav 4th E/P40)

70. Ans. (b) Ankylosis of temporomandibular joint

(Ref: Ajay Yadav 4th E/P39)

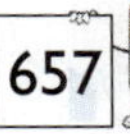

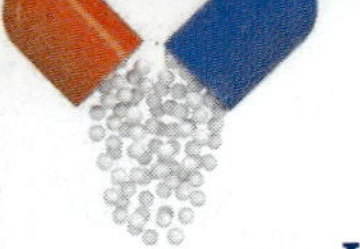

Indications of Blind Nasal Intubation

- Ankylosis of temporomandibular joint
- Trismus
- Neck contractures

71. Ans. (b) Fracture cervical spine

(Ref: Mohan Manual of ICU procedures/P17)

Both nasal and oral intubation	Nasal intubation
Intact gag reflex Unstable cervical spine Transaction of trachea High risk of laryngospasm (epiglottitis, laryngitis)	Basilar skull fracture CSF rhinorrhea Nasal polyps, abscess, adenoids Bleeding disorders

72. Ans. (d) Increased thyromental distance

(Ref: Miller's Anesthesia 8th E/P1669)

73. Ans. (d) Base of skull fracture

(Ref: Ajay Yadav 4th E/P38)

Contraindications of nasal intubation
Basilar skull fracture
CSF rhinorrhea
Nasal polyps, abscess, adenoids
Bleeding disorders

74. Ans. (a) To maintain airway patency during GA

(Ref: Miller's Anesthesia 8th E/P1665)

75. Ans. (a) Lorazepam

(Ref: Miller's Anesthesia 8th E/P841)

- Benzodiazepines like midazolam, lorazepam and diazepam can be used for induction of anesthesia.
- Other uses of benzodiazepines in anesthesia are for premedication, sedation and prophylaxis of postoperative nausea and vomiting (PONV).
- Overall the benzodiazepine of choice in anesthesia is midazolam as it has fastest onset of action.
- Dexmeditomidine is not used for induction of anesthesia as it requires high doses which can cause severe hypotension.

76. Ans. (a) Give atropine

(Ref: Miller's Anesthesia 8th E/P3209)

- The drug of choice for treatment of bradycardia in infants and children is epinephrine by intravenous or intraosseous route (1:10,000). The dose is 0.01 mg/kg and is repeated every 3-5 minutes.
- Epinephrine can also be given by endotracheal route at doses 0.1 mg/kg (1:1000).
- If patient does not respond to epinephrine, then atropine at doses of 0.2 mg/kg is used.
- If patient does not respond to both epinephrine and atropine then transcutaneous cardiac pacing is done.

77. Ans. (a) Ketamine followed by Intubation and GA

(Ref: Miller's Anesthesia 8th E/P849)

- **Due to cardiostimulatory effect ketamine is the preferred IV anesthetic agent of choice in hypovolemic and hemorrhagic shock.**
- **As this is a clear case of hemorrhagic shock, ketamine should be initiated followed by general anesthesia.**

78. Ans. (b) Propofol

(Ref: Miller's Anesthesia 8th E/P831)

Anesthetic Agents Associated with Pain on:

- Intravenous injection: Propofol
- Intraarterial injection: Thiopentone

79. Ans. (a) Remifentanyl, midazolam, propofol

(Ref: Miller's Anesthesia 8th E/P830)

- Propofol is the intravenous anesthetic agent of choice for:
  - Day care surgery (recovery faster than thiopental)
  - Total intravenous anesthesia (TIVA)
  - Sedation in ICU
  - Surgery and in patients susceptible to malignant hyperthermia.
- Remifentanyl is shortest acting opioid and midazolam is shortest acting benzodiazepine and hence also preferred in day care surgery.

80. Ans. (a) Propofol

(Ref: Miller's Anesthesia 8th E/P830)

81. Ans. (a) Ketamine

(Ref: Miller's Anesthesia 8th E/P850)

Contraindications of Ketamine

- Epilepsy
- Schizophrenia
- Glaucoma
- Ocular injury
- Ischemic heart disease
- Vascular aneurysms

82. Ans. (c) Ketamine

(Ref: Miller's Anesthesia 8th E/P849)

83. Ans. (c) Etomidate

(Ref: Goodman Gilman 12th E/P538)

Etomidate is Preferred for Induction in

- Old patients
- Cardiovascular disorders (aneurysm, cardiomyopathy, CAD, aortic stenosis)
- Altered hemodynamic states (splenic rupture, hemorrhagic shock)

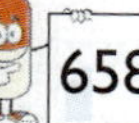

84. Ans. (c) Ketamine

(Ref: Goodman Gilman 13th E/P391)

- All IV anesthetic agent cause pain on injection except ketamine.
- Maximum pain is caused by propofol.
- Pain on accidental intraarterial injection is caused by thiopentone.

85. Ans. (b) Ketamine

(Ref: Goodman Gilman 13th E/P389)

86. Ans. (c) Redistribution of the drug from sites in the CNS

(Ref: Morgan's 5th E/P170)

87. Ans. (a) Myoclonus and adrenal suppression

(Ref: Morgan's 5th E/P185)

88. Ans. (c) Thiopentone

(Ref: Goodman Gilman 12th E/P535)

89. Ans. (c) Hyperactive airways

(Ref: Miller's Anesthesia 8th E/P849)

- Ketamine causes bronchodilation due to its sympathomimetic effect and hence preferred in case of reactive airway diseases for induction.
- Halothane has similar effect and is preferred for maintenance.

90. Ans. (c) Propofol

(Ref: Miller's Anesthesia 8th E/P830)

91. Ans. (b) Ketamine

(Ref: Miller's Anesthesia 8th E/P848)

- Ketamine causes bronchodilation due to its sympathomimetic effect and hence preferred in case of reactive airway diseases for induction.
- Halothane has similar effect and is preferred for maintenance.

92. Ans. (a) Ketamine

(Ref: Miller's Anesthesia 8th E/P847)

- Ketamine primarily acts by inhibiting NMDA subtype of glutamate receptors in the association area of cortex and thalamus which produces **dissociative anesthesia and strong analgesia respectively**.
- In this dissociative or cataleptic state patient appears awake with preserved reflexes (corneal, laryngeal and pharyngeal) but is detached from the surrounding with eyes open.

93. Ans. (a) Acute intermittent porphyria

(Ref: Goodman Gilman 12th E/P535)

Acute intermittent Porphyria can be seen with drugs like:

Drugs causing acute intermittent porphyria

- Barbiturates
- Etomidate
- Halothane
- Cocaine
- Lidocaine
- Prilocaine
- Clonidine
- Metoclopromide
- Hyoscine
- Diclofenac
- Ranitidine

94. Ans. (b) Etomidate

(Ref: Goodman Gilman 12th E/P538)

95. Ans. (c) Ketamine

(Ref: Miller's Anesthesia 8th E/P849)

96. Ans. (b) Althesin

(Ref: Ajay Yadav 4th E/P93)

Althesin is a steroid derivative associated with side effects like

- Anaphylaxis
- Raised intracranial tension

97. Ans. (b) Propofol

(Ref: Goodman Gilman 12th E/P537)

Excitatory effects characterized by involuntary movements are seen with propofol and thiopentone > methohexital like

- Choreiform movements
- Opisthotonus

98. Ans. (c) Ketamine

(Ref: Goodman Gilman 12th E/P535-38)

99. Ans. (a) Etomidate

(Ref: Goodman Gilman 12th E/P538)

100. Ans. (b) Good analgesic action

(Ref: Miller's Anesthesia 8th E/P849)

- Ketamine produces strong analgesia by inhibiting glutamate receptors in the thalamus.
- Thus it can be used in low doses for pain in post-operative period, cancer, neuropathy, fibromyalgia, migraine and phantom limb.
- Other options are incorrect as all kinds of pressure like blood pressure, ICP and IOP are increased.

101. Ans. (c) Ketamine

(Ref: Miller's Anesthesia 8th E/P848)

102. Ans. (b) Ketamine

(Ref: Miller's Anesthesia 8th E/P849)

- DIC is associated with bleeding and hypotension and hence ketamine should be preferred for induction as it stimulates sympathetic system which increases cardiac output and blood pressure.

103. Ans. (c) Ketamine

(Ref: Miller's Anesthesia 8th E/P848)

- **Intraoperative wheezing can be seen due to bronchospasm, secretions etc.**
- **Since ketamine is a bronchodilator it can be used in this case.**

104. Ans. (c) 2.5%

(Ref: Goodman Gilman 12th E/P535)

Percentage of Barbiturates Used

Thiopental sodium	2.5%
Thiamylal	2%
Methohexital	1%

105. Ans. (b) Propofol

(Ref: Miller's Anesthesia 8th E/P830)

- Propofol is the intravenous anesthetic agent of choice for:
  - Day care surgery (recovery faster than thiopental)
  - Total intravenous anesthesia (TIVA)
  - Sedation in ICU
  - Surgery and in patients susceptible to malignant hyperthermia.

106. Ans. (d) Ketamine

(Ref: Miller's Anesthesia 8th E/P850)

- **Ketamine increases muscle tone and hence should be avoided in patients with malignant hyperthermia.**

107. Ans. (a) Propofol

(Ref: Goodman Gilman 12th E/P534)

Plasma Protein Binding

Propofol	**98% (Maximum)**
Barbiturates	85%
Etomidate	76%
Ketamine	**27% (Minimum)**

108. Ans. (b) Decreases cerebral metabolism and decreases intracranial tension

(Ref: Goodman Gilman 12th E/P535)

109. Ans. (c) Ketamine

(Ref: Miller's Anesthesia 8th E/P847)

- Ketamine stimulates limbic system, which causes **hallucinations and emergence reaction**.
- Emergence reaction seen during awakening from ketamine anesthesia is characterized by vivid dreams, sensation of floating out of body, illusions, confusion and euphoria. The drug of choice for treatment of same is benzodiazepines.

110. Ans. (d) Ketamine

(Ref: Miller's Anesthesia 8th E/P848)

- Apart from this it also has stimulatory effect on sympathetic and opioid receptors and inhibitory effect on muscarinic receptors.
- Sympathetic receptor stimulation **stimulates heart (tachycardia)** and causes vasoconstriction (increase in blood pressure) and bronchodilation.

111. Ans. (a) Ketamine

(Ref: Miller's Anesthesia 8th E/P848)

Ketamine causes **bronchodilation** and hence is preferred IV anesthetic agent in **reactive airway disease like bronchial asthma** and **status asthmaticus**.

112. Ans. (b) Ketamine

(Ref: Miller's Anesthesia 8th E/P849)

- Since ketamine has cardiostimulatory effect and increases blood pressure it is IV anesthetic agent of choice in **shock (hypovolemic, hemorrhagic, septic), DIC** and preferred in cardiac tamponade, restrictive pericarditis and **cyanotic congenital heart diseases with right to left shunt** also.
- In cyanotic congenital heart disease, systemic vasoconstriction limits the right to left shunting.

113. Ans. (d) Ketamine

(Ref: Miller's Anesthesia 8th E/P850)

114. Ans. (b) Ketamine

(Ref: Miller's Anesthesia 8th E/P850)

115. Ans. (d) Etomidate

(Ref: Goodman Gilman 12th E/P538)

116. Ans. (d) All of the above

(Ref: Goodman Gilman 12th E/P536-538)

- Pain on intravenous injection is caused by maximum with propofol followed by other drugs like barbiturates (methohexital > thiopental) and etomidate.
- Pain on intraarterial injection is caused by thiopental sodium.

117. Ans. (a) Hypertension

(Ref: Miller's Anesthesia 8th E/P850)

- **Ketamine stimulates sympathetic system and increases blood pressure and hence should be avoided in hypertensive patients.**

118. Ans. (c) Ketamine

(Ref: Miller's Anesthesia 8th E/P845)

- Ketamine was synthesized by Stevens but first used clinically by Corssen and Domino.
- It is a **phencyclidine** with high lipid solubility and poor plasma protein binding; hence It has a very high volume of distribution.

119. Ans. (b) Infants >neonates > adults

(Ref: Ajay Yadav 4th E/P59)

- MAC decreases with age, however its maximum at the age of 6 months.
- Hence in the given options its maximum with infants > neonates > adults.

120. Ans. (b) Nitrous oxide

(Ref: Ajay Yadav 4th E/P65)

- Absorption and secretion of CSF is decreased by thiopentone and increased by halothane and ketamine.
- Nitrous oxide has no effect on CSF absorption or secretion.

121. Ans. (b) Combined with nitrous oxide

(Ref: Ajay Yadav 4th E/P66)

Induction is Faster with

- Agent having low blood gas partition coefficient
- Patient with decreased residual volume – As more gas will be passed on to the pulmonary circulation at a faster rate.
- Left to right shunt – As more blood will be diverted to pulmonary circulation that will lead to faster delivery of anesthetic agents to brain.

122. Ans. (c) Sevoflurane

(Ref: Miller's Anesthesia 8th E/P402)

Inhalational agents	Increase in ICP
Halothane	+++++++++ (Maximum)
Sevoflurane	**+ (Minimum)**
Nitrous oxide	+
Isoflurane	++
Desflurane	++

123. Ans. (a) Nitrous oxide

(Ref: Ajay Yadav 4th E/P65)

124. Ans. (c) Slow induction and slow recovery

(Ref: Ajay Yadav 4th E/P66)

- Xenon overall has least blood gas partition coefficient and thus has fastest induction and recovery.
- Though it is not commonly used due to its high cost.

125. Ans. (a) Desflurane

(Ref: Goodman Gilman 13th E/P394)

- Desflurane > Isoflurane are respiratory irritant drugs that can cause cough and laryngospasm.
- Hence these are not preferred for induction of anesthesia, rather used in maintenance.

126. Ans. (c) Sevoflurane

(Ref: Goodman Gilman 12th E/P564)

127. Ans. (a) Halothane

(Ref: Goodman Gilman 12th E/P543)

- Halothane has a tocolytic effect and hence is used for internal version and manual removal of placenta.

128. Ans. (c) Halothane

(Ref: Goodman Gilman 12th E/P542)

Preferred Bronchodilators in Asthma

Induction: Ketamine
Maintenance: Halothane

129. Ans. (a) Minimum alveolar concentration

(Ref: Miller's Anesthesia 8th E/P767-68)

Minimum Alveolar Concentration (MAC)

- 1 MAC is the minimum alveolar concentration that prevents movement in response to surgical stimulation in 50% of patients. It is described in percentage of agent required in alveolar air to produce the above effect. Sevoflurane has a MAC of 2%; this means out of 100% space in alveoli 2% should be occupied by sevoflurane to produce effect in 50% patients. Thus to produce effect in 100% patients 2 MAC is required, i.e. 4% of sevoflurane in the alveolar space.
- Comparing MAC to pharmacodynamics, it is like the minimum dose required for a particular effect, hence **MAC is a measure of potency of inhalational agents.**

130. Ans. (c) Diethyl ether

(Ref: Goodman Gilman 12th E/P527)

- Ether was first used as anesthetic agent by Crawford Long.
- Ether was first used for public demonstration by WTG Morton.

131. Ans. (b) Speed of induction and recovery

(Ref: Ajay Yadav 4th E/P60)

Blood Gas Partition Coefficient

- Blood gas partition coefficient is the ratio of solubility of inhalational anesthetic agent in blood to gas.
- When an inhalational anesthetic agent is started it diffuses out of alveoli into pulmonary capillaries and depends upon its solubility it takes time to saturate in blood. An agent with high solubility in blood will take more time and vice versa. After the blood is saturated the inhalational agent starts to exert a partial pressure and this is responsible for anesthetic effect by acting on CNS. Thus a drug with high solubility in blood takes more time to exert a partial pressure and hence effect is delayed. Similarly on discontinuation of drug, effect is terminated after the free agent plus the one soluble in blood is exhaled or metabolized; thus for agents with high solubility in blood, recovery is also slower.
- Thus agents with high blood gas partition coefficient have slower induction and recovery and agents with low blood as partition coefficient have faster induction and recovery.

132. Ans. (c) N_2O

(Ref: Ajay Yadav 4th E/P64)

133. Ans. (a) Halothane

(Ref: Goodman Gilman 12th E/P543)

- A metabolite of halothane called as trifluoroacetyldehyde can acetylate liver proteins and cause hepatic necrosis.

134. Ans. (b) Hepatitis

(Ref: Goodman Gilman 12th E/P543)

135. Ans. (a) Diffusion hypoxia

(Ref: Ajay Yadav 4th E/P62)

Concentration Effect, Second Gas Effect and Diffusion Hypoxia

- A low blood gas partition coefficient of nitrous oxide produces effects like concentration effect, second gas effect and diffusion hypoxia.
- It diffuses immediately out of alveoli into capillaries and creates a negative pressure in the alveoli which draws more nitrous oxide from the cylinder; this is known as **concentration effect**.
- This negative pressure can pull oxygen or other volatile agents also into the alveoli; this is known as **second gas effect**.
- After nitrous oxide is discontinued, the alveoli are flooded back with nitrous oxide from the capillaries; this is called as **diffusion hypoxia**. Diffusion hypoxia is prevented by administering **100% oxygen to the patient for five minutes** before discontinuation of nitrous oxide. These effects are seen only with nitrous oxide, as it is the only agent used at high concentration.

136. Ans. (b) Nitrous oxide

(Ref: Ajay Yadav 4th E/P62)

137. Ans. (d) Entonox

(Ref: Ajay Yadav 4th E/P24)

138. Ans. (b) Methoxyflurane

(Ref: Ajay Yadav 4th E/P72)

139. Ans. (a) Succinylcholine + halothane

(Ref: Goodman Gilman 12th E/P543)

- Anesthetic agents like halothane and muscle relaxant like succinylcholine stimulate ryanodine receptors and cause malignant hyperthermia.
- The drug of choice for same is dantrolene.

140. Ans. (b) Sevoflurane

(Ref: Goodman Gilman 12th E/P546)

Uses of Sevoflurane

- Sevoflurane has a low blood gas partition coefficient and hence causes a faster induction and recovery; thus preferred in day care surgery.
- As it is non-pungent it does not cause cough and laryngospasm and is the inhalational induction agent of choice in infants and children.
- It maintains a normal heart rate and does not increases oxygen demand; hence preferred in myocardial ischemia.
- It causes least increase in intracranial pressure and hence preferred in neurosurgery.

141. Ans. (a) Ether

(Ref: Ajay Yadav 4th E/P71)

142. Ans. (c) Isoflurane

(Ref: Goodman Gilman 12th E/P543)

143. Ans. (c) Methoxyflurane

(Ref: Ajay Yadav 4th E/P71)

144. Ans. (d) 6

(Ref: Ajay Yadav 4th E/P59)

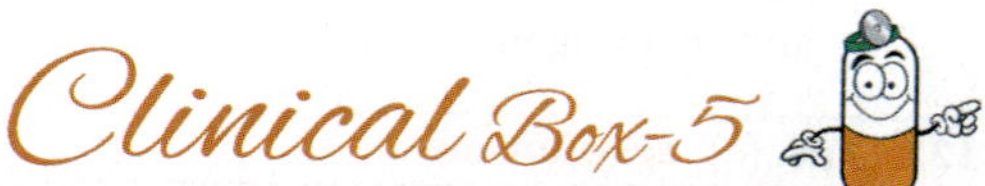

Inhalational agent	MAC	Blood gas partition coefficient	Odor
Nitrous Oxide	104	0.47	Nil
Halothane	0.75	2.5	Sweet
Enflurane	1.58	1.9	Nil
Isoflurane	1.28	1.4	Irritant
Desflurane	6.0	0.45	Pungent
Sevoflurane	2.05	0.65	Nil
Methoxyflurane	0.2	12	Nil
Xenon	71	0.14	Nil

145. Ans. (b) Reversal of anesthesia

(Ref: Ajay Yadav 4th E/P65)

146. Ans. (b) N_2O

(Ref: Ajay Yadav 4th E/P65)

- Nitrous oxide inactivates vitamin B_{12} and its deficiency resulting in peripheral neuropathy, megaloblastic anemia and subacute combined degeneration of spinal cord.
- It can diffuse into cavities and accumulate and hence contraindicated in patients with pneumothorax, pneumoperitoneum, volvulus, laparoscopic procedures ocular surgery and middle ear surgery.
- It can increase homocysteine, which increases vascular inflammation and thrombosis. Other side effects associated are methemoglobinemia, pulmonary edema and laryngospasm (due to impurities).

147. Ans. (d) Desflurane

(Ref: Ajay Yadav 4th E/P63)

Fluoride Content is

- Maximum in **Methoxyflurane**
- Minimum with **Desflurane**

148. Ans. (c) Trielene

(Ref: Ajay Yadav 4th E/P73)

- Tachypnea is seen with trielene > ether.

149. Ans. (c) Trielene

(Ref: Ajay Yadav 4th E/P73)

Trilene reacts with sodalime in closed circuit to produce toxic compounds:

- Dicholoroacetylene causes neurotoxicity involving fifth cranial nerve most commonly
- Phosgene causes ARDS.

150. Ans. (a) Isoflurane

(Ref: Ajay Yadav 4th E/P63)

- Fluoride content is least with desflurane followed by isoflurane.
- Halothane produces fluoride only in anaerobic conditions.

151. Ans. (d) N_2O

(Ref: Ajay Yadav 4th E/P61)

Among the given agents N_2O has the least blood gas partition coefficient and hence will be associated with fstest induction and recovery.

152. Ans. (c) Trielene

(Ref: Ajay Yadav 4th E/P73)

- All agents decrease myocardial contractility except ether which increases contractility due to release of catecholamines.
- Trielene does not have any effect on myocardial contractility.

153. Ans. (c) N_2O

(Ref: Ajay Yadav 4th E/P63)

154. Ans. (a) Halothane

(Ref: Goodman Gilman 12th E/P542)

- Halothane sensitizes heart to catecholamines and hence it is contraindicated in patients with pheochromocytoma.
- Premature ventricular contractions and ventricular tachycardia can be seen with halothane if used with epinephrine.

155. Ans. (d) Desflurane

(Ref: Ajay Yadav 4th E/P61)

- Desflurane has the least blood gas partition coefficient and hence associated with fastest induction as well as recovery.

156. Ans. (b) Halothane

(Ref: Wylie and Churchill Davidson's A Practise of Anaesthesia, 5th ed/P198-206)

157. Ans. (c) Halothane

(Ref: Goodman Gilman 12th E/P543)

- Bandle contraction ring is seen in case of obstructed labour for which halothane can be used due to its tocolytic effect.

158. Ans. (a) Nitrous oxide

(Ref: Ajay Yadav 4th E/P64)

159. Ans. (d) 36.5°C

(Ref: Ajay Yadav 4th E/P64)

Properties of Nitrous Oxide

Boiling Point	-89°C
Critical temperature	36.5°C
Molecular weight	44
MAC	104%

160. Ans. (a) 50:50

(Ref: Ajay Yadav 4th E/P65)

161. Ans. (b) Xenon

(Ref: Miller's Anaesthesia 8th Ed/P666-667)

162. Ans. (c) Minimum alveolar concentration

(Ref: Ajay Yadav 4th E/P58)

163. Ans. (a) N_2O

(Ref: Ajay Yadav 4th E/P65)

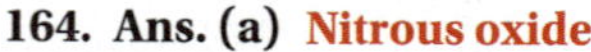

164. Ans. (a) Nitrous oxide

(Ref: Ajay Yadav 4th E/P65)

165. Ans. (b) Halothane

(Ref: Goodman Gilman 12th E/P543)

- Postoperative chills and shivering can be seen with halothane due to a decrease in the core temperature of the body.
- Drugs used for treatment of same are pethidine (DOC) and tramadol.

166. Ans. (d) It is nephrotoxic at high doses

(Ref: Ajay Yadav 4th E/P70)

167. Ans. (d) Nitrous oxide

(Ref: Ajay Yadav 4th E/P65)

- All inhalational agents undergo metabolism in liver except nitrous oxide which is excreted unchanged by lungs and hence preferred in patients with liver disease.

168. Ans. (a) Slow induction and recovery

(Ref: Goodman Gilman 12th E/P543)

- Overall xenon has the least blood gas partition coefficient and hence has fastest induction and recovery.

169. Ans. (b) Enflurane

(Ref: Goodman Gilman 12th E/P544)

170. Ans. (b) Ether

(Ref: Ajay Yadav 4th E/P71)

171. Ans. (a) Halothane

(Ref: Goodman Gilman 12th E/P542)

172. Ans. (b) Nitrous oxide

(Ref: Goodman Gilman 12th E/P547)

173. Ans. (c) Methoxyflurane

(Ref: Ajay Yadav 4th E/P72)

174. Ans. (b) Nitrous oxide

(Ref: Ajay Yadav 4th E/P65)

175. Ans. (a) Methoxyflurane

(Ref: Ajay Yadav 4th E/P72)

176. Ans. (b) Halothane

(Ref: Ajay Yadav 4th E/P59)

177. Ans. (c) Lowers ICT, hence preferred in CNS surgeries

(Ref: Goodman Gilman 12th E/P542)

- Halothane increases cerebral blood flow and ICP and hence contraindicated in neurosurgery.

178. Ans. (c) Isoflurane

(Ref: Goodman Gilman 12th E/P543)

- The agent which undergoes maximum metabolism is methoxyflurane followed by halothane, followed by others (methoxyflurane > halothane > enflurane > isoflurane > desflurane).
- Hence isoflurane undergoes least metabolism among given options and is least hepatotoxic.

179. Ans. (b) Doesn't release histamine

(Ref: Goodman Gilman 13th E/P182)

180. Ans. (c) Blocks Ach receptors

(Ref: Goodman Gilman 13th E/P179)

181. Ans. (b) Sugammadex

(Ref: Goodman Gilman 13th E/P187)

- Sugammadex is a gamma cyclodextrin which encapsulates the muscle relaxants and removes them from neuromuscular junction and plasma.
- It is used for emergency reversal of rocuronium and vecuronium.

182. Ans. (c) Inhibition of acetylcholine receptors

(Ref: Goodman Gilman 12th E/P258)

- d-tubocurare is a nondepolarizing muscle relaxant which competitively blocks the nicotinic acetylcholine receptors in the neuromuscular junction.
- Suxamethonium and decamethonium are depolarizing muscle relaxants which act by depolarizing post synaptic membrane followed by inactivation of sodium channels.

183. Ans. (a) Ulnar nerve

(Ref: Ajay Yadav 5th E/P64)

The most common muscle used to assess effect of muscle relaxants is adductor pollicis which is supplied by ulnar nerve.

184. Ans. (b) Dantrolene sodium

(Ref: Goodman Gilman 12th E/P264)

- Depolarizing muscle relaxants like succinylcholine and nondepolarizing uscle relaxants like pipecuronium and mivacurium act on the neuromuscular junction.
- Dantrolene acts by inhibiting ryanodine receptors in the endoplasmic reticulum.

185. Ans. (b) Neuromuscular blockers

(Ref: Goodman Gilman 12th E/P267)

186. Ans. (a) Atracurium

(Ref: Goodman Gilman 12th E/P263)

187. Ans. (b) Atracurium

(Ref: Goodman Gilman 12th E/P263)

- Atracurium undergoes ester hydrolysis (60%) and spontaneous degradation known as Hofmann elimination (40%), in which it is converted into a tertiary amine.
- Hence it is the muscle relaxant of choice in hepatic failure, renal failure, myastrhenia gravis, old age and new born.

188. Ans. (b) Succinylcholine

(Ref: Goodman Gilman 12th E/P260)

- Persistent depolarization of post synaptic membranes with Sch can cause hyperkalemia and contraction of muscles leading to side effects mentioned below.

Increased muscle contraction	Fasciculations Masseter spasm **Myalgia** Muscle damage – Raised myoglobin and CPK
Increased abdominal muscle contraction	Increased intragastric pressure
Increased oxygen consumption and carbon dioxide production due to muscle contraction cause cerebral vasodilation	Increased ICP
Increased tonic myofibrils contraction and dilation of choroidal blood vessels	Increased IOP
Increased catecholamine release	Increased blood pressure Ventricular tachyarrhythmia
Depolarization of muscles	Hyperkalemia
Cardiac muscarinic receptor stimulation	Sinus bradycardia Junctional rhythms
Stimulation of ryanodine receptor	Malignant hyperthermia

189. Ans. (a) Head and neck

(Ref: Goodman Gilman 12th E/P261)

- The central muscles with abundant blood supply like diaphragm, larynx and muscles of head and neck have fastest onset and offset of action. The peripheral muscles like that of hands like adductor pollicis have slowest onset and offset of action.
- The peripheral muscles are more sensitive to NDMR as compared to central muscles like diaphragm.

190. Ans. (b) Suxamethonium

(Ref: Goodman Gilman 12th E/P268)

191. Ans. (c) 2 years

(Ref: Smith's Fundamentals of Anesthesia 3rd E/P619)

192. Ans. (a) Atracurium

(Ref: Miller's Anesthesia 8th E/P986)

- There is correlation between total body weight and duration of action of atracurium.
- The duration of action is prolonged when atracurium is given based on ideal body weight.

193. Ans. (a) Monitoring neuromuscular function

(Ref: Miler's Anesthesia 8th E/P997)

- The muscular response can be recorded by kinemography (KMG), electromyography (EMG) and acceleromyography (AMG).
- KMG measures the electrical response in a piezoelectric film attached to the muscle. EMG measures the evoked electrical response of muscle. AMG measures the acceleration of muscle response.

194. Ans. (d) It occurs due to deficiency of cholinesterase

(Ref: Goodman Gilman 12th E/P267)

- Scoline apnea is seen due to deficiency of pseudo cholinesterase and not cholinesterase.
- It is a pharmacogenetic condition and hence can be inherited.
- Patients usually do not die if ventilation is continued till spontaneous respiration is established.

195. Ans. (c) No histamine release

(Ref: Ajaya Yadav 4th E/P101)

Cis-atracurium as Compared to Atracurium is Associated with:

- No histamine release
- Five times more potency
- Five times lesser laudanosine production

196. Ans. (b) Atracurium

(Ref: Ajay Yadav 4th E/P101)

- Laudanosine is produced by atracurium > cis-atracurium and hence atracurium is a better answer.

197. Ans. (a) Sodium Channels

(Ref: Goodman Gilman 12th E/P260)

- Suxamethonium is a depolarizing muscle relaxant, i.e. it acts by acting on the N_M subtype of nicotinic receptors on neuromuscular junction.
- This leads to opening of sodium channels and influx of sodium which causes depolarization of muscles.

198. Ans. (a) Atracurium

(Ref: Goodman Gilman 12th E/P263)

Atracurium is primarily eliminated by Hoffman's elimination, i.e. spontaneous degradation.

199. Ans. (b) Suxamethonium

(Ref: Goodman Gilman 12th E/P260)

200. Ans. (a) Produces bradycardia

(Ref: Ajay Yadav 4th E/P97)

Persistent depolarization of post synaptic membranes can cause hyperkalemia and contraction of muscles leading to side effects mentioned below.

Increased muscle contraction	Fasciculations Masseter spasm Myalgia Muscle damage – Raised myoglobin and CPK
Increased abdominal muscle contraction	Increased intragastric pressure
Increased oxygen consumption and carbon dioxide production due to muscle contraction cause cerebral vasodilation	Increased ICP
Increased tonic myofibrils contraction and dilation of choroidal blood vessels	Increased IOP
Increased catecholamine release	Increased blood pressure Ventricular tachyarrhythmia
Depolarization of muscles	Hyperkalemia
Cardiac muscarinic receptor stimulation	**Sinus bradycardia** Junctional rhythms
Stimulation of ryanodine receptor	Malignant hyperthermia

201. Ans. (d) Pancuronium

(Ref: Ajay Yadav 4th E/P99)

- Mivacurium and atracurium are benzylisoquinoline compounds which can cause histamine release and hence are contraindicated in bronchospastic disorders like bronchial asthma and COPD.
- Succinylcholine has been reported to cause bronchial asthma in some patients.
- Hence pancuronium is the best possible answer here.

202. Ans. (c) Pancuronium

(Ref: Goodman Gilman 12th E/P264)

203. Ans. (a) Dantrolene

(Ref: Miller's Anesthesia 8th E/P983)

- Dantrolene acts by inhibiting ryanodine receptors in the endoplasmic reticulum of muscles, which leads to decreased calcium release and muscle relaxation.
- Hence it is called as a directly acting muscle elaxant, i.e. acts on the muscles.

204. Ans. (c) Mivacurium

(Ref: Goodman Gilman 12th E/P264)

- Mivacurium is metabolized by pseudocholinesterase in plasma and hence is shortest acting available NDMR.
- It is the NDMR of choice for day care surgery.

205. Ans. (b) Suxamethonium

(Ref: Ajay Yadav 4th E/P97)

206. Ans. (a) Hypertension

(Ref: Ajay Yadav 4th E/P99)

Benzylisoquinolinium Compounds

- This group has drugs like d-tubocurare, doxacurium, mivacurium, atracurium and gantacurium.
- This class is notorious for causing histamine release and autonomic ganglionic block, which is maximum with d-tubocurare and hence is not used.
- Since these drugs can cause histamine release, hence are contraindicated in bronchospastic disorders like bronchial asthma and COPD.
- Histamine release can also cause hypotension and flushing.

207. Ans. (a) Doxacurium

(Ref: Goodman Gilman 12th E/P264)

- Doxacurium is most potent and longest acting NDMR with a duration of action of 120 minutes.
- Succinylcholine is the shortest and fastest acting muscle relaxant overall.
- Rocuronium is fastest acting NDMR.
- Rapacuronium is shortest acting available NDMR.
- Gantacurium is the shortest acting NDMR, but under trial.

208. Ans. (d) Atracurium

(Ref: Ajay Yadav 4th E/P99)

209. Ans. (a) Atracurium

(Ref: Ajay Yadav 4th E/P101)

210. Ans. (c) Curare

(Ref: Ajay Yadav 4th E/P99)

211. Ans. (d) Neostigmine

(Ref: Ajay Yadav 4th E/P103)

Reversal Agents

- ACHE inhibitors like edrophonium and neostigmine are routinely used for reversal of muscle relaxants. The details of this class is discussed in the chapter of autonomic nervous system.
- Sugammadex is a gamma cyclodextrin which encapsulates the muscle relaxants and removes them from plasma and neuromuscular junction. It is used for emergency reversal of rocuronium and vecuronium. It can cause hypersensitivity and bradycardia.

212. Ans. (c) Ryanodine receptor

(Ref: Goodman Gilman 12th E/P268)

213. Ans. (d) Pancuronium

(Ref: Ajay Yadav 4th E/P99)

Classification of Muscle Relaxants

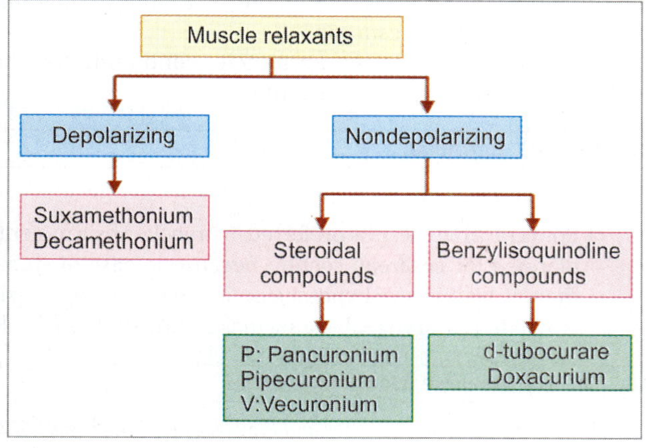

214. Ans. (c) Doxacurium

(Ref: Ajay Yadav 4th E/P99)

215. Ans. (a) Inhibiting calcium release from smooth muscle cells

(Ref: Goodman Gilman 12th E/P268)

216. Ans. (c) Pancuronium

(Ref: Goodman Gilman 12th E/P264)

- Doxacurium is the longest acting muscle relaxant with a duration of 120 minutes.
- Pancuronium is the second longest acting NDMR with a duration of 85–100 minutes.

217. Ans. (a) Rocuronium

(Ref: Goodman Gilman 12th E/P264)

218. Ans. (b) Pancuronium

(Ref: Goodman Gilman 12th E/P264)

- All NDMRs are excreted primarily by kidney (maximum with pancuronium) except with rocuronium which are excreted by liver.
- Vecuronium is excreted almost equally by liver and kidney.
- Atracurium and cis-atracurium undergo spontaneous degradation, i.e. Hoffman's elimination.

219. Ans. (d) Centrally acting Muscle relaxant

(Ref: Ajay Yadav 4th E/P102)

220. Ans. (c) Succinylcholine

(Ref: Godman Gilman 12th E/P264)

221. Ans. (b) Mivacurium

(Ref: Goodman Gilman 12th E/P264)

222. Ans. (a) Tetanic fade

(Ref: Goodman Gilman 12th E/P265)

223. Ans. (a) Atracurium

(Ref: Ajay Yadav 4th E/P101)

- Laudanosine in prodeuced by atracurium > cis-atracurium
- Hence atracurium is a better answer here.

224. Ans. (d) Succinylcholine

(Ref: Ajay Yadav 4th E/P97)

225. Ans. (c) Vecuronium

(Ref: Goodman Gilman 12th E/P264)

- All NDMRs are excreted primarily by kidney (maximum with pancuronium) except with rocuronium which are excreted by liver.
- Vecuronium is excreted almost equally by liver and kidney. Hence is relatively safe in renal disease.

226. Ans. (a) Ach cholinesterase activity derangement

(Ref: Miller's Anesthesia 8th E/P1136)

- Patients with atypical pseudocholinesterase due to genetic variability are unable to metabolize Sch and hence there is prolonged apnea.
- Dibucaine number is used to find out the amount of normal enzyme; dibucaine a local anesthetic inhibits 80% of normal enzyme but only 20% of abnormal enzyme. If it is said that the dibucaine number in a patient is 80, it means dibucaine inhibits 80% of normal enzyme.

Dibucaine number	Pseudocholinesterase type	Response to Sch
70–80	Homozygous typical	Normal
50–60	Heterozygous atypical	Abnormal
20–30	Homozygous atypical	Abnormal

227. Ans. (c) 80

(Ref: Miller's Anesthesia 8th E/P1136)

228. Ans. (a) Mivacurium

(Ref: Goodman Gilman 12th E/P264)

229. Ans. (c) Adductor pollicis

(Ref: Goodman Gilman 12th E/P265)

For neuromusclural blockade monitoring

- Most common muscle used : Adductor pollicis
- Most ideal muscle is : Orbicularis oculi

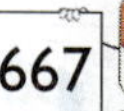

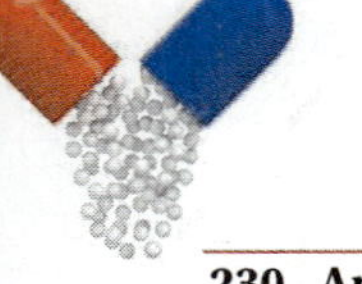

230. Ans. (d) Masseter spasm

(Ref: Goodman Gilman 12th E/P268)

231. Ans. (a) Tizanidine

(Ref: Ajay Yadav 4th E/P102)

232. Ans. (c) Rocuronium

(Ref: Ajay Yadav 4th E/P100)

233. Ans. (a) Glycopyrrolate

(Ref: Ajay Yadav 4th E/P234)

- Glycopyrrolate is an anticholinergic drug used to prevent secretions in almost every patient prior to surgery as a part of preanesthetic medications.
- Glycopyrrolate is preferred as It is a quarternary amine and hence does not cross the blood brain barrier.

234. Ans. (b) Retrograde amnesia

(Ref: Goodman Gilman 12th E/P552-53)

- Benzodiazepines cause anterograde amnesia and sedation.
- Since both are desirable in anesthesia, benzodiazepines like midazolam and lorazepam are routinely used in anesthesia as preanesthetic medications.

235. Ans. (c) Pethidine

(Ref: Miller's Anesthesia 8th E/P902)

- A decreased core temperature is responsible for post operative shivering, for which the drug of choice is pethidine.
- Other drugs that can be used are tramadol, clonidine, dexmeditomidine, ketanserin, nefopam, physostigmine and magnesium sulphate.

236. Ans. (d) All of the above

(Ref: Ajay Yadav 4th E/P47)

237. Ans. (a) Fentanyl

(Ref: Goodman Gilman 12th E/P507)

238. Ans. (b) Remifentanil

(Ref: Miller's Anesthesia 8th E/P1698)

Opioids Used in Spinal Anesthesia:

- Morphine
- Sufentanil
- Fentanyl

239. Ans. (d) Noscapine

(Ref: Goodman Gilman 12th E/P485)

240. Ans. (c) C type

(Ref: Miller's Anesthesia 8th E/P 1033)

Sequence of block in nerve fibres in response to local anesthetics:
A (gamma>delta>beta>alpha) > B > C

241. Ans. (a) Absolutely contraindicated in coagulation disorder

(Ref: Ajay Yadav 5th E/P165)

- The needle given in the picture is a dura cutting one used in spinal anesthesia.
- Spinal anesthesia is absolutely contraindicated in patients of coagulation disorder.

242. Ans. (b) Epidural

(Ref: Ajay Yadav 5th E/P204)

- Epidural Anesthesia is preferred in preeclampsia patients planned for cesarean section because in case of spinal there is high risk of hypotension and general anesthesia is avoided as laryngeal edema makes intubation difficult.

243. Ans. (c) Reverse Bainbridge reflex

(Ref: Hemming's Pharmacology and Physiology for Anesthesia/P377)

- Bainbridge reflex: An increase in blood volume in heart causes atrial stretch and the atrial stretch receptors inhibit parasympathetic activity in the heart causing tachycardia.
- Reverse Bainbridge reflex: A decrease in blood volume in heart conversely can cause bradycardia. This can be seen by a decrease in preload due to venodilation caused by spinal and epidural anesthesia.
- Bezold-Jarisch reflex: When noxious stimuli in the ventricles stimulate chemoreceptors and mechanoreceptors a triad of hypotension, bradycardia and coronary artery dilation is seen. It is usually seen with associated hypovolemia when a small systolic volume stimulates mechanoreceptors.
- Cardiac accelerator nerve fiber arise from T1 to T4 and its block cause bradycardia. Since in this case it is a block at T6 level it can be ruled out.

244. Ans. (b) Lumbar puncture

(Ref: Miller's Anesthesia 8th E/P1702)

245. Ans. (c) Ligamentum flavum

(Ref: Miller's Anesthesia 8th E/P1700)

246. Ans. (a) T4

(Ref: Miller's Anesthesia 8th E/P1693)

Level of block required for surgical procedures

Surgical Procedure	Level of block
Upper abdominal surgery **Cesarean delivery**	**T4**
Transurethral resection of prostate (TURP) Hip surgery	T10
Foot and ankle surgery	L2

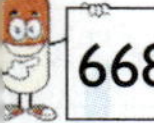

247. Ans. (d) Patient on antihypertensive medication

(Ref: Ajay Yadav 4th E/P138)

Mnemonics

Contraindication of Spinal and Epidural Anesthesia

- **S :** Stenotic valvular heart disease
- **H :** Hypovolemia
- **A :** Anticoagulation/Antiaggregant therapy
- **R :** Raised ICP
- **P :** Platelet count < 80,000
- **Injection:** Infection at local site

248. Ans. (c) Supplementation of fluid

(Ref: Miller's Anesthesia 8th E/P1712)

249. Ans. (b) It is most cardiotoxic local anesthetic

(Ref: Goodman Gilman 12th E/P572)

- Most cardiotoxic local anesthetic is bupivacaine and not lignocaine.
- Lidocaine blocks sodium channels both in closed and open state.
- It has a high first pass metabolism and hence for systemic use as in case of arrhythmia, needs to be given by intravenous route.

250. Ans. (a) Exaggerated lumbar lordosis

(Ref: Miller's Anesthesia 8th E/P1703)

Reasons for Decreased Local Anesthetic Requirement in Pregnancy:

- In pregnancy an increased abdominal pressure causes epidural veins engorgement and a decreased subarachnoid space and CSF volume.
- In pregnancy there is increased local anesthetic diffusion across the membranes due to decrease in serum bicarbonate and elevated CSF ph.
- There is increased sensitivity of the nerves to local anesthetics due to elevated progesterone levels.

251. Ans. (c) 7 mg/kg

(Ref: Ajay Yadav 4th E/P123)

Safe dose of local anesthetics	
Lidocaine	Without adrenaline: 3 mg/kg or 200 mg **With adrenaline: 7 mg/kg or 500 mg**
Bupivacaine	2 mg/kg
Chlorprocaine Procaine	12 mg/kg or 1000 mg
Tetracaine	3 mg/kg
Prilocaine	8 mg/kg
Mepivacaine	4.5 mg/kg
Etidocaine	4 mg/kg
Dibucaine	1 mg/kg

252. Ans. (b) Neuraxial analgesia

(Ref: Miller's Anesthesia 8th E/P1703)

253. Ans. (a) Bupivacaine

(Ref: Goodman Gilman 12th E/P573)

254. Ans. (c) Spinal anesthetic with 15 mg bupivacaine

(Ref: Morgan's 5th E/P967, 943)

255. Ans. (c) Epidural

(Ref: Miller's Anesthesia 8th E/P1241)

- Continuous Epidural Anesthesia is the first choice for patients with preeclampsia during labour, vaginal delivery and cesarean section.
- Preeclampsia patient has a risk of severe airway edema, which makes intubation difficult.
- Continuous Epidural Anesthesia can improve uteroplacental perfusion and also decrease catecholamine secretions.

256. Ans. (b) 48 hours

(Ref: Miller's Anesthesia 8th E/P1712)

Post Spinal Headache is

- Initiated within 48 hours
- Resolves within 7 days

257. Ans. (a) Prilocaine

(Ref: Miller's Anesthesia 8th E/P1045)

- Local anesthetics preferred for topical anesthesia commonly are lidocaine, dibucaine, tetracaine, cyclonine, hexylcaine and benzocaine.
- These drugs are used for anesthesia of mucous membranes or denuded skin.
- Spray of lidocaine and tetracaine are used in intubation, bronchoscopy and esophagoscopy.

258. Ans. (b) Upper limb surgeries

(Ref: Miller's Anesthesia 8th E/P1041)

259. Ans. (d) Dibucaine

(Ref: Ajay Yadav 4th E/P124)

260. Ans. (a) Na^+ channel inhibition

(Ref: Godman Gilman 12th E/P565)

261. Ans. (c) Clotting disorders

(Ref: Ajay Yadav 4th E/P138)

262. Ans. (c) Bier's block

(Ref: Miller's Anesthesia 8th E/P1684)

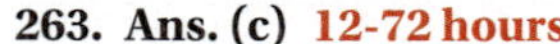

263. Ans. (c) 12-72 hours

(Ref: Miller's Anesthesia 8th E/P1712)

264. Ans. (a) Ischial tuberosity

(Ref: `Miller's Anesthesia 8th E/P2343)

265. Ans. (d) Chlorprocaine

(Ref: Ajay Yadav 4th E/P124)

Local Anesthetic:

- Longest acting - Dibucaine
- Shortest acting - Chlorprocaine

266. Ans. (c) High block

(Ref: Miller's Anesthesia 8th E/P1703)

267. Ans. (a) A

(Ref: Miller's Anesthesia 8th E/P1037)

Factors Affecting Local Anesthetic Effect

- Type of fiber: The orders of sensitivity of fibers is type A > B > C. In fiber type A the order is gamma > delta > beta and alpha.
- pH: Local anesthetics are weak bases and hence added with bicarbonate, which makes them unionized or lipid soluble; in this form they can traverse through the lipid barrier, but in the neurons they turn into ionized form and inhibit sodium channels. In ischemic and infected tissues as the medium is acidic, local anesthetics are less effective.
- Addition of vasoconstrictors: Epinephrine (5 μg/ml or 1:200,000) as a vasoconstrictor increases duration of action and decreases toxicity of local anesthetics. Local anesthetics with epinephrine is contraindicated in some conditins mentioned below.
- Onset and duration of action depends on the site of injection. Fastest onset and shortest duration of action is seen with subarachnoid and subcutaneous injection, whereas slowest onset and longest duration of action is seen brachial plexus block.

268. Ans. (a) Procaine

(Ref: Ajay Yadav 4th E/P124)

- Shortest acting local anesthetics are chlorprocaine < procaine.

269. Ans. (a) Lidocaine

(Ref: Miller's Anesthesia 8th E/P1711)

- Cauda equine syndrome is a side effect of local anesthetics administered by spinal route.
- It is usually seen with high doses of local anesthetic like 5% lidocaine.

270. Ans. (a) Infiltration anesthesia

(Ref: Miller's Anesthesia 8th E/P1042)

Infiltration Anesthesia

- Infiltration anesthesia is performed by injecting the local anesthetics directly into the tissue of interest.
- The local anesthetics preferred are lidocaine, procaine and bupivacaine.
- It is used for minor procedures like CLW suturing and hydrocele operation.

271. Ans. (d) Total intravenous anesthesia

(Ref: Miller's Anesthesia 8th E/P1041-43)

272. Ans. (d) Diazepam

(Ref: Goodman Gilman 12th E/P572)

- Side effects of lidocaine are mostly neurological like drowsiness, tinnitus, dizziness and twitching, seizure and coma.
- In genetically susceptible patients it can also cause malignant hyperthermia.
- Treatment of neurological side effects is supportive and for seizures benzodiazepines are the drug of choice.

273. Ans. (b) Procaine

(Ref: Ajay Yadav 4th E/P118)

Classification of local anesthetics	
Amides	**Esters**
Lidocaine	**Procaine**
Articaine	Cocaine
Mepivacaine	Chlorprocaine
Bupivacaine	Benzocaine
Prilocaine	Tetracaine
Etidocaine	
Ropivacaine	

274. Ans. (b) Bupivacaine

(Ref: Miller's Anesthesia 8th E/P1045)

275. Ans. (c) Saddle block

(Ref: Ajay Yadav 4th E/P139)

276. Ans. (d) Bupivacaine

(Ref: Goodman Gilman 12th E/P573)

- As bupivacaine is the most cardiotoxic local anesthetic it is contraindicated in IVRA or Bier's block.
- Drugs preferred for IVRA are lidocaine > prilocaine.

277. Ans. (a) Outside the dura

(Ref: Miller's Anesthesia 8th E/P1703)

278. Ans. (b) Forceps delivery

(Ref: Miller's Anesthesia 8th E/P2343)

- Pudendal nerve block can be used for procedures around perineum.
- For vaginal delivery with forceps and for episiotomy it is preferred; a trans vaginal approach is preferred taking ischial spine as anatomical land mark and then needle is passed through vaginal mucosa towards ischial spine and after passing through sacrospinous ligament drug is injected.

279. Ans. (c) Ischial spine

(Ref: Miller's Anesthesia 8th E/P2719)

280. Ans. (a) Local anesthesia

(Ref: Miller's Anesthesia 8th E/P1590)

281. Ans. (d) 6

(Ref: Complication in Spinal Anaesthesia By Alparslan Apan and Ozgun Cuvas Apan/Chap-7)

282. Ans. (a) 0.5%

(Ref: Miller's Anesthesia 8th E/P1704)

Duration of procedure	LA of choice	Dextrose concentration
Short	Lidocaine 0.5% or 5%	7.5 %
Intermediate to long	**Bupivacaine 0.5%** or 0.75%	8.25%
Long	Tetracaine 0.25% or 1%	5 %
Diagnostic block	Procaine 10%	5%

283. Ans. (d) 5%

(Ref: Miller's Anesthesia 8th E/P1704)

284. Ans. (d) 5%

(Ref: Miller's Anesthesia 8th E/P1704)

285. Ans. (b) 2% Xylocaine

(Ref: Miller's Anesthesia 8th E/P1044)

286. Ans. (c) 7-10 days

(Ref: Miller's Anesthesia 8th E/P1712)

287. Ans. (c) No motor paralysis

(Ref: Miller's Anesthesia 8th E/P1704)

288. Ans. (b) Prilocaine

(Ref: Goodman Gilman 12th E/P573)

- Prilocaine is metabolizd to o-toludine which causes methemoglobinemia and hence its use is mostly limited to dental procedures.
- Since neonates are more sensitive to toxic effect of methemoglobinemia, prilocaine is not used.

289. Ans. (a) Digital block

(Ref: Ajay Yadav 4th E/P120)

Mnemonics

Contraindications to use of LA with Epinephrine

- **B :** Block of areas with end arteries e.g. Digital block
- **H :** Hypertension, Hyperthyroidism, with Halothane
- **I :** Intravenous regional anesthesia
- **M :** Myocardial ischemia

290. Ans. (c) Aγ

(Ref: Miller's Anesthesia 8th E/P1037)

- The orders of sensitivity of fibers is type A > B > C.
- In fiber type A the order is gamma > delta > beta and alpha.

291. Ans. (b) Bicarbonate

(Ref: Goodman Gilman 12th E/P569)

292. Ans. (c) Cocaine

(Ref: Goodman Gilman 12th E/P570)

- Cocaine inhibits reuptake of NE in the synapse and this NE by acting of alpha receptors of blood vessels can cause vasoconstriction.
- Hence cocaine is not used along with epinephrine.

293. Ans. (d) Block the influx of sodium into the cell

(Ref: Miller's Anesthesia 8th E/P1029)

Local anesthetics inhibit voltage gated sodium channels and hence block influx of sodium into the neurons.

294. Ans. (a) Less cardiotoxic than lignocaine

(Ref: Goodman Gilman 12th E/P573)

295. Ans. (a) Vasoconstriction

(Ref: Goodman Gilman 12th E/P572)

296. Ans. (b) Pain

(Ref: Miller's Anesthesia 8th E/P1037)

- The orders of sensitivity of fibers is type A > B (preganglionic sympathetic) > C (Temperature). In fiber type A the order is gamma (muscle tone) > delta (Pin prick/pain) > beta (touch) and alpha (motor).
- Thus the sequence of block in local anesthesia is muscle tone > pin prick/pain > touch > motor > preganglionic sympathetic > temperature.

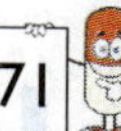

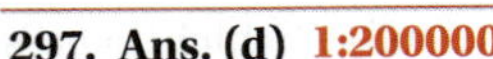

297. Ans. (d) 1:200000

(Ref: Miller's Anesthesia 8th E/P1040)

298. Ans. (d) Bupivacaine

(Ref: Miller's Anesthesia 8th E/P1045)

299. Ans. (b) Bupivacaine

(Ref: Miller's Anesthesia 8th E/P2342)

Bupivacaine and ropivacaine are preferred local anesthetic of choice for epidural analgesia in labor as they have a higher sensory to motor block ratio as compared to other drugs like lidocaine.

300. Ans. (b) 2.5 % lignocaine and 2.5% prilocaine

(Ref: Miller's Anesthesia 8th E/P1045)

- For application on intact skin eutectic mixture of local anesthetic (EMLA), i.e. lidocaine (2.5%) and prilocaine (2.5%) is preferred.
- An eutectic mixture has a melting point lesser than individual drugs and hence the mixture is in oil form at room temperature.
- The cream is applied 45-60 minutes before the procedure with an occlusive dressing. It is preferred for circumcision, venipuncture, cannulation and skin grafting.

301. Ans. (a) Bupivacaine

(Ref: Miller's Anesthesia 8th E/P1031)

Bupivacaine precipitates with bicarbonate and hence these should not be combined.

302. Ans. (c) Makes the injection less painful

(Ref: Goodman Gilman 12th E/P1040)

- Epinephrine (5 μg/ml or 1:200,000) as a vasoconstrictor increases duration of action and decreases toxicity of local anesthetics.
- Pain on injection is decreased by addition of bicarbonate.

303. Ans. (b) Slow idioventricular rhythm

(Ref: Katzung 11th E/P448)

304. Ans. (b) Pia and arachnoid

(Ref: Miller's Anesthesia 8th E/P1700)

305. Ans. (c) Dura-arachnoid membrane

(Ref: Miller's Anesthesia 8th E/P1700)

Resistance is felt at the ligamentum flavum and dura, whereas pop is felt after passing through the dura.

306. Ans. (c) Increase on lying down & relieved by sitting or standing

(Ref: Miller's Anesthesia 8th E/P1712)

307. Ans. (d) Low volume headache

(Ref: Miller's Anesthesia 8th E/P1715)

308. Ans. (c) Caudal block

(Ref: Miller's Anesthesia 8th E/P1710)

- Caudal block is a type of epidural anesthesia used in children for perineal, anal, rectal, genital and urethral surgeries.
- Child is positioned in left lateral decubitus position and after sacral hiatus is identified a Tuhoy's needle is inserted with an angle of 45 degrees to sacrum till it enters the caudal space.

309. Ans. (c) Position of patient before the injection

(Ref: Miller's Anesthesia 8th E/P1703)

Factors determining height of block in epidural anesthesia	
More important factors	Less important factors
Dose	**Patient position**
Volume	Weight
Age	Height
Pregnancy	
Level of injection	

310. Ans. (c) Sympathetic preganglionic

(Ref: Miller's Anesthesia 8th E/P1688)

- The sequence of block of nerves in spinal anesthesia is different from local anesthesia in tissues (A>B>C).
- In spinal anesthesia the sequence is B (preganglionic sympathetic) > C (Temperature) > A.
- The sequence of block in A fibers is A delta (Pin prick) > A beta (touch) > A alpha (motor).
- The sequence of block is temperature > pin prick > touch > motor. The order of reversal of block is opposite, i.e. motor > touch > pin prick > temperature.

311. Ans. (d) Prilocaine

(Ref: Goodman Gilman 12th E/P573)

312. Ans. (b) 25-100 mg

(Ref: Miller's Anesthesia 8th E/P1697)

Duration of procedure	LA of choice	Safe dose in mg
Short	Lidocaine 0.5% or 5%	50-100
Intermediate to long	**Bupivacaine 0.5%** or 0.75%	4-5
Long	Tetracaine 0.25% or 1%	5-15
Diagnostic block	Procaine 10%	50-200

313. Ans. ALL

(Ref: Miller's Anesthesia 8th E/P1690)

314. Ans. (a) Succinylcholine, (b) Methoxyflurane and (c)Pancuronium

(Ref: Miller's Anesthesia 8th E/P986-87)

315. Ans. (a) Lidocaine is used for awake intubation, (b) Bupivacaine more cardiotoxic and longer acting than lidocaine, (c) Intralipid is used for cardiotoxicity of bupivacaine and (d) Ropivacaine- used in peripheral nerve block

(Ref: Goodman Gilman 13th E/P405)

316. Ans. (a) Succinylcholine is short acting muscle relaxant, (b) Succinylcholine is used for rapid-sequence induction in full stomach patients and (d) Rocuronium can be used for rapid-sequence induction

(Ref: Goodman Gilman 13th E/P183)

317. Ans. (b) In day care surgery, halothane is most commonly used inhalational agent

(Ref: Goodman Gilman 13th E/P395)

318. Ans. (a) Caffeine, (b) Blood patch, (d) Hydration, (e) Sumatriptan

(Ref: Miller's Anesthesia 8th E/P1172)

Management of Post Dural Headache

- Analgesics
- Sumatriptan
- Hydration
- Intravenous caffeine
- Autologous blood patch
- Supine positioning

319. Ans. (c) Reversal of muscle relaxants

(Ref: Miller's Anesthesia 8th E/P1014)

- Sugammadex is a gamma cyclodextrin which encapsulates the muscle relaxants and removes them from plasma and neuromuscular junction.
- It is used for emergency reversal of muscle relaxants like rocuronium and vecuronium.

320. Ans. (a) Halothane, (b) Succinylcholine

(Ref: Goodman Gilman 12th E/P542)

Drugs Causing malignant hyperthermia

Inhalational agents	Muscle relaxants	Local anesthetics
Halothane – Most common Sevoflurane Desflurane Methoxyflurane Isoflurane	Suxamethonium – Overall most common Decamethonium	Lidocaine

321. Ans. (b) Seizure, (c) Masseter spasm, (d) Metabolic acidosis

(Ref: Ajay Yadav 4th E/P115)

322. Ans. ALL

(Ref: Miller's Anesthesia 8th E/P2767)

Drugs used in induction of anesthesia

- Propofol: Most commonly used drug
- Thiopental
- Etomidate
- Methohexital
- Ketamine
- Benzodiazepines: Midazolam is benzodiazepine of choice for induction, however diazepam and lorazepam can also be used.

323. Ans. (c) Intralipids, (e) Epinephrine

(Ref: Miller's Anesthesia 8th E/P1048)

- Currently antiarrhythmic drugs like bretylium, amiodarone and lidocaine are not advised in bupivacaine toxicity.
- Rather the ACLS advised drugs like atropine and epinephrine are used along with cardioversion for ventricular fibrillation.
- Lipid emulsion is also advised for treatment of cardiotoxicity.

324. Ans. (b) Gender, (c) Weight, (d) Height, (e) Underlying condition of patient

(Ref: Ajay Yadav 5th E/P235)

325. Ans. (a) Non cuffed tube is used in pediatric age group, (b) Made of PVC and disposable, (c) Can be put either oral or nasal according to different situations, (e) More tendency to go to right bronchus thereby decreasing left lung ventilation

(Ref: Ajay Yadav 5th E/P43-47)

326. Ans. ALL

(Ref: Ajay Yadav 5th E/P43-47)

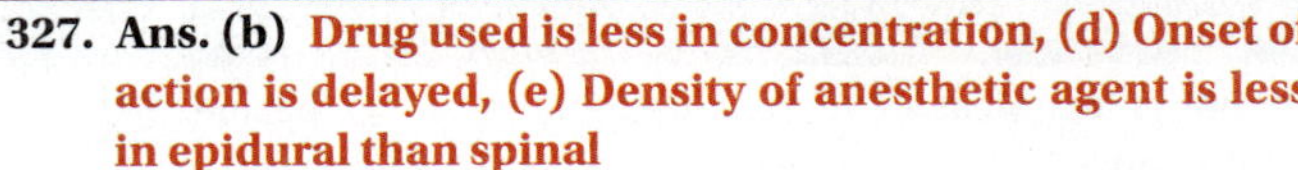

327. Ans. (b) Drug used is less in concentration, (d) Onset of action is delayed, (e) Density of anesthetic agent is less in epidural than spinal

(Ref: Ajay Yadav 5th E/P166)

Difference Between Spinal and Epidural Anesthesia

Spinal Anesthesia	Epidural Anesthesia
• Simple and cheap procedure • Rapid onset of action • Reliable • Side effects like hypotension, headache etc. • Limited duration of action • Higher concentration of LA used • Lesser amount of LA required • Good quality block • Lesser chances of intravascular injection and total spinal block • Low failure chances	• Complex and costly procedure • Delayed onset of action • Less reliable • No hypotension and headache • Can be used for longer duration • Lower concentration of LA used • Large amount of LA required • Patchy block • High chances of intravascular injection and total spinal block • High failure chances

328. Ans. (a) Atracurium, (c) Enflurane, (d) Pethidine

(Ref: Goodman Gilman 12th E/P544-55)

329. Ans. (a) Environment friendly, (c) Low blood solubility, (d) Inert, (e) Stable

(Ref: Goodman Gilman 12th E/P547-48)

330. Ans. (b) Pressure gradient, (e) Density of gas

(Ref: Ajay Yadav 5th E/P29)

Flow of gas through tubes depends on

- Pressure gradient and density of gas in case of high flow rate (turbulent)
- Pressure gradient and viscosity of gas in ca of low flow rate (laminar)

331. Ans. (c) CO_2, (d) Cyclopropane, (e) Nitrous oxide

(Ref: Ajay Yadav 5th E/P26)

332. Ans. (a) Boiling point is <23°C, (b) Chemically it is Flourinated methyl ethyl ether, (c) It increases the effect of muscle relaxant

(Ref: Goodman Gilman 12th E/P545)

- Desflurane is difluoromethyl 1-fluoro-2,2,2-trifluoromethyl ester.
- It has a boiling point less than 23 oC.
- It has a mild muscle relaxant effect.
- Almost all inhalational agents can cause malignant hyperthermia and its maximum with halothane.
- Desflurane has higher MAC than isoflurane and hence desflurane is less potent than isoflurane.

333. Ans. (a) Mallampati grading, (c) Thyromental distance, (d) Teeth arrangement

(Ref: Miller's Anesthesia 8th E/P1669)

Mnemonics

Indicator of Difficult Laryngoscopy/Intubation

S : Short thyromental distance, short neck
M : Mallampati class III and IV, Mouth opening small
A : Arched, high palate
L : Long upper incisors
L : Limited cervical mobility
Palate : Prominent overbite

334. Ans. (d) Sodium bicarbonate is given to correct alkalosis

(Ref: Ajay Yadav 4th E/P115)

335. Ans. (b) Used to assess patient condition to tolerate anaesthesia & surgery, (d) Relieves anxiety of patient, (e) Help in planning anaesthesia technique

(Ref: Ajay Yadav 5th/53,194,225; Morgan Anaesthesia 5th/ 296-97; Lee13th/3; Miller Anaesthesia 7th/1001-10)

336. Ans. (a) N_2O-increases efficacy of other inhalational agents, (c) Sevoflurane is agent of choice in children

(Ref: Goodman Gilman 12th E/P541-547)

337. Ans. (d) Thiopentone triggers

(Ref: Ajay Yadav 4th E/P115)

338. Ans. (a) Most common used size for adult male is 8-8.5, (b) Most common used size for adult female is 7-7.5, (d) In children cuffed tube is not used

(Ref: Ajay Yadav 4th E/P37)

339. Ans. (d) Hypotension is most common side effect

(Ref: Miller's Anesthesia 8th E/P1713)

340. Ans. (d) Atracurium

(Ref: Ajay Yadav 4th E/P101)

341. Ans. (a) Burn, (b) Spinal cord injury, (c) Muscular dystrophy, (d) Tetanus

(Ref: Ajay Yadav 4th E/P97)

342. Ans. (a) Sodium thiopentone, (c) Mannitol, (e) Propofol

(Ref: Goodman Gilman 12th E/P535-38)

343. Ans. (a) GABA-A receptor, (c) NMDA receptor

(Ref: Goodman Gilman 12th E/P529)

- All anesthetic agents act by stimulating glycine and GABA receptors. The site of action for GABA is in the α subunit, whereas for benzodiazepines is between α and γ subunits and for all general anesthetics is located on the β subunit.

- Only ketamine, cyclopropane, N_2O and xenon act by opening potassium channel and by inhibiting NMDA receptors.

344. Ans. (e) In regional block i.v. injection is used

(Ref: Miller's Anesthesia 8th E/P1041)

345. Ans. None

(Ref: Miler's Anesthesia 8th E/P1662)

346. Ans. (d) Mapleson E

(Ref: Miller's Anesthesia 8th E/P791)

347. Ans. (a) SIMV, (c) CPAP

(Ref: Miller's Anesthesia 8th E/P3065-66)

Modes of ventilation used for weaning are:

- SIMV
- PSV
- CPAP

348. Ans. (b) Ketamine

(Ref: Goodman Gilman 12th E/P539)

- Ketamine increases intraocular pressure and hence is contraindicated in patients with ocular surgery.
- Propofol has antiemetic effect and hence would be preferable in this condition.

349. Ans. (a) Performed for postoperative analgesia, (d) Pneumothorax may occur as a complication

(Ref: Miller's Anesthesia 8th E/P1042)

- Intercostal nerve block is done for relaxation and anesthesia of abdominal wall and is used for post-operative analgesia and rib fractures.
- It is associated with maximum systemic absorption. The drug is injected in the mid or posterior axillary line at inferior border of rib.
- Pneumothorax is a complication that can be associated.

350. Ans. (b) It is the inhalational agent of choice for controlled hypotension, (d) Cardiac stable agent

(Ref: Goodman Gilman 12th E/P543)

Isoflurane is anesthetic agent of choice in	Cause
Cardiac surgery	Maintains cardiac output
Controlled hypotension	Vasodilation

351. Ans. (a) Neck is extended, (b) Direction of pressure should be backward & upward, (c) Preoxygenation with 100% oxygenation for 3-4 minute is mandatory

(Ref: Miller's Anesthesia 8th E/P2430)

- Cricoid pressure is applied until endotracheal tube is placement and cuff inflation is confirmed.
- The chin of the patient is elevated without cervical spine displacement and then cricoid cartilage is pushed posteriorly towards the esophagus.
- It impairs laryngoscopic view and hence is contraindicated in patients of cardiac arrest.
- Preoxygenation with 100% oxygen is not always mandatory.

352. Ans. (b) Artificial Manual Breathing Unit

(Ref: Ajay Yadav 4th E/P41)

353. Ans. (c) Mepivacaine, (e) Bupivacaine

(Ref: Miller's Anesthesia 8th E/P1045)

354. Ans. (b) Halothane, (c) Suxamethonium

(Ref: Goodman Gilman 12th E/P542)

Drugs Causing Malignant Hyperthermia

Inhalational Agents	Muscle Relaxants	Local Anesthetics
• Halothane – Most common	• Suxamethonium – Overall most common cause	• Lidocaine
• Sevofluane	• Decamethonium	
• Desflurane		
• Methoxyflurane		
• Isoflurane		

355. Ans. (a) Blood : gas partition coefficient is 0.14, (b) Minimum alveolar concentration is high, (c) Minimal hemodynamic effect, (d) Heavier than air

(Ref: Goodman Gilman 12th E/P547-48)

- Xenon is a noble and inert gas with viscosity and density more than air. It has least blood gas partition coefficient and hence causes fastest induction and recovery. Though it has a high MAC of 71 only second to that of nitrous oxide.
- Antagonism of NMDA receptors produces anesthesia whereas potassium channel opening causes analgesia.
- It is the most ideal gas as has limited effect on CVS, CNS and respiratory system. It can also be used in place of nitrous oxide as oxygen carrier.
- However it is not widely used, as it cannot be synthesized and needs to be extracted from air; this considerably increases costing. Since it has more density than air, it increases resistance to flow and can cause difficult breathing in airway disorders. Nausea and vomiting is more common than propofol.

356. Ans. (c) Ether

(Ref: Ajay Yadav 4th E/P71)

357. Ans. (a) Enflurane, (d) Sevoflurane

(Ref: Goodman Gilman 12th E/P544-45)

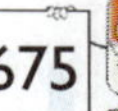

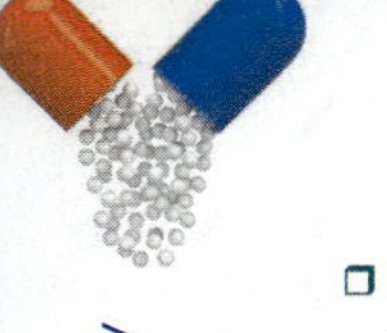

- Enflurane can cause epilepsy at normal doses whereas sevoflurane at high doses.

358. Ans. (d) E

(Ref: Ajay Yadav 4th E/P24)

359. Ans. (a) Shorter acting than tetracaine

(Ref: Ajay Yadav 4th E/P124)

- *Dibucaine is the most potent and longest acting local anesthetic.*
- *A dibucaine number of 80 indicated adequate quantity of pseudocholinesterase.*

360. Ans. (a) Tachycardia, (c) Excessive sweating (e) ↓ed O_2 saturation

(Ref: Ajay Yadav 4th E/P115)

361. Ans. (e) In malignant hyperthermia $ETCO_2$ decreases

(Ref: Miller's Anesthesia 8th E/P1554)

Uses of capnography
• Confirmation of intubation: Capnography is the surest method.
• Disconnection indicator
• Alveolar ventilation indicator
• Cardiac output indicator
• Indicator of pulmonary embolism: Fall in capnogram
• **Diagnosis of malignant hyperthermia: End tidal CO_2 is highly raised and can be > 100 mm Hg**
• Indicator of ET tube displacement/obstruction or ventilator failure: Flat capnogram

362. Ans. All

(Ref: Miller's Anesthesia 8th E/P1049)

- Hypercapnia, acidosis and hypoxia potentiate the systemic toxic effects of local anesthetics.
- In pregnancy and old age the sensitivity to local anesthetics increase and hence patients are at higher risk of toxicity.
- As most local anesthetics are excreted by kidney, toxicity increases in renal failure.

363. Ans. (a) Rapid induction and recovery, (b) Low potency, (d) Non-explosive, (e) Heavier than air

(Ref: Goodman Gilman 12th E/P547-48)

364. Ans. (a) Helium is an inert gas, (d) Reduces work of breathing, (e) Mixture of He & O_2

(Ref: Goodman Gilman 12th E/P560)

Helium

- Helium is an inert gas stored in brown colored cylinders. Heliox is 79% helium plus 21% oxygen stored in brown cylinders with white shoulders.
- As helium is lighter than air and viscosity is higher than air and has a low density, heliox is used in case of airway obstruction to decrease turbulence.
- Low solubility is the reason for its use in diving; nitrogen is also used but it causes narcosis.
- High thermal conductivity makes it ideal for use in laser surgery.

365. Ans. (a) Enflurane interacts with sodalime, (d) Ketamine acts through GABA-A receptors

(Ref: Ajay Yadav 4th E/P69)

366. Ans. (b) Epinephrine

(Ref: Miller's Anesthesia 8th E/P1048)

- Currently antiarrhythmic drugs like bretylium, amiodarone and lidocaine are not advised for treatment of bupivacaine toxicity.
- Rather the ACLS advised drugs like atropine and epinephrine are used along with cardioversion for ventricular fibrillation.
- Lipid emulsion is also advised for treatment of cardiotoxicity.

367. Ans. (b) Can be used in porphyria, (d) Used in day care surgery

(Ref: Goodman Gilman 12th E/P537)

368. Ans. (b) Mapleson type D, (c) Can be used for spontaneous respiration, (d) Can be used for controlled ventilation, (e) Coaxial

(Ref: Ajay Yadv 4th E/P30)

- Type D circuit: It is also known as Bain's circuit. As compared to type A in this one is a coaxial circuit in which there are separate tubes for the inhaled and exhaled gases and hence there is no mixing. Since the chance of hypoxia are lesser, it is the semiclosed circuit of choice for controlled ventilation. Though it can be also used for spontaneous ventilation.

369. Ans. (a) More reliable than face mask, (c) Alternative to Endotracheal tube (E.T.T), (d) Does not require laryngoscope & visualization

(Ref: Miller's Anesthesia 8th E/P1663)

370. Ans. (b) Pin is present on machine

(Ref: Miller's Anesthesia 8th E/P755)

- The pin is present on the yoke assembly of anesthesia machine.
- The holes for the pins are present on the cylinder.

371. Ans. (b) C/I in coagulopathies, (d) Venous return decreases

(Ref: Miller's Anesthesia 8th E/P1713)

372. Ans. (b) Isoflurane, (d) Desflurane

(Ref: Goodman Gilman 12th E/P543-44)

373. Ans. (c) Aspiration of gastric contents

(Ref: Miller's Anesthesia 8th E/P1655)

374. Ans. (c) Mivacurium, (d) Butarphanol, (e) Buprenorphine

(Ref: Miller's Anesthesia 8th E/P1041)

375. Ans. (a) Thipentone, (d) Etomidate

(Ref: Goodman Gilman 12th E/P535-38)

Drugs Causing Acute Intermittent Porphyria
• Barbiturates
• Etomidate
• Halothane
• Cocaine
• Lidocaine
• Prilocaine
• Clonidine
• Metoclopromide
• Hyoscine
• Diclofenac
• Ranitidine

376. Ans. (a) Mivacurium

(Ref: Ajay Yadav 4th E/P99)

377. Ans. (b) Thiopentone

(Ref: Goodman Gilman 12th E/P535)

378. Ans. (a) LMA, (b) Endotracheal tube, (c) Combitube

(Ref: Miller's Anesthesia 8th E/P1659-1665)

379. Ans. (a) Ligamentum flavum, (b) Duramater, (c) Supraspinous ligament

(Ref: Miller's Anesthesia 8th E/P1700)

380. Ans. (b) Etomidate, (d) Ketamine

(Ref: Goodman Gilman 12th E/P535-38)

- Etomidate has no effect on the cardiovascular system.
- Ketamine due to release of catecholamines causes myocardial stimulation.

381. Ans. (b) Fibreoptic bronchoscopy

(Ref: Miller's Anesthesia 8th E/P1670)

- **Endotracheal tube placement confirmation is best by fibreoptic bronchoscopy but is rarely used.**
- **More commonly used is capnography.**

382. Ans. (a) Dantrolene, (b) Cooling, (d) Discontinue inhalational anesthesia, (e) Give O_2 therapy with 100% O_2

(Ref: Ajay Yadav 4th E/P115)

383. Ans. (a) Succinylcholine & halothane predisposes, (b) Dantrolene useful in all cases, (d) Propofol is safe, (e) Muscle biopsy is diagnostic

(Ref: Ajay Yadav 4th E/P115)

384. Ans. (a) Atracurium, (b) Cisatracurium, (e) Mivacurium

(Ref: Ajay Yadav 4th E/P101)

- Most muscle relaxants are excreted by kidney and hence contraindicated in renal failure.
- Vecuronium is excreted by both liver and kidney and hence safe in renal failure.
- Atracurium and cisatracurium are eliminated by Hoffman's elimination and hence also safe in renal failure.

385. Ans. (a) Sevoflurane

(Ref: Goodman Gilman 12thE/P546)

386. Ans. (a) Cylinder is a part of high pressure system, (c) O_2 flush delivers > 35 lts

(Ref: Ajay Yadav 4th E/P24)

387. Ans. (a) Available in 8 sizes, (b) Intubation can be done, (c) Size 1 for neonates, (d) Size 3 for adults

(Ref: Miller's Anesthesia 8th E/P1662)

LMA Sizes (8)	
Age Group	Size
Neonate	1
Infant 5 – 10 kg	1.5
Children 10 – 20 kg	2
Children 20 – 30 kg	2.5
Children or Adult 30 – 50 kg	3
Adult 50 – 70 kg	4
Adult > 70 – 100 kg	5
Adult > 100 kg	6

388. Ans. (a) Pin index 3,5; (b) Blue in colour, (c) Stored as liquid, (d) MAC 105

(Ref: Ajay Yadav 4th E/P24)

389. Ans. (b) Ketamine

(Ref: Miller's Anesthesia 8th E/P847)

390. Ans. (e) Benzodiazepines

(Ref: Miller's Anesthesia 8th E/P1047)

CNS toxicity which presents as seizures with local anesthetics can be treated with benzodiazepines.

391. Ans. (a) O_2, (b) CO, (c) N_2O, (d) Cyclopropane

(Ref: Ajay Yadav 4th E/P24)

392. Ans. (a) 2%, (b) 4%, (c) 5%, (d) 10%, (e) 1%

(Ref: Miller's Anesthesia 8th E/P1042-45)

Lidocaine uses	Concentration (%)
Topical	Ointment: 2.5 – 5 Solution: 2 – 4 Jelly: 2 Suppositories: 10 Aerosol: 10
Spinal	1.5 5
Epidural	1 – 2
Major nerve block	1 – 2
Minor nerve block	1

393. Ans. (b) Short half life, (c) More potent than Alfentanyl

(Ref: Lee synopsis 12th/188-89; Wylie Anesthesilogy 7th / 556)

394. Ans. (d) Medium granules size

(Ref: Miller's Anesthesia 8th E/P790)

- There are various factors that can affect CO_2 absorption; these are
  - Surface area of granules: Smaller is the size of granules more is the area exposed to gas and more is CO_2 absorption.
  - Airway resistance: Smaller is the size of granules more is airway resistance and lesser is CO_2 absorption. Hence to maintain a higer surface area exposure with lesser resistance a medium size of 4-8 mesh is preferred for granules.
  - Channeling: Passage of gas through the gaps in between the granules is called channeling, which can decrease CO_2 absorption.

395. Ans. (a) Atracurium, (b) Cis-atracurium

(Ref: Ajay Yadav 4th E/P101)

396. Ans. (a) Non - irritant, (c) It antagonises bronchospasm, (d) Vasodilator

(Ref: Goodman Gilman 12th E/P541)

397. Ans. (a) Vecuronium, (b) Doxacurium, (d) Rocuronium, (e) Mivacurium

(Ref: Ajay Yadav 4th E/P99-101)

398. Ans. (b) Mixture of local anesthesia, (d) Used in children

(Ref: Miller's Anesthesia 8th E/P1045)

- For application on intact skin eutectic mixture of local anesthetic (EMLA), i.e. lidocaine (2.5%) and prilocaine (2.5%) is preferred.
- An eutectic mixture has a melting point lesser than individual drugs and hence the mixture is in oil form at room temperature.
- The cream is applied 45-60 minutes before the procedure with an occlusive dressing.
- It is preferred for circumcision in children, venipuncture, cannulation and skin grafting.

399. Ans. (d) Propofol

(Ref: Goodman Gilman 13th E/P350)

400. Ans. (b) Isoflurane

(Ref: Ajay Yadav 4th E/P59)

401. Ans. (c) Xenon

(Ref: Ajay Yadav 4th E/P66)

402. Ans. (a) Ligamentum flavum

(Ref: Miller's Anesthesia 8th E/P1700)

403. Ans. (a) Blocking sodium gated channel

(Ref: Goodman Gilman 13th E/P405)

404. Ans. (c) NSAIDs

(Ref: Miller's Anesthesia 8th E/P1195)

- Opioids are rarely associated with anaphylaxis.
- Antibiotics are the third most common cause of anaphylaxis in anesthesia, but it would be seen in the beginning as antibiotics are given before anesthesia.
- NSAIDs are given towards the end of surgery and hence anaphylaxis at end of generak anesthesia can be seen due to NSAIDs. Other differential diagnosis includes latex and colloid induced anaphylaxis which can also be seen towards end of general anesthesia.
- Benzodiazepines are used as premedication and hence anaphylaxis would be seen in the beginning of general anesthesia or even before.

405. Ans. (a) Ligamentum flavum

(Ref: Miller's Anesthesia 8th E/P1700)

- After the place for spinal anesthesia is selected on back, local anesthetic is applied and then needle is inserted at 10-15 degrees of a cephalad angle through skin, subcutaneous tissue, supraspinous ligament and interspinous ligament until a resistance is felt while piercing through ligamentum flavum and dura mater.

406. Ans. (d) Ischemia of lower limbs

(Ref: Miller's Anesthesia 8th E/P1710-14)

407. Ans. (a) Alkalinize the LA

(Ref: Ajay Yadav 4th E/P120)

408. Ans. (c) Capnography may not detect esophageal intubation during cardiac arrest

(Ref: Miller's Anesthesia 8th E/P1670)

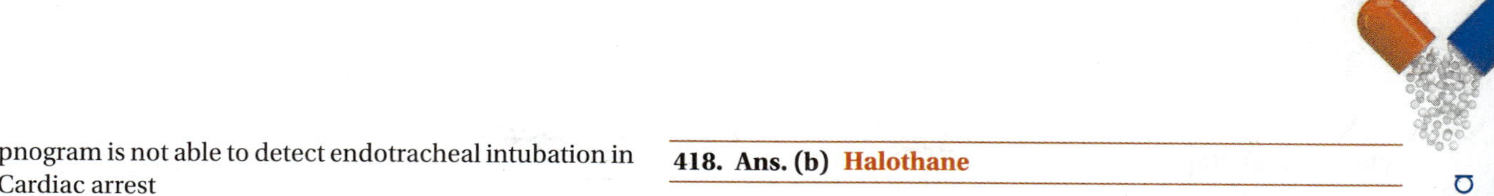

Capnogram is not able to detect endotracheal intubation in
- ❒ Cardiac arrest
- ❒ Severe bronchospasm
- ❒ Hemodynamic collapse
- ❒ Equipment malfunction

409. Ans. (b) Succinylcholine

(Ref: Ajay Yadav 4th E/P97)

410. Ans. (a) Ondansetron

(Ref: Miller's Anesthesia 8th E/P2970)

411. Ans. (d) Non rebreathing face mask with oxygen reservoir

(Ref: Ajay Yadav 4th E/P43)

Oxygen delivery devices	Percentage of oxygen delivered
Venturi Mask	60%
Oxygen Mask	60%
Rebreathing Mask	100%
Nonrebreathing Mask	80%
Nonrebreathing mask with reservoir	95%
Nasal Cannula	44%

412. Ans. (d) Drug entering into subarachnoid space

(Ref: Miller's Anesthesia 8th E/P1713)

- ❒ Drug entering into subarachnoid space can cause a high level block T1 to T4, causing block of cardiac accelerator fibers and hence associated with hypotension.
- ❒ Similarly high level block can cause respiratory depression also.

413. Ans. (a) Thiopentone

(Ref: Goodman Gilman 12th E/P535)

- ❒ Thiopentone maintains a normal intracranial pressure and hence would be preferred in this case of head trauma.
- ❒ Other drugs mentioned in the options can increase intracranial pressure and hance are contraindicated.

414. Ans. (d) Sevoflurane

(Ref: Goodman Gilman 12th E/P546)

415. Ans. (c) Neuroaxial block analgesia

(Ref: Miller's Anesthesia 8th E/P1704)

416. Ans. (a) Body may loose heat by conduction

(Ref: Miller's Anesthesia 8th E/P1623)

Heat loss during surgery is primarily by
- ❒ Conduction
- ❒ Radiation

417. Ans. (a) Mapelson A

(Ref: Miller's Anesthesia 8th E/P791)

418. Ans. (b) Halothane

(Ref: Goodman Gilman 12th E/P541)

- ❒ Halothane is 60-80% excreted unchanged by lungs, whereas rest is metabolized by liver.
- ❒ Rest are excreted unchanged by lungs to the extent of 99% and only 1% undergoes metabolism.

419. Ans. (c) Ketamine

(Ref: Miller's Anesthesia 8th E/P847)

- ❒ Ketamine causes an increase in intracranial pressure, cerebral blood flow and cerebral oxygen consumption.

420. Ans. (b) Ketamine

(Ref: Miller's Anesthesia 8th E/P847)

421. Ans. (c) Bupivacaine

(Ref: Miller's Anesthesia 8th E/P1031)

422. Ans. (d) Deepen plane of anesthesia

(Ref: Stoelting coexisting diseases 5th E/Chapter 9)

Wheezing can be seen due to weaning off of the anesthetic effect and the best thing to do is deepen the plane of anesthesia.

423. Ans. (d) Patient on antihypertensive medication

(Ref: Ajay Yadav 4th E/P136)

424. Ans. (a) Bilaterally done, (b) Diarrhea and hypotension are common side effects

(Ref: Ajay Yadav 4th E/P129)

425. Ans. (d) Hydration by crystalloids infusion

(Ref: Miller's Anesthesia 8th E/P1712)

The incidence of headache can be decreased by using a small bore and atraumatic needle (dura separating), removing the stylet prior to needle and by placing the needle bevel in long axis of neuraxis.

426. Ans. (c) Succinylcholine

(Ref: Ajay Yadav 4th E/P97)

427. Ans. (a) Diaphragm

(Ref: Ajay Yadav 4th E/P96)

428. Ans. (b) Treated with warm saline

(Ref: Miller's Anesthesia 8th E/P1638)

429. Ans. (c) Sevoflurane

(Ref: Miller's Anesthesia 8th E/P789)

- ❒ Maximum CO production - Desflurane
- ❒ Minimum CO production – Sevoflurane and halothane

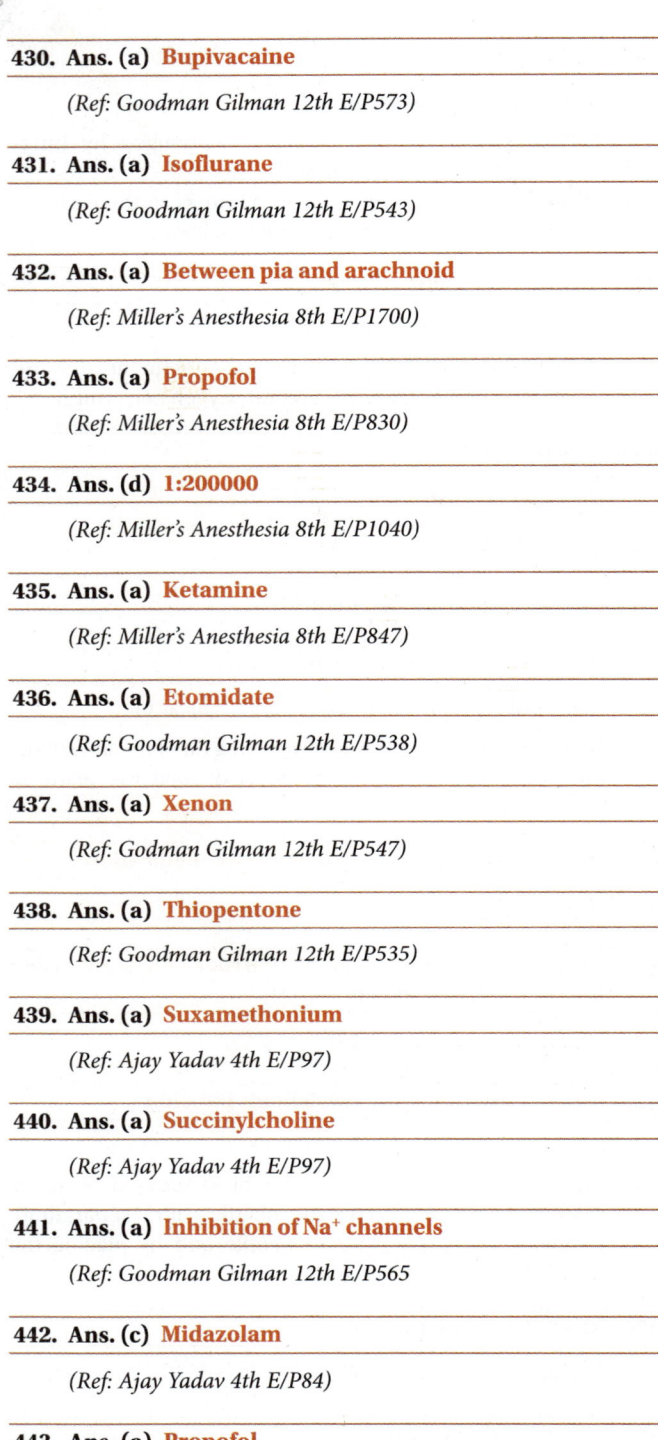

430. Ans. (a) Bupivacaine

(Ref: Goodman Gilman 12th E/P573)

431. Ans. (a) Isoflurane

(Ref: Goodman Gilman 12th E/P543)

432. Ans. (a) Between pia and arachnoid

(Ref: Miller's Anesthesia 8th E/P1700)

433. Ans. (a) Propofol

(Ref: Miller's Anesthesia 8th E/P830)

434. Ans. (d) 1:200000

(Ref: Miller's Anesthesia 8th E/P1040)

435. Ans. (a) Ketamine

(Ref: Miller's Anesthesia 8th E/P847)

436. Ans. (a) Etomidate

(Ref: Goodman Gilman 12th E/P538)

437. Ans. (a) Xenon

(Ref: Godman Gilman 12th E/P547)

438. Ans. (a) Thiopentone

(Ref: Goodman Gilman 12th E/P535)

439. Ans. (a) Suxamethonium

(Ref: Ajay Yadav 4th E/P97)

440. Ans. (a) Succinylcholine

(Ref: Ajay Yadav 4th E/P97)

441. Ans. (a) Inhibition of Na^+ channels

(Ref: Goodman Gilman 12th E/P565

442. Ans. (c) Midazolam

(Ref: Ajay Yadav 4th E/P84)

443. Ans. (a) Propofol

(Ref: Miller's Anesthesia 8th E/P830)

- Propofol has a very short duration of action due to its high lipid solubility, which causes high redistribution.

444. Ans. (a) Myasthenia gravis

(Ref: Ajay Yadav 4th E/P98)

- In myasthenia gravis there are anti N_M antibodies which competitively inhibit N_M receptors and hence decreases effect of succinylcholine.

445. Ans. (a) Potency

(Ref: Ajay Yadav 4th E/P59)

446. Ans. (a) Pin index system

(Ref: Miller's Anesthesia 8th E/P755)

447. Ans. (a) Suxamethonium

(Ref: Goodman Gilman 12th E/P264)

448. Ans. (d) CMV

(Ref: Miller's Anesthesia 8th E/P30641)

449. Ans. (a) Venturi Mask

(Ref: Ajay Yadav 4th E/P43)

450. Ans. (a) Nitrous oxide

(Ref: Goodman Gilman 12th E/P546-47)

451. Ans. (b) Succinylcholine

(Ref: Goodman Gilman 12th E/P268))

452. Ans. (c) Ketamine

(Ref: Miller's Anesthesia 8th E/P848)

453. Ans. (a) Succinylcholine

(Ref: Goodman Gilman 12th E/P268)

454. Ans. (a) Propofol

(Ref: Miller's Anesthesia 8th E/P830)

455. Ans. (a) Nitrous oxide

(Ref: Goodman Gilman 12th E/P547)

456. Ans. (b) Epidural anesthesia

(Ref: Miller's Anesthesia 8th E/P1703)

457. Ans. (b) Patient on aspirin

(Ref: Ajay Yadav 4th E/P136)

Mnemonics

Contraindication of Spinal and Epidural Anesthesia

S : Stenotic valvular heart disease
H : Hypovolemia
A : Anticoagulation therapy
R : Raised ICP
P : Platelet count < 80,000
Injection : Infection at local site

458. Ans. (d) It inhibits salivation

(Ref: Ajay Yadav 4th E/P71)

459. Ans. (d) Endotracheal intubation

(Ref: Ajay Yadav 4th E/P37)

Endotracheal intubation decreases the dead space by 70 ml.

460. Ans. (a) CPAP

(Ref: Miller's Anesthesia 8th E/P3068)

461. Ans. (a) Ketamine

(Ref: Miller's Anesthesia 8th E/P848)

462. Ans. (a) Atracurium

(Ref: Ajay Yadav 4th E/P101)

463. Ans. (a) Atracurium

(Ref: Ajay Yadav 4th E/P101)

464. Ans. (a) Halothane

(Ref: Goodman Gilman 12th E/P542)

465. Ans. (c) SIMV

(Ref: Miller's Anesthesia 8th E/P 3065-66)

Patient-ventilator asynchrony can be seen with:

- ACMV
- SIMV

466. Ans. (a) Isoflurane

(Ref: Goodman Gilman 12th E/P543)

467. Ans. (b) Propofol

(Ref: Miller's Anesthesia 8th E/P831)

468. Ans. (b) Ketamine

(Ref: Miller's Anesthesia 8th E/P848)

469. Ans. (d) Sevoflurane

(Ref: Ajay Yadav 4th E/P70)

Sevoflurane decreases portal blood flow but increases hepatic artery blood flow and hence maintains the total hepatic blood flow as compared to other agents.

470. Ans. (d) Pethidine

(Ref: Miller's Anesthesia 8th E/P902)

471. Ans. (c) Adequacy of collateral circulation in the hand

(Ref: Miller's Anesthesia 8th E/P1349)

472. Ans. (d) Suxamethonium

(Ref: Goodman Gilman 12th E/P264)

473. Ans. (a) Thiopentone sodium

(Ref: Goodman Gilman 12th E/P268)

474. Ans. (d) Enflurane

(Ref: Goodman Gilman 12th E/P544)

475. Ans. (b) Ketamine

(Ref: Miller's Anesthesia 8th E/P847)

476. Ans. (c) Etomidate

(Ref: Goodman Gilman 12th E/P538)

477. Ans. (c) Induction by Propofol, Maintenance by N_2O and O_2

(Ref: Goodman Gilman 12th E/P546)

478. Ans. (d) Non-depolarising agents triggers malignant hyperthermia

(Ref: Goodman Gilman 12th E/P268)

479. Ans. (a) Hyperkalemia

(Ref: Goodman Gilman 12th E/P268)

480. Ans. (d) All of the above

(Ref: Goodman Gilman 12th E/P268)

481. Ans. (b) 2 mg/kg

(Ref: Ajay Yadav 4th E/P81)

482. Ans. (a) NMDA receptor

(Ref: Miller's Anesthesia 8th E/P845)

483. Ans. (d) Acute intermittent porphyria

(Ref: Goodman Gilman 12th E/P535)

484. Ans. (d) Associated with photophobia

(Ref: Miller's Anesthesia 8th E/P1712)

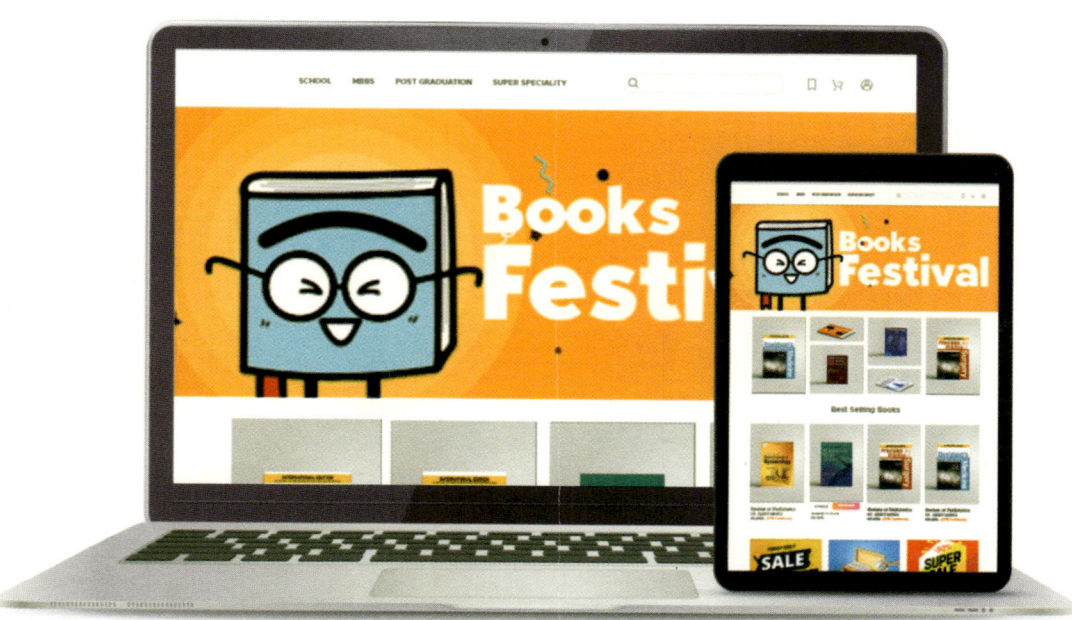

Salient Features

- A never before 'Fun and Learn Approach' to study a bland subject like pharmacology. The book retains the same flavor in studying the subject, as the author's classes.
- The content has been thoroughly revised and updated as per the recent developments.
- An Integrated Approach of Understanding has been followed in the book with Conceptual Boxes highlighting the Interrelation of Pharmacology with other Clinical and Non-clinical Subjects.
- Further details related to drugs have been summarized in Clinical Boxes.
- All chapters now contain Classifications of Various Drug Classes to strengthen the Basic Understanding of the readers.
- Recent Guidelines in Management of Tuberculosis, Leprosy and HIV have been incorporated.
- Antimalarial, Anti-leprosy and Anti-HIV Vaccines have also been discussed.
- A detailed chart on Autonomic Nervous System Drugs has been included for quick revision.

About the Author

Ranjan Kumar Patel, *MD Pharmacology*, is a renowned faculty of Pharmacology in India as well as Visiting Faculty in various Medical Colleges based in the countries, like China, Russia, Ukraine, Philippines and many European countries as well. He completed his MD in Pharmacology from University College of Medical Sciences and GTB Hospital, Delhi. Being a topper in AIPG, he opted for Pharmacology which shows his immense love for the subject. His eloquent speaking style and passion for teaching make him very popular amongst the students. He organizes his own classes in pharmacology all over India known as CPR (Conceptual Pharmacology Revision). Every year thousands of students are benefitted from his lectures and achieve their desired goals.

Join Author's **Facebook Discussion Group** – www.facebook.com/Dr Ranjan's Pharmacology Discussion and Updates

Students' Review about the 4th Edition of the Book

Just amazing and unbelievable... can't imagine pharma can be written so nicely with diagram, flowchart, concept, and many more.. lots of respect for the author...loved the book...a must read book.
Anonymous ★★★★★

Well, always a fan of Ranjan sir book.. Autonomic system ... general pharmacology at its best.....new updates with recent drugs
Shubhda Singh ★★★★★

Very nicely written. Good presentation.It has all the latest updates. Saves time before exams
Sohail Khan ★★★★★

This book is very descriptive. It has all the necessary contents that are required for preparation of PG Entrance Exams. It can also be used for university exams. We can get an in-depth idea which will be the base for studying entire pharmacology.
Varshini V. M. ★★★★★

Pharmacology Book not only covers pharmacology but medicine and physiology as well. No doubt book is well written in simple language, beautiful explanation and wonderful drawing by sir. I am fan of sir and this book. I also love presentation of this book.. This book already doing well in market.
Manav Babbar ★★★★★

I am a fan of Ranjan sir's lectures and this book is again a wonderful work by him. Pharmacology has been presented beautifully with concepts helping for easy recall during the exams. Superb!
George Zacharia ★★★★★

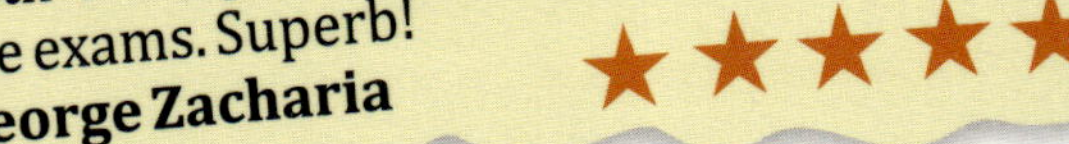
ISBN: 978-93-89941-96-8

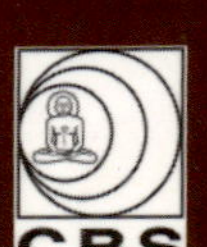

CBS Publishers & Distributors Pvt. Ltd.
4819/XI, Prahlad Street, 24 Ansari Road, Daryaganj, New Delhi 110 002, India
E-mail: delhi@cbspd.com, cbspubs@airtelmail.in: **Website:** www.cbspd.com
New Delhi | Bengaluru | Chennai | Kochi | Kolkata | Mumbai | Pune
Hyderabad | Nagpur | Patna | Vijayawada